Concepts for Nursing Practice
Content Organization

Sexuality and Reproduction

Health and Illness Concepts

Cognitive Function

Maladaptive Behavior

Attributes and Roles of Nurse

Care Competencies

Professional Nursing and Health Care Concepts

Health Care Delivery

Health Care Infrastructures

Alphabetical Listing of Concepts

CONCEPTS *for* NURSING PRACTICE

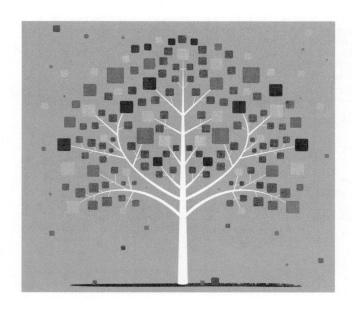

Jean Foret Giddens, PhD, RN, FAAN
Professor and Executive Dean
RWJF Executive Nurse Fellow
College of Nursing
University of New Mexico
Albuquerque, NM

ELSEVIER

3251 Riverport Lane
St. Louis, Missouri 63043

CONCEPTS FOR NURSING PRACTICE
Copyright © 2013 by Mosby, an imprint of Elsevier, Inc.

VST ISBN: 978-0-323-08376-8
KNO ISBN: 978-0-323-22372-0

Notice

Knowledge and best practice in this field are constantly changing. As new research and experience broaden our knowledge, changes in practice, treatment, and drug therapy may become necessary or appropriate. Readers are advised to check the most current information provided (i) on procedures featured or (ii) by the manufacturer of each product to be administered, to verify the recommended dose or formula, the method and duration of administration, and contraindications. It is the responsibility of the practitioner, relying on their own experience and knowledge of the patient, to make diagnoses, to determine dosages and the best treatment for each individual patient, and to take all appropriate safety precautions. To the fullest extent of the law, neither the Publisher nor the Author assumes any liability for any injury and/or damage to persons or property arising out of or related to any use of the material contained in this book.

The Publisher

Library of Congress Cataloging-in-Publication Data

Concepts for nursing practice / [edited by] Jean Foret Giddens.
   p. ; cm.
Includes bibliographical references.
VST ISBN 978-0-323-08376-8 (pbk. : alk. paper)
KNO ISBN: 978-0-323-22372-0 (pbk. : alk. paper)
I. Giddens, Jean.
[DNLM: 1. Nursing Process. 2. Nursing Care. 3. Nursing. WY 100.1]
610.73—dc23

2012007240

Director, eContent Solutions: Robin Carter
Content Development Specialists: Angela Perdue, Shephali Graf
Publishing Services Manager: Jeff Patterson
Design Direction: Karen Pauls
Cover Art: Copyright© 2012 by Michael Austin c/o theispot.com

Printed in the United States of America

Last digit is the print number: 9 8 7 6 5 4 3 2

Dr. Giddens earned a Bachelor of Science in Nursing from the University of Kansas, a Master of Science in Nursing from the University of Texas at El Paso, and a Doctorate in Education and Human Resource Studies from Colorado State University. Dr. Giddens has 25 years' experience in associate degree, baccalaureate degree, and graduate degree nursing programs in New Mexico, Texas, and Colorado. She is an expert in concept-based curriculum development and evaluation as well as innovative strategies for teaching and learning. Dr. Giddens is the author of multiple journal articles, nursing textbooks, and electronic media, and serves as an education consultant to nursing programs throughout the country.

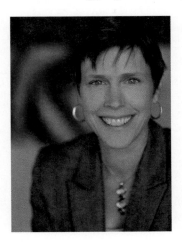

ACKNOWLEDGEMENTS

Developing and writing *Concepts for Nursing Practice* has truly been an amazing collaboration of nurse educators from across the country. I extend my gratitude and appreciation to the contributors and reviewers for sharing their expertise and wisdom. I also am grateful to my colleagues at Elsevier—particularly Robin Carter, who has been a supporter, advocate, and friend over a number of years. Lastly, I extend deep appreciation to my husband Jay—for without your friendship, love, and support I could not accomplish such work.

Lyda C. Arevalo-Flechas PhD RN
Assistant Professor
John A. Hartford Foundation
Claire M. Fagin Fellow
St. David's School of Nursing
Texas State University
San Marcos, TX

Gail E. Armstrong, DNP,
    ACNS-BC, CNE
Assistant Professor
University of Colorado College of Nursing
Denver, CO

Jan Belden, MSN, RN-BC, FNP-BC
Certified Pain Management Nurse
Loma Linda University Medical Center
Loma Linda, CA

Deb Bennett-Woods, EdD, FACHE
Director, Center for Ethics and Leadership
    in the Health Professions
Rueckert-Hartman College for Health
    Professions, Regis University
Denver, CO

Janet Prvu Bettger, ScD, FAHA
Assistant Professor
Duke University School of Nursing
Durham, NC

Janice M. Bissonnette, PhD,
    RN-NP, MScN
Advanced Practice Nurse/Joint Appointee
The Ottawa Hospital Renal Transplantation/
    The University of Ottawa
Ottawa, ONT

Lynne Buchanan, PhD,
    MSN, APRN-NP, BC
Associate Professor
University of Nebraska Medical Center
    College of Nursing
Adult Health and Illness Department
Omaha, NE

Susan Caplan, PhD, MSN, APRN-BC
Assistant Professor and Specialty Director,
    Family Nurse Practitioner Program
College of Nursing, Rutgers University
Newark, NJ

Barbara M. Carranti, MS, RN, CNS
Clinical Assistant Professor
LeMoyne College
Syracuse, NY

Michelle A. Cole, MSN, RN, CPN
Instructor of Nursing
Sacred Heart University
Fairfield, CT

Helen B. Connors, PhD, RN, FAAN
Professor/Associate Dean
University of Kansas School of Nursing
Executive Director KU Center for Health
    Informatics
Kansas City, KS

Kathleen DeLeskey, DNP,
    RN, CNE, CPAN
Associate Professor of Nursing
Lawrence Memorial/Regis College Center
    of Excellence
Medford, Weston, MA

Kelley Edds, MSN, CNP
Nursing Faculty
Caplan University
Davenport, IA

Robert Elgie, MSN, RN, BC
Clinical Educator
University of New Mexico College of
    Nursing
Albuquerque, NM

Linda Felver, PhD, RN
Associate Professor
Oregon Health & Science University,
    School of Nursing
Portland, OR

Louise K. Fleming, MSN, RN
Clinical Instructor
UNC Chapel Hill School of Nursing
Chapel Hill, NC

Jean Foret Giddens, PhD, RN, FAAN
Professor and Executive Dean
RWJF Executive Nurse Fellow
College of Nursing
University of New Mexico
Albuquerque, NM

Debra Hagler, PhD, RN,
    ACNS-BC, CNE, ANEF
Clinical Professor
College of Nursing and Health Innovation,
    Arizona State University
Phoenix, AZ

Ingrid C. Hendrix, BA, MILS
Nursing Services Librarian
Health Services Library and Informatics
    Center, University of New Mexico
Albuquerque, NM

Nancy Hoffart, PhD, RN
Founding Dean and Professor
Alice Ramez Chagoury School of Nursing
Byblos, Lebanon

Barbara I. Holmes Damron,
    PhD, RN, FAAN
Director, Office of Community Partnerships
    & Cancer Health Disparities
University of New Mexico Cancer Center
Associate Professor
Robert Wood Johnson Foundation
Nursing & Health Policy Collaborative
University of New Mexico College of
    Nursing
Albuquerque, NM

Jaclynn S. Huse, PhD, RN, CNE
Professor of Nursing
Southern Adventist University
Collegedale, TN

Teresa Keller, PhD, RN
Associate Professor
School of Nursing
New Mexico State University
Las Cruces, NM

Kim K. Kuebler, DNP, RN, ANP-BC
Assistant Clinical Professor
Sacred Heart University
Fairfield, CT

Martha Langhorne, MSN,
    RN, FNP, AOCN
Nurse Practitioner
Binghamton Gastroenterology
Binghamton, NY

Kathie Lasater, EdD, RN, ANEF
Associate Professor
Oregon Health & Science University
Portland, OR

Sharon Lewis, PhD, RN, FAAN
Research Professor
Castella Distinguished Professor
University of Texas Health Science Center
    at San Antonio
San Antonio, TX

Judy Liesveld, PhD, CPNP
Assistant Professor
University of New Mexico College of
    Nursing
Albuquerque, NM

Yvonne M. Masters, JD, BSN, RN
Clinical Instructor, Legal Nurse Consultant
Arizona State University, Dignity Health
Phoenix, AZ

Carolyn R. McKenzie, PhD, RN
Clinical Assistant Professor
The University of North Carolina at Chapel
    Hill
Chapel Hill, NC

Denise Miner-Williams,
    PhD, RN, CHPN
Research Assistant Professor
University of Texas Health Science Center
    San Antonio
San Antonio, TX

Frances Donovan Monahan,
    PhD, RN, ANEF
Faculty RN to BSN Program University of
    Arkansas at Little Rock
Faculty Excelsior College
Albany, NY

Ann Nielsen, MN, RN
Assistant Professor
Oregon Health and Science University
Portland, OR

Barbara H.M. Pascoe, MA, RN, BA
Director of Maternity, Gynecology, and
    Pediatrics
Concord Hospital
Concord, NH

Chris Pasero, MS, RN-BC, FAAN
Pain Management Educator and Clinical
    Consultant
El Dorado Hills, CA

Nancy J. Peckenpaugh, MSEd,
    RD, CDN, CDE
Registered Dietician and Certified Diabetes
    Educator
Lifetime Nutrition Services
Ithaca, NY

Shannon E. Perry, PhD, RN, FAAN
Professor Emerita
San Francisco State University
San Francisco, CA

Sue Popkess-Vawter, PhD, RN
Professor of Nursing
University of Kansas School of Nursing
Kansas City, KS

Nancy Ridenour, PhD,
    APRN, BC, FAAN
Dean and Professor
University of New Mexico College of
    Nursing
Albuquerque, NM

L. Jane Rosati, EdD, MSN, RN-BC
Assistant Chair of the ADN Program
Daytona State College
Daytona Beach, FL

Carolyn E. Sabo, EdD, RN, CNE
Professor, School of Nursing
University of Nevada, Las Vegas
Las Vegas, NV

Jodene Scheller, PhD, MSN, RN
Professor, Nursing
Lewis and Clark Community College
Godfrey, Illinois

Pamela N. Schultz, PhD, RN
Professor, Associate Dean and Director of
    the School of Nursing
New Mexico State University
Las Cruces, NM

Gwen Sherwood, PhD, RN, FAAN
Professor and Associate Dean for Academic
    Affairs
University of North Carolina at Chapel Hill
    School of Nursing
Chapel Hill, NC

Debra J. Smith, MSN, RN, CNE
Instructor
University of New Mexico, College of
    Nursing
Albuquerque, NM

Amy Szoka, MSN, RN
Assistant Professor
Daytona State College
Daytona Beach, FL

Jenny E. Vacek, MSN, RN
Instructor
University of New Mexico College of
    Nursing
Albuquerque, NM

Judith J. Warren, PhD, RN,
    BC, FAAN, FACMI
Director of Nursing Informatics for KU
    Center for Health Informatics
University of Kansas School of Nursing
Kansas City, KS

Susan F. Wilson, PhD, RN, CNE
Associate Professor
University of Alaska Anchorage
Anchorage, AK

P.J. Woods, PhD, MBA, RN
Associate Professor
Nursing Administration Concentration
    Coordinator
University of New Mexico, College of
    Nursing
Albuquerque, NM

Jan Lamarche Zdanuk, DNP,
    APRN, FNP-BC, CNS, CWS,
    FACCWS, FAANP
Doctor of Nursing Practice
Visiting Physician's Association
South University
Assistant Professor
College of Nursing
Fort Worth, TX

Kristen D. Zulkosky, PhD, RN, CCRN
Nursing Instructor
Lancaster General College of Nursing and
    Health Sciences
Lancaster, PA

REVIEWERS

Elizabeth C. Arnold, PhD, RN, PMHCNS-BC
Associate Professor
University of Maryland School of Nursing
Baltimore, MD

Lisa A. Bagnall, MSN, CCRN, CNL
Courtesy Assistant Clinical Professor
University of Florida
Gainesville, FL

Janet Prvu Bettger, ScD
Assistant Professor
Duke University School of Nursing
Durham, NC

Audrey J. Bopp, MSN, RN, CNS
Assistant Professor
University of Northern Colorado
Greeley, CO

Debra Brady, PhD, RN
Associate Professor & Education Chair
University of New Mexico
Albuquerque, NM

Lynne Buchanan, PhD, MSN, APRN-NP, BC
Associate Professor
University of Nebraska Medical Center
College of Nursing
Adult Health and Illness Department
Omaha, NE

Annette M. Conklin, PhD(c), MSN, OCN, CNE
Faculty
Holy Family University
Philadelphia, PA

Shirlee Proctor Davidson, MSN, RN
Associate Professor
Santa Fe Community College
Santa Fe, NM

Hazel A. Dennison, DNP, RN, APNc, CPHQ
Advanced Practice Nurse
Virtua Health System
Marlton, NJ

Wende N. Fedder, DNP-c, RN, MBA, FAHA
Clinical Director
Alexian Brothers Hospital Network
Elk Grove Village, IL

Nelda Godfrey, PhD, RN, ACNS-BC
Associate Dean, Clinical Associate Professor
University of Kansas School of Nursing
Kansas City, KS

Jessica Greni, MSN, RN
Nursing Instructor
University of Nebraska Medical Center-
Kearney Division
Kearney, NE

Kathy Hammond, MS, RN, BSN, BSHE, RD, LD
Corporate Education and Development
Gentiva Health Services, Inc.
Atlanta, GA

Robbyn Harry-Ieremie, MSN, RN
Psychiatric Nurse
Kent State University
Cleveland, OH

Jaclynn S. Huse, PhD, RN, CNE
Professor of Nursing
Southern Adventist University
Collegedale, TN

Susan R. Kell, BSN, RN
Director
Kindred Hospital Tucson
Tucson, AZ

Teresa Keller, PhD, RN
Health Policy, Nursing Administration
New Mexico State University
Albuquerque, NM

Lucina Kimpel, PhD, RN
Assistant Professor of Nursing
Grand View University
Des Moines, IA

Kim K. Kuebler, DNP, RN, ANP-BC
Assistant Clinical Professor
Sacred Heart University
Fairfield, CT

Maria E. Lauer, MSN, RN, CNE
Nursing Instructor
Thomas Edison State College
Trenton, NJ

Claranne Mathiesen, MSN, RN, CNRN
Assistant Professor Nursing
East Stroudsburg University
East Stroudsburg, PA

Frances Donovan Monahan, PhD, RN, ANEF
Faculty RN to BSN Program University of
Arkansas at Little Rock
Faculty Excelsior College
Albany, NY

Mary Courtney Moore, PhD, RN, RD, MSN, BSN
Research Associate Professor
Vanderbilt University School of Medicine
Nashville, TN

Audrey Nelson, PhD, RN
Associate Professor
University of Nebraska Medical Center,
College of Nursing
Omaha, NE

Barbara H.M. Pascoe, MA, RN, BA
Director of Maternity, Gynecology and
Pediatrics
Concord Hospital
Concord, NH

Renee Diane Pennington, MSN, PMHNP-BC
Psychiatric Nurse Practitioner
Recovery Resources
Cleveland, OH

Carolyn E. Sabo, EdD, RN, CNE
Professor, School of Nursing
University of Nevada—Las Vegas
Las Vegas, NV

Lisa A. Ruth-Sahd, DEd, RN, MSN, CCN, CCRN
Associate Professor of Nursing
York College of Pennsylvania
York, PA

Jeanne Saunders, EdD, MSN, RN-BC
Professor
Daytona State College
Daytona Beach, FL

Winni Tucker, MSN, ARNP
Professor
Daytona State College
Daytona Beach, FL

Joanne Warner, PhD, RN
Dean and Professor
University of Portland
Portland, OR

Nurse educators are faced with a myriad of challenges as they prepare graduates to provide safe care in increasingly complex health care environments. There is an ever-increasing body of knowledge, new evidence for best practices, and shifts in the type of patients and settings in which nurses will provide care. To prepare our students for these realities, nurse educators must design curricula and courses that provide opportunities for students to search, retrieve, critique, and synthesize information for making situated clinical judgments, in other words, to think conceptually.

It is in this context that *Concepts for Nursing Practice* arrives in a timely manner to guide students and faculty to meet the challenges of learning to be a nurse. For *students*, this book is a source that truly and fully explains concepts, and will encourage learning for clinical application, not memorization, thereby facilitating thinking and eliminating information saturation. Students will be able to develop their own clinical frameworks in which to embed new knowledge throughout their career. *Faculty* who assign this book will be inspired to streamline their courses and eliminate redundant "content" in the program, and will easily guide students to link concepts learned in the classroom to clinical practice.

The book is exquisitely designed to focus on health problems across all patient populations while integrating care competencies, such as patient safety, and health care delivery concepts, such as care coordination. The concepts in the book follow a consistent framework, thus reinforcing a thinking process for students. The concepts provide succinct descriptions of pathophysiology accompanied by easy-to-understand illustrations; boxed material highlights important nursing actions, and explanations regarding how concepts are interrelated across the lifespan. A table in each concept identifies significant health problems that arise from health disruptions related to the concept(s); each concept concludes with a model case of a clinical exemplar.

Health care systems will increasingly depend on nurses who can integrate clinical data to provide safe and high-quality nursing care. This book will provide the solid foundation of knowledge and application that students need in order to be prepared for success in their educational and professional careers.

Diane M. Billings, EdD, RN, FAAN
Chancellor's Professor of Nursing
Indiana University School of Nursing
Indianapolis, Indiana

Wisdom means keeping a sense of the fallibility of our views and opinions, and of the uncertainty and instability of the things we most count on.

Gerard Brown

INTRODUCTION TO CONCEPTUAL LEARNING

Conceptual learning is increasingly viewed as a major trend for the future of education—not in nursing alone, but across numerous disciplines. This belief is based on the premise that *concepts* can be used effectively as unifying classifications or principles for framing learning while knowledge increases exponentially.

So, what is a *concept*? Simply stated, a concept is an organizing principle, or a classification of information. A concept can be limited or complex in scope, and can be useful as a basis for education from preschool through doctoral education. In advanced applications, concepts are considered building blocks or the foundation for theory.

By gaining a deeper understanding of a core set of concepts, a student can recognize and understand similarities and recurring characteristics, which can be applied more effectively than memorized facts. Teaching conceptually turns traditional learning upside down, focusing on generalities (concepts) and then applying this understanding to specifics (exemplars), instead of the traditional educational approach that focuses more heavily on content and facts.

HOW THIS BOOK IS ORGANIZED

The conceptual approach in nursing involves an examination of concepts that link to the delivery of patient care. There are multiple concepts applicable to nursing practice. This book does not attempt to present all nursing concepts, nor does it suggest the featured concepts chosen are the most important. However, the 53 concepts featured in this book are commonly seen in nursing literature or representative of important practice phenomena; they are the concepts that apply to the broadest group of patients of various ages and across various health care settings. A simplified concept analysis format using consistent headings is intentionally used for the presentation of concepts in this book so that students will find the approach intuitive and, at the same time, an understanding of more formalized conceptual analyses will be fostered. Three overarching groups of concepts or *units* are featured:

- **Patient Profile Concepts (Unit One)**—concepts that help us understand the individuals for whom we care
- **Health and Illness Concepts (Unit Two)**—concepts that help us make sense of the multiple health conditions experienced by our patients across the lifespan
- **Professional Nursing and Health Care Concepts (Unit Three)**—concepts that guide our professional practice in the context of health care

These three overarching units are further categorized into *themes*, into which concepts are organized to provide a structured framework. This structured approach promotes a thorough understanding of individual concepts and their important context within related health care concepts.

Each concept provides a full spectrum of information with separate subheadings for concept definition, risk factors, health assessment, context of the concept to nursing and health care, interrelated concepts, model cases, and examples (exemplars) of concepts in practice. Each piece helps build an understanding of the concept as a whole, which in turn will promote the development of clinical judgment, a key outcome if nursing students are to practice effectively in today's complex health care environment.

FEATURES

Concept discussions include holistic concept diagrams that help visualize conceptual processes, along with *interrelated concepts* diagrams. These illustrations encourage students to build important associations among interrelated concepts. *Model cases,* or representative patient cases, and, where appropriate, contrary cases provide specific patient scenarios along with a succinct case analysis that ties the context of patient care to the concept.

An extensive list of *exemplars* (boxes at the end of every concept chapter) is based on incidence and prevalence across the lifespan and clinical settings. Using a custom technology, direct links to selected exemplars have been embedded into a core collection of Elsevier Pageburst Digital Textbooks. This option of linking directly to a curated list of exemplars in a set collection of titles allows for a seamless user experience by uniting concepts to priority exemplars. Although instructors have complete flexibility to choose those concepts and exemplars best suited to their particular institution, these direct links are provided to allow quick access to those exemplars likely to be used in the majority of cases.* *Interactive review questions* incorporated into a self-assessment student testing engine are provided as an additional feature of this book's Evolve website (http:/evolve.elsevier.com/Giddens/concepts). These 250 student questions include multiple-choice and multi-select questions to simulate the NCLEX™ Examination testing experience, along with correct answer options and rationales.

---

*These links will be released and updated in phases, shortly following the initial release of the title.

Additional material to support faculty is included on the *Evolve Instructor Resources* site. These instructor resources include the following for each concept: definition, key points, outline, media resources, nursing skills correlated with the concept, interrelated concepts, priority concepts, active learning activities, simulation suite connections from Elsevier's Simulation Learning System (a simulation tool available separately for programs employing simulated patient mannekins in their curricula), 250 PowerPoint slides, and 400 new concept-based test bank questions.

CONCLUSION

Why use a conceptual approach? One reason is it is very likely there will continue to be an exponential generation of new knowledge and information in all areas of our world; health care and nursing are no exception. It is literally impossible for anyone to know all information within the discipline of nursing. The study of nursing concepts provides the learner with an understanding of essential components associated with nursing practice without becoming saturated and lost in the details for each area of clinical specialty. If concepts are understood deeply, links can be made when these are applied in various areas of nursing practice.

Another reason the conceptual approach for learning is important is for future advancement of our discipline. This book, influenced by the work of Virginia Carrieri-Kohlman, Ada Lindsey, and Claudia West, serves as a guide to learning about concepts and their application in clinical nursing practice. The conceptual approach for learning, clinical practice, and research efforts are needed to continue to build substantive knowledge to the discipline of nursing. Carrieri-Kohlman and colleagues suggested that the conceptual approach "generates a spirit of inquiry,"[1] which is essential to ensure the continued development of professional nursing practice.

I sincerely welcome user feedback since this represents a first step on a new journey and, as such, it is a journey that embraces change and learning.

Let the journey begin!

Jean Foret Giddens

REFERENCE

1. Carrieri-Kohlman V, Lindsey AM, West CM: *Pathophysiologic phenomena in nursing: human response to illness*, ed 3, St Louis, 2003, Elsevier.

CONTENTS

UNIT 3   PROFESSIONAL NURSING AND HEALTH CARE CONCEPTS

Patient Profile Concepts

Historically, health care has been delivered in a disease-centered model. In such a model, nearly all treatment-related decisions are made by the physician based on the underlying disease or condition, the physician's clinical experience, and the results of diagnostic tests. Health care providers control and direct care with little input from patients regarding their desires or their concerns about the impact of the treatment plan on their lives. Patients were apprised of the plan as opposed to discussing options for disease management.[1] Individuals who did not follow the recommendations of their physicians or nurses were considered noncompliant.

Health care has actively been moving away from this disease-centered perspective towards a patient-centered model of health care. In a patient-centered model, patients and their families are active participants in their care. Health care services are designed to meet the needs and wishes of the individual as a unique person, considering personal preferences. In such a model, the health care professionals counsel and provide advice related to health care decisions, based on their clinical expertise and evidence.

The delivery of patient-centered care involves establishing a partnership between the patient and health care professionals and ensuring that health care decisions take into account the unique needs and preferences of the patient.[2] Fundamental to this is the ability to understand the distinct attributes of each and every patient. For the successful delivery of patient-centered care, it is essential for nurses to understand the concepts presented in this unit. The two themes within this unit include *Attributes and Resources* and *Personal Preferences.*

Attributes and Resources include concepts associated with unique attributes (characteristics) associated with each patient. The concepts *Development* and *Functional Ability* are critical to consider for each and every patient encounter; these concepts direct all nursing care decisions, ranging from attaining optimal patient interaction to assessing the patient, delivering health care interventions, understanding the impact of coexisting health-related conditions, and providing patient education strategies. *Family Dynamics* as a concept is included within this theme because of the important role families have in health care decisions and it is important to consider how the family is impacted by one or members who become ill.

Personal Preferences as a theme include concepts that influence an individual's attitudes and preferences regarding health care. Concepts within this theme include *Culture, Motivation,* and *Adherence.* These are basic concepts to understand because they help explain the decision making and behavior of patients, and inform providers of strategies necessary to reach decisions that are mutually acceptable and agreeable to patients and providers.

REFERENCES

1. Agency for Healthcare Research and Quality: Expanding patient centered care to empower patients and assist providers, *Research in action,* ed 5, Bethesda, Md, 2002, U.S. Department of Health and Human Services.
2. Institute of Medicine: *Crossing the quality chasm: a new health system for the 21st century,* Washington, DC, 2001, National Academies Press.

1

Development

Frances D. Monahan

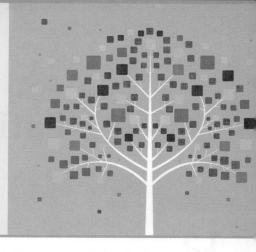

A basic characteristic of human life is change. Development is a gradual, qualitative change in which an individual's abilities expand and increase in complexity according to a dynamic, predictable sequence that begins at conception and continues over the lifespan until death.[1-3] The ability to provide patient-centered, quality care requires nurses to be able to assess an individual's developmental level and then provide care appropriate for that level. It is also important for nurses to recognize when expected developmental stages are not being met, so that collaborative interventions can be initiated.

DEFINITION(S)

Development refers to *the sequence of physical, psychosocial, and cognitive developmental changes that take place over the human lifespan.*[3] Development does not occur as an isolated phenomenon. Rather, it occurs as a simultaneous and ongoing interrelationship with three processes of change: growth, differentiation, and maturation. *Growth* is a quantitative change in which an increase in cell number and size results in an increase in overall size or weight of the body or any of its parts. *Differentiation* is the process by which initially formed cells and structures become specialized. This is a qualitative change from simple to complex in which broad global function becomes refined and specific. *Maturation,* also a qualitative change, is associated with the process of aging. Maturation enables cells to function or to operate at a higher level. Thus maturation increases adaptability and competence in new situations.[3] Development, as well as the interrelated processes of growth, differentiation, and adaptation, is the result of genetics, environmental factors, culture, and family values.[3-5]

There are several other terms that are related to development. *Developmental level* refers to the position of an individual in the sequence of development. *Developmental milestones* are a set of functional skills or age-specific tasks that most children can complete at a certain age range.[1,6] These milestones provide a basis for developmental assessment because they serve as major markers in tracking the emergence of motor, social, cognitive, and language skills. Unique sets of skills and competencies that need to be mastered at each developmental stage in order for the individual to cope with the environment are called *developmental tasks.*[7] Developmental tasks are broad in scope and are, to a significant degree, determined by culture.[8] They may relate to the individual or to the family. Examples of developmental tasks are toilet training and adjusting to the loss of a spouse.[9]

The order of skill development is more important than the chronological age at which each occurs because although development is ongoing, its speed varies. Each individual has a unique developmental pace. Periods of accelerated and decelerated growth occur in the organism as a whole and in its subsystems. For example, while a growth spurt is occurring in one area such as gross motor skills, little growth may be seen other areas such as language skills. Rate and level of development in all areas are related to the physiological maturity of the nervous, muscular, and skeletal systems and the range of skills and the age at which each skill is acquired vary greatly. Thus age-related developmental expectancies or norms are always based on an age range—never an exact point in time when specific skills will be achieved.[1,3,6] The term *developmental age* is used to describe developmental progress. It is stated as age and is determined by standardized measurements of body size, motor function, psychosocial function, and performance on mental and aptitude tests. *Developmental arrest* is the cessation of one or more phases of development before it reaches normal completion. When this occurs in utero, a congenital anomaly results.[10]

SCOPE AND CATEGORIES

Scope

The scope of the concept correlates with developmental lifespan stages—from infancy to death. Across all the dimensions previously described, normal human development is

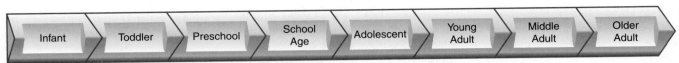

FIGURE 1-1 Scope of Development Concept Across the Lifespan.

organized and progressive and follows a predictable sequence. Based on this sequence, stages of development have been identified. The traditional stages of development are infant, toddler, preschool, school age, adolescent, young adult, middle adult, and older adult (Figure 1-1).

These stages identify characteristics found in the majority of individuals within a stated age range. Although individuals vary in the time of onset of each stage and in the length of time spent in each stage, the sequence itself does not vary.

Development is also characterized by susceptible periods. These are points in the lifespan when there is greater susceptibility to positive or negative influences with resulting beneficial or detrimental effects.[7] An example of the latter is the finding that young children appear to be particularly vulnerable to environmental hazards and exhibit marked detrimental effects from such exposures.[15]

Categories

Development is a complex concept representing five major categories: physical, social/emotional, cognitive, communication, and adaptive (Figure 1-2).

Physical Development

Physical development refers to the growth and changes in body tissues and organ systems and the resultant changes in body proportions. Physical development is bilateral and symmetrical, progressing in direction cephalocaudally (from head to tail) and proximodistally (from midline to periphery). It also progresses from gross motor to fine motor skills in a process called refinement. Gross motor skills involve the use of large muscles to move about in the environment. They include sitting, standing, walking, running, maintaining balance, and changing positions. Fine motor skills involve the use of small muscles in a very precise manner. Activities that constitute fine motor skills include using the hands to eat, draw, dress, play, and write.[10,11]

Social/Emotional Development

Social and emotional development pertains to personality, emotion, and behavior; this phase of development involves interacting with others; having relationships with family, friends, and teachers; and cooperating and responding to the feelings of others. This also refers to maintaining emotional control.[12]

Cognitive Development

The cognitive dimension relates to the sensory reception, processing, and use of information about the environment and objects in the environment, as well as understanding the relationships between self and this information. These processes underlie the development of thinking skills, which include learning, understanding, problem solving, reasoning, and remembering. Ultimately, cognitive abilities enable moral and spiritual development.[1]

Communication Development

Speech is the spoken expression of language. The three components of speech are articulation, which refers to the pronunciation of sounds; voice, which refers to the production of sound by the vocal cords; and fluency, which refers to the rhythm of speech. Language is a set of rules shared by a group of people that allows the communication of thoughts, ideas, and emotions. Receptive language function is the ability to understand what others say. Expressive language function is the ability to express completely one's own thoughts, ideas, and emotions.[13]

Adaptive Development

Adaptive development refers to the acquisition of a range of skills that enable independence at home and in the community. Adaptive skills are learned and include self-care activities such as dressing/undressing, eating/feeding, toileting, and grooming; management of one's immediate environment; and functional behaviors within the community such as crossing the street safely, going to the store, and following rules of politeness when interacting with others.[14]

THEORETICAL LINKS

Several theories comprehensively address the different dimensions of development and developmental level. Four of the classic theories presented in this concept analysis

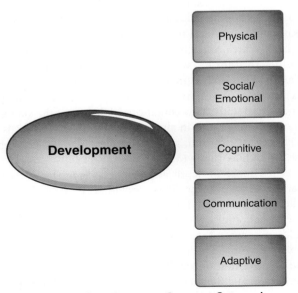

FIGURE 1-2 Development Concept Categories.

include Freud's theory of psychosexual development, Erikson's eight stages of psychosocial development, Piaget's theory of cognitive development, and Kohlberg's theory of moral development.

Freud's Theory of Psychosexual Development

The term psychosexual, as used by Freud, refers to any sensual pleasure. Freud believed that at different ages, particular areas of the body provide the chief source of sensual pleasure and that experiences with these pleasure centers significantly impacts the development of personality.

Freud described three components of the personality: id, ego, and superego. The id is inborn and the most primitive. It is unconscious, instinct driven, and concerned with instant gratification. The ego is the conscious mind driven by the reality principle. Within the structure of reality, the ego finds rational and acceptable ways to satisfy basic instincts. It blocks the irrational impulses of the id and uses a variety of defense mechanisms to protect against excessive anxiety. The superego is the conscience, the internalization of moral standards. It prevents the expression of unacceptable instincts and hence functions to maintain the social order. Freud further identified five stages of personality development (Table 1-1). Each of these stages has associated conflicts that must be resolved. Under stress, individuals may regress temporarily to an earlier stage. If resolution is not satisfactorily achieved, the individual may become fixated in the stage and personality development will be arrested.[16,17]

Erikson's Theory of Psychosocial Development

Erikson's theory of psychosocial development covers the entire lifespan and is an expansion and refinement of Freud's theory of psychosexual development. Erikson's theory identifies eight stages of life between birth and death. Each stage has a particular identified task in the form of a conflict that must be resolved (Table 1-1).[16,18]

Piaget's Theory of Cognitive Development

Piaget's theory of cognitive development seeks to explain how children organize their world and learn to think. Cognitive development is viewed as progressing from illogical to logical, from concrete to abstract, and from simple to complex. It is a product of inborn intellectual capacity, nervous system maturation, perceptual ability, and exposure to new experiences that serve as stimuli for cognitive development. The theory identifies four general periods; each is comprised of a number of stages that are age related and sequential. The four general periods and major characteristics of each are presented in Table 1-1.[12,19]

Kohlberg's Theory of Moral Development

Kohlberg's theory expands on Piaget's cognitive theory to address the development of moral reasoning across the lifespan. According to Kohlberg, when a conflict in universal values occurs, a moral choice must be made. This choice is based on moral reasoning, which is postulated to develop progressively over three levels; each level is comprised of two stages (Table 1-1). Moral reasoning depends on cognitive skills but is not definitively linked to specific developmental stages.[20]

CONTEXT TO NURSING AND HEALTH CARE

Development, as a concept, has implications for nursing practice across all populations and health care settings. First, recognition of risk and developmental assessment is essential to the early identification of developmental problems. Subsequent management therefore is critical to the health status of individuals. Second, knowledge of an individual's developmental level in the physical, social/emotional, cognitive, communication, and adaptive dimensions is essential to planning and implementing effective individualized patient care.

Risk Recognition

Developmental delay occurs in all social classes and in all ethnic groups, although it is most commonly identified among pediatric populations (infancy through adolescents).[21,22] Several types of risk exist, including the following:

- **Prenatal:** genetic conditions leading to developmental disabilities or delays, congenital infections, and prenatal exposure to illicit drugs and/or alcohol
- **Birth risk:** prematurity, low birth weight, birth trauma, cerebral palsy
- **Social:** poverty, parenting difficulties, abuse and neglect, environmental exposure to toxins, adverse living conditions
- **Health status:** chronic illness (e.g., congenital heart disease, cancer, brain injury, cystic fibrosis), injuries or conditions requiring prolonged bed rest, multiple/prolonged hospitalizations[11]

Developmental Assessment
Infants and Children

Screening for developmental problems primarily occurs as a part of well-child health visits.[21] In addition, the use of parent report developmental screening tools is encouraged. The most commonly used measure of developmental status used by health care professionals is the Denver II test. The Denver II is designed for use with children from 1 month to 6 years of age and has been standardized for minority populations. It assesses gross motor, fine motor-adaptive, language, and personal-social skills. Two limitations in the use of the Denver II are that it may result in an excessive number of referrals for further evaluation and, conversely, may fail to detect cerebral palsy in a child's first year.[3,9,23]

When more in-depth assessment of language is needed than what the Denver II test provides, the Early Language Milestones Scale (ELM Scale-2)[24] may be used to assess auditory visual, auditory receptive, and expressive language in children between the ages of 1 month and 3 years. Examples of parent report developmental screening tools are the Ages and Stages Questionnaire (ASQ),[9] the Parents Evaluation of Developmental Status (PEDS), and the Learn the Signs/Act Early Interactive Milestones Checklist program sponsored by

TABLE 1-1 DEVELOPMENTAL THEORIES

THEORIST	STAGE/AGE	TASKS
Freud[17]	Oral (birth to 1 yr)	Primary source of pleasure is from oral activities such as sucking, biting, chewing, and vocalizing.
	Anal (1-3 yr)	Primary source of pleasure is associated with anal region and capacity to withhold or expel feces. Toilet training is a critical experience.
	Phallic stage (3-6 yr)	Genitalia become a source of interest as differences between sexes are recognized and explored.
	Latency (6-12 yr)	Energy is focused on acquisition of knowledge and skills.
	Genital stage (puberty and older)	Maturation of reproductive organs and release of sex hormones; genitalia are primary source of tension and pleasure. Friendships and marriage are important.
Erikson[23]	Trust vs mistrust (birth to 1 yr)	Biological needs are predominant. Infant learns to trust or mistrust that needs will be met. This learning begins with receiving or not receiving oral satisfaction. Ultimately infant learns to trust or mistrust people and world. Positive resolution results in hope.
	Autonomy vs sense of shame and doubt (1-3 yr)	Self-control and making choices begin and lead to development of self-confidence. Shame and/or doubt develop when punishment is severe or choices are not allowed. Positive resolution results in self-control and will power.
	Initiative vs guilt (3-6 yr)	Environment is actively explored; new roles are tried out through fantasy and imitation of adults. Development of conscience begins. Guilt may result from conflict between desire to explore and limits set and/or punishment given. Positive resolution results in purpose and direction.
	Industry vs inferiority (6-11 yr)	Focus is on working with peers and learning productive skills valued by society. Behaves according to rules and responds overwhelmingly to praise. If skills are too difficult or learning is not supported, a sense of inadequacy and inferiority results. Positive resolution results in a sense of competence.
	Identity vs role confusion (11-18 yr)	Matures sexually; experiences feelings of indecisiveness; begins to plan for future and separation from family. Establishes a sense of personal identity based on past experiences. Positive resolution results in devotion and fidelity.
	Intimacy vs isolation (18-25 yr)	Commits to relationships and career; participates in community acting with adult freedom and responsibility. Positive resolution results in affiliation and love.
	Generativity vs self-absorption and stagnation (25-65 yr)	Personal and social involvement expands with production of children, ideas, services, or products. Concern for future generations expressed through parenting, teaching, and guiding. Positive resolution results in productivity and caring.
	Integrity vs despair (65 yr to death)	Adjusts to life changes and losses. Finds order, meaning, and value in life as it is and was. Positive resolution results in wisdom.
Piaget[35]	Period I: sensorimotor (birth to 2 yr)	Reflexes predominate at birth followed by occurrence of repetitive behaviors and then imitative behaviors; gradually relates to external environment but focused on sensations and actions that affect self; object permanence.
	Period II: preoperational (2-7 yr)	Focus is egocentric; thinks everyone sees world as he or she does; gradually begins to reason about concrete and observable; sees only one aspect of situation at a time. Intuitive reasoning occurs by end of this period.
	Period III: concrete operations (7-11 yr)	Concrete problems can be solved; concepts such as right and left and relative size are understood; grasps cause and effect; aware of people having different views. Able to sort, classify, organize information. Reasoning is inductive and different aspects of a situation can be considered simultaneously.
	Period IV: formal operations (11 yr to adult)	Thinking is logical and abstract ideas can be considered; reasoning is deductive and future oriented.

Continued

TABLE 1-1	DEVELOPMENTAL THEORIES—cont'd	
THEORIST	**STAGE/AGE**	**TASKS**
Kohlberg[20]	Level I: preconventional level (18 mo to 5 yr)	Perceived consequences (i.e., reward or punishment) determine actions. *Stage 1: Punishment and Obedience Orientation* Absolute obedience to rules and authority is essential or punishment, which is proof the child is wrong, will result. *Stage 2: Instrumental Relativist Orientation* Child perceives that authorities may differ about what is right; child's action is based on meeting his or her own needs and occasionally needs of others. Punishment does not mean child is wrong, but in meeting own needs is to be avoided.
	Level II: conventional level (6-12 yr)	Concerned with how actions will affect relationship with others; wants to fulfill internalized expectations of family and society. *Stage 3: Good Boy-Nice Girl Orientation* Approval is desired and obtained by "being nice," that is, by having good motives and showing concern, respect, gratitude, trust, and loyalty in relationships with others. *Stage 4: Society-Maintaining Orientation* Focus expands to include concerns with duty, respect for authority, and maintaining place in society.
	Level III: postconventional (12-19 yr)	Individuals define moral principles, which balance basic individual rights and responsibilities with rules and regulations of society for themselves. *Stage 5: Social Contract Orientation* Laws are seen as agreements by society about basic rights and values. There is concern about what societal values should be and laws are seen as able to be changed to better reflect them. *Stage 6: Universal Ethical Principle Orientation* Focus moves beyond basic rights and democratic process to abstract, universal, consistent, and comprehensive ethical principles that will result in most just agreements. Principles are self-chosen through a decision of conscience.

the CDC National Center on Birth Defects and Developmental Disabilities.[25] This program provides on-line milestone checklists for ages 1 month through 5 years. The checklist for the child's age is selected and the child's name and age are entered. The parent then checks off the behaviors that apply to the child and can print the list for reference.

There is a great deal of detailed information and tools to assess development available from pediatric and growth and development textbooks and from reliable websites such as the Center for Disease Control (http://www.cdc.gov/ncbddd/act early/milestones/). It is important for nurses to ensure that parents understand that screening tools do not provide a diagnosis. Diagnosis requires a thorough neurodevelopmental history and physical examination.[26] Developmental delay, which is suggested by screening, is a symptom, not a diagnosis.

Adolescents

Routine physical examinations monitor continued physical and sexual development into the adolescent years. In addition, the HEADSS Adolescent Risk Profile may be used.[27] HEADSS is a screening tool that assesses *h*ome, *e*ducation, *a*ctivities, *d*rugs, *s*ex, and *s*uicide for the purpose of identifying high-risk adolescents and the need for anticipatory guidance.

Adults

In adulthood, physical examinations continue to monitor normal developmental patterns. Physical characteristics of individuals are assessed relative to age and in older females reproductive organs are monitored for the normal decline in size and function. Screening tools designed for use with adults include the Recent Life Changes Questionnaire, the Life Experiences Survey,[12] and the Stress Audit, all of which aim to identify those in need of guidance relative to stress and coping.[23]

Older Adults

After adulthood, there is little focus on developmental assessment until individuals reach the older adult stage, unless an adult has a serious mental or physical illness or injury. When this is the case, the focus is on functional assessment (or functional ability)—that is, an assessment of an individual's ability to carry out basic activities of daily living (BADLs) and instrumental activities of daily living (IADLs).[28] BADLs include skills such as hygiene, toileting, eating, and ambulating. IADLs are skills that are needed to function independently and include preparing meals, shopping, taking medications, traveling within the community, and maintaining finances.

MODEL CASE

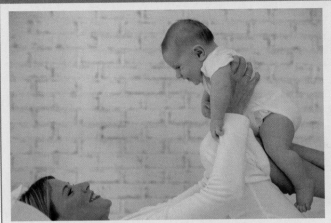

A first-time mother brings her 3-month-old daughter to the well-baby clinic. When the nurse asks the mother if she has any problems or concerns with the baby, the mother responds "I'm worried because she is still so small and she lifts her head up when she is on her stomach but she doesn't turn over from stomach to side. My neighbor says her grandchild was starting to turn over when she was about four months old and my friend's baby who is just about the same age weighs a pound and a half more than mine."

As part of the assessment, the nurse gathers the following information:
- Length at birth: 46 centimeters (cm) (18.4 inches)
- Current length: 54 cm (21.6 inches)
- Birth weight: 2786 grams (g) (6 pounds [lb], 2 ounces [oz])
- Current weight: 4736 g (10 lb, 7 oz)
- Social behavior: face appears expressive with eye and mouth movements
- Movement: kicks when placed on back; opens and shuts hands; holds head and chest up when prone; pushes down on legs when feet placed on solid surface
- Vision: follows a moving object
- Hearing and speech: turns head toward sound; babbles

Based on knowledge of development, the nurse recognizes the physical growth (based on birth weight and length, compared to current weight and length is within norms for female infants and the major 3-month milestones are met; no indication of developmental delay in the development of social behavior, movement, vision, hearing, or speech.

The nurse reviews the assessment findings with the mother and explains that the child is within expected norms. The nurse also explains general principles of development, (stressing the importance of sequence as opposed to age and individual developmental pace) and developmental milestones, emphasizing that children normally differ in size, growth, and speed of development. The nurse also provides the mother a list for reference and tracking and stresses that reports of others children are not always accurate and that children normally differ in size, growth, and speed of development.

Functional assessment is described in greater detail in the Functional Ability concept. In the case of serious mental or physical disease or injury, the adult is also assessed for emotional regression because of the frequency of regression to an earlier level of emotional expression.

Developmental Delay

A problem associated with failure to meet the expected developmental level is referred to as a developmental delay. The legal definition of developmental delay varies, but usually involves a delay of at least 2.5 standard deviations in one or more areas of development, including physical development (growth and fine/gross motor skills), cognitive (intellectual), communication (speech and language), social/emotional (social skills and emotional control), and adaptive development (self-management skills).[29] Specific types of developmental delays are presented in the Exemplar section and Box 1-1.

Care Delivery
Presence of Developmental Delay

Early identification and early intervention are among the most important points when developmental delay is present. Generally speaking, regardless of the type of delay, the earlier the intervention, the better the outcome.

Management of developmental delay truly requires intradisciplinary collaboration. Early intervention services can include one or more of the following services: nursing, medicine, physical therapy, occupational therapy, psychological intervention, individual and/or family counseling, nutritional consulting, speech and language services, audiology services, and assistive technologies.

The concern of the professional nurse with development as part of his or her practice is underscored by the NANDA-I nursing diagnostic categories of *Delayed Growth and Development* and *Risk for Delayed Development*.[30] *Delayed Growth and Development* is defined as "Deviations from age-group norms."[31] The definition of *Risk for Delayed Development* is "At risk for delay of 25% or more in one or more of the areas of social or self-regulatory behavior or cognitive, language, gross or fine motor skills."[31] The Nursing Outcomes Classification (NOC) contains development-related outcomes such as *Development: late adulthood,* which is defined as the cognitive, psychosocial, and moral progression from 65 years of age and older.[32] Similarly, the Nursing Interventions Classification (NIC) contains interventions related to development.[33] An example of one of these NIC interventions is *Developmental enhancement: adolescent*, which is defined as facilitating optimal physical, cognitive, social, and emotional growth of individuals during the transition from childhood to adulthood.

Absence of Developmental Delay

Knowledge of the individual's developmental level is critical to nursing care even when no developmental problems exist. Developmental level impacts every aspect of care. It

Causes

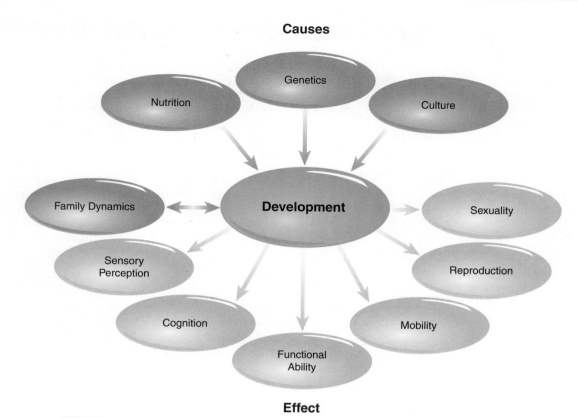

Effect

FIGURE 1-3 Cause and Effects Model of Development and Interrelated Concepts.

determines appropriate communication, teaching levels and techniques, safety provisions, assistance with activities of daily living, and approaches to therapeutic interventions. Developmental level also determines need for anticipatory guidance and health promotion interventions. To provide appropriate information on recommended health screenings, immunizations, and chemoprophylaxis as well as counseling on health topics such injury prevention, cigarette smoking, alcohol and drug abuse, diet, exercise, and sexual behavior, the developmental level of the individual must be known.

INTERRELATED CONCEPTS

The human person is an integrated whole. For clarity and ease, various dimensions, systems, and parts of the person may be discussed and examined separately but the whole person is more than simply the sum of its parts. It follows therefore that concepts used to describe the human person do not represent isolated phenomena but rather phenomena that interrelate with one another. The strength and direction of the impact of one conceptual phenomenon on another vary with the central concept under consideration. The interrelated concepts are presented in Figure 1-3. Concepts representing major influencing factors and hence determinants of development are **Genetic** endowment, **Nutrition, Environment,** and **Culture** with its unique variations in practices and expectations. These appear in green at the top of the diagram and their influence on development is indicated by the arrow

pointing in the direction of the concept. **Family dynamics** is a concept with a clearly reciprocal relationship with **Development.** This is represented by the purple oval with a double-headed arrow. The concepts identified in blue at the bottom of the diagram are those most significantly impacted by development. The relationship is indicated by an arrow pointing from developmental level to each of the concepts.

EXEMPLARS

Conditions resulting from problems in development are many and varied. They may affect any of the developmental dimensions: physical, social/emotional, cognitive, communication, or adaptive. Further, they may result in a specific problem or deficit primarily affecting one aspect of one dimension, or they may be pervasive or global, affecting many aspects of all dimensions. Causes of developmental problems are similarly complex. A small number of them are clearly identified as genetic or chromosomal problems but the causes of the vast majority are unknown, with numerous environmental conditions proposed as probable factors in their occurrence. Developmental problems may be diagnosed in utero (e.g., Down syndrome diagnosed via amniocentesis, congenital heart disease diagnosed on sonogram), they may be diagnosed at birth, or they may become evident with age and ongoing development (e.g., mental retardation, learning disabilities, and autism).[11] With advances in science and technology, causes of developmental disorders should be

BOX 1-1 EXEMPLARS OF DEVELOPMENT

Physical Developmental Delay
- Angelman's syndrome
- Bladder exstrophy
- Chronic kidney disease
- Cleft lip/palate
- Congenital heart disease
- Cystic fibrosis
- Developmental hip dysplasia
- Down syndrome
- Fragile X syndrome
- Hydrocephaly
- Klinefelter's syndrome
- Prader-Willi syndrome
- Spina bifida and other neural tube defects
- Turner's syndrome

Social/Emotional Developmental Delay
- Autism
- Asperger's syndrome
- Childhood (Pediatric) disintegrative disorder not otherwise specified (PDD-NOS)
- Dysfunctional attachments
- Failure to thrive

- Generalized anxiety disorder
- Obsessive-compulsive disorder (OCD)
- Reactive attachment disorder
- (Rett syndrome?)
- Separation anxiety disorder

Cognitive Developmental Delay
- ADD
- ADHD
- Fetal alcohol syndrome

Communication Developmental Delay
- Central auditory processing disorder (CAPD)
- Deafness
- Expressive language disorder
- Receptive language disorder

Adaptive Developmental Delay
- Blindness
- Cerebral palsy
- Developmental dyspraxia
- Duchenne's muscular dystrophy
- Oppositional defiant disorder

more easily identified and understood and earlier diagnosis with increased accuracy and ease should be possible.

Developmental anomaly is a term used to refer to any congenital defect whereas developmental disability refers to any type of pathological condition that occurs before the age of 22 and persists throughout the life of the individual.[34] Thus a developmental anomaly may or may not be a developmental disability. A developmental delay is a significant lag in a child's biophysical, psychosocial, or cognitive development in comparison with norms.[29] It is estimated that at least 8% of all children from birth to 6 years have developmental problems and delays in one or more areas of development. Global delay refers to lag in all developmental areas—speech and language, gross and fine motor skills, and personal and social development.[26] The term developmental deficit is used to refer to a specific weakness as opposed to a global delay. A developmental crisis is an episode of severe stress resulting from inability to complete a psychosocial task and progress to the next stage. Examples of the variety of developmental problems grouped according to the dimension of development most blatantly affected are presented in Box 1-1.

ACCESS EXEMPLAR LINKS ON pageburst

REFERENCES

1. Santrock JW: *Life-span development*, ed 12, New York, 2008, McGraw-Hill.
2. Feldman RS: *Development across the life-span*, ed 6, Englewood Cliffs, NJ, 2010, Prentice-Hall.
3. Hesselgrave J: Developmental influences on child health promotion. Chapter 5 in Hockenberry JJ, Wilson D, editors: *Wong's nursing care of infants and children*, ed 9, St Louis, 2011, Mosby.
4. Seidel HM, Ball JW, Dains JE, et al: *Mosby's guide to physical examination*, ed 6, St Louis, 2007, Mosby.
5. Haith M, Benson J: *Encyclopedia of infant and early childhood development*, St Louis, 2008, Elsevier.
6. Sigelman CK, Rider EA: *Lifespan human development*, Belmont, Calif, 1998, Wadsworth.
7. Perry SE, Hockenberry MJ, Lowdermilk DL, et al: *Maternal-child nursing care*, ed 4, St Louis, 2010, Mosby.
8. Trawick-Smith J: *Early childhood development: a multicultural perspective*, ed 4, Upper Saddle River, NJ, 2006, Pearson Education.
9. Wilson SF, Giddens JF: *Health assessment for nursing practice*, ed 4, St Louis, 2009, Mosby.
10. Chamley C: *Developmental anatomy & physiology of children*, New York, 2005, Churchill Livingstone.
11. Kliegman R: *Nelson's textbook of pediatrics*, ed 18, New York, 2007, Saunders.
12. Sarason JG, Johnson JH, Siegal JM: Assessing the impact of life changes: development of life experiences survey, *J Consult Clin Psychol* 46:932–946, 1978.
13. American Speech-Language-Hearing Association: *Your child's communication development: kindergarten through fifth grade* Retrieved from, asha.org/public/speech/development/language-speech.htm.
14. LaBerge M, Gale T: *Adaptive behavior scales for infants and early childhood. Gale encyclopedia of public health*, Gale Cengage, Farmington Hills, MI, 2006, The Gale Group Inc. Retrieved from www.healthline.com/galecontent/adaptive-scales-for-infants-and-early-childhood/5.
15. Etzel RA: Developmental milestones in children's environmental health, *Environ Health Perspect* A420–A421, Oct 2010.
16. Crain W: *Theories of development*, ed 6, Englewood Cliffs, NJ, 2010, Prentice-Hall.

17. Freud S: *The ego and the id and other works*, Vol 19, London, 1966, Hogarth Press and the Institute of Psychoanalysis. Strachy J, translator.

18. Erikson EH: *Childhood and society*, ed 2, New York, 1963, Norton.

19. Singer DG, Revenson TA: *A Piaget primer: how a child thinks*, New York, 1996, Penguin Books.

20. Kohlberg L: *The philosophy of moral development: moral stages and the idea of justice*, San Francisco, 1981, Harper & Row.

21. Leifer G: *Introduction to maternity & pediatric nursing*, St Louis, 2007, Mosby.

22. Whitley PP: Developmental, behavioural and somatic factors in pervasive developmental disorders: preliminary analysis, *Child Care Health Dev* 30(1):5–11, 2004.

23. Estes MEZ: *Health assessment & physical examination*, ed 4, Farmington Hills, MI, 2010, U.S. Delmar Cengage Learning.

24. Caplan J, Gleason JR: Test-retest and interobserver reliability of the Early Language Milestone Scale, ed 2 (ELM Scale-2), *J Pediatr Health Care* 7:212–219, 2006.

25. CDC National Center on Birth Defects and Developmental Disabilities, Division of Birth Defects and Developmental Disabilities: *Developmental stage interactive checklists*. Retrieved from www.cdc.gov/ncbddd/actearly/interactive/checklists.html.

26. Tervo R: Identifying patterns of developmental delays can help diagnose neurodevelopmental disorders, *Pediatric Perspectives*, Vol 12, No. 3, St Paul, Minn, July 2003, Gillette Children's Specialty Healthcare. Retrieved from www.gillettechildrens.org/fileUpload/Vol12No3.pdf.

27. Neinstein LS, Gordon CM, Katzman DK, et al, editors: *Adolescent health care: a practical guide*, ed 5, New York, 2007, Lippincott Williams & Wilkins.

28. Kozier B, Erb G, Berman A, et al: *Fundamentals of nursing concepts, process, and practice*, ed 7, Upper Saddle River, NJ, 2004, Pearson/Prentice Hall.

29. *What is a developmental disability?* Developmental Disabilities Resource Center, Lakewood, Colo. 2010, Retrieved from ddrcco.com/dddef.asp.

30. NANDA-I: *Nursing diagnoses: definitions and classification, 2009-2010*, Philadelphia, 2009, Author.

31. Ackley BJ, Ladwig GB: *Nursing diagnosis handbook*, ed 8, St Louis, 2008, Mosby.

32. Moorhead S, Johnson M, Maas M: *Nursing outcomes classification (NOC)*, ed 3, St Louis, 2004, Mosby.

33. McCloskey-Dochterman JC, Bulechek GM: *Nursing interventions classification (NIC)*, ed 4, St Louis, 2004, Mosby.

34. Department of Health and Human ServicesCenters for Disease Control: *Developmental disabilities*, 2004. Retrieved from cdc.gov/ncbddd/dd/.

35. Piaget J: *The theory of stages in cognitive development*, New York, 1969, McGraw-Hill.

Functional Ability

Frances D. Monahan

Traditionally, *health* has been seen as freedom from disease and *health care* has focused on the treatment of disease and prevention of death. A challenge to this view occurred with the World Health Organization's definition of health as a "state of complete physical, mental and social well-being, not merely the absence of disease or infirmity."[1] Gradually over the ensuing years, this idea of health has been accepted, expanded, and refined. The result is that today quality of life is seen as an inherent element of health as evidenced by one of the four overarching goals of *Healthy People 2020*, namely, to attain *high-quality*, longer lives free of preventable disease, disability, injury, and premature death.[2] A key factor in quality of life, and therefore in health, is an individual's ability to function. This is recognized in the Institute of Medicine (IOM) report *Crossing the quality chasm: a new health system for the 21st century*, which emphasizes that a goal of the U.S. health care system is "to improve the health and functioning of the people of the United States."[3] Thus the concept of functional ability has implications for collaborative health care across all populations and settings.

DEFINITION(S)

Functional ability refers to the individual's ability to perform the normal daily activities required to meet basic needs; fulfill usual roles in the family, workplace, and community; and maintain health and well-being.[4] It is the product of development and learning. Specifically, it reflects the adaptive dimension of development, which is concerned with the acquisition of a range of skills that enable independence in the home and in the community. For the purposes of this concept analysis, functional ability is defined as *the physical, psychological, cognitive, and social ability to carry on the normal activities of life*. Functional ability may differ from functional performance, which refers to the actual daily activities carried out by an individual. Functional impairment, disability, or handicap refers to varying degrees of an individual's inability to perform the tasks required to complete normal life activities without assistance.

SCOPE AND CATEGORIES

Scope

On the broadest level, the scope of functional ability occurs along a continuum ranging from complete independence to complete dependence (Figure 2-1). A person's position on this continuum varies across the lifespan and is influenced by developmental and biological factors, including current state of health, as well as by psychological, sociocultural, environmental, and politicoeconomic factors. Changes in functional level may be temporary (such as recovering from an illness or injury) or long term. An individual with full functional ability can independently meet all necessary life activities without any sort of assistance or use of assistive devices. Dependence refers to the amount of assistance needed to meet life activities; assistance can be in the form of care from another person, from assistive services, or from an adaptive device.

Categories

Functional ability is a complex concept that represents the interaction of the physical, psychological, cognitive, and social domains of the human person (Figure 2-2). Two basic categories of functional ability are the basic activities of daily living (BADLs or ADLs) and the instrumental activities of daily living (IADLs). The BADLs relate to personal care and mobility and include eating as well as hygienic and grooming activities such as bathing, mouth care, dressing, and toileting. IADLs are more complex skills that are essential to living in the community. Examples of IADLs are managing money, grocery shopping, cooking, house cleaning, doing laundry, taking

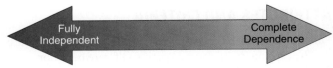

FIGURE 2-1 Scope of Concept. Functional ability ranges from full independence in daily activities to full dependence in daily activities.

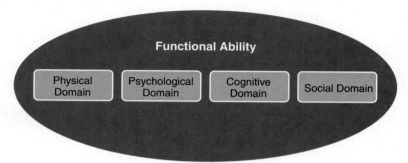

FIGURE 2-2 Categories of Functional Ability.

medication, using the telephone, and accessing transportation. BADLs and IADLs are essential to independent living.[5]

Alterations in functional ability occur as primary or secondary problems. Primary problems are those in which the ability to perform a particular function never developed. Secondary problems, on the other hand, occur after functional ability has been attained. Thus secondary problems represent a loss of functional ability.

Lifespan Considerations

Functional ability changes across the lifespan as a function of development (occurring predominantly during the infant, toddler, preschool, school age, adolescent, and young adult developmental stages) although changes in environment, lifestyle, and technology require some continued development of functional skills across the entire lifespan. In infants and young children, expected development of functional ability is indicated by achievement of developmental milestones and developmental tasks. Specialized age-appropriate tests of development are used when indicated to determine developmental delays (see Development Concept). During young and middle adulthood, identification of new problems with functional ability relies primarily on routine observations of health care providers, self-report, and report of family or others. For older adults, functional status ordinarily refers to the safe, effective performance of ADLs essential for independent living.[6] For this age group, intentional screening focused on factors known to contribute to a decline in functional ability is essential. A comprehensive, interprofessional assessment, focused on observed functional decline or changes in cognition, should be performed for individuals with multiple medical problems as well as frail elderly persons living in the community. Functional assessment requires evaluation of vision and hearing, mobility, continence, nutrition, cognition, affect, home environment, and social support, as well as BADLs and IADLs.[7]

ATTRIBUTES AND CRITERIA

Functional ability has two dimensions that serve as attributes:
1. The capacity to perform a specific self-care behavior
2. The actual performance of the behavior

At any given time an individual with the capacity to perform a self-care activity may not complete that activity because of cultural, environmental, or personal choice factors. Functional ability is further characterized by gradations of capacity or performance. It is not simply a matter of whether the individual *can* or *does* perform the activity, but instead under what circumstances, with what type and amount of assistance, and in what length of time and with what degree of effort the person *can* or *does* perform the activity. All aspects of this concept analysis are based on these attribute principals.

THEORETICAL LINKS

Functional ability is important to all individuals because it is a major contributing factor to quality of life. It allows independence and participation in activities that are fulfilling to human nature. Functional ability is also important to health care providers and health care financers because it can indicate the existence and severity of disease, signal the need for services, monitor success of treatment/disease progression, and facilitate cost-effectiveness in the provision of care.[8]

A model of nursing with the concept of functional ability as a cornerstone is the *Roper-Logan-Tierney Model of Nursing*. According to this model, 12 activities of daily living are central to human life; these are presented in Box 2-1. This model was developed in Edinburgh and is used throughout Europe as well as in many other parts of the world to guide nursing education and practice by providing a framework to organize and individualize care. It has a focus on health rather than illness and promotes care directed toward health promotion and wellness. Ongoing patient assessment and facilitation of

BOX 2-1	THE 12 ACTIVITIES OF DAILY LIVING ACCORDING TO THE ROPER-LOGAN-TIERNEY MODEL OF NURSING[9]
Maintaining a safe environment	Personal cleansing and dressing
Breathing	Maintaining body temperature
Communication	Working and playing
Mobilizing	Sleeping
Eating and drinking	Expressing sexuality
Eliminating	Dying

independence in the patient's normal activities of living are central to the model.[9,10]

CONTEXT TO NURSING AND HEALTH CARE

Functional ability is a critical consideration in virtually all areas of health care and to all members of the health care team representing interprofessional interest. It is a critical element in discharge planning from health care facilities. Successful transition is dependent on the functional level in combination with supportive services such as home care services, inpatient or outpatient rehabilitation services, or placement in a long term care facility. In the rehabilitation setting, the focus is on restoring functional ability and evaluating the functional outcomes of treatment by means of a functional assessment. For long-term care services, functional impairment—defined as needing assistance with a minimum of two or three ADLs—is a common eligibility criterion.[11]

Nursing practice has three major dimensions of concern relative to an individual's functional ability: (1) risk recognition, (2) functional assessment, and (3) planning and delivery of individualized care appropriate to level of functional ability.

Risk Recognition

Risk recognition is essential to the early identification of functional deficiencies and subsequent management. This is critical to the health status of individuals because research has shown that functional deficits are associated with poor health outcomes whereas good functional ability is associated with positive outcomes. For example, a study of stroke patients revealed that major predictors of independence 5 months after stroke were independent living status and independent in ADLs.[12]

There are multiple risk factors for impaired functional ability because of the multiple variables that impact function, including developmental abnormalities, physical or psychological trauma or disease, social and cultural factors including beliefs and perceptions of health, and physical environment. Research has repeatedly documented age,[12] cognitive function,[13] and level of depression[14] as risk factors for and predictors of functional impairment. Comorbidities and socioeconomic factors have also been implicated. Preclinical disability, defined as task modification without report of difficulty in performing a specific activity, has also been found to be an important predictor of future functional decline and disability in the elderly. In a study of postpartum women, those with postpartum depression (PPD) were 12 times less likely to achieve prepregnancy functional levels than those without PPD. Postpartal depression predicted lower personal, household, and social functioning, but without deficit in infant care.[15] Sudden onset of functional decline is often indicative of acute illness or worsening of a chronic disease.

Risk reduction should be the focus of care for patients with identified risks. Teaching about factors associated with maintenance of high-level functional ability is required. These factors include well-balanced nutrition, physical activity, routine health checkups, stress management, regular participation in meaningful activity, and avoidance of tobacco and other substances associated with abuse.[6] In addition, patients need teaching and guidance to develop effective action plans designed to decrease their specific risks.

Functional Assessment

Comprehensive functional assessment is a time-intensive, interprofessional effort requiring use of multiple assessment tools. Comprehensive functional assessment is indicated under specific circumstances. As discussed with the Development concept, children who are delayed in meeting developmental milestones and accomplishing developmental tasks are referred for assessment across domains of development including that of adaptive behavior, which is analogous to functional ability. Comprehensive assessment of functional ability in older adults is indicated when the individual has demonstrated a loss of functional ability; has experienced a change in mental status; has multiple health conditions; or is a frail elderly person living in the community. Screening for functional deficits in older adults should be a part of routine care[16] just as screening for meeting developmental milestones is for children.

An individual's performance of activities of daily living is basic to functional assessment. ADLs as indicators of functional ability evolved in the late 1950s with the identification of a group of basic physical activities, the performance of which was to be used to evaluate the success of rehabilitation programs. A decade later, instrumental activities of daily living were identified as indicators of ability to live independently in the community. This led to the use of ADLs as a measure of need and eligibility for long-term care and other support services and to the development of an array of assessment tools.

Assessment Tools

The two basic types of assessment tools are self-report and performance-based. Self-report tools provide information about the patient's perception of functional ability whereas performance-based tools involve actual observation of a standardized task, completion of which is judged by objective criteria. Performance-based assessments are preferred because they avoid potential for inaccurate measurement inherent in self-report. They also can measure functional ability with repetition and with consideration of time on task. Potential problems with self-report measures of functional activity stem from the effect of an individual's personal characteristics and preferences as well as environmental factors. Interpretation of what is meant by the question can vary from person to person. Even when vocabulary is correctly understood, the phrasing of the question can lead to an ambiguous response. For example, if a person is asked "Can you…?" the answer is based on the person's perception of his or her ability to perform the task not necessarily on actual ability. Thus overstatements of ability may occur because of a lack of awareness that gradual changes in ability have occurred. Understatements of ability are possible when an individual has not attempted to

TABLE 2-1   EXAMPLES FUNCTIONAL ASSESSMENT TOOLS

FUNCTIONAL ASSESSMENT TOOL	FUNCTION ASSESSED/ TARGET POPULATION
Barthel Index[31]	Activities of Daily Living
FIMTM Instrument	Self-care, sphincter control, transfers, locomotion, communication,
Functional Independence Measure[32]	and social cognition
Dartmouth COOP Functional Health Assessment Charts[33]	Adults: comprehensive functional and social health
	Adolescent: comprehensive functional and social health
NGAGED (Now, Growth & Development, Activities of Daily Living, General Health, Environment, and Documentation)[34]	Children ages 2-12 with physical disabilities: assesses engagement in life activities: personal, family, social, and school parameters
Functional Activities Questionnaire (FAQ)™[35]	Older adults: assesses IADLs
Folstein Mini-Mental Status Examination (MMSE)[36]	Older adults: cognitive function
Minimum Data Set (MDS) for Nursing Facility Resident Assessment and Care Screening[37]	Nursing home residents
Functional Assessment Screening in the Elderly (FASE)[37]	Older adults: functional disability
Functional Status Scale (FSS)[38]	Hospitalized children
The Edmonton Functional Assessment Tool[39]	Cancer patients: functional performance
24-Hour Functional Ability Questionnaire (24hFAQ)[41]	Outpatient postoperative patients: functional ability
Geriatric Depression Scale[42]	Older adults: depression
Inventory of Functional Status after Childbirth[43]	Postpartum women: functional status

perform the activity in question because of culture or preference or mistakenly believes that he or she is unable to perform the task. Ability can also be overreported or underreported by individuals based on personal reasons. Pride and the desire to be seen as self-sufficient, fear of losing independence, and fear of long-term care placement are common reasons for overstatement of ability, especially among elders.

Meaningful measurement of functional ability also has to address the areas of dependency and difficulty. Dependency refers to the amount of assistance needed to function, whether it involves the assistance of an adaptive device or another person. *No assistance, partial assistance,* or *total assistance* are examples of common options related to dependency used when scoring functional assessment tools. Common scoring options related to difficulty are *some, a lot,* or *unable to perform.* In addition to functional assessment tools that focus on complex, multidimensional abilities like ADLs, there are tools designed to assess a specific area of function such as mental status, mobility status, or hand function. There are also tools designed for use with specific populations[17-20] and age groups.[21-24] Examples of the wide variety of functional assessment tools are presented in Tables 2-1. Table 2-2 presents questions and observations associated with functional assessment.

Care Delivery

Knowledge of an individual's functional level in the physical, social/emotional, cognitive, and communication dimensions is essential to planning and implementing effective patient care. Functional level determines the patient's need for assistance as well as the type and amount of assistance required. It guides the nurse in helping with activities while ensuring use of adaptive equipment and maximizing the patient's independent function. This goal of optimal independent function along with the prevention of functional decline is essential to the improvement of health-related quality of life (HRQoL),

which as an outcome of care is an objective for individuals of all ages with chronic illness or disability.[25]

Management of functional activity impairment involves a multidisciplinary effort. Early intervention can include one or more of the following services: nursing, medicine, physical therapy, occupational therapy, psychological intervention, individual and/or family counseling, nutritional consulting, speech and language services, audiology services, home health or homemaker assistance, community services (such as day care), support groups, and assistive technologies. When functional activity is impaired early intervention is critical because, in general, the earlier the intervention, the better the outcome.[26]

The concern of the professional nurse with functional activity as part of his or her practice is underscored by the NANDA-I nursing diagnostic categories related to Self-Care Deficit and Impaired Mobility[27] as well as the Nursing Outcomes Classification (NOC) outcomes[28] and the Nursing Interventions Classification (NIC) interventions related to self-care and mobility.[29] Table 2-3 presents these diagnostic categories, outcomes, and interventions.

INTERRELATED CONCEPTS

The human person is a complex integrated whole that is greater than the sum of its parts. It follows therefore that concepts used to describe aspects of the human person represent interrelated rather than isolated phenomena. The strength and direction of the impact of one conceptual phenomenon on another vary with the central concept under consideration. Because functional activity depends on the interplay of multiple elements within the physical, psychological, social, and cognitive dimensions, and because it allows for purposeful interaction with the environment, a multitude of concepts can be identified as influencing and/or being influenced by it.

TABLE 2-2   GUIDE TO FUNCTIONAL ASSESSMENT SCREENING[45-49]

FUNCTIONAL ASSESSMENT COMPONENT	SAMPLE QUESTIONS	OBSERVATIONS/EXAMINATIONS
Vision	Do you have any difficulty seeing? Do you wear glasses or contact lens? Do you use any special equipment to help you see such as a high-intensity light or magnifying glass? When was your last eye exam?	Observe for signs of impaired vision during interaction with patient: turning head to one side in an effort to see better; nonapplicable comments about room seeming dark; feeling for items Have patient hold a magazine or newspaper and read a line of print Have patient read a wall clock or sign at a distance
Hearing	Do you have difficulty hearing? Does anyone tell you that you are hard of hearing? Do you have to ask people to repeat what they say? Can you hear well in crowds? Can you hear when the area is noisy?	Note patient's apparent hearing during your interaction with him or her Rub your thumb and forefinger together in front of each of patient's ears; patient should easily hear the sound
Mobility	Do you have any trouble moving? Do you feel steady when you walk? Do you use anything to help you walk? Do you have trouble getting out of bed? Do you have difficulty sitting down or standing up?	Observe patient's general movements; look for obvious limitation of movement in any body part Have patient put hands together behind neck and then behind waist to assess external and internal rotation of shoulder Assess lower extremity function, balance, and gait by asking patient to arise from a straight-back chair, stand still, walk across room (about 10 feet), turn, walk back, and sit down Note ability to stand up and sit down; balance when sitting, standing, and walking; gait; and ability to turn
Fall history	Have you had any falls? Have you had any near falls? Do you take any precautions against falling?	
Continence	Do you ever lose control of your bowels? Do you ever lose control of your urine and wet yourself? Do you wear any type of protective pad or underclothes in case of an accident with urine or bowels?	
Nutrition	Have you gained or lost 10 pounds in the last 6 months without trying? What do you typically eat in a day? Do you have difficulty chewing or swallowing? When was your last dental visit?	Note general appearance as related to nutritional status: well nourished, undernourished, emaciated Obtain weight Determine body mass index (BMI)
Cognition	Do you have any trouble with your memory?	Note patient's ability to respond appropriately to questions and directions Three-item recall at 1 minute; if patient fails this test, follow with MMSE
Affect	Do you often feel anxious or overstressed? Do you often feel sad or down?	Note patient's expression and if this matches mood
Home environment	Who do you live with? What type of house do you have: single home, multiple family, apartment? How many floors does the home have? Are there stairs you must use?	
Social participation	What keeps you busy all day? How often do you go out? How often do you have company?	
ADLs (basic and instrumental)	Use a reliable, valid assessment tool to assess function related to grooming, toileting, dressing, eating, walking, shopping, meal preparation, housekeeping, travel/driving, money management.	

TABLE 2-3	ACTIVITIES OF DAILY LIVING: NANDA-I DIAGNOSTIC CATEGORIES, NOC OUTCOMES, AND NIC INTERVENTIONS		
NANDA-I DIAGNOSTIC CATEGORY[50]	**DEFINITION[51]**	**NOC OUTCOME[52]**	**NIC INTERVENTIONS[52]**
Bathing Self-Care Deficit	Impaired ability to perform or complete bathing activities for self	Self-Care: Activities of Daily Living (ADL), Bathing, Hygiene	Self-Care Assistance: Bathing/Hygiene
Dressing Self-Care Deficit	Impaired ability to perform or complete dressing activities for self	Self-Care: Activities of Daily Living (ADL), Dressing, Hygiene, Grooming	Self-Care Assistance: Dressing/Grooming
Feeding Self-Care Deficit	Impaired ability to perform or complete self-feeding activities	Self-Care: Activities of Daily Living (ADL), Eating	Self-Care Assistance: Feeding
Toileting Self-Care Deficit	Impaired ability to perform or complete for self toileting activities	Self-Care: Activities of Daily Living (ADL), Toileting	Self-Care Assistance: Toileting
Impaired Physical Mobility	Limitation in independent, purposeful physical movement of the body or of one or more extremities	Ambulation Ambulation: Wheelchair, Mobility Self-Care: Activities of Daily Living Transfer Performance	Exercise Therapy: Ambulation, Joint Mobility, Positioning
Impaired Wheelchair Mobility	Limitation of independent operation of wheelchair within environment	Ambulation: Wheelchair	Exercise Therapy: Muscle Control Positioning: Wheelchair

Nursing Diagnoses–Definitions and Classification 2012-2014. Copyright © 2012, 1994-2012 by NANDA International. Used by arrangement with Blackwell Publishing Limited, a company of John Wiley & Sons, Inc.

Figure 2-3 depicts the most prominent of these interrelationships. Concepts representing major influencing factors and hence determinants of functional ability are **Development, Cognition,** and **Culture,** with its unique variations in practices and expectations. These appear at the top of the diagram and their influence on functional activity is indicated by the arrow pointing in the direction of this concept. **Family dynamics, Motivation,** and **Coping** as well as the physiologically focused concepts of **Mobility, Nutrition, Sensory perception, Gas exchange,** and **Perfusion** have a clearly reciprocal relationship with functional activity. These concepts surround either side of the concept with double-headed arrows because of their mutual interaction with it. The concepts of **Elimination** and **Sexuality** are shown at the very bottom of the figure with arrows pointing from functional activity to them because of the primarily unidirectional relationship of these concepts.

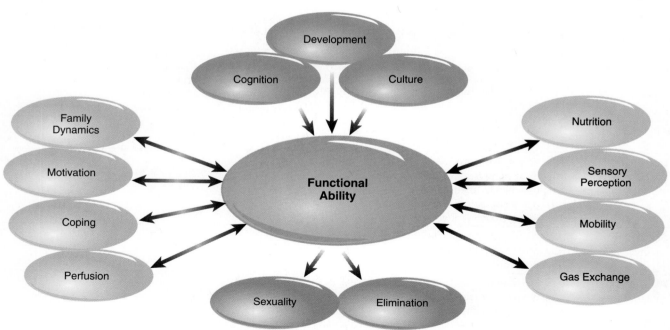

FIGURE 2-3 Functional Ability and Interrelated Concepts.

MODEL CASE

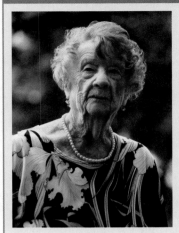

Mrs. Rose Finney is an 85-year-old woman with ovarian cancer. She presented at the oncology clinic for a scheduled appointment 6 weeks after surgical removal of her ovaries, uterus, a section of large bowel, and as much tumor mass as possible from other areas of her abdomen. The purpose of the visit was a postoperative checkup and planning for chemotherapy. Mrs. Finney was accompanied by a niece with whom she had stayed while recovering from the surgery. The niece lives out of state and the patient will be returning to her own home following this follow-up appointment. At this visit, the nurse interviewed the patient to obtain detailed self-report information related to functional ability. The information gathered is presented below.

- Alert, well-groomed, well-spoken, fiercely independent elderly woman recuperating remarkably well from extensive surgery
- Uncontrolled glaucoma with limited vision in one eye; 20/80 vision with glasses in other eye
- Slightly hard of hearing

- Arthritis in fingers along with lack of strength makes some tasks difficult (e.g., opening jars, using telephone)
- Uncertain walking outdoors, particularly in unfamiliar areas and when ground uneven; no assistive devices
- Medication: Synthroid every morning for 47 years
- Never married, no children
- Lives alone in a single home; bedroom on first floor but laundry facilities and garage are on basement level
- Does not drive
- Only living relatives in addition to the niece are two nephews: one lives out of state and other lives ½ hour away
- Telephone contact with closer nephew daily, occasional visits and trips for shopping and other errands
- Three friends in neighborhood, each of whom calls or visits on average every 2 weeks

Case Analysis

Mrs. Finney is at risk for falls as a result of unsteadiness, poor vision, and stair use in her home. In the event of an accident, she is at risk for inability to call for help as a result of living alone and having limited strength, poor eyesight, and arthritis, which makes telephone dialing difficult. Mrs. Finney needs reliable transportation for care appointments and for grocery shopping. Her poor eyesight also makes her at risk for problems with medication compliance during the chemotherapy treatment regimen. Additional monitoring will also be needed because of the risk of associated side effects as a result of chemotherapy.

EXEMPLARS

As discussed earlier, alterations in functional ability occur as primary or secondary problems. Primary problems are those in which the ability to perform a particular function never developed. Secondary problems, on the other hand, occur after functional ability has been attained. Thus secondary problems represent a loss of functional ability.

Alterations in functional ability, whether primary or secondary, may affect one very specific area of function or may be global and affect widespread function. Impaired functional ability is often complex and may involve an array of environmental as well as individual factors. Furthermore, similar alterations in function can be the result of very different causes.

■■■ BOX 2-2   EXEMPLARS OF FUNCTIONAL ABILITY

Causes of Primary Problems
- Angelman's syndrome
- Autism spectrum disorder
- Cerebral palsy
- Down syndrome
- Duchenne's muscular dystrophy
- Fetal alcohol syndrome
- Hypoplastic limb
- Malnutrition
- Receptive or expressive language disorder

Causes of Secondary Problems
- Alzheimer's disease
- Blindness
- Brain injury

- Cardiovascular disease
- Chronic pain
- Chronic fatigue
- Chronic obstructive pulmonary disease
- Deafness
- Malnutrition
- Multiple sclerosis
- Osteoarthritis
- Parkinson's disease
- Rheumatoid arthritis
- Schizophrenia
- Spinal cord injury
- Skeletal fracture
- Stroke

Causes of primary problems of functional ability may be genetic in origin (i.e., the result of a congenital defect) or may be a result of trauma, disease, or negative environmental factors occurring during the early years of development. Often, however, as with many developmental problems, the cause is unclear.

Secondary problems of functional activity are more commonly identifiable as the result of aging, disease, trauma, or negative environmental factors. Sudden onset of functional decline is a sign of acute disease such as pneumonia, urinary tract infection, or fluid and electrolyte imbalance. Alternatively, it can be a sign of worsening chronic disease such as diabetes, chronic obstructive pulmonary disease (COPD), or heart failure.[30] Depending on the extent of alteration in functional ability, the problem may be termed an impairment, a disability, or a handicap. Examples of specific causes of primary and secondary problems of functional activity are presented in Box 2-2.

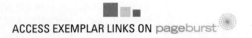

ACCESS EXEMPLAR LINKS ON pageburst

REFERENCES

1. World Health Organization: The constitution of the World Health Organization, *WHO Chronicle* 1:6–24, 1947.
2. U.S. Department of Health and Human Services: *Healthy People 2020*. Retrieved from www.health.gov/healthypeople.
3. Institute of Medicine, Committee on Quality of Health Care in America: *Crossing the quality chasm: a new health system for the 21st century*, Washington, DC, 2001, National Academies Press.
4. American Thoracic Society: *Quality of life resource*, 2007. Retrieved from www.qol.thoracic.org/sections/key-concepts/functional-status.html.
5. Goldman L, Ausiello D, editors: *Cecil medicine*, ed 23, Philadelphia, 2008, Saunders.
6. Potter PA, Perry AG: *Fundamentals of nursing*, ed 7, St Louis, 2009, Mosby.
7. Lachs MS, Feinsttein AR, Cooney LM, et al: A simple procedure for general screening for functional disability in elderly patients, American College of Physicians, *Ann Intern Med* 12(9):699–706, 1990.
8. Min LC, Wenger NS, Reuben DB, et al: A short functional survey is responsive to changes in functional status in vulnerable older people, *J Am Geriatr Soc* 56(10):1932–1936, 2008.
9. Roper N, Logan WW: *The Roger-Logan-Tierney model of nursing: based on activities of living*, London, 2004, Elsevier/Churchill-Livingstone.
10. Allegoode M, Tomey AM: *Nursing theorists and their work*, ed 7, St Louis, 2010, Mosby.
11. Geron SM: Functional ability. *Encyclopedia of aging*, 2002. Accessed March 24, 2011, at www.encyclopedia.com.
12. Hankey GJ: *Stroke*, ed 2, London, 2007, Churchill Livingstone.
13. Royall DR, Lauterbach EC, Kaufer D: The Committee on Research of the American Neuropsychiatric Association: The cognitive correlates of functional status: a review from the Committee on Research of the American Neuropsychiatric Association, *J Am Geriatr Soc* 55:1705–1711, 2007.
14. Van der Weele GM, Gussekloo J, De Waal MM, et al: Co-occurrence of depression and anxiety in elderly subjects aged 90 years and its relationship with functional status, quality of life and mortality, *Int J Geriatr Psychiatr* 24(6):595–601, 2009.
15. Posmontier B: Functional status outcomes in mothers with and without postpartum depression, *J Midwifery Womens Health* 53(4):310–318, 2008.
16. Bierman AS: Functional status: the sixth vital sign, *J Gen Intern Med* 16(11):785–786, 2001.
17. Hogue SL, Reese PR, Colopy M, et al: Assessing a tool to measure patient functional ability after outpatient surgery, *Anesth Analgesia* 91(1):97–106, 2000. Retrieved from ncbi.nlm.nih.gov/pubmed/10866894.
18. Hudak PL, Amadio PC, Bombardier C: Development of an upper extremity outcome measure: the DASH (disabilities of the arm, shoulder and hand) [corrected]. The Upper Extremity Collaborative Group (UECG), *Am J Ind Med* 29(6):602–608, 1996. erratum in *Am J Ind Med* 30(3):372, 1996.
19. Leidy NK: Functional status and the forward progress of merry-go-rounds: toward a coherent analytical framework, *Nurs Res* 43:196–202, 1994.
20. Pfeffer RI, Kurosaki TT, Harrah CH Jr, et al: Measurement of functional activities in older adults in the community, *J Gerontol* 37(3):323–329, 1982. Reprinted with permission of The Gerontological Society of America, 1030 15th St NW, Suite 250, Washington, DC 20005, via Copyright Clearance. Retrieved from ncbi.nlm.nih.gov/pubmed/7069156.
21. Center for Functional Assessment Research at SUNY Buffalo: *Guide for the uniform data set for medical rehabilitation for children (WeeFIM), Version 4.0*, Buffalo, NY, 1993, State University of New York at Buffalo.
22. Odetola F: Assessing the functional status of children, *Pediatrics* 124(1):e163–e165, 2009. (doi:10.1542/peds.2009-0859).
23. Pollack MM, Holubkov R, Glass P, et al: Eunice Kennedy Shriver National Institute of Child Health and Human Development Collaborative Pediatric Critical Care Research Network. Functional status scale: a new pediatric outcome measure, *Pediatrics* 124(1):e18–e28, 2009.
24. Wasson JH, Kairys SW, Nelson EC, et al: A short survey for assessing health and social problems of adolescents, *J Fam Pract* 38:489–494, 1994.
25. Wilson IB, Cleary PD: Linking clinical variables with health-related quality of life, *JAMA* 59-65:1995, 1995.
26. Lubkin IM, Larsen PD: *Chronic illness impact and intervention*, ed 6, Boston, 2006, Jones and Bartlett.
27. NANDA-I: *Nursing diagnoses: definitions and classification, 2009-2010*, Philadelphia, 2009, Author.
28. McCloskey-Dochterman JC, Bulechek GM: *Nursing interventions classification (NIC)*, ed 4, St Louis, 2004, Mosby.
29. Moorhead S, Johnson M, Maas M: *Nursing outcomes classification (NOC)*, ed 3, St Louis, 2004, Mosby.
30. Krevesic DM, Mezey M: Assessment of function. In Mezey M, Fulmer T, Abraham I, editors: *Geriatric nursing protocols for best practice*, ed 2, New York, 2003, Springer.
31. Neal LJ: Current functional assessment tools, *Home Healthcare Nurse* 16(11):762–772, 1996.
32. Turner-Stokes T, et al: The UK FIM+FAM: development and evaluation, *Clin Rehabil* 13:277–287, 1999. Retrieved from www.Radcliffeoxford.com/books/samplechapter/2668/Gupta-section%2002C-146Fe2aOrdz.pdf.

33. Nelson E, Wasson J, Kirk J, et al: Assessment of function in routine clinical practice: description of the COOP chart method and preliminary findings, *J Chron Dis* 40(suppl 1): 55S–63S, 1987.

34. Guillet SE: Assessing the child with disabilities, *Home Healthcare Nurse* 16:402–409, 1998.

35. McDowell I, Newell C: Functional disability and handicap. *Measuring health: a guide to rating scales and questionnaires*, ed 2, New York, 1996, Oxford University Press.

36. Kurlowicz L, Wallace M: The mini mental status examination. *Try this: best practices in nursing care to older adults from the Hartford Institute for Geriatric Nursing* No. 3, July 1999. Retrieved April 5, 2011, from www.CNA-nurses.ca/CNAdocuments/pdf/toolkit/evidence/mini_mental_status_examination.pdfJuly 1999.

37. Estes MEZ: *Health assessment & physical examination*, ed 4, Farmington Hills, MI, 2010, U.S. Delmar Cengage Learning.

38. Pollack MM, Holubkov R, Glass P, et al: Eunice Kennedy Shriver National Institute of Child Health and Human Development Collaborative Pediatric Critical Care Research Network. Functional status scale: a new pediatric outcome measure, *Pediatrics* 124(1):e18–e28, 2009.

39. The Edmonton Functional Assessment Tool: preliminary development and evaluation for use in palliative care, *Neuropsychiatr Clin Neurosci* 19:249–265, 2007.

40. Hogue SL, Reese PR, Colopy M, et al: Assessing a tool to measure patient functional ability after outpatient surgery, *Anesth Analgesia* 91(1):97–106, 2000. Retrieved from ncbi.nlm.nih.gov/pubmed/10866894.

41. Goldman L, Ausiello D, editors: *Cecil medicine*, ed 23, Philadelphia, 2008, Saunders.

42. Posmontier B: Functional status outcomes in mothers with and without postpartum depression, *J Midwifery Womens Health* 53(4):310–318, 2008.

43. Hudak PL, Amadio PC, Bombardier C: Development of an upper extremity outcome measure: the DASH (disabilities of the arm, shoulder and hand) [corrected]. The Upper Extremity Collaborative Group (UECG), *Am J Ind Med* 29(6):602–608, 1996. erratum in *Am J Ind Med* 30(3):372, 1996.

44. Seidel HM, Ball JW, Dains JE, et al: *Mosby's guide to physical examination*, ed 6, St Louis, 2007, Mosby.

45. Estes MEZ: *Health assessment & physical examination*, ed 4, Farmington Hills, MI, 2010, U.S. Delmar Cengage Learning.

46. Goldman L, Ausiello D, editors: *Cecil medicine*, ed 23, Philadelphia, 2008, Saunders.

47. Nelson E, Landgraf JM, Hays RD, et al: The functional status of patients: how can it be measured in physicians' offices? *Med Care* 28:1111–1126, 1990.

48. Lachs MS, Feinsttein AR, Cooney LM, et al: A simple procedure for general screening for functional disability in elderly patients, American College of Physicians, *Ann Intern Med* 12(9):699–706, 1990.

49. NANDA-I: *Nursing diagnoses: definitions and classification, 2009-2010*, Philadelphia, 2009, Author.

50. Ackley BJ, Ladwig GB: *Nursing diagnosis handbook*, ed 8, St Louis, 2008, Mosby.

51. McCloskey-Dochterman JC, Bulechek GM: *Nursing interventions classification (NIC)*, ed 4, St Louis, 2004, Mosby.

52. Moorhead S, Johnson M, Maas M: *Nursing outcomes classification (NOC)*, ed 3, St Louis, 2004, Mosby.

3

Family Dynamics

Shannon E. Perry

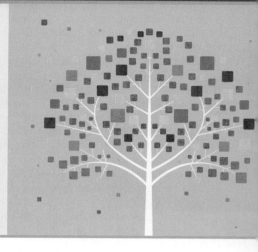

The *family* has been viewed traditionally as the primary unit of socialization, the basic structural unit within a community. A family consists of (1) parents and their children, (2) those related by blood such as ancestors and descendants, or, in a less restricted definition, (3) any group living together as if they were related by blood. A family is who they say they are.

There are a variety of family configurations: the nuclear family, married-parent families, extended families, married-blended families, cohabiting-parent families, single-parent families, no-parent families, and same-sex families. The interaction among family members will vary in each of these configurations. The more numerous the family members, the more complex will be the interactions among the family members (Figure 3-1).

Because families are the foundation of social context, nurses must have an understanding of and appreciation for the ways in which family dynamics influence the delivery of health care to individuals. This concept presents family dynamics and includes definitions and examples of the application of this concept to professional nursing practice.

DEFINITION(S)

For the purposes of this concept analysis, the term *family dynamics* is defined as "interrelationships between and among individual family members" or "the forces at work within a family that produce particular behaviors or symptoms."[1] The dynamic is created by the way in which a family lives and interacts with one another. That dynamic—whether positive or negative, supportive or destructive, nurturing or damaging—changes who people are and influences how they view and interact with the world outside of the family. A number of culturally sensitive tools have been developed to assess or measure family dynamics (Table 3-1). These and other models are often used in studies of family dynamics.

Influences on family dynamics are many and varied. These include such factors as the family configuration, relationship between the parents, number of children in the family, parental absence, chronic illness, disability, substance abuse, physical abuse, death, culture, socioeconomic status, unemployment, family values, and parenting practices.

When examining family dynamics, ages within the family should be considered. A grandparent will likely have views different from their grandchildren. The history of the people in the family is important. When a couple marry, they bring with them the culture and norms of their family of origin. This will influence the family dynamics. The role each member plays in the family is significant; it may be important to change roles to increase understanding among family members and decrease resentment.

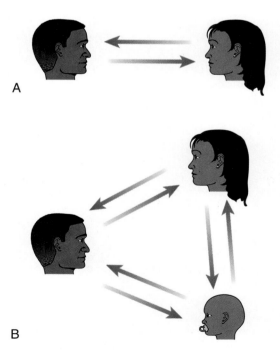

FIGURE 3-1 Complexity of Relationships.

TABLE 3-1   MODELS AND TOOLS TO ASSESS FAMILY DYNAMICS

MODEL	PURPOSE/DESCRIPTION
Calgary Family Assessment Model[a]	A multidimensional framework with three major categories: structural, developmental, and functional. Is embedded in larger worldviews of postmodernism, feminism, and biology of cognition. Theory foundation of model includes systems, cybernetics, communication, and change. Diversity issues are included.
Circumplex Model of Marital & Family Systems[b]	Family model grounded in systems theory. Includes dimensions of *family cohesion* (emotional bonding that couple and family members have toward one another), *flexibility* (amount of change in its leadership, role relationships, and relationship rules), and *communication* (includes family as a group in relation to listening skills, speaking skills, self-disclosure, clarity, continuity tracking, and respect and regard).
Family Adaptability and Cohesion Evaluation Scales (FACES IV)[c]	Updated version of self-report scale designed to assess full range of cohesion and flexibility dimensions of Circumplex Model.
Dyadic Adjustment Scale[d]	Self-report 32-item questionnaire administered to both members of a couple. Scales include *dyadic consensus, dyadic satisfaction, affectional expression,* and *dyadic cohesion.*
Chinese Family Assessment Instrument (C-FAI)[e]	Self-report measure to assess family functioning in Chinese populations. Contains five dimensions: (1) *mutuality,* (2) *communication and cohesiveness,* (3) *conflict and harmony,* (4) *parental concern,* and (5) *parental control.*
Family Dynamics Measure II (FDM II)[f]	Based on eight bipolar dimensions of Barnhill.[g] First six of dimensions were selected for inclusion: (1) *individuation versus enmeshment;* (2) *mutuality versus isolation;* (3) *flexibility versus rigidity;* (4) *stability versus disorganization;* (5) *clear communication versus unclear or distorted communication;* and (6) *role compatibility versus role conflict.*

[a]Wright LM, Leahey M: Nurses and families. *A guide to family assessment and intervention,* ed 5, Philadelphia, 2009, FA Davis.
[b]Olson DH, Gorall DM: Circumplex model of marital and family systems. In Walsh F, editor: *Normal family processes,* ed 3, New York, 2003, Guilford.
[c]Olson DH: Circumplex model of family systems, *J Fam Ther* 22(2):144-167, 2000.
[d]Spanier G: Measuring dyadic adjustment: new scales for assessing the quality of marriage and similar dyads, *J Marriage Fam* 38(1):15-28, 1976.
[e]Shek DTL: Assessment of family functioning Chinese adolescents: the Chinese Family Assessment Instrument. In Singh NN, Ollendick T, Singh AN, editors: *International perspectives on child and adolescent mental health,* pp 297-316, Amsterdam, 2002, Elsevier.
[f]Lasky P, Buckwalter KC, Whall A et al: Developing an instrument for the assessment of family dynamics, *West J Nurs Res* 7(1):40-57, 1985.
[g]Barnhill LR: Healthy family systems, *Fam Coordinator* 28:94-100, 1979.

Quality of Relationships

Relationships within a family may be healthy: loving and respectful, with members supporting each other, providing nurturance and assistance, and forming a unit within society. They support each other within the family and within the larger community.

Family interactions can be *dysfunctional* "because of physical, mental, or situational problems of one or more family members."[1] A husband may berate his wife for perceived shortcomings or denigrate a child for having difficulty with school. Siblings may squabble and place blame for incidents. In some instances, a parent and siblings may abuse one child. Observing dysfunctional interactions by parents can lead children to imitate those negative behaviors.

Roles of Family Members

Within the family, individuals assume or are assigned roles: spouse, parent, child, sibling, grandchild, disciplinarian, leader, scapegoat, nurturer, enabler, hero, and so on. Healthy families are able to adapt and adjust. Roles may change over time—for example, as children grow and develop, crises are encountered, illnesses develop, or family members leave home. It may be difficult for family members, especially children, to understand roles, changes in roles and the way those changes affect the balance of relationships within the family, and the effects of one family member's actions on the remainder of the family.

SCOPE AND CATEGORIES

The emphasis in nursing today is on providing family-centered care. Wherever nurses practice, they will work with families and observe family dynamics across the lifespan. Family dynamics occur between couples, with parents and children, and with extended family members. As implied by the word "dynamic," the interactions between family members are fluid and change with growth and development and by circumstances. Family therapists, marriage and family counselors, social workers, and those working with victims of intimate partner violence and child abuse all encounter patients experiencing a breakdown in healthy family dynamics.

Scope—Positive to Negative or Dysfunctional

The dynamics change between a married couple when their first child is born; this is because the dynamics in a triad are more complex than those in a dyad (see Figure 3-1), and further increases in complexity occur when additional children are born. Extended family relationships add to the complexity as do divorce, remarriage, and stepchildren. In times of illness and stress, family interactions may change—sometimes for the better and sometimes for the worse. Family members can express concern for the ill member; extended family may gather and provide assistance and support. Old quarrels can be resolved; hurts can be forgiven; love can be expressed; and memories can be shared. At other times, quarrels can arise over past slights, the perceived or real burdens of caregiving, and the strain on family finances. Ill family members can become more demanding, feeling they deserve special treatment and care. Death must be faced, burial details settled, and assets divided.

Dysfunctional families and families exhibiting maladaptive behavior tax the nurse's ingenuity and resourcefulness. Although the primary concern of the nurse is the patient, in a broader sense, the whole family is the patient. Nurses can, at times, role model more appropriate interactions or provide suggestions for improving communication and interactions among family members. At other times, when maladaptive or dysfunctional behaviors are observed, the nurse can intervene and refer to other professionals or specialists as appropriate.

ATTRIBUTES AND CRITERIA

Defining attributes of family dynamics include the following:
- Family, however that is defined, is involved.
- Communication, verbal or nonverbal, among family members must occur.
- Interactions among family members are fluid, flexible, and changeable (dynamic) (Figure 3-2).

The family, whether a couple or a multigenerational group, communicates and interacts. The more members involved, the greater the complexity of interaction and communication. Communication and interaction are dynamic and changing and can be positive or negative. Positive interactions and communications are growth-producing and produce cohesion. Negative interactions and communications are divisive and disruptive and lead to dysfunction and alienation.

THEORETICAL LINKS

Family Systems Theory

Wright and Leahy[2] describe systems theory as allowing nurses to "view the family as a unit and thus focus on observing the interaction among family members rather than studying family members individually." Key characteristics of the family systems theory are that (1) a family system is part of a larger suprasystem and is composed of many subsystems, (2) the family as a whole is greater than the sum of its individual members, (3) a change in one family member affects all family members, (4) the family is able to create a balance between change and stability, and (5) family members' behaviors are best understood from a view of circular rather than linear causality.[2]

Because a change in one family member affects all family members, a change in family dynamics occurs. For example, when Tama, a mother of three children, gave birth to her fourth child, the father and the siblings of the baby experienced change, and the relationships among the members of the family changed. The father, Peter, has to assume additional responsibilities for care of the family while the mother recuperates from the birth. He can prepare meals and do laundry; he can assume some care of the newborn. Siblings must share their mother's love and time with this new member; sibling rivalry may occur. The family attempts to balance this change and restore stability. As the newborn is incorporated into the family, the siblings resume their previous activities.

Because one family member changes, the family changes, and in turn this change affects the member who changed

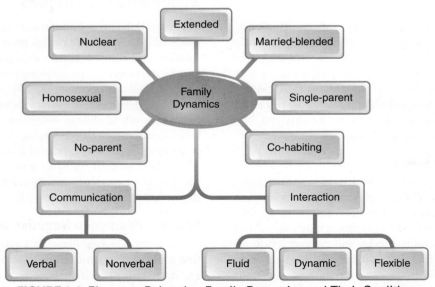

FIGURE 3-2 Elements Related to Family Dynamics and Their Qualities.

(circular causality). The mother is now the mother of four children with the additional responsibilities entailed in caring for a newborn and three other children while maintaining her relationship with her partner.

Structural-Functional Theory

The origins of structural-functional theory are in social anthropology.[3,4] In this theory, the family is a social system. Family members have specific roles such as the father role, mother role, and daughter or son role. Maintaining equilibrium between complementary roles is accomplished through family dynamics. This permits the family to function within the family unit and in society. Some families establish rigid boundaries and outsiders are kept at a distance. Some families may be isolated and may find that in times of crisis their resources are inadequate. Other families maintain open boundaries and give and accept assistance when needed. Some reciprocal relationships within the family can be detrimental, such as designating one member as the family scapegoat or viewing another family member as weak or dependent. Another family member may be identified as the strong or responsible one and undue expectations may be placed upon that member.

Family Stress Theory

The ways in which families react to stress is the focus of this theory.[5] Stress of families can be studied in the contexts in which the family is living, both internal and external. Events that the family can change or control (e.g., family structure, psychological defenses, and philosophical values and beliefs) comprise the internal context. The time and place in which a family finds itself and over which the family has no control (e.g., culture of the larger society, time in history, economic state of society, maturity of the individuals involved, success of the family in coping with stressors, and genetic inheritance) comprise the external context.

Tama and Peter have a strong sense of family, are supportive of each other, and value family (internal context). They were prepared to cope with the stress on family finances incurred by the addition of the fourth child. However, at 6 weeks of age the baby was diagnosed with pyloric stenosis and required hospitalization and surgery. This created additional stress on the family—concern about the health of the baby, separation of the mother and infant from the family during the hospitalization, and increased strain on finances. The maternal grandmother assisted with the care of the children while the infant was hospitalized, introducing a different level of relationship and increasing the number of interactions within the family. Peter and his mother-in-law do not always agree on child-rearing activities, meal preparation, or discipline, which creates additional stress.

The number of grandparents raising grandchildren has increased significantly over the last several decades. Custody of grandchildren creates multiple challenges for grandparents. The stresses accompanying child-rearing may negatively influence the health of the grandparents; however, their health is critical to their ability to parent.[6] Nursing interventions can improve the health and role functions of grandparents.

Family Life Cycle (Developmental) Theory

Families pass through stages. Relationships among family members move through transitions. Although families have roles and functions, a family's main value is in relationships that are irreplaceable. Developmental stresses can disrupt the life cycle process.[7]

The family of Tama and Peter went through stages of dating and marriage, to a couple, to parents of one child, and now to parents of four children. Tama and Peter's exclusive relationship expanded to include their firstborn. When the second child was born, the firstborn had to relinquish his role as an only child and develop a relationship with his sibling. The complexity of relationships increased exponentially as the size of the family increased.

Children grow and develop within the family and expand the cycle of their relationships through play groups, school, church, and social club activities.

CONTEXT TO NURSING AND HEALTH CARE

The family influences and is influenced by other people and institutions and plays a pivotal role in health care. Understanding family dynamics and how these dynamics relate to health is important to nurses for the provision of quality nursing care.[8] The family, whether present or absent, influences the patient, either positively or negatively.

Conducting a Family Assessment

The Calgary Family Assessment Model (CFAM)[2] is widely used by nurses to assess families. Wright and Leahy[2] caution that the nurse must recognize that such an assessment is based on "the nurse's personal and professional life experiences, beliefs, and relationships with those being interviewed." The assessment is not "the truth" about the family but is just one perspective at one point in time.

The model is used to ask the family questions about themselves in order to gain understanding of the structure, development, and function at a point in time. Not all questions within the subcategories are asked at the first interview and not all questions are appropriate for all families. While individuals are interviewed, the focus of a family assessment is on the interaction among the individuals in the family.

The three major categories of the CFAM are structural, developmental, and functional.[2] There are several subcategories for each category. In this brief explanation of the model, only the major categories will be addressed. Sample questions used in an assessment are included. Consult the Wright and Leahey text for a full explanation of the model.

Structural Assessment

Assessment of the structure of the family includes determining the members of the family, the relationship among family members in contrast to relationships with those outside the

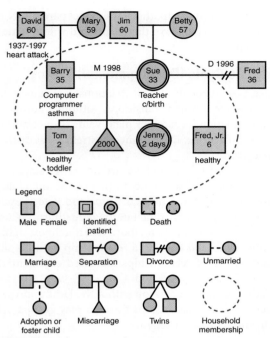

Legend

Male Female   Identified   Death
                 patient

Marriage   Separation   Divorce   Unmarried

Adoption or   Miscarriage   Twins   Household
foster child   membership

FIGURE 3-3 Example of an Ecomap that Describes Social Relationships and Depicts Available Supports. (From Lowdermilk DL, Perry SE, Cashion K, et al: *Maternity and women's health care,* ed 10, St Louis, 2012, Elsevier; Figure 2-5, p 23.)

family, and the context of the family. Questions to assess the structure include the following:

- Who is in your family?
- Does anyone else live with you?
- Has anyone moved out recently?
- Is there anyone you think of as family who does not live with you?[2]

Genograms and ecomaps (Figure 3-3) are useful tools to outline the family's internal and external structures. These tools can be hand drawn; in addition, some computer programs are available to construct genograms.

Developmental Assessment

Most nurses are knowledgeable about the stages of child development and adult development and there is increasing literature about development during senior years. However, family development is more than concurrent development of individuals in a family. Family development is different from family life cycle. Family development takes into consideration the vicissitudes of living with both predictable and unpredictable events whereas family life cycle describes the typical trajectory followed by most families. The CFAM uses family life cycle to organize the assessment of family development.[2]

The following are sample questions for families in later life:

- When you review your life, what aspects did you enjoy the most?
- What aspects generate the most regret?
- As your health is declining, what plans have you made for your care or that of others in your family who are in ill health?

Functional Assessment

Functional assessment addresses how individuals actually behave in relation to one another.[2] The two basic aspects of family functioning are instrumental and expressive. Instrumental aspects include routine activities of daily living such as preparing meals, eating, sleeping, doing laundry, and changing dressings. Expressive aspects include communication (emotional, verbal, nonverbal, circular), problem solving, roles, influence and power, beliefs, and alliances and coalitions.[2] The categories are not used to define a family's emotional health; it is the family's judgment of whether they are functioning well that is important.

Questions such as the following can be asked:

- Whose role is it to see that Granddad takes his medicine?
- Whose turn is it to bathe Granddad?
- Why is Jimmy not helping to take care of Granddad?
- How can we get Jimmy to help with the caretaking?

If the family is having trouble coping with instrumental issues, often expressive issues exist. However, the family can cope with instrumental issues and still have expressive issues. Thus assessment of both is essential.

Examples and Nursing Interventions
Dysfunctional Family Dynamics

When Andrew was admitted to the coronary care unit, his wife, Barbara, was overheard berating him for not taking better care of himself and leaving her with four children to raise. Outside the unit Barbara scolded the children for "worrying your father to death."

An appropriate nursing intervention would be to take Barbara aside and show empathy for her concerns about the health and survival of Andrew. The nurse could request that the physician spend some time with Barbara to provide her with a prognosis and suggestions for dealing with the anxiety she must feel. Referral to a social worker might assist Barbara to express her anxiety around her children in a more appropriate way.

When Alyssa was diagnosed with breast cancer and a radical mastectomy was performed, she spent much of her time before and after surgery comforting her husband and father, who had great difficulty accepting the diagnosis and facing the issue of mortality associated with a diagnosis of cancer. The nurse observed no family member or friend providing encouragement or support for Alyssa.

The nurse could spend time with Alyssa, expressing her empathy and answering Alyssa's questions. The nurse could volunteer to contact any friends or family members who would be supportive of Alyssa's condition. A member of a cancer-survivor group such as Reach to Recovery is often helpful because members have an understanding of exactly what Alyssa is experiencing.

April arrived at the emergency department with significant bruising on her arms and legs, a black eye, and a forearm that is obviously broken. She is moaning and crying with pain. She is accompanied by her husband, Ronnie. He informed the nurse that April is clumsy and fell down the stairs. He hovers over her solicitously and refuses to leave her side when requested by the nurse. When the nurse tries to take a history, Ronnie interrupts and answers all the questions for April.

The nurse should suspect intimate partner violence (IPV) and endeavor to speak to April alone. For example, she can accompany April to the women's restroom where Ronnie would not be present. She could ask April about IPV and assure her that no one deserves to be abused. She can provide April with phone numbers of organizations or persons who assist women experiencing IPV. The nurse may support April in contacting the police.

While Herman was dying of renal failure, his children argued loudly outside his room about who would be responsible for the hospital bills and burial costs.

After suggesting that the family move further away from Herman's room, the nurse can recommend that the family consult a social worker to deal with the financial implications of the hospitalization and the death of their father. In the meantime, spending time with their father and assuring him of their love and support are more therapeutic for both the family and the father. A hospice worker may be useful in helping the family deal with the death of their father.

Positive Family Dynamics in the Expanding Family

A nurse caring for Tama during her labor and birth assists Peter to coach and support Tama. She ascertains how the children have been prepared for the birth of the baby, and encourages Peter to bring the children to the birth center to visit their mother and meet the new baby. She provides teaching about sibling rivalry, breastfeeding, and postpartum recovery; encourages rest and good nutrition; offers exercises that will assist in recovery; and includes Peter and the siblings in appropriate teaching. She observes interactions among the family, identifies any obvious difficulties, and makes recommendations and referrals as appropriate.

Negative Family Dynamics in the Expanding Family

Donna is in labor with her second pregnancy. She is single and has a 2-year-old daughter who is staying with her mother. The father of the baby, Robert, is not the father of Donna's 2-year-old daughter. Donna confided that Robert "Does not really like to have somebody else's kid around so she leaves the 2 year old with her mother most of the time, which is fine since her mother does not like Robert." The father of the 2 year old has not seen his daughter since she was 3 months old. Currently, Robert is at work but plans to come to the hospital when his shift ends, "but he will probably go have a beer with his buddies first." Robert and Donna live in a one-bedroom apartment. Donna works as a waitress in a local cafe but had to quit work near the end of the pregnancy and "Robert wasn't very happy about that. He says we can't afford a baby and he doesn't want to get married." "My mom is after me to get married; at least the baby and I could be covered by Robert's health insurance." Donna has no other support during labor. The nurse becomes her support person and maintains a constant presence during labor. She encourages Donna and between contractions, talks about how a 2 year old will respond to a baby, encourages breastfeeding, listens as Donna shares her concerns about her relationship with Robert and his relationship with her mother and her 2 year old, and suggests referral to a social worker.

Family Dynamics Following a Diagnosis of Breast Cancer

A diagnosis of breast cancer can change family dynamics. The family must make decisions and strive to cope with the changes engendered by the diagnosis, treatment, and prognosis. Commonly the women in the family are the ones who carry the greatest responsibility for maintaining family balance and harmony.[2] Communication is the foundation of good relationships. In a study of perception of family functioning among family members of women who had breast cancer, Biffi and Mamede[9] found that both male and female family members became closer and had similar perceptions of the family identity and the adaptation to change. Sons and daughters assumed a problem-coping stance and attempted to help. Female relatives were important in the provision of support. Clear communication among family members relieved tension and encouraged family interactions.[10]

To support the woman dealing with breast cancer and its treatment, nursing care must be family-centered and all members of the family included to the extent that they and the woman desire. The family can be informed of their crucial role in the recovery of the breast cancer survivor and suggestions provided for ways to provide support. Communication with the woman and among the family can be encouraged. When a breakdown in communication is observed, the nurse can facilitate opportunities for family interactions to clarify misunderstandings. When there is a true breakdown in communications that negatively affects the woman, referral to a mental health professional may be recommended.

Psychiatric Treatment and Family Dynamics

Complex family issues often occur in conjunction with hospitalization for psychiatric conditions. High levels of collaboration among the referring provider, the patient, and the family contribute to the success of therapy. Medical family therapy can help patients and their families make systemic changes that will reduce the likelihood of rehospitalization for psychiatric concerns.[10] Nurses working in psychiatric settings participate in individual and group therapy sessions; they may also participate in medical family therapy. Inclusion of the family in the plan of care is crucial for increasing the possibility of integrating the patient back into the family upon discharge from the psychiatric facility.

Adolescence and Family Dynamics

In a study of subjective well-being (SWB) of adolescents and family dynamics, the researchers found that SWB of adolescents is positively related to their perceptions of family dynamics.[11] The more stable the family, the higher the

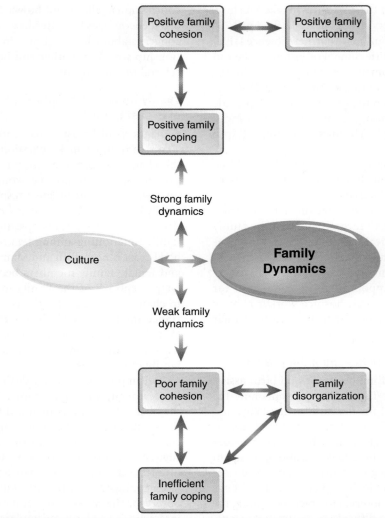

FIGURE 3-4 Interrelated Concepts and Their Relationship to Family Dynamics.

self-esteem and the more positive the attitude of the adolescent. In contrast, the parent's perception of family dynamics had little or no relation to the well-being of the adolescent.[11] Thus, because the perceptions of adolescents and their families may differ, it is incumbent upon nurses working with adolescents to ascertain perceptions of all family members before providing support or attempting interventions.

Teen parenting poses a special challenge. Most teen parents continue to live with their families. This affects the multigenerational structure of the family. Despite negative stereotypes about adolescent fathers, most fathers want involvement with the infant.[12] In a study of pregnant Latina adolescents' transition to parenthood, East and Chien[13] found that family conflict declined soon after birth but increased in the second half of the first year. The adolescents and their siblings perceived a significant increase in family cohesion whereas the mother perceived a significant decrease. Preparation for parenthood by adolescents predicted an increase in family conflict and a decrease in family cohesion, suggesting that the increasing independence and autonomy of the female adolescent created conflicts with her mother.

INTERRELATED CONCEPTS

The following concepts are related to family dynamics. Figure 3-4 illustrates how these concepts are related.

Family cohesion—"the emotional bonding that couple and family members have toward one another."[14] The five levels of cohesion range from *disengaged/disconnected* to *somewhat connected* to *connected* to *very connected* to *enmeshed/overly connected*. The three levels of balanced cohesion are hypothesized to lead to optimal family functioning whereas the extreme levels are seen as problematic for relationships over time.

Family coping—"family actions to manage stressors that tax family resources."[15] Indicators of family coping include confronting family problems, involving family members in decision making, using family-centered stress reduction activity, and seeking family assistance when appropriate.

Family disorganization—"breakdown of a family system which may be associated with parental overburdening or loss of significant others who served as role models for

MODEL CASE

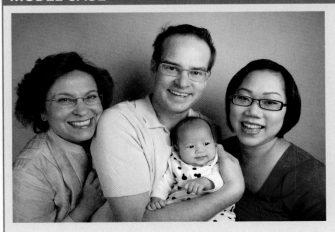

Tama and Peter have been married 11 years. They met in high school and dated for 2 years after graduation before receiving permission from Tama's parents to marry. They have four children, ages 9, 6, 2, and the newborn. The 9-year-old and 6-year-old children are in school during the day. They have exhibited a great deal of interest in the baby and like to "help" Tama by fetching diapers, holding the baby, and rocking the bassinet when the baby cries. The 2 year old has become more "clingy" since the baby was born and has reverted to crying for her pacifier. Tama's mother, Maria, exerts a strong influence in Tama's life. As the only child, born after two miscarriages, Tama holds a special place in her parents' lives. Peter, however, was the oldest of four boys in his family; he is a mechanic and works in a local garage. Peter's father and three younger brothers run the family printing business in a neighboring city.

Peter's parents pride themselves on not interfering in their sons' family affairs, but the boys sometimes express resentment that Peter moved away, has his own job, and does not help in the family business. Tama's mother has spent time with the family after the birth of each of the children and has helped with household chores such as cleaning the house and preparing meals as well as entertaining the children. Peter appreciates her assistance but has told Tama that her mother is "too bossy." Peter's family came to meet the baby but stayed only a short time, stating that they must return to the family business. While Peter's family visited, they spent time talking to Peter but spent little time with Tama or the baby.

Tama and Peter try to make time every day for conversation without the children. They feel that their couple relationship is very important but could be lost in the day-to-day care of four children. They agree on most things, but Tama wishes that Peter would not work such long hours. Peter says he must work overtime to support the family. As a consequence of his long hours at work, the care and discipline of the children and the care of the household are largely Tama's responsibility.

Case Analysis

Peter and Tama are in the stage of "families with young children" in the "family life cycle" whereas their parents are in the stage of "families in later life." Positive family dynamics include the time Tama and Peter spend together; negative dynamics can occur if the concern about Peter's long work hours and limited time in instrumental activities in the household and with childcare escalates. The 2 year old exhibits some sibling rivalry; the older children have a more positive relationship with the baby. Positive dynamics are present between Tama and her mother; some negativity exists between Peter and his mother-in-law. There is excellent instrumental and expressive support from Tama's mother but limited or none from Peter's family. Some negative dynamics between Peter and his brothers occurs in relation to Peter's independence from the family business. Overall, this is a healthy family with many examples of positive family dynamics. Peter and Tama need to continue talking to resolve some negative overtones related to his work hours. Communication with the extended family may improve dynamics. As the 2 year old adjusts to the baby, more mature behavior will develop.

CONTRARY CASE

Belinda is a nurse at a local public health center. She has worked in this setting for 7 years and has developed excellent rapport with a number of diabetic patients, considering them "her family." She meets with the patients in a group regularly, advises them in their striving to maintain and improve their health, leads them in a group discussion, and refers them to a nutritionist or dietitian as necessary. The patients refer to Belinda as a good problem solver and the majority of the group has shown improvement in glucose control, nutrition, and weight loss.

Although the elements of communication and interaction exist and are manifested in group dynamics, this is not an example of family dynamics. The patients in the group do not live together nor consider themselves a family. They are a group for the sole purpose of improving their health and Belinda is a great facilitator in that effort.

children or support systems for family members. Family disorganization can contribute to the loss of social controls that families usually impose on their members."[1] Family disorganization can contribute to negative family dynamics. When John, a 45-year-old insurance salesman, died unexpectedly of an acute myocardial infarction, Jeanette, his 40-year-old wife, and their three children were devastated. Jeanette's social drinking escalated in an effort to cope with John's death. The children began experiencing behavioral problems in school that Jeanette did not feel capable of correcting. Evenings were spent quarreling with and among the children while Jeanette drank herself to sleep.

> ## ■■ BOX 3-1   EXEMPLARS OF FAMILY DYNAMICS
>
> **Changes to Family Dynamics**
> - Aging of family members
> - Caregiver role for family member
> - Change in socioeconomic status of family
> - Chronic illness of family member
> - Death of family member
> - Divorce/remarriage
> - Disability of family member
> - End-of-life care
> - Expanding family (birth or adoption of an infant; blended family)
> - Traumatic injury of family member
>
> **Negative/Dysfunctional Family Dynamics**
> - Absent extended family
> - Child abuse
> - Codependency (related to substance abuse by a family member)
> - Interfering in-laws
> - Intimate partner violence
> - Marital infidelity
> - Placing blame for birth of a preterm infant or for death of a young child by SIDS*
> - Sibling rivalry
> - Teenage runaway

*SIDS, Sudden infant death syndrome.

Family functioning—"capacity of the family system to meet the needs of its members through developmental transitions."[15] In many studies of family functioning, family dynamics is the variable of interest. The quality of family functioning is related to the quality of the communication and interactions, which help the family grow and meet the needs of the family members.

Culture—shared beliefs and values of a group that are passed from generation to generation. Culture has a direct effect on health behaviors. Beliefs, values, and attitudes that are culturally acquired may influence perceptions of illness, health care seeking behavior, and response to treatment.[16]

EXEMPLARS

Positive and negative exemplars of family dynamics provide opportunity to see the great variety of situations in which family dynamics can be observed (Box 3-1). The importance of understanding family dynamics when caring for families should lead the nurse to study the factors involved, to practice observation of families, and to learn appropriate intervention techniques.

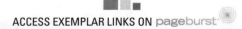

ACCESS EXEMPLAR LINKS ON pageburst

REFERENCES

1. *Mosby's medical dictionary*, ed 8, St Louis, 2009, Elsevier.
2. Wright LM, Leahy M: *Nurses and families. A guide to family assessment and intervention*, ed 5, Philadelphia, 2009, FA Davis.
3. Malinowski F: *The dynamics of cultural change*, New Haven, Conn, 1945, Yale University Press.
4. Radcliffe-Brown A: *Structure and function in a primitive society*, New York, 1952, Free Press.
5. Boss P: *Family stress management*, ed 2, Thousand Oaks, Calif, 2002, Sage.
6. Kelley SJ, Whitley DM, Campos PE: Grandmothers raising grandchildren: results of an intervention to improve health outcomes, *J Nurs Scholarship* 42(4):379–386, 2010.
7. McGoldrick M, Carter B, Garcia-Preto N: *The expanded family life cycle: individual, family and social perspectives*, ed 4, Englewood Cliffs, NJ, 2010, Prentice-Hall.
8. White MA, Elder JH, Paavilainen E, et al: Family dynamics in the United States, Finland and Iceland, *Scand J Caring Sci* 24(1):84–93, 2010.
9. Biffi RG, Mamede MV: Perception of family functioning among relatives of women who survived breast cancer: gender differences, *Rev Latino-Am Enfermagem* 18(2):269–277, 2010.
10. Anderson RJ, Huff NL, Hodgson JL: Medical family therapy in an inpatient psychiatric setting: a qualitative study, *Families Systems Health* 26(2):164–180, 2008.
11. Rask K, Åstedt-Kurki P, Paavilainen E, et al: Adolescent subjective well-being and family dynamics, *Scand J Caring Sci* 17:129–138, 2003.
12. Savio Beers LA, Hollo RE: Approaching the adolescent-headed family: a review of teen parenting, *Curr Probl Pediatr Adolesc Health Care* 39(9):216–233, 2009.
13. East PL, Chien NC: Family dynamics across pregnant Latina adolescents' transition to parenthood, *J Fam Psychol* 24(6):709–720, 2010.
14. Olson DH, Gorall DM: Circumplex model of marital and family systems. In Walsh F, editor: *Normal family processes*, ed 3, New York, 2003, Guilford.
15. Moorhead S, Johnson M, Maas M: *Nursing outcomes classification (NOC)*, St Louis, 2004, Mosby.
16. Lowdermilk DL, Perry SE, Cashion K, et al: *Maternity and women's health care*, ed 10, St Louis, 2012, Elsevier.

Culture

Susan Caplan

Human beings need to construct meaning from their experiences and this construction or created reality is known as culture.[1] The concept of culture is a critical aspect of understanding human behavior[2] and, in particular, is a critical part of understanding how to provide person-centered nursing care.

DEFINITION(S)

For the purposes of this concept analysis, culture is defined as *a pattern of shared attitudes, beliefs, self-definitions, norms, roles, and values that can occur among those who speak a particular language, or live in a defined geographical region.*[3] These dimensions guide such areas as social relationships; expression of thoughts, emotions, and morality; religious beliefs and rituals; and use of technology.

A discussion of culture includes the sub-concepts of enculturation, acculturation, assimilation, biculturalism, ethnicity, and ethnic identity. *Enculturation* is the process by which a person learns the norms, values, and behaviors of a culture, similar to socialization. *Acculturation* is the process of acquiring new attitudes, roles, customs, or behaviors as a result of contact with another culture. Both the host culture and the culture of origin are changed as a result of reciprocal influences. Unlike acculturation, *assimilation* is a process by which a person gives up their original identity and develops a new cultural identity by becoming absorbed into the more dominant cultural group.[4] Usually in assimilation, the dominant group imposes their values on the minority group, with the assumption that the less dominant group must change. In assimilation, the less dominant group does not have a choice about what aspects of a culture it wishes to adopt. In the case of *biculturalism,* the individual has a duel pattern of identification and chooses which aspects of the new culture he/she wishes to adopt and which aspects of their original culture he/she wishes to retain.

Ethnicity refers to a common ancestry that leads to shared values and beliefs. It is transmitted over generations by the family and community. Ethnicity is a powerful determinant of one's identity, known as *ethnic identity*. Race is sometimes thought of in biological terms (for some people, it has a biological meaning) based on the belief that there exist hereditary physical differences among people that define membership in a particular group.[5] However, there are no genetic characteristics that distinguish one group of people from another and, in fact, there are more genetic differences among people who are labeled "Black" than there are differences between "Blacks" and people labeled "White."[5] As stated by Haney Lopez in 1994, "It is clear that even though race does not have a biological meaning, it does have a social meaning which has been legally constructed."[5,pp6,7]

SCOPE AND CATEGORIES

The concept of culture is very broad and influences the shared beliefs, values, and behaviors of a group. Cultural norms impact all aspects of life including everything from interpersonal relationships, family dynamics, and child-rearing practices to gender roles, dietary preferences, communication, dress, and religious practices. Cultural norms also significantly influence how people make decisions about treatment preferences, medication adherence, self-care, and perceptions of illness, which in turn affects nursing care and health care delivery. The scope of these influences, in the context of health and illness, is illustrated in Figure 4-1. Kleinman (1988),[6] a medical anthropologist, makes the distinction between the Western biomedical model of disease and traditional models of illness. Disease is a response to physiological causes explained by pathophysiology and manifested by symptoms and signs.[7] In contrast, traditional health beliefs define illness in terms of mind, body, and spiritual and social connections.[8] Therefore, all illnesses reflect the influence of the environment, including an individual's cultural experiences.

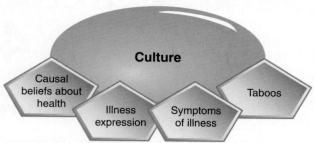

FIGURE 4-1 Scope of Culture Related to Health Care.

Causal Beliefs About Illness

In the health care context, cultural differences can result in different explanations for illness.[9,10] In non-Western cultures, explanatory models of illness might include natural causes (e.g., bacteria, viruses, climate, and environmental irritants), the social world (e.g., punishment for individual behaviors or negative social interactions), or the supernatural world (e.g., ancestral spirits, deities). Western cultures are more likely to endorse solely biomedical causation theories.[10,11] Karasz and McKinley[12] studied cultural differences in causal explanations of fatigue. They compared the illness representations of upper middle class European-American women in New York City and Southeast Asian immigrant women from Queens. They found that European-American women endorsed more biomedical explanations for the medically unexplained symptom of fatigue, such as chronic fatigue syndrome and depression. For the European-American women in this study, fatigue was also attributed to lack of fulfillment or "not getting to do what one wants to do." In contrast, Southeast Asian women had a concept of the body that was ayurvedic, a traditional Indian medical belief that is concerned with balance of essential energies. They believed fatigue was related to weak blood, anemia, and lack of energy attributable to poor nutrition or blood loss from childbirth. They also did not believe that lack of fulfillment of one's personal desires could cause fatigue. The Southeast Asian women were much more likely to attribute fatigue to specific situations or family problems, such as too much household work.

Symptoms of Illness

The symptoms of an illness may vary depending on how a culture understands and perceives the illness. Throughout the world, depression and other mental illnesses are primarily experienced in bodily terms of backaches, headaches, and fatigue, rather than disturbances in mood and affect.[13,14] It is currently believed that both somatic and psychological forms of expressing emotions are equally valid and meaningful, depending upon the sociocultural context.[15] Cultural differences in expression of emotion and the value a culture places on modulating emotions can also result in differences in the way symptoms are expressed. In some cultures, it is acceptable to verbalize that one is in pain, whereas in other cultures the verbalization of pain is seen as a sign of weakness or lack of control.

Illness Expression

The manifestation of illness can be unique for different cultures. These "culture-bound syndromes"[16] occur in specific societies and are considered diagnostic categories for aggregated symptoms. For example, ataque de nervios is a Latino-Caribbean culture-bound syndrome that usually occurs in response to a specific stressor and is characterized by disassociation or trance-like states, crying, uncontrollable spasms, trembling, or shouting.[17,18] Shenjing shuairuo or "weakness of nerves" in Chinese culture is described in the *Chinese Classification of Mental Disorders* as a condition caused by a decrease in vital energy that reduces the function of the internal organ systems and lowers resistance to disease.[19] Its symptoms include fatigue, weakness, dizziness, and memory loss.[16] Also known as neurasthenia throughout Asia, the *International Classification of Diseases and Related Disorders* defines this disorder as characterized primarily by extreme fatigue after mental effort and bodily weakness of persistent duration.[20] Neurasthenia is a more socially acceptable illness label in Asia than depression, which might be considered a more stigmatizing mental illness.[21] Although many Americans would not consider anorexia nervosa or bulimia to be culture-bound syndromes, they conform to the definition of culture-bound syndrome,[22] because a major risk factor for the illness is the social pressure to be thin and media messages equating beauty and thinness that are more prevalent in Westernized, developed countries.[22-24]

Taboos

In many cultures certain illnesses or behaviors that may be characteristic of illnesses are highly stigmatized, and are often not revealed to health care providers. A patient may deny the existence of socially disapproved symptoms and/or decide not to seek treatment. This is particularly true for mental illnesses, behavioral disorders in children, sexually transmitted infections, and heritable and potentially fatal illnesses.

ATTRIBUTES AND CRITERIA

There are several attributes related to the concept of culture, in other words, conditions common to all cultures. These include that *culture is learned* through families and other group members; *culture is changeable* and adaptive to new conditions; and cultural values, beliefs, and behaviors are *shared* by all within a group.

Culture is Learned

Culture may be transmitted to individuals during childhood and adolescence by the process of socialization or enculturation. However, a culture is not limited to members who share the same country of origin or ethnicity and may not be determined solely in childhood, but may encompass any group who shares certain roles and values, norms, and attitudes, sometimes referred to as subcultures. Subcultures can include members of racial and ethnic minorities; people of indigenous or aboriginal heritage; professions, such as nursing; people of different socioeconomic levels, such as the "culture of poverty"[25,26]; individuals who are bisexual, gay, or lesbian or transgender; individuals affiliated with particular religious or spiritual groups; age groups, such as teenagers or the elderly; and persons with disabilities. Culture is determined by self-identification and most people identify with a mix of cultures.

Changing and Adapting

Since the beginning of man's history, culture has been constantly changing as people adapt to environmental and technical innovations and in response to globalization and influences of diverse cultural groups.[22,27] Population migration occurs as a result of regional overpopulation, changes in economic circumstances, occurrence of catastrophic events (such as earthquakes, floods, or famines), and the existence of religious or ethnic conflicts. These migration processes result in ongoing encounters between individuals of different cultures, with subsequent changes in both groups, or acculturation.[28]

Shared Beliefs, Values, and Behaviors

Language, rituals, customs (such as holiday celebrations), dietary practices, and manner of dress are among the most overt attributes of culture that are readily apparent to non–group members. Some of the more subtle attributes of culture, such as values, relationship to authority, social interactions, gender roles, and orientation towards the present or future, are probably the attributes of culture that are most relevant to health care and communication. These kinds of cultural attributes were examined in several landmark studies by Hofstede[29,30] in his research. His research yielded five dimensions of these attributes. Four of the five dimensions, plus religiosity, have particular significance for health care and are presented in the following sections.

Individualism Versus Collectivism

This attribute places value on the degree of closeness and the structure of social relationships, and whether loyalties belong to immediate families or to the extended family or clan. The differences in these interpersonal interactions can be thought of as interdependent versus independent and are reflected in the concept of self. Western Europe and the United States are characteristic of individualist societies. Child-rearing practices and a "family model of independence" produce a separated or independent sense of self.[31,pp20,32] The self is distinct and separate from the "non-self," which includes the environment and social worlds.[33] Collectivistic cultures foster development of an interdependent self-concept. People who have an interdependent sense of self consider their social worth in relation to others. The value of collectivism or interdependence in self-concept is most clearly exemplified by Asian cultures, but it also applies to African, Latin American, some southern European cultures, and some minority cultures within the United States.[31,34] Cultural differences in social practices are apparent in the differences in colloquialisms heard in the United States and Japan. In the United

States, "the squeaky wheel gets the grease," whereas in Japan, "the nail that stands out gets pounded down."[34,p224] One sees evidence of these cultural differences in health care in the manner in which people decide on obtaining treatments and medical care. For independent cultures an individual will put him/herself first in the case of a life-threatening illness, whereas, even in such dire situations, members of collectivist cultures may still consult other family members for the best course of action.

Power Distance

Power distance is the acceptance of an unequal distribution of power as legitimate or fair versus illegitimate from the point of view of the less powerful. In cultures that value a more equal distribution of power, people have the expectation that their opinions will be heard and equally valued. People who are less powerful have the right to criticize those in power. In contrast, in cultures in which a greater power distance is observed, people are unlikely to overtly challenge or disagree with people in positions of authority, because such power is the result of longstanding formal and hierarchical arrangements. People from cultures with greater inequality of power distance may be unwilling to disagree with or question the authority of a health care provider, whereas people from cultures where there is an expectation of equality of relationships may not be hesitant in expressing their wishes and needs for their own health care. Therefore, when a nurse provides nutritional education to the patient who is from a culture that values greater power distance, it might appear that the patient is willing to accept all the nurse's suggestions, when further prompting might elicit additional questions or concerns of the patient.

Masculinity Versus Femininity

Masculinity versus femininity describes how gender roles are distributed and how greatly male and female roles differ. Some societies place greater value on masculine attributes (as defined by Western culture), such as achievement, material success, and recognition, versus more feminine attributes, such as harmonious relationships, modesty, and taking care of others. In some cultures only men can enact masculine roles, whereas in other cultures gender roles are more flexible. In cultures with more fixed gender roles, women are usually given the role of caretaker for aging relatives and may suffer the stresses of caregiver strain.

Long-Term Versus Short-Term Orientation

Long- versus short-term orientation is the degree to which a culture is oriented to the future and long-term rewards versus the degree to which a culture is oriented to the past or present.[35,36] Long-term oriented cultures favor thrift, perseverance, and adapting to changing circumstances. Short-term oriented cultures are oriented to the present or past and emphasize quick results; they favor respect for tradition and fulfillment of social obligations, although status is not a major issue in relationships and leisure time is important. Among the most long-term oriented countries are China,

Hong Kong, Taiwan, and Japan, whereas the United States, Great Britain, Canada, and the Philippines are among the most short-term oriented countries.[36]

It is important to note that not everyone in a country will share the same values and that individuals within a culture will vary on cultural attributes. In a health care context, long-term orientation might be illustrated by the case of Mr. Donovan, a 52-year-old male of Irish and Italian heritage, who visits the company-sponsored clinic of a large brokerage firm where he is a financial analyst. "I'm here for my annual flu shot, and to schedule a colonoscopy, and I'd like to discuss PSA testing. I've been reading that the test is now somewhat controversial, but I certainly don't want to put myself at risk by not being screened." An individual with a short-term orientation might resemble Mr. Molinari, a 56-year-old male of Irish and Italian heritage. He goes to a clinic today for back pain, which is interfering with his job as a housepainter. The nurse practitioner evaluates his back pain and reminds him that he should come in for a routine physical and that he should schedule a colonoscopy. "No," he replies to that suggestion. "If it ain't broke, don't fix it."

Religiosity

Another cultural dimension is religiosity, which varies according to how much religion permeates one's day-to-day existence, and to what degree religious practices can be separated from nonreligious practices. Individuals from cultures that are more secular, or less identified with religious institutions, may behave similarly to Mr. Wentworth, a 45-year-old, third-generation American of Ukrainian, German, and English heritage. He is terminally ill with colon cancer. He has undergone several chemotherapy and radiation treatments, but his cancer has metastasized and his health care providers have told him that his cancer is too advanced to warrant further treatment. He was told he has less than 6 months to live and has been referred to hospice for palliative care. Mr. Wentworth says he will absolutely not consider palliative care. "I'm gonna beat this thing. I've read about a clinic in the Southwest that offers alternative treatments. I'm going there. I'm gonna win." In contrast, some cultures believe that religion is religious practices and beliefs are enmeshed with and encompass most aspects of culture.[37] Mrs. Farah, a 45-year-old, first-generation immigrant Somali woman, is terminally ill with cervical cancer. She has undergone several chemotherapy and radiation treatments, but her health care providers have told her that her cancer is too advanced to warrant further treatment. Mrs. Farah is very grateful for the care she has received. She is slowly accepting her imminent death, and is helped by her faith in Allah. She knows she has no control over her illness at this point and believes it is "God's will." She begins to make plans with extended family and her husband for the care of her children.

THEORETICAL LINKS

The importance of culture and its influence on human behavior has not always been an accepted theoretical premise. Theories of human behavior have been dominated by the underlying premise of the "psychic unity" of humankind, a theory that states that all human social behavior is derived from evolution.[38] Scientists who believe in these concepts claim that through evolution and natural selection, certain genes in the species that enhance survival are most likely to be passed down from one generation to the next and these genes specify cognitive functioning and the manner in which people perceive the world.[39] Therefore, thoughts, behaviors, and emotions develop universally and account for such diverse behaviors as favoring relatives (i.e., altruism), creating and following rules, or adopting specific beliefs about religion and warfare.[40] Language, culture, and religion are incidental to or and outgrowth of these genetically-determined behavioral processes. Karasz and McKinley[12] refer to "the 'culture-free' approach of traditional health psychology."

More recently, behavioral geneticists have shown us how the social environment has a major influence on how genes are expressed. Although there might be inherent biological factors that produce emotions and behavior, genes interact with the environment to produce differences in emotional responses.[41] Moreover, the biological determinism of traditional psychology was challenged when assumptions derived under experimental laboratory conditions were evaluated in a real world context. Cultural psychologists and medical and nursing anthropologists have rectified the limited worldview of traditional science, with its culture-free categories.

Leininger's Theory of Culture Care Diversity and Universality

Berry, a cross-cultural psychologist, and Leininger, a nurse anthropologist and the leading theorist in culture care, emphasized the importance of understanding human behavior in the context of culture.[42-44] They applied the concepts of "emic" and "etic," which referred to an approach to understanding behaviors. The term *emic* refers to an approach to understanding culture from within (i.e., the insider's viewpoint) whereas *etic* refers to the application of constructs external to a culture, to discover universal characteristics common to all cultures. The assumption of universality can also imply an imposition of an outsider's values, rules, and understanding to another culture or subculture. The concepts of *emic* and *etic* are essential aspects of Leininger's theory of Culture Care Diversity and Universality.[45]

The central tenet of this theory is that both *etic* and *emic* approaches could lead to more responsive approaches to caring, the most important focus of nursing. To provide meaningful and holistic care, social structure factors, such as religion, economics, education, technology, ethnic background, and history, have to be taken into account because these factors have major influences on health, well-being, and illness.[46] This comprehensive approach to nursing formed the basis of Leininger's development of transcultural nursing, the "formal area of humanistic and scientific knowledge and practices focused on holistic culture care...to assist individuals or groups to maintain or regain their health (or well-being)."[46,p84]

Interprofessional Theory of Social Suffering

Arthur Kleinman echoes Leininger's themes of the multifactorial approach to understanding illness.[47] Kleinman's interprofessional theory of social suffering states that relationships and social interactions shape our illness experiences and collective perceptions of the existential experiences of suffering. Memories of trauma and suffering exist collectively and are transmitted through shared experiences and learning. All illnesses are a form of social suffering, mediated by cultural and political institutions. Technological advances can treat an individual's disease, but do not address the root causes of illness: poverty and the global political economy. Tuberculosis, depression, sexually transmitted infections, substance abuse, domestic violence, post-traumatic stress disorders, and acquired immunodeficiency syndrome (AIDS) are not individual problems, but a reflection of social structure and inequities. Kleinman believes it is important to understand the individual's cultural interpretation of illness and suffering. These cultural representations of suffering and the response to it comprise the diversity of human responses to illness and pain. In some cultures, silent endurance is valued, whereas other cultures rail against unjust Gods.[47,ppix-xiv] Some cultures place a high priority on the well-being and health of its members, whereas other societies are characterized by greater inequities in the health status of its populations.

CONTEXT TO NURSING AND HEALTH CARE

Many nursing students have asked, "Why is there such an emphasis on culture in health care? That's all we keep hearing about." Culture is an essential aspect of health care because of the increasing diversity of the United States. In 2008 the U.S. population was estimated at 304 million. In that year, the non-Hispanic White population of the United States represented 67% of the total population.[48] By 2050 that number will decrease to 50%. Half of the population will be comprised of people who identify themselves as belonging to a racial or ethnic minority population, including Black, Asian, and Pacific Islander; American Indian, Eskimo, and Aleut; and Hispanic. In 2008 approximately 12% of the United States population, or 36 million people, had a disability.[49] Persons with disabilities identify themselves as part of a culture based on shared life experiences; this identification has led to music, publications, and media products unique to that culture, as well as to the disability rights movement to address discrimination in housing, employment, and health care. An estimated 4% of the U.S. population ages 18 to 44 years identified themselves as lesbian, gay, bisexual, or transgender.[50] Persons who are lesbian, gay, bisexual, or transgender experience societal discrimination, societal stigma, and human rights abuses that have led to higher rates of mental illness in addition to higher rates of human immunodeficiency virus (HIV) and sexually transmitted infections.[51,52]

Health Care Disparities

This increasing cultural diversity in the United States has resulted in the national health objective proposed in *Healthy People 2020*: achieving the highest level of health for all people by addressing societal inequalities and "historical and contemporary injustices."[53] One of the major goals of *Healthy People 2020* is the elimination of health care disparities. *Healthy People 2020* defines a health disparity as "a particular type of health difference that is closely linked with social, economic, and/or environmental disadvantage. Health disparities adversely affect groups of people who have systematically experienced greater obstacles to health based on their racial or ethnic group; religion; socioeconomic status; gender; age; mental health; cognitive, sensory, or physical disability; sexual orientation or gender identity; geographic location; or other characteristics historically linked to discrimination or exclusion."[54] The goal of eliminating health care disparities is closely allied with nursing's basic tenet of social justice, which is the belief that all people deserve quality health care and access to care is a basic human right.[55]

One of the major factors in lower quality care for ethnic and racial minorities is patient–health care provider miscommunication attributable to stereotyping, prejudice, or discrimination.[56] To improve quality of care and optimize the treatment of all people, *Healthy People 2020* emphasizes the need to provide culturally competent health care services and to improve health literacy and health education among non–English-speaking populations.

Cultural Competency in Nursing

Cultural competence is an expected component of nursing education and professional nursing practice. Culturally competent care means conveying acceptance of the patient's health beliefs while sharing information, encouraging self-efficacy, and strengthening the patient's coping resources.[57] The scope and standards of nursing practice specifically identify cultural competency as it relates to assessment, outcomes identification, planning, and implementation.[55] Cultural competency is more of an imperative now as we begin to understand that health care provider's unconscious biases contribute to disparities in treatment,[58] even though nurses and physicians continue to deny that their own behavior is a factor in health care inequalities.[59]

As a nursing student, you might be thinking, "YES, but we are taught how to communicate with our patients and if I treat everyone with respect and understanding, isn't that sufficient?" Well, no. By treating everyone the same, we are not providing quality care because we are ignoring societal factors that contribute to worse health outcomes among vulnerable populations. It is true that communicating respectfully is an essential aspect of communication and every patient is an individual with unique needs. However, failure to recognize the fact that people identify themselves as members of certain groups who have shared experiences of social injustice and who are currently treated differently in health care will result in an inability to understand some of the most essential human experiences of our patients.[60]

Now, you may be saying to yourself, "Yes, I understand cultural competency is important, but really, there are so many other things that we need to learn as nurses."

Leininger informs us that nurses are struggling more than ever to keep up with technology, new procedures, and treatments.[46,p74] This emphasis places greater value on the medical model and physician expectations that nurses perform medical tasks to treat and cure disease. Rubin defines expert nursing as the ability to recognize qualitative distinctions between patients.[61] The ability to make qualitative distinctions, or to be able to understand differences in the patient's life experiences, requires empathy. Nurses who lack this ability have a lack of clinical knowledge, because the nurse does not understand the individual's self-perceptions of how he/she came to feel that way. In a cultural sense, this could be illustrated by the description of one nursing student's health assessment and history taking. She writes, "His parents are from India and he practices Hinduism. He goes to Mosques regularly and is a lot like my patient from Sudan, who is also very religious and celebrates Ramadan." This assumption of similarity between Muslim and Hindu practices and the confusion between the two evidences an inability to make qualitative distinctions in a person's history, or to really attempt to understand that person's experience of religion. Individualized care or "patient centered" care is facilitated by cultural competence that respects and acknowledges patient's values, needs, and preferences.[62]

How does a nurse become culturally competent? The process of cultural competence consists of four interrelated constructs: self-awareness, cultural knowledge, cultural skill, and cultural desire; the pivotal construct is cultural desire.

Self Awareness, Knowledge, and Skills

Self-awareness, knowledge, and skills are the broad components of cultural competency.[63-65] Self-awareness involves identifying and understanding one's own cultural identity. You might think about some aspects of your own cultural identity. Did you grow up with people of the same ethnic background as yourself? Did you gather with extended family and engage in traditional activities? Do members of your family make frequent visits to their country of origin or old neighborhood? Do you participate in ethnic cultural events? Do you speak another language? Do you have pride in your cultural background?

Perhaps you are saying to yourself, "But I grew up in an area where everyone is the same as I am, and we don't have traditions from the countries where my great grandparents came from and we just eat normal American food and celebrate the same holidays as everyone else. *I don't have any cultural identification.*" If you feel that way, ask yourself, what about the place you grew up? Is it like every other place in the United States? What about the meals you prepare? Does everyone in America celebrate the same holidays? Are all Americans the same? What are my own values and beliefs? What are my own biases?

Biases not only are negative stereotypes but also can be any tendency to act, think, or feel in a certain way towards other people. For example, you may believe that Vietnamese people are hardworking, they want their children to do well in school, they expect that their children show respect to their parents, and they stick together. Many nurses believe, "But that really doesn't apply to me, because I know that even if I personally don't like someone or something they've done, I will treat everyone in a professional manner and will treat everyone the same." Nurses grow up with the values and beliefs of their cultures and the society around them. Perhaps you believe that abortion is wrong, that it is immoral to have same-sex relationships, that people with depression could really snap out of it if they wanted to, that people with substance abuse do not have a mental illness; they make choices. Perhaps you feel angry that some people receive health benefits that are "free" and are paid for by your tax dollars. After all, you work hard to earn money, "Why can't they?" How come all of those refugees who have moved into my community get Medicaid and can get medications that I can barely afford? Is it possible to separate all of these feelings from our practice? Many studies in many fields say that those feelings carry over into the care we provide.

Even when one's own values and beliefs are directed against a particular group of people, they may still reflect the biases of the dominant cultural group. For example, nurses from independent cultures will develop nursing objectives based on the cultural value of autonomy—developing one's own potential and maintaining one's independence—and equate "more" of such traits with better health. A patient from a more interdependent, collectivist culture might not share such values. For this patient, it might be expected that he/she is dependent on other family members in times of ill health. Moreover, the family's needs and desires might be valued more highly than obtaining one's own personal goals. The use of the concept of "self esteem" as part of a nursing diagnosis may reflect the bias that the self is construed similarly in all cultures. As Markus and Kitayama[34] explain, in interdependent cultures, the essence of self is defined by one's relationships to others, rather than the inner self. Internal attributes such as desires, abilities, and personality traits are viewed as situation dependent and, therefore, unreliable. Self is not a constant, but is fluid and changes according to the situation or the relationship. It is important for the nurse to assess the patient's own values and definition of health and to develop mutually agreed upon nursing care plans.

Cultural Desire

A pivotal construct is cultural desire. Desire to understand people who are different from yourself provides the means for overcoming one's biases and their effect upon care. Desire leads to knowledge. Knowledge as a domain of cultural competency does not imply learning facts about every culture, but rather exposing one's self to other cultures and being motivated to learn. Knowledge can be acquired by reading journals that represent different groups; visiting ethnic neighborhoods and sampling different foods; learning a foreign language; attending a community meeting in a different neighborhood; speaking with someone from another culture; walking into botánicas, ethnic grocery stores, or herb shops; attending a service at a mosque or synagogue; speaking with a hospital translator; going to a gay pride march or Puerto Rican day parade; or reading a novel about someone growing up in another culture.

Skills are acquired by practice in communication. There are many resources available to learn basic medical terminology on the Web, including Internet and smartphone applications that serve as translators. There are also assessment questions designed to understand the sociocultural contexts of people's health care needs. The RESPECT model, based on a series of eight questions developed by Kleinman,[66] provides a blueprint to develop skills needed to become culturally competent.[67] RESPECT is an acronym for Respect, Explanatory model, Sociocultural context, Power, Empathy, Concerns and fears, and Therapeutic alliance/trust. *Respect* and *empathy* are attitudes that demonstrate to the patient that his/her concerns are valued and he/she is understood. The nurse can further assess for the patient's *explanatory model*, or understanding of what is the cause of his/her illness; and the *sociocultural context*, which are factors in a person's life that may contribute to the current state of health and expectations for treatment, such as poverty, stress, and social support. *Power* refers to the importance of acknowledging that the patient is in a vulnerable position and that there is a difference between patients and health care providers in terms of access to resources, knowledge level, and control over outcomes. The loss of power and control that a patient faces can contribute to *concerns and fears* about treatment, illness outcomes, and the future. Bearing in mind the meaning of these concepts in the nursing relationship enhances communication and assessment skills between patient and nurse and creates a *therapeutic alliance and trust*.

INTERRELATED CONCEPTS

Several concepts within this textbook are closely related to the concept of culture; those specifically featured include family dynamics, communication, and coping. These are shown in Figure 4-2.

Family dynamics are definitely intricately tied to one's culture. Culture affects family dynamics in terms of the ways in which people cope with stress, the manner in which sick family members receive care, and the beliefs about sharing information with outsiders about a family member's illness. Culture determines beliefs about appropriate child-rearing practices. For many cultures, the dominant practice in America of letting an infant cry him/herself to sleep to learn how to self-soothe may be construed as a form of neglect, particularly for people of cultures that believe in sharing a bed with an infant. Some cultures would not understand that behaviors that fit into the diagnostic definition of attention-deficit/hyperactivity disorder (ADHD) would be considered a disease, rather than a normal variation of childhood exuberance. There are differences in viewpoints about genetic screening and prenatal testing, with people of some cultures believing that one accepts what God provides.

The concept **Communication** is closely related to culture because communication patterns, both verbal and nonverbal, are determined by cultural norms. Degree of eye contact, personal space, and the acceptability of touch all vary by cultures. Culture dictates the nature of relationships and the degree of hierarchy and structure in relationships. In some cultures, a high degree of formality and reserve is expected when addressing people of greater social status, whereas in other cultures there is less stratification by age or social standing and it is acceptable to be direct and open with everyone. Similarly, in some cultures personal revelations or discussion of family problems is taboo, whereas in other cultures there are no such restrictions on communication.

Coping mechanisms and ways of dealing with life's difficulties are, to a large extent, culturally determined. Cultural belief systems form the basis of a coping strategy by creating a redefinition of negative circumstances.[68] These belief systems may encompass religious beliefs and religiosity, which may have a beneficial effect on health by fostering positive emotions such as hope, gratitude, and reverence.[69] Religiosity may result in decreased symptoms of distress and may help with coping by decreasing loneliness and fostering cultural identity.[70]

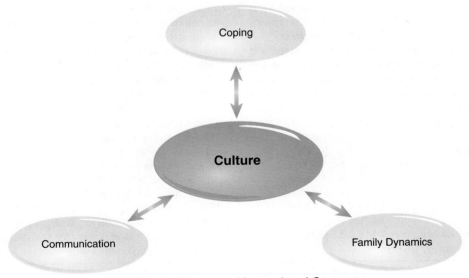

FIGURE 4-2 Culture and Interrelated Concepts.

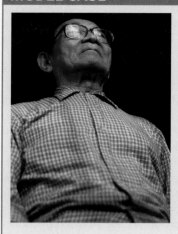

Ms. Faye, a nurse on the rehabilitation unit of a nursing home in New York, has been assigned to Mr. Wong, a 78-year-old male from mainland China, who has been admitted for rehabilitation following total hip replacement surgery and is expected to be discharged back to his senior housing community in four weeks. Ms. Faye is concerned about Mr. Wong's weight loss and reports from the nursing and rehabilitation staff that he is too tired to attend physical therapy. He is not meeting his goals for rehabilitation.

Ms. Faye reads the nursing assistant's reports for the past week and sees that he is only eating about one third of his meals. She studies his medical record and learns that Mr. Wong emigrated from China at the age of 38, worked as a short-order cook in a Chinese restaurant, and speaks only Cantonese. He has a son and daughter-in-law and two grandchildren who live in San Francisco. His wife is deceased.

Ms. Faye sees that labs were drawn to evaluate his nutritional status and determine physiological causes of weight loss. After reading the health record, she notes that Mr. Wong's lab results are normal and there is no evidence of an underlying disease process that would explain his weight loss.

She speaks to the social worker, Mr. Magioncalda, who has had a chance to interview Mr. Wong in more depth. She wonders aloud why Mr. Wong never learned English after living here for so long. Mr. Mangioncalda explains that like most Chinese Americans of his age, Mr. Wong lived in an ethnic neighborhood enclave with other Chinese Americans who only spoke Cantonese, and he worked between 10 and 12 hours a day, precluding the opportunity to learn English.

This insight into the life of Mr. Wong caused Ms. Faye to think about what other judgments or misconceptions she might have about people from China. "Well," she thought to herself, "it is hard to figure out what they're feeling, because they don't seem to express their emotions the way most people I know do."

She realizes that she has not yet seen Mr. Wong's son and wonders if perhaps Mr. Wong is depressed because his son is not visiting him and not meeting his expectation that his son will take care of him. Ms. Faye believes that Chinese people are hardworking, they want their children to do well in school, they expect their children to show respect to their parents and they stick together. Ms. Faye requests that the occupational therapy assistant, Ms. Lee, who also serves as the Cantonese translator, accompany her to talk to Mr. Wong. She and Ms. Lee knock and enter his room, where he is lying on the bed. Ms. Faye greets him and asks Ms. Lee to tell Mr. Wong that she would like to ask him a couple of questions.

First, Ms. Faye asks Ms. Lee to ask Mr. Wong if he is in pain. Mr. Wong responds softly, "no."

Ms. Faye proceeds to ask Ms. Lee to ask Mr. Wong if he is depressed or anxious.

Mr. Wong wonders why such a young woman is looking at him so directly and asking him very personal questions. He is even somewhat annoyed, because he would not allow himself to become depressed, even if he was going through a very difficult time.

Without looking at the two women, he responds that he is fine.

Ms. Faye asks Ms. Lee to translate that if he needs anything, he should let her know.

She walks away with Ms. Lee, thinking, "It is just like I thought. He is not going to tell me what he is feeling."

Ms. Lee, as if reading her mind, says "Elderly Chinese people believe that they must be stoic about pain and there is a stigma about talking about any mental health problems."

This explanation had not occurred to Ms. Faye, who decides maybe she should learn a little more about Chinese culture. She realizes that it is important to learn about the Chinese elderly because this is one of the fastest growing subpopulations in the United States. She reads more about Chinese culture and as she suspected, the Chinese family structure is very important. It is influenced by Confucianism, which emphasizes interdependence and harmonious family relationships. Family relationships are defined by prescribed roles, hierarchy, and traditional obligations. Parents expect their children to take care of them and many sons never leave their families out of a sense of duty. Ms. Faye wondered how living in the United States might have affected traditional relationships. She reads some more articles and is surprised to learn that through the process of acculturation many Chinese elderly in the United States no longer feel quite as strongly that their children are responsible for taking care of them; the Chinese elderly are more self-reliant but also rely upon a network of neighbors to help them, particularly when children are far away. Ms. Faye decided to take a different approach with Mr. Wong.

Learning that Mr. Wong might be more comfortable talking to another man, Ms. Faye asks Mr. Chou, a nurse and trained translator, to speak with Mr. Wong. This time she asks Mr. Chou to ask about Mr. Wong's family, and if his son was planning on visiting him. Having read that Mr. Wong is not accustomed to communicating with direct eye contact, she keeps her eyes averted. Mr. Wong responds that his son is a very busy cardiac surgeon in San Francisco and has not been able to take time off from work, but he and his family should be arriving in two days. Ms. Faye then asks Mr. Chou to ask Mr. Wong if something is bothering him. Mr. Wong reports that his neighbor, who is his best friend, is in the hospital after having suffered a stroke and he has not been able to visit him. He is very worried about him, but was unable to navigate New York's subway system without someone to accompany him. Since his friend had a stroke three weeks ago, he has lost his appetite and just feels exhausted. Ms. Faye suggests that maybe when his son arrives with his family, they can take him to the hospital to visit his friend. Mr. Wong replies that he does not want to be a bother to his son. Ms. Faye asks Mr. Chou to tell Mr. Wong that she would advise the family that it is important for Mr. Wong's health to see his friend. Mr. Wong nodded in agreement.

MODEL CASE—cont'd

Encouraged by that response, Ms. Faye decided to learn more about the culture. She learned that illness was viewed holistically and was believed to be caused by an imbalance of yin and yang and a disruption of the flow of vital energies. Certain foods were used during periods of illness, when "hot" or "yang" foods might be preferred because of their healing properties. Because of hot and cold theories of illness, or simply from long-established custom, an elderly Chinese patient might be reluctant to drink cold water and might prefer hot tea. She also learned that many Chinese immigrants experience depression from the stress of adjusting to a new culture, loss of family and traditions, loss of social status, and memories of severe deprivation or political violence in their countries of origin. However, as in many cultures, people may not consider their symptoms of depression to be a mental illness and therefore may express their symptoms of depression in terms of bodily complaints such as fatigue and pain.

The next time Ms. Faye went on rounds to give Mr. Wong his medication, she brought hot tea instead of the usual cold water. Mr. Wong is sitting up in bed, speaking animatedly with his family, who have just come to visit. He is happily eating some Congee, a rice porridge sprinkled with ground pork, that his family brought him. She introduces herself to the family in English and greets Mr. Wong with "Ni hao ma?" ("Hello, how are you?"), a phrase that she learned from the translator. Mr. Wong looked at her, surprised, but nodded his head to indicate that he was okay. She handed him his medicine and the hot tea, which he willingly accepted.

She then asks if he is experiencing any pain, "Ni xian zai tong ma?" Mr. Wong nods his head no. His daughter-in-law explained that he does appear to be in pain when he moves, but he does not want to take any pain medication because he believes he will become addicted. Ms. Faye explains that the medication he has been prescribed, ibuprofen, is not addicting. He nods his head in agreement. Ms. Faye gives him the ibuprofen and asks the family if they can take him to see his friend. The family agrees and Ms. Faye leaves the room to make arrangements for his transportation.

The next day, Ms. Faye is working the night shift. Neither Mr. Chou nor Ms. Lee is working that shift, so Ms. Faye enters Mr. Wong's room with his medication and a Chinese Pain Scale. Mr. Wong points to the numbers on the scale, indicating that his pain is well-controlled with the ibuprofen. She then opens a Chinese translator that she has downloaded into her cell phone and types "Is there anything else I can help you with?" and she hands him the phone. He types back in Cantonese, "Yes, please play the CD that my family has brought me." She turns on the CD and for the first time, he smiles happily as she says good-bye.

BOX 4-1 EXEMPLARS OF CULTURE

Health Care Practices/Beliefs
- Symptoms of illness
- Identification of illness
- Causal beliefs
- Treatment preferences
- Personal control over illness
- Beliefs about consequences of illness/preventive care
- Diet/nutrition
- Religious healing practices
- Alternative/complementary medicine

Developmental/Family Roles
- Birthrights
- Child-rearing practices
- Gender roles
- Rites of passage

- Family structure
- Death and dying
- Caregiver roles

Patient-Provider Communication
- Eye contact
- Personal space
- Touch
- Body posture
- Power distance/relationship to authority
- Taboos
- Social desirability
- Acceptability of revealing personal information
- Language preference and usage
- Greetings and leave takings
- Expression of emotions

EXEMPLARS

There are multiple exemplars of culture and they are best presented from the context of health care practices and beliefs, developmental and family roles, and patient-provider communication. The exemplars are presented in Box 4-1.

REFERENCES

1. Shweder RA: Cultural psychology—what is it? In Stigler JW, Shweder RA, Herdt G, editors: *Cultural psychology*, Cambridge, 1990, Cambridge University Press, pp 1–43.
2. Geertz C: *The interpretation of cultures*, New York, 1973, Basic Books.
3. Triandis HC: The psychological measurement of cultural syndromes, *Am Psychol* 51(4):407–415, 1996. Retrieved from http://dx.doi.org/10.1037/0003-066X.51.4.407.
4. Cengage G: Acculturation. In Breslow L, editor: *Encyclopedia of public health, 2002, eNotes.com*, 2006, Retrieved Jan 14, 2011, from www.enotes.com/public-health-encyclopedia/acculturation.

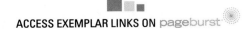

ACCESS EXEMPLAR LINKS ON pageburst

5. Haney Lopez IF: *The social construction of race: some observations on illusion, fabrication, and choice,* 29 Harvard Civil Rights-Civil Liberties Law Review 1-62, 6-7, 11-17, Winter 1994.

6. Kleinman A: *Rethinking psychiatry: from cultural category to personal experience,* New York, 1988, Free Press.

7. Huff RM: Cross-cultural concepts of health and disease. In Huff RM, Kline MV, editors: *Promoting health in multicultural populations,* Thousand Oaks, Calif, 1999, Sage Publications, pp 23–39.

8. Baer RD, Clark L, Pederson C: Folk illnesses. In Loue S, editor: *Handbook of immigrant health,* New York, 1998, Plenum Press, pp 183–202.

9. Huff RM, Kline MV: Health promotion in the context of culture. In Huff RM, Kline MV, editors: *Promoting health in multicultural populations,* Thousand Oaks, Calif, 1999, Sage Publications, pp 3–21.

10. Rivera SV: Latino cultural beliefs of the causes of a medical and a psychological illness, *Dissert Abstr Int Sect B Sci Eng* 62(2-B):1096, 2001.

11. Klonoff EA, Landrine H: Culture and gender diversity in commonsense beliefs about the causes of six illnesses, *J Behav Med* 17(4):407–418, 1994.

12. Karasz A, McKinley PS: Cultural differences in conceptual models of everyday fatigue: a vignette study, *J Health Psychol* 12(4):613–626, 2007.

13. Escobar JI, Hoyos Nervi C: Gara MA: Immigration and mental health: Mexican Americans in the United States, *Harvard Rev Psychiatr* 8(2):64–72, 2000.

14. Kleinman A: Depression, somatization and the "new Cross-Cultural Psychiatry," *Soc Sci Med* 11:3–10, 1977.

15. U.S. Department of Health and Human Services: *Mental health: culture, race and ethnicity—a supplement to mental health: A report of the Surgeon General* U.S. Public Health Service No. 01–3613, Rockville, Md, 2001, Substance Abuse and Mental Health Services Administration.

16. American Psychiatric Association (APA): *Diagnostic and statistical manual of mental disorders,* ed 4, Washington, DC, 1994, The Association.

17. Guarnaccia PJ, Lewis-Fernandez R, Marano MR: Toward a Puerto Rican popular nosology: Nervios and Ataque de Nervios, *Cult Med Psychiatr* 27(3):339–366, 2003.

18. Guarnaccia PJ, Lewis-Fernandez R, Martinez Pincay I, et al: Ataque de Nervios as a marker of social and psychiatric vulnerability: results from the NLAAS, *Int J Soc Psychiatr* 56:298–309, 2010. doi: 10.1177/0020764008101636.

19. Chinese Medical Association and Nanjing Medical University: *Chinese classification of mental disorders, Second Edition, Revised (CCMD-2-R),* Nanjing, 1995, Dong Nan University Press.

20. World Health Organization: *International classification of diseases and related disorders (ICD-10),* Geneva, 1992, Author.

21. Schwartz PY: Why is neurasthenia important in Asian cultures? *West J Med* 176(4):257–258, 2002.

22. Lopez SR, Guarnaccia PJ: Cultural psychopathology: uncovering the social world of mental illness, *Annu Rev Psychol* 51:571–598, 2000.

23. Jacobi C, Hayward C, de Zwaan M, et al: Coming to terms with risk factors for eating disorders: application of risk terminology and suggestions for a general taxonomy, *Psychol Bull* 130:19–65, 2004.

24. Taylor CB, Bryson SW, Altman TM, et al: Risk factors for the onset of eating disorders in adolescent girls: results of the McKnight longitudinal risk factor study, *Am J Psychiatr* 160:248–254, 2003.

25. Lewis O: *The children of Sanchez: autobiography of a Mexican family,* New York, 1961, Random House.

26. Moynihan DP: *The Negro family: the case for national action, Office of Policy Planning and Research, United States Department of Labor,* 1965. Retrieved from www.dol.gov/oasam/programs/history/webid-meynihan.htm.

27. Committee on Cultural Psychiatry Group for the Advancement of Psychiatry: *Cultural assessment in clinical psychiatry,* Washington, DC, 2002, American Psychiatric Publishing.

28. Redfield R, Linton R, Herskovits MJ: Memorandum for the study of acculturation, *Am Anthropol* 38:149–152, 1936.

29. Hofstede G: *Culture's consequences: international differences in work-related values,* Beverly Hills, Calif, 1980, Sage Publications.

30. Hofstede G: Empirical models of cultural differences. In Bleichrodt N, Drenth P, editors: *Contemporary issues in cross-cultural psychology,* Lisse, Netherlands, 1991, Swets & Zeitlinger Publishers, pp 4–20.

31. Kagitcibasi C: Individualism and collectivism. In Berry JW, Segall MH, Kagitcibasi C, editors: *Handbook of cross-cultural psychology, Volume 3: Social behavior and applications,* ed 2, Needham Heights, Mass, 1997, Allyn & Bacon.

32. Mesquita B: Emotions in collectivist and individualist contexts, *J Personality Soc Psychol* 80(1):68–74, 2001.

33. Landrine H, Klonoff EA: Culture and health-related schemas: a review and proposal for interdisciplinary integration, *Health Psychol* 11(4):267–276, 1992.

34. Markus HR, Kitayama S: Culture and the self: implications for cognition, emotion, and motivation, *Psychol Rev* 98:224–253, 1991.

35. Hofstede G: *Culture and organizations: software of the mind,* New York, 1997, McGraw-Hill.

36. Hofstede G, Bond MH: The Confucius connection: from cultural roots to economic growth, *Organiz Dyn* 16:5–21, 1988.

37. Matsumoto D, Yoo SH: Toward a new generation of cross-cultural research, *Perspect Psychol Sci* 1(3):234–250, 2006.

38. Tooby J, Cosmides L: Evolutionary psychology and the generation of culture, part I: theoretical considerations, *Ethnol Sociobiol* 10:29–49, 1989.

39. Wilson EO: *Sociobiology: the new synthesis,* Cambridge, Mass, 1975, Harvard University Press.

40. Fukuyama F: *The origins of political order: from prehuman times to the French Revolution,* New York, 2011, Farrar, Straus and Giroux.

41. Caspi A, Moffitt TE, Morgan J, et al: Maternal expressed emotion predicts children's antisocial behavior problems: using monozygotic-twin differences to identify environmental effects on behavioral development, *Dev Psychol* 40(2):149–161, 2004.

42. Berry JW: On cross-cultural comparability, *Int J Psychol* 4:119–128, 1969.

43. Berry JW: Imposed etics-emics-derived etics: the operationalization of a compelling idea, *Int J Psychol* 24:721–735, 1989.

44. Leininger MM: Leininger's theory of nursing: culture care diversity and universality, *Nurs Sci Q* 1:152–160, 1988.

45. Leininger MM: *Culture care diversity and universality, a theory of nursing,* New York, 1991, National League for Nursing Press.

46. Leininger M, McFarland MR: *Transcultural nursing: concepts, theories, research and practices,* ed 3, New York, 2002, McGraw-Hill.

47. Kleinman A, Das V, Locke M: *Introduction in social suffering,* London, 1997, University of California Press.

48. U.S. Census Bureau: American FactFinder, United States: *American Community Survey. American Community Survey 1-year estimates, ACS demographic and housing estimates,* 2008. Retrieved from http://factfinder.census.gov.

49. U.S. Census Bureau: American FactFinder, United States: *American Community Survey. American Community Survey 1-year estimates, Selected social characteristics in the United States,* 2008. Retrieved from http://factfinder.census.gov.

50. Mayer KH, Bradford JB, Makadon HJ, et al: Sexual and gender minority health: what we know and what needs to be done, *Am J Public Health* 98:989–995, 2008.

51. McLaughlin KA, Hatzenbuehler ML, Keyes KM: Responses to discrimination and psychiatric disorders among Black, Hispanic, female, and lesbian, gay, and bisexual individuals, *Am J Public Health* 100:1477–1484, 2010.

52. Centers for Disease Control and Prevention (CDC): *HIV and AIDS among gay and bisexual men,* Atlanta, Sept 2010, Author. Available from www.cdc.gov/nchhstp/newsroom/docs/Fast Facts-MSM-FINAL508COMP.pdf.

53. U.S. Department of Health and Human Services: Office of Minority Health, National Partnership for Action to End Health Disparities. *The national plan for action draft as of February 17, 2010, Chapter 1: Introduction,* 2010a. Retrieved from www.minorityhealth.hhs.gov/npa/templates/browse.aspx?&;lvl=2&lvlid=34.

54. U.S. Department of Health and Human Services: The Secretary's Advisory Committee on National Health Promotion and Disease Prevention Objectives for 2020. *Phase I report: recommendations for the framework and format of Healthy People 2020. Section IV, Advisory committee findings and recommendations,* 2010b. Available atwww.healthypeople.gov/hp2020/advisory/PhaseI/sec4.htm#_Toc211942917.

55. American Nurses Association: *Nursing scope and standards of practice,* ed 2, Silver Spring, Md, 2010, Author.

56. U.S. Department of Health and Human Services: Office of Minority Health, National Partnership for Action to End Health Disparities, *Health disparities,* 2010c. Retrieved from www.minorityhealth.hhs.gov/npa/templates/browse.aspx?lvl=1&;lvlid=13.

57. Caplan S, Paris M, Whittemore R, et al: Correlates of religious, supernatural and psychosocial causal beliefs about depression among Latino immigrants in primary care, *Ment Health Relig Cult* 13(7):1469–9737, 2010.

58. Van Ryn M, Fu SS: Paved with good intentions: do public health and human service providers contribute to racial/ethnic disparities in health? *Am J Public Health* 93(2):248–255, 2003.

59. Clark-Hitt R, Malat J, Burgess D, et al: Doctors' and nurses' explanations for racial disparities in medical treatment, *J Health Care Poor Underserved* 21(1):386–400, 2010.

60. Brown CR, Mazza GJ: *Healing into action,* Washington, DC, 1997, National Coalition Building Institute.

61. Rubin J: Impediments to the development of clinical knowledge and ethical judgment in critical care nursing. In Benner P, Tanner C, Cheslan C, editors: *Expertise in nursing practice: caring, clinical judgment, and ethics,* ed 2, New York, 2009, Springer, pp 171–198.

62. Institute of Medicine (IOM): *Health professions education: a bridge to quality,* Washington, DC, 2003, National Academies Press.

63. Betancourt JR: Cross-cultural medical education: conceptual approaches and frameworks for evaluation, *Acad Med* 78(6):560–569, 2003.

64. Campinha-Bacote J: A culturally conscious approach to holistic nursing. Program and abstracts of the American Holistic Nurses Association 2005 Conference, King of Prussia, Pa, June 16–19, 2005.

65. Cavillo E, Clark L, Ballantyne JE, et al: Cultural competency in baccalaureate nursing education, *J Transcult Nurs* 20:137–145, 2009. doi: 10.1177/1043659608330354.

66. Kleinman A: *Patients and healers in the context of culture,* Berkeley, Calif, 1980, University of California Press.

67. Mostow C, Crosson J, Gordon S, et al: Treating and precepting with RESPECT: a relational model addressing race, ethnicity, and culture in medical training, *J Gen Intern Med* 25(suppl 2):146–154, 2010.

68. Folkman S, Lazarus RS: The relationship between coping and emotion: implications for theory and research, *Soc Sci Med* 26:309–317, 1988.

69. Emmons RA: Emotion and religion. In Paloutzian RF, Park CL, editors: *Handbook of the psychology of religion and spirituality,* New York, 2005, Guilford Press, pp 235–252.

70. Rosmarin DH, Krumrei E, Andersson G: Religion as a predictor of psychological distress in two religious communities, *Cognitive Behav Ther* 38:54–64, 2009.

5

Motivation

Kristen Zulkosky and Jaclynn Huse

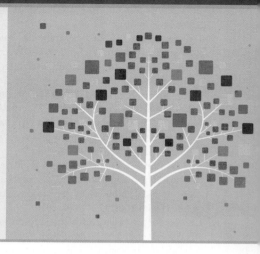

Health care professionals employed in a wide range of health-related settings have the unique opportunity to work with patients who are experiencing life-changing events such as pregnancy, diagnoses of acute or chronic diseases, and the aging process. These types of events evoke a plethora of emotions ranging from happiness and euphoria to desperation and despair. It is during these susceptible or vulnerable situations that health care professionals have the chance to impact a patient's understanding of this life-changing process and educate the patient on preventative health measures, the potential of reversing the disease process, or perhaps preservation of the quality of life. Understanding the concept of motivation, rather than just the definition, offers nurses the opportunity to appreciate their patient with a deeper level of understanding and to design a patient-centered plan of care that encourages the patient to desire the healthiest path and motivates the patient to persevere with his/her choices.

The concept of motivation explains the influences on people's beliefs and actions. Beyond the simple definition, motivation continues to mystify most scholars because of the differing assumptions and terminology. One of the problems with understanding the concept of motivation is that it seems intangible—we cannot see it; we cannot touch it. However, motivation is important for several reasons, one of which is that motivation improves and facilitates learning.[1] Learning is a key component when it comes to inspiring change and designing patient-centered education. Additionally, motivation explains why, within the health care environment, some patients may thrive and others fail to comply with expert opinions and advice. The goal of this concept analysis is to analyze and clarify the concept of motivation by providing a more thorough definition and by discussing the various types of motivation. The attributes of motivation along with the theoretical underpinnings will be explored. The ways in which motivation relates to nursing and the interrelated concepts are identified in this concept. A model case, a contrary case, and exemplars of this concept are also presented and discussed.

DEFINITION(S)

On the surface, the definition of motivation seems rather simplistic—"to stimulate toward action"[2]—or, in other words, motivation implies "the energy and direction of action."[3] In reality, the concept of motivation is rather complex—much like an intricate spider web—because there are so many influential factors that impact a person's energy and direction of action.

Bandura[4,p228] stated that "*motivation encompasses self-regulatory processes involving the selection, activation, and sustained direction of behavior toward certain goals.*" Ajzen[5] further elaborates that the motivation to behave in a certain manner is impacted by beliefs about the consequences of the behavior, the normal expectations of other influential people, and the amount of control the individual has in making the decisions. The perceived level of individual control and self-determination has a powerful impact on motivating an individual to perform or behave in a certain manner.[5-8] In health care it is imperative that nurses have a broad understanding of the concept of motivation in order to provide patients with a motive to maintain health or alter unhealthy lifestyles.

SCOPE AND CATEGORIES

Scope

The concept of motivation can be described along a continuum. A person who feels uninspired to act can be characterized as unmotivated; conversely, someone who is eager to act and meet a goal is considered motivated.[9] People can report different amounts of motivation and also different kinds of motivation (see Figure 5-1).

Ryan and Deci[10] stated that people "vary not only in the *level* of motivation (i.e., how much motivation), but also in the *orientation* of that motivation (i.e., what type of motivation)." The orientation of motivation focuses on the "underlying attitudes and goals that give rise to action, that is, it concerns the *why* of actions."[10,p54] For example,

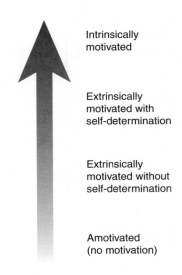

Intrinsically
motivated

Extrinsically
motivated with
self-determination

Extrinsically
motivated without
self-determination

Amotivated
(no motivation)

FIGURE 5-1 Scope of Motivation.

patients can be highly motivated to learn about a new disease process out of curiosity and interest or, alternatively, because they want the approval of the nurse and family. Patients can also be motivated to learn how to administer insulin because they understand the potential implications of a high blood sugar. In these examples, the patients may all have the same level or amount of motivation and similar outcomes but the focus of the motivation varies. There are two major types of motivation based on the goals that inspire people to act. Intrinsic motivation refers to "doing something because it is inherently interesting or enjoyable, and extrinsic motivation refers to doing something because it leads to a separable outcome."[10,p55]

Intrinsic motivation and extrinsic motivation are highly influenced by personal attributes such as age and cognitive level, environmental factors such as accessibility to physical resources and health care facilities, and relationships with family, friends, and the community. Figure 5-2 illustrates how these characteristics influence intrinsic and extrinsic factors that determine motivation.

Intrinsic Motivation

When people are intrinsically motivated, they act a certain way because of feelings of enjoyment and competence rather than because of obligations, pressures, or rewards.[9,11,12] This phenomenon was first observed with animal experiments where it was noted that many organisms exhibit curiosity-driven behaviors without an associated award or reinforcement. The behaviors appeared to occur for the sole purpose of having a positive experience connected with extending one's capabilities. The same can be seen in humans. From birth onward, humans are energetic, inquisitive, and curious to learn; and they do not require rewards or incentives to act. This behavior is a critical element in cognitive, social, and physical development as one grows in knowledge and skills. It not only is limited to childhood but also is a noteworthy phenomenon of human nature

that ultimately influences performance, persistence, and well-being.

Interestingly, intrinsic motivation exists within people; however, it also exists between people and certain activities. People are "intrinsically motivated for some activities and not others, but not everyone will be intrinsically motivated for any particular task."[10,p56]

Extrinsic Motivation

In contrast to intrinsic motivation, external motivation relies on attainment of an award or independent outcome.[10] There are two types of external motivation that relate to the degree of autonomy. Patients who participate in physical therapy sessions because they feel pressured by their families are extrinsically motivated; therefore, their behavior is not self-determined. Conversely, patients can demonstrate extrinsic motivation and self-determination when they choose to participate in physical therapy sessions because they realize that it will help them return home and live independently.[9] Both examples involve a means to improve health, but the latter instance contains a feeling of choice whereas the former involves compliance with an external control. Both examples "represent intentional behavior, but the two types of extrinsic motivation vary in their relative autonomy."[10,p60]

Amotivated

When patients' behavior "lacks intentionality and a sense of personal causation" they are classified as amotivated.[10,p61] Amotivation occurs because patients do not value an activity, do not feel competent to complete it, or do not believe it will obtain a desired outcome. Amotivation may also be the result of cognitive or emotional dysfunction. Considering the above physical therapy example, if patients do not believe that therapy sessions will help the recovery process, they are viewed as amotivated.[10]

Categories

The scope of motivation is influenced by a host of factors including four major categories. The following section will describe and explain each of these categories and demonstrate how each category is utilized in the popular NBC television program, "The Biggest Loser"—a show in which morbidly obese contestants arrive at a health/fitness ranch in order to be motivated to change their lives.

Achievement Motivation

The self-satisfaction obtained from achieving a goal can serve as motivation.[12] For example, contestants on "The Biggest Loser" undergo an extensive health analysis by the program's physician. The program airs segments that show the physician talking to the contestant and presenting graphic displays that illustrate all of the contestant's body fat or a life calculator that estimates the contestant's actual "inner body age"—usually decades older than the person's actual birth age. Contestants react in horror and dismay because they had no idea how much of an impact their poor lifestyle habits were having on the inside of their bodies. Most of these frightening

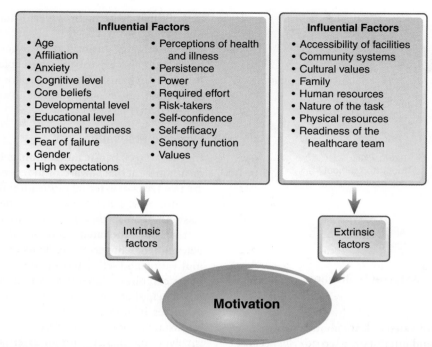

FIGURE 5-2 Relationships Between Intrinsic and Extrinsic Factors and Motivation.

conversations serve as a motivation strategy within itself that leads to increased vigor in the gym and compliance with the dieting strategy.

Together with the physician and personal trainers, a personalized health care plan is devised with moderate goals that the contestant should strive for on a weekly basis in order to reach the ultimate goal—complete physical health by the end of the contestant's stay on the ranch. The self-satisfaction comes from stepping on the scale every week and seeing the pounds disappear and from repeated visits to the physician that demonstrate that important healthy changes are happening internally. Each weekly victory serves as an achievement motivation for the contestant.

In the health care field, it is important to recognize that patients will feel like they want to achieve a goal and that the goal is attainable. It is up to the health care providers to help design patient-centered goals that are considered "moderately hard" tasks because these are the types of goals that patients will believe they can actually achieve. According to McClelland,[13] if the overall goal is too simple, the patient may feel that there really is no challenge because just about anyone could achieve that goal, leaving the patient feeling less motivated to try. In contrast, if the goal is too difficult, the patient may perceive that he/she will never be able to accomplish it and the patient will quit trying to achieve the goal.

Power Motivation

Some people feel the need to be successful in competition and the idea of winning or being number one serves as a powerful influence on motivation. People who tend to be motivated by power tend to be more assertive and aggressive

in nature.[12] Contestants on "The Biggest Loser" are in an actual weight loss competition—it is not just about personal victories but also defeating other contestants in order to remain the single champion of the show and win $250,000. A wide range of personality types are displayed within the contestants and there are always one or two contestants who are portrayed as "Game Players"; that is, their motivation for being on the show is to just win the show rather than really making important lifestyle changes. This is demonstrated in contestants who face weekly temptation events in which they have the opportunity to gain power over the game if they will just eat a pizza or a box of doughnuts. Many contestants resist the urge to eat their favorite foods, but there are always one or two contestants who would like to have control over the game and possibly their own fate in making it to the final rounds of the competition by giving in to the temptation in order to increase their odds of winning the overall game.

As a nurse, it is important to understand that the power motive can serve a particular personality type very well. If a patient is more assertive and aggressive, goals should be designed that help the patient feel like he/she can win the competition—even if it is a one-man competition. Utilizing the patient's assertiveness and aggressiveness can be considered a strength when thoughtful consideration has been given into helping this person accomplish his/her goals.

Affiliative Motivation

Affiliative motivation is defined as "a nonconscious concern for establishing, maintaining, and restoring close personal relationships with others."[14] Individuals with high affiliative motivation tend to display opposite characteristics of those who thrive on high power motivation. In general, people who respond to affiliative motivation are more likely to be nonassertive and more dependent on others.[12,13]

Often on "The Biggest Loser" contestants are battling devastating personal loss and tragedy and they explain how these shattering events led them to not care anymore about their own personal appearance and/or health because the intimacy and belonging that they once experienced has been destroyed. One particular contestant shared how within one single moment her husband and two small children were all killed in a car accident and how she began seeking food and overeating as a solace for her broken heart. She described her family as her affiliative motivation and without them she felt like her relevance and motivation for living and caring had been lost.

Nurses are going to work with patients who have experienced a plethora of emotions. Understanding their dependency on other people and their strong need for feeling a connection or bond can help the nurse determine what strategy would best encourage a healthy lifestyle. Motivation is not a singular entity; it is multifaceted. Motivation can come from physical, psychological, spiritual, and cultural factors. Nurses need to understand the relevance of each of these factors for their individual patients.

Avoidance Motivation

Anxiety, which is fear of the unknown, and fear, which is object related, are powerful, distressing emotions that can motivate a person to behave in a certain manner. Anxiety and fear of failure, rejection, success, power, and other phobias are rationales often presented as an individual's motivation to achieve a desired goal.[12] This type of individual is willing to do just about anything to prevent harm to himself or herself.

In "The Biggest Loser" the physician talks to the obese contestant and offers graphics and charts that show just how much internal bodily damage has occurred as a result of the contestant's sedentary lifestyle and poor dietary habits. Seeing images that depict how much fat they are carrying or their projected date of death serves as a powerful motivator by invoking fear into these people. Many of the contestants are very young parents who want to see their children grow up; they want to walk their daughter down the aisle at her wedding, see their son graduate, and become grandparents. The conversation with the physician elucidates the actuality of the contestant's condition and creates anxiety and fear of survival. Many of these contestants use these physician visits as motivation, and by the end of the show many contestants have been able to discontinue taking diabetic, blood pressure, and cholesterol medications because they won the overall battle.

In a health care setting, patients will also be faced with truths that are difficult to accept and quite overwhelming. Judgment must be exercised in determining how much information a patient or family can handle at one time. Nurses will have the opportunity to assess and evaluate these vulnerable situations and create valuable educational experiences

---

BOX 5-1	**ATTRIBUTES OF MOTIVATION**

- Self-determination
- Desire
- Compelled
- Aspiration
- Preference for challenge
- Energizing force
- Persistence
- Internal dispositions

---

so that the patient can experience hope and work towards a brighter future.

ATTRIBUTES AND CRITERIA

The defining attributes of a concept are those characteristics that appear frequently throughout the literature[15] and constitute a "*real* definition" beyond a dictionary explanation of a concept that "merely substitutes one synonymous expression for another."[16,p91] The defining attributes of motivation include self-determination,[17,18] desire,[19] compelled, aspiration,[20,21] preference for challenge, energizing force,[22] persistence,[17,22] and internal dispositions.[23] Attributes are presented in Box 5-1.

Motivation is influenced by a host of factors (see Table 5-1). First, characteristics that strongly influence motivation include the personal traits of the individual. These characteristics include age; developmental, cognitive, and educational levels; emotional readiness; actual or perceived state of health or illness; gender; sensory function;[24] core beliefs and values;[5,24] self-confidence; and the amount of effort required to succeed.[25] According to Richards and Digger,[24] individuals must also have a grasp of the complexity and urgency of the situation in order to be motivated to make changes. From a cognitive standpoint, the ability to think, remember, and process information can influence motivation.[26] Motivation may also be influenced by positive factors such as high expectations of one's own ability to achieve,[27] curiosity,[25] power, and the need for affiliation.[12] Negative factors such as anxiety,[12,24,25] the need to find the cause to a predicament,[28] or fear of failure can influence or discourage achievement-oriented behavior.[27]

Characteristics of the environment that influence motivation include human and physical resources, such as an individuals' perception of the accessibility of the health care facility and the psychological availability and readiness of the health care system.[24] In addition, the task itself in relation to level of difficulty, ambiguity, and rate of progression influences motivation.[25]

Relationship factors include the powerful influences of family and community systems, cultural expectations and customs, and the individuals' role within the community.[5,24] Emotional ties such as love, intimacy, sexual gratification, and a need for acceptance and an affiliation with others can motivate individuals to perform in a certain manner.[12]

TABLE 5-1   INFLUENTIAL CHARACTERISTICS ON MOTIVATION

Personal Traits
- Age
- Developmental, cognitive, and educational levels
- Emotional readiness
- Actual or perceived state of health or illness
- Gender
- Sensory function
- Core beliefs and values
- Self-confidence
- Effort required to succeed
- High expectations
- Curiosity
- Power
- Anxiety
- Urgency to find a cause to a predicament
- Fear of failure

Environmental Factors
- Available human and physical resources
- Accessibility of health care facility
- Psychological availability and readiness of health care system
- Level of difficulty and ambiguity of task
- Rate of progression

Relationships
- Powerful influences of family and community systems
- Cultural expectations and customs
- Individuals' role within community
- Emotional ties such as love, intimacy, and sexual gratification
- Need for acceptance and an affiliation with others

THEORETICAL LINKS

The concept of motivation is primarily linked to biological and psychological theories. Biological theories attempt to explain that motivation is a result of a person experiencing a physiological need or deficit. This deficit serves as motivation for the person to make necessary changes to eliminate the deficiency.[29] In contrast, field theories explain that action-oriented choices—voluntary decisions rather than automatic biological function—serve as a cognitive motivator to increase satisfaction and diminish discomfort.[29] Both of these theories have contrasting perspectives on the origins of motivation but neither is comprehensive; therefore cognitive theories were developed with the intention to have a more holistic perspective on motivation. Cognitive theorists did not dismiss the importance of biological and environmental influences; rather, they recognized that these were just two components of motivation and that evaluation of the cognitive process, including self-efficacy, beliefs, emotion, and other factors, influenced motivation.[29] The following theoretical linkages are organized according to these three major categories.

Biological Theories

In the 1930s, Clark Hull constructed the Drive Reduction Theory of Motivation in an attempt to explain motivation from a biological perspective.[30] His theory is derived from the concept of homeostasis and that the body has many compensatory mechanisms that function in order to maintain a biological balance. Borrowing from the field of biology, Hull postulated that motivation could be considered within the same light—that motivation originated with a biological imbalance and that an internal drive or motivation would eliminate the deficiency within the person.[30]

In 1943 Abraham Maslow proposed the humanistic Theory of Human Motivation through the conceptualization of the hierarchy of human needs. The fundamental proponent of his theory was that a person must feel satisfied that essential physiological needs such as food, water, oxygen, and shelter must be met before the individual will feel compelled or motivated to strive for higher needs such as safety, loving and belonging, self-esteem (which includes confidence), self-respect, and respect of others. Meeting all of these needs leads to the pinnacle of self-actualization. According to Maslow, conscious or unconscious motivation is primarily multifactorial and can be strongly influenced by cultural differences.[31,32]

Field Theories

Kurt Lewin,[20,21] considered "the father of social psychology," attempted to explain the importance of understanding psychology and its relationship to motivating particular behaviors. In his proposed Field Theory, Lewin suggested that influences of an individual's total situation must be taken into account. Furthermore, this theory elaborates on how important it is to take into context the value placed upon a specific goal and the probability that an individual will follow through and achieve that goal.[29]

Highly influenced by previous philosophers such as Hull, John Atkinson[27] developed the Theory of Achievement Motivation in order to explain individual differences in motivation. Atkinson found that individuals will be positively or negatively motivated to achieve a goal based upon their perception of their ability or lack of ability to reach that goal. He viewed individuals as rationale human beings who understood the value associated with making choices that would maximize individual satisfaction.[33] Atkinson[27] found that individuals with high levels of the need to achieve had a stronger expectation of success and that this served as a stronger motivator than the fear of failure. Atkinson later collaborated with David McClelland, who elaborated further on the significance of how achievement, power, the need for affiliation, and avoidance motives influence individual behavior.[12]

Cognitive Theories

Prochaska and DiClemente[34] developed the Transtheoretical Model of Change (also known as the Stages of Change model). Through longitudinal studies it was found that people move through five stages in the change process. The model explains and predicts how and when people will reject poor health care choices and adopt healthy ones.[35]

This model defines the five stages of change based on beliefs of readiness to change: precontemplation (deny the problem and not think about change); contemplation (recognize the advantages of changing and think about change within 6 months); preparation (intend to change in the next 60 days); action (actively make changes); and maintenance (sustain action for 6 months and work to prevent relapse). For most people, the change process is spiral, not linear, with periods of relapse before attaining a permanent behavior change.[36,37] Although the model does not include the construct motivation, it uses *levels* of readiness to change as an indicator of the level of individual motivation.[29]

Social Learning Theory[38,39] describes how behaviors are learned and focuses on the learning that occurs within a social context. The theory states that people learn from one another, and it includes concepts such as observational learning, imitation, and modeling. Motivation is a necessary ingredient for modeling to occur because learners must want to demonstrate what they have learned. People will take action if they believe they have control over an outcome, view few external environmental barriers, and have a strong sense of self-efficacy. The level of self-efficacy is the single, most important element that moves people into action.[39]

John Keller[40] spent 2 decades developing and testing a model that incorporates the motivation concept with instructional teaching. To recognize and solve issues with learning about motivation, he developed a model to find a more effective way to understand the major influences on motivation. His theory integrates concepts from other theories such as social learning, environmental theories, and cognitive dissonance theory. The motivation theory is not proposed to stand-alone but rather supplement other instructional theories.[41]

Keller proposed four conditions that must be met before a person is motivated to learn. Attention, relevance, confidence, and satisfaction (ARCS) are the conditions that, when integrated, motivate someone to learn. Attention strategies are used when arousing and sustaining curiosity and interest; relevance strategies link the person's needs, interests, and motives; confidence strategies help people develop a positive expectation for successful achievement; satisfaction strategies provide extrinsic and intrinsic reinforcement for effort. Keller believes that in an instructional situation, the learning task needs to be presented in a way that is engaging and meaningful to the learner, and in a way that promotes positive expectations for the successful achievement of learning objectives.[41]

Deci and colleagues[7] offered the contemporary, humanistic Self-Determination Theory in an effort to demonstrate the relevance of how behavior can be an outcome of two distinct motivating features. First, when a behavior is self-determined, the individual perceives that the motivation is internal and that he/she is in full control of his/her behaviors. In contrast, when a behavior is considered controlled, an individual feels the pressure externally, such as from families, peers, and coworkers. Both of these opposing forces lead to motivation.

CONTEXT TO NURSING AND HEALTH CARE

Although the majority of frameworks on motivation were written in the context of psychology, practicing nurses in all specialties of nursing would benefit from a greater understanding of how to motivate positive patient behavior. In addition, a complete understanding of motivation makes the nurse more acutely aware of influences that can be detrimental to the healing of individuals, families, and communities so that he/she will be better prepared to intervene on society's behalf.

Motivation is situation specific and can change depending on the person, the goal, or the context. Being motivated to read a book or learn a new skill depends on the book or skill. If two people are given the same skill to complete, they both will respond differently. The motivated person will surpass the less motivated person even though they may both have the same capabilities. When people are not motivated to complete a task, their behavior is accompanied by various reactions such as boredom, distraction, and frustration. Motivating others can be challenging but it is important when helping people obtain goals related to health care.[1,42]

Nurses need to be cognizant of the personal, relationship, and environmental characteristics that influence motivation. Some characteristics such as age and gender are nonmodifiable whereas others are changeable, and these are the influential factors that nurses can manipulate to effect positive patient outcomes. For example, if a person is anxious, the nurse can help decrease the feelings of anxiety or advocate for a prescribed treatment. In addition, if the assigned task involves many elements, it is important for the nurse to break it into smaller more manageable pieces. Through these nursing interventions, the nurse may positively affect the person's health care outcome.

INTERRELATED CONCEPTS

Self-Efficacy

The history of self-efficacy begins within Bandura's Social Learning Theory,[43] which was renamed Social Cognitive Theory in 1986. One of Bandura's major concepts in his theory is self-efficacy. Self-efficacy is defined as:

people's judgments of their capabilities to organize and execute courses of action required to attain designated types of performance. It is concerned not with the skills one has but with judgments of what one can do with whatever skills one possesses.[44,p391]

According to theory and research,[45] self-efficacy makes a difference in how people feel, think, and behave and in their intentions to become motivated. In terms of feeling, a low sense of self-efficacy is associated with stress, depression, anxiety, and helplessness. Such individuals may experience low self-esteem and become pessimistic about their accomplishments and personal development. In terms of thinking, a strong sense of efficacy facilitates cognitive processes and performance in a variety of settings, including quality of decision making and academic achievement. When it comes to behaving, self-efficacy can influence people's choice of activities. Self-efficacy levels can increase or hamper motivation. People with high self-efficacy approach difficult tasks as challenges and do not try to avoid them. According to Bandura,[43,p1176] "People's self-efficacy beliefs determine their level of motivation, as reflected in how much effort they will exert in an endeavor and how long they will persevere in the face of obstacles."

Bandura[43,p1175] explains the importance of self-efficacy as beliefs that function as "an important set of proximal determinants of human motivation, affect, and action." These beliefs constitute a form of action through motivational, cognitive, and affective intervening processes. An example of a cognitive process pertains to setting personal goals. The higher level of perceived self-efficacy, the higher levels of goals people set for themselves, which leads to a higher level of commitment to the goals.

Intentions

Intentions are defined as "a course of action that one intends to follow" or "an aim that guides action."[2] Furthermore, Ajzen[5] defines intention as "an indication of a person's readiness to perform a given behavior, and it is considered to be the immediate antecedent of behavior."

According to Ajzen,[5] the Theory of Planned Behavior delineates three separate influential factors that impact intentions. First, an individual's beliefs about a particular behavior will directly influence the person's attitude about that behavior. In turn, attitude has a direct impact on the person's intentions to behave in a certain manner. Second, the perceived behavioral expectations (normative beliefs) of family, friends, coworkers, and health care providers influence an individual's motivation to comply with the perceived social pressure from these groups (subjective norm) to behave in a certain way. It is this subjective norm that directly influences intention. Third, control beliefs, which are perceived factors that encourage or discourage performance of a behavior, influence the individual's perceived behavioral control that he/she has the ability to actually perform a particular behavior. Combined, attitude, pressure from influential groups, and an individuals' belief in their own ability to accomplish a certain task influence the individual's intention to actually go forward and behave in a certain manner. From a health care standpoint, all three of these factors can have a direct influence on an individual's motivation to actually put forth the effort to achieve his/her goals and lifestyle changes.

Compliance and Control

The term compliance is defined as "the degree of constancy and accuracy with which a patient follows a prescribed regimen, as distinguished from adherence or maintenance."[2] Compliance to a prescribed regimen consists of observable behaviors and can be directly measured whereas motivation is a "precursor to action that can be measured through behavioral consequences or results."[46,p169] In comparison, compliance equals achievement of goals or an end unto itself whereas motivation factors are a means unto an end.

Compliance can be conveyed negatively because the patient is in a submissive role with little input to a prescribed regimen whereas the health care provider is in an authoritative role who dictates the plan of care. This concept violates the philosophy of patient-centered care in which a patient should be able to make his/her own health care choices and be given the opportunity to not necessarily follow a predetermined plan set by health care professionals.[46] When patients do not follow directions given by the health care team, they are labeled noncompliant, which is a subjective term. This term eliminates the ethical principle of autonomy that should be inherent in health care treatment plans.

The term "locus of control" is related to compliance with therapeutic regimens. People can be categorized as having an internal locus of control if they are self-directed and believe they have control over events. Conversely, a person with an external locus of control believes that others have control over events and influence health outcomes. "Internals" believe in controlling their own destiny while "externals" believe that fate is a prevailing force that determines their destiny. If two people have a family history of heart disease, the internal will

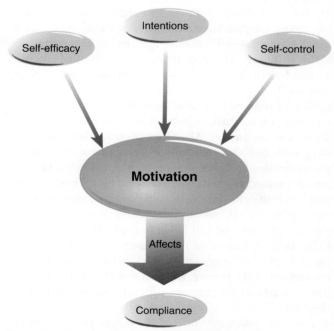

FIGURE 5-3 Relationships Between Motivation and Interrelated Concepts.

MODEL CASE

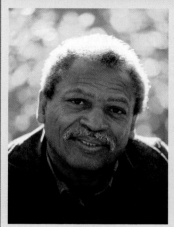

John is a 56-year-old African-American male with a history of hypertension, obesity, hyperlipidemia, and a family history of heart disease. He does not follow a low-fat diet or exercise regularly. He takes one blood pressure medication sporadically. John was admitted to the hospital with chest pain after shoveling snow. He was diagnosed with a myocardial infarction and received a coronary angioplasty. In addition, John's blood glucose level was elevated and he was diagnosed with new-onset diabetes mellitus. John's health care provider informed him that he needed to lose weight, eat a more healthy diet, exercise at least three times a week for 40 minutes, take medications regularly, attend cardiac rehabilitation sessions, and follow-up with health care provider visits. John knew he needed to make changes in his life despite having a family history of heart disease or he may not survive his next cardiac event. John's belief shows he has an internal locus of control.

Consequently, John decided to attend his cardiac rehabilitation sessions to help improve his lifestyle. At his first appointment, John was interviewed by his cardiac rehab nurse, Kathy, and completed a learning needs assessment to determine what he knew about exercise, diet, and medications. Kathy asked John what goals he wanted to set for himself while helping him set realistic goals. She found out what resources John needed to achieve his goals. Kathy asked John to bring his wife to the next appointment to review John's nutritional needs because she is the main meal preparer in the house.

At John's second visit, he and his wife, Sally, learned how to decrease the sugar, salt, and fat in his diet to better control his diabetes and to decrease his hypertension and cholesterol level. Sally was willing to eliminate the fried foods she cooked and add more baked foods. John and Sally decided to join the local gym and begin an exercise program together because they both needed to lose weight. They met other people with similar health issues who successfully learned to modify their lifestyle. Through role modeling they were motivated to adhere to the treatment regimen.

After 3 weeks of attending the gym for the prescribed three times per week and decreasing the amount of calories and fat he ate, John lost 9 pounds. Kathy praised John on his success and encouraged him to meet his additional goals. John became intrinsically motivated as he lost weight, which makes him determined to adhere to his treatment plan.

John continued attending his cardiac rehab sessions to gain more knowledge about his heart disease and how to maintain a healthier lifestyle. After 6 weeks, John returned to his health care provider for a check-up. John's cholesterol and blood glucose levels decreased and he lost a total of 15 pounds. His health care provider was very impressed with John's progress, which encouraged him to lose more weight. John completed his cardiac rehabilitation sessions and set new goals with Kathy's assistance before he was discharged.

After 6 months, John returned to his health care provider, who reported that John's cholesterol level was trending down and his blood glucose level was within normal limits. The health care provider decided John no longer needed to take his oral antidiabetes medication. In addition, John lost a total of 40 pounds, which improved his quality of life. John could walk up a flight of stairs without becoming short of breath. John continues to control his diabetes and heart disease with diet and exercise. He looks forward to playing with his new grandson because now he knows he can be the active grandpa he always wanted to be. John's level of self-efficacy is high and he is very happy with his motivation to stay healthy.

CONTRARY CASE

Using the previous case all items remain the same in the contrary case except, after being discharged from the hospital John does not follow the suggestions of his health care providers. John feels so overwhelmed with the amount of information Kathy presents to him at his first cardiac rehabilitation session that he misses his second appointment. John tells Kathy at his first meeting that his dad died of heart disease and he will too no matter what he eats and how much he exercises. John's beliefs show an external locus of control because he thinks that he cannot control his own fate. John returns to his health care provider when he needs medication refills. He continues to eat foods that are not

heart healthy and tells his health care provider he does not have time to exercise. John's health care provider pressures John into going back to cardiac rehabilitation. John's wife also demands that John complete the cardiac rehab program. John makes a second appointment and meets with Kathy again. Despite John's participation in cardiac rehab he is extrinsically motivated and has a behavior that is not self-determined. He is not motivated to change his lifestyle and is attending cardiac rehab because of the pressures of his health care provider and wife. Instead of seizing the opportunity to take control of his health and stay alive, John does the opposite and becomes amotivated.

respond by eating healthy, exercising, and not smoking while the external will do nothing because heart disease runs in the family and nothing can prevent it from developing.[46] Both the internal and the external locus of control will directly impact a person's intentions to become motivated to comply with a specified medical regimen.

There are many influential factors that persuade motivation. As the three interrelated concepts have depicted, one's ability to feel that he/she is capable of achieving a goal and his/her perception of who actually has control over a particular situation will impact the person's intentions to be motivated to comply with a specific medical regimen (see Figure 5-3). Having

BOX 5-2   EXEMPLARS OF MOTIVATION

AREA IMPACTED BY MOTIVATION	INTRINSIC MOTIVATION	EXTRINSIC MOTIVATION WITH SELF-DETERMINATION	EXTRINSIC MOTIVATION WITHOUT SELF-DETERMINATION	AMOTIVATED
Medication management	Takes medications regularly because they ↑ energy and ↓ pain.	Takes medication to prolong life.	Takes medications to appease an insistent health care provider.	Fails to take medications on a regular basis.
Exercise/treatment	Participates in PT because of enjoyment of exercises.	Participates in PT sessions because it helps person return home and live independently.	Participates in PT sessions because of feeling pressure from family.	Does not participate in PT sessions.
Health promotion	Attends prenatal visits because of personal learning that occurs.	Attends prenatal visits because of benefits for baby.	Attends prenatal visits because significant other insists.	Does not attend prenatal visits.
Health promotion	Quits smoking because it is satisfying to ↓ risk of cancer.	Quits smoking to ↓ admissions to hospital.	Attempts to quit smoking because of family pressure.	Does not quit smoking.

a broad understanding of influential factors allows the nurse to develop a patient-centered plan of care that is designed to maximize attaining health and compliance within the patient.

EXEMPLARS

There are endless examples of motivation. The three areas in which the large majority of clinical situations fall are medication management, treatment modalities, and health promotion strategies. Box 5-2 presents examples of each of these areas on the motivation continuum described earlier.

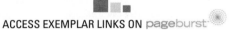

ACCESS EXEMPLAR LINKS ON pageburst

REFERENCES

1. Wlodkowski R: *Enhancing adult motivation to learn*, San Francisco, 1999, Jossey-Bass.
2. Online Etymology Dictionary: *Motivate*, n.d. Retrieved Jan 6, 2011, from Dictionary.com, http://dictionary.reference.com/browse/motivate.
3. Ryan RM, Lynch MF, et al: Motivation and autonomy in counseling, psychotherapy, and behavior change: a look at theory and practice, *Counsel Psychol* 39(193):193–260, 2011.
4. Bandura A: *Self-efficacy: the exercise of control*, New York, 1997, WH Freeman.
5. Ajzen I: *Attitudes, personality, and behavior*, ed 2, Berkshire, England, 2005, Open University Press.
6. Deci EL, Koestner R, Ryan RM: Extrinsic rewards and intrinsic motivation in education: reconsidered once again, *Rev Educ Res* 71(1):1–27, 2001.
7. Deci EL, Vallerand RJ, Pelletier LG, et al: Motivation and education: the self-determination perspective, *Educ Psychol* 26(3&4):325–346, 1991.
8. Ryan RM, Deci EL: Intrinsic and extrinsic motivations: classic definitions and new directions, *Contemp Educ Psychol* 25:54–67, 2000.
9. Hallams S, Baker K: The development of a questionnaire to assess motivation in stroke survivors: a pilot study, *New Zealand Journal of Physiotherapy* 37(2):55–60, 2009.
10. Ryan RM, Deci EL: Intrinsic and extrinsic motivations: Classic definitions and new directions, *Contemporary Educational Psychology* 25:54–67, 2000.
12. Ryan RM, Deci EL: Self-determination theory and the facilitation of intrinsic motivation, social development, and well-being, *Am Psychol* 55(1):68–78, 2000.
13. McClelland DC: *Human motivation*, Melborne, 1987, Cambridge University Press.
14. Ratzburg WH: *Motivating organizational members: McClelland's achievement motivation theory*, n.d. Retrieved Jan 31, 2011, from the Motivating Organization Members website, http://jam3c.tripod.com/index.html.
15. Walker LO, Avant KC: *Strategies for theory construction in nursing*, ed 4, Upper Saddle River, NJ, 2005, Pearson Prentice Hall.
16. Rodgers BL: Concept analysis: an evolutionary view. In Rodgers BL, Knafl KA, editors: *Concept development in nursing: foundations, techniques, and applications*, ed 2, Philadelphia, 2000, Saunders, pp 77–102.
17. Engin E, Cam O: Validity and reliability study of the Turkish psychiatric nurses of job motivation scale, *J Psychiatr Ment Health Nurs* 16:462–472, 2009.
18. Haggar M, Chatzisarantis NLD, Hein V, et al: Teacher, peer and parent autonomy support in physical education and leisure-time physical activity: a trans-contextual model of motivation in four nations, *Psychol Health* 24(6):689–711, 2009.
19. Sitzmann T, Brown KG, Ely K, et al: A cyclical model of motivational constructs in web-based courses, *Military Psychol* 21:534–551, 2009.
20. Lewin K: Field theory and learning. In Henry NB, editor: *The forty-first yearbook of the National Society for the Study of Education: Part II—the psychology of learning*, Chicago, 1942, The University of Chicago Press, pp 215–242.
21. Lewin K: Field theory and experiment in social psychology. In Cartwright D, editor: *Field theory in social science: selected theoretical papers*, New York, 1951, Harper & Brothers Publishers, pp 130–154.

22. Gilmore L, Cuskelly M: A longitudinal study of motivation and competence in children with Down syndrome: early childhood to early adolescence, *J Intellect Disabil Res* 53(5):482–492, 2009.

23. MacLean N, Pound P: A critical review of the concept of patient motivation in the literature on physical rehabilitation, *Soc Sci Med* 50:495–506, 2000.

24. Richards E, Digger K: Compliance, motivation, and health behaviors of the learner. In Bastable SB, editor: *Nurse as educator: principles of teaching and learning for nursing practice*, ed 3, Sudbury, Mass, 2008, Jones and Bartlett , pp 199–228.

25. Drillings M, O'Neil HF Jr: Introduction to motivation: theory and research. In O'Neal HF Jr, Drillings M, editors: *Motivation: theory and research*, Hillsdale, NJ, 1994, Lawrence Erlbaum Associates Inc. Publishing, pp 1–12.

26. Driscoll M: *Psychology of learning for instruction*, ed 3, Boston, 2005, Pearson Publishing.

27. Atkinson JW: *An introduction to motivation*, Princeton, NJ, 1964, D. Van Nostrand.

28. Graham S: Classroom motivation from an attributional perspective. In O'Neal HF Jr, Drillings M, editors: *Motivation: theory and research*, Hillsdale, NJ, 1994, Lawrence Erlbaum Associates Inc. Publishing, pp 31–48.

29. Dunsmore S, Goodson P: Motivation for healthy behavior: a review of health promotion research, *Am J Health Educ* 37(3):170–183, 2006.

30. Hull CL: *Principles of behavior*, New York, 1943, Appleton, Century, Crofts.

31. Maslow AH: A theory of human motivation, *Psychol Rev* 50:370–396, 1943.

32. Maslow AH: *Toward a psychology of being*, New York, 1962, D. Van Nostrand.

33. Weiner B: *Human motivation: metaphors, theories, and research*, Thousand Oaks, Calif, 1992, Sage.

34. Prochaska JO, DiClemente CC: Stages and processes of self-change of smoking: toward an integrative model of change, *J Consult Clin Psychol* 51:390–395, 1983.

35. DiNoia J, Prochaska JO: Dietary stages of change and decisional balance: a meta-analytic review, *Am J Health Behav* 34:618–634, 2010.

36. Prochaska JM, Prochaska JO, Cohen FC, et al: The transtheoretical model of change for multi-level interventions for alcohol abuse on campus, *J Alcohol Drug Educ* 47(3):34–50, 2004.

37. Prochaska JO, Wright JA, Velicer WF: Evaluating theories of health behavior change: a hierarchy of criteria applied to transtheoretical model, *Appl Psychol Int Rev* 57(4):561–588, 2008.

38. Bandura A: Human agency in social cognitive theory, *Am Psychol* 44:1175–1184, Sept 1989.

39. Bandura A: Social cognitive theory: an agentic perspective, *Annu Rev Psychol* 52:1–26, 2001.

40. Keller J: Development and use of the ARSC model of instructional design, *J Instruct Dev* 10(3):2–10, 1987.

41. Keller JM, Kopp TW: An application of the ARCS model of motivational design. In Reigeluth CM, editor: *Instructional theories in action: lessons illustrating selected theories and models*, Hillsdale, NJ, 1987, Lawrence Erlbaum Associates, pp 289–320.

42. Wlodkowski R, Ginsberg M: *Teaching intensive and accelerated courses*, San Francisco, Calif, 2010, Jossey-Bass.

43. Bandura A: *Self-efficacy: the exercise of control*, New York, 1977, WH Freeman.

44. Bandura A: *Social foundations of thought and action: a social cognitive theory*, Englewood Cliffs, NJ, 1986, Prentice-Hall.

45. Bandura A: *Self-efficacy in changing societies*, New York, 1995, Cambridge University Press.

46. Bastable SB, Dart MA: Developmental stages of the learner. In Bastable SB, editor: *Nurse as educator: principles of teaching and learning for nursing practice*, ed 3, Sudbury, Mass, 2008, Jones and Bartlett, pp 147–198.

6

Adherence

Janice M. Bissonnette

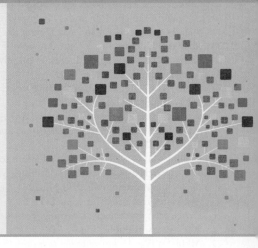

dherence is the patient profile concept of interest in this section and has numerous definitions across health care, which can also have contradictory meanings.[1-10] In nursing, the concept of adherence is more closely associated with patient-centered care and the work required by nurses to support a patient's long-term adherence to treatment.[10,11] This concept analysis provides the most common definitions of adherence as well as examples of the way this concept is applied in practice.

DEFINITION(S)

The North American Nursing Diagnosis Association International (NANDA-I) defines adherence behavior as a self-initiated action taken to promote wellness, recovery, and rehabilitation.[12] Haynes[13] defined adherence as the extent to which patients follow the instructions they are given for prescribed treatments. Christensen[14] offered an alternative definition, in keeping with a less paternalistic approach. Adherence in this context is patient focused and is defined as the extent to which a person's actions or behavior coincides with advice or instruction from a health care provider intended to prevent, monitor, or ameliorate a disorder.

Cohen,[15] in a concept analysis of adherence related to the nursing practice of patients with cardiovascular disease, defined adherence as "persistence in the practice and maintenance of desired health behaviours and is the result of active participation and agreement." Adherence is also associated with terms such as compliance, concordance, obedience, observance, conformity, acceptance, cooperation, mutuality, persistence, and therapeutic alliance.[16-19] The concept of adherence became more prominent in nursing literature in the late 1990s.[7,20]

Before the late 1990s, compliance was the more commonly used term to describe a patient's behavior related to following a recommended treatment.[21,22] The definition of compliance behavior as an outcome for nursing diagnostic categories is distinctly different from that for adherence behavior. In this context, compliance behavior is "the action taken on the basis of professional advice to promote wellness, recovery, and rehabilitation."[12,p458] The concept compliance was the primary descriptor for a patient's obedience to prescribed treatments.[22] David Sackett[23] is one of the original and major researchers in medical compliance, and published randomized clinical trial results of strategies for improving medication compliance in patients with hypertension. The majority of compliance research published from the 1970s to the 1980s was from physicians or behavioral scientists and contained no input from nursing.[22,23] Nursing became involved in the debate over compliance as a measurable behavior through the works of Marston.[24]

Variation and debate exist on how to define adherence, how it differs from compliance or concordance, and how the behavior of adherence relates to patients, health care professionals, and system factors.[2,7,8,25-28] The historical transition and change in terminology from compliance to adherence, and more recently concordance, requires a reclarification of "adherence" as a concept for nursing practice.[10,11,29,30] In nursing practice, it is important to determine if the concept of adherence, as a profile of the patient's behavior, provides an effective way of characterizing the behavior individuals demonstrate or experience in response to a prescribed treatment regimen.

SCOPE AND CATEGORIES

The scope of adherence essentially ranges from a total lack of adherence to complete adherence (Figure 6-1). The degree of adherence within this range includes the patient's intentional or rationale decision to stop the medication, or change the dose or frequency of the medication.[17,31] Also included in this range is the patient's unintentional change in medication-taking behavior, which represents a nonpurposeful overlooking of taking the medication.[32,33] The same applies for health

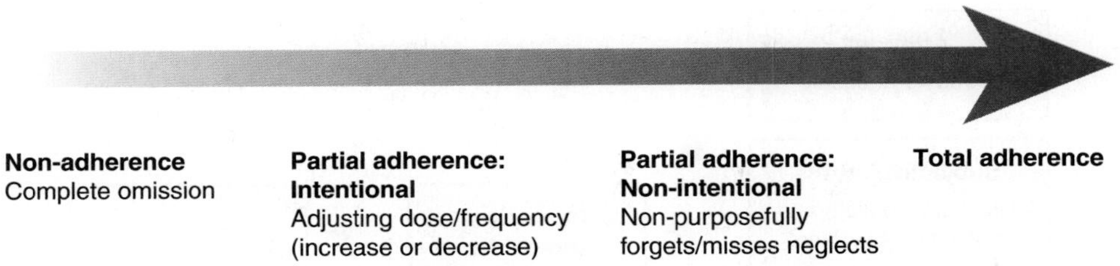

Non-adherence	Partial adherence:	Partial adherence:	Total adherence
Complete omission	**Intentional**	**Non-intentional**	
	Adjusting dose/frequency	Non-purposefully	
	(increase or decrease)	forgets/misses neglects	

FIGURE 6-1 Scope of the Concept Adherence.

promotion activities—for example, reducing the amount of recommended exercise, increasing the amount of recommended salt in the diet on weekends, or not attending physician's appointments. Despite the potential for any degree of nonadherence to influence a patient's disease control or health, it is unclear where within this range patients become most at risk for negative outcomes.[33]

The primary situation preceding the evaluation of a patient's adherence behavior is the recommendation or prescription of a treatment by a health care professional. Most often, however, the focus is on the patient's adherence to long-term medications or treatments and health promotion activities in the face of chronic disease.[27] Other adherence regimens include those associated with weight loss, exercise, smoking cessation, and diet or fluid restrictions. The theme underlying the patient's total or positive adherent behavior suggests the patient views/believes the professional to be a trusted and knowledgeable source concerning recommended treatment for the disease or health state in question. The action or behavior of adherence assumes some degree of willingness on the part of the patient to accept all or part of the prescription or recommendation. What is not clear with the behavior of adherence is the degree to which the patient agreed with or was involved in the prescription or recommendation.

Within health care, the consequences of nonadherence fall into three areas: patient related, health professional related, and health care system related.[13,29] Patient-related consequences include (a) increased mortality and morbidity, (b) conflict, (c) attributional uncertainty, (d) embarrassment, and (e) changes in quality of life.[30] Health professional related consequences include (a) ambivalence, (b) misinterpretation, (c) avoidance, (d) decisional conflict, and (e) empathy.[34-36] Health care system related consequences include increased cost and health care service use.[27,29]

Nurses are present in the majority of health care settings in which patients receive treatment recommendations. This provides a good opportunity to assess, integrate, and reinforce treatment adherence strategies with patients.

ATTRIBUTES AND CRITERIA

The attributes of adherence support identification of situations or behaviors that are best characterized by using the concept of adherence. The cluster of attributes comprises the real life definition of a concept, as opposed to the dictionary definition.[37] A number of attributes are associated with the concept of adherence (Box 6-1).

In the context of a number of nursing diagnoses, adherence behavior is the anticipated outcome. For example, for the diagnosis of *Health-Seeking Behaviors,* defined as "the state in which an individual in stable health is actively seeking ways to alter personal health habits, and/or the environment in order to move toward a higher level of health,"[12,p162] adherence behavior is the outcome. The nursing diagnosis of *Individual Management of Therapeutic Regimen, Effective,* defined as "a pattern of regulating and integrating into daily living a program for treatment of illness and its sequelae that are satisfactory for meeting specific health goals,"[12,p179] adherence behavior is the outcome. Thirdly, the nursing diagnosis of *Noncompliance,* defined as "the extent to which a person's and/or caregiver's behaviour coincides or fails to coincide with a health-promoting or therapeutic plan agreed upon by the person (and/or family, and/or community) and health care professional or in the presence of an agreed-upon, health-promoting or therapeutic plan, person's or caregiver's behaviour is fully or partially non-adherent and may lead to clinically effective, partially effective or ineffective outcomes"[12,p210] again adherence behavior is the anticipated outcome.

BOX 6-1 **ATTRIBUTES OF ADHERENCE**[14]

- Decisional conflict
- Predictability
- Personal experience
- Power conflict
- Agreement
- Alignment

THEORETICAL LINKS

Social psychologists have developed a number of behavioral approaches to guide the assessment of a patient's medication-taking behavior and the overall enhancement of adherence behavior. The social cognition models are the most common theories underpinning the behavior change associated with adherence or nonadherence.[14,37-43] The more common theories in this category include the Theory of Planned Behavior[41] and the Health Belief Model.[43] The primary outcome in each of these models is a specific health behavior based on a deliberate process of decision making. The patient's preexisting intentions, beliefs, or degree of confidence in his/her success influences the decision-making process.

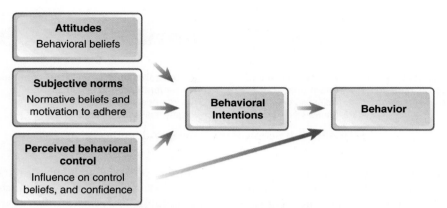

FIGURE 6-2 The Theory of Planned Behavior.

Theory of Planned Behavior (TPB)

The Theory of Planned Behavior proposes a model about how human action is guided.[41,44] It predicts the occurrence of a specific behavior if that behavior is intentional. As depicted in Figure 6-2, the model integrates the variables of attitude (e.g., behavioral beliefs), subjective norms (e.g., normative beliefs and motivation), and perceived behavioral control (e.g., influence and confidence of control beliefs), which predict the intention to perform the behavior. In this model intentions precede the actual behavior.

The key assumptions of TPB relate to the prediction of whether a person **intends** to do something. The predicators are the patient's attitude (i.e., if the patient is in agreement with completing the treatment), the subjective norm (i.e., the amount of social pressure the patient feels to proceed with the treatment), and the perceived behavioral control (i.e., the level of control the patient feels he/she has over the treatment or choice of treatment). By influencing or enhancing these three "predictors," nurses can increase the chance that the individual will intend to proceed with a recommended or prescribed treatment, and then actually do it.[41,44]

For example, a patient presents to a nurse clinician in a diabetes clinic with elevated fasting glucose and hemoglobin A_{1c} (HbA$_{1c}$) measurements. Will the patient tell the nurse that the elevated measurements are attributable to the fact that he has not been taking his insulin regularly or following his diet? The answer to this question depends on whether the patient **intends** to do so. In other words, it is not an automatic, habitual, or thoughtless action. The intention, in turn, depends on the following considerations:

- Whether, overall, the patient has a positive or negative **attitude** to revealing his nonadherent behavior
- To what extent the patient perceives that he experiences social pressure to adhere to healthy lifestyle practices for control of his diabetes and associated health risks, including whether the patient believes:
  - The nurse wants to know how he manages his diabetes
  - Family/friends/significant others would approve of him telling the nurse (normative beliefs)
  - These people's opinions are important to the patient

- Whether the patient finds it **difficult** to discuss his diabetes self-management and adherence with the nurse, and that this will result in an appropriate treatment plan

The final behavior is predicted by the degree to which each of the above components influences the patient's intention to act.

The Health Belief Model

The Health Belief Model (HBM) first conceptualized beliefs as predictors of preventive health behavior to help explain the failure of some individuals to use these behaviors.[43] The theory hypothesizes that people are likely to initiate a health-related behavior to the extent that they (a) perceive that they could become ill or be susceptible to the problem (e.g., perceived susceptibility), (b) believe that the illness has serious outcomes or will disrupt their daily functioning (e.g., perceived severity), (c) believe that the required recommendation will be effective in reducing symptoms (e.g., perceived benefits), and (d) believe that there are few barriers to initiating the recommendation (e.g., perceived barriers).[43]

For example, using the same scenario previously described, a patient presents to a nurse clinician with elevated fasting glucose and HbA$_{1c}$ measurements. Will the patient tell the nurse the elevation is because he has not been taking his insulin regularly or following his diet? The answer to this question depends on the patient's perceptions of susceptibility, risk, benefits, and barriers. Engaging in a conversation of insulin adherence, in turn, depends on the following factors:

- Whether the patient perceives his diabetes as severe and his perceptions of susceptibility to the health risks associated with diabetes
- The extent to which the patient perceives that insulin therapy and diet control are beneficial in the control of his diabetes and reduction of risk factors
- Whether the patient perceives barriers exist with the use of insulin therapy and diet control

The extent or degree of these perceptions influences the patient's engagement in the behavior—or in this case whether he participates in a conversation on his insulin-taking behavior.

CONTEXT TO NURSING AND HEALTH CARE

Evangelista[7] reviewed the literature on adherence and compliance from all health disciplines in an attempt to distinguish between the everyday health care practice use and that associated with scientific use. Adherence is a dynamic concept, influenced in part by the social context of its use. The social or disciplinary context of interest for the purpose of this section is nursing practice, with identification of interrelations between and with other health disciplines. Similar inductive approaches have been applied by nurse researchers for the analysis of such concepts as chronic pain,[45] symptom clusters,[46] conflict in nursing work environments,[47] and adaptive systems.[48] Understanding the perspective and use of adherence from each discipline is fundamental for clarification of the concept and for identification of contextual variations.[49,50] The following sections present the major characteristics of the concept of adherence emerging from the disciplines of nursing, mental health, general medicine, and pharmacy.

Nursing

Before the introduction of the concept adherence, Marston,[24] as one of the first nursing authors to enter the compliance debate, raised concerns about medicine's multiple definitions of compliance in addition to the lack of objective compliance measures. Marston[24] encouraged nurses to participate in the debates related to compliance to improve the nursing knowledge of compliance from a more holistic nurse-patient perspective. In 1973, NANDA accepted noncompliance as a nursing diagnosis. The new diagnostic category reflected little recognition of the impact on nursing practice, but resulted more in response to the medically based literature.[47,51]

Kim[50] suggested the diagnostic taxonomies for nursing appeared to unify communication and documentation between nurses, but did not add to the development of nursing science because of the lack of association with an explanatory framework. From 1973 to present, members of NANDA-I, supported by additional nursing authors, pursued the removal of noncompliance from this diagnostic nomenclature because the term emphasized a paternalistic obligation to follow orders.[50-53] Interestingly, as discussed earlier, the nursing diagnosis of noncompliance remains in use, with adherence behavior as the expected outcome

Mental Health

Adherence to therapies is a key component of care in mental health settings.[1,38,39,42] Estimates of medication nonadherence for patients with mental disease are 24% to 90%, with one in four patients experiencing psychosis associated with nonadherence.[35,36,39,54] Adherence and compliance continue to be described as interchangeable concepts in the mental health literature.[38,39] An important theme identified from the mental health literature was the association between the patient's nonadherence and the patient's feelings of embarrassment when questioned about the nonadherence.[54-56] Hui[35] reported an underrecognition by mental health clinicians of both the patient's nonadherent behavior and the patient's associated feelings of embarrassment. No formally recognized diagnostic category for nonadherence exists in the *Diagnostic and Statistical Manual of Mental Disorders, edition 4, text revision (DSM-IV-TR)*. Nonadherence became a symptom of mental illness as opposed to a distinct entity.

General Medicine

In the general medicine literature, adherence and compliance are synonymous. Adherence is most frequently associated with efforts to develop a statistically based measurement to predict presence or risk of adherence and correlation to a health outcome or disease-specific outcomes.[13,26] The chronic disease states most commonly studied for nonadherence rates include asthma, diabetes, human immunodeficiency virus (HIV)/acquired immunodeficiency syndrome (AIDS), transplantation, cardiovascular disease, hypertension, epilepsy, and cancer.[5,6,8,13,16] Research within these disease states attempts to provide answers to the questions of how to best predict, measure, or intervene for nonadherent patient behavior.[13]

Pharmacy

The health care discipline of pharmacy very much mirrors the general medicine literature. Pharmacology research focuses on the development of measurement tools for nonadherence, with reference to pharmacist-led interventions to improve patient adherence as a means of achieving therapeutic goals.[1,57,58] The most common formal definition was from Haynes and colleagues.[13] Some authors did describe the general intent of using the term adherence to reflect a more active, voluntary, and collaborative relationship between the patient and health care provider, but continued to use compliance and adherence interchangeably.[55,58]

INTERRELATED CONCEPTS

Three principles that provide measures of adherence are compliance, persistence, and concordance. These principles are described in the following paragraphs. Additionally, several concepts featured in this textbook influence the degree of adherence. These include **Motivation, Culture, Development, Cognition, Family dynamics,** and **Function** (Figure 6-3).

Compliance or "obedience" with a prescribed treatment attributes an undertone of blame towards the patient when the patient's behavior does not meet with health professionals' expectations.[4,59] The definition for medication compliance, developed by the International Society for Pharmacoeconomics and Outcomes Research (ISPOR) group, is "the extent to which a patient acts in accordance with the prescribed interval and dose of a dosing regimen."[58,p46] In this context, compliance is the behavior of conforming to treatment for a recommended length of time. The World Health Organization[27] attempted to change this undertone by introducing adherence as an alternative to the more paternalistic concept

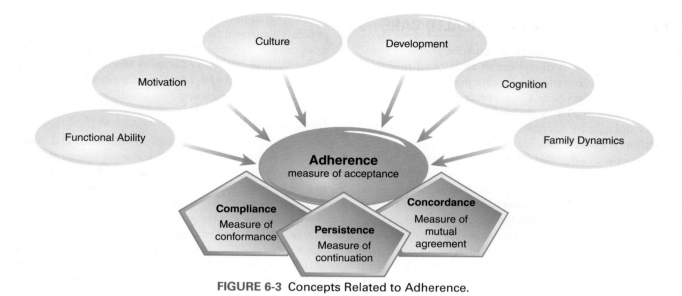

FIGURE 6-3 Concepts Related to Adherence.

MODEL CASE

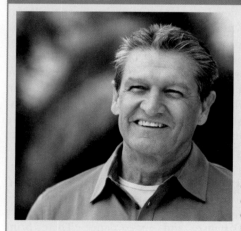

Martin Herrera is a 65-year-old male admitted to the cardiology unit for a non–ST-elevated myocardial infarction (non-STEMI). Mr. Herrera is now 3 days post stent insertion, and is preparing for discharge the next day. Prior medical history for Martin includes known coronary artery disease, anterior wall MI 2 years ago, hyperlipidemia, hypertension, and metabolic syndrome. In addition, Martin continues to smoke, although he has reduced his smoking to 20 cigarettes per day. In preparing Mr. Herrera for discharge, the nurse reviews his discharge medications, medication-taking behavior before admission, and specific cardiovascular disease (CVD) risk reduction strategies (e.g., weight control, exercise, smoking cessation). Martin admitted to not taking his medications on a regular basis, often missing them 2 to 3 days a week. The most common reason given by Martin was forgetfulness and "it won't make a difference anyways."

To begin the assessment of adherence, it is first important to clarify with the patient (a) his beliefs and perceptions about his health risk status, (b) his existing knowledge about CVD risk reduction, (c) any prior experience with health care professionals, and (d) his degree of confidence with controlling the disease. Clarification of these areas reveals the following: (a) Martin believes that because he has a very strong family history of CVD, noting his father died at age 66 and his brother at age 60, nothing he does will change the final outcome; (b) Martin states he saw a video while in the hospital and was given a bunch of pamphlets, but does not really remember any specifics; in addition, he has never participated in a smoking cessation program; (c) he is seen by a cardiologist every 12 months, but did not attend his last appointment because he was told if he did not quit smoking the cardiologist was transferring him for follow-up by his family physician; and (d) Martin states he tried to quit smoking but was only able to reduce to 10 cigarettes a day and feels he is unlikely to smoke any less.

Analysis

This case study illustrates the concept of adherence in the context of a nursing assessment for CVD risk reduction. According to the TPB, Mr. Herrera's attitude, beliefs, and perceptions influence his intention to adhere to his recommended medications and treatment plan. The comments made by Martin suggest a negative attitude towards his ability to control the disease outcomes or benefits of recommended treatments and a lack of confidence with lifestyle changes (e.g., smoking cessation). The nurse can focus on these particular assumptions and work with Mr. Herrera to develop a better understanding of his disease severity and progression as well as the benefits of recommended treatments. To improve Martin's adherence to treatment, it will be important to help him develop reminder strategies that fit into his lifestyle and support long-term adherence (e.g., persistence, agreement), and to address Martin's misperceptions of the benefits of medications and lifestyle change to control CVD progression (e.g., decisional conflict, knowledge alignment).

of compliance. Adherence purportedly suggests the patient's agreement to prescribed recommendations rather than passive cooperation in obedience to them.[27] Some authors describe the main function of such terms as compliance and adherence as ideological, in that these terms serve as a framework from which health care professionals convey their ideas concerning how patients should behave.[29,62-64]

The concept of **Persistence** appears primarily within the context of chronic disease management therapies.[59] In contrast to compliance, medication persistence is the time from initiation to discontinuation of a recommended or prescribed treatment.[59] In nursing practice, the patient's degree of persistence is of most value when assessing the patient's adherence behavior. Confirming how often a patient renews or refills his/her prescriptions is a measurement of the patient's persistence with continuation of the treatment.

Concordance is the most recent conceptual term added in an attempt to more accurately reflect the behavior of adherence and suggests that patients and health care professionals come to a mutually agreed upon regimen through a process of negotiation and shared decision making.[24,60] The behavior of concordance reflects development of an alliance with patients based on realistic expectations.[65]

EXEMPLARS

In moving beyond the ideological and semantic debate, the practical reality of not following a recommended course of treatment, particularly in chronic illness, remains a major cause of poor health outcomes and increased health care costs.[27,28] In 2003 the World Health Organization launched a global initiative to improve worldwide rates of adherence to therapies commonly used in treating chronic conditions. Adherence rates with prescribed regimens in chronic illness average 50%, ranging from zero to 100% depending on the method of measurement.[27]

The most common exemplar for adherence is medication-taking behavior. Medication-taking behavior is associated with short- and long-term medication regimens (Box 6-2). Health care practitioners are all familiar with many patients not completing a full course of antibiotics because they feel better. According to the WHO, nonadherence with long-term medications is an ongoing problem that results in serious health risks.[27] The total cost of nonadherence is estimated to be $100 billion annually for the health care system in the United States.[66] Results of a systematic review by Cramer[16] found adherence and persistence with cardiovascular and glucose lowering medications is poor. In this review, only 59% of patients took medication for greater than 80% of the expected therapy days.

Additional adherence behavior exemplars include diet and preventative health activities (see Box 6-2). In the context of chronic illness such as chronic kidney disease, patients face a long-term commitment to dietary restrictions (e.g., fluid, sodium, protein) and challenges with ongoing exercise. Nonadherence rates are estimated between 50% and 80% for chronic disease management and lifestyle changes.[27] If patients do not perceive any benefit from changing their behavior, sustaining the change becomes very difficult. Health care professionals, such as nurses, can influence adherence behavior by supporting patients' knowledge development, using negotiation for realistic and mutually agreed upon goal setting.[10,52]

SUMMARY

The historical and present day use of compliance, adherence, and concordance continues to reflect the power structure within the social system of health care. In their ongoing attempt to develop and maintain a power hold, nursing has confronted this power structure without having a clear understanding of its impact on nursing practice. Very few researchers to date have explored the health care professional's perceptions and understanding of adherence, and none has focused on nursing alone. It is hard to know if this is an intentional or rationale avoidance considering the complexity of adherence as a concept. The question that now comes to mind is the following: Do we need to rethink how we see or explore the phenomena and concern with patients' "obedience" with treatment recommendations?

If asked, patients would not label themselves as nonadherent, noncompliant, nonconcordant, or disobedient. When

---

BOX 6-2 CLINICAL EXEMPLARS OF ADHERENCE BEHAVIOR

Medication Management
Short-Term Medication Treatment
- Antibiotics
- Anticoagulants

Long-Term Medication Treatment
- Antihypertensive agents
- Antirejection medications
- Birth control
- Cholesterol lowering agents
- Insulin

Diet
- Diabetic diet
- Low cholesterol diet
- Renal diet
- Sodium restrictions

Preventative Health Activities
- Annual influenza vaccination
- Regular exercise
- Smoking cessation
- Use of sunscreen

confronted with questions of nonadherent behavior, patients admit to feeling blamed and accused, stating very few attempts were being made by nurses or physicians to understand the context or basis of decisions to "non-adhere."[4,14] As with the notion of informed consent, if patients understand the consequences of nonadherence, do we have the right to make a judgment on that individual's choice? After 40 years of studying compliance and adherence, with no clear development of guidance on how to best intervene, perhaps now is the time to be acceptant of this as a phenomenon of human nature with no one solution or one investigational approach.[11,67,68]

Concepts that are similar yet different, such as adherence, compliance, and concordance, often share empirical or measurable indicators that make differentiation more difficult.[66] Research attempting to provide an objective measure of these concepts reveals variability in identifying a gold standard measure as well as limited success in interventional efficacy directed at improving adherence rates.[13,14] There remains an inconsistent definition of adherence as it relates to health care recommendations, which has led to the ongoing labeling of patients as nonadherent or noncompliant.

Despite the possible replacement of adherence with the new language of persistence or concordance, Russell[10] noted that the understanding of what is best for patients' lives is seldom addressed in the literature. Nursing plays a major role in supporting patients' acceptance and adjustment to the impact of illness on their lives. Adherence from a patient-centered approach supports the goal of nursing by advocating for what is best in the context of each patient's life. The concept analysis of adherence as a separate and distinct phenomenon provides the first step to identifying if a patient-centered approach applies to the current concept use of adherence, and implications on how nursing might best achieve that goal.

The concept analysis approach serves as a preliminary step to broadening nurses' appreciation for the complexity of adherence as a patient behavior.[67] This analytical process represents an integration of what we know about adherence. As the "Achilles' heel"[14] of modern health, the debate and concern with patient nonadherence persist. A concept analysis of adherence provides the opportunity to clarify its historical context as well as implications for future impact on nursing knowledge.

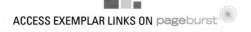

ACCESS EXEMPLAR LINKS ON pageburst

REFERENCES

1. Akerblad A, Bengtsson F, Ekselius L, et al: Effects of an educational compliance enhancement programme and therapeutic drug monitoring on treatment adherence in depressed patients managed by general practitioners, *Int Clin Psychopharmacol* 18(6):347–354, 2004.
2. Bissonnette J: A concept analysis: adherence, *J Adv Nurs* 63(6):634–643, 2008.
3. Buchmann W: Adherence: a matter of self-efficacy and power, *J Adv Nurs* 26:132–137, 1997.
4. Carpenter R: Perceived threat in compliance and adherence research, *Nurs Inquiry* 12(3):192–199, 2005.
5. Dunbar-Jacob J, Mortimer-Stephens MK: Treatment adherence in chronic disease, *J Clin Epidemiol* 54:S57–S60, 2001.
6. De Geest S, Dobbels R, Fluri C, et al: Adherence to the therapeutic regimen in heart, lung and heart-lung transplant recipients, *J Cardiovasc Nurs* 20(55):S85–S95, 2005.
7. Evangelista LS: Compliance: a concept analysis, *Nurs Forum* 34(1):5–11, 1999.
8. Gray R, Wykes T, Cournay K: From compliance to concordance: a review of the literature on interventions to enhance compliance with antipsychotic medication, *J Psychiatr Ment Health Nurs* 9:277–284, 2002.
9. Murphy N, Canales M: A critical analysis of compliance, *Nurs Inquiry* 8(3):173–181, 2001.
10. Russell S, Daly J, Hughes E, et al: Nurses and 'difficult' patients: negotiating non-compliance, *J Adv Nurs* 43(3): 281–287, 2003.
11. Lehane E, McCarthy G: Medication non-adherence—exploring the conceptual mire, *Int J Nurs Pract* 15:25–31, 2009.
12. Johnson M, Bulechek G, McCloskey-Dochterman J, et al, editors: *Nursing diagnoses, outcomes, & interventions: NANDA, NOC, and NIC linkages*, St Louis, 2001, Mosby.
13. Haynes RB, Yoa X, Degani A, et al: Interventions to enhance medication adherence (review), *Cochrane Database Systemat Rev* (issue 4), 2005.
14. Christensen AJ: *Patient adherence to medical treatment regimens: bridging the gap between behavioral science and biomedicine*, New Haven, Conn, 2004, Yale University Press.
15. Cohen SM: Concept analysis of adherence in the context of cardiovascular risk reduction, *Nurs Forum* 44(1):25–36, 2009.
16. Cramer JA, Benedict A, Muszbek N, et al: The significance of compliance and persistence in the treatment of diabetes, hypertension and dyslipidaemia: a review, *Int J Clin Pract* 62:76–87, 2008.
17. Donovan JL, Blake DR: Patient non-compliance, deviance or reasoned decision making? *Soc Sci Med* 34:507–513, 1992.
18. Kontz M: Compliance redefined and implications for home care, *Holistic Nurs Pract* 3:54–56, 1989.
19. Kyngäs H, Duffy M, Kroll T: Concept analysis of compliance, *J Clin Nurs* 9:5–12, 2000.
20. Playle JF, Keeley P: Non-compliance and professional power, *J Adv Nurs* 27:304–311, 1998.
21. Dracup A, Meleis AJ: Compliance: an interactional approach, *Nurs Res* 31:31–36, 1982.
22. Sackett DL, Haynes RB: *Compliance with therapeutic regimens*, Baltimore, Md, 1976, The Johns Hopkins University Press.
23. Sackett DL, Haynes RB, Gibson ES, et al: Randomized clinical trial of strategies for improving medication compliance in primary hypertension, *Lancet* 1:1205–1207, 1975.
24. Marston MV: Compliance with medical regimens: a review of the literature, *Nurs Res* 19(4):312–333, 1970.
25. Bissell P, May C, Noyce P: From compliance to concordance: barriers to accomplishing a re-framed model of health care interactions, *Soc Sci Med* 58:851–862, 2004.
26. Farmer K: Methods for measuring and monitoring mediations regimen adherence in clinical trials and clinical practice, *Clin Ther* 21(6):1074–1090, 1999.
27. Sabaté E: *Adherence to long-term therapies: evidence for action*, Geneva, 2003, World Health Organization.

28. Simpson S, Eurich D, Majumdar S, et al: A meta-analysis of the association between adherence to drug therapy and mortality, *BMJ*, 2006. doi: 10.1136/bmj.38875.675486.55.

29. Stevenson F, Cox K, Britten N, et al: A systematic review of the research on communication between patients and health care professionals about medicines: the consequences for concordance, *Health Expect* 7:235–245, 2004.

30. Vermeire E, Hearnshaw H, Van Royen P, et al: Patient adherence to treatment: three decades of research. A comprehensive review, *J Clin Pharm Ther* 26:331–342, 2001.

31. Crow J: Intentional non-adherence, *Pract Nurse* 26(6):12–17, 2003.

32. Crow J: Unintentional non-adherence, *Pract Nurse* 26(5):28–34, 2003.

33. Lehane E, McCarthy G: Intentional and unintentional medication non-adherence: a comprehensive framework for clinical research and practice? A discussion paper, *Int J Nurs Stud* 44:1468–1477, 2007.

34. Wilson HS, Hutchinson SA, Holzemer WL: Reconciling incompatibilities: a grounded theory of HIV medication adherence and symptom management, *Qual Health Res* 12(10):1309–1322, 2002.

35. Hui C, Chen E, Kan C, et al: Anti-psychotics adherence among out-patients with schizophrenia in Hong Kong, *Keio J Med* 55(1):9–14, 2006.

36. Hui C, Chen E, Kan C, et al: Detection of non-adherent behaviour in early psychosis, *Austral N Z J Psychiatr* 40(5):446–451, 2006.

37. Rodgers BL: Concept analysis: an evolutionary view. In Rogers BL, Knafl KA, editors: *Concept development in nursing: foundations, techniques and applications*, ed 2, Philadelphia, 2000, Saunders, pp 77–102.

38. Kamali M, Kelly B, Clarke M, et al: A prospective evaluation of adherence to medication in first episode schizophrenia, *Eur Psychiatr J Assoc Eur Psychiatr* 21(1):29–33, 2006.

39. Pratt S, Mueser K, Driscoll M, et al: Medication nonadherence in older people with serious mental illness: prevalence and correlates, *Psychiatr Rehabil J* 29(4):299–310, 2006.

40. Dunbar-Jacob J: Models for changing patient behavior, *Am J Nurs* 107(6):20–25, 2007.

41. Ajzen I, Fishbein M: *Understanding attitudes and predicting social behavior*, Englewood Cliffs, NJ, 1980, Prentice-Hall.

42. Sajatovic M, Valenstein M, Blow FC, et al: Treatment adherence with antipsychotic medications in bipolar disorder, *Bipolar Disord* 8(3):232–241, 2006.

43. Rosenstock IM: Historical origins of the health belief model. In Becker MH, editor: *The health belief model and personal health behavior*, Thorofare, NJ, 1974, Charles B. Slack, pp 1–8.

44. Ajzen I: The theory of planned behavior, *Organiz Behav Hum Decision Processes* 50:179–211, 1991.

45. Breen J: Transitions in the concept of chronic pain, *Adv Nurs Sci* 24(4):48–59, 2002.

46. Kim HS, McGuire D, Tulman L, et al: Symptom clusters: concept analysis and clinical implications for cancer nursing, *Cancer Nurs* 28(4):270–282, 2005.

47. Almost J: Conflict within nursing work environments: concept analysis, *J Adv Nurs* 53(4):444–453, 2006.

48. Holden L: Complex adaptive systems: concept analysis, *J Adv Nurs* 52(6):651–657, 2005.

49. Rodgers BL: Concepts, analysis and the development of nursing knowledge: the evolutionary cycle, *J Adv Nurs* 14(4):330–335, 1989.

50. Kim HS: Structuring the nursing knowledge system: a typology of four domains, *Schol Inquiry Nurs Pract* 1(2):99–110, 1987.

51. Bakker RH, Kasterman MC, Dassen TW: Non-compliance and ineffective management of therapeutic regimen: use in practice and theoretical implications. In Rant MJ, LeMone P, editors: *Classification of nursing diagnoses: proceedings of the twelfth conference/North American Nursing Diagnoses Associations*, CINHAL Information Systems, 1997, Glendale, Calif, pp 196–201.

52. Bradley-Springer L: Prevention: the original adherence issue, *J Assoc Nurses AIDS Care* 9(3):17–18, 1998.

53. Kim MJ, Moritz DA: *Classification of nursing diagnoses: proceedings of the third and fourth national conferences*, New York, 1982, McGraw-Hill.

54. Nose M, Barbui C, Tansella M: How often do patients with psychosis fail to adhere to treatment programmes? A systematic review, *Psychol Med* 33(7):1149–1160, 2003.

55. Akerblad A, Bengtsson F, Von Knorring L, et al: Response, remission and relapse in relation to adherence in primary care treatment of depression: a 2-year outcome study, *Int Clin Psychopharmacol* 21(2):117–124, 2006.

56. Pope M, Scott J: Do clinicians understand why individuals stop taking lithium? *J Affective Disord* 74(3):287–291, 2003.

57. Chisholm MA: Enhancing transplant patients' adherence to medication therapy, *Clin Transplant* 16(1):30–38, 2000.

58. Raynor DK, Nicolson M, Nunney J, et al: The development and evaluation of an extended adherence support programme by community pharmacists for elderly patients at home, *Int J Pharm Pract* 8(3):157–164, 2000.

59. Cramer JA, Burrell A, Fairchild CJ, et al: Medication compliance and persistence: terminology and definitions, *Value Health* 11(1):44–47, 2008.

60. Fraser S: Concordance, compliance, preference or adherence, *Patient Pref Adher* 4:95–96, 2010.

61. Lutfey K, Wishner W: Beyond "Compliance" is "Adherence": improving the prospect of diabetes care, *Diabetes Care* 22:635–639, 1999.

62. Evangelista LS, Dracup K: A closer look at compliance research in heart failure patients in the last decade, *Prog Cardiovasc Nurs* 15(3):97–103, 2000.

63. Britten N: Prescribing and the defense of clinical autonomy, *Soc Health Illness* 23(4):478–496, 2001.

64. Trostle JA: Medical compliance as an ideology, *Soc Sci Med* 27:1299–1308, 1988.

65. Jones G: Prescribing and taking medicines: concordance is a fine theory but is mostly not being practiced, *Br Med J* 327:819, 2003.

66. Julius R, Novitsky M, Dubin W: Medication adherence: a review of the literature and implications for clinical practice, *J Psychiatr Pract* 15(1):34–44, 2009.

67. Hupcey J, Penrod J: Concept analysis: examining the state of the science, *Res Theory Nurs Pract Int J* 19(2):197–208, 2005.

68. Wagner GJ, Rabkin JG: Measuring medication adherence: are missed doses reported more accurately than perfect adherence? *AIDS Care* 12(4):405–408, 2000.

UNIT 2

Health and Illness Concepts

The provision of health care is geared toward three general goals: to promote health, to prevent disease, and to treat illness when it arises. These do not represent three separate and competing goals, but rather these goals characterize the health and illness continuum and apply to all people across the lifespan. The concepts presented in Unit 2 are related to these goals within the context of the patients who receive our care.

Health and illness concepts are complex and represent a multitude of health-related conditions. These concepts are presented similarly and include concept definition, scope of concept, risk factors, physiologic processes and consequences, assessment, collaborative management, a model case, interrelated concepts, and clinical exemplars. Presented from a lifespan and health-continuum perspective, these concepts focus on the commonalities of conditions represented, as opposed to specific disease conditions. For each concept, nurses should understand the concept and notice situations that place an individual at risk for less than optimal function; further, nurses should know how to recognize alterations when they occur, and have a general understanding of interventions both to promote optimal health and to restore health if an alteration occurs.

A total of 8 themes are used to organize the 28 concepts in this unit. Because of the wide range of health conditions represented by these concepts, this is the largest of the three units within this textbook. The following eight themes are included in this unit:

- *Homeostasis and Regulation:* concepts that are associated with controlling and integrating multiple body systems so that physiologic control and balance can be maintained. Concepts within this theme include Fluid and electrolyte balance, Acid-base balance, Thermoregulation, Cellular regulation, Intracranial regulation, Glucose regulation, Nutrition, and Elimination.
- *Oxygenation and Hemostasis:* concepts that are represent optimal perfusion of oxygenated blood to body tissues. Concepts included within this theme are Perfusion, Gas exchange, and Clotting.
- *Sexuality and Reproduction:* concepts associated with sexual responses and human reproduction. Specifically, this theme is represented by two concepts: Reproduction and Sexuality.
- *Protection and Movement:* concepts that represent various levels of protection mechanisms and purposeful movement necessary for survival. Concepts include Immunity, Inflammation, Infection, Mobility, Tissue Integrity, Sensory Perception, and Pain.
- *Coping and Stress Tolerance:* concepts associated with the physiologic response to body stressors. The two concepts within this theme are Stress and Coping.
- *Emotion:* concepts associated with emotional well-being and threats to emotional well-being. The concept Mood and effect and the concept Anxiety represent this theme.
- *Cognitive Function:* concepts that represent an interaction of physiologic and neuropsychosocial processes associated with cognitive and mental information processing. Concepts represented include Cognition and Psychosis.
- *Maladaptive Behavior:* concepts that represent physiologic and psychosocial issues that manifest with challenging behaviors. This theme is represented by two concepts: Addiction and Personal violence.

Fluid and Electrolyte Balance

Linda Felver

Fluid in the body circulates in the blood and lymph vessels, surrounds the cells, and provides the environment inside cells in which they perform their cellular chemistry. The amount, concentration, and composition of the fluid in the body influence function at all levels from the cell to the whole person. The body continuously adjusts the characteristics and location of its fluid through specific physiologic processes that nurses must understand in order to assist individuals to maintain or restore their fluid and electrolyte balance and function optimally. This concept presents a conceptual analysis of fluid and electrolyte balance, including the recognition and management of fluid and electrolyte imbalances when they occur.

DEFINITION(S)

Fluid and electrolyte balance is defined as the *process of regulating the extracellular fluid volume, body fluid osmolality, and plasma concentrations of electrolytes.* Fluid is water plus the substances dissolved and suspended in it. Important characteristics of fluid are its volume (amount) and its degree of concentration (osmolality). Electrolytes are substances that are charged particles (ions) when they are placed in water. Examples of electrolytes are sodium ions (Na^+), potassium ions (K^+), calcium ions (Ca^{++}), and magnesium ions (Mg^{++}). In health care settings, people often omit the word "ion" when discussing electrolytes, referring to potassium ions as "potassium," for example. All body fluids contain electrolytes; body fluids in different locations normally contain different concentrations of electrolytes that are necessary for optimal function.

Fluid and electrolyte balance is a dynamic interplay between three processes: fluid and electrolyte intake and absorption; fluid and electrolyte distribution; and fluid and electrolyte output. *Fluid and electrolyte intake and absorption* are addition of fluid and electrolytes to the body (intake) and their movement into the blood (absorption). *Fluid and electrolyte distribution* is the process of moving fluid and electrolytes between the various body fluid compartments. These fluid compartments include inside the cells *(intracellular)* and

outside the cells *(extracellular)*. The extracellular compartment includes fluid between the cells *(interstitial)* and fluid inside blood vessels *(vascular).*[1] *Fluid and electrolyte output* is removal of fluid and electrolytes from the body, through normal or abnormal routes.

Fluid and electrolyte balance is a dynamic interplay because fluid and electrolyte output occurs continuously. Intake of fluid and electrolytes influences output to some degree, but it can easily become less than or more than output. Fluid and electrolyte distribution can shift rapidly when conditions change. Optimal fluid and electrolyte balance keeps the volume, osmolality, and electrolyte concentrations of fluid in the various body fluid compartments within their normal physiologic ranges.

SCOPE AND CATEGORIES

Scope

From the most abstract perspective, the concept of fluid and electrolyte balance is quite simple: one either has optimal balance or disrupted balance (an imbalance). Fluid and electrolyte imbalances can be either too little, too much, or misplaced. As the discussion of fluid and electrolytes unfolds in this concept, this will become more clear.

Conceptually, *fluid balance* has two aspects: extracellular volume and osmolality; *electrolyte balance* requires separate consideration. Extracellular fluid volume, body fluid osmolality, and plasma electrolyte concentrations each can be visualized as a continuum with three categories: optimal balance and two types of disrupted balance (Figure 7-1). The term imbalance often is used to indicate disrupted fluid or electrolyte balance.

Optimal Fluid and Electrolyte Balance

Optimal fluid and electrolyte balance occurs when both of these characteristics are present:
- Fluid and electrolyte intake and absorption match the fluid and electrolyte output.

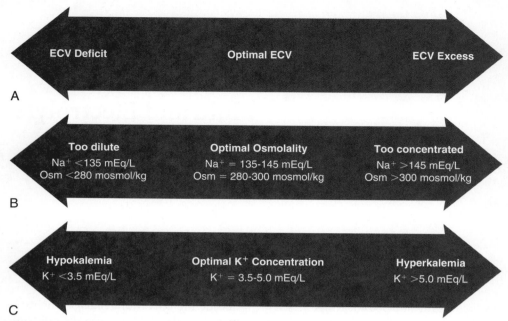

FIGURE 7-1 Scope of Fluid and Electrolyte Balance. A, Scope of extracellular fluid volume (ECV) balance. **B,** Scope of body fluid osmolality balance. **C,** Scope of electrolyte balance. Potassium (K^+) is used as an example.

- Volume, osmolality, and electrolyte concentrations of fluid in the various body fluid compartments are within their normal ranges.

Extracellular Fluid Volume Imbalances

As their name indicates, extracellular fluid volume (ECV) imbalances are abnormal amounts of fluid in the extracellular compartment (vascular plus interstitial). Fluid that has the same effective concentration as normal body fluid is called isotonic fluid.[2] Normal extracellular fluid (ECF) is isotonic Na^+-containing fluid. The Na^+ is necessary to hold the water in the extracellular compartment.

There are two types of ECV imbalances. ECV deficit is too little Na^+-containing isotonic fluid in the extracellular compartment; ECV excess is too much Na^+-containing isotonic ECF. With ECV imbalances, the amount of isotonic fluid changes, but its concentration remains the same unless an osmolality imbalance is present at the same time.

Osmolality Imbalances

Osmolality imbalances are changes in the degree of concentration of body fluid. If osmolality changes, it equilibrates rapidly between ECF and intracellular fluid as a result of osmotic shifts of water across cell membranes. Although osmolality can be measured directly, in many clinical settings it is tracked using the serum Na^+ concentration, which usually rises or falls in parallel with osmolality.[3] Na^+ stays in the ECF when water moves into or out of cells, which is why the serum Na^+ concentration changes when the osmolality changes.

There are two types of osmolality imbalances. Hypernatremia (increased serum Na^+ concentration) indicates that body fluids are too concentrated (osmolality is too high). Hyponatremia (decreased serum Na^+ concentration) indicates that body fluids are too dilute (osmolality is too low). Osmolality imbalances can occur alone or with ECV imbalances. The combination of ECV deficit and hypernatremia is known as clinical dehydration.[4]

Electrolyte Imbalances

Electrolyte imbalances are abnormal plasma concentrations of electrolytes such as K^+, Ca^{++}, and Mg^{++}. Although Na^+ also is an electrolyte, its concentration reflects the osmolality as discussed previously. Electrolyte concentrations are measured from blood samples and do not necessarily correlate with the concentrations inside cells.

There are two types of electrolyte imbalances: plasma concentration deficits and excesses. Names of electrolyte imbalances are constructed from a prefix that indicates whether the concentration is too low *(hypo-)* or too high *(hyper-)*; a combining form that indicates the specific electrolyte involved (e.g., *-kal-* for K^+, *-calc-* for Ca^{++}, *-magnes-* for Mg^{++}); and the suffix *-emia* that signifies "in the blood". Electrolyte imbalances can occur alone or with ECV and/or osmolality imbalances.

RISK FACTORS

Optimal fluid and electrolyte balance is necessary for physiologic function for all individuals, regardless of race, culture, age, or socioeconomic status. Nurses can deduce logically the individual risk factors for fluid and electrolyte imbalances by considering the dynamic interplay of the processes involved in fluid and electrolyte balance. Individuals at greatest risk are the very young, the very old, those with serious injury, or those with significant health conditions.

Because so many different disease processes and behaviors can disrupt fluid and electrolyte balance, it is more useful to think about risk factors in terms of what the disease or behavior is causing rather than focus on the disease itself. Practically speaking, there are only three overarching risk factors; all fluid and electrolyte imbalances involve at least one of the following risk factors (Figure 7-2):

- Fluid and electrolyte output *greater than* intake and absorption
- Fluid and electrolyte output *less than* intake and absorption
- Altered fluid and electrolyte distribution

Fluid and Electrolyte Output Greater than Intake and Absorption

To maintain optimal fluid and electrolyte balance, output must be matched by appropriate intake, and the intake must be absorbed (Figure 7-2, *A*). Individuals whose fluid and electrolyte output is greater than intake and absorption are at high risk for developing the imbalances ECV deficit, increased osmolality (hypernatremia), and various plasma electrolyte deficits. Two situations cause output to exceed intake and absorption (Figure 7-2, *B*):

- Normal output but deficient intake or absorption
- Increased output not balanced by increased intake

Normal Output but Deficient Intake or Absorption

Body fluid output through urine, feces, skin, and respirations combined is dilute Na^+-containing fluid. Therefore daily intake of some Na^+ and considerable water is necessary to maintain optimal fluid balance. Although the kidneys are able to reduce their fluid output to some degree in response to decreased fluid intake, some renal output is obligatory, as is water output through the skin and respiration.[5] When intake is less than normal output, the fluid imbalance a person develops depends on the type of fluid that is deficient. For example, people who do not drink enough water to match their water output can make their body fluids too concentrated (osmolality too high; hypernatremia). See hypernatremia in Box 7-1 for examples.

Deficient electrolyte intake and absorption with normal output can cause plasma electrolyte deficits such as hypokalemia or hypomagnesemia. Box 7-1 lists specific causes of electrolyte deficits due to normal output but decreased intake or absorption.

Increased Output Not Balanced by Increased Intake

Another situation in which fluid and electrolyte output becomes greater than intake arises when output increases but intake does not increase enough to balance it. For example, diarrhea increases output of Na^+, water, and K^+. During diarrhea, an intake of Na^+, water, and K^+ that does not balance the increased output creates high risk for ECV deficit, increased osmolality (hypernatremia), and hypokalemia.[6] Box 7-1 has other examples of imbalances due to increased output not balanced by increased intake. To prevent these imbalances, fluid and electrolyte intake must increase to balance increased output.

Fluid and Electrolyte Output Less than Intake and Absorption

When fluid and electrolyte output is less than intake and absorption, the risk is for a different set of imbalances: ECV excess, decreased osmolality (hyponatremia), and plasma electrolyte excesses. Two situations cause intake to be greater than output (Figure 7-2, *C*):

- Output less than excessive or too rapid intake
- Decreased output not balanced by decreased intake

Output Less than Excessive or Too Rapid Intake

Even people who have normal renal function may overwhelm their output capacity by excessive or very rapid intake of fluid and electrolytes. This situation most commonly occurs with intravenous (IV) infusions. Any person receiving IV fluid is at risk for developing fluid and electrolyte imbalances from excessive or too rapid infusion of the solution, even if the infusion is intended to replace a fluid or electrolyte deficit. The specific imbalance that develops depends on the type of IV solution being administered.[7] Nurses need to be especially alert when infusing IV solutions that contain K^+, because hyperkalemia caused by too rapid infusion can cause dangerous cardiac dysrhythmias.[8]

Excessive oral intake that overwhelms normal output mechanisms also is possible. The most common example is mild ECV excess that occurs when people eat salty foods and drink water. They may notice tight rings or shoes and overnight weight gain, which resolve in a day or two as the kidneys excrete the excess Na^+ and water. People who have conditions that cause chronic ECV excess, such as compensated heart failure or end-stage chronic renal failure, often follow low-Na^+ diets to avoid exacerbating their ECV excess.

When people drink a lot of water without salt, they normally produce less antidiuretic hormone and their kidneys excrete the extra water. However, massive rapid oral intake of water can overwhelm renal water excretion capacity and make body fluids too dilute (osmolality too low; hyponatremia).[9,10] See hyponatremia in Box 7-1 for specific examples. Oral intake of electrolyte-rich foods by people who have normal renal function usually is not problematic because the kidneys excrete any excess.

Decreased Output Not Balanced by Decreased Intake

People who have oliguria from any cause have decreased output of fluid and electrolytes and their intake must be decreased as well to prevent imbalances. For example, people who have oliguric renal disease develop ECV excess, hyperkalemia, and hypermagnesemia unless their intake is decreased appropriately.[6] See other examples in Box 7-1.

Combining excessive or too rapid intake of fluid and electrolytes with decreased output creates a potentially dangerous situation in which imbalances can develop rapidly. An IV solution that infuses in excess amounts or too rapidly into an individual who is oliguric can cause life-threatening

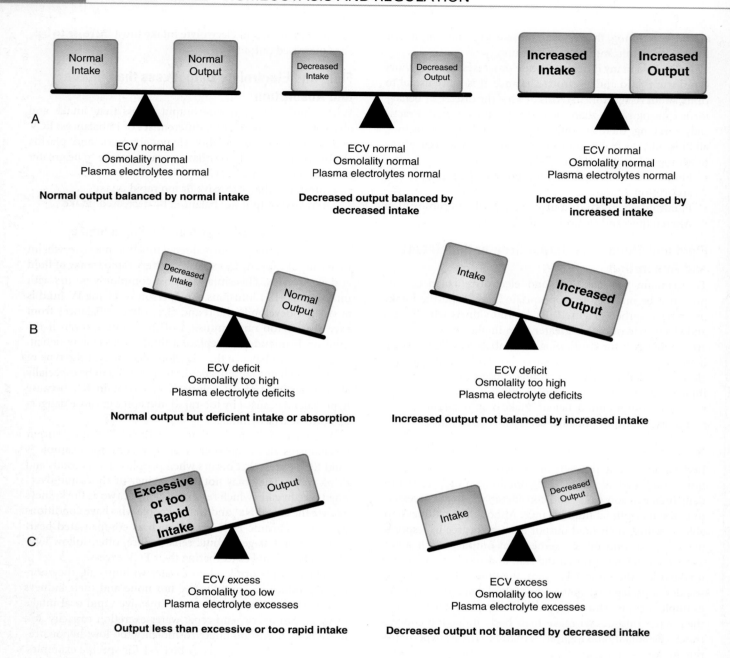

FIGURE 7-2 Optimal and Disrupted Balance of Fluid and Electrolytes. **A,** Optimal balance with fluid and electrolyte output balanced by intake. **B,** Imbalance from fluid and electrolyte output greater than intake and absorption. **C,** Imbalance from fluid and electrolyte output less than intake and absorption. **D,** Imbalance from altered fluid and electrolyte distribution.

BOX 7-1 CAUSES OF DISRUPTED FLUID AND ELECTROLYTE BALANCE

ECV Deficit (Too Little Extracellular Volume)
Normal Output but Deficient Intake of Na⁺ and Water
- Lack of access to Na⁺ and water

Increased Output Not Balanced by Increased Intake of Na⁺ and Water
- Vomiting
- Acute or chronic diarrhea from any cause, including laxative abuse
- Draining GI fistula, gastric suction, or intestinal decompression
- Hemorrhage or burns
- Overuse of diuretics
- Lack of aldosterone (adrenal insufficiency, Addison's disease)

Rapid Fluid Shift from ECV into a Third Space
- Acute intestinal obstruction
- Ascites that develops rapidly

ECV Excess (Too Much Extracellular Volume)
Output Less than Excessive or Too Rapid Intake of Na⁺ and Water
- Excessive IV infusion of Na⁺-containing isotonic solution (0.9% NaCl, Ringer's)
- High oral intake of salty foods and water with renal retention of Na⁺ and water

Decreased Output Not Balanced by Decreased Intake of Na⁺ and Water
- Oliguria (e.g., acute kidney injury, acute glomerulonephritis, end-stage renal disease)
- Aldosterone excess (e.g., cirrhosis, chronic heart failure, primary hyperaldosteronism)
- High levels of glucocorticoids (e.g., corticosteroid therapy, Cushing's disease)

Hypernatremia (Body Fluids Too Concentrated; Osmolality Too High)
Normal Output but Deficient Intake of Water
- No access to water or inability to respond to or communicate thirst (e.g., aphasia, coma, infancy)
- Tube feeding without additional water intake

Increased Output Not Balanced by Increased Intake of Water
- Vomiting or diarrhea with replacement of Na⁺ but not enough water
- Diabetes insipidus (lack of antidiuretic hormone)

Hyponatremia (Body Fluids Too Dilute; Osmolality Too Low)
Output Less than Excessive or Too Rapid Intake of Water
- IV 5% dextrose in water (D_5W) infusion with excess rate or amount
- Rapid oral ingestion of massive amounts of water (e.g., child abuse, club initiation, psychiatric disorders)
- Overuse of tap water enemas or hypotonic irrigating solutions
- Massive replacement of water without Na⁺ during vomiting or diarrhea

Decreased Output Not Balanced by Decreased Intake of Water
- Excessive antidiuretic hormone

Hypokalemia (Plasma K⁺ Deficit)
Normal Output but Deficient K⁺ Intake
- Prolonged anorexia or diet lacking K⁺-rich foods
- No oral intake plus IV solutions not containing K⁺

Increased Output Not Balanced by Increased K⁺ Intake
- Vomiting
- Acute or chronic diarrhea from any cause, including laxative abuse
- Use of K⁺-wasting diuretics or other drugs that increase renal K⁺ excretion
- Excessive aldosterone effect (e.g., large amounts of black licorice, cirrhosis, chronic heart failure, primary hyperaldosteronism)
- High levels of glucocorticoids (e.g., corticosteroid therapy, Cushing's disease)

Rapid K⁺ Shift from ECF into Cells
- Alkalosis, excessive beta-adrenergic stimulation, or excessive insulin

Hyperkalemia (Plasma K⁺ Excess)
Output Less than Excessive or Too Rapid K⁺ Intake
- IV K⁺ infusion with excess rate or amount
- Massive transfusion (>8 units) of stored blood

Decreased Output Not Balanced by Decreased K⁺ Intake
- Oliguria (e.g., severe hypovolemia, circulatory shock, acute kidney injury, end-stage renal disease)
- Use of K⁺-sparing diuretics, angiotensin-converting enzyme (ACE) inhibitors, or other drugs that decrease renal K⁺ excretion
- Lack of aldosterone (e.g., adrenal insufficiency, Addison's disease)

Rapid K⁺ Shift from Cells into ECF
- Lack of insulin or acidosis due to mineral acids
- Massive sudden cell death (e.g., crushing injuries, tumor lysis syndrome)

Hypocalcemia (Plasma Ca⁺⁺ Deficit)
Normal Output but Deficient Ca⁺⁺ Intake or Absorption
- Diet lacking Ca⁺⁺-rich foods
- Poor Ca⁺⁺ absorption (e.g., chronic diarrhea, lack of vitamin D)

Increased Output Not Balanced by Increased Ca⁺⁺ Intake and Absorption
- Steatorrhea (binds Ca⁺⁺ in GI secretions as well as dietary Ca⁺⁺)

Ca⁺⁺ Shift from ECF into Bone or Physiologically Unavailable Form
- Hypoparathyroidism
- Large load of citrate from massive blood transfusion (binds Ca⁺⁺)

Continued

BOX 7-1   CAUSES OF DISRUPTED FLUID AND ELECTROLYTE BALANCE—cont'd

- Alkalosis (more Ca^{++} binds albumin) or elevated plasma phosphate level
- Acute pancreatitis (Ca^{++} binds necrotic fat in abdomen)

Hypercalcemia (Plasma Ca^{++} Excess)
Output Less than Excessive Ca^{++} Intake and Absorption
- Vitamin D or Ca^{++} overdose (includes shark cartilage supplements)

Decreased Output Not Balanced by Decreased Ca^{++} Intake
- Use of thiazide diuretics

Ca^{++} Shift from Bone into ECF
- Hyperparathyroidism
- Cancers that secrete bone-resorbing factors

Hypomagnesemia (Plasma Mg^{++} Deficit)
Normal Output but Deficient Mg^{++} Intake or Absorption
- Diet lacking Mg^{++}-rich foods
- Poor Mg^{++} absorption (e.g., chronic diarrhea, ileal resection, chronic alcoholism)

Increased Output Not Balanced by Increased Mg^{++} Intake and Absorption
- Prolonged vomiting, gastric suction, or draining GI fistula
- Steatorrhea (binds Mg^{++} in GI secretions as well as dietary Mg^{++})
- Use of diuretics or other drugs that increase urinary Mg^{++}

Mg^{++} Shift into Physiologically Unavailable Form
- Large load of citrate from massive blood transfusion (binds Mg^{++})
- Alkalosis (more Mg^{++} binds albumin)

Hypermagnesemia (Plasma Mg^{++} Excess)
Output Less than Excessive Mg^{++} Intake and Absorption
- Overuse of Mg^{++}-containing laxatives or antacids

Decreased Output Not Balanced by Decreased Mg^{++} Intake
- Chronic oliguric renal disease

ECV excess (Na^+-containing fluid) or hyperkalemia (K^+-containing fluid).[5,6,8]

Altered Fluid and Electrolyte Distribution

Alterations of distribution, the process of moving fluid and electrolytes between their various compartments, can create a fluid imbalance and two types of electrolyte imbalances (Figure 7-2, *D*):
- Rapid shift of ECF into a "third space" can create ECV deficit.
- Electrolyte shift from ECF into its electrolyte pool causes plasma electrolyte deficits.
- Electrolyte shift from its electrolyte pool into ECF causes plasma electrolyte excesses.

Rapid ECF Shift into "Third Space"

The term "third space" refers to a location where ECF accumulates abnormally (becomes misplaced) that is neither the vascular nor the interstitial compartment. The peritoneal cavity is an example of a third space. ECF accumulating in the peritoneal cavity creates ascites. Rapid shift of ECF into a third space can cause ECV deficit. If the shift occurs gradually, there is time for the ECV to be replenished without causing symptomatic ECV deficit.

Electrolyte Shift from ECF into Its Electrolyte Pool

The electrolytes K^+, Ca^{++}, and Mg^{++} have low concentrations in the ECF and high concentrations in other locations, such as inside cells or in bone, that are called electrolyte pools. Many factors influence distribution of these electrolytes between the ECF and their electrolyte pools, with some factors moving electrolytes from the ECF into their pools and others moving them in the opposite direction. Abnormal concentrations of these factors that shift electrolytes into their pools can cause

plasma electrolyte deficits.[6] See hypokalemia, hypocalcemia, and hypomagnesemia in Box 7-1 for specific examples.

Electrolyte Shift from Its Electrolyte Pool into ECF

The factors that distribute electrolytes between the ECF and electrolyte pools can be altered in a way that shifts electrolytes from their pools into the ECF, causing plasma electrolyte excesses.[6] See hyperkalemia and hypercalcemia in Box 7-1 for specific examples.

PHYSIOLOGIC PROCESSES AND CONSEQUENCES

Understanding the physiologic processes of fluid and electrolyte balance provides the foundation for understanding the consequences of disrupting them.

Physiologic Processes of Fluid and Electrolyte Balance

The three physiologic processes whose interplay creates fluid and electrolyte balance were defined at the beginning of this concept: fluid and electrolyte intake and absorption; fluid and electrolyte distribution; and fluid and electrolyte output. This discussion describes these processes in more detail.

Fluid and Electrolyte Intake and Absorption

The most common route of fluid and electrolyte intake is oral. Other routes include IV administration and less common avenues such as insertion into the rectum, introduction through nasogastric or other tubes into the gastrointestinal tract, instillation into body cavities, and infusion into subcutaneous tissues (hypodermoclysis)[11,12] or bone marrow (intraosseous).[13] The amount and type of intake can be manipulated deliberately to maintain fluid and electrolyte balance. Habit and thirst are the strongest influences on oral fluid intake.[14,15] The most important stimulus to thirst is increased osmolality of body fluids, although angiotensin II and arterial baroreceptor stimulation during severe hypovolemia also trigger thirst.[16,17] The thirst sensation is blunted in older adults.[15]

Fluid and electrolytes that enter the body by all routes except intravenous (IV) must be absorbed. IV fluid and electrolytes do not need absorption because they enter the bloodstream directly. Absorption is especially important to consider for oral intake of the electrolytes Ca^{++} and Mg^{++}, which have specialized absorption mechanisms in the intestines. Ca^{++} absorption in the duodenum, its most important absorptive site, is dependent on adequate availability of vitamin D.[1] Having a healthy intestinal epithelium in the terminal section of the ileum is necessary for Mg^{++} absorption. If fluid and electrolytes are not absorbed, they remain in the gastrointestinal (GI) tract and leave the body in the feces.

Fluid and Electrolyte Distribution

After fluid and electrolytes enter the blood, they are distributed to various body compartments. Normal fluid and electrolyte distribution is necessary for optimal function. The process of filtration distributes the ECF between the two major extracellular compartments: vascular and interstitial. The process of osmosis distributes water between ECF and cells because of osmotic forces. Numerous factors distribute electrolytes between the ECF and electrolyte pools.[6]

Fluid distribution between vascular and interstitial compartments. Fluid distribution between the vascular and interstitial compartments occurs by *filtration,* the net result of simultaneous opposing forces at the capillary level. Two forces tend to move fluid out of capillaries and two other forces tend to move fluid into capillaries.[3] The forces that are stronger at any particular time determine which way the fluid moves. *Hydrostatic pressure* pushes fluid out of its compartment. Capillary blood hydrostatic pressure (a relatively strong force) pushes fluid out of the capillaries; interstitial fluid hydrostatic pressure (a relatively weak force) pushes fluid out of the interstitial compartment back into capillaries. *Colloid osmotic pressure,* caused by large protein particles in the fluid, pulls fluid into its compartment. Thus, capillary blood colloid osmotic pressure (normally a relatively strong force) pulls fluid into the capillaries; interstitial fluid colloid osmotic pressure (normally a very weak force) pulls fluid out of the capillaries into the interstitial compartment. With normal fluid distribution, the net result of these opposing forces filters some of the ECF from capillaries into the interstitial compartment at the arterial end of capillaries, bringing oxygen and nutrients to cells. At the venous end of the capillary, some interstitial fluid filters back into the capillary, carrying waste products to be excreted.

Changes in the forces that cause too much fluid to filter into the interstitial compartment create too much interstitial fluid, which is called *edema.* ECV excess causes edema by increasing capillary blood hydrostatic pressure. Other causes of edema, such as inflammation and hypoalbuminemia, alter the four opposing forces in other ways.

Water distribution between ECF and intracellular fluid. The structure of cell membranes allows water to cross the membrane readily but Na^+ enters with difficulty. This is the reason that cell membranes are called *semipermeable.* The process of *osmosis* is movement of water across a semipermeable membrane that separates compartments with different concentrations of particles. As noted previously, the osmolality of a fluid is its degree of concentration. Technically, it is the number of particles per kilogram of water.[3] Osmosis occurs almost instantaneously when the osmolality changes on one side of the semipermeable cell membrane. This rapid equilibration keeps the ECF and intracellular fluid at the same osmolality.

If the ECF becomes too concentrated (hypernatremia), as from increased water output that is not replaced by intake, it has increased osmolality. Osmosis pulls water rapidly from cells, causing them to shrivel. The shriveling of brain cells causes the nonspecific signs of impaired cerebral function seen with hypernatremia. Conversely, if the ECF becomes too dilute (hyponatremia), as from excessive water intake that is not removed by output, it has decreased osmolality. Water moves rapidly into cells, causing them to swell. Swollen brain cells also cause impaired cerebral function, the basis of the signs and symptoms of hyponatremia.[3]

Electrolyte distribution. With the exception of Na^+, which has a high ECF concentration that reflects osmolality, electrolytes have low concentrations in the ECF compared to their concentrations in electrolyte pools.[5] The K^+ pool is inside cells, where its concentration is 30 times higher than that in the ECF.[18] Bone is an important Ca^{++} pool. Mg^{++} pools include inside cells and bones. Physiologically inactive forms of Ca^{++} and Mg^{++} bound to albumin or organic anions such as citrate also can be considered electrolyte pools.

Numerous opposing factors influence distribution of electrolytes between the ECF and the electrolyte pools. For example, two hormones influence Ca^{++} distribution: parathyroid hormone (PTH) from the parathyroid glands and calcitonin from the thyroid.[1] Calcitonin moves Ca^{++} into bone; PTH shifts Ca^{++} from bone into the ECF.[19] Unusual amounts of factors that shift electrolytes can alter their distribution and cause plasma electrolyte deficits or excesses. Box 7-1 lists specific examples under the electrolyte imbalances. Although these distribution shifts may not change whole body electrolyte concentration, they cause signs and symptoms by changing the ratio of electrolytes inside and outside cells or the amount of physiologically active electrolyte.[20]

Fluid and Electrolyte Output

The normal excretory routes of fluid and electrolyte output are urine, feces, through the skin, and respiration. Some of the normal routes of fluid and electrolyte output are regulated physiologically to maintain optimal balance, but those regulatory mechanisms can be overwhelmed. The regulated routes are urine, sweat, and, to some degree, feces. Other output routes, including insensible water exiting through skin and lungs, are mandatory, regardless of fluid balance.[5] Abnormal routes of fluid and electrolyte output include emesis, hemorrhage, drainage through tubes or fistulas, and other routes of fluid and electrolyte loss often seen in clinical situations.[6] These abnormal output routes do not have physiologic regulatory mechanisms.

Renal excretion provides the largest output of fluid and electrolytes in normal circumstances. The hormones aldosterone and natriuretic peptides (not discussed in this concept analysis) regulate renal excretion of Na^+ and water (isotonic fluid), whereas antidiuretic hormone (ADH) regulates excretion of water.[9] Aldosterone increases renal excretion of K^+ directly and probably Mg^{++} indirectly.

Aldosterone. The adrenal cortex secretes aldosterone in response to angiotensin II, one of the components of the renin-angiotensin system. When the ECV is low, the resulting decreased blood flow through the renal arteries increases release of renin, formation of angiotensin I, and then formation of angiotensin II, thus increasing secretion of aldosterone. Aldosterone acts on the kidneys to remove Na^+ and water from the renal tubules and return it to the blood, which expands the ECV.[1] This mechanism restores ECV to normal. However, other stimuli can increase renin release, such as decreased cardiac output from heart failure. The resulting elevated aldosterone secretion can cause ECV excess by retaining excessive amounts of Na^+ and water. The liver cells normally metabolize aldosterone, which stops its action. Decreased renin release or damage to the adrenal cortex will decrease aldosterone secretion, thus increasing renal Na^+ and water excretion. Aldosterone is the major hormonal regulator of ECV.[1]

Aldosterone also facilitates renal excretion of K^+. Increased concentration of plasma K^+ stimulates aldosterone secretion, which causes the kidneys to excrete more K^+ and helps return plasma K^+ concentration to normal. If plasma K^+ concentration decreases, aldosterone secretion is suppressed and the kidneys excrete less potassium. Another influence on renal excretion of K^+ is the amount of flow in the distal nephrons where K^+ is secreted into renal tubular fluid. More flow in the distal nephrons increases K^+ output in urine.[3,21] This situation is clinically important with osmotic diuresis and with use of potassium-wasting diuretics, both of which can cause hypokalemia.

Cortisol and other glucocorticoids have some aldosterone-like action on the kidneys. Conditions that cause deficient or excessive secretion of aldosterone or cortisol cause ECV imbalances and may cause plasma K^+ concentration imbalances as well.[3]

Antidiuretic hormone (ADH). ADH regulates renal excretion of water but not Na^+. Its name describes its action on the kidneys; the antidiuretic effect removes water from the renal distal tubules and collecting ducts and returns it to the blood, which dilutes the ECV and other body fluids. The posterior pituitary normally releases ADH at a level that maintains osmolality (degree of concentration) within normal limits. When body fluids become too concentrated (osmolality too high), osmosensitive cells in the hypothalamus trigger more release of ADH from the posterior pituitary. Increased renal action of ADH retains more water and dilutes body fluids back to their normal osmolality.[1,22] On the other hand,

when body fluids become too dilute (osmolality too low), the osmosensitive cells in the hypothalamus suppress release of ADH from the posterior pituitary. Less ADH action on the kidneys allows more water excretion in the urine and concentrates body fluids back to their normal osmolality. The serum Na^+ concentration usually reflects the osmolality of body fluids. Conditions that cause excessive or deficient ADH release cause plasma Na^+ concentration imbalances.[3,23]

Physiologic Consequences of Disrupted Fluid and Electrolyte Balance

Disruptions of fluid and electrolyte balance have different physiologic consequences, depending on the type of imbalance. ECV and K^+, Mg^{++}, and Ca^{++} concentration imbalances can interfere with perfusion and oxygenation. Osmolality imbalances impair cerebral function. K^+, Mg^{++}, and Ca^{++} concentration imbalances impair neuromuscular function.[6]

Impaired Perfusion and Oxygenation

A normal volume of ECF is necessary to provide tissue perfusion and oxygenate cells. Moderate or severe ECV deficit reduces tissue perfusion by decreasing arterial blood pressure (BP). Very severe ECV deficit leads to hypovolemic shock, a condition that severely impairs perfusion and oxygenation.[24] ECV excess also can impair oxygenation. Edema fluid from ECV excess pushes cells farther from capillaries, creating a larger distance for oxygen to diffuse before it reaches cells. This subtle change is part of the reason for delayed healing of injuries to edematous tissue. A more dramatic example of impaired oxygenation from ECV excess is pulmonary edema that arises from sudden or very severe ECV excess.[24,25] Fluid in the alveoli interferes with gas exchange and thus oxygenation.

K^+, Mg^{++}, and Ca^{++} concentration imbalances can cause cardiac dysrhythmias, some of which can impair perfusion by reducing cardiac output.[24,26,27] Severe hyperkalemia causes cardiac arrest.

Impaired Cerebral Function

The previous discussion of distribution of water between ECF and intracellular fluid explained that osmolality imbalances cause shriveling (hypernatremia) or swelling (hyponatremia) of cells. Impaired cerebral function occurs with either condition.[3] The usual cerebral impairment with osmolality imbalances is decreased level of consciousness (LOC), which occurs on a continuum from drowsiness to coma. Seizures may occur if the osmolality changes very rapidly, rises very high, or falls very low.[28] The brain cell dysfunction caused by osmolality imbalances is reversible with well-managed return of osmolality to normal, avoiding rapid changes that can injure fragile brain structures.[29]

Impaired Neuromuscular Function

Plasma concentration imbalances of K^+, Ca^{++}, and Mg^{++} impair neuromuscular function, although they impair it in different ways. The ratio of K^+ inside to outside cells is a major determinant of resting membrane potential of muscle cells.[3] Plasma K^+ deficit and excess change the resting membrane potential of skeletal muscle by altering that ratio. Although the state of the resting potential is different in hypokalemia and hyperkalemia, the effect on skeletal muscles is similar: flaccid muscle weakness.[3,8]

Extracellular Ca^{++} concentration is a major determinant of the speed of ion fluxes through the membranes of nerve and muscle cells. Mg^{++} suppresses release of the neurotransmitter acetylcholine at neuromuscular junctions. Plasma concentration imbalances of Ca^{++} and Mg^{++} impair neuromuscular function by altering these processes. Plasma deficits of Ca^{++} and Mg^{++} increase neuromuscular excitability, which is why hypocalcemia and hypomagnesemia have similar signs and symptoms: muscle twitching and cramping, hyperactive reflexes, and seizures if very severe. In contrast, plasma excesses of Ca^{++} and Mg^{++} decrease neuromuscular excitability, causing similar manifestations of muscle weakness, depressed reflexes, and lethargy.[6]

ASSESSMENT

Assessments for fluid and electrolyte imbalances often occur in the context of other conditions that cause such imbalances. Nurses can use the risk factors for these imbalances to guide their assessment.

History

Because many of the presenting signs and symptoms of fluid and electrolyte imbalances have other causes, taking a careful history is important. The standard questions for history taking will not be repeated here, but are expected. In addition to focus on the renal, endocrine, or other conditions that may cause the fluid or electrolyte imbalance, the history must include questions regarding fluid and electrolyte intake and output. Recent vomiting or diarrhea should be explored as to frequency and quantity, as well as the type and quantity of water, Na^+, and K^+ replacement. Medication history, including dietary supplements, is an important focus because numerous medications influence fluid and electrolyte balance.[3,6,8]

Examination Findings

Clinical manifestations of fluid and electrolyte imbalances often are part of a larger clinical picture of the underlying disease process that caused the imbalance. For example,

the ankle edema, bounding pulse, and distended neck veins caused by ECV excess in individuals who have left-sided heart failure will be noted as part of the wider cardiac, respiratory, and functional examination. However, the quadriceps muscle weakness and constipation of hypokalemia in these individuals may escape detection until the manifestations become severe, unless they are assessed specifically.

Astute clinicians incorporate assessment for the individual's most likely fluid and electrolyte imbalances into every physical assessment, rather than waiting until the signs and symptoms become severe. For example, a person who has chronic diarrhea needs assessment for ECV deficit, hypernatremia, hypokalemia, hypocalcemia, and hypomagnesemia in addition to assessments related to the cause of the diarrhea and its consequences on skin integrity.[6]

Tables 7-1 and 7-2 present signs and symptoms of fluid and electrolyte imbalances. These manifestations arise from the physiologic consequences described earlier in this concept analysis. Interpretation of assessment findings may be complicated by the presence of acid-base imbalances (see Acid-Base Concept).

Diagnostic Tests

Diagnosis of ECV deficit and excess usually is made on the basis of history and clinical examination. Laboratory tests performed on blood samples provide the definitive diagnosis for osmolality and electrolyte imbalances. Normal ranges are provided in Tables 7-1 and 7-2.

CLINICAL MANAGEMENT

Primary and secondary prevention strategies as well as interventions for people who have fluid and electrolyte imbalances occur in all clinical settings.

Primary Prevention

Primary prevention of fluid and electrolyte imbalances is based on the principle that intake must balance output to maintain optimal fluid and electrolyte balance. For example, teaching people to replace body fluid output from vomiting or diarrhea with Na^+-containing fluid can prevent ECV deficit. Similarly, teaching individuals who take potassium-wasting diuretics how to increase their dietary K^+ intake and

TABLE 7-1	CLINICAL MANIFESTATIONS OF DISRUPTED FLUID BALANCE		
EXTRACELLULAR VOLUME IMBALANCE		**OSMOLALITY IMBALANCE**	
TOO LITTLE VOLUME (ECV DEFICIT)	**TOO MUCH VOLUME (ECV EXCESS)**	**TOO DILUTE (HYPONATREMIA)**	**TOO CONCENTRATED (HYPERNATREMIA)**
Sudden weight loss, skin tenting, dry mucous membranes, vascular underload: rapid thready pulse, postural BP drop, lightheadedness, flat neck veins when supine, oliguria, syncope, shock if severe	Sudden weight gain, dependent edema, vascular overload: bounding pulse, distended neck veins when upright, dyspnea, pulmonary edema if severe	Impaired cerebral function: decreased LOC, nausea, seizures if severe; serum Na^+ <130 mEq/L	Impaired cerebral function: decreased LOC, thirst (not older adults), seizures if severe; serum Na^+ >145 mEq/L

the importance of taking prescribed K^+ supplements helps prevent hypokalemia. Teaching for people who have oliguric renal disease focuses on decreasing their intake of Na^+, K^+, and Mg^{++} because their output is decreased.[5]

In addition to teaching people how to maintain optimal fluid and electrolyte balance, nurses engage in primary prevention in clinical settings when they see risk factors for various imbalances and intervene to modify intake or output appropriately. For example, nurses provide accessible fluids at a patient's preferred temperature as an independent nursing intervention; they request an order for an antiemetic or antidiarrheal medication as a collaborative intervention.

Secondary Prevention (Screening)

Screening to detect disrupted fluid and electrolyte balance is not performed in the general population except as part of a routine physical exam that would include assessment for physical signs of ECV excess or deficit and standard laboratory tests including measurement of serum Na^+, K^+, and Ca^{++} levels.

Collaborative Interventions

Because fluid and electrolyte intake is easier to modify than output, interventions to restore optimal fluid and electrolyte balance often focus on intake.

Fluid and Electrolyte Support

ECV deficit, hypernatremia, and plasma electrolyte deficits are treated by fluid or electrolyte replacement and by treatment of any underlying cause. ECV deficit requires isotonic Na^+-containing fluid; hypernatremia requires water; electrolyte deficit usually requires replacement of the deficient electrolyte.[3,8] A person who has clinical dehydration will need both isotonic Na^+-containing fluid and extra water. These fluids and electrolytes can be administered orally, by IV infusion, or through other routes, depending on patient status and the resources of the setting. Nursing responsibilities during fluid and electrolyte replacement include safely administering the replacement, measuring fluid intake and

output, monitoring for complications of therapy, and teaching patients and families regarding the therapy.

Treatments for ECV excess, hyponatremia, and plasma electrolyte excesses usually involve some type of restriction: Na^+ restriction for ECV excess, water restriction for hyponatremia, and decreased intake of the electrolyte that is excessive.[3,8,30] Nurses need to be sure that people know the reason for the restriction and receive culturally appropriate teaching regarding how to change their diet or fluid intake. In addition to the appropriate restrictions, medications may be used to treat ECV excess, hyponatremia, and plasma electrolyte excesses.

Medication Management

In addition to the fluid and electrolyte replacements mentioned earlier, people who have disrupted fluid and electrolyte balance may receive other medications. Depending on the situation, these medications are directed toward various goals: treat the underlying cause (e.g., antiemetic for imbalances due to vomiting or vasopressin for ADH deficiency); increase the output of fluid or electrolytes (e.g., diuretics for ECV excess or severe hyperkalemia); shift electrolytes into their pools to decrease plasma concentration (e.g., insulin and glucose for acute hyperkalemia or calcitonin for acute hypercalcemia)[31]; or counteract life-threatening effects of the imbalance (e.g., calcium salts to counteract the effect of hyperkalemia on cardiac function).[31,32] In addition, medications that can contribute to the individual's fluid and electrolyte imbalances must be discontinued or their dosage should be modified.

Independent Nursing Interventions

Independent nursing interventions to provide safety and comfort are foundational for people who have fluid and electrolyte imbalances. For example, safety is high priority for patients with decreased level of consciousness from osmolality imbalances or substantial muscle weakness from severe hypokalemia. Comfort measures are especially important for people who need to restrict fluid or Na^+. People who have fluid restrictions

TABLE 7-2	CLINICAL MANIFESTATIONS OF DISRUPTED ELECTROLYTE BALANCE				
PLASMA K^+ IMBALANCES		**PLASMA Ca^{++} IMBALANCES**		**PLASMA Mg^{++} IMBALANCES**	
HYPOKALEMIA	**HYPERKALEMIA**	**HYPOCALCEMIA**	**HYPERCALCEMIA**	**HYPOMAGNESEMIA**	**HYPERMAGNESEMIA**
Bilateral ascending flaccid muscle weakness, abdominal distention, constipation, postural hypotension, polyuria, cardiac dysrhythmias; serum K^+ <3.5 mEq/L	Bilateral ascending flaccid muscle weakness, cardiac dysrhythmias, cardiac arrest if severe; serum K^+ >5.0 mEq/L	Increased neuromuscular excitability: positive Chvostek's and Trousseau's signs, muscle cramps, twitching, hyperactive reflexes, carpal and pedal spasms, tetany, seizures, laryngospasm, cardiac dysrhythmias; serum total Ca^{++} <9 mg/dL (4.5 mEq/L)	Decreased neuromuscular excitability: anorexia, nausea, constipation, muscle weakness, diminished reflexes, decreased LOC, cardiac dysrhythmias; serum total Ca^{++} >11 mg/dL (5.5 mEq/L)	Increased neuromuscular excitability: positive Chvostek's and Trousseau's signs, insomnia, hyperactive reflexes, muscle cramps and twitching, nystagmus, tetany, seizures, cardiac dysrhythmias; serum Mg^{++} <1.5 mEq/L	Decreased neuromuscular excitability: flushing, diaphoresis, diminished reflexes, hypotension, decreased LOC, muscle weakness, respiratory depression, bradycardia, cardiac dysrhythmias; serum Mg^{++} >2.5 mEq/L

frequently are uncomfortable from thirst. Interventions such as performing frequent oral hygiene, lubricating the lips, keeping fluids out of sight, providing the allowed liquids in insulated containers, and instructing people to swish fluids in their mouths before swallowing promote comfort during fluid restriction. Individuals who need to restrict Na^+ intake because of chronic ECV excess can be comforted with the knowledge that salt taste often changes after a few weeks of salt restriction, so that the food that seems tasteless at first probably will have enjoyable flavor in a few weeks. Assistance with learning about herbs and spices also is useful for these individuals.

Nurses use many different interventions to facilitate oral intake of Na^+-containing fluid for people who have mild ECV

deficit or oral water intake for people with mild hypernatremia. For example, they can make fluids available frequently, provide them at the individual's preferred temperature, and assist individuals to keep their own intake records. Increased fluid intake also is important for individuals with hypercalcemia to prevent renal damage. Teaching people how to prevent fluid and electrolyte imbalances in the future by balancing output with appropriate intake is extremely important. Box 7-2 summarizes nursing interventions for people with disrupted fluid and electrolyte balance.

INTERRELATED CONCEPTS

The concept fluid and electrolyte balance has many interrelationships with other concepts discussed in this book. Fluid and electrolyte balance and **Acid-base balance** are closely related; changes in one of them can cause changes in the other and situations such as vomiting and diarrhea can lead to both. **Nutrition** greatly influences fluid and electrolyte intake. **Elimination** creates fluid and electrolyte output; elimination alterations such as oliguria and diarrhea can disrupt fluid and electrolyte balance. Fluid and electrolyte imbalances can influence **Perfusion** and **Gas exchange** (ECV imbalances), **Cognition** (osmolality imbalances), and **Mobility** (electrolyte imbalances that cause muscle weakness). These interrelationships are illustrated in Figure 7-3.

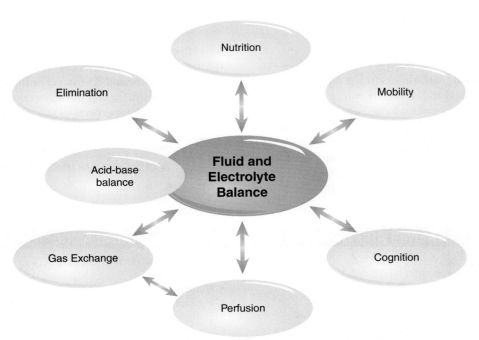

FIGURE 7-3 Fluid and Electrolyte Balance and Interrelated Concepts.

MODEL CASE

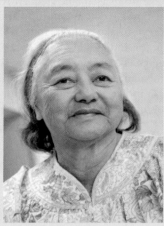

Mrs. Malone, age 83, lives in an apartment with her cat. She has hypertension, hyperlipidemia, and chronic left-sided heart failure, which are managed with the diuretic furosemide, KCl, several other medications, and dietary Na^+ restriction. Mrs. Malone volunteers at a nearby elementary school, where earlier in the week several students were sent home sick after vomiting. Mrs. Malone developed vomiting and diarrhea. Although the vomiting stopped, the diarrhea persisted. She drank more water than usual, ate rice and dry toast, and stopped taking her KCl to avoid upsetting her stomach. After 2 days of diarrhea, Mrs. Malone became lightheaded when she got out of bed and had difficulty standing up after using the toilet because her legs were so weak. She telephoned her nurse practitioner (NP), who advised her to drink some broth with salt in it as well as some orange juice. Mrs. Malone needed considerable teaching regarding the importance of Na^+ intake to replace her increased Na^+ output in diarrhea, but eventually she did agree to try the rehydration schedule her NP advised. After checking back by telephone later in the day and learning that Mrs. Malone was no longer lightheaded but still had "weak legs," the NP advised Mrs. Malone to restart her KCl, continue drinking orange juice, and make an appointment to have her plasma K^+ concentration checked.

Case Analysis

Mrs. Malone had chronic heart failure. Her reduced cardiac output and other mechanisms of heart failure increased activation of her renin-angiotensin-aldosterone system, causing more renal retention of Na^+ and water and creating chronic ECV excess. To counteract her decreased Na^+ and water output, she used the prescribed furosemide, a K^+-wasting diuretic that increases Na^+ and water output. Because this diuretic also increases K^+ output, Mrs. Malone also took KCl to increase her K^+ intake. She adhered to her Na^+-restricted diet because she had learned that Na^+ kept water in her body and "made her ankles swell more" (her understanding of ECV excess). When Mrs. Malone developed increased Na^+, water, and K^+ output from vomiting and diarrhea, her intake did not increase appropriately, so she developed ECV deficit (lightheaded upon standing) and hypokalemia (bilateral quadriceps weakness). Learning about the vomiting and diarrhea, her NP asked appropriate assessment questions over the telephone to elicit these symptoms and planned appropriate fluid and electrolyte replacement therapy. The NP taught Mrs. Malone the reason for the temporarily increased Na^+ intake, even though she usually followed a Na^+-restricted diet, and asked Mrs. Malone to make a follow-up appointment.

EXEMPLARS

An exemplar of optimal fluid and electrolyte balance is a person of any age whose fluid and electrolyte output is balanced by appropriate type and amount of intake and whose fluid and electrolyte distributions are normal. This person has ECV, osmolality, and plasma electrolyte values within the normal range.

Box 7-3 lists exemplars of disrupted fluid and electrolyte balance. Using the general individual risk factors presented earlier in this concept, nurses can understand the risk factors for each exemplar. For example, hypokalemia can occur from normal output but deficient K^+ intake, increased output not balanced by increased K^+ intake, or rapid K^+ shift from ECF into cells. Specific causes of each exemplar are organized in Box 7-1 under these general individual risk factors.

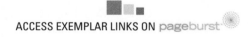

ACCESS EXEMPLAR LINKS ON pageburst

BOX 7-3 EXEMPLARS OF FLUID AND ELECTROLYTE IMBALANCE

Fluid Imbalances
- Extracellular fluid volume deficit (ECV deficit)
- ECV excess
- Hypernatremia (increased osmolality)
- Hyponatremia (decreased osmolality; water intoxication)
- Dehydration (ECV deficit plus hypernatremia)

Electrolyte Imbalances
- Hypokalemia
- Hyperkalemia
- Hypocalcemia
- Hypercalcemia
- Hypomagnesemia
- Hypermagnesemia

REFERENCES

1. Hall JE: *Guyton and Hall textbook of medical physiology*, ed 12, Philadelphia, 2011, Saunders/Elsevier.
2. Caon M: Osmoles, osmolality and osmotic pressure: clarifying the puzzle of solution concentration, *Contemp Nurs* 29(1):92, 2008.
3. Rose BD: *Clinical physiology of acid-base and electrolyte disorders*, ed 6, New York, 2011, McGraw-Hill.
4. Bryant H: Dehydration in older people: assessment and management, *Emerg Nurs* 15(4):22, 2007.
5. Metheney NM: *Fluid and electrolyte balance: nursing applications*, ed 5, Sudbury, Mass, 2012, Jones and Bartlett Learning.
6. Felver L: Fluid and electrolyte homeostasis and imbalances. In Copstead LC, Banasik JL: *Pathophysiology*, ed 4, St Louis, 2010, Saunders/Elsevier.
7. Kanda K, Nozu K, Kaito H, et al: The relationship between arginine vasopressin levels and hyponatremia following a percutaneous renal biopsy in children receiving hypotonic or isotonic intravenous fluids, *Pediatr Nephrol* 26:99, 2011.
8. Goldstein MB, et al: *Fluid, electrolyte and acid-base physiology: a problem-based approach*, ed 4, St Louis, 2010, Saunders/Elsevier.
9. Ali N, Imbriano LJ, Maesaka JK: A 66-year-old male with hyponatremia. Psychogenic polydipsia, *Kidney Int* 76:233, 2009.
10. Yalcin-Cakmakli G, Karli Oguz K, Shorbagi A, et al: Hyponatremic encephalopathy after excessive water ingestion prior to pelvic ultrasound: neuroimaging findings, *Intern Med* 49:1807, 2010.
11. Mongardon N, Le Manach Y, Tresallet C, et al: Subcutaneous hydration: a potentially hazardous route, *Eur J Anaesth* 25:771, 2008.
12. Pershad J: A systematic data review of the cost of rehydration therapy, *Appl Health Econ Health Policy* 8:203, 2010.
13. Rouhani S, Meloney L, Ahn R, et al: Alternative rehydration methods: a systematic review and lessons for resource-limited care, *Pediatrics* 127:e748, 2011.
14. Johnson A: Psychobiology of thirst and salt appetite, *Med Sci Sports Exercise* 39(8):1388, 2007.
15. Price KA: Hydration in cancer patients, *Curr Opin Suppor Palliative Care* 4:276, 2010.
16. Gerhardt RT, Shaffer BM, Dixon P, et al: Diagnostic and predictive values of thirst, angiotensin II, and vasopressin during trauma resuscitation, *Prehosp Emerg Care* 14:317, 2010.
17. Thornton SN: Thirst and hydration: physiology and consequences of dysfunction, *Physiol Beh* 100:15, 2010.
18. Unwin RJ, Luft FC, Shirley DG: Pathophysiology and management of hypokalemia: a clinical perspective, *Nature Rev Nephrol* 7(2):75, 2011.
19. Wu SD, Gao L: Is routine calcium supplementation necessary in patients undergoing total thyroidectomy plus neck dissection? *Surg Today* 41:183, 2011.
20. Ho KM, Leonard A: Risk factors and outcome associated with hypomagnesemia in massive transfusion, *Transfusion* 51:270, 2011.
21. Palmer BF: A physiologic-based approach to the evaluation of a patient with hypokalemia, *Am J Kidney Dis* 56:1184, 2010.
22. Liu J, Sharma N, Zheng W, et al: Sex differences in vasopressin V2 receptor expression and vasopressin-induced antidiuresis, *Am J Physiol Renal Physiol* 300:F433, 2011.
23. Shapiro DS, Sonnenblick M, Galperin I, et al: Severe hyponatraemia in elderly hospitalized patients: prevalence, aetiology and outcome, *Intern Med J* 40:574, 2010.
24. Felver L: *Cardiac nursing*, ed 6, Philadelphia, 2010, Lippincott.
25. Murray JF: Pulmonary edema: pathophysiology and diagnosis, *Int J Tuberculosis Lung Dis* 15:155, 2011.
26. Clausen T: Hormonal and pharmacological modification of plasma potassium homeostasis, *Fundamen Clin Pharmacol* 24:595, 2010.
27. Osadchii OE: Mechanisms of hypokalemia-induced ventricular arrhythmogenicity, *Fundamen Clin Pharmacol* 24:547, 2010.
28. Halawa I, Andersson T, Tomson T: Hyponatremia and risk of seizures: a retrospective cross-sectional study, *Epilepsia* 52:410, 2011.
29. Kaplan LJ, Kellum JA: Fluids, pH, ions and electrolytes, *Curr Opinion Crit Care* 16:323, 2010.
30. Wakil A, Atkin SL: Serum sodium disorders: safe management, *Clin Med* 10:79, 2010.
31. Mahoney BA, Smith WAD, Lo D, et al: Emergency interventions for hyperkalaemia, *Cochrane Database Syst Rev*, (Issue 2) Art. No, CD003235, 2005.
32. Shingarev R, Allon M: A physiologic-based approach to the treatment of acute hyperkalemia, *Am J Kidney Dis* 56:578, 2010.

Acid-Base Balance

Linda Felver

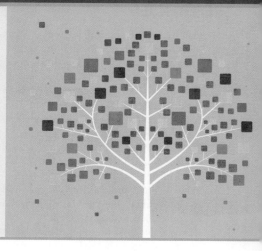

The human body requires precise control of multiple physiologic processes for optimal function. The concentration of hydrogen ions in body fluids influences cellular function and thus organ, system, and whole person function. An abnormal hydrogen ion concentration impairs cellular and organ function and can be fatal. The body maintains the hydrogen ion concentration within the normal range by continuously making adjustments through specific processes. Nurses providing care to acutely and chronically ill patients must understand these processes in order to optimize their function. This concept presents an analysis of acid-base balance, including the recognition and management of acid-base imbalances when they occur.

DEFINITION(S)

For the purposes of this concept analysis, acid-base balance is defined as *the process of regulating the pH, bicarbonate concentration, and partial pressure of carbon dioxide of body fluids.* The definitions of acid and base are the foundation for the concept of acid-base balance. An *acid* is a substance that releases hydrogen ions (H^+) and a *base* is a substance that takes up H^+. The most important base in the body is bicarbonate (HCO_3^-). The pH of a solution, technically defined later in this concept analysis, is a measure of its degree of acidity. A low pH means the solution is acidic; a high pH means it is basic (alkaline).

Acid-base balance is a dynamic interplay between three processes: acid production or intake, acid buffering, and acid excretion. *Acid production* is generation of acid through cellular metabolism. Our cells continuously generate two kinds of acid during metabolism: carbonic acid (H_2CO_3) and metabolic acids. Although the chemical structures of metabolic acids vary, both normal and abnormal types of cellular metabolism generate metabolic acids. Occasionally, *acid intake* occurs, which involves entry into the body of acids or substances that the body converts to acids (acid precursors). *Acid buffering* is a process by which body fluids resist large changes in pH when acids or bases are added or removed. Body fluids normally have buffers, which are pairs of chemicals that take up H^+ or release it to keep pH in the normal range. *Acid excretion* is removal of acid from the body. These concepts are described in greater detail later in this concept analysis.

Acid-base balance is described as a dynamic interplay because acid production is occurring constantly, the body fluids constantly have cellular acids added to them that must be buffered to preserve function, and the acid excretion mechanisms must function continuously to keep acids from accumulating in the body. Optimal acid-base balance keeps the pH of the blood and body fluids within the normal physiologic range (7.35 to 7.45).

SCOPE AND CATEGORIES

Scope

Considered conceptually, the scope of acid-base balance is on a continuum from acidotic (low pH) on one end, optimal balance (normal pH and other parameters) in the middle, and alkalotic (high pH) on the other end (Figure 8-1). These link to the three categories of acid-base balance: optimal acid-base balance and two types of disrupted acid-base balance: acidosis (too much acid) and alkalosis (too little acid). The term acid-base imbalance often is used to indicate disrupted acid-base balance.

Optimal Acid-Base Balance

When optimal acid-base balance is occurring, the buffers are not overwhelmed by the amount of acid that is generated and acid excretion keeps pace with acid production. The blood pH and other measures of acid-base status are in the normal range (7.35 to 7.45).

Acidosis (Too Much Acid)

In a situation of too much acid, the buffers have been overwhelmed and body fluids have too much acid. Acid excretion is not able to keep up with acid production or intake.

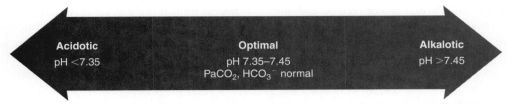

FIGURE 8-1 Scope of Concept. Acid-base balance ranges from optimal balance to acidotic and alkalotic imbalances.

Conditions of too much acid are called *acidosis* and are given an additional descriptor that explains whether there is too much carbonic acid or too much metabolic acid. Because the lungs excrete carbonic acid, the condition of too much carbonic acid is called *respiratory acidosis*. Similarly, because the kidneys excrete metabolic acid, the condition of too much metabolic acid is called *metabolic acidosis*. In some cases of metabolic acidosis, the base bicarbonate has been lost from the body, which causes relatively too much metabolic acid. In situations of too much acid, the pH is below the normal range (or in the low part of the normal range) and some other measures of acid-base status are abnormal. These laboratory values are explained in the Assessment section.

Alkalosis (Too Little Acid)

In situations of too little acid, the buffers also are not able to keep the pH in the normal range and body fluids do not have enough acid. Too much of the base bicarbonate has been added to the buffer system or acid excretion is greater than acid production. Conditions of too little acid are called *alkalosis,* either *respiratory alkalosis* when there is too little carbonic acid or *metabolic alkalosis* when there is too little metabolic acid. In these situations of too little acid, the pH is above the normal range (or in the high part of the normal range) and some other measures of acid-base status are abnormal. The Assessment section explains these measures.

RISK FACTORS

All individuals, regardless of race, culture, age, or socioeconomic status, need optimal acid-base balance for physiologic function. Acid-base imbalances usually occur as a consequence of another underlying condition. Nurses can deduce logically the risk factors for acid-base imbalance by considering the processes whose dynamic interplay creates acid-base balance. Those at greatest risk for acid-base imbalances are individuals who have at least one of these risk factors:

- Excessive production or intake of metabolic acid
- Altered acid buffering due to loss or gain of bicarbonate
- Altered acid excretion
- Abnormal shift of H$^+$ into cells

Excessive Production or Intake of Metabolic Acid

The cells are capable of making excessive amounts of metabolic acid that overwhelm the acid buffering and excretory capacities. A common clinical example of too much metabolic

acid due to acid production is diabetic ketoacidosis, in which abnormal cellular metabolism caused by lack of insulin produces ketoacids faster than the kidneys are able to excrete them.[1] Diabetic ketoacidosis is a type of metabolic acidosis. Other high-risk populations for ketoacidosis are people who do not have enough carbohydrate intake and people who abuse alcohol. In addition to production of excessive metabolic acid within the body, excessive intake of acid or acid precursors also causes metabolic acidosis. Although metabolic acidosis from intake of acid or acid precursors is less common, it is significant clinically in populations such as small children who accidentally ingest boric acid (intended for ant poisoning); individuals who overdose on aspirin (acetylsalicylic acid); or people who drink methanol or antifreeze (acid precursor).[2]

In summary, risk factors for excessive production or intake of metabolic acid include the risk factors for ketoacidosis or poisoning with acids or substances the body converts to acid. All of these situations place people at risk for metabolic acidosis. The cells cannot stop producing metabolic acid, so decreased acid production is not a risk factor.

Altered Acid Buffering Due to Loss or Gain of Bicarbonate

The base bicarbonate is a component of the major buffer system that buffers metabolic acids. It is possible to lose or gain bicarbonate and thus alter the buffering capacity. People who lose a lot of bicarbonate, such as through prolonged diarrhea, lose buffering capacity and have relatively too much metabolic acid. Thus bicarbonate loss causes metabolic acidosis.[3] Conversely, gaining a lot of bicarbonate, such as by ingesting baking soda (sodium bicarbonate) as an antacid or by receiving excessive intravenous (IV) sodium bicarbonate, alters the normal balance of buffer chemicals, which creates too little metabolic acid. Thus bicarbonate gain causes metabolic alkalosis.[4] In summary, risk factors for altered acid buffering include prolonged diarrhea[5] and excessive sodium bicarbonate intake in people of any age. These conditions place them at risk for metabolic acidosis or metabolic alkalosis.

Altered Acid Excretion

Cellular metabolism generates two types of acid that are excreted by two different organ systems. For this reason, altered acid excretion occurs in many disease processes that affect lung and kidney function. Carbonic acid excretion occurs by gas exchange in the lung alveoli followed by exhalation; thus it is possible to decrease or increase carbonic acid excretion. People at high risk for decreased carbonic acid excretion have acute or chronic respiratory diseases or other conditions that interfere with alveolar ventilation.[6] The cells continue producing carbonic acid, but the respiratory system is unable to excrete enough of it. The result is respiratory acidosis, too much carbonic acid. For example, people who have type B chronic obstructive pulmonary disease (COPD) (chronic bronchitis) have decreased carbonic acid excretion due to structural changes in their lungs and excessive mucus production that obstructs airflow. They develop chronic respiratory acidosis. So do people of any age who have severe acute respiratory conditions such as asthma or bacterial pneumonia. Infants and small children have increased risk of respiratory acidosis with acute conditions because their airways have such small diameters.

Although decreased carbonic acid secretion is the most common problem with carbonic acid secretion, it is possible to excrete excessive carbonic acid through hyperventilation.[7] This situation causes too little carbonic acid, creating respiratory alkalosis. High-risk populations for too little carbonic acid due to hyperventilation include people who are hypoxic, are experiencing acute pain, or are upset and anxious. These conditions that cause respiratory alkalosis tend to be more short term than many causes of respiratory acidosis.

Excretion of metabolic acid also may be altered, either decreased or increased. People who have prolonged oliguria for any reason cannot excrete enough of the metabolic acid that their cells continue to produce. Thus they develop metabolic acidosis. These high-risk populations include people of any age with acute or chronic oliguric renal disease[8] and those with circulatory shock. Infants have immature kidneys that are not yet fully effective in excreting metabolic acid; older adults often have reduced ability to excrete a metabolic acid load. These difficulties in excreting metabolic acid make them vulnerable to metabolic acidosis, especially in conjunction with increased acid production or intake.

Increased excretion of metabolic acid through the kidneys can occur in people with excessive aldosterone; however, the most common condition involving excessive removal of metabolic acid from the body is vomiting,[9] which removes hydrochloric acid. Vomiting also triggers bicarbonate retention by the kidneys, which alters buffering capacity and contributes to the resulting metabolic alkalosis.

In summary, risk factors for altered acid excretion include respiratory or other conditions that interfere with the ability to excrete enough carbonic acid; conditions causing hyperventilation that excretes too much carbonic acid; kidneys that are unable to excrete enough metabolic acid; and situations in which the kidneys or repeated episodes of vomiting remove too much metabolic acid from the body.

Abnormal Shift of H⁺ into Cells

Factors that shift substantial numbers of H^+ into cells can cause too little acid to be in the blood. The most common example in this category of risk factors is hypokalemia (abnormally low plasma potassium concentration).[1] When hypokalemia is present, some potassium ions (K^+) leave cells and hydrogen ions (H^+) enter cells to maintain a balance of electrical charge. The result is too little metabolic acid in the blood, known as metabolic alkalosis. The primary risk factor for abnormal shift of H^+ into cells is hypokalemia. Risk factors for hypokalemia are discussed in the Fluid and Electrolyte Balance concept.

PHYSIOLOGIC PROCESSES AND CONSEQUENCES

A firm grasp of the physiologic processes that comprise acid-base balance makes it possible to understand the consequences when these processes are disrupted.

Physiologic Processes of Acid-Base Balance

The processes whose dynamic interplay is involved in acid-base balance were defined at the beginning of this concept analysis. These processes are acid production, acid buffering, and acid excretion. This discussion explains their function in more detail. The process is illustrated in Figure 8-2.

Acid Production

As mentioned previously, cellular metabolism continuously generates carbonic acid and metabolic acids. Increased cellular metabolism produces more of these acids.

Carbonic acid production. Cellular metabolism generates carbonic acid (H_2CO_3) in the form of carbon dioxide (CO_2) and water (H_2O). The enzyme carbonic anhydrase in erythrocytes and other cells facilitates the conversion either way, depending on the location in the body. In the tissues, where CO_2 is abundant because it is being produced, the excess of CO_2 in the blood drives the equilibrium toward making H_2CO_3. H_2CO_3 is a weak acid, which means that it dissociates (separates into H^+ and HCO_3^-) only partially in solution.

$$CO_2 + H_2O \rightleftharpoons H_2CO_3 \rightleftharpoons H^+ + HCO_3^-$$

Bicarbonate in the blood is transported to the lung capillaries, where the CO_2 level is low because CO_2 diffuses into the alveoli and is exhaled. Carbonic anhydrase in the lungs converts H_2CO_3 back to CO_2 and H_2O, the form in which it is excreted through exhalation.

Metabolic acid production. Metabolic acid, the other type of acid produced by cellular metabolism, is a general term that includes all acids except carbonic acid. Examples of metabolic acid are citric acid, pyruvic acid, and lactic acid. Cells can produce abnormal metabolic acids, such as the ketoacid beta-hydroxybutyric acid, when cellular metabolism is disrupted or incomplete. The symbol that represents all metabolic acids is HA. The A indicates anion, which means negatively charged particle. Some, but not all, of these molecules dissociate into H^+ and A^-, because they are weak acids. Metabolic acid moves from the cells that produce it into the body fluids, where it is buffered before it reaches the kidneys where it is excreted.

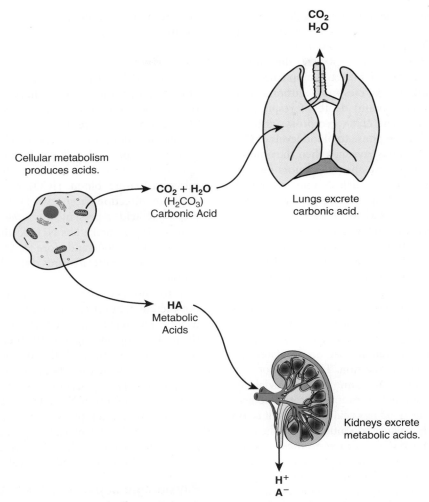

FIGURE 8-2 Acid Production and Excretion. (From Potter PA, Perry AG: *Fundamentals of nursing*, ed 8, St Louis, 2013, Mosby Elsevier.)

Acid Buffering

Buffers help keep the pH of the blood and other body fluids in the normal range in spite of the metabolic acid continuously produced by the cells. A buffer is a pair of chemicals, consisting of a weak acid and its base, that are in equilibrium in a solution. These two parts of a buffer system must be present in a specific ratio to keep the pH normal. The most important buffer in the extracellular fluid is the bicarbonate buffer system, which consists of carbonic acid (the weak acid) and bicarbonate (its base). When the bicarbonate:carbonic acid ratio is 20:1, the blood pH is in the normal range. If the ratio changes significantly, the blood pH becomes abnormal.

The bicarbonate buffer system buffers metabolic acid that is produced by cells or ingested. The bicarbonate portion of the buffer combines with the H^+ from the metabolic acid, to make carbonic acid:

$$H^+ + HCO_3^- \rightleftharpoons H_2CO_3$$

This process could decrease the available bicarbonate and increase the concentration of carbonic acid, but normally the 20:1 ratio of bicarbonate to carbonic acid is restored immediately because the lungs excrete the carbonic acid as carbon dioxide and water. Most of the function of bicarbonate buffers in normal physiology is buffering metabolic acid. They cannot buffer carbonic acid, because that is part of the buffer. If too much metabolic acid is present, the plasma bicarbonate concentration will decrease below its normal range because so much bicarbonate was used in buffering.

In abnormal circumstances in which there is too little metabolic acid present, the carbonic acid portion of the bicarbonate buffer system will release H^+. This process simultaneously raises the bicarbonate concentration and may restore the pH. However, if entirely too little metabolic acid is present, the plasma bicarbonate concentration will increase above its normal range. Thus the plasma bicarbonate concentration is an indicator of the metabolic acid status in the blood.

Acid Excretion

The two types of acid produced by cellular metabolism differ in that one is converted to gases and the other is not. The lungs excrete the gaseous form and the kidneys excrete the other acid.

Carbonic acid excretion. The lungs serve as the excretory organ for carbonic acid. The lungs are not able to excrete metabolic acid because it cannot be converted into a gaseous form. Changes in respiratory rate and depth alter the amount of carbonic acid that is excreted. Hyperventilation (increased rate and depth of respiration) excretes more carbonic acid; hypoventilation (decreased rate and depth of respiration) excretes less carbonic acid. The chemoreceptors influence respiratory rate and depth in response to blood levels of CO_2 and H^+ and, in some situations, oxygen. When the amount of CO_2 increases in the blood, the chemoreceptors increase the respiratory rate and depth,[10] which excretes more CO_2 and H_2O (carbonic acid) and helps restore the CO_2 level to its normal range. If the blood has too little CO_2, the chemoreceptors decrease the respiratory rate and depth, which enables CO_2 level to rise to its normal range because the cells constantly are producing it. These are examples of *correction:* fixing the problem and returning the blood values to their normal range.

Because chemoreceptors respond to H^+ concentration as well as to blood levels of CO_2, they modify respiratory rate and depth in response to the level of metabolic acid as well as carbonic acid. If too much metabolic acid accumulates, the chemoreceptors trigger hyperventilation. This does not correct the problem because the lungs cannot excrete metabolic acid, but increased respirations remove more carbonic acid from the body, making the blood less acidic. The result is too little carbonic acid to help balance too much metabolic acid. The technical term for this process is *compensation:* moving the pH toward its normal range while making other blood values abnormal. If too little metabolic acid is present, the chemoreceptors cause hypoventilation.[11] This compensatory process moves the pH down toward its normal range by allowing too much carbonic acid to help balance the too little metabolic acid.

Metabolic acid excretion. The kidneys excrete metabolic acid but are unable to excrete carbonic acid. They have several mechanisms for excreting metabolic acid. Glomerular filtrate that enters the renal tubules contains HCO_3^- from blood. Cells that line the renal proximal tubules perform chemical processes that essentially take H^+ from the blood and secrete it into renal tubular fluid while moving HCO_3^- the opposite direction, from the renal tubules into blood.[12] The $A-$ portion of metabolic acids enters renal tubular fluid in the proximal tubules as well.

Secretion of metabolic acid into the renal tubules adds free H^+ to the fluid, which potentially could damage renal cells. However, many of these H^+ combine with other molecules in the renal tubular fluid, and they no longer influence the pH. For example, renal tubular fluid contains buffers, especially phosphate buffers that were filtered at the glomerulus. Many of the secreted H^+ are buffered; buffered H^+ in urine are called *titratable acidity.*[1] Additional free H^+ bind to ammonia (NH_3) that renal tubular cells produce when additional metabolic acid needs to be excreted. The H^+ no longer are free but are part of ammonium ions (NH_4^+), which do not contribute to the pH. NH_4^+ ions do not return to the cells but remain in the renal tubular fluid and are excreted in the urine.

$$H^+ + NH_3 \rightleftharpoons NH_4^+$$

By adjusting their H^+ secretion rate and the amount of ammonia they make, the kidneys are able to excrete more or less metabolic acid, which assists in maintaining optimal acid-base balance. If too much metabolic acid is present in the blood, the kidneys increase their secretion of H^+ and make more NH_3. These mechanisms correct the problem by removing more HA from the blood and simultaneously increasing blood HCO_3^- concentration (moves the opposite direction from the H^+). Similarly, if too little metabolic acid is present, the kidneys decrease their secretion of H^+ and make less NH_3 so that more metabolic acid remains in the blood and more HCO_3^- is excreted in the urine. These corrective mechanisms normalize the pH by fixing the problem.

If too much carbonic acid accumulates, the kidneys cannot excrete it, but they can excrete more metabolic acid than usual.[13] This renal response to decreased pH compensates for the problem by causing too little metabolic acid in the blood, which somewhat balances the too much carbonic acid. Similarly, if the pH increases because there is too little carbonic acid, the renal compensatory response is less secretion of H^+ and less generation of NH_3. The resulting increase of metabolic acid is an attempt to balance the lack of carbonic acid, normalizing the pH by making other blood values abnormal. Table 8-1 summarizes the corrective and compensatory responses to disrupted acid-base balance.

Physiologic Consequences of Disrupted Acid-Base Balance

Acid-base imbalances trigger compensatory mechanisms, as described in the previous section. The time course of those mechanisms has important clinical implications. In addition to triggering compensatory mechanisms, pH changes impair cellular and organ function.

Time Course of Compensatory Mechanisms

Disruptions of acid-base balance cause the blood pH to move outside its normal range. In these situations, the buffers have been overwhelmed and the acid excretion mechanisms must work to keep pH from reaching the fatal limits. If the pH falls abnormally low from too much acid, both the lungs and the kidneys will excrete more acid, even though only one of these organs will be excreting the type of acid that is excessive. The other organ is compensating. Depending on the time course and the severity of the problem, the disruption may be uncompensated, partially compensated, or fully compensated.

As explained in the previous section, if a problem with the respiratory system disrupts acid-base balance and the lungs are unable to correct it, renal compensatory mechanisms adjust the pH toward normal. It takes several days for renal compensatory mechanisms to become clinically significant;[1,14] therefore a short-lived respiratory acidosis or

TABLE 8-1 **RESPIRATORY AND RENAL RESPONSES TO DISRUPTED ACID-BASE BALANCE**		
STIMULUS	**RESPIRATORY RESPONSE**	**RENAL RESPONSE**
Too much carbonic acid (respiratory acidosis)	*Cause:* Hypoventilation *Correction:* Hyperventilation	*Compensation:* Increased secretion of H^+ More NH_3 production
Too little carbonic acid (respiratory alkalosis)	*Cause:* Hyperventilation *Correction:* Hypoventilation	*Compensation:* Decreased secretion of H^+ Less NH_3 production
Too much metabolic acid (metabolic acidosis)	*Compensation:* Hyperventilation	*Cause:* More metabolic acid than kidneys can excrete *Correction:* Increased secretion of H^+ More NH_3 production
Too little metabolic acid (metabolic alkalosis)	*Compensation:* Hypoventilation	*Cause:* More bicarbonate than kidneys can excrete (too little metabolic acid) *Correction:* Decreased secretion of H^+ Less NH_3 production

alkalosis will not become compensated. Rapid treatment of an acute respiratory acidosis will correct the problem before renal compensation can occur. On the other hand, people who have chronic respiratory acidosis or an acute episode that lasts several days do develop some degree of renal compensation, either partial or full. Episodes of respiratory alkalosis occur from hyperventilation and usually do not last long enough for renal compensation to occur.

Analogously, if a problem with the kidneys disrupts acid-base balance and the kidneys are unable to correct it, respiratory compensatory mechanisms adjust the pH toward normal.[14] Respiratory compensation begins a few minutes after the pH becomes abnormal, so it is common to have some degree of compensation for a disruption of acid-base balance that involves too much or too little metabolic acid. When the disruption is severe, it will be only partially compensated.[15] In cases of metabolic alkalosis (too little metabolic acid), compensatory hypoventilation is limited by the respiratory drive for oxygen, so that full compensation usually does not occur. It is important to realize that even if compensatory mechanisms do not return pH to the normal range, they do prevent pH from becoming more abnormal.

Impaired Cellular and Organ Function

Disruptions of acid-base balance alter cell function, especially in the brain. The disorders involving carbonic acid, respiratory acidosis and alkalosis, generally cause more neurologic signs and symptoms than those involving metabolic acid, metabolic acidosis and alkalosis.[1] This difference occurs because CO_2 from carbonic acid crosses the blood-brain barrier easily and changes the pH of cerebrospinal fluid rapidly. Metabolic acid and HCO_3^- cross the blood-brain barrier with difficulty and produce fewer neurologic manifestations or cause them more slowly.

The enzymes inside cells work most effectively when pH is normal. Abnormal extracellular pH can cause intracellular pH to change, especially with respiratory acidosis and alkalosis. The resulting change in enzyme activity contributes to cell dysfunction. Acidosis decreases the level of consciousness (LOC). With alkalosis, initial excitation may occur, followed by decreased LOC if the pH increase becomes more severe. In addition to cerebral dysfunction that changes LOC and may cause other neurologic manifestations, dysfunction of cardiac cells may cause dysrhythmias.[16]

ASSESSMENT

Disruptions of acid-base balance nearly always result from other conditions. For this reason, assessments of acid-base status usually are performed in the context of other conditions.

History

Clinical manifestations associated with disrupted acid-base balance often are due to an underlying condition and associated fluid and electrolyte imbalances. Acid-base imbalances themselves cause nonspecific signs such as decreased LOC that have many possible causes. It is critical that nurses consider presenting symptoms in the context of other current health conditions. The history focuses on the respiratory, renal, or other conditions that could cause the acid-base problem. The standard questions for any history apply and will not be repeated here. Other areas to explore in the history include the following: a recent history of vomiting or diarrhea (repeated vomiting causes metabolic alkalosis; prolonged diarrhea causes metabolic acidosis); use of heartburn or indigestion medications (a few days of baking

TABLE 8-2   CLINICAL MANIFESTATIONS OF DISRUPTED ACID-BASE BALANCE

| | TOO MUCH ACID | | TOO LITTLE ACID | |
| | TOO MUCH CARBONIC ACID (RESPIRATORY ACIDOSIS) | TOO MUCH METABOLIC ACID (METABOLIC ACIDOSIS) | | TOO LITTLE METABOLIC ACID (METABOLIC ALKALOSIS) |
TYPE OF PROBLEM			**TOO LITTLE CARBONIC ACID (RESPIRATORY ALKALOSIS)**	
Common clinical findings	Headache Decreased LOC Hypoventilation (cause of problem) Cardiac dysrhythmias If severe: hypotension	Decreased LOC Hyperventilation (compensatory mechanism) Abdominal pain Nausea and vomiting Cardiac dysrhythmias	Excitation and belligerence, lightheadedness, unusual behaviors; followed by decreased LOC if severe Perioral and digital paresthesias, carpopedal spasm, tetany Diaphoresis Hyperventilation (cause of problem) Cardiac dysrhythmias	Excitation followed by decreased LOC if severe Perioral and digital paresthesias, carpopedal spasm Hypoventilation (compensatory mechanism) Signs of volume depletion and hypokalemia if present
Blood gas findings	Blood gases: pH decreased (or low normal if fully compensated); $Paco_2$ increased; HCO_3^- increased from compensation	Blood gases: pH decreased (or low normal if fully compensated); $Paco_2$ decreased from compensation; HCO_3^- decreased	Blood gases: pH increased; $Paco_2$ decreased; HCO_3^- decreased if compensation	Blood gases: pH increased; $Paco_2$ increased from compensation; HCO_3^- increased

soda/sodium bicarbonate ingestion can cause metabolic alkalosis); recent attempts to lose weight and methods employed (high-fat, low-carbohydrate diet or fasting predisposes to starvation ketoacidosis); use of medications, dietary supplements, and alcohol.[17]

Examination Findings

Unless the acid-base imbalance is severe, specific signs and symptoms of disrupted acid-base balance often are overshadowed by the clinical manifestations of the underlying cause. For example, in a person who has type B COPD (chronic bronchitis), the dyspnea and excessive mucus production usually are more obvious than the mild drowsiness from partially compensated respiratory acidosis. With severe acute asthma, the chest tightness, coughing, wheezing, use of accessory respiratory muscles, and poor oxygenation typically overshadow the manifestations of acute respiratory acidosis. People who have end-stage renal disease experience many clinical manifestations from this chronic oliguric condition that predominate over lethargy from the metabolic acidosis that may occur between dialysis sessions, unless it becomes severe.

With substantial rapid changes of pH, such as with ketoacidosis, dramatic changes in LOC can overshadow the signs and symptoms of the underlying condition. For example, a person who develops diabetic ketoacidosis typically will have been experiencing the polyuria, polydipsia, polyphagia, and weight loss of hyperglycemia before the onset of ketoacidosis. These manifestations often are realized only in retrospect, after abdominal pain and decreased LOC from the

ketoacidosis have become the focus of attention and the metabolic acidosis is resolved.

Table 8-2 presents signs and symptoms of the various disruptions of acid-base balance. These manifestations arise from the impaired cellular and organ function described earlier in this concept analysis. Decreased level of consciousness occurs on a continuum from decreased attention span and drowsiness on one end to stupor and coma on the other. Interpretation of assessment findings may be complicated by the presence of fluid and electrolyte imbalances (see Fluid and Electrolyte Concept).

Diagnostic Tests

Arterial blood gas measurement is the definitive test for acid-base balance.[18,19] This section provides the conceptual basis for interpreting them. The commonly used values are pH, $Paco_2$, HCO_3^- concentration, and base excess. The partial pressure of oxygen in arterial blood (Pao_2) and the saturation of oxygen in arterial blood (Sao_2), which are measures of oxygenation, will not be discussed here.

pH

The pH is defined technically as the negative logarithm of the H^+ concentration. H^+ ions arise from dissociation of acids, both carbonic acid and metabolic acid. The H^+ concentration is very small and awkward to write[10]; for that reason, the pH is calculated. The pH scale ranges from 1 to 14, with a pH of 7 being neutral. Because pH is a negative logarithm, a low pH indicates a solution that is acidic (has a high H^+ concentration). A high pH indicates a solution that is alkaline (has a low H^+ concentration). The pH of the blood has a normal range of 7.35 to 7.45 in adults, which is slightly alkaline. The normal range is lower in neonates and infants. In clinical settings, the term *acidemia* is used when the pH drops below the lower limit of normal (becomes *acidotic*). Even though the blood still may be slightly alkaline (above 7.0), it is more acidic than the normal range. The term *alkalemia* denotes a blood pH that is above the normal range (becomes *alkalotic*).

$Paco_2$

$Paco_2$ is the partial pressure of CO_2 in the arterial blood. It indicates how well the lungs are excreting carbonic acid (CO_2 and H_2O). The normal range of $Paco_2$ is 35 to 45 mm Hg (4.7 to 6.0 kilopascals [kPa]) for adults (lower in infants). Increased $Paco_2$ level indicates CO_2 accumulation in the blood (too much carbonic acid) caused by primary or compensatory hypoventilation; decreased $Paco_2$ level indicates excessive CO_2 excretion (too little carbonic acid) caused by primary or compensatory hyperventilation.

HCO_3^- Concentration

The serum HCO_3^- concentration indicates how well the kidneys are excreting metabolic acid.[20] The normal adult range is 22 to 26 mEq/L (22-26 mmol/L); the range is lower in infants. Increased HCO_3^- concentration indicates that the blood has too little metabolic acid; decreased HCO_3^- concentration indicates that the blood has too much metabolic acid.

Base Excess

Base excess, which normally ranges from −2 to +2 mmol/L, is an indicator of how well the buffers are managing metabolic acid. Values below −2 mmol/L (negative base excess) indicate too much metabolic acid; values above +2 mmol/L indicate too little metabolic acid. When people develop metabolic acidosis, clinicians may calculate other values, such as the anion gap and strong ion difference, to assist in diagnosing the specific cause.[21-23]

CLINICAL MANAGEMENT

Clinical management of acid-base balance encompasses all clinical settings with primary and secondary prevention as well as interventions for people with acid-base imbalances.

Primary Prevention

The primary prevention for disrupted acid-base balance focuses on prevention of the major risk factors previously discussed rather than on prevention of disrupted acid-base balance itself. For example, prevention of respiratory diseases helps to prevent risk factors for accumulating too much carbonic acid. Thus efforts to convince people not to begin smoking or to assist them to stop smoking, although targeted directly at prevention of respiratory disease, also indirectly prevent disruption of acid-base balance. Similarly, careful diabetes teaching and management help prevent ketoacidosis as well as other potential complications of diabetes. Teaching people how to lose weight safely without totally eliminating

carbohydrates can help prevent starvation ketoacidosis as well as achieve weight management goals. Poison prevention efforts can help prevent excessive ingestion of acids or acid precursors. Instruction regarding hand hygiene and safe food storage helps prevent diarrhea and vomiting, two common risk factors for disrupted acid-base balance. In summary, most of the primary prevention strategies aimed at specific disease processes and behaviors detrimental to health in general also help prevent disrupted acid-base balance that can arise from these risk factors.

Secondary Prevention (Screening)

Screening to detect disrupted acid-base balance is not performed in the general population.

Collaborative Interventions

Patients experiencing acid-base imbalance require aggressive collaborative management aimed at treating the underlying condition. If left untreated, acid-base imbalances can be fatal.

Most medical and nursing management is directed at the disease process that disrupts acid-base balance. Generally speaking, collaborative interventions to manage acid-base imbalances caused by an underlying respiratory condition include respiratory support. Likewise, collaborative interventions to manage acid-base imbalances caused by an underlying metabolic condition usually include fluid and electrolyte support.

Respiratory Support

People who have too much or too little carbonic acid usually receive some type of respiratory support, such as airway management and oxgen therapy. For example, with primary respiratory acidosis (too much carbonic acid), the focus of collaborative interventions is treatment of the disease process that is impairing alveolar ventilation. By treating the underlying cause of the disruption, acid-base balance may return to normal, or at least to a more stable state. People who are hyperventilating develop respiratory alkalosis (too little carbonic acid). Collaborative interventions for these people focus on treating the underlying factor (e.g., hypoxia, acute pain, or acute anxiety) that drives the hyperventilation. Hyperventilation that is a compensatory response to metabolic acidosis (too many metabolic acids) should be allowed to continue while the metabolic acidosis is treated.

Fluid and Electrolyte Support

People whose acid-base balance is disrupted by too much or too little metabolic acid usually receive fluid and electrolyte support as part of collaborative interventions to treat the underlying problem. For example, providing insulin and fluids to treat diabetic ketoacidosis removes the original problem and normalizes acid-base balance. Dialysis for a person who accumulates too much metabolic acid from oliguric renal disease treats multiple aspects of the condition, including the disrupted acid-base balance.

Very low pH can be fatal; therefore in situations of very severe metabolic acidosis in which pH is dangerously low, the collaborative focus may expand to adjusting the pH itself.

BOX 8-1   **FRAMEWORK FOR NURSING INTERVENTIONS FOR PEOPLE WITH DISRUPTED ACID-BASE BALANCE**

Provide safety and comfort.
Support compensatory mechanisms.
Administer collaborative interventions:
    Treatment of the underlying cause
    Adjustment of the pH (controversial)
Monitor for complications of therapy.
Teach how to avoid in the future (if appropriate) or when to seek help (if chronic).

The most common agent used for pH adjustment is intravenous (IV) sodium bicarbonate, but its use is controversial.[24-26] Administration of IV sodium bicarbonate may cause extracellular fluid volume (ECV) excess, delay renal excretion of ketoacids, or even lead to metabolic alkalosis from excessive administration. Monitoring for signs and symptoms of these complications, in addition to monitoring the patient's acid-base balance, is crucial.

Independent Nursing Interventions

Independent nursing interventions provide safety and comfort for people who have disrupted acid-base balance. Safety is high priority for patients with decreased LOC. In addition, interventions can promote compensatory mechanisms. For example, patients who are hyperventilating in compensation for metabolic acidosis need careful positioning to facilitate chest expansion and frequent oral care to prevent drying and cracking of their lips and oral mucous membranes. Another important type of intervention is teaching people how to prevent disruptions of acid-base balance or when to seek help

if they have chronic problems. Box 8-1 summarizes nursing interventions for people with disrupted acid-base balance.

INTERRELATED CONCEPTS

Numerous concepts discussed in this book have interrelationships with acid-base balance. For example, **Fluid and electrolyte balance** and acid-base balance are closely related because changes in one of them can cause changes in the other. **Oxygenation, Perfusion,** and **Nutrition** facilitate optimal acid-base balance by allowing normal acid production, whereas alterations such as ischemia, hypoxia, starvation, and high-fat, low-carbohydrate diets can disrupt that process. Similarly, **Elimination** facilitates optimal acid-base balance through acid excretion, whereas changes such as oliguria and diarrhea can disrupt acid-base balance. An individual who has disrupted acid-base balance can experience altered cognition. These interrelationships are illustrated in Figure 8-3.

EXEMPLARS

An exemplar of optimal acid-base balance is a healthy person of any age. This person's acid production is balanced by acid excretion with adequate buffering. Optimal acid-base balance also can occur in a person with acute or chronic illness (e.g., osteoporosis) that does not seriously impair respiratory, gastrointestinal, endocrine, or renal function.

As explained previously, many disease processes can disrupt acid-base balance. Box 8-2 lists exemplars of disrupted acid-base balance. The exemplars under each imbalance are organized under general causes that provide a framework for remembering the exemplars. For example, respiratory acidosis (too much carbonic acid) can arise from alveolar

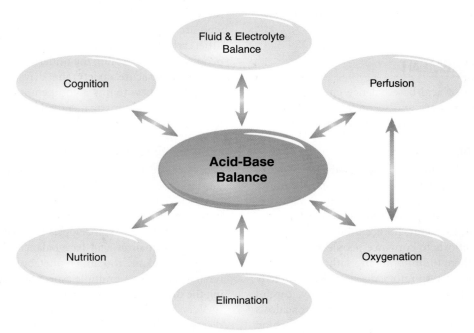

FIGURE 8-3 Acid-Base Balance and Interrelated Concepts.

MODEL CASE

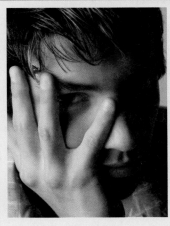

Kevin Harney, age 14, did not appear for breakfast when his mother called him. "That's unusual," she thought. "He has been so hungry lately. And he is so skinny, he really needs the food!" She found Kevin lying on his bed, breathing rapidly and deeply. He responded slowly with one or two words at a time to her increasingly frantic questions. Some of his answers did not make sense. Kevin's parents took him to the nearest emergency department, where his laboratory tests showed arterial blood pH 7.20, $Paco_2$ 21 mm Hg (2.8 kPa), serum HCO_3^- concentration 8 mEq/L (8 mmol/L), and glucose concentration 450 mg/dL (25 mmol/L). Kevin was diagnosed with diabetic ketoacidosis (DKA) arising from previously undiagnosed type 1 diabetes. During Kevin's hospitalization, interventions focused initially on intensive collaborative management of his disrupted acid-base balance with insulin and IV fluid to treat the diabetes. As a safety intervention, Kevin was positioned on his side to prevent aspiration if he vomited. During this phase of management, attention also was given to supporting his parents, explaining that Kevin's unusual breathing pattern actually was beneficial to him and letting his mother assume the task of protecting Kevin's lips by keeping them lubricated. Careful monitoring of blood values and physical assessment parameters was used to follow his progress and modify therapy when his condition changed. As Kevin began to be more responsive and stable, the focus of nursing interventions expanded to teaching Kevin and his parents about type 1 diabetes, how to manage it, and how to recognize the signs of hyperglycemia. Although not directed specifically at acid-base balance, this teaching helped prevent future episodes of diabetic ketoacidosis through disease management.

Case Analysis

Kevin developed diabetic ketoacidosis, a type of metabolic acidosis (too much metabolic acid), from a combination of excessive production and decreased excretion of metabolic acid. Because of his type 1 diabetes, Kevin's pancreas no longer was able to secrete insulin. The resulting metabolic problems included hyperglycemia and incomplete metabolism of fat that generated large amounts of ketoacids (increased acid production). Although Kevin did not have kidney disease, his kidneys were unable to excrete enough ketoacids to prevent their accumulation. An initial osmotic diuresis from hyperglycemia often decreases the extracellular fluid volume (ECV) and decreases glomerular filtration rate, causing oliguria when the ECV becomes low. Oliguria decreased the excretion of the ketoacids, contributing to their accumulation. As his blood pH decreased, Kevin's chemoreceptors triggered compensatory hyperventilation. Kevin's arterial blood gas values demonstrate his disrupted acid-base balance: decreased pH (acidosis from too much acid), decreased $Paco_2$ (carbonic acid removed by compensatory hyperventilation), and decreased HCO_3^- concentration (used in buffering the excess metabolic acids). Interventions directed at treating Kevin's diabetes and promoting safety, comfort, and teaching provided effective care.

■■■ BOX 8-2 EXEMPLARS OF ACID-BASE BALANCE

Respiratory Acidosis (Too Much Carbonic Acid)
Alveolar Hypoventilation
- Type B COPD (chronic bronchitis)
- End-stage type A COPD (emphysema)
- Severe asthma episode
- Bacterial pneumonia
- Pulmonary edema

Ineffective Respiratory Pump
- Guillain-Barré syndrome

Central Suppression of Respiration
- Opioid overdose

Metabolic Acidosis (Too Much Metabolic Acid)
Excessive Production or Intake of Metabolic Acid
- Diabetic ketoacidosis
- Starvation ketoacidosis
- Alcoholic ketoacidosis
- Lactic acidosis (from tissue anoxia)
- Thyroid storm
- Aspirin overdose

Decreased Excretion of Metabolic Acid
- Oliguria from any cause

Loss of Bicarbonate
- Prolonged diarrhea
- Draining intestinal or pancreatic fistula

Respiratory Alkalosis (Too Little Carbonic Acid)
Hyperventilation
- Acute hypoxia
- Acute pain
- Acute anxiety or emotional distress
- Central stimulation of respirations by inflammation from head injury or meningitis

Metabolic Alkalosis (Too Little Metabolic Acid)
Gain of Base (Bicarbonate)
- Excessive ingestion or infusion of $NaHCO_3$
- Diuretic therapy (contraction alkalosis)

Excessive Excretion of Metabolic Acid
- Repeated vomiting
- Mineralocorticoid excess

hypoventilation, ineffective neuromuscular action of the chest respiratory pump, or suppression of the neural drive from the brainstem that triggers respirations. Nurses can use these categories to understand specifically how the exemplars cause respiratory acidosis. In addition, they can generalize their knowledge to other conditions that cause respiratory acidosis by similar mechanisms. Box 8-2 provides these general categories for each acid-base imbalance.

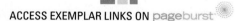

ACCESS EXEMPLAR LINKS ON pageburst

REFERENCES

1. Rose BD: *Clinical physiology of acid-base and electrolyte disorders*, ed 6, New York, 2011, McGraw-Hill.
2. Gilbert C, Baram M, Marik PE: Continuous venovenous hemodiafiltration in severe metabolic acidosis secondary to ethylene glycol ingestion, *S Med J* 103:846, 2010.
3. Kimia AA, Johnston P, Capraro A, et al: Occurrence of metabolic acidosis in pediatric emergency department patients as a data source for disease surveillance systems, *Pediatr Emerg Care* 26:733, 2010.
4. Grotegut C, Dandolu V, Katari S, et al: Baking soda pica: a case of hypokalemic metabolic alkalosis and rhabdomyolysis in pregnancy, *Obstet Gynecol* 107:484, 2006.
5. Bar A, Riskin A, Iancu T, et al: A newborn infant with protracted diarrhea and metabolic acidosis, *J Pediatr* 150:198, 2007.
6. Ucgun I, Metintas M, Moral H, et al: Predictors of hospital outcome and intubation in COPD patients admitted to the respiratory ICU for acute hypercapnic respiratory failure, *Resp Med* 100:66, 2006.
7. Abbiss C, Nosaka K, Laursen P: Hyperthermic-induced hyperventilation and associated respiratory alkalosis in humans, *Eur J Appl Physiol* 100:63, 2007.
8. Yaqoob MM: Acidosis and progression of chronic kidney disease, *Curr Opinion Nephrol Hypertens* 19:489, 2010.
9. McCauley M, Gunawardane M, Cowan M: Severe metabolic alkalosis due to pyloric obstruction: case presentation, evaluation, and management, *Am J Med Sci* 332:346, 2006.
10. Hall JE: *Guyton and Hall textbook of medical physiology*, ed 12, Philadelphia, 2011, Saunders/Elsevier.
11. Giovannini I, Greco F, Chiarla V, et al: Exceptional nonfatal metabolic alkalosis (blood base excess +48 mEq/Liter), *Intens Care Med* 31:166, 2005.
12. Boron WF: Acid-base transport by the renal proximal tubule, *J Am Soc Nephrol* 17:2368, 2006.
13. de Seigneux S, Malte H, Dimke H, et al: Renal compensation to chronic hypoxic hypercapnia: downregulation of pendrin and adaptation of the proximal tubule, *Am J Physiol* 292:F1256, 2007.
14. Adrogué HJ, Madias NE: Secondary responses to altered acid-base status: the rules of engagement, *J Am Soc Nephrol* 21:920, 2010.
15. Ward S: Ventilatory control in humans: constraints and limitations, *Exp Physiol* 92:357, 2007.
16. Felver L: *Cardiac nursing*, ed 6, Philadelphia, 2010, Lippincott.
17. Liamis G, Milionis HJ, Elisaf M: Pharmacologically-induced metabolic acidosis: a review, *Drug Safety* 33:371, 2010.
18. Edwards SL: Pathophysiology of acid base balance: the theory practice relationship, *Intens Crit Care Nurs* 24:28, 2007.
19. Kramer BJ, Raymond MK: Arterial blood gases, *RN* 72(4):22, 2009.
20. Schoolwerth A, Kaneko T, Sedlacek M, et al: Acid-base disturbances in the intensive care unit: metabolic acidosis, *Sem Dialysis* 19:492, 2006.
21. Dubin A, Menises MM, Masevicius FD, et al: Comparison of three different methods of evaluation of metabolic acid-base disorders, *Crit Care Med* 35:1264, 2007.
22. Kraut JA, Madias NE: Serum anion gap: its uses and limitations in clinical medicine, *Clin J Am Soc Nephrol* 2:162, 2007.
23. Nagaoka D, Nassar AP Jr, Maciel AT, et al: The use of sodium-chloride difference and chloride-sodium ratio as strong ion surrogates in the evaluation of metabolic acidosis in critically ill patients, *J Crit Care* 25:525, 2010.
24. Beveridge CJE, Wilkinson AR: Sodium bicarbonate infusion during resuscitation of infants at birth, *Cochrane Database Sys Rev* 1:CD004864, 2006. doi: 10.1002/14651858.CD004864.pub2.
25. Kraut JA, Madias NE: Consequences and therapy of the metabolic acidosis of chronic kidney disease, *Pediatr Nephrol* 26:19, 2011.
26. Lawn CJ, Weir FJ, McGuire W: Base administration or fluid bolus for preventing morbidity and mortality in preterm infants with metabolic acidosis, *Cochrane Database Sys Rev* 2:CD003215, 2005. doi: 10.1002/14651858.CD003215.pub2.

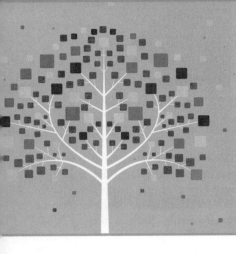

Thermoregulation

L. Jane Rosati and Amy Szoka

The human body has the capability of regulating body temperature at a near constant value, a process known as thermoregulation. Temperature regulation is critical for optimal physiologic function. Thermoregulation is a foundational nursing concept; thus it is essential that nurses apply this concept into nursing practice.

DEFINITION(S)

Optimal physiologic function of the human body occurs when a near-constant core temperature is maintained. Normal body temperature ranges from 36.2° to 37.6° C (97.0° to 100° F), or an average of 37° C (98.6° F).[1] Fluctuation outside this range is an indication of a disease process, strenuous or unusual activity, or extreme environmental exposure. Thermoregulation is defined as *the process of maintaining core body temperature at a near constant value.*[1] The term *normothermia* refers to the state in which body temperature is within the "normal" range. The term *hypothermia* refers to a body temperature below normal range (<36.2° C) and *hyperthermia* refers to a body temperature above normal range (>37.6° C). An extremely high body temperature is referred to as *hyperpyrexia.*

SCOPE AND CATEGORIES

Scope

Thermoregulation is an aspect of homeostasis that balances heat gain and heat loss. Body temperatures can range from above normal to below normal; thus the scope of this concept will be considered in this way (see Figure 9-1). Physiologic adjustments to body temperature are controlled by the hypothalamus—often considered the thermostat center of the body. The nurse uses the average target temperature of 37° C (98.6° F) to assess this state.

Hyperthermia

Hyperthermia occurs when the body temperature rises above 37.6° C with an unchanged hypothalamic set point. Heat-related conditions occur when the body's natural ability to

dissipate heat is interrupted, resulting in a rise in body temperature that exceeds heat loss. This can occur as a result of several factors, including environment (temperature, humidity, lack of air movement), genetic abnormality, injury to the hypothalamus, and pharmacologic agents.

Fever also represents an elevation of body temperature, but differs from hyperthermia because it is associated with an increase in the hypothalamic set point caused by the release of interleukin-1 and tumor necrosis factor from white blood cells. Fever is usually associated with an inflammatory process but can also be caused by drugs and tumors. Fever is one of the most common presenting symptoms in clinical practice. The differentiation between hyperthermia and fever is not based on the body temperature, but rather the underlying cause.

Hypothermia

Hypothermia occurs when the body temperature falls below 36.2° C and is further classified as mild (34° to 36° C or 93.2° to 96.8° F); moderate (30° to 34° C or 86° to 93° F); or severe (<30° C or <86° F). Hypothermia may be either accidental or therapeutic. Accidental hypothermia results from environmental exposure or as a complication from serious systemic disorders. Therapeutic hypothermia is intentionally induced to reduce metabolism and thereby preserve tissue by preventing tissue ischemia.

RISK FACTORS

All individuals have the potential to develop problems associated with thermoregulation. Risk factors can be described in terms of both populations at risk and individual risk factors. Recognition of risk factors is essential so that appropriate preventive measures can be initiated.

Populations at Risk

Although all humans are at risk for alterations in thermoregulation, certain population groups have significantly greater risk—particularly the very young and the very old.

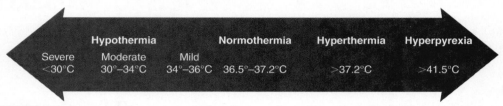

FIGURE 9-1 Scope of Thermoregulation Ranges from Hypothermia, to Normothermia, to Hyperthermia.

Infants and Young Children

Infants (particularly premature infants) have undeveloped temperature regulation capacity. Infants usually produce sufficient body heat, but lack the ability to conserve heat produced; a large surface area relative to body mass makes them susceptible to excessive temperature loss.[2] In addition, because of limited subcutaneous fat, infants are not as well insulated compared to adults. Immediately after birth, infants are particularly susceptible to hypothermia, requiring immediate measures to provide warmth. Low birth weight and poorly nourished infants and children are also at greater risk for hypothermia. The inability to independently take measures to correct changes in temperature—such as adding or removing clothing, adding or removing a blanket, or adjusting a thermostat—also places infants and children at risk. They are completely dependent on the appropriate actions of caregivers for maintenance of a normothermic temperature range.

Older Adults

The elderly experience fluctuations in temperature because of a diminished ability to regulate body temperature. As the body ages, the sweat glands decrease in number and efficiency. Other age-related factors—such as reduced circulation, a decreased vasoconstrictive response, reduced shivering response, slower metabolic rate, and reduced physical activity—all contribute to a less effective thermoregulatory response.[3] The elderly also have a reduced perception of heat and cold; thus they may not recognize when to take appropriate action in a timely manner. Elderly who lack resources to stay warm or cool in temperature extremes are also at risk for thermodysregulation.

Other Population Groups

Other population groups at risk for imbalance in thermoregulation include those who reside in very cold or hot climates and the poor (low socioeconomic status), who may lack resources for adequate clothing, heating, and cooling. The homeless population (because of their frequent exposure to the elements and lack of adequate shelter) is particularly at high risk for hyperthermia or hypothermia.

Studies analyzing heat-related deaths emphasize the previously mentioned risk factors. Statistics from the Centers for Disease Control and Prevention (CDC) show a total of 3442 deaths resulted from exposure to extreme heat between 1999 and 2003.[4] The majority of deaths occurred among those age 65 and older; the two states with the highest average

annual hyperthermia-related death rate were Arizona and Nevada.[5] An alarming number of heat-related deaths among children have resulted from being left in vehicles, where life-threatening temperatures develop quickly.[6] Since 1998 there have been 494 such deaths involving children ranging in age from 5 days to 14 years old.[5]

Population-based risk factors for deaths associated with hypothermia are also reflected in studies. The CDC reported a total of 646 hypothermia-related deaths in 2002.[7] Hypothermic deaths more commonly affect persons ages 65 years or older with the majority population being unmarried men.[7] Although geographic areas with cold climates have a higher incidence of hypothermia, this occurs in all 50 states. The states with highest deaths associated with hypothermia include Alaska, Montana, Wyoming, and New Mexico.[4]

Individual Risk Factors

Individual risk factors are unique to an individual. A person's age and the climate where the person lives are risk factors described previously. Other individual risk factors include impaired cognition, underlying health conditions, genetics, and environmental exposure.

Impaired Cognition

Individuals with impairments in cognition (either acute or chronic) are at risk for imbalanced temperature because of the potential inability to recognize dangerous environmental exposures or the inability to react appropriately. For example, older adults with dementia may not select appropriate clothing when going outdoors, or may wander outdoors without an awareness of their actions. As another example, individuals may experience cognitive impairment attributable to substance abuse. Persons under the influence are at risk because sensory alterations affect judgment or there may be a loss of consciousness, thus increasing the risk for environmental exposure. Alcohol acts as a vasodilator—dilation of surface blood vessels leads to loss of body heat. Unfortunately, the drinker feels warm and may not engage in self-protective behaviors. Alcohol as a common underlying factor in hypothermic deaths attests to this point.[7]

Underlying Health Conditions

Individuals with preexisting medical conditions (such as congestive heart failure, diabetes, or gait disturbance) are at increased risk for hypothermia because their bodies have a reduced ability to generate heat. They may also be less likely to recognize symptoms of hypothermia and less likely to seek shelter from the cold because of these comorbidities.[5] Individuals who have experienced traumatic brain injury are at risk for problems with thermoregulation, particularly if the area of the brain damaged leads to hypothalamic dysfunction.[1] Individuals who undergo surgical procedures are also at risk for hypothermia, particularly if the procedure is long.

Body heat is largely fueled by food intake and fat provides insulation; poor nutritional status makes an individual at increased risk for hypothermia. Poor hydration increases risk for hyperthermia because of the need for body fluids associated with perspiration.

Genetics

A less common risk factor for impaired thermoregulation is genetic predisposition. The classic example of this is malignant hyperthermia, a condition associated with an inherited autosomal dominant pattern. Malignant hyperthermia is often considered a surgical complication because it is commonly discovered after a patient is given a general anesthetic. This condition is actually a biochemical chain reaction triggered by commonly used general anesthetics and succinylcholine.

Recreational or Occupational Exposures

Individuals may suffer impairments in thermoregulation as a consequence of participating in recreational activities or working in conditions associated with temperature extremes. Strenuous activity in high ambient temperatures, particularly with high humidity, can lead to hyperthermia. Winter recreational activities such as hiking, snowmobiling, and skiing can lead to hypothermia if an individual has inadequate clothing for the activity or if the individual becomes lost or injured. Cold water exposure also quickly leads to hypothermia, particularly if the air temperature is also cold.[8]

PHYSIOLOGIC PROCESSES AND CONSEQUENCES

Thermoregulation occurs through a dynamic and complex physiologic process controlled by the hypothalamus that balances heat loss and gain. Compensatory and regulatory actions maintain a steady core temperature. When a person sits or stands, walks or runs, digests food, or even changes his or her respiratory rate, regulation of body functions takes place as the body compensates. A basic review of heat production, heat conservation, and heat loss is foundational to an understanding of thermoregulation.

Heat Production and Conservation

Body heat is continually produced through metabolic activity by chemical reactions occurring in the cells. The greatest amount of heat is produced by muscles and through metabolic activity in the liver. Metabolic activity involves the ingestion and metabolism of food and the basal metabolic rate (BMR)—or the energy required to maintain the body at rest. Basal metabolic rate tends to be higher among younger individuals and decreases as the body ages. The amount of heat produced is affected by food consumption, physical activity, and hormone levels. The contraction of muscles produces heat through muscle tone and shivering. Chemical thermogenesis occurs as a result of epinephrine release, which increases metabolic rate. In addition to heat production, the body conserves heat through peripheral vasoconstriction. Essentially this process shunts warm blood away from the superficial body tissues and skin surfaces and increases muscle activity to minimize heat loss.

Heat Loss

Not only does the body continually produce heat through metabolic activity, but also it continuously loses heat. Heat loss occurs as a result of multiple mechanisms including radiation, conduction, convection, vasodilation, evaporation, reduced muscle activity, and increased respiration. These processes are an important basis for treatment strategies when heat loss is desired.

Heat loss to *radiation* occurs through a process of electromagnetic waves that emit heat from skin surfaces to the air. The degree of heat loss through radiation is directly related to the difference between ambient air temperature, skin temperature, and exposure. *Conduction* is a transfer of heat through direct contact of one surface to another; warmer surfaces lose heat to cooler surfaces. A loss of heat by air currents (caused by wind or a fan) moving across the body surface is referred to as *convection*.[3] Warmer air at the body surface is replaced by the cooler air, resulting in cooling of the skin surface. Wet skin or clothing accelerates this process.

In addition to radiation, conduction, and convection, heat loss can occur through other physiologic compensatory mechanisms. Heat loss can be increased through peripheral *vasodilation,* which brings a greater volume of blood to the body surface. Increased heat loss occurs by conduction (explained above). This process is not effective, however, if ambient air temperature is greater than body temperature. A reduction in muscle tone and muscle activity occurs as another mechanism to minimize heat production. This process explains the fatigue or "washed out" feeling experienced in hot weather or after sitting in a hot tub for a period of time.[3] Perspiration is yet another mechanism involved with heat loss; this process is explained by evaporation of moisture from the skin surface. This provides a significant source of heat reduction and normally accounts for 600 ml of water loss per day. In extreme heat, an individual can lose as much as 4 L of fluids in an hour; for this reason, replacement of fluids and electrolytes is essential to prevent dehydration. Heat is also lost during the process of respiration. Cool ambient air is inhaled and warmed in the respiratory tract and by the microcirculation within the alveoli. The warmed air is then exhaled. For this reason, elevated respiratory rates are seen among individuals with elevated temperature and lower respiratory rates are seen in individuals with hypothermia.

Temperature Control

Temperature control is mediated by the hypothalamus through hormonal control. The hypothalamus is located below the thalamus in an area of the brain called the

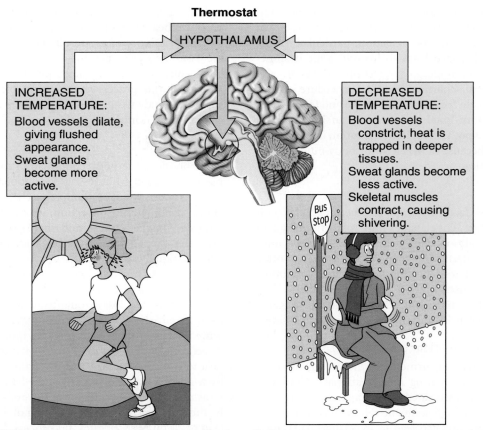

Thermostat

HYPOTHALAMUS

INCREASED TEMPERATURE:
Blood vessels dilate, giving flushed appearance.
Sweat glands become more active.

DECREASED TEMPERATURE:
Blood vessels constrict, heat is trapped in deeper tissues.
Sweat glands become less active.
Skeletal muscles contract, causing shivering.

FIGURE 9-2 Temperature Regulation. The hypothalamus controls body temperature and signals for mechanisms to increase heat production or to facilitate heat loss. (From Herlihy B: *The human body in health and illness,* ed 4, St Louis, 2011, Elsevier.)

diencephalon. This is a small but important part of the brain located between the midbrain and the cerebrum (Figure 9-2).

Thermoregulation involves a negative feedback system, which reverses or opposes a change in a controlled condition.[9] Multiple thermoreceptors are located throughout the body. Peripheral thermoreceptors (located in the skin) and central thermoreceptors (located in the spinal cord, abdominal organs, and hypothalamus) provide skin and core temperature information to the hypothalamus. The hypothalamus activates a series of responses to lower or raise body temperature based on information received by the thermoreceptors.

When the thermoreceptors signal a drop in body temperature, the hypothalamus initiates a series of heat-producing and heat-conserving mechanisms through endocrine and sympathetic nervous system connections. Thyrotropin (or thyroxine)-stimulating hormone–releasing hormone (TSH-RH) is secreted by the hypothalamus, which in turn stimulates the anterior pituitary to release thyroid-stimulating hormone (TSH). TSH acts on the thyroid gland to release thyroxine (T_4), which activates the adrenal medulla to cause the release of epinephrine into the blood. Epinephrine increases heat production by increasing the metabolic rate, stimulating glycolysis, and causing vasoconstriction (see Figure 9-2). The hypothalamus also stimulates the sympathetic nervous

system, which triggers the adrenal cortex to increase muscle tone and initiate a shivering and vasoconstriction response.

When the thermoreceptors signal an increase in body temperature, the same mechanisms are reversed (the classic feature of a negative feedback system). The release of TSH-RH is discontinued (thus stopping the T_4 and epinephrine responses) and the sympathetic nervous system is signaled to induce vasodilation, decrease muscle tone, and initiate sweat production (see Figure 9-2). Sweat glands rapidly produce and release increased levels of perspiration; heat dissipates from the body as sweat evaporates from its surface.[10]

Pathophysiologic Consequences
Hyperthermia

A significant rise in body temperature leads to many physiologic changes that can be fatal as a result of cardiovascular collapse and damage to the nervous system. Mentioned previously, one compensatory response to elevation in body temperature is sweating—a measure that helps to cool the body. Excessive and prolonged sweating coupled with a sustained high body temperature can result in sodium loss and dehydration if fluid replacement does not occur. Over time, excessive body temperature can lead to hypotension, tachycardia, and decreased cardiac output, progressing to reduced perfusion and coagulation within the microcirculation and cardiovascular collapse. Sustained high core body temperature coupled with reduced perfusion leads to cerebral edema, central nervous system degeneration, and renal necrosis.

Hypothermia

The physiologic consequences of hypothermia are dependent on the severity and duration of exposure. As core body temperature decreases, compensatory mechanisms including shivering (muscle contraction to simulate warmth) and vasoconstriction (to reduce heat loss) occur. However, because prolonged vasoconstriction would lead to peripheral tissue ischemia, intermittent reperfusion of peripheral tissues occurs. Prolonged hypothermia eventually leads to reduced perfusion in the microcirculation attributable to increased viscosity of the blood and reduced blood flow and coagulation. Also, the vasoconstrictive efforts controlled by the hypothalamus eventually fail, causing vasodilation and thus accelerating the loss of body heat. Individuals experiencing significant hypothermia have been known to remove clothing because of reduced cognition and because the vasodilation can create a false warming sensation. The first evidence of cell damage can be seen microscopically when swelling is observed in the cell.[11] As body temperature falls further below 28° C, ice crystals actually form on the inside of the cell, causing cellular rupture.[11]

ASSESSMENT

Body temperature is included in nearly all assessments because this provides baseline information about homeostasis and general health. When problems associated with thermoregulation present, a history and examination are warranted.

History

Typically, a history does not include specific questions related to normal body temperature or thermoregulation. However, in the event of thermoregulation imbalance, a history provides valuable information needed to understand the problem. The age, health history, family history (for malignant hyperthermia), and social history provide necessary information to establish risk factors. Additional questions include presence of recent injury, illnesses, or environmental exposure. If there has been recent environmental exposure, the type of exposure, severity, and length of exposure should be determined.

Presenting symptoms related to hyperthermia can include weakness, nausea, vomiting, syncope, change in cognition, muscle cramps, and a report of "feeling hot." Additional symptoms may be "feeling cold" or shivering, altered mental status, lethargy, and complaints of clumsiness or lack of coordination.

Examination Findings
Vital Signs

Nursing assessment for alterations in thermoregulation begins with a set of vital signs. Some older adults may have temperature variances lower than the established adult temperature.[12] A common way to measure temperature is by the oral route or using a temporal thermometer. However, when an individual has hyperthermia or hypothermia, the most reliable means available for assessing core temperature is a rectal temperature, which is considered the standard of practice. A lubricated probe is inserted into the rectal canal at a depth of 1 to 1.5 inches in the adult and 0.5 to 1 inch in the child. In the critical care setting, the pulmonary artery catheter may be used to measure core temperature. Additional core temperature sites include the esophagus, tympanic membrane, and urinary bladder.

Other vital sign measurements are important when assessing an individual with hyperthermia or hypothermia because of compensatory mechanisms. The heart rate and respiratory rate increase with hyperthermia and are decreased in hypothermia. Blood pressure may not be noticeably changed with mild variations in body temperature; however, hypotension and eventual cardiovascular collapse occur with severe hypothermia and hyperthermia.

Examination Findings: Hyperthermia

Although the general appearance of an individual experiencing hyperthermia varies (depending on the underlying cause and the degree of temperature elevation), several common clinical findings are observed. Vasodilation occurs, causing the skin to appear flushed and warm or hot to touch. If the sweat mechanism has been activated, the individual will be diaphoretic, although this finding may be absent. Patients will often present with dry skin and mucous membranes, decreased urinary output, and other signs of dehydration and electrolyte imbalance. Because of the effects of high body temperature on the brain and central nervous system, seizures may occur and the patient's cognitive status may range from slightly confused or delirious to coma.

Examination Findings: Hypothermia

The clinical presentation of hypothermic patients also varies, depending on the severity of the condition. Peripheral vasoconstriction causes the skin to feel cool and have slow capillary refill; skin color is pale and becomes cyanotic. Muscle rigidity and shivering is typically present in an effort to generate heat. The shivering response diminishes or ceases when the core temperature drops to 30° C. Cognition is affected because of a gradual reduction in cerebral blood flow. A person may experience poor coordination and sluggish thought processes at 34° C; this progresses to confusion and eventually stupor and coma by the time the temperature drops to 30° C. Dysrhythmias (such as atrial and ventricular fibrillation) may occur due to myocardial irritability. As hypothermia progresses, the metabolic rate declines and perfusion of blood is significantly reduced, leading to diminished urinary function, coma, and cardiovascular collapse.[13]

CLINICAL MANAGEMENT
Primary Prevention

Most cases of hyperthermia and hypothermia are preventable by reducing risk. The nurse's role in primary prevention is through patient education. Avoidance of exposure to temperature extremes is an obvious way to prevent problems associated with thermoregulation. When this is unavoidable, planning is essential to ensure adequate resources are available. Primary prevention measures include environmental control and shelter, appropriate clothing for different conditions, and physical activity.

Environmental Control and Shelter

Maintaining optimal ambient temperature in the home or having adequate shelter during temperature extremes is essential. If a home does not have air conditioning in the summer months, opening windows and using fans are encouraged. If home heating is inadequate during cold weather, patients should be advised to wear additional clothing and use blankets for additional warmth. Wind drafts should be blocked and curtains hung at windows to improve insulation.

Community resources, including homeless shelters, can be used to assist those who are unable to stay cool during warm months and warm during the cold months. Individuals can also be encouraged to go to public buildings such as indoor shopping malls or libraries, where ambient temperatures are usually adequately regulated. For those exposed to the elements, seeking adequate shelter can be lifesaving. Shelter includes finding shade and ideally a breeze when temperatures are high and avoiding the wind and precipitation when temperatures are low.

Appropriate Clothing

The selection of appropriate clothing is another primary prevention strategy. Although this applies for both types of temperature extremes, adequate clothing is essential to prevent hypothermia with cold temperatures. Evaporate heat loss is five times greater when clothing is wet; thus dry clothing is essential. A newborn is susceptible to rapid heat loss directly after birth and hypothermia may result. Immediately after delivery, the infant should be dried quickly, wrapped in blankets, and moved to a heated environment. Care should be taken to limit the time the infant's skin is wet (e.g., bathing, wet diapers or clothing).

Patients should be taught to dress in layers, and cover the head. New parents should be instructed about heat loss in newborns and young children; dressing the infant and child appropriately for the weather and adequate regulation of temperature in the home are essential. When environmental temperature is low, infants should be provided with a hat to guard against heat loss, just as the elderly patient may need a sweater or clothing with long sleeves for comfort. The elderly may need to be reminded to dress in clothing appropriate for the weather.

Physical Activity

Physical activity increases body temperature. Increasing physical activity helps to warm the body when exposed to low temperatures and can prevent hypothermia. When temperatures are elevated, physical exertion increases risk for hyperthermia because the heat gains may exceed heat loss. For this reason, individuals should be encouraged to limit physical exertion during high temperatures to reduce risk. Maintaining adequate hydration and nutrition also reduce risk.

Collaborative Interventions

Management of the patient with altered thermoregulation is dependent on the core body temperature and the overall physical condition of the individual. Generally, infants and young children, the elderly, and individuals in poor health not only have greater risk factors but also have less physical capacity for physiologic compensation when changes in core body temperature occur.

Hyperthermia

The underlying cause of the elevated body temperature should be identified (e.g., a fever associated with an inflammatory process or hyperthermia associated with exposure). Regardless of the cause, the goal is to minimize cardiovascular and neurologic complications associated with excessive body temperature. Care of the individual whose temperature has exceeded 37° C should include removal of excess blanketing and clothing while observing for continued signs of hyperthermia (increased respiration, increased or decreased perspiration, high fever, seizures). Signs and symptoms that persist beyond 1 hour require further intervention. Hydration with parenteral fluids, nutritional support, and other palliative measures to reduce core temperature should be implemented. Cool packs may be placed in the axillary and groin areas; a cooling blanket or lukewarm bath may also facilitate temperature reduction. Care should be taken to not induce shivering. More aggressive cooling efforts include gastric or colonic lavage with cool fluids.

The presence of fever is considered an expected finding with a systemic inflammatory response. Mild to moderate fever generally does little harm and may actually have beneficial effects to counteract the inflammation. However, complications such as dehydration and increased metabolic demand can occur.[14] Symptomatic relief of persistent or intermittent fevers can be treated with antipyretics such as nonsteroidal antiinflammatory drugs (NSAIDs) (e.g., naproxen or ibuprofen) and acetaminophen. Aspirin is also useful in reducing fever but should be used with caution; aspirin is not recommended for children because of the risk of Reye syndrome. The use of a drug called dantrolene sodium can reverse the effects of malignant hyperthermia. Intracellular calcium levels are elevated in malignant hyperthermia; dantrolene counteracts this abnormality by reducing muscle tone and metabolism. Administration of dantrolene intravenously has dramatically reduced the mortality rate of malignant hyperthermia.[15]

Hypothermia

The goal of managing hypothermic patients is to raise the body temperature to the normal range. An initial step is to remove the individual from the cold. If hypothermia is mild, passive and active external rewarming measures are indicated. Passive measures include dry warm clothing, warm drinks, and exercise, and these may be sufficient. However, active rewarming measures may be necessary and include

CLINICAL NURSING SKILLS FOR THERMOREGULATION

- Assessment
- External warming devices
  - Warm blankets
  - Administer warm oral fluids
- Active core warming
  - Warm intravenous fluids
  - Heated humidified oxygen
  - Warm fluid lavage
- Cooling measures
  - Cool water bath
  - Cool intravenous fluids
  - Cool fluid lavage
  - Cooling blankets

providing warm blankets or heating pads, drawing a warm water bath, and placing the patient in a heated environment.

When core body temperature falls below 30° C, active core rewarming measures are indicated—meaning there is an application of heat directly to the core. Core rewarming should be done slowly and carefully to minimize the risk of triggering dysrhythmias; thus continuous cardiac monitoring and core body temperature observation are necessary. Active core rewarming strategies include infusion of warm intravenous solutions, gastric lavage with warm fluid, peritoneal lavage with warm fluid, and inhalation of warmed oxygen. If hypothermia is severe, cardiopulmonary bypass or arteriovenous rewarming may be indicated.[8]

INTERRELATED CONCEPTS

A large number of concepts are clearly interrelated to thermoregulation. Those that have greatest importance are presented in Figure 9-3.

Intracranial regulation. The hypothalamus regulates body temperature. Any injury to the brain can damage or impair function of the hypothalamus. Traumatic brain injury, with its associated cerebral edema, ischemia, energy failure, oxidative stress, and neuronal death, may directly affect the temperature control center.[16] Often, when injury occurs to the brain or spinal cord, there is interruption of the sympathetic nervous system that prevents peripheral temperature sensations from reaching the hypothalamus. During this period of disruption the body has decreased ability to sweat or shiver below the level of the lesion. A condition of *poikilothermism* results—known as the adjustment of the body temperature to the room temperature.[9] A variety of interventions are used to treat brain and spinal cord injury including external control of thermoregulation by induced hypothermia.

Perfusion. Perfusion is impacted by body temperature. Measures to minimize or maximize heat loss include vasodilation and vasoconstriction within the blood vessels; severe extremes in body temperature can result in cardiovascular collapse.

Tissue integrity. The skin plays an important role in body temperature regulation. The skin acts as a protective layer to reduce heat loss. Additionally, thermoreceptors in the skin alert all individual to extremes in temperatures, thus preventing injury.

Nutrition. Metabolism of nutrients provides the body with fuel needed for the generation of heat and body activities. Malnutrition increases risk for hypothermia because of an inability to generate adequate heat.

Fluids and electrolytes. Perspiration is an essential component of thermoregulation. Efficient perspiration requires adequate fluid balances. Fluid and electrolyte imbalances can occur when excessive body temperature exhausts available fluids for perspiration.

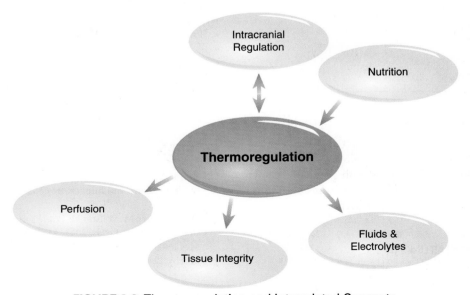

FIGURE 9-3 Thermoregulation and Interrelated Concepts.

MODEL CASE

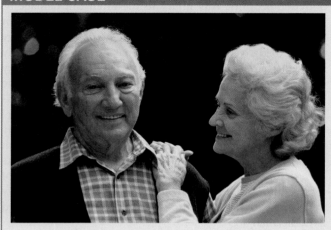

Tom Anderson is an 86-year-old white male who lives with his 82-year-old wife of 64 years in their home in upstate New York. Over the past few years, Mrs. Anderson has noticed a decline in her husband's mental status. Early on a January morning, Mrs. Anderson was awaked at 4 AM by the doorbell. When she opened the door, a neighbor was standing with her husband who was wearing nothing but his pajamas. The neighbor explained he saw Tom wandering outside on the snowy street. Tom was shivering uncontrollably and confused; the outdoor temperature was only 19° F. Mrs. Anderson immediately called 911 and had her husband transported to the hospital.

Upon arrival to the emergency department (ED), Mr. Anderson was assessed by the ED nurse, who noted the following assessment findings:

- Mental status: confused; not oriented to person, place, or time
- Vital signs: temperature, 33.1° C rectally; pulse, 62 beats/min; respirations, 12 breaths/min; blood pressure, 100/62 mm Hg
- Skin: pale, cyanosis around lips and extremities
- Uncontrollable shivering

The nurse immediately placed Tom in a dry gown, covered him with a warm blanket, and placed him in a warm room. The findings were immediately reported to the physician; the nurse initiated the following orders of the physician:

- Stat electrocardiogram (ECG) followed by continuous cardiac monitoring
- Continuous vital sign and pulse oximeter monitoring
- Start IV of 1000 ml of 0.9% normal saline to run over 8 hours; solution to be warmed to 98.6° F
- Cover patient with warming blanket set at 98.6° F
- Apply warm oxygen at 3 L/min via nasal cannula
- Blood draw for hemoglobin and hematocrit, electrolytes, blood gases, blood urea nitrogen (BUN) and creatinine, blood glucose, and toxicology screen

After several hours in the ED, Tom's core body temperature slowly rises to 35.4° C; he has stabilized but remains confused. He is admitted to the medical unit for further evaluation.

Case Analysis

The case illustrates several aspects of this concept. Risk factors include age, climate, limited cognition, and environmental exposure. The clinical findings were consistent with hypothermia. The treatment measures center on passive and active rewarming interventions.

◼◼◼ BOX 9-1   EXEMPLARS OF THERMOREGULATION

Hyperthermia
- Brain injury
- Environmental exposure
- Fever
- Heat exhaustion
- Heatstroke
- Hyperthyroidism
- Infection: bacterial/viral
- Malignant hyperthermia
- Thyroid storm

Hypothermia
- Brain injury
- Environmental exposure
- Frostbite
- Preterm infant

EXEMPLARS

There are several conditions associated with changes in body temperature. These are presented in Box 9-1 as conditions associated with hyperthermia and hypothermia.

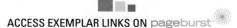

ACCESS EXEMPLAR LINKS ON pageburst

REFERENCES

1. Braine M: The role of the hypothalamus, part 1: the regulation of temperature and hunger, *Br J Neurosci Nurs* 5(2):66–72, 2009.
2. Hockenberry M, Wilson D: *Wong's nursing care of infants and children*, ed 9, St Louis, 2011, Mosby/Elsevier.
3. McCance K, Huether S: *Pathophysiology*, ed 6, St Louis, 2010, Mosby/Elsevier.

4. Centers for Disease Control and Prevention: *Heat-related deaths—United States, 1999-2003*, 2011. Retrieved from www.cdc.gov/mmwr/preview/mmwrhtml/mm5529a2.htm.

5. Centers for Disease Control and Prevention: *Hypothermia-related deaths—United States, 1999-2002 and 2005*, 2011. Retrieved from www.cdc.gov/mmwr/preview/mmwrhtml/mm5510a5.htm.

6. Department of Geosciences: *Hyperthermia deaths of children in vehicles*, 2011. Available at http://ggweather.com/heat/.

7. Centers for Disease Control and Prevention: Hypothermia-related deaths, United States, 2003, *MMMR Wkly Rep* 53(8):172–173, 2004.

8. Lewis S, Dirksen S, Heitkemper M, et al: *Medical-surgical nursing: assessment and management of clinical problems*, St Louis, 2011, Mosby/Elsevier.

9. Thibodeau G, Patton K: *Structure and function of the body*, ed 13, St Louis, 2008, Elsevier.

10. McLafferty E, Farley A, Hendry C: Prevention of hypothermia, *Nurs Older People* 21(4):34–38, 2009.

11. Hildebrandt B, Wust P, Ahlers O: The cellular and molecular basis of hyperthermia, *Crit Rev Oncol/Hematol* 43:33–56, 2002.

12. Lu S, Dai Y: Normal body temperature and the effects of age, sex, ambient temperature and body mass index on normal oral temperature: a prospective, comparative study, *Int J Nurs Stud* 46:661–668, 2008.

13. Miller CA: *Nursing for wellness in older adults*, Philadelphia, 2009, Lippincott Williams & Wilkins, pp 530–538.

14. National Cancer Institute: 2010. *Fever*. Retrieved from www.cancer.gov/cancertopics/pdq/supportivecare/fever/HealthProfessional/page1.

15. Malignant Hyperthermia Association of the United States (MHAUS): *Emergency therapy for malignant hyperthermia*, 2008. Retrieved from http://medical.mhaus.org/PubData/PDFs/treatmentposter.pdf.

16. Adamides A, Winter C, Lewis P, et al: Current controversies in the management of patients with severe traumatic brain injury, *ANZ J Surg* 76(3):163–174, 2006.

10

Cellular Regulation

Barbara Damron and Jean Giddens

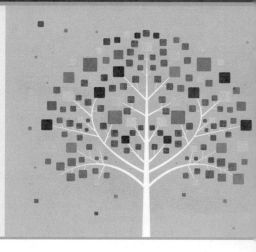

> *The cell is always speaking—the secret is to learn its language.*
>
> **Andrew S. Bajer, Cell Biologist**

Cells are the smallest form of life; they are the functional and structural units of all living things. The regulation of cellular activity—across the lifespan of the cell and between individual cells—is an intricate and accurate process. To keep our bodies healthy and running smoothly, cells are constantly working, changing, sending and responding to chemical cues, and correcting mistakes whenever possible. However, because of a variety of factors, mistakes within this process can occur, leading to cellular changes. Unfortunately, changes in cellular regulation can significantly impact biophysical health, psychosocial health, and functional status. Nurses should be familiar with the scope and process of cellular regulation, the consequences of altered cellular regulation, and the health care priorities to implement when conditions of altered cellular regulation develop.

DEFINITION(S)

The term cellular regulation refers to all functions carried out within the cells to maintain homeostasis, including their responses to extracellular signals (e.g., hormones, neurotransmitters) and the way each cell produces an intracellular response.[1] Included within these functions is cellular *replication* and *growth*. Common terms used to describe detailed aspects of cellular reproduction and growth include *proliferation* and *differentiation*. *Proliferation* refers to the reproduction of new cells through cell division. *Differentiation* refers to the acquisition of a specific cell function; this is a normal process by which a less specialized cell becomes a more specialized cell type. These terms are further described later in this chapter. Another important term associated with this concept is *neoplasia*, an abnormal and progressive multiplication of cells, leading to the formation of a neoplasm. A *neoplasm* (also known as a tumor) refers to new and abnormal tissue growth that is uncontrolled and progressive. The two categories of neoplasms are *benign* and *malignant* (or cancerous).

SCOPE AND CATEGORIES

The concept of cellular regulation is very broad and represents all aspects of cellular functioning. Several of the basic functions that cells have in common include creating fuel for the body, manufacturing proteins, transporting materials, and disposing of wastes. Included in cellular regulation is cellular division and reproduction, which is strictly controlled for normal cells. The scope of this concept analysis will focus on the *cellular growth and reproduction* aspect of cellular regulation, ranging from optimal cellular growth and reproduction to errors in replication and growth resulting in neoplasia. The development of pathologic conditions as a result of neoplasia depends on the location, growth rate, and characteristics of the neoplastic tissue.

RISK FACTORS

As mentioned previously, cellular regulation is a normal and expected physiologic process. However, problems associated with excessive growth and/or inappropriate cellular reproduction are common. An estimated 1,596,670 new cancer cases (excluding basal and squamous cell skin cancers) will be diagnosed in 2011 with an estimated 571,950 cancer deaths.[2] Among men, the three most common new cancer sites are prostate, lung/bronchus, and colon/rectum; for women the top three sites are breast, lung/bronchus, and colon/rectum. Lung cancer is the most common cause of death among men and women followed by breast and colorectal among women and prostate and colorectal cancers among men. An estimated 11,210 children will be diagnosed with cancer in 2011. Leukemia and cancers affecting the brain or central nervous system are the most common childhood cancers; combined, they represent more than 50% of all new cases in children.[3]

Age

One of the greatest risk factors for cancer is advanced age. The probability of developing invasive cancer increases exponentially as a person ages. For example, between ages 40 and 59, the probability of developing cancer (among those who were previously cancer free) is 8% for men and 9% for women. The probability increases to 30% for men and 25% for women age 70 and older.[2] It is estimated that 75% of new cancer diagnoses occur among those ages 55 and older. In contrast, cancer among children is relatively rare, representing less than 1% of all new cancer cases.

Smoking

Another clear risk factor for cancer is smoking. At least 30% of all cancer-related deaths and 87% of all lung cancer deaths can be attributed to smoking. Smoking increases the risk for many other cancers, including those involving the nasopharynx, nasal cavity, lip, oral cavity, pharynx, esophagus, pancreas, ovary, kidney, and bladder as well as colorectal cancers and some leukemias. Smoking is also a major risk factor for cardiovascular disease and death. Because of smoking's association with two major causes of death, smoking cessation is a major health policy agenda.[4,5]

Nutrition and Physical Activity

In addition to smoking, poor nutrition and a sedentary lifestyle—along with excessive weight—represent significant risk factors. In fact, more than 30% of all cancers are attributed to these risk factors combined, which is equal to smoking. Being overweight or obese is associated with increased risk for developing cancers and cancer recurrence. Weight loss has been shown to reduce cancer risk, although the exact mechanism is not well understood. Increased physical activity is believed to decrease cancer risk both by reducing obesity through improved energy metabolism and by improving the circulation of hormones that affect cellular reproduction and growth.[2]

Carcinogens

Environmental carcinogens are associated with the development of many cancers. As mentioned earlier, smoking is the most important of all carcinogens. Other environmental carcinogens play a less important role, but are worth mentioning—these include sun exposure; environmental pollutants in the air, water, soil, or food (such as radon or asbestos); or a consequence of medical treatments (such as medications and radiation). Although exposure to these other carcinogens is thought to account for only 6% of cancer deaths, a large number of people are affected (an estimated 34,320 in 2011)[2] and most of these cases occur disproportionately among lower income workers and communities, contributing to cancer disparities within the population.

Genetic Risk

Several general risk factors for cancer are known. Only a small percentage of cancers (about 5%) have a strong hereditary risk, meaning that a person has inherited a genetic alteration that is associated with developing certain types of cancer. Several familial risks are well documented—first-degree relatives and the development of breast cancer is an example.

Racial and Socioeconomic Disparities

When cancer death rates are evaluated across populations, certain racial groups have higher risk. For years the differences were attributed to biologic differences, but this link is actually not clear. Such differences may actually be partly explained by social disparities, such as the ability to obtain recommended screenings.[6] When educational and socioeconomic variables are controlled, racial differences are much less significant.

PHYSIOLOGIC PROCESSES AND CONSEQUENCES

Normal Cellular Reproduction and Growth

Cellular replication is an incredibly efficient process with millions of cells generated daily over the course of one's life. New cells are formed through a process of cell division, a process referred to as proliferation. The rate of proliferation varies according to the tissue involved. For example, rapid proliferation occurs within epithelial cells, bone marrow, and the gastrointestinal (GI) tract while slow proliferation occurs in muscles, cartilage, and bone.

There are two kinds of normal cell division: mitosis and meiosis. *Mitosis* is essentially a duplication process: two genetically identical "daughter" cells are produced from a single "parent" cell. Mitosis takes place in cells in all parts of the body, keeping tissues and organs in optimal working order. Normal cells capable of mitosis divide for only one of two reasons: to develop normal tissues or to replace lost or damaged normal tissues. *Meiosis* is quite different, generating daughter cells that are distinct from one another and from the original parent cell. Essentially all cells undergo mitosis, but only a few special cells are capable of meiosis—those that will become eggs in females and sperm in males. Basically, mitosis is for growth and maintenance and meiosis is for sexual reproduction.

Replication

Cellular replication is activated in the presence of cellular degeneration and death or on the basis of physiologic need—that is, new cells are created at the same rate as old cells die. The determination and timing of cellular division are strictly controlled by molecular "stop" and "go" signals. For example, when a wound occurs injured cells send go signals to the surrounding cells, which respond by growing and dividing and in time sealing over the wound. Conversely, stop signals are initiated when a cell is in a nutrient-poor environment. However, stop and go signals can function abnormally. A go signal can be produced when it should not be, and a stop signal can be ignored—and could result in uncontrolled growth and neoplasia. It takes more than one incorrect stop or go signal for neoplasia to occur; the human body is quite efficient at protecting its essential systems, and it usually requires multiple errors for healthy cells to turn malignant.[7]

With normal reproduction, cells proceed through a cycle (known as the cell cycle) that is produced by mitosis and that lasts until the cell undergoes its own mitosis and splits in two. This is done in an orderly progression whereby certain steps need to precede others in order for the process to work. The cell cycle is divided into distinct phases: G1 (gap 1), S (synthesis), G2 (gap 2), and M (mitosis, or division). The cell must leave the resting state, G0, in order to enter the cell cycle. G1 through G2 is known as interphase, during which chromosomes (the genetic material) are copied and cells typically double in size. During the M phase, mitosis (or cellular division) occurs, leading to the formation of an identical cell. Entering the cell cycle is an irreversible act and commits the cell to eventual mitosis. Cells can become trapped in any stage of the cell cycle, but they do not reverse the process and go backwards to G0. The most fundamental aspect of cell-cycle control is the regulation of entry and exit.

Differentiation

Most mature normal cells are functionally and morphologically differentiated. *Differentiation* means that a cell acquires functions that are *different* from those of the original type. This is a normal process by which a less specialized cell develops or matures to possess a more distinct form and function; it becomes a more specialized cell type. *Morphology* refers to the science of structure and form without regard to function. Each cell type has a specific morphology and at least one specific function. All normal cells contain the total amount of genetic material that is appropriate for the species. Even though all normal cells contain a full complement of human genes, not all genes are active in every cell.

Surveillance of Cellular Replication and Growth

Normal cellular replication and growth requires accurate cell signaling. Signaling is similar to a complex communication system, sending critical blueprint information within the cell (intracellular coding) and among cells (from one cell to another). Signaling occurs in multiple steps throughout the cell cycle. There are many factors that can negatively impact cellular signaling such as genetic mutations and protein abnormalities. When a signaling mistake is made, surveillance mechanisms usually recognize the error and either repair or destroy the cell, preventing replication of the error. This process maintains accurate replication.

Abnormal Cellular Replication and Growth and Consequences

Despite the efficiency of cellular reproduction and growth, mistakes can occur at several points within the cell cycle. As stated previously, usually surveillance factors recognize incorrect coding or replication and destroy cells that have been incorrectly produced. However, when a signaling

TABLE 10-1	COMPARISON OF BENIGN AND MALIGNANT NEOPLASMS	
CHARACTERISTIC	**BENIGN**	**MALIGNANT**
Encapsulated	Usually	Rarely
Differentiated	Normally	Poorly
Metastasis	Absent	Capable
Recurrence	Rare	Possible
Vascularity	Slight	Moderate to marked
Mode of growth	Expansive	Infiltrative and expansive
Cell characteristics	Fairly normal; similar to parent cells	Cells abnormal, become more unlike parent cells

From Lewis SL et al: *Medical surgical nursing*, ed 8, St Louis, 2011, Mosby/Elsevier.

mistake remains undetected or when repair is incomplete or ineffective (known as surveillance failure), cellular mutations can occur and can lead to neoplasia, and the formation of neoplasms. Comparisons between benign and malignant neoplasms are presented in Table 10-1.

Benign Neoplasm

Benign neoplastic cells arise from normal differentiated cells. They tend to retain most of the morphologic and functional characteristics of the normal cells from which they arose. They do, however, represent groups of abnormal cells with excessive growth. Benign cells are capable of mitosis, but are not capable of metastasis. Examples of common benign neoplastic tissues include endometriosis, nevi, and hypertrophic scars.

Benign tumors are generally far less concerning than are malignant tumors because they do not invade adjacent tissue or metastasize. However, benign tumors can result in significant health consequences. A benign tumor can obstruct or press on other body structures, resulting in pain, physiologic dysfunction, or even death attributable to their continued presence and growth. As an example, a benign enlargement of the prostate gland pushes inward on the urethra, making it gradually more difficult to void. If left untreated, urinary retention results and can lead to other complications such as urinary tract infections and pyelonephritis. Benign brain tumors are troubling because the enlarged tumor compresses brain structures and leads to various manifestations of neurologic dysfunction, depending on the size and location of the tumor. Some benign tumors are visible and can impact the physical appearance of an individual—lipomas are one example.

Malignant Neoplasm

A malignant neoplasm (cancer) is a disease of the cell that is characterized by abnormal function, growth, and dissemination of affected cells. An alteration within the cell cycle leads to excessive cell proliferation (reproduction rapidly and repeatedly of new parts, as by cell division), poor differentiation, and a longer than typical cell lifespan. Malignant neoplastic cells arise from normal differentiated cells, but over time and with errors in replication, they lose normal cell characteristics and acquire new characteristics. Unfortunately, the new characteristics that persist typically give the malignant cell an advantage and allow it and its offspring to thrive and survive, even when surrounded by unfavorable conditions. In cell culture, malignant cells are considered to be immortal. The farther along the continuum of malignancy a cancer cell is, the less it has in common with the parent tissue from which it arose. Multiple factors are associated with the development of each type of cancer and occur in an orderly process involving several stages over a period of time.[8] The stages include initiation, promotion, and progression.

- **Initiation stage:** This first stage is an irreversible mutation of a gene that may lead to malignant transformation. The cell may appear somewhat abnormal, but it is still able to carry out its original functions. The mutation at this point does not impair the cell's ability to replicate; otherwise, the cell would die.
- **Promotion stage:** To become malignant, the cell must enter this stage. There is usually a latency period between initiation and promotion; many factors influence the length of the latency period. The promoting agent stimulates the growth and division of a cell; it does not act on the deoxyribonucleic acid (DNA) directly. Promoting elements have a threshold—a minimum dose that is required before they stimulate the growth of the cancer cell.
- **Progression:** This is the final stage in the natural history of the development of cancer and refers to the series of changes that lead to an undifferentiated cell. Included in this stage is increased growth rate of the tumor, increased invasive ability of the tumor, and metastasis—the spread of the cancer to other sites in the body. During metastasis, certain cells in the tumor undergo genetic changes that allow them to migrate to and remain in distant organs, as well as establish a blood supply.

Malignant tumors are programmed to spread, invade, and destroy normal tissue. Like any other tissue, cancer tumors require oxygen and nutrition to sustain the rapid growth. While the tumor grows, it forms blood vessels to provide the tumor nourishment. This process, known as tumor angiogenesis, facilitates further growth and invasion capability. Typically, blood vessels formed within the tumor are friable (fragile) and break easily, leading to bleeding and anemia.[9] While the tumor increases in size and metastasizes, it literally acts like a parasite, robbing normal body tissues of nutrients and oxygen and destroying invaded tissues. Unless treatment is successful, the result is fatigue, weight loss, pain, organ failure, and death.

Despite the fact that many cancers are curable, people often associate the term cancer with pain and death. Thus several psychosocial consequences are associated with a diagnosis of cancer; among the most common are fear, stress, and anxiety. When a tumor is first discovered, patients and their family members often experience tremendous stress for days to weeks during the diagnostic process. Often, the fear of the unknown is reportedly worse than the diagnosis itself. Some individuals cope with this process through a mechanism of denial whereas others become very proactive and interested in every aspect of the diagnostic and/or treatment process. When a child is diagnosed with cancer, the entire family (child, parents, and siblings) is impacted. Parents often exhibit depression, stress, and anxiety; children commonly experience fear, anger, guilt, and grief, often expressed through behavioral changes.[10]

In addition to fear and anxiety, several other psychosocial consequences of cancer occur. Changes in family dynamics are common. Financial challenges often occur as a result of medical expenses and reduced or lost income associated with diagnostic and treatment processes. Changes in self-image and self-identify, particularly for those who experience significant role change or changes in physical appearance as a result of the disease process, can lead to alterations in interpersonal relationships and the development of mood disorders. The psychosocial effects of cancer are particularly pronounced for cancer survivors and their families when cancer reoccurs.[11]

ASSESSMENT

Assessment involves the collection of data gained from a health history, physical examination, and diagnostic studies. It is not the intention of this chapter to describe the process of assessment, nor is it the intention to describe the specific findings of all problems associated with cellular reproduction and growth because these are highly variable based on the tissue, organ, or system involved. However, several presenting symptoms or clinical findings serve as "red flags"—findings that are unusual and worthy of further investigation. Nurses should have an awareness of the significance of these symptoms and findings.

History

Initially, individuals are usually asymptomatic when neoplasms begin to develop. While the tumor grows, an individual may become aware of its presence or notice symptoms caused by the tumor. The most common presenting complaints include discovery of a lump, mass, or lesion as well as concerns regarding symptoms (such as unusual or unexplained bleeding, pain, cough, or fatigue), changes in appearance (such as the skin or an area of the body), or signs associated with alterations in major body functions (such as changes in appetite, weight, mental status, swallowing, or elimination). Often, symptoms are vague and the nurse should conduct a symptom analysis to collect as much information as possible. This would include questions regarding the duration of the symptom as well as its location, characteristics, aggravating factors, relieving factors, and treatments undertaken if any.[12] In addition to documenting the symptoms, these questions also provide early information about the patient's coping and/or potential denial. A medical history, a family history, and a psychosocial history are taken to provide additional information that may prove to be valuable (for example, a previous or family history of cancer, a history of smoking).

Examination

When a patient presents with a specific symptom (as noted earlier) that raises concern, the examination can be targeted to learn more about the presenting problem. However, patients do not always experience symptoms; thus the nurse should always maintain vigilance for possible indicators when conducting any physical exam. Abnormal findings that could suggest the presence of a neoplasm include visible lesions, physical asymmetry, palpable masses, and the presence of blood (pelvic exam or guaiac test for occult blood).[12]

Diagnostic Tests

A diagnostic workup is indicated when a symptom, examination finding, or screening test suggests the presence of a tumor. The following tests are those most commonly used in the detection and diagnosis of tumors.

Radiographic Tests

Radiographic tests provide an image of tumors so that size and location can be assessed. The most common radiographic tests used for the diagnostic process related to cellular regulation include radiographs (x-rays), magnetic resonance imaging (MRI), computed tomography (CT) or radioisotope scans, ultrasound, and diagnostic mammography.[13]

Direct Visualization

Some tumors can be evaluated by insertion of a lighted scope into a lumen or body cavity (e.g., colonoscopy, endoscopy, sigmoidoscopy). These tests not only provide visualization but also allow procurement of samples for pathologic analysis.

Laboratory Tests

Several laboratory tests are useful in the diagnostic process. Perhaps the two most useful tests associated with the diagnostic process are the complete blood count (CBC) and the chemistry panel. Although these are not diagnostic in themselves for neoplasms, they can provide information about overall health status and potentially important clues of the presence of neoplasms. For example, an undiagnosed malignancy might first be detected in an individual with unexplained anemia or changes in white blood cells. A limited number of genetic/tumor markers can be detected in the blood and some of these are helpful in determining risk. As an example, *BRCA1* and *BRCA2* genes are linked to breast cancer.[2]

Pathology

The term *pathology* refers to the study of disease. From the perspective of diagnostic study, pathology refers to the examination of tissues and cells. It is the only definitive way to determine if tumor cells are malignant or benign. Pathologic evaluation of the tissue also provides valuable information needed to treat the tumor such as the tissue type (histology) and the degree of differentiation (grade) of the tumor.

Cytology is the microscopic study of cells. Because this relates to diagnostic testing for cellular regulation, cells are obtained either through an aspiration technique (called aspiration biopsy cytology) or from a smear, washing, or scraping. The cells are then evaluated for characteristics of malignancy.

Biopsy involves removal of tissue for pathologic review. Incisional biopsy involves the removal of part of the tumor for evaluation while excisional biopsy is the removal of the entire tumor for tissue pathology evaluation. Different biopsy approaches are done based on the location and tissue to be evaluated. These include through the skin (percutaneous), through a scope (endoscopic), or directly during surgery. Percutaneous and endoscopic biopsy procedures are often facilitated with stereotactic approaches—a process in which exact points within the body can be located precisely.[13]

Classification: Grading and Staging

If a malignant tumor is found, clinical staging is done as part of the diagnostic workup. This includes determining the size of the tumor, the location of the tumor, and the presence or absence of metastasis. Grading includes determining the origin of the malignancy based on the tissue type and anatomic site, the histologic grade of the tumor (that is, the degree of differentiation), and the extent of disease classification.

Grading Cellular Differentiation

Grading is the measure of the degree of differentiation of neoplasms. Some pathology grading systems apply only to malignant neoplasms (cancer); others apply also to benign neoplasms. The neoplastic grading is a measure of cell *anaplasia* (lack of differentiation) in the sampled tumors arising from the *hyperplasia* (excessive proliferation of cells) of normal tissue. Several grading systems classify the microscopic cell appearance abnormality, including the American Joint Commission on Cancer[14] (Box 10-1), the Gleason Score[15] (used to grade prostate cancer), the Bloom-Richardson grading system[16] (used to grade breast cancer), and the Fuhrman system[17] (used to grade kidney cancer). A cancer cell that is well differentiated is more like the normal cell; one that is poorly differentiated is usually a more advanced cancer, with less form and function of the original normal cell.

Clinical Staging

A consistent mechanism used for clinical staging for most cancers is the TNM Classification System.[14] The staging is based on three factors: **T**umor size and invasiveness; presence or absence of regional spread to lymph **N**odes; and **M**etastasis

---

BOX 10-1   GRADING SYSTEM OF THE AMERICAN JOINT COMMITTEE ON CANCER

- GX—Grade cannot be assessed
- G1—Well differentiated (low grade)
- G2—Moderately differentiated (intermediate grade)
- G3—Poorly differentiated (high grade)
- G4—Undifferentiated (high grade)

to distant organs (Table 10-2). Although the TNM Classification System is used for the majority of cancers, not all cancers can be staged in this way because of variability in the growth and distribution of malignant cells. Examples include leukemias and brain cancers.

COLLABORATIVE CARE

Primary Prevention

The cornerstone of primary prevention to reduce cancer risk is participating in regular physical activity, eating a balanced diet, and avoiding smoking and excessive sun exposure.[18] Combined, these risk factors account for nearly 60% of all cancers.[2] Six major topic areas associated with reducing cancer risk are found within *Healthy People 2020*, including Cancer History, Tobacco Use, Nutrition, Weight Status, Oral Health, and Genomics. Although not common, another primary prevention strategy is prophylactic surgery as advised by the patient's provider. As an example, a woman with multiple risk factors including the presence of the *BRCA1* genetic marker might elect to have a bilateral mastectomy to prevent the development of breast cancer.

The nurse has an instrumental role in primary prevention through patient education and community-based interventions aimed at reducing these risks. It is especially important to target children and young adults so that healthy behaviors begin early in life.

Secondary Prevention (Screening)

The goal of secondary prevention is early disease detection so that prompt treatment can be initiated. It is important to note that screening and diagnosis are two separate entities. Individuals who have positive screening tests are referred for a full diagnostic workup to determine the course of treatment needed, if any.

There are multiple types of cancer screening and a discussion of each is beyond the scope of this chapter. General principles of screenings include easy to reach/see/detect, reliability, and cost-effectiveness. Examples of common screening tests for cancer include a two-way mammography for breast cancer, prostate-specific antigen test for prostate cancer, and colonoscopy and guaiac test for occult blood in the stool for colon cancer. The U.S. Preventive Services Task Force establishes screening recommendations for the general population based on evidence;[19] because these are based on the latest scientific evidence, screening recommendations periodically change. Nurses have an important role associated with screening through patient education and the performance of many screening tests; thus it is critical for nurses to maintain an awareness of changes to screening recommendations.

Collaborative Interventions

Interventions for neoplasia are addressed in terms of treatment goals, which include cure, control, and palliation/end-of-life care. The following interventions may be used in various sequences.

Surgery

Surgery is the oldest method of cancer treatment. In addition to primary treatment, classic applications of surgery include diagnosis, staging, and cytoreduction (debulking). Surgery may also be used to prevent cancer, to relieve the symptoms of cancer (palliation), and to enhance functional and cosmetic outcomes. Although primary surgical resection is usually intended as a cure, surgery is frequently combined with other treatment modalities to improve cure rates and increase disease-free intervals. These additional therapies are called *adjuvant*, and may include chemotherapy or radiation therapy.[20,21]

Nursing care associated with the patient undergoing surgical procedures for any aspect of cancer (prevention, cure, palliation, reconstruction) includes patient education, pre- and

TABLE 10-2	TNM CLASSIFICATION SYSTEM
Primary Tumor (T)*	
TX	Tumor cannot be measured
T0	No evidence of primary tumor (tumor cannot be found)
Tis	Tumor in situ, meaning malignant cells only within superficial layer of tissue; no extension into deeper tissue
T1	Description of primary tumor based
T2	on size and/or invasion into nearby
T3	structures; the higher the T number,
T4	the larger the tumor and/or the more it has grown into nearby tissues
Regional Lymph Nodes (N)†	
NX	Nearby lymph nodes cannot be evaluated
N0	No evidence of cancer cells in regional lymph nodes
N1	Description of size, location, and/or
N2	number of lymph nodes involved;
N3	the higher the N number, the more extensive the lymph node involvement
Metastases (M)‡	
MX	Metastases cannot be evaluated
M0	No evidence of metastases can be found
M1	Description of extent of metastasis; the
M2	higher the M number, the more
M3	extensive the metastasis
M4	

*Describes the primary (original) tumor based on size (measured in centimeters).
†Describes whether or not the cancer has spread into regional (nearby) lymph nodes.
‡Describes whether or not the cancer has metastasized (spread) to other parts of the body.
From American Cancer Society: www.cancer.org/.

postoperative care, infection prevention, pain management, nutritional education, and psychosocial care.

Radiation Therapy

Radiation therapy is a local treatment for cancer and is used throughout the disease trajectory; it can take the form of either palliative or potentially curative treatment. Radiation is essentially considered packets of energy in the form of photons (such as x-rays and ultraviolet light) or particles (such as protons, neutrons, alpha-particles, and electrons).[22] When these packets of energy penetrate into the tissue and the cells, ionization can induce direct biologic damage within the cells. Radiation therapy may be delivered in several ways. The most common delivery system is external beam therapy using a linear accelerator. Another delivery system is brachytherapy, which provides high doses of radiation to a limited volume of tissue.[23] Radioactive materials are placed in or near the treatment site and radiation is administered by high-dose rate (HDR) or low-dose rate (LDR).[24] The nursing management of patients receiving either external beam radiation therapy or brachytherapy largely involves patient education and the management of symptoms associated with the therapies.

Chemotherapy

While the use of chemotherapy in the management of cancer dates back to the 1500s when heavy metals were used to treat a variety of cancers, modern chemotherapy began in the 1950s following World War II, when certain groups of chemicals, called alkylating agents, were recognized as having anti–cell growth effects. The word "chemotherapy" in general means treatment with chemicals; however, the term *chemotherapy* has evolved to mean the systemic treatment of cancer.[25] The purpose of treating cancer cells with chemotherapy is to prevent these cells from multiplying, invading, and metastasizing to distant sites. Unlike surgery or radiation therapies, which are local and regional treatments, chemotherapy is a systemic treatment that enables drugs to reach the site of the tumor as well as distant sites.[26,27]

Cancer chemotherapy is based upon the cell cycle. The cell cycle of the cancer cell is qualitatively the same as that of normal cells, and most chemotherapeutic drugs are classified according to the specific phase of the cell cycle in which they exert their cytotoxic effects. The role of the nurse in cancer chemotherapy is vast, pivotal, and rewarding. The nurse is responsible for the handling and administration of chemotherapeutic agents, the management of side effects, the assessment and education of the patient, and the management of psychosocial issues. Typically, nurses become chemotherapy certified through the Oncology Nursing Society before administering chemotherapy.

Hormonal Therapy

Another effective form of cancer treatment uses hormonal agents. The primary use of these agents is in the treatment of hormonally responsive cancers, such as breast, prostate, or endometrial cancers. Before the development of hormonal therapy, patients with these types of cancers would have been treated with an ablative surgical procedure (e.g., castration, adrenalectomy, oophorectomy) that would limit the production of hormones. Current approaches to treatment may include the use of hormonal agonists or antagonists, depending on the nature of the disease process. Hormonal therapies are very specific in their ability to block specific receptors and various feedback loops; these therapies were therefore the first form of targeted therapy.[28]

Targeted Therapy

Targeted therapies encompass the molecular and genetic biology of cancer, therefore creating a poignant need for nurses to understand cancer treatment from the perspective of basic cell functioning, the concept presented in this chapter. The signaling pathways that control the cellular processes are the basis upon which targeted therapy operates. Targeted therapies work differently from chemotherapy by interfering with the specific molecules involved in the processes of carcinogenesis, tumor growth, and metastasis. Molecular targeted therapies are directed at blocking any of the signaling processes responsible for the growth and spread of cancer cells.[29]

Biologic Therapy

Biotherapy (previously known as immunotherapy) refers to the modulation of the immune response. Biologic response modification, immunotherapy, and immune system modulation are some of the many terms that have been used through the years to represent the same therapeutic approach.[30] Biotherapy is generally used as a global term to describe the use of biologic agents to activate the immune system and treat cancer. It also includes biologic approaches that manipulate the immune system, such as gene therapy.[31] Biotherapy is sometimes considered the fourth treatment modality for patients with cancer (along with surgery, radiation therapy, and chemotherapy). Biologic agents are substances that are extracted or produced from biologic material. Biologic response modifiers are the agents used in biotherapy. Biotherapy includes treatments affecting other biologic responses such as growth and differentiation factors, chimeric molecules, and agents that influence the ability of tumor cells to metastasize.[32] Included within the category of biologic response modifiers are colony-stimulating factors, gene therapy, monoclonal antibodies, nonspecific immunomodulating agents, angiogenesis inhibitors, and vaccines.

The role of the nurse in providing quality care to patients receiving biotherapy includes side effect management, patient education, and psychosocial support. There are frequently economic issues for the patient receiving biotherapy.

Bone Marrow and Hematopoietic Stem Cell Transplantation

Hematopoietic stem cells are found in the bone marrow. These stem cells eventually proliferate into mature erythrocytes, leukocytes, and platelets. Hematopoietic stem cell transplantation is the process of replacing diseased, destroyed, or nonfunctioning hematopoietic cells (i.e., the bone marrow) with normally functioning, healthy hematopoietic progenitor cells, also called stem cells.[33,34] Bone marrow transplantation can be autologous (using one's own marrow), allogeneic (the donor is a matched sibling or family donor or unrelated donor), or syngeneic (the donor is an identical twin). Replacing diseased marrow is usually done for the purpose of cure or quality-of-life years gained. There are multiple and complicated issues with bone marrow transplantation and nurses working with bone marrow transplant patients need specialized training.

One of the most rapid changes in transplantation medicine has been the shift from bone marrow to peripheral and umbilical cord blood as a viable stem cell source. This treatment option involves the transfusion of stem cells (collected from peripheral blood) into a patient for the purpose of cure or quality-of-life years gained. The donor sources are either autologous (self) or allogeneic (other donor) and, as with bone marrow transplantation, numerous disease are treated with this approach. The nurse has roles similar to those of nurses involved in bone marrow transplantation.

Symptom Management Resulting from Cancer and Cancer Treatment

Individuals who have advanced cancer and those who undergo cancer treatment experience multiple complications, adverse effects, and side effects; thus nursing interventions are geared toward managing these complications. Psychosocial support is also an important component in cancer care. Supporting the individual and family members through the identification of coping mechanisms and resources is essential. Specific complications and adverse effects associated with all the treatment modalities previously discussed are beyond the scope of this chapter. The most common and important

complications/side effects are briefly presented in the Interrelated Concepts section that follows.

INTERRELATED CONCEPTS

Cellular regulation is closely related to many concepts presented in this textbook. The interrelated concepts can be associated with the process of the disease itself, a consequence of the treatment, or both. The most important interrelated concepts are presented in Figure 10-1 and briefly described in the following list.

Nutrition. Many cancer patients experience protein and calorie malnutrition. Cancerous cells rob nutrients from the body to sustain the rapid cellular growth and expansion. Additionally, because of significant side effects, many individuals undergoing cancer treatment lose weight from reduced or lost appetite, nausea, stomatitis, or an inability to eat as part of the disease process.[8,24,26]

Immunity. Compromised immune functioning commonly results as a consequence of disease or as a side effect among those who take chemotherapy agents or undergo radiation therapy.[8,24,26]

Infection. Immunodeficiency leads to a significant risk for infection—in fact, infection is a common cause of death for patients with cancer. Immunodeficiency often masks common signs and symptoms of infection. This can be fatal if there is a delay in recognition and treatment.[8,24,26]

Pain. Pain is a very common symptom associated with cancer. Of all cancer symptoms, pain is among the most feared. Pain is a complex symptom to manage because of the wide variability in pain perception, an individual's unique interpretation of the pain, past pain experiences, cultural influences on pain perception, and response to treatment.

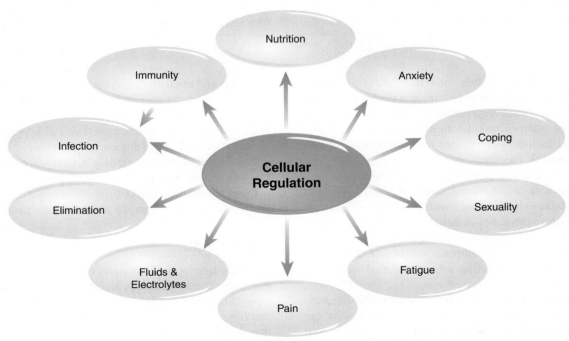

FIGURE 10-1 Cellular Regulation and Interrelated Concepts.

MODEL CASE

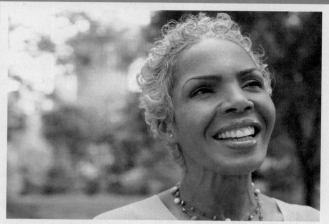

Katrina Wells, a 54-year-old African-American female, works a sedentary job in telecommunications; it is a job that has limited health care benefits. She has been overweight most of her life (beginning in early adolescence) and has never engaged in physical activity on a regular basis. Katrina became pregnant with her first child at age 16 and never finished high school. Because of limited finances, Katrina only seeks health care when she is ill.

Through a community outreach program, Katrina met a nurse, Lydia Robinson, who helped her gain access to basic preventive health care services; because of the advice of the nurse and the support of the services, Katrina agreed to have a screening mammogram. Katrina heard about mammography exams from women at work and understood it was a test for breast cancer. A radiologist reviewing the mammography films discovered a small mass in Katrina's left breast, in the upper outer quadrant near the axilla. Katrina was contacted by the radiologist and was told she had an abnormal mammography result and that she needed to return to the imaging center for further workup. Katrina, not knowing what this meant, asked if she had cancer. She was told that cancer was a possibility, and further testing was needed to determine if this was the case.

Katrina was upset with this information and was not sure she wanted any more tests. Her mother had breast cancer and she watched her mother lose her breast and hair, and she was very sick from the medications. Katrina became fearful of a similar outcome and decided the best course of action was to ignore the mammography results. She did not return to the imaging center on the scheduled day. When contacted by the scheduler, Katrina responded that she could not get off work and was too busy. Lydia Robinson, the nurse at the community outreach program, reached out to Katrina and helped her understand the need for the workup.

Over the next 4 weeks, Katrina underwent several diagnostic tests as part of her diagnostic workup. Each step of the way, Lydia helped Katrina by explaining the process and providing emotional support. The diagnostic mammogram and ultrasound examination of the breast revealed a 7.4-mm lesion. A needle biopsy was performed, which confirmed a diagnosis of breast cancer. Katrina was referred to a surgical and medical oncologist at the local cancer center for treatment. An oncology clinical nurse specialist at the cancer center met with Katrina at the time of her first oncology appointment to begin helping her through the treatment process.

Case Analysis

This case exemplifies several aspects of cellular regulation gone awry. Katrina had several important risk factors for cancer: obesity, sedentary lifestyle, family history of cancer, and limited access to health care. Health policy initiatives for community outreach programs have been instituted to reduce cancer disparities; without these initiatives, it is unlikely Katrina would have been screened. Katrina experienced common fears and anxiety associated with a diagnostic workup for cancer. The nurse helped Katrina cope with these fears and assisted Katrina throughout the diagnostic process. A caring atmosphere exemplified by the health care providers at the cancer center is just as important as the physical care they provide.

Unfortunately, pain is often underassessed and undertreated.[35] Pain can result when a tumor is pushing on other organs and as a consequence of tissue destruction. National standards for interprofessional approaches for cancer pain management include a combination of pharmacologic and nonpharmacologic measures.

Fatigue. Fatigue is a common symptom associated with cancer. Known as *cancer-related fatigue (CRF)*, the primary cause is thought to be associated with high levels of circulating inflammatory cytokines. A multitude of other contributing factors to CRF include side effects to medications (such as chemotherapy), anemia, anorexia, weight loss, depression, and general organ dysfunction often associated with later-stage cancer.[36]

Elimination. The effects of chemotherapy and radiation therapy often cause diarrhea. Also, bowel obstructions can occur as a result of the disease process (in the case of colorectal cancer) or an enlarged prostate can block urinary flow.

Fluids and electrolytes. Several fluid and electrolyte imbalances can occur as a result of cancer and cancer treatment. Third spacing of fluids, dehydration, syndrome of inappropriate antidiuretic hormone secretion, and hypercalcemia are common with advanced disease.

Additional concepts including **Anxiety, Mood and affect, Coping,** and **Sexuality** are interrelated to this concept because of the psychosocial impact (including changes in body image) associated with the diagnostic and treatment process.

EXEMPLARS

There are hundreds of examples of abnormal cellular reproduction and growth; in fact, there are more than 200 different types of cancer alone. It is beyond the scope of this chapter to describe all types of abnormalities related to cellular regulation; however, some of the most common are presented in Box 10-2. Specific and accurate information related to each

■■■ BOX 10-2   EXEMPLARS OF CELLULAR REGULATION

Benign Tumors
- Adenoma
- Benign prostate hypertrophy
- Benign brain tumor
- Fibroma
- Lipoma
- Meningioma
- Papilloma
- Rhabdomyoma

Malignant Tumors

Carcinoma and Adenocarcinoma (Originate from Skin, Glands, Mucous Membrane Lining of Respiratory, Gastrointestinal, and Genitourinary Tracts)
- Breast cancer
- Prostate cancer
- Lung cancer
- Colon cancer

Sarcoma (Originates from Muscle/Bone/Connective Tissues)
- Chondrosarcoma
- Ewing's sarcoma
- Fibrosarcoma
- Kaposi sarcoma
- Rhabdomyosarcoma
- Osteosarcoma

Lymphomas (Originates from Lymph System)
- Hodgkin's lymphoma
- Non-Hodgkin's lymphoma

Leukemia (Originates from Hematopoietic System)
- Chronic lymphocytic leukemia (CLL)
- Chronic myeloid leukemia (CML)
- Acute lymphocytic leukemia (ALL)*
- Acute myeloid leukemia (AML)*

*Common among children.

of these exemplars is readily available in nursing and medical textbooks, as well as on select websites, such as those of the American Cancer Society (www.cancer.org/) and the National Cancer Institute (www.cancer.gov/).

■■■
ACCESS EXEMPLAR LINKS ON pageburst

REFERENCES

1. Rosenberg SA: Principles of surgical oncology: general issues. In DeVita VT, Hellman S, Rosenberg SA, editors: *Cancer: principles & practice of oncology*, Philadelphia, 2005, Lippincott Williams & Wilkins.
2. American Cancer Society: *Cancer facts and figures*, Atlanta, 2011, Author.
3. National Cancer Institute: *Fact sheet: childhood cancers*, 2008. Retrieved from www.cancer.gov/cancertopics/factsheet/Sites-Types/childhood.
4. Secretan B, Straif K, Baan R, et al: A review of human carcinogens—part E: tobacco, areca nut, alcohol, coal smoke, and salted fish, *Lancet Oncol* 10(11):1033–1034, 2009.
5. U.S. Department of Health and Human Services (USDHHS): *The health consequences of smoking—a report of the Surgeon General*, Rockville, Md, 2004, USDHHS, Public Health Service, Centers for Disease Control and Prevention, Center for Chronic Disease Prevention and Health Promotion, Office on Smoking and Health.
6. Centers for Disease Control and Prevention, *Health disparities in cancer*, 2011. Retrieved from www.cdc.gov/cancer/healthdisparities/.
7. U.S. Department of Health and Human Services: *Inside the cell* NIH Pub No. 05–1051, Rockville, Md, Sept 2005, USDHHS, National Institutes of Health, National Institute of General Medical Sciences.
8. Cady J, Jackowski JA, et al: Cancer. In Lewis SL, editor: *Medical-surgical nursing*, ed 8, St Louis, 2011, Mosby/Elsevier.
9. McCance K, Huether S: *Pathophysiology: the biologic basis for disease in adults & children*, ed 8, St Louis, 2010, Mosby/Elsevier.
10. Peek G, Melnyk BM: Coping interventions for parents of children newly diagnosed with cancer: an evidence review with implications for clinical practice and future research, *Pediatr Nurs* 36(6):306–313, 2010.
11. Vivar CG, Navidad C, Canga A, et al: The psychosocial impact of recurrence on cancer survivors and family members: a narrative review, *J Adv Nurs* 65(4):724–736, 2009.
12. Wilson S, Giddens J: *Health assessment for nursing practice*, ed 4, St Louis, 2009, Mosby/Elsevier.
13. Pagana KD, Pagana TJ: *Mosby's diagnostic and laboratory test reference*, ed 10, St Louis, 2011, Mosby/Elsevier.
14. Edge SB, Bryd DR, Compton CC, et al: *AJCC cancer staging manual*, ed 7, New York, 2009, Springer.
15. Egevad L, Granfors T, Karlberg L, et al: Prognostic value of the Gleason Score in prostate cancer, *Br J Urol* 89(6):538–542, 2002.
16. American Cancer Society: *How is breast cancer diagnosed?* Retrieved from www.cancer.org/Cancer/BreastCancer/DetailedGuide/breast-cancer-diagnosis.
17. National Cancer Institute: *Tumor grade.* Retrieved from www.cancer.gov/cancertopics/factsheet/detection/tumor-grade.
18. U.S. Department of Health and Human Services: *Healthy People, 2020.* Accessed at www.healthypeople.gov.
19. U.S. Preventive Services Task Force: *Recommendations.* Retrieved from www.uspreventiveservicestaskforce.org/recommendations.htm.
20. Lester J: Surgery. In Langhorne ME, Fulton JS, Otto SE, editors: *Oncology nursing*, ed 5, St Louis, 2007, Mosby/Elsevier, pp 337–345.
21. Payne Y: Surgical therapy. In Newton S, Hickey M, Marrs J, editors: *Mosby's oncology nursing advisory: a comprehensive guide to clinical practice*, St Louis, 2009, Mosby/Elsevier, pp 139–140.
22. Connell PP, Martel MK, Hellman S: Principles of radiation oncology. In DeVita VT, Hellman S, Rosenberg SA, editors: *Cancer: principles & practice of oncology*, Philadelphia, 2005, Lippincott Williams & Wilkins.

23. Strohl R: Radiation therapy. In Newton S, Hickey M, Marrs J, editors: *Mosby's oncology nursing advisory: a comprehensive guide to clinical practice*, St Louis, 2009, Mosby/Elsevier, pp 140–142.

24. Aistars J: Radiation therapy. In Langhorne ME, Fulton JS, Otto SE, editors: *Oncology nursing*, ed 5, St Louis, 2007, Mosby/Elsevier, pp 346–361.

25. Chu D: Drug development. In DeVita VT, Hellman S, Rosenberg SA, editors: *Cancer: principles & practice of oncology*, Philadelphia, 2005, Lippincott Williams & Wilkins.

26. Otto S: Chemotherapy. In Langhorne ME, Fulton JS, Otto SE, editors: *Oncology nursing*, ed 5, St Louis, 2007, Mosby/Elsevier, pp 362–376.

27. Wells JH, Murphy M: Chemotherapy. In Newton S, Hickey M, Marrs J, editors: *Mosby's oncology nursing advisory: a comprehensive guide to clinical practice*, St Louis, 2009, Mosby/Elsevier, pp 183–196.

28. Orbaugh K: Hormonal therapy. In Newton S, Hickey M, Marrs J, editors: *Mosby's oncology nursing advisory: a comprehensive guide to clinical practice*, St Louis, 2009, Mosby/Elsevier, pp 314–316.

29. Remer S: Targeted therapy. In Newton S, Hickey M, Marrs J, editors: *Mosby's oncology nursing advisory: a comprehensive guide to clinical practice*, St Louis, 2009, Mosby/Elsevier, pp 287–297.

30. Rothaermel JM, Baum B: Biological response modifiers. In Newton S, Hickey M, Marrs J, editors: *Mosby's oncology nursing advisory: a comprehensive guide to clinical practice*, St Louis, 2009, Mosby/Elsevier, pp 161–172.

31. DeMeyer E, Stein B: Biotherapy. In Miaskowski C, Buchsel P, editors: *Oncology nursing: assessment and clinical care*, St Louis, 1999, Mosby.

32. Appel CP: Biotherapy. In Langhorne ME, Fulton JS, Otto SE, editors: *Oncology nursing*, ed 5, St Louis, 2007, Mosby/Elsevier, pp 377–387.

33. Keller C: Bone marrow and stem cell transplant. In Langhorne ME, Fulton JS, Otto SE, editors: *Oncology nursing*, ed 5, St Louis, 2007, Mosby/Elsevier, pp 388–401.

34. Mitchell SA: Hematopoietic stem cell transplantation. In Newton S, Hickey M, Marrs J, editors: *Mosby's oncology nursing advisory: a comprehensive guide to clinical practice*, St Louis, 2009, Mosby/Elsevier, pp 142–160.

35. Oncology Nurses Society: *Cancer pain management*. Retrieved from www.ons.org/Publications/Positions/Pain/.

36. Hawthorn M: Fatigue in patients with advanced cancer, *Int J Palliat Nurs* 16(11):536–541, 2010.

Intracranial Regulation

Debra J. Smith

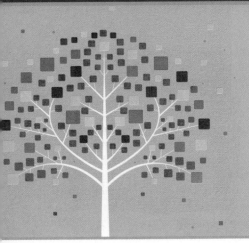

The brain is a highly complex organ that processes internal and external stimuli and controls body functions. As the largest component of the central nervous system, the brain lies within the cranium and is protected by the skull. The Intracranial Regulation (ICR) concept includes normal and abnormal processes of cranial function.

DEFINITION(S)

The term *cranium* refers to the collective bone structure of the head—also known as the skull.[1] The prefix *intra-* refers to within. Thus the term intracranial refers to those components that lie within the skull, which include the brain, circulatory system, and dura mater. *Regulation* is a term that refers to compliance and maintenance of balance. In the case of ICR, it is referring to maintaining a balance to promote an environment that is conducive to optimal brain functioning. The concept of ICR includes anything that affects the contents of the cranium and impacts the regulation of maintaining an optimally functioning brain. For the purpose of this concept analysis ICR is defined as *mechanisms or conditions that impact intracranial processing and function.* Though the brain receives input from outside the cranium, specifically through the peripheral nervous system and the spinal cord component of the central nervous system, this concept does not include problems with the peripheral nervous system or spinal cord. ICR focuses on those conditions that specifically affect the contents of the cranium. As will be discussed further, there are many variables that can upset this balance with potentially devastating results.

SCOPE AND CATEGORIES

Scope

The scope of this concept ranges from normal to impaired function. There are several categories that describe impairment or dysfunction associated with ICR. These include problems associated with perfusion, neurotransmission, and pathologic processes. These categories are briefly described next, and the pathologic consequences of these impairments are detailed in the sections that follow.

Categories

Perfusion

For the brain to function optimally, there must be a consistent supply of blood, delivering oxygen and nutrients. Intracerebral perfusion can be disrupted in a number of different conditions such as internal blockage of a vessel, severe hypotension, or loss of vessel integrity attributable to damage or excessive external pressure on a vessel that exceeds perfusion pressure. For example, an ischemic stroke is the result of inadequate perfusion past the thrombus or embolus. Perfusion can also be disrupted as the result of an intracranial hemorrhage, such as a subdural hematoma or subarachnoid hemorrhage caused by a traumatic brain injury (TBI). A disruption of cerebral perfusion leads to a wide variety of ICR problems depending on the area of the brain that is affected and the length of time before perfusion is restored.

Neurotransmission

Optimal functioning of the brain is dependent on the transmission of nerve impulses across neuronal synapses by neurotransmitters. Normal transmission requires fully functioning neurons, nerves, and neurotransmitters. Presynaptic neurons release neurotransmitters that travel to postsynaptic neurons. Neurotransmitters can be either excitatory or inhibitory. There are many components of this process that can be disrupted. Degenerative diseases (see Pathology section) disrupt brain functioning by the loss of neurons, which also disrupts neurotransmission. The concentration of the neurotransmitter acetylcholine is reduced in Alzheimer's disease secondary to the destruction of acetylcholine-secreting neurons. Neurotransmitters can be affected by drugs and toxins, which can modify their function or block their attachment to receptor sites on the postsynaptic membrane. For example, heroin binds to presynaptic endorphin receptors and reduces pain by blocking the release of the neurotransmitter that causes pain.[2] Seizures are aberrant neuronal activity that can manifest clinically as disrupted motor control, sensory perception, behavior, and/or autonomic function.

Pathology

There are many pathologic states that disrupt intracranial functioning and regulation. Pathology of the brain can take many forms, such as brain tumors, degenerative diseases, and inflammatory conditions.

Many degenerative diseases of the brain are exemplars of the ICR concept. Alzheimer's disease is a degenerative process that results in the loss of neurons primarily in the gray matter of the brain. Parkinson's disease is a result of damage to the basal ganglia, and Huntington's disease is a degeneration of striatal neurons. Though the degenerative process varies with each of these diseases, the result is the same—disruption of brain function and regulation.

The most common inflammatory conditions of the brain are abscesses, meningitis, and encephalitis. Although the etiology varies with each condition, the result is an inflammatory response that can result in disrupted cerebral function and regulation.

RISK FACTORS

All populations are potentially at risk for problems with ICR, because there are such a wide variety of conditions included in this concept. Depending on the condition, some populations are at a higher risk. ICR problems related to degenerative pathology have a higher incidence in the elderly population. Injury-related ICR problems are more commonly seen in the adolescent and young adult age groups. The leading causes of TBI are falls and motor vehicle accidents.[3] Falls are more of an issue with the very young and elderly populations; and because of risk-taking behavior, motor vehicle accidents are more prevalent in the young adult population.

Personal risk factors are dependent on the cause of injury or pathology. For example, the risk factors for stroke include age, hypertension, diabetes, smoking, obesity, and cardiovascular disease. Some of the degenerative pathologic conditions have a strong genetic component, and put certain individuals at higher risk.

PHYSIOLOGIC PROCESSES AND CONSEQUENCES

There are several unique physiologic processes in place to protect and preserve critical brain functions. When there is impaired blood flow, compromised neurotransmission, and damage to brain tissue from trauma or other pathologic conditions, pathophysiologic consequences occur. The expected physiologic functions and consequences of impaired intracranial regulation are discussed.

Expected Physiologic Function
Cranial Vault/Skull

The skull is composed of multiple bones that act as a rigid, noncompliant protective covering of the brain. Within the skull are three components: brain tissue (80%), blood (10%), cerebrospinal fluid (CSF) (10%). Intracranial pressure (ICP) is the sum of the pressure exerted by these three volumes in the skull. In adults, ICP is normally ≤15 mm Hg; ≥20 mm Hg is considered intracranial hypertension (ICH). Normal ICP is somewhat lower in children and newborns.[4] Sutures are ossified by age 12 years, with no expansion of the skull after 5 years old.[5] Before the sutures are entirely closed, there is some room for expansion in the case of cerebral edema and increasing ICP.

Because the total volume inside the skull cannot change, a change in one component necessitates a change in another. This interrelationship of volume and compliance of the three cranial components is known as the Monro-Kellie doctrine.[6]

Blood-Brain Barrier

Between the arterial and venous network of the brain is a unique capillary system called the blood-brain barrier (BBB), consisting of a tight layer of endothelial cells. This restrictive barrier makes it difficult for neurotoxic substances to pass into the brain. This barrier may become compromised secondary to decreased perfusion.[7]

Meninges

There are three layers of protective membranes that surround the brain and spinal cord: dura mater, arachnoid layer, and pia mater. The area between the arachnoid layer and pia mater is referred to as the subarachnoid space, which contains CSF. ICR problems are frequently referred to in relation to the meningeal layer location—for example, subarachnoid hemorrhage, subdural hematoma, or epidural hematoma. Meningitis is an inflammatory condition of the meninges.

Glucose

Because the brain cannot store glucose, a constant supply is needed to maintain optimal functioning. Areas of the brain that are particularly sensitive to hypoglycemia are the cerebral cortex, hippocampus, and cerebellum. Prolonged hypoglycemia may cause widespread neuronal injury.[8] Children, who have smaller glycogen stores, are particularly susceptible to hypoglycemia, which can adversely affect brain tissue.

Hyperglycemia (glucose level >126 mg/dl) can also cause problems by augmenting brain injury in acute stroke. Some of the deleterious effects of hyperglycemia are worsened ischemic damage, an increased infarction size, and increased BBB permeability. The optimal glucose range is being studied, but yet to be determined.[9]

Autoregulation

Cerebral blood flow (CBF) is normally maintained at a relatively constant rate by intrinsic cerebral mechanisms referred to as autoregulation. Autoregulation adjusts regional CBF in response to the brain's metabolic demands by changing the diameter of cerebral blood vessels. Cerebral arterial walls are thinner than those in the systemic circulation because of a lack of smooth muscle and a decreased thickness of the tunica media. They also do not have the ability to develop collateral circulation in response to ischemia. Autoregulation allows the cerebral circulation to deliver a constant supply of blood despite wide fluctuations in systemic blood pressure. It becomes impaired when the mean arterial pressure (MAP) is <70 mm Hg or >170 mm Hg, if intracranial pressure (ICP) is >40 mm Hg, or as a result of localized or global cerebral injury.[7]

Cerebral Spinal Fluid

CSF is produced at a rate of approximately 20 ml/hour, circulates within the subarachnoid space, and then is absorbed into the venous system. It acts to cushion and support the brain and other structures of the central nervous system and provides nutrients. CSF analysis provides useful diagnostic information related to certain nervous system conditions (see Diagnostic Tests).

Hyperventilation

Another protective mechanism in response to increasing cerebral volume is spontaneous hyperventilation. Carbon dioxide is a potent vasodilator. Hyperventilation is a compensatory mechanism that causes vasoconstriction, which reduces cerebral blood volume and ICP.

Physiologic Consequences of Impaired Intracranial Regulation

Cerebral Edema

Cerebral or brain parenchymal edema occurs for many reasons. Box 11-1 shows common causes of cerebral edema. It is a symptom that is common to many ICR conditions. Cerebral edema may be classified as vasogenic, cytotoxic, or interstitial. Regardless of the classification or origin of cerebral edema, the result is an increase in brain size that will negatively affect perfusion and oxygenation to the brain. As discussed next, signs and symptoms will become evident to varying degrees based on the location and amount of cerebral edema.

Increased Intracranial Pressure

Elevated ICP is a potentially devastating complication of neurologic injury. Pathologic ICP is present at sustained pressures ≥20 mm Hg. Several conditions may cause increased ICP, such as traumatic brain injury (TBI), ruptured aneurysm, central nervous system (CNS) infections, hydrocephalus, and brain tumors. Symptoms of increased ICP include headache, decreased level of consciousness, and vomiting. Signs may include cranial nerve VI palsies, papilledema, and periorbital bruising; a late sign may be the manifestation of Cushing's triad (see Intracranial Pressure [ICP] Monitoring).[6] The untoward consequence of increased ICP is impaired perfusion (see Measurement of Cerebral Perfusion Pressure).

Brain Tumors

A tumor can occur in any part of the brain and spinal cord. Brain tumors are most commonly a result of metastasis from another primary site outside the brain. Clinical

---

BOX 11-1 CAUSES OF CEREBRAL EDEMA

Mass Lesions
- Brain abscess
- Brain tumor (primary or metastatic)
- Hematoma (intracerebral, subdural, epidural)
- Hemorrhage (intracerebral, cerebellar, brainstem)

Head Injuries and Brain Surgery
- Contusion
- Hemorrhage
- Posttraumatic brain swelling

Cerebral Infection
- Meningitis
- Encephalitis

Vascular Insult
- Anoxic and ischemic episodes
- Cerebral infarction (thrombotic or embolic)
- Venous sinus thrombosis

Toxic or Metabolic Encephalopathic Conditions
- Lead or arsenic intoxication
- Hepatic encephalopathy
- Uremia

From Lewis SL, Dirksen SR, Heitkemper MM et al: *Medical-surgical nursing: assessment and management of clinical problems,* ed 8, St Louis, 2011, Mosby/Elsevier.

---

manifestations will depend on the size and location of the tumor.

ASSESSMENT

History

A thorough history should be solicited from the patient or a family member if the patient is unable to provide information. Patient presentation will help direct the practitioner to the most relevant areas of inquiry. Information in a history that provides data about intracranial function can relate to multiple systems. Asking pertinent questions will provide clues to the examiner of ICR problems and will help to focus the physical examination. Potential ICR areas on which to focus include the following:

- Numbness, paralysis, tingling, neuralgia
- Loss of consciousness, dizziness, fainting, confusion
- Changes in recent or remote memory
- Changes in vision, hearing, balance, gait
- Speech problems (expressive and/or receptive)
- Chewing/swallowing problems
- Muscle weakness or loss of bowel or urinary control
- Onset of unexplained tremors or other motion disturbances
- Unexplained, severe headache
- Vomiting
- Symptom onset
- History of head injury

Physical Examination Findings

Objective examination findings that convey neurologic status are found throughout a physical examination. Specific signs of dysfunction vary depending on the ICR problem. There are many age-related degenerative changes that occur in the central nervous system (CNS). When assessing an older adult, it is important to distinguish between these expected changes and changes potentially related to an ICR problem that could improve with appropriate treatment. Findings common to most conditions are a change in mental status and motor function. Some of the more common examination techniques and tools will be discussed next, but are not all-inclusive.

Mental Status

A complete mental status examination includes thorough assessment of the individual in the following categories: general description, emotional state, experiences, thinking, sensorium, and cognition. Depending on the patient's presenting condition, the nurse will decide which components of the exam are relevant.[10] If it is not practical or necessary to do a complete mental status exam, the Mini-Mental Status Examination is an option, which is a simplified scored form of the cognitive portion of the mental status examination. It consists of 11 questions and takes only 5 to 10 minutes to administer.[11]

A subtle change in cognitive and motor functioning occurs in the very old.[12] When assessing an elderly patient, it is essential to determine the patient's baseline neurologic functioning in order to establish if there are significant changes.

Glasgow Coma Scale

The Glasgow Coma Scale (GCS) was developed by Teasdale and Jennett in 1974[13] to give a standardized numeric score of the neurologic patient assessment. This is a widely used measurement tool that consists of three components: eye opening, verbal response, and motor response. Although this is an objective measurement tool, there is room for subjective interpretation of assessment findings. To minimize subjectivity and support consistency, when transferring care of a patient, nurses should complete the GCS together and agree on the values. Changes in the GCS will help to determine treatment methods and priorities. Table 11-1 shows an example of the Glasgow Coma Scale. A coma is characterized by the total absence of arousal and awareness lasting greater than 1 hour. Generally, for adults a GCS score ≤8 is considered a coma; for children it is considered a GCS score ≤5. Clinical signs that correlate with poor prognosis after coma include the score for the motor component of GCS, the length of time in a coma, and signs of brainstem damage.[14]

Cranial Nerves

As the name implies, the cranial nerves originate in the cranium; therefore assessment of the cranial nerves should be included in a thorough neurologic assessment. Abnormal findings will help to locate the affected area of the brain.

TABLE 11-1 GLASGOW COMA SCALE

APPROPRIATE STIMULUS	RESPONSE	SCORE
Eyes Open Approach to bedside Verbal command Pain	Spontaneous response	4
	Opening of eyes to name or command	3
	Lack of opening of eyes to previous stimuli but opening to pain	2
	Lack of opening of eyes to any stimulus	1
	Untestable*	U
Best Verbal Response Verbal questioning with maximum arousal	Appropriate orientation, conversant; correct identification of self, place, year, and month	5
	Confusion; conversant, but disorientation in one or more spheres	4
	Inappropriate or disorganized use of words (e.g., cursing), lack of sustained conversation	3
	Incomprehensible words, sounds (e.g., moaning)	2
	Lack of sound, even with painful stimuli	1
	Untestable*	U
Best Motor Response Verbal command (e.g., "raise your arm, hold up two fingers") Pain (pressure on proximal nail bed)	Obedience of command	6
	Localization of pain, lack of obedience but presence of attempts to remove offending stimulus	5
	Flexion withdrawal, *flexion of arm in response to pain without abnormal flexion posture	4
	Abnormal flexion, flexing of arm at elbow and pronation, making a fist	3
	Abnormal extension, extension of arm at elbow usually with abduction and internal rotation of arm at shoulder	2
	Lack of response	1
	Untestable*	U

*Added to the original scale by some centers.

From Lewis SL, Dirksen SR, Heitkemper MM et al: *Medical-surgical nursing: assessment and management of clinical problems,* ed 8, St Louis, 2011, Mosby/Elsevier.

Assessment procedures can be found in nursing assessment textbooks.

Intracranial Pressure (ICP)

The earliest sign of increased ICP is a change in level of consciousness. Another early sign is headache. Headache characteristics associated with increased ICP include nocturnal awakening, pain worsened by cough/defecation, recurrent and localized, progressive increase in frequency or severity.[15] Vomiting, usually not preceded by nausea, is often a nonspecific sign of increased ICP.

Infants have less specific symptoms of increased ICP, such as irritability, bulging fontanel, lethargy, flat affect, and poor feeding. Retinal hemorrhage in children with increased ICP should raise suspicion of nonaccidental head trauma. Infants with elevated ICP may develop macrocephaly, split sutures, or a bulging fontanel.[4]

ICP is measured using a catheter placed in one of the following locations in the cranium: intraventricular, intraparenchymal, subarachnoid, or epidural (Figure 11-1). The most common placement is in the lateral ventricle. Patients must be in an intensive care environment for this type of monitoring. Most commonly, ICP monitoring is done in trauma patients with a closed head injury. Some other indications include stroke, intracerebral hemorrhage, hydrocephalus, and subarachnoid hemorrhage. Guidelines for management of severe head injury recommend that ICP monitoring is indicated in comatose head injury patients with a GCS score of 3 to 8 and with an abnormal computerized tomography (CT) scan. The goal of care is to keep ICP <20 mm Hg.[16]

If hydrocephalus is present, a ventriculostomy may be used to remove CSF. There are catheters available that are able to monitor ICP, drain CSF, and measure brain oxygenation. In children, a "sun setting" appearance of the eyes is evident.[4]

The relationship between ICP and blood pressure was first recognized and described by Cushing in 1901[13] and is useful in explaining the late signs of increased ICP. Cushing's triad is an ominous late sign of increased ICP and an indication of impending herniation. The triad consists of hypertension (with widened pulse pressure), bradycardia, and changes in respiratory pattern in the presence of increased ICP. Pupil and vision changes may become apparent as edema impinges on cranial nerves II, III, IV, and/or VI.

Measurement of Cerebral Perfusion Pressure

Cerebral blood flow increases with hypercapnia and hypoxia. Ischemia results from inadequate cerebral perfusion or increased cerebral oxygen consumption. To maintain adequate perfusion, it is necessary to optimize cerebral perfusion pressure (CPP), which is calculated by subtracting the ICP from the mean arterial pressure (MAP). When CPP is <60 mm Hg, cerebral blood flow is compromised and autoregulation is impaired.[6] CPP should be kept between 60 and 70 mm Hg in patients with elevated ICP to avoid ischemic injury. CPP >70 mm Hg should be avoided because of an increased risk for adult respiratory distress syndrome.[15]

Normal CPP range for children is not well established, but is likely lower than that of adults because systolic blood pressure is lower in children. Appropriate CPP values are probably 50 to 60 mm Hg.[4]

The National Institutes of Health Stroke Scale (NIHSS)

This scale is an example of one type of specific tool for nurses to use when assessing a patient following stroke. This scale, composed of 11 items, has been widely used and validated. The NIHSS score on admission has been correlated to stroke outcome and is recommended for all patients with suspected stroke.[9,17]

Diagnostic Tests

When an ICR problem is suspected, time is of the essence. Diagnostic tests that can quickly give the most pertinent information are recommended initially.

Neuroimaging Studies

Imaging studies are essential to obtain in patients presenting with sudden neurologic deterioration, and may also be utilized with nonemergent conditions such as suspected brain tumor. A noncontrast computed tomography (CT) or magnetic resonance imaging (MRI) scan should be performed as quickly as possible to determine the origin of a neurologic injury. Current guidelines recommend a head CT for all TBI patients with a GCS of 14 or lower, which can detect skull fractures, intracranial hematomas, and cerebral edema.[18] There are advanced CT and MRI technologies available, such as magnetic resonance angiography (MRA) and positron emission tomography (PET), that are able to distinguish between brain tissue that is irreversibly infarcted and potentially salvageable, which will help when deciding appropriate treatment.

The number of CNS neurons decreases in the geriatric patient, with a resulting decrease in brain weight and size. This change is seen primarily in the frontal lobe and will appear as atrophy on CT scan or MRI. There is also decreased adherence of the dura mater to the skull, fibrosis, thickening of the meninges, and an increase in the subarachnoid space.

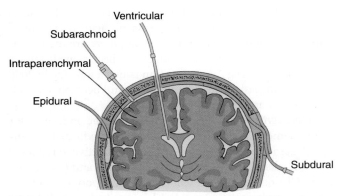

FIGURE 11-1 Coronal Section of Brain Showing Potential Sites for Placement of ICP Monitoring Devices. (From Lewis SL, Dirksen SR, Heitkemper MM et al: *Medical-surgical nursing: assessment and management of clinical problems,* ed 8, St Louis, 2011, Elsevier.)

Skull Radiograph

Depending on the mechanism of action and patient presentation, a skull x-ray may be ordered to detect fractures, bone erosion, calcification, and/or abnormal vasculature.

Electroencephalogram (EEG)

An EEG measures and records the brain's electrical activity through multiple electrodes placed on the scalp. Video EEG monitoring refers to continuous EEG monitoring over a prolonged period of time while simultaneously recording the patient's movements and activity. This monitoring combination is useful in diagnosing and localizing the area of seizure origin. By ruling out seizures, the EEG is also helpful in identifying psychogenic nonepileptic seizures, also known as pseudoseizures (emotional or stress related in origin).

Brain Biopsy

To determine the type and stage of a brain tumor, a biopsy is performed, usually during a surgical procedure. Preliminary histologic type can usually be determined quickly in the operating room; then the tumor is sent to pathology for complete analysis and final determination.

Lumbar Puncture

The lumbar puncture (spinal tap) may be indicated when infection is suspected. A lumbar puncture should be deferred until after the head CT scan if intracranial hypertension is suspected because herniation may be precipitated by increasing the pressure gradient.

CLINICAL MANAGMENT

Primary Prevention

Primary prevention strategies are intended to maintain optimal health and prevent injury or disease. This applies to intracranial regulation in many ways. Leading a healthy lifestyle, which includes stopping smoking, maintaining a healthy weight, controlling blood pressure, and exercising, can decrease the risk of vascular disease impacting the cerebral arteries. This is linked to risk reduction for stroke. Injury prevention measures such as proper use of seat belts and/or helmets, knowledge of firearm safety, and participation in violence prevention programs reduce the risk of TBI. *Healthy People 2020*[19] has identified the following three objectives specifically related to the prevention/reduction of brain injury:

- Reduce fatal traumatic brain injuries.
- Reduce hospitalization for nonfatal traumatic brain injuries.
- Reduce emergency department visits for nonfatal traumatic brain injuries.

Secondary Prevention (Screening)

There are no true screening tests available related to ICR. In the event of injury or the presence of clinical findings suggesting intracranial dysfunction, specific diagnostics tests are initiated to determine a cause.

Collaborative Interventions

There are many interventions related to caring for patients with ICR issues. A few common examples, not covering all possible interventions, will be discussed. The overarching goal of caring for patients is to prevent secondary injury (damage to the vulnerable adjacent tissues) by improving cerebral perfusion; this is primarily achieved by decreasing cerebral edema and ICP, which will improve oxygenation to prevent cell death.

Pharmacotherapy

Osmotic diuretics. Osmotic diuretics create an osmolar gradient that draws water across the BBB, leading to a decrease in interstitial volume and a subsequent decrease in ICP. Mannitol is the agent used most commonly to achieve ICP control in a variety of conditions, and has been shown to improve cerebral blood flow. Hypertonic saline is increasingly being used, but the research has not clearly determined the volume, tonicity, or most effective method of administration.[18]

Sedatives. Sedatives can decrease ICP by reducing metabolic demand. Propofol (Diprivan) is frequently used in the intensive care unit (ICU) setting because it has a short half-life and is easily titrated, permitting frequent neurologic assessment. Barbiturate coma is sometimes used as a final effort in the case of uncontrolled increased ICP, but there is little clinical evidence to support its use.[18] Benzodiazepines, such as lorazepam (Ativan), are another sedative option.

Analgesics. Pain increases oxygen demand; therefore in addition to controlling pain for patient comfort, it should be controlled to avoid compromising sufficient oxygen delivery to ischemic neuronal cells. The use and choice of sedative agents should be individualized according to specific clinical circumstances and provider expertise. Short-acting narcotics, such as fentanyl or morphine, are generally preferable to allow for periodic neurologic assessments.

Antiepileptics. Seizures can exacerbate or cause increased ICP and increase oxygen demand. Antiepileptics may be used as a prophylactic or treatment measure. The incidence of posttraumatic seizures may be as high as 30% in severe TBI patients.[18] These medications act by stabilizing nerve cell membranes and preventing the distribution of the epileptic discharge. Initial seizure management of TBI patients includes phenytoin (Dilantin) or valproic acid (Depakote).[17] Patient education is important because there are many serious side effects associated with antiepileptic medications. The Food and Drug Administration issued a warning in 2008 related to the risk of suicidal thoughts and behaviors associated with 11 antiepileptic medications.[20]

Glucocorticoids. Glucocorticoids may be indicated for use in some ICR problems and are contraindicated in others. Dexamethasone (Decadron) may be effective in reducing cerebral edema related to tumors, abscesses, and CNS infections. Glucocorticoids are associated with a poor outcome in treating moderate to severe head injury and should not be used in this patient population.[15]

Antipyretics. Fever may worsen the outcome after stroke and severe head injury by aggravating secondary brain injury caused by increased metabolic demand. Normothermia should be maintained through the use of antipyretic medications, such as acetaminophen, or by implementation of other treatment modalities such as mechanical cooling.

Anti-hypertensive medications. Depending on the ICR condition, anti-hypertensive medications may be detrimental or beneficial. Mean arterial pressure must be adequate to maintain sufficient CPP to limit secondary injury. Because of this, higher systemic blood pressures are tolerated in patients with ICR conditions that impair CPP. In these patients, anti-hypertensive medications are not recommended, and medications may be initiated in order to sufficiently raise the systemic pressure, particularly if the ICP is elevated. Several studies have shown that lowering the systemic blood pressure in patients with acute ischemic stroke has been associated with clinical deterioration. Conversely, reducing blood pressure in patients with a hemorrhagic stroke may be beneficial by minimizing further bleeding and continued vascular damage.[9]

Labetalol (Trandate) is usually the first drug of choice if pharmacologic therapy is necessary in the acute phase. It allows rapid and safe titration to the goal blood pressure. Other first-line agents include transdermal nitroglycerin paste and intravenous nicardipine (Cardene).[9]

Antiparkinsonian medications. Antiparkinsonian medications attempt to restore the balance of dopamine through one of several mechanisms, depending on drug type. The most effective drugs, called dopaminergic drugs, replace dopamine, or mimic its action in the brain. Another group of drugs delays the breakdown of dopamine, thus increasing the level in the brain.

Levodopa (Sinemet) is the most commonly used antiparkinsonian medication; it is converted to dopamine in the CNS, where it serves as a neurotransmitter. To minimize the side effects of dopamine in the periphery, another medication is administered with levodopa. In the United States this drug is carbidopa, which prevents the conversion of levodopa to dopamine until it reaches the brain.

Dopamine agonists mimic the effect of dopamine by stimulating the same cells as dopamine. Examples are pramipexole (Mirapex), ropinirole (Requip), and bromocriptine (Cycloset). Monoamine oxidase B (MAO-B) is an enzyme that breaks down levodopa in the brain. MAO-B inhibitors prolong the effectiveness of dopamine and also levodopa. The most common example of this type of medication is selegiline (Carbex).

Cholinesterase inhibitors. Cholinesterase inhibitors are prescribed to patients with mild to moderate dementia to make acetylcholine more available, improving cortical function. Examples include donepezil (Aricept), rivastigmine (Exelon), and galantamine (Reminyl). In moderate to severe dementia, an *N*-methyl-D-aspartate (NMDA) receptor antagonist, such as memantine (Namenda), may have a neuroprotective function as well as decrease dementia symptoms. It does not, however, slow progression of the disease.[21]

Surgery

Many types of cranial surgery are available to address ICR problems. Some examples are craniotomy, craniectomy, and shunt and stereotactic procedures.

A *decompressive craniectomy* removes the rigid confines of the skull, allowing for expansion of the cranial contents and lowering the ICP. Potential complications of this surgery may include herniation through the skull defect, spinal fluid leakage, wound infection, and epidural and subdural hematoma.

A *craniotomy* may be performed to remove a lesion or tumor, to repair a damaged area, or to relieve pressure and/or drain blood secondary to epidural, subdural, or intracerebral hematomas.

Frequently the origin of seizures is located in either the hippocampus or the amygdala, which is located in the temporal lobe of the brain (see Diagnostic Tests: EEG). If seizures are found to arise from these areas, a temporal lobectomy surgery is performed to resect the identified area. This surgery is becoming more common and has been successful in obtaining seizure control.

Stereotactic procedures allow precise localization of a specific area of the brain and may be utilized for dissection or to obtain a biopsy (Figure 11-2).

Shunt procedures place an artificial pathway for excessive CSF to be drained from an area of the brain to an extracranial location using a tube or implanted device. Accumulation of CSF may be due to overproduction, obstruction, or problems with normal reabsorption. Placement of a ventriculoperitoneal shunt is a common example of this type of procedure.

Ongoing Assessment

With prevention of secondary injury being the goal of patient care, it is of upmost importance to recognize changes in the patient's condition early. For this reason, thorough and frequent neurologic assessment is critical in the care of a patient with ICR problems. A complete neurologic assessment includes

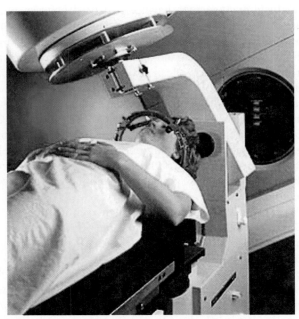

FIGURE 11-2 Stereotactic Frame. (From Lewis SL, Dirksen SR, Heitkemper MM et al: *Medical-surgical nursing: assessment and management of clinical problems*, ed 8, St Louis, 2011, Mosby/Elsevier.)

determination of level of consciousness (LOC) and measurement of GCS score along with motor and cognitive functioning.

Vital signs should be monitored consistently on all patients with an ICR problem. The frequency will be dictated by the condition and acuity of the patient. Assessment should be frequent enough to detect significant changes early so that the appropriate interventions can be implemented to prevent patient deterioration (see Cushing's triad under Intracranial Pressure Monitoring).

ICP/CPP Monitoring

As discussed earlier, it is imperative that the brain receive a constant, adequate blood supply to optimize brain functioning. Severely head-injured patients should receive continuous ICP and CPP monitoring. If these values are not optimal, there are several possible collaborative and nursing interventions available. Most guidelines recommend that treatment for elevated ICP should be initiated when ICP is >20 mm Hg.

Interventions to Lower ICP

Positioning. The intracranial venous system consists of canals and sinuses, and, unlike the peripheral venous system, lacks valves. Interventions promoting venous outflow from the head decrease cerebral volume, and help to lower ICP. Such interventions include head-of-bed elevation and proper alignment of the head and neck with the body. Head-of-bed elevation of 30 degrees is usually recommended to decrease ICP. It is also important to keep the head and neck midline (to prevent compression of jugular veins) and to limit hip flexion. Head-of-bed elevation potentially could decrease cerebral perfusion, by increasing venous return. Therefore head-of-bed elevation is recommended as long as the CPP remains at an appropriate level.

Activity management. Balance is needed between being efficient and not increasing oxygen demand when providing nursing care. Clustering of many nursing tasks at once will increase oxygen demand and may compromise cerebral perfusion. Distribution of care procedures over a longer time frame is preferable.

Airway management. Endotracheal suctioning stimulates coughing, which increases ICP. Patients with increased ICP should undergo endotracheal suctioning only when suctioning is indicated; in addition, these patients may need to be sedated before the procedure. Careful assessment is necessary to maintain an adequate airway and minimize complications of increased ICP.

Hyperventilation. Prophylactic hyperventilation ($Paco_2$ ≤25 mm Hg) in TBI is not recommended because it decreases perfusion, which will negatively impact oxygen delivery. Hyperventilation is recommended only as a temporary measure to reduce elevated ICP.[15] A 1 mm Hg change in $Paco_2$ is associated with a 3% change in cerebral blood flow.[6] Hyperventilation can also increase extracellular lactate and glutamate levels, which may contribute to secondary brain injury.[18]

Bowel management. Constipation increases intraabdominal pressure and causes straining when defecating, thereby raising ICP. Stool softeners or laxatives may be necessary to minimize these untoward effects on ICP.

Nutrition Management

Nutrition management is a high priority when caring for patients with ICR conditions. The nurse needs to advocate for an early dietary consultation in order to ensure prompt and adequate nutrition to facilitate healing. Depending on the ICR impairment and patient condition, enteral or parenteral feeding will be appropriate. Swallowing function should be assessed before initiation of enteral feeding for certain patients, particularly following a stroke.

Patient Education

Patient education is always a primary nursing function, which is no exception when caring for patients with ICR conditions. Education should be focused on all levels of health promotion (see Primary Prevention and following section, Rehabilitation). Problems involving the brain can have devastating and long-lasting effects. Nursing is uniquely qualified and available to assist patients and their families throughout the course of their care.

Rehabilitation

Particularly after a stroke or head injury, rehabilitation is an important part of patient care. The focus is on returning the patient to optimal functioning. The composition of the rehabilitation team will depend on the patient's needs, which may include speech therapy, physical therapy, and occupational therapy along with medical and nursing care as needed. As soon as the patient is stabilized in the acute care setting, rehabilitation should begin. It may take months to years to determine how much function will be regained.

INTERRELATED CONCEPTS

Many concepts are closely related to ICR; the concepts with the strongest linkages are depicted in Figure 11-3. **Cognitive function** is dependent on an optimally functioning

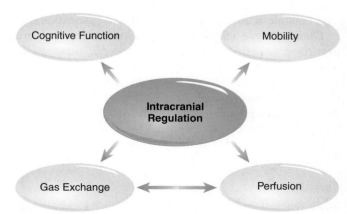

FIGURE 11-3 Intracranial Regulation and Interrelated Concepts.

brain. If ICR is disrupted, depending on the area of the brain affected, cognitive function may be impaired either temporarily or permanently. The degree of cognitive function impairment is dependent on the number of neuronal cells affected. Similarly, **Mobility** is frequently affected by ICR problems with the most common example being a cerebrovascular accident (CVA). **Perfusion and oxygenation** have been discussed thoroughly and are intimately involved with ICR. Without adequate perfusion and oxygenation the brain cannot function. Other concepts that may be related, but not included in the diagram, include **Clotting, Interpersonal violence,** and **Pain.**

MODEL CASE

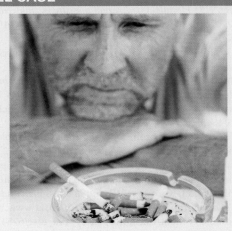

Mr. James Hobson is a 69-year-old male with a history of hypertension that is fairly well controlled on medication. He has been smoking 1 or 2 packs of cigarettes a day for the past 52 years and has a body mass index of 37.3. He awoke yesterday morning complaining of blurry vision and some weakness on the left side of his body. He thought he had just slept wrong so he was not concerned. Later in the morning he was having trouble walking and his wife convinced him to call his physician. The physician's office called 911, and Mr. Hobson was transported to the nearest hospital.

Upon arrival to the emergency department the physical exam findings were: HR 112 beats/min, BP 172/90 mm Hg, RR 24 breaths/min, O_2 Sat 90%, leg arm and leg weakness (3/5), and somewhat decreased sensation. He was awake and responding to questions appropriately, though slowly. The following diagnostics tests were ordered: noncontrast CT (NCCT) of the head; ECG; CBC with platelets, cardiac enzymes, and troponin; electrolytes; BUN; creatinine; glucose; PT/INR; and PTT. A NCCT will exclude or confirm the presence of hemorrhage. The sensitivity of a NCCT to show ischemia increases after 24 hours. This patient's CT scan did not show any signs of hemorrhage. Currently, thrombolytics are administered to treat an ischemic stroke within 3 hours of symptom onset. Studies are underway to evaluate the safety and efficacy of extending this window to 4½ hours. Because it was unclear exactly when the symptoms began, the decision was made not to administer a thrombolytic.

Case Analysis

A cerebrovascular accident (CVA) is an excellent exemplar of the ICR concept. The condition originates inside the cranium, which affects functioning within and outside the cranium. Sudden loss of focal brain function is the core feature of the onset of ischemic stroke.[9] Because of a clot (thrombotic or embolic), perfusion is compromised to areas of the brain distal to the blockage. Clinical manifestations will vary depending on the ischemic area of the brain. Other conditions may mimic a stroke presentation (seizures, syncope, migraine, hypoglycemia), so it is important to perform appropriate diagnostic testing early. A thorough history is imperative to determine onset of symptoms as early as possible, since this will determine treatment and time is of the essence—particularly in the case of an ischemic stroke. A CT scan or MRI will determine if a stroke has occurred and its origin—hemorrhagic or ischemic.

CONTRARY CASE

Mr. Anthony Williams, a 52-year-old male, noticed the following symptoms over a period of several months: progressive weakness of his arms, difficulty swallowing, and constipation. At first he attributed his symptoms to stress at work, but with a progression of symptoms he began to wonder if he had suffered a stroke. After a complete workup with his physician, Mr. Williams was diagnosed with amyotrophic lateral sclerosis (ALS), a progressive neurologic disorder characterized by loss of motor neurons in the spinal cord.

Contrary Case Analysis

This is not an exemplar of ICR because with ALS, electrical and chemical messages that originate in the brain do not reach the muscles. Motor function is affected, but the brain is functioning properly. Although the symptoms may be similar to those in other ICR exemplars, this exemplar does not fit the definition of the ICR concept.

EXEMPLARS

ICR concept exemplars are listed by category in Box 11-2. Though exemplars are listed under a specific category, there are instances when an exemplar could fit under more than one category. For example, brain tumors can be considered *Pathology* and can also cause problems with *Neurotransmission*. Similarly, if a brain tumor is large enough and exerts enough pressure, it can also disrupt *Perfusion*. The categories are not meant to be all-inclusive or exclusive, but a suggested organization framework for ICR conditions.

ACCESS EXEMPLAR LINKS ON **pageburst**

BOX 11-2   EXEMPLARS OF INTRACRANIAL REGULATION

Perfusion
Ischemic Stroke
- Embolic stroke
- Thrombotic stroke

Hemorrhagic Stroke
- Intracerebral hemorrhage
- Ruptured aneurysm
- Subarachnoid hemorrhage

Head Injury
- Epidural hematoma
- Skull fractures
- Subdural hematoma
- Traumatic brain injury

Neurologic Transmission
- Epilepsy
- Seizure

Pathology
Brain Neoplasm
- Benign brain tumor
- Malignant brain tumor

Degenerative Conditions
- Alzheimer's disease
- Dementia
- Huntington's disease
- Multiple sclerosis
- Parkinson's disease

Inflammatory Conditions
- Bacterial meningitis
- Brain abscess
- Encephalitis
- Viral meningitis

REFERENCES

1. *Stedman's medical dictionary for the health professions and nursing*, ed 6, Philadelphia, 2008, Lippincott Williams & Wilkins.
2. Lewis SL, Dirksen SR, Heitkemper MM, et al: *Medical-surgical nursing: assessment and management of clinical problems*, ed 8, St Louis, 2011, Mosby/Elsevier.
3. Centers for Disease Control and Prevention (CDC): *Leading causes of TBI.* Accessed Dec 27, 2010, at www.cdc.gov/TraumaticBrainInjury/causes.html.
4. Brasher WK: *Elevated intracranial pressure in children.* Accessed Nov 27, 2010, at. www.uptodate.com/online/content/topic.do?topicKey=ped_emer/5819.
5. Ball JW, Bindler R, Cowen KJ: *Child health nursing*, ed 2, New York, 2010, Pearson.
6. Smith ER, Amin-Hanjani S: *Evaluation and management of elevated intracranial pressure in adults.* Accessed Nov 27, 2010, at www.uptodate.com/online/content/topic.do?topicKey=cc_neuro/4543.
7. Eigsti J, Henke K: Anatomy and physiology of neurological compensatory mechanisms, *Dimens Crit Care Nurs* 25:5, 2006.
8. Kumar V, Abbas AK, Fausto N: *Robbins and Cotran pathologic basis of disease*, ed 7, Philadelphia, 2005, Elsevier/Saunders.
9. Oliveira-Filho J, Koroshetz WJ: *Initial assessment and management of acute stroke.* Accessed Nov 27, 2010, at www.uptodate.com/online/content/toic.do?topicKey=cva_dise/6754.
10. Stuart GW: *Principles and practice of psychiatric nursing*, ed 9, St Louis, 2009, Mosby/Elsevier.
11. *Mini-Mental Status Examination (MMSE).* Accessed Dec 29, 2010, at www.nmaging.state.nm.us/pdf_files/Mini_Mental_Status_Exam.pdf.
12. Ebersole P, Hess P, Touhy TA, et al: *Toward healthy aging: human needs & nursing response*, ed 7, St Louis, 2008, Mosby/Elsevier.
13. May K: The pathophysiology and causes of raised intracranial pressure, *Br J Nurs* 18:15, 2009.
14. Stevens RD, Bhardwaj A: Approach to the comatose patient, *Crit Care Med* 34:1, 2006.
15. Brain Trauma Foundation: *Guidelines for acute medical management of severe traumatic brain injury of infants, children and adolescents*, 2003. Accessed Dec 27, 2010, at www.braintrauma.org/pdf/protected/guidelines_pediatric.pdf.
16. Brain Trauma Foundation: *Guidelines for the management of severe traumatic brain injury*, ed 3, 2007. Accessed Dec 27, 2010, at www.braintrauma.org/pdf/protected/Guidelines_Management_2007w_bookmarks.pdf.
17. *National Institute of Health Stroke Scale (NIHSS).* Accessed Dec 28, 2010, at www.ninds.nih.gov/doctors/NIH_Stroke_Scale.pdf.
18. Phan N, Hemphill JC: *Management of acute severe traumatic brain injury.* Accessed Nov 27, 2010, at www.uptodate.com/online/content/topic.do?topicKey=medneuro/4782.
19. *Healthy People 2010.* U.S. Department of Public Health. Available at www.healthypeople.gov:2020.
20. U.S. Food & Drug Administration: *Suicidal thoughts and behavior: anti-epileptic drugs— overview.* Available at www.fda.gov/Drugs/DrugSafety/DrugSafetyPodcasts/ucm077078.htm.
21. Press D, Alexander M: *Treatment of dementia.* Accessed Feb 22, 2011, at www.uptodate.com/contents/treatment-of-dementia?source=search_result&selectedTitle=3%7E150.

Glucose Regulation

Nancy J. Peckenpaugh

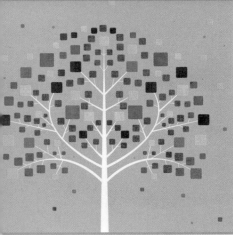

Glucose, with its carbon component, is fundamental to the process of human life. The metabolism of glucose at the cellular level is largely influenced by the body's regulatory processes through hormonal and metabolic enzymes. The need for glucose is particularly true of the neurologic system, with the brain and nerves being dependent on glucose for energy needs. Carbohydrates, used for metabolism, are essential for human life; when glucose metabolism becomes impaired, serious health consequences can occur. Because this concept represents a foundational basis of health, the nurse must possess a solid understanding of glucose regulation including the ability to recognize and respond to situations in which this process is impaired.

DEFINITION(S)

Glucose metabolism represents a very complex physiologic process by which glucose is utilized by the body. Glucose metabolism is influenced by multiple variables, but the ultimate end result on a cellular level is the use of glucose for energy—or adenosine triphosphate (ATP)—synthesis. The efficiency of glucose metabolism is reflected in circulating blood glucose levels. The concept glucose regulation refers to *the process of maintaining optimal blood glucose levels.*

Several additional key terms related to this concept are important to mention. *Glycogen* is the storage form of glucose. Most glycogen is stored in the liver. The term *glycogenolysis* refers to the physiologic process of breaking down glycogen to increase blood glucose concentration to an optimal level. This process is facilitated by *counter-regulatory hormones.* Specifically, counter-regulatory hormones (e.g., glucagon, epinephrine, cortisol, growth hormone, and norepinephrine) lead to utilization of glycogen stores; levels of these hormones are also increased with stress-related conditions, both physical (such as pain, illness, and injury) and emotional, and are therefore often referred to as stress hormones. Another hormone, insulin, is produced by the beta-cells in the pancreas and is the only hormone that allows transfer of blood glucose

into body cells, thus decreasing blood glucose concentration to an optimal level after ingestion of carbohydrates. The term *insulin resistance* refers to a state in which the body cells resist the action of insulin. Insulin resistance is an underlying problem in many conditions that contribute to impaired glucose metabolism and regulation. One final definition basic to an understanding of glucose regulation is *gluconeogenesis.* This is a process in which nitrogen is cleaved from protein sources (dietary or lean muscle tissue), resulting in the creation of glucose. Gluconeogenesis is required if blood glucose and glycogen stores are insufficient. Gluconeogenesis can also occur with stress conditions, from hormonal changes, or from use of steroid medications, with resulting increased risk of loss of muscle mass.

SCOPE AND CATEGORIES

The scope of glucose regulation can conceptually be represented by the categories of normal/optimal regulation and impaired regulation. Normal blood glucose (BG) levels range between 70 and 140 mg/dl at all times (both preprandial and postprandial); this state is referred to as *euglycemia.* Impaired regulation can be further categorized by the etiology of extra- or intracellular processes and is reflected in abnormally high or low blood glucose levels. *Hyperglycemia* is the term used to describe a state of elevated blood glucose levels, generally defined as greater than 100 mg/dl in the fasting state or greater than 140 mg/dl postprandial. On the other end of the spectrum, *hypoglycemia* refers to a state of insufficient or low blood glucose levels, defined as less than 70 mg/dl. Figure 12-1 shows the spectrum of glucose metabolism and regulation: hypoglycemia, euglycemia, and hyperglycemia.

RISK FACTORS

In the healthy individual, glucose regulation occurs with little attention given to the process. All individuals, however, can potentially develop impaired glucose regulation. Diabetes is

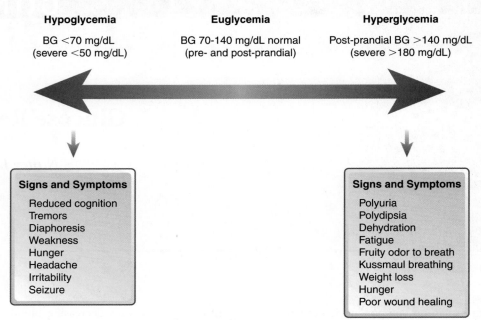

FIGURE 12-1 The Spectrum of Glycemia.

the most well-known example of impaired glucose regulation. There are nearly 26 million individuals in the United States with diabetes and another 79 million with pre-diabetes.[1] *Pre-diabetes* is defined as a state of hyperglycemia that is not high enough to meet the criteria for diabetes. The following sections highlight some patient populations and risk factors that place patients at increased risk for impaired glucose regulation (see also Box 12-1).

Infants and Elderly

Two known populations at increased risk of impaired glucose metabolism are the very young and very old. Infants who are large for gestational age (LGA) are at increased risk for hypoglycemia shortly after birth. An antenatal maternal 1-hour oral glucose tolerance test (OGTT) is advised for women who have delivered a LGA neonate, with a single elevated 1-hour value of 180 mg/dl or greater increasing the risk of neonatal hypoglycemia.[2] The prevalence of neonatal hypoglycemia is also higher among infants whose mothers had diabetes during pregnancy.[3] The hypoglycemia is generally attributed to neonatal hyperinsulinemia as a result of exposure to elevated glucose levels in utero. Small for gestational age (SGA) and premature infants are at risk of

hypoglycemic states because of increased energy needs and insufficient glycogen stores.

Older adults as a group are at greater risk for impaired glucose metabolism because of a reduction in lean muscle mass, where most glucose is metabolized. This is often accompanied with reduced insulin production and resulting reduced capacity to regulate and metabolize glucose concentration. For this reason, the elderly are at increased risk for hyperglycemia.

Racial/Ethnic Groups

Certain racial and ethnic populations have greater genetic predisposition to insulin resistance, leading to type 2 diabetes. This susceptibility is believed to be related to the genetics of having a "thrifty gene" that would have allowed survival, historically, during cycles of famine. In the United States, populations with greatest tendencies for diabetes, according to the Centers for Disease Control and Prevention, are African Americans (age-adjusted percentile of 8.6%), Hispanic/Latino (8% with Puerto Ricans and Mexican Americans having the highest rate), and Asian Americans (6.3%) as compared to 5.3% among Whites.[4] The U.S. Department of Health and Human Services estimates American Indians

---

BOX 12-1   RISK FACTORS FOR IMPAIRED GLUCOSE UTILIZATION

Genetic Predisposition
- At-risk population
- Strong family history of type 2 diabetes

Environmental Factors
- Poor diet with high glycemic load meals, high saturated fat, low fiber intake
- Inactivity

Metabolic Syndrome
- Central obesity
- Hypertension
- Dyslipidemia
- Pre-diabetes
- Gout/PCOS

have about three times the rate of white Americans.[5] Pacific Islander Americans and Eskimos also have high rates of diabetes. Insulin resistance, however, is found around the world, and is not limited to these known high-risk populations. Other racial and ethnic groups, particularly those of Northern European descent, have a genetic tendency for the autoimmune form of diabetes, type 1. Other autoimmune disorders are found in increased frequency among persons with type 1 diabetes, such as celiac disease and autoimmune thyroid disorders.[6]

Genetic Risk Factors

Persons with a family history of diabetes, obesity, and low levels of high-density lipoprotein (HDL) cholesterol are at increased risk of insulin resistance and type 2 diabetes.[7] A family history of medical conditions related to insulin resistance increases other family members' risk of type 2 diabetes. This includes a family history of factors associated with metabolic syndrome including hypertension and polycystic ovary syndrome (PCOS).[8] Gout is also found in persons at genetic risk for insulin resistance.[9] Mitochondrial diseases can have a genetic basis and mitochondrial dysfunction is linked with some variants of type 2 diabetes.[10] Research is rapidly progressing on the genetics of diabetes. Currently there are at least 40 known genetic markers, including *HLA* genes, associated with the risk of diabetes.[11,12] Ultimately, insulin resistance is the common feature associated with metabolic syndrome and type 2 diabetes.[13]

Lifestyle Risk Factors

There are a number of lifestyle choices that exacerbate a predisposition to insulin resistance. This includes a poor diet with a high intake of saturated and trans fatty acids (with the excess caloric intake leading to obesity) and a low fiber intake. An inapproriate intake of carbohydrates will also adversely impact glucose metabolism regardless of the presence of insulin resistance or type 2 diabetes. Lack of physical activity contributes to insulin resistance. However, diminished fuel utilization within lean muscle tissue necessary for exercise contributes to the sedentary lifestyle of persons with metabolic syndrome[14] that serves to reinforce insulin resistance.

Medical Risk Factors

Many medical conditions are associated with impaired glucose regulation—diabetes and metabolic syndrome are most notable. Many other medical conditions interfere with oral intake, creating the need for enteral or parenteral nutrition that may impact glucose regulation. Gastrointestinal problems can lead to malabsorption and resulting nutrient deficiencies required for cellular metabolism of glucose. This includes the recently recognized effect of vitamin D deficiency—insulin resistance and the development of autoimmune diseases such as type 1 diabetes. Vitamin D deficiency is further related to suppressed insulin production.[15]

Glucose regulation is impaired with altered hormonal states. Increased need for insulin is found with infection and other high-stress conditions such as traumatic injury, cancer, and surgery. Hypothyroidism suppresses glucose utilization whereas hyperthyroidism increases the need for carbohydrate as a fuel substrate. Persons with various forms of heart or nerve disease that result in impaired circulation, and therefore reduced blood flow, will have reduced glucose provision to cells.

Pharmocotherapy

Several medications can lead to impaired glucose regulation, placing many individuals at risk for hyperglycemia and hypoglycemia. Table 12-1 presents common medications and the associated impact on blood glucose concentration.

PHYSIOLOGIC PROCESSES AND CONSEQUENCES

To help maintain glucose homeostasis, a variety of hormones are required. Insulin is the only hormone produced that lowers elevated blood glucose (BG) levels after carbohydrate intake. There are several counter-regulatory hormones required to raise BG if levels begin to wane or if needed in anticipation of increased needs (e.g., the "fight or flight" reaction). These work counter to insulin to allow glucose to be formed initially from the breakdown of glycogen stores in the liver and muscles through the process of glycogenolysis. When this system works efficiently a person will never know it is occurring. Problems arise when the BG-regulating hormones are either deficient or excessive, or when the timing of production is not balanced with BG needs. The following

TABLE 12-1	NONDIABETIC MEDICATION CLASSES AND IMPACT ON BLOOD GLUCOSE LEVEL
MEDICATION CLASS*	BLOOD GLUCOSE CONCENTRATION IMPACT
ACE inhibitors	↓
Antiarthritics	↓↑
Antibiotics	↓↑
Antiepileptics	↑
Antifungals	↑
Antimanics	↑
Antineoplastics	↓↑
Antipsychotics, second generation	↑
Antiviral agents	↓↑
Beta-blockers	↓↑
Bronchodilators	↑
CoQ$_{10}$ (with concomitant insulin)	↓
Corticosteroids	↑
Estrogen	↓↑
Immunosuppressants	↓↑
Laxatives (carbohydrate based)	↑
MAO inhibitors	↓
Potassium-depleting diuretics	↑
Proton pump inhibitors	↑

*CoQ_{10}, Coenzyme Q_{10}; *MAO,* monoamine oxidase.

BOX 12-2   CONSEQUENCES OF HYPERGLYCEMIA AND HYPOGLYCEMIA

Hyperglycemia
- Long-term known complications: nerve damage with diminished circulation (peripheral vascular disease [PVD]) and loss of sensation (risk of amputation), kidney disease, eye disease (retinopathy)
- Short-term complications: dehydration with falls, poor skin integrity/pressure ulcers, constipation, increased risk of clot formation (myocardial infarction/cerebrovascular accident [MI/CVA])

Hypoglycemia
- Severe complications: seizures, unconsciousness, cell damage/death
- Possible links to: obesity (cortisol/hunger), migraines, seizure activity among persons without diabetes, psychosis, aggression/violence

---

is a brief review of the etiology and impact of altered glucose regulating hormones.

Hyperinsulinemia, as generally found with insulin resistance, is felt to contribute to atherosclerosis[16] and many forms of cancer[17] with reduced risk found among persons taking the insulin-sensitizing agent metformin.[18] Hyperinsulinemia promotes hypertension through its role in reducing elasticity of blood vessels.[19] Reinforcing this influence on hypertension is the recognition that reducing carbohydrate intake can lower blood pressure levels.[20,21] Hyperinsulinemia is generally the cause of elevated triglyceride levels and lowered HDL cholesterol levels.

In regard to counter-regulatory hormones, glucagon is the first to be produced in response to cellular deficiency of glucose. An excess amount of glucagon production can lead to nausea, and may explain why some persons experience nausea in the morning after the overnight fast. There is limited research on glucagon's role in morning sickness of pregnancy. However, populations with a high risk of insulin resistance have a higher frequency of hyperemesis than women with Caucasian heritage.[22] Hyperinsulinemia inhibits the production of glucagon with the resulting tendency toward the secondary release of cortisol and epinephrine (adrenaline) to raise glucose levels if hypoglycemia develops. Cortisol levels can increase from a variety of causes other than hypoglycemia, such as poor sleeping habits, chronic stress, pain, and illness. Because cortisol is a counter-regulatory hormone, chronic sleep deprivation and stress lead to hyperglycemia. It is also related to central obesity as found with Cushing's disease.[23]

Epinephrine production is increased if glucagon and cortisol are insufficient to raise cellular glucose levels. Symptoms associated with epinephrine release include increased heart rate, which can be problematic with preexisting cardiac disease. It is related to symptoms of physical tremors, and symptoms are quite common among the population.

The counter-regulatory hormonal response required to prevent or to correct hypoglycemia has been associated with neurologic diseases. This includes a possible association of increased cortisol and homocysteine levels in conjunction with reduced levels of folate, vitamin B$_{12}$, and the docosahexaenoic acid (DHA) form of omega-3 fatty acid as contributors to the neuropathology of psychosis.[24] Elevated cortisol levels and abnormal glucose tolerance are found with schizophrenia.[25,26] Migraines may be related to

hypoglycemia, or hyperinsulinemia itself may be the precipitating factor.[27,28]

Physiologic Impact and Consequences of Hyperglycemia

Hyperglycemia has both short-term and long-term consequences. Significant elevations in blood glucose levels lead to the classic symptoms of hyperglycemia (see Figure 12-1) and include *polyphagia* (excess oral intake), attributable to cells not being adequately fueled with consequent increased hunger, along with *polydipsia* (excess thirst) and consequent *polyuria* (excess urination) when the renal glucose threshold of 180 mg/dl is exceeded. Increased risk of urinary incontinence occurs with polyuria.

Another potential consequence of hyperglycemia is dehydration. Dehydration occurs because of excessive water loss from the osmotic effect of excessive glucose in the urine (this links to the renal threshold mentioned previously). Risk of falls increases with dehydration because the body is less able to sense its positioning. Severe dehydration within the brain causes confusion, and if not corrected in a timely manner can lead to coma. This latter condition is called hyperosmolar nonketotic syndrome or HNKS. Fortunately, HNKS is now fairly rare because of routine screening of glucose levels, and home blood glucose monitoring.

Individuals with long-standing or chronic hyperglycemia, as found with poorly controlled diabetes or impaired glucose tolerance (elevated postprandial blood glucose levels not high enough for the diagnosis of diabetes), are at risk for developing several significant physiologic complications associated with end-organ disease attributable to angiopathy (damage to blood vessels). Chronic elevations of blood glucose concentration damage the basement membrane of small blood vessels and impair adequate oxygenation to the tissues. These are known microvascular effects and directly lead to damage to the eye (retinopathy and ultimate blindness if not treated) and the kidney (chronic kidney disease that can lead to end-stage renal disease unless blood glucose level and blood pressure are controlled). It is believed that the polyol pathway as related to chronic hyperglycemia leads to nerve damage (neuropathy). Peripheral neuropathy can be extremely painful, but will also lead to loss of nerve sensation.

Chronic hyperglycemia further damages medium and larger blood vessels, leading to hypertension and cardiovascular and peripheral vascular disease. Cardiometabolic syndrome is a term that recognizes the increased risk of cardiac disease found with metabolic syndrome. A reduction in the risk of complications associated with hyperglycemia has been demonstrated unequivocally through the landmark study known as the Diabetes Control and Complications Trial (the DCCT study), which has provided lasting positive impact on the health of the original research subjects.[29,30]

Physiologic Impact and Consequences of Hypoglycemia

Hypoglycemia is generally attributed to use of exogenous insulin or the sulfonylurea form of oral hypoglycemic agents, which increases endogenous insulin production. Severe hypoglycemia causing unconsciousness is certainly a concern with the potential for cellular death or loss of life, but even lesser degrees of hypoglycemia can invoke adverse outcomes. This includes reduced cognition resulting in increased motor vehicle accidents[31] and has been linked with increased risk of dementia among older persons.[32] The combination of hypoglycemia and stress is a known causative agent of irritability and sometimes anger and aggression.

Other consequences related to excess levels of insulin and hypoglycemia include seizures[33] and peripheral neuropathy with exposure to BG less than 50 mg/dl.[34] The A_{1c} laboratory measurement (the current accepted terminology for hemoglobin A_{1c}, or glycated hemoglobin, which provides an average blood glucose reading over 3 months) is advised to be higher for persons with reduced symptoms of hypoglycemia, such as with young children, the elderly, and persons taking certain medications, such as beta-blockers. This is due to a lower A_{1c} value generally being related to unrecognized hypoglycemia episodes.

Labile Blood Glucose Levels

A known outcome of labile BG (both hyper- and hypoglycemia), generally referred to as uncontrolled diabetes, is an increased incidence of depression. This may be due to altered cellular metabolism as well as increased cortisol production[35] related to hypoglycemia. Hyperglycemia, with reduced circulation and oxygen delivery to tissues as body fluids become thick and viscous, may also contribute to depression. Further, treatment goals for diabetes can reinforce depression, and it is advised that individualized care for diabetes be provided to lessen the psychologic consequences.[36]

Chronic hypoglycemia leads to the condition of hypoglycemia unawareness in which the counter-regulatory hormonal response is blunted. This occurs in type 1 diabetes and is often referred to as "brittle diabetes" when severe fluctuations of BG levels occur, often on a daily basis and without major symptoms to the person. This generally is not innate to the individual's physiology, but rather to problems with insulin dosing, as discussed at the end of the chapter.

To a large degree, the impact of the body's processes to contend with and overcome adverse effects of inadequate glucose availability is largely unknown. There is limited research in the area of hypoglycemia except as it relates to diabetes. For persons with reactive hypoglycemia or symptoms related to a strong counter-regulatory hormonal system, the impact is very real. Often persons may learn to avoid the symptoms of hypoglycemia by eating larger meals that "hold" them longer or by eating a candy bar to abate the symptoms. This can promote weight gain and worsen preexisting insulin resistance, further promoting impaired glucose regulation.

ASSESSMENT

History

Conducting a nursing history provides an opportunity for the nurse to uncover data associated with risk factors or specific conditions known to impact glucose metabolism and regulation. The history includes personal medical history and family history of markers including central obesity, diabetes, hypertension, cardiovascular disease, and cancer at a minimum. As mentioned previously, an adverse effect of several medications is changes in glucose metabolism (Table 12-1). Thus it is important to note these in the history as well.

The history needs to include a review of symptoms. Assessing whether the classic symptoms associated with impaired glucose regulation are present helps determine the degree of impaired metabolism (polyphagia, polydipsia, or polyuria). An increase in weight supports the assessment of polyphagia, but weight loss may occur despite excess caloric intake because of *glycosuria* (loss of glucose through the urine). The symptoms related to hypoglycemia should also be determined and include assessment of the occurrence of diaphoresis, tremors, headaches, seizures, irritability, and reports of changes in behavior/cognition. It may help to identify persons at risk for psychologic disorders because these disorders are related to impaired glucose metabolism, such as schizophrenia and depression as previously discussed.

Examination Data

There are several examination findings that are associated with impaired glucose regulation. Mental status and cognition are negatively impacted in significant hypoglycemic states. Anthropometric measurements such as height and weight are needed to determine body mass index (BMI). Obesity is defined as BMI >30. Waist to hip measurement ratio is indicated for persons with more normal BMI levels, but who carry excess weight centrally (men waist/hip ratio >1.0; women >0.8 indicates central obesity). Waist measurement alone is also useful with >40 inches being defined as central obesity for men and >35 inches for women. Mentioned previously, individuals with obesity are at risk for impaired glucose regulation.

There are several physical findings common among individuals with long-standing states of impaired glucose metabolism. Acanthosis nigricans, a darkening of the skin that is sometimes referred to as "dirty neck syndrome" because this is often the site of observation, or cutaneous papillomas (skin tags) are associated with hyperinsulinemia. Common cardiovascular complications can be potentially identified through blood pressure measurement (hypertension) and examination of the lower extremities for evidence of peripheral vascular disease (poor perfusion and chronic wounds). Examination of the extremities should also include assessment of alterations in sensation to evaluate for neuropathy. Assessing visual acuity and inspection of intraocular structures (with an ophthalmoscope) may provide important information associated with retinopathy.

Diagnostic Tests

Diagnostic testing is an essential component associated with assessment for impairments in glucose regulation and metabolism. Laboratory tests can help reveal the etiology of impaired glucose metabolism, measure and assess blood glucose management, and evaluate consequences of impaired glucose metabolism on other disease conditions.

Glucose Screening and Assessment

Measurement of fasting blood glucose concentration is generally used for screening and monitoring of impaired glucose metabolism—with >100 mg/dl indicative of prediabetes or impaired fasting glucose, ≥126 mg/dl on two occasions indicative of diabetes, or any blood glucose measurement >200 mg/dl with signs and symptoms of diabetes being conclusive. Urine dips may also still be used, but are not sensitive enough to assess elevated blood glucose levels <180 mg/dl. As screening tools, either the fasting blood glucose or the urine dips can fail to diagnose diabetes. An A_{1c} measurement can better diagnose impaired glucose tolerance and diabetes as related to elevated postprandial blood glucose levels. As a result of increased standardization and reliability of A_{1c} test results, the A_{1c} is now used as a diagnostic tool with a reading ≥6.5% indicative of diabetes. Goals for A_{1c} measurements are generally less than 8% for all persons and <7% for persons at low risk of hypoglycemia and/or with expected life expectancy >5 years. If there is no risk of hypoglycemia a normal A_{1c} <5.7% may be optimal, but this should be determined on a case-by-case basis. The A_{1c} test, however, is not infallible. It can be falsely low in the presence of anemia and falsely high in patients who have renal disease.

The most reliable measure of blood glucose metabolism to diagnose diabetes is the 2-hour oral glucose tolerance test (OGTT).

Assessing Autoimmune Diabetes

Assessment of antibodies is used to confirm type 1 diabetes mellitus. The most common test is the GAD (glutamic acid decarboxylase) antibody test. A C-peptide test (an indirect measure of insulin levels) and fasting insulin level may also be measured to help determine the quantity of residual insulin production.

Monitoring and Management of Blood Glucose

Blood glucose meters, in which finger-stick capillary glucose levels are measured, have been used since the 1980s. Most BG meters today are calibrated to read equivalent to plasma glucose, as in a laboratory setting (10% higher reading). Because blood glucose concentration fluctuates throughout the day, self-monitoring of blood glucose (SMBG) best allows daily evaluation of blood glucose level, but can also be used to assess blood glucose management decisions related to carbohydrate intake and medications. Self-monitoring may be done with a blood glucose meter or may also involve the newer technology of a continuous glucose monitor that can reveal blood glucose concentration changes that occur every 5 minutes. Finger-stick readings are the most predominant form of glucose monitoring in health care settings.

Lipid Analysis

The most common lipid assessments include measurements of total cholesterol, HDL cholesterol, and triglycerides. From these results, the low-density lipoprotein (LDL) cholesterol level is calculated, which is referred to as calculated LDL. Lipid goals are LDL <100 mg/dl (<70 mg/dl if there is preexisting cardiovascular disease), HDL >40 mg/dl (>50 mg/dl for women), and triglycerides <150 mg/dl, although optimal triglycerides may be <100 mg/dl as found with type 1 diabetes in which there is no hyperinsulinemia. Triglyceride levels generally reflect hyperinsulinemia although an individual with newly diagnosed type 1 diabetes may have temporary elevations of triglycerides. HDL levels indicate level of insulin sensitivity—insulin resistance with low levels of HDL and insulin sensitivity with high levels of HDL.

Microalbuminuria

An early indication of renal disease and risk of diabetes, if not already overt, is protein loss in the urine, measured by the amount of albumin. When loss of albumin into the urine is severe with levels >300 mcg/dl, multiple adverse outcomes occur because the innumerable body proteins required for physiologic function will be compromised.

C-Reactive Protein

C-reactive protein (CRP) testing can be undertaken to help assess inflammation, felt to be an underlying etiology of insulin resistance. Controlling the inflammatory process can be challenging, but is a goal in achieving optimal health status.

CLINICAL MANAGEMENT

Primary Prevention

Primary prevention measures for optimal glucose regulation center around a healthy lifestyle. The general message of including regular physical activity with "10,000 steps" or equivalent, such as ≥150 minutes exercise per week or 30 to 60 minutes exercise on most days, can greatly reduce the risk of conditions related to impaired glucose regulation and promote improved cellular metabolism. Humans ultimately are complex machines and, as such, are meant to move. Primary prevention further includes avoiding excess caloric intake and striving for a healthy weight. MyPlate.gov and the *2010 Dietary Guidelines* should be promoted; these emphasize consuming a diet high in whole grains, fruits and vegetables that are deep orange in color, leafy green vegetables, and legumes/beans along with low-fat milk and a variety of lean protein sources. These foods contribute to optimal cellular metabolism through provision of vitamin, minerals, and appropriate amounts of macronutrients and kilocalories needed for health; in addition, lower sodium guidelines can help lower blood pressure and reduce the risk of cardiovascular disease.

Secondary Prevention (Screening)

The ABC Campaign addresses goals for A_{1c}, Blood pressure, and Cholesterol management. *Healthy People 2020* reinforces these goals of A_{1c} <7% as well as control of blood pressure and lipid levels. *Healthy People 2020* has several other management goals aimed at reducing the number of lower extremity amputations and the death rate among persons with diabetes through a variety of measures that include increasing the proportion of adults with diabetes who self-manage blood glucose level at least daily, who have glycosylated hemoglobin measurements at least twice per year, who have annual urinary microalbumin measurements, who receive formal diabetes education, and who have annual dental, foot, and dilated eye examinations.[37]

Collaborative Interventions

Diabetes education is aimed at including the person with diabetes within the health care team. The various health care professionals can all provide insight into management decisions, but the person with diabetes is the individual who is involved in applying daily decision making, even in institutional settings, such as adherence to carbohydrate intake goals. If oral hypoglycemic agents or injections of insulin are utilized, the nurse should be aware of signs and symptoms of hypoglycemia (see Figure 12-1 and Box 12-2).

Correcting hypoglycemia without inducing a rebound hyperglycemic state is undertaken with the *15/15 rule*. It was shown through the DCCT study, as described previously, that 15 g of quick-acting carbohydrate can raise blood glucose levels by 50 "points" (mg/dl). Retesting blood glucose level with a finger-stick measure in 15 minutes can verify correction of hypoglycemia. If hypoglycemia is not corrected in 15 minutes, the process is repeated until euglycemia is achieved (15 g of quick-acting carbohydrate followed by a repeat finger-stick in 15 minutes). The exception to the *15/15 rule* is when severe hypoglycemia has occurred, in which 30 g of quick-acting carbohydrate can be provided for the conscious individual (with an expected BG rise of 100 points); for the unconscious individual with hypoglycemia, either intravenous dextrose or glucagon injection may be given. The person receiving a glucagon injection needs to be rolled onto his or her side or face-down; this position change will help reduce the risk of aspiration because severe nausea and vomiting may be associated with the administration of high-dosage glucagon.

Increasingly, nurses are being given more responsibility in insulin provision. Nurses have had an ability to "hold insulin" if felt warranted because of concerns of hypoglycemia. Nurses

are now expected to understand how glucose regulation occurs with the different types of diabetes, how diabetes medications are effective, how to apply insulin-to-carbohydrate based on a predetermined ratio for prandial insulin requirements as described more fully in the section on Insulin Usage, how to correct hyperglycemia with additional correction insulin, and how to appropriately correct hypoglycemia. Using a basal/bolus insulin regimen is described below.

Nutrition Therapy

Once an individual is identified as having or being at high risk of impaired glucose regulation, a diet history should be obtained and educational needs determined. Intervention strategies should be developed in conjunction with the individual to assess his or her needs, readiness, and ability to alter lifestyle. Advising inclusion of low-glycemic load meals every 3 to 4 hours or a simpler message of eating smaller, frequent meals is appropriate. This is education that all health care providers can reinforce for optimal health and well-being.

When diabetes has developed, there is a need to further individualize treatment. Preprinted diet sheets, for example, are typically ineffective and interfere with provider/patient communication. A registered dietitian who is also a certified diabetes educator (RD, CDE) can best provide medical nutrition therapy for the goal of euglycemia. This team approach, in which the patient is part of the team, can serve to prevent long-term complications, such as renal disease, and short-term conditions, such as management of pressure ulcers.

Using Pattern Management to Promote Euglycemia

A person with pre-diabetes or diabetes can benefit with regular screening of A_{1c} levels as well as finger-stick glucose measurement for postprandial effects. Knowledge of postprandial finger-stick readings can guide both patients and health care providers in determining carbohydrate tolerance. This is one form of pattern management, and monitoring meal-related BG excursions can help in decisions for treatment through diet and/or medications.

For most persons with insulin resistance, reactive hypoglycemia, or type 2 diabetes, a range of up to 50 to 60 g of carbohydrate per meal is generally well tolerated, especially if the meal is low in glycemic index. Occasionally a person is very insulin resistant with inability to tolerate even reasonable amounts of carbohydrate. For such persons, or for those with insufficient insulin production to override the cellular insulin resistance, medications are in order. Insulin may be required to control BG level even though there may be normal or elevated levels of endogenous insulin production.

Oral Hypoglycemic Agents

If medical nutrition therapy, increased physical activity, and weight loss are not sufficient to achieve euglycemia, oral agents may be used by the person with type 2 diabetes. These include insulin sensitizers for those persons in whom insulin resistance is the primary issue or insulin secretagogues for persons who have insufficient insulin production for their needs, but with expected ability to release more insulin. Although not intended to be insulin-sensitizer agents, it has been recognized that statins for cholesterol management and angiotensin-converting enzyme (ACE) inhibitors, a type of blood pressure medication, promote insulin sensitivity.

The hormone incretin is now recognized to have a role in maintaining insulin levels. Incretin mimetics are now being used to promote endogenous insulin use. Although incretin mimetics are injectable, they are not insulin.

Insulin Usage

Historically, short-acting "R" or regular insulin was used to cover meal intake, and strict diet regimens using the food exchange system were employed. With the advent of the landmark DCCT study, the approach changed to carbohydrate counting. It was found in the DCCT study that a more predictable BG outcome could be obtained if prandial meal coverage (bolus) insulin based on total carbohydrate intake was utilized with an optimal ratio of insulin to carbohydrate. Unfortunately, even more than 15 years later, most health care providers do not prescribe insulin adjustment based on carbohydrate counting, despite this approach being advocated by the American Diabetes Association and the American Medical Directors Association. Instead of using this proactive approach to prevent postprandial hyperglycemia, the reactive approach of sliding-scale insulin based on premeal BG levels has predominated. The outcome of the sliding-scale approach is that if premeal BG level is at target, no meal coverage for carbohydrate intake is given, often resulting in hyperglycemia that is not addressed until the next meal and finger-stick reading.

The sliding scale, as determined by the attending health care provider, assumes a typical intake of carbohydrate, and thus is a higher quantity than an insulin correction factor (described later in this section). If the person eats more or less carbohydrate than usual, the sliding-scale approach tends to promote either hyper- or hypoglycemia. The sliding-scale approach should be discontinued.[38,39] Hospitals, long-term care (LTC) centers, and other health care settings can either print the carbohydrate quantity of menu items on meal tickets or have the carbohydrate content consistently managed via food portions served as arranged by a registered dietitian. In an institutional setting, the use of a basal/bolus insulin regimen rather than a sliding-scale approach has been shown to be effective in lowering average BG level while having no increased risk of hypoglycemia over a 4-year period.[40]

Pattern management based on carbohydrate counting can be effective in stabilizing BG level with reduced frequency of hypo- and hyperglycemia, and is now the recommended approach. In this approach, assessments of finger-stick readings, grams of carbohydrate consumed, and the number of insulin units used help to verify the needed ratio of insulin to carbohydrate intake. Typically, most adults who are insulin sensitive (who tend to be thin with high HDL cholesterol levels) require 1 unit per every 15 g of carbohydrate, or 1 carb serving. A very active adult with insulin sensitivity or a young child may need as little as 1 unit for every 30 g of carbohydrate

whereas an obese, insulin-resistant individual may need as much as 1 unit for every 2 or 3 g of carbohydrate intake. The target pattern is for the 3- to 4-hour postprandial BG excursion to be within 30 points of the premeal reading. Generally after this period there is little deviation in BG level if a rapid-acting analogue insulin is used. If there is a consistent pattern of hyper- or hypoglycemia by this time period, or by the next meal, the amount of insulin or carbohydrate can be adjusted up or down as needed. Once a ratio is determined, this will generally apply to other meals, although exceptions do occur. For example, the dawn phenomenon causes the early morning BG level to rise through increased production of cortisol and growth hormone, both counter-regulatory hormones. With breakfast, as a consequence, there is often a decreased tolerance to carbohydrate intake with increased need for insulin (endogenous or exogenous).

An insulin correction factor may be needed to correct hyperglycemia in addition to using the insulin-to-carbohydrate ratio. Again, this is different from the usual sliding scale with the amount of insulin needed to correct hyperglycemia being less than that typical with a sliding scale. The *1800 rule* predicts the drop in BG level for each 1 unit of extra insulin beyond the bolus insulin needed to cover meal carbohydrate intake. The insulin correction factor is determined by dividing the total daily dose (TDD) of insulin units (both long-acting basal insulin and rapid-acting meal bolus insulin) into the number 1800. For example if a person is taking a usual TDD of 100 units, the predicted insulin correction factor is 18 (1800/100 = 18). In other words, each additional unit of insulin taken will drop the BG level by 18 points. Another person may only be taking 10 units of TDD insulin, which predicts 1 extra unit of rapid-acting insulin would drop the BG 180 points (1800/10 = 180). The insulin correction factor is also referred to as the insulin sensitivity factor.

> ### CLINICAL NURSING SKILLS FOR GLUCOSE REGULATION
>
> - Assessment
>   - Blood glucose monitoring
>   - Dietary teaching
> - Medication Administration

INTERRELATED CONCEPTS

Glucose regulation affects and is affected by most, if not all, physiologic processes. As the primary energy substrate, all life processes are dependent on normal glucose metabolism and regulation. Figure 12-2 shows some of the most important interrelated concepts; these relationships are described next.

Two of the most obvious interrelated concepts are **Nutrition** and **Mobility**. Mentioned previously, proper nutrition and regular physical activity are needed for optimal regulation of glucose concentration and management of conditions in which regulatory mechanisms are impaired. In this case, nutrition and physical activities are viewed not only as preventive measures but also as part of the treatment strategy in disease states.

Long term consequences of hyperglycemia lead to micro- and macrovascular changes (**Perfusion**), reduced renal function (**Elimination**), and changes in vision and peripheral sensation (**Sensory perception**). Lung disease and impaired circulation can lead to reduced oxygenation and glucose utilization, resulting in suppressed cellular metabolism and potentially cell death. Hypermetabolic states such as cancer increase the need for glucose, but increased insulin production or provision is required.

Patient profile concepts of **Family dynamics, Adherence, Motivation,** and **Culture influence** the ability of the individual to make behavioral changes needed for optimal health promotion or disease management. Family relationships can suffer when attempts to regulate the diet of one individual have an adverse impact on mealtime that affects other family members. This can result in mealtime-associated stress if optimal family dynamics are not present. Eating disorders generally have a basis in psychologic function that is influenced by the internal family level of functioning as well as by external influences such as the media or individual cohorts. Food availability impacts glucose regulation through the ability of an individual to access appropriate carbohydrate intake that influences optimal cellular metabolism.

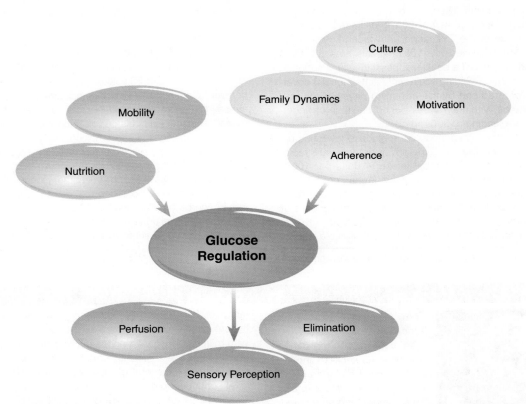

FIGURE 12-2 Glucose Regulation and Interrelated Concepts. Nutrition and mobility *(green)* are biophysical concepts that impact glucose regulation directly. Patient profile concepts *(yellow)* impact behaviors associated with health promotion and disease management. The rose-colored ovals represent Health and Illness concepts with long-term consequences to poor glucose regulation.

MODEL CASE 1

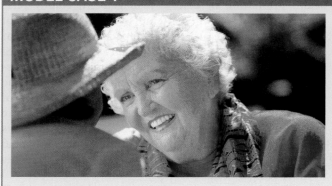

Ms. Karen Farley is a 74-year-old female who lives in a long-term care (LTC) center. She has a diagnosis of type 2 diabetes and obesity. She was initially administered a sulfonylurea form of oral antidiabetic agent (OAD) of 20 mg daily and had maintained an A_{1c} value in the 7% range until recently when the A_{1c} measurement increased to >10%. At this time her OAD is discontinued and use of a peakless, basal insulin is added at 20 units every evening. Sliding-scale rapid-acting insulin coverage has been ordered stat by the attending physician on four separate occasions within a 1-week period because of finger-stick (FS) glucose readings >300 mg/dl.

Because Ms. Farley experienced wide glucose level fluctuation patterns from meal to meal, the physician ordered a rapid-acting bolus insulin based on meal intake (4 units per 100% oral [po] intake, 3 units per 75% po intake, 2 units per 50% po intake, and 1 unit for 25% po intake) and her FS glucose readings were increased to four times a day. After a few weeks of glucose measurements between 70 and 180 mg/dl, the frequency of FS glucose readings was reduced to twice a day.

However, her levels again became elevated. Her fasting FS blood glucose readings began ranging between 133 and 237 mg/dl; thus her basal insulin dosage was increased by 10%, per standard protocol, to 22 units. The increased basal insulin was ordered since fasting FS readings were high ranging from 133 to 237 mg/dl. An insulin correction factor is determined to be 1 unit per 50 point drop in blood glucose to correct hyperglycemia. This was determined based on the *1800 rule* (1800 ÷ Total Daily Dose of 34 units of basal (22 units) and bolus insulin (12 units/day at 100% po) resulting in the quotient 52.9). The orders for the insulin correction dose is to add the additional insulin to the postprandial bolus meal coverage insulin at 1 unit for FS 150–200 mg/dl, 2 units for 201–250 mg/dl, and higher. Finally, an insulin sensitizer form of OAD was added. A follow-up A_{1c} measurement 3 months later is found to be at target, which is <8.0% (for her advanced age), and the majority of FS measurements are <170 mg/dl.

Case Analysis

With a diagnosis of type 2 diabetes, Ms. Farley is generally at low risk for hypoglycemia because of the underlying insulin resistance. Her increased FS values are found in the history taking to be related to a number of factors including the counter-regulatory stress-related hormones attributable to a recent ear infection, chronic shoulder pain, history of colon cancer, and perhaps the stress of stopping cigarette smoking. Her insulin production may also be declining, as is expected with the progression of type 2 diabetes. With the addition of the insulin sensitizer along with the basal/bolus insulin correction regimen, there was improved BG control. In fact, as compared to the previous reactive sliding-scale insulin approach, Ms. Farley had three times as many FS readings at target level and a reduced frequency of hyperglycemia that allowed her A_{1c} measurements to improve from >10% to <8%.

MODEL CASE 2

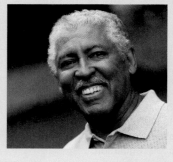

Tom Welty is a 64-year-old African-American male who was hospitalized for dehydration attributable to uncontrolled type 1 diabetes (with a history of A_{1c} values in the 10% range) and end-stage renal disease (ESRD) requiring dialysis. While in the hospital, Mr. Welty begins a sliding-scale insulin regimen to correct hyperglycemia along with routine 70/30 insulin of 24 units at 0730 and 18 units at 1630 after having experienced a severe hypoglycemic episode with basal/bolus insulin.

Tom is then discharged to a LTC facility because of inability for self-care. The physician who prescribed 70/30 insulin with sliding-scale coverage continues to be Tom's attending physician in the LTC facility, and does not want to use a basal/bolus approach because of concerns of hypoglycemia. The diabetes committee reviews Tom's finger-stick (FS) blood glucose readings and finds labile numbers with a 0730-hour FS range of 74–329 mg/dl, a 1130-hour FS range of 43–365 mg/dl, a 1630-hour FS range of 88–276 mg/dl, and a 2200-hour FS range of 73–165 mg/dl. Tom subsequently develops severe hypoglycemia, which is noted as the result of another resident with mild dementia alerting the nursing station that Tom seems drunk. His FS level at that time (1730 hour) was found to be 47 mg/dl. Despite oral glucose treatment, his blood glucose level continues to decline as low as 28 mg/dl; following administration of a tube of instant glucose, the blood glucose level rises to 64 mg/dl.

The following morning Tom is sent to the hospital because of severe blood glucose level fluctuations with a 0600 FS measurement of 312 mg/dl. He returns from the hospital with a smaller dose of 70/30 insulin twice a day, but continues to have blood glucose readings that fluctuate—with a pattern of significant drop in FS values by lunchtime and hyperglycemia by dinnertime. The attending physician agrees to basal/bolus insulin calculated at 0.3 unit/kg body weight of total daily dose (TDD) of insulin. Half of this dose is administered as a basal insulin and the balance is divided for bolus meal coverage based on the percentage of meal consumed. Per the *1800 rule,* the insulin correction factor is calculated to be 1:100, written as FS 200–300 mg/dl with 1 extra unit rapid-acting insulin, and upwards. After several days, the FS glucose level returns to normal, and is once again mostly at target, but with a range of 152–292 mg/dl throughout the day.

MODEL CASE 2—cont'd

Case Analysis

Tom, with type 1 diabetes, has a low BMI and is very insulin sensitive. He requires replacement insulin, but because of his insulin sensitivity he does not need a large dose. Having ESRD, insulin is not readily cleared via his kidneys and can therefore accumulate in his system, further promoting hypoglycemia. Because of a history of chronic hypoglycemia, Tom has few recognizable symptoms. The use of 70/30 insulin was not physiologically sound for Tom because the dosage cannot be increased to cover fasting hyperglycemia without causing hypoglycemia when the peak effect of the long-acting insulin occurs, which is typically near lunchtime but can range from as soon as 3 hours to as late as 6 to 8 hours after injection. Using a basal/bolus regimen is optimal, and can be provided either with injections or with an insulin pump. Relying on FS readings, rather than A_{1c} measurements, is a more objective measure of blood glucose control because of Tom's dialysis treatment.

■■ BOX 12-3 EXEMPLARS OF GLUCOSE REGULATION

Hyperglycemia
- Conditions of excess counter-regulatory hormones
- Cushing's syndrome
- Cystic fibrosis
- Diabetes, type 1
- Diabetes, type 2
- Endogenous correction of hypoglycemia
- Gestational diabetes
- Gout
- Hemochromatosis
- Hypertension
- Infection
- Insulin resistance
- Pancreatitis
- Pheochromocytoma
- Polycystic ovarian syndrome
- Somogyi effect
- Stress response (injury/pain)

Hypoglycemia
- Conditions of inadequate counter-regulatory hormones
- Endogenous hyperinsulinemia
- Gastroparesis
- Glycogen storage diseases
- Insulinoma
- Insulin treatment
- Liver failure
- Prematurity
- Starvation

EXEMPLARS

As mentioned throughout the chapter, there are multiple conditions that are associated with glucose metabolism problems. These are presented in Box 12-3.

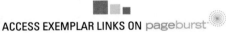

ACCESS EXEMPLAR LINKS ON pageburst

REFERENCES

1. American Diabetes Association: Alexandria, Va, 2011.
2. Schaefer-Graf UM, Rossi R, Bührer C, et al: Rate and risk factors of hypoglycemia in large-for-gestational-age newborn infants of nondiabetic mothers, *Am J Obstet Gynecol* 187(4):913–917, 2002.
3. Maayan-Metzger A, Lubin D, Kuint J: Hypoglycemia rates in the first days of life among term infants born to diabetic mothers, *Neonatology* 96(2):80–85, 2009.
4. Centers for Disease Control and Prevention, Center for Health Statistics, Division of Health Interview Statistics: *Data from the National Health Interview Survey,* Oct 15, 2010.
5. U.S. Department of Health and Human Services, Agency for Healthcare Research and Quality (AHRQ), Rockville, Md, 2010.
6. Ergür AT, Oçal G, Berberoğlu M, et al: Celiac disease and autoimmune thyroid disease in children with type 1 diabetes mellitus: clinical and HLA-genotyping results, *J Clin Res Pediatr Endocrinol* 2(4):151–154, 2010.
7. Wilson PW, D'Agostino RB, Fox CS, et al: Type 2 diabetes risk in persons with dysglycemia: The Framingham Offspring Study, *Diabetes Res Clin Pract* 92(1):124–127, 2011.
8. Ewens KG, Jones MR, Ankener W, et al: FTO and MC4R gene variants are associated with obesity in polycystic ovary syndrome, *PLoS One* 6(1):e16390, 2011.
9. Mitu F, Drăgan MV: Hyperuricemia and the metabolic syndrome, *Rev Med Chir Soc Med Nat Iasi* 113(4):1001–1005, 2009.
10. Ren J, Pulakat L, Whaley-Connell A, et al: Mitochondrial biogenesis in the metabolic syndrome and cardiovascular disease, *J Mol Med* 88(10):993–1001, 2010.
11. McCarthy MI: Dorothy Hodgkin lecture 2010. From hype to hope? A journey through the genetics of type 2 diabetes, *Diabet Med* 28(2):132–140, 2011.
12. Tipu HN, Ahmed TA, Bashir MM: Human leukocyte antigen class ii susceptibility conferring alleles among non-insulin dependent diabetes mellitus patients, *J Coll Physic Surg Pak* 21(1):26–29, 2011.
13. Gallagher EJ, Leroith D, Karnieli E: Insulin resistance in obesity as the underlying cause for the metabolic syndrome, *Mt Sinai J Med* 77(5):511–523, 2010.
14. Chomentowski P, Coen PM, Radiková Z, et al: Skeletal muscle mitochondria in insulin resistance: differences in intermyofibrillar versus subsarcolemmal subpopulations and relationship to metabolic flexibility, *J Clin Endocrinol Metab* 96(2):494–503, 2010.
15. Courbebaisse M, Souberbielle JC, Prié D, et al: Non phospho-calcic actions of vitamin D, *Med Sci (Paris)* 26(4):417–421, 2010.

16. Parapid B, Saponjski J, Ostojić M, et al: The degree of coronary atherosclerosis as a marker of insulin resistance in non-diabetics, *Srp Arh Celok Lek* 138(7-8):436–443, 2010.

17. Gallagher EJ, Fierz Y, Ferguson RD, et al: The pathway from diabetes and obesity to cancer, on the route to targeted therapy, *Endocr Pract* 14:1–30, 2010.

18. Anisimov VN: Metformin for aging and cancer prevention, *Aging (Albany NY)* 2(11):760–774, 2010.

19. Chaudhary K, Buddineni JP, Nistala R, et al: Resistant hypertension in the high-risk metabolic patient, *Curr Diab Rep* 11(1):41–46, 2010.

20. Appel LJ, Sacks FM, Carey VJ, et al: OmniHeart Collaborative Research Group. Effects of protein, monounsaturated fat, and carbohydrate intake on blood pressure and serum lipids: results of the OmniHeart randomized trial, *JAMA* 294(19):2455–2464, 2005.

21. Shah M, Adams-Huet B, Garg A: Effect of high-carbohydrate or high-cis-monounsaturated fat diets on blood pressure: a meta-analysis of intervention trials, *Am J Clin Nutr* 85(5):1251–1256, 2007.

22. Vikanes A, Grjibovski AM, Vangen S, et al: Variations in prevalence of hyperemesis gravidarum by country of birth: a study of 900,074 pregnancies in Norway, 1967-2005, *Scand J Public Health* 36(2):135–142, 2008.

23. Whitworth JA, Williamson PM, Mangos G, et al: Cardiovascular consequences of cortisol excess, *Vasc Health Risk Manag* 1(4):291–299, 2005.

24. Kale A, Naphade N, Sapkale S, et al: Reduced folic acid, vitamin B_{12} and docosahexaenoic acid and increased homocysteine and cortisol in never-medicated schizophrenia patients: implications for altered one-carbon metabolism, *Psychiatr Res* 175(1-2):47–53, 2010.

25. Walker EF, Brennan PA, Esterberg M, et al: Longitudinal changes in cortisol secretion and conversion to psychosis in at-risk youth, *J Abnorm Psychol* 119(2):401–408, 2010.

26. Kirkpatrick B, Miller BJ, Garcia-Rizo C, et al: Is abnormal glucose tolerance in antipsychotic-naive patients with nonaffective psychosis confounded by poor health habits? *Schizophr Bull*, 1–5, 2010 Jun 17. http://schizophreniabulletin.oxfordjournals.org/content/early/2010/06/17/schbul.sbq058.full.pdf+html.

27. Jacome DE: Hypoglycemia rebound migraine, *Headache* 41(9):895–898, 2001.

28. Cavestro C, Rosatello A, Micca G, et al: Insulin metabolism is altered in migraineurs: a new pathogenic mechanism for migraine? *Headache* 47(10):1436–1442, 2007.

29. Diabetes Control and Complications Trial/Epidemiology of Diabetes Interventions and Complications (DCCT/EDIC) Research Group: Modern-day clinical course of type 1 diabetes mellitus after 30 years' duration: the Diabetes Control and Complications Trial/Epidemiology of Diabetes Interventions and Complications and Pittsburgh Epidemiology of Diabetes Complications Experience (1983-2005), *Arch Intern Med* 169(14):1307–1316, 2009.

30. Kilpatrick ES, Rigby AS, Atkin SL: The Diabetes Control and Complications Trial: the gift that keeps giving, *Nat Rev Endocrinol* 5(10):537–545, 2009.

31. Campbell LK, Gonder-Frederick LA, Broshek DK, et al: Neurocognitive differences between drivers with type 1 diabetes with and without a recent history of recurrent driving mishaps, *Int J Diabetes Mellit* 2(2):73–77, 2010.

32. Whitmer RA, Karter AJ, Yaffe K, et al: Hypoglycemic episodes and risk of dementia in older patients with type 2 diabetes mellitus, *JAMA* 301(15):1565–1572, 2009.

33. Lapenta L, Di Bonaventura C, Fattouch J, et al: Focal epileptic seizure induced by transient hypoglycaemia in insulin-treated diabetes, *Epileptic Disord* 12(1):84–87, 2010.

34. Ozaki K, Sano T, Tsuji N, et al: Insulin-induced hypoglycemic peripheral motor neuropathy in spontaneously diabetic WBN/Kob rats, *Comp Med* 60(4):282–287, 2010.

35. Goekoop JG: A multidimensional description and validation of two subtypes in the field of endogenous and melancholic depression, *Tijdschr Psychiatr* 50(3):159–170, 2008.

36. Saatci E, Tahmiscioglu G, Bozdemir N, et al: The well-being and treatment satisfaction of diabetic patients in primary care, *Health Qual Life Outcomes* 8:67, 2010.

37. U.S. Department of Health and Human Services: *Healthy People 2020,* 200 Independence Ave, SW, Washington, DC 20201.

38. Bray B: Transitioning and adjusting insulin analog therapy in elderly patients, *Consult Pharm* Suppl B:17–23, 2008.

39. Hirsch IB: Sliding scale insulin—time to stop sliding, *JAMA* 301(2):213–214, 2009.

40. Murphy DM, Vercruysse RA, Bertucci TM, et al: Reducing hyperglycemia hospitalwide: the basal-bolus concept, *Jt Comm J Qual Patient Safety* 35(4):216–223, 2009.

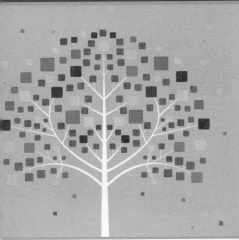

13

Nutrition

Nancy J. Peckenpaugh

The science of nutrition is related to the process by which food nutrients affect processes of growth and development, cellular function and repair, and maintenance or promotion of health status. It encompasses the requirements and functions of the macronutrients and micronutrients for optimal physiologic functioning to promote short-term and long-term health and prevent or alleviate complications associated with chronic disease. Nutritional status has an impact on a variety of health conditions and diseases. On the other hand, health conditions and diseases can adversely affect nutritional status through issues of ingestion, digestion, absorption, metabolism, and homeostasis of cellular and serum levels of nutrients. Because nutrition is directly linked to health, this represents a fundamental concept for nursing practice.

DEFINITION(S)

The concept of nutrition is complex, involving a number of physiologic processes. For the purpose of this concept analysis, nutrition is defined as *the science of optimal cellular metabolism and its impact on health and disease.* There are a number of terms essential to an understanding of this concept that merit definition. *Macronutrients* are the *kilocalorie (kcal) (energy)* sources of carbohydrates, proteins, and fats. Alcohol is a source of kilocalories, but is not considered a macronutrient. *Micronutrients* include vitamins and minerals. Water is also an essential nutrient for physiologic processes. *Phytochemicals* are plant compounds that are thought to have health-protecting qualities—such as antioxidant and immune-boosting properties. Examples of phytochemicals include lutein (associated with the green color of vegetables) and lycopene (found in high amounts in tomato products). *Malnutrition* is a general term that refers to conditions in which there is either undernutrition (e.g., insufficient protein ingestion or inadequate kilocalorie intake) or imbalanced nutrition (e.g., excess kilocalorie intake, as found with obesity, or excess consumption of certain vitamins or minerals that results in metabolic deficiency of others). *Sarcopenia* is

a relatively new term, being coined in 1989 to describe the condition of loss of muscle mass and strength. Research continues to explore the causes of loss of muscle strength.[1,2] Generalized edema includes *anasarca,* the condition of massive fluid overload, and can be adversely influenced through *hypoalbuminemia,* the condition of too little protein in the blood.

SCOPE AND CATEGORIES

Nutritional status can be viewed as either optimal or suboptimal (or malnutrition). An optimal nutritional status is one in which all nutrients are available, in balanced amounts, for cellular metabolism and physiologic function. Malnutrition can be categorized as insufficient or excessive quantity or quality of macronutrients or micronutrients. The scope of this concept is represented on a continuum with malnutrition on both ends (undernutrition and overnutrition) and optimal nutrition in the middle (Figure 13-1). Health status and nutrition are integral to one another—that is, poor nutritional status negatively impacts health, and poor health status can negatively impact nutritional status (Figure 13-2).

RISK FACTORS

All individuals potentially are at risk for malnutrition. Some risk factors are common to population groups and some are based on unique individual attributes.

Populations at Risk
Age
The two ends of the age continuum—the very young and very old—represent population groups in which nutrition is a common concern. The very young are at risk because of immature organ development and total reliance on others for feeding. Particularly at risk for altered nutrition are premature infants because of impaired oral intake with potential reliance on parenteral or tube feeding; in addition, inadequate

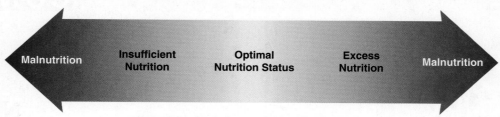

FIGURE 13-1 Scope of Nutrition Concept.

nutritional knowledge by the caregiver can further contribute to altered nutritional status in this population group.[3,4] The elderly in general are at risk for altered nutrition attributable to a number of factors, such as reduced organ function, interactions of multiple medications, and increased isolation with its adverse impact on appetite and interest in preparing nutritious meals. The elderly who are institutionalized are at even greater risk because of institutional feeding issues, such as therapeutic diet restrictions or regulated mealtimes, along with generalized poorer health status requiring assistance with activities of daily living (ADLs). Other physiologic risk factors among the elderly population include poor appetite unrelated to social isolation[5] and severely altered physiology. Physiologic contributors to malnutrition in the elderly can range from obvious frailty (with a body mass index [BMI] <21 associated with a high risk of mortality despite nutritional intervention)[6] to less discernible conditions such as impaired gastrointestinal function related to neurologic disease. Sarcopenia has been estimated to occur in more than 50% of persons older than age 75.[7]

Race/Ethnicity

Many nutritional risks plague certain racial groups more than others. Vitamin D deficiency is more frequently found among persons of African heritage[8] and has increased in prevalence, especially among the infants of breastfeeding African-American mothers.[9] Type 2 diabetes is more frequently found in populations whose heritage can be traced to regions nearer the equator (see Glucose Regulation concept), typically referred to as the minority population in the United States. The same holds true with risk of obesity, although lifestyle factors as found with the Western diet influence the expression of both obesity and type 2 diabetes. Other conditions associated with metabolic syndrome (see Glucose Regulation concept) are further found in higher frequency in

minorities, especially hypertension (HTN).[10] Increased risk of diseases related to Northern heritage include type 1 diabetes, celiac disease, and some neurodegenerative disorders such as Huntington's chorea.[11]

Socioeconomic Status

Risk factors for malnutrition as related to excess or inadequate intake of macronutrients and micronutrients include external forces of food insecurity and food availability. The prevalence of obesity has been found to be directly related to a limited number of neighborhood supermarkets but greater numbers of convenience grocery stores and fast-food restaurants.[12] Insufficient finances to purchase unrefined foods can contribute to excess intake of macronutrients while limiting the intake of micronutrients needed for optimal cellular metabolism. Lack of exposure to a variety of foods at home or in other settings such as schools and restaurants can result in limited food preferences.

Individual Risk Factors
Genetics

Many conditions that impact nutrition are linked to genetics. Inherited metabolic defects include phenylketonuria (PKU); individuals with PKU are deficient in the enzyme responsible for the metabolism of the amino acid phenylalanine, resulting in accumulation of phenylalanine in blood and tissues. Brain damage occurs unless a low-phenylalanine diet is followed throughout the lifetime of the affected individual. Other inherited metabolic defects include galactosemia and maple syrup urine disease. Fructose intolerance may be genetic or acquired as well as having obvious or limited symptoms.[13] Some genetic conditions eventually lead to nutritional challenges. For example, in cystic fibrosis thick secretions block pancreatic ducts, eventually leading to impaired digestion and absorption of fats and fat-soluble vitamins.

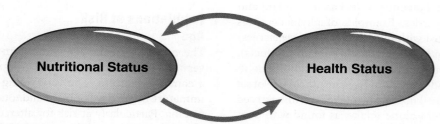

FIGURE 13-2 Nutritional Status Impacts Health Status, and Health Status Impacts Nutritional Status.

Lifestyle and Patterns of Eating

Lifestyle will affect patterns of eating and ultimately nutritional status. Factors that affect lifestyle include interpersonal relationships, learned stress-coping mechanisms, and alterations in mood. Weight gain from dating and marriage can occur when food habits change to match those of the partner. Family food offerings can positively influence nutritional intake, such as avoidance of high-fat and high-sugar foods with emphasis on inclusion of a variety of vegetables, fruits, whole grains, lean meats, and low-fat milk; such food choices can occur either in families dieting for weight loss or in families simply interested in good nutrition in general. Family influences that can negatively impact nutritional status include lack of home-prepared meals, eating meals on the run, food restrictions (as with food allergies, dislikes, or preferences to avoid certain foods, as with a vegan diet), or food insecurity issues related to family finances. The influence of peers, as frequently seen in adolescence, can have a profound impact on food choices; examples include choosing salty and sugary snacks as opposed to healthy foods or eating at fast-food restaurants with peer pressure to order super-sized portions. Coping mechanisms may revolve around eating comfort foods or may result in reduced food intake, such as the diminished appetite often found with depression. Mood can increase oral intake negatively, such as rewarding oneself for a job well-done with a sugary dessert, or positively, such as willingness to practice good, healthy eating and exercise habits.

Culturally, there are a wide range of foods that can meet nutritional needs. With regard to protein intake, as long as all nine essential amino acids are provided in adequate amounts within a 24-hour period, the body, primarily the liver, is able to produce needed structural, metabolic, and carrier proteins required for life processes. Sources of protein vary worldwide, ranging from primarily the milk of various mammals; to worms and insects; to eel, carp, and raw fish; to beans, rice, and corn; to organ meats; or to the more common Western diet of red meat and potatoes (or, more recently, hamburgers and french fries).

Personal choice related to food intake can be considered an internal force. For example, adherence to a vegan diet (because of a belief system) combined with inadequate knowledge or restricted food preferences may limit the intake of essential amino acids or vitamin B_{12}, calcium, and vitamin D, which can affect physiologic function.[14] All infants of vegan breastfeeding mothers who exhibit hypotonia, failure-to-thrive, developmental delay, microcephaly, or megaloblastic anemia should be screened for vitamin B_{12} deficiency.[15,16] Inadequate vitamin B_{12} is associated with neurologic damage as well as anemia and osteoporosis.[17] Vitamin D deficiency is a well-known factor in reduced calcium absorption, affecting bone health, but evidence also indicates lack of calcium with normal vitamin D levels is associated with rickets as well.[18] Calcium and vitamin D levels tend to be low in a vegan diet unless fortified foods or supplements are used. Without adequate intake of all essential amino acids, which is challenging in a vegan diet, protein deficiency can occur. On a positive note, a vegan diet can reduce cholesterol levels and reduce cancer risk.[19]

Medical Conditions

Impaired oral intake. Cleft palate impacts an infant's sucking ability, thereby limiting successful breastfeeding. Pain from dental caries and loss of teeth can impair ability to chew. A person with dysphagia generally requires altered food and beverage consistency (e.g., mechanical soft/ground meat, puree consistency, or thickened liquids) to regulate the rate in which food passes through the pharynx and esophagus. Consequently, nutrient intake can be compromised because food with altered consistency may seem less palatable; in addition, persons with dysphagia often have severe neurologic damage affecting swallowing. Impaired sense of smell will result in diminished, altered, or loss of taste that can impact food choices and intake (see Table 13-1). Psychologic reasons for limited food intake include anorexia nervosa.[20] Diet regimens, such as consumption of a very-low-carbohydrate diet or starvation (e.g., anorexia nervosa), will have physiologic consequences, one of them being scurvy. This is because vitamin C is only provided in fruits and vegetables, such as potatoes, which are significant sources of carbohydrates.[21]

Impaired digestion. Lactose intolerance is a common digestive problem that includes symptoms of abdominal bloating and diarrhea. Although lactose intolerance may be genetic, any insult to the gastrointestinal (GI) tract can result in reduced levels of the digestive enzyme lactase and consequent inability to digest lactose. However, this condition may be temporary until the GI tract returns to health. Other digestive problems include gastroparesis, a form of autonomic neuropathy that causes reduction in the ability of the stomach to transfer food contents into the small intestine because of reduced peristalsis. Gastric resection further limits intake because of the small size of the stomach pouch. This can result in intentional weight loss (e.g., as with bariatric surgery) but also can lead to unintentional compromised nutritional status, such as zinc deficiency from limited ability to consume adequate sources in the form of meat.[22,23]

Inadequate stomach acidity, as can occur with excessive antacid use, can limit the ability to metabolize and utilize a variety of nutrients. Vitamin B_{12} deficiency can occur as a result of the reduced gastric acidity associated with use of proton pump inhibitors, and supplementation is often warranted.[24]

Problems with digestion can continue throughout the small intestinal tract. Dumping syndrome, as commonly found after any form of gastric surgery, but especially with the form of bariatric surgery that bypasses the pyloric sphincter, causes insufficient digestion through rapid passage of food into the intestinal tract. This can result in severe abdominal pain as well as diarrhea, and may further reduce intake of food in an attempt to avoid the symptoms; dumping syndrome is associated with malnutrition.[25] Damage to the intestinal tract, as found with inflammatory bowel diseases or surgical resection from

TABLE 13-1   IMPACT OF MEDICAL CONDITIONS ON RISK OF MALNUTRITION

MEDICAL CONDITIONS OR STATES	IMPACT ON NUTRITIONAL STATUS
Oral/GI problems with limited protein-calorie intake (e.g., sensory issues, allergies, dental problems, dysphagia) Impaired intestinal absorption of proteins (diarrhea/malabsorption: e.g., celiac disease, Crohn's disease, short-bowel syndrome, bariatric surgery) Hepatic disease with impaired protein synthesis CKD with proteinuria and macroalbuminuria; nephrotic syndrome Cancer with increased metabolic needs Burns with loss of protein in body fluids	Hypoalbuminemia/impaired protein nutrition
Hypoalbuminemia (lack of carrier proteins) Hyperphosphatemia (ESRD)* Malabsorption/diarrhea Hypoparathyroidism Hypomagnesemia Vitamin D deficiency	Hypocalcemia
Hyperparathyroidism Hyperthyroidism Adrenal insufficiency Cancer Hypervitaminosis A and D	Hypercalcemia
Wound healing protocol with excess supplementation of zinc	Copper deficiency anemia
GI bleed	Iron deficiency anemia/microcytic anemia
Hemochromatosis Hepatic disease	Iron overload
Gastrectomy Pernicious anemia/lack of intrinsic factor Primary hypothyroidism Achlorhydria	Vitamin B$_{12}$ deficiency
Epilepsy with use of antiseizure medications ESRD and dialysis treatments Edema/HTN with K$^+$-depleting diuretics Malabsorption/diarrhea Hepatic disease Pancreatitis	Folic acid deficiency/megaloblastic anemia Hypomagnesemia
CKD with limited ability to convert to active form Malabsorption	Vitamin D deficiency
Hypoalbuminemia ESRD with dialysis Alcoholic cirrhosis/hepatic disease Inflammatory bowel disease Sickle cell anemia	Zinc deficiency

*ESRD, End-stage renal disease.

the malabsorptive forms of bariatric surgery, will result in deficiency of a variety of micro- and macronutrients with resulting adverse health outcomes depending on the site of malabsorption.[26-28]

Disorders of metabolism. A variety of conditions increase the metabolic rate, and consequently caloric needs. Conditions of hypermetabolism include cancer, severe burns, chronic obstructive pulmonary disease (COPD), Parkinson's disease, and autoimmune deficiency syndrome (AIDS), and people with these conditions may find it difficult to meet increased needs without enteral or parenteral nutrition. Hyperthyroidism will also increase caloric needs, but is a condition that is correctable. Suppressed metabolism, as found with hypothyroidism, can lead to obesity and elevated levels of lipids and glucose.

Organ damage will affect the metabolism of nutrients; for example, hepatic disease adversely impacts the ability to reassemble amino acids into the various proteins needed for physiologic function. In the common condition chronic kidney disease (CKD), nutritional status is adversely impacted through a variety of mechanisms. Protein is lost through the urine and can cause hypoalbuminemia that, in turn, can lead to impaired skin integrity, impaired wound healing, suppressed immunity, sarcopenia, and generalized edema (such as found with anasarca), attributable to altered osmotic pressure. While CKD progresses, phosphorous levels can increase and lead to hypocalcemia. Renal disease will further reduce nutrient levels, such as vitamin D because of impaired ability to metabolize vitamin D_2 into the active D_3 form. With lowered vitamin D status, bone health is impacted because vitamin D is required to absorb calcium into bones. Bone-mineral disease is common with CKD. The kidneys are involved in producing red blood cells; therefore in patients with CKD, anemia can develop that is unresponsive to iron intake because of insufficient erythropoietin levels, a protein-based hormone. Iron deficiency anemia, however, may be found with CKD because of the loss of carrier proteins. Even medical nutrition therapy (MNT) in managing CKD disease can have adverse nutritional consequences attributable to limitations on food intake and corresponding nutrients with protein and potassium restrictions. This is especially true when CKD is compounded with an acute illness.[29] Any condition of organ damage can adversely impact nutritional status as shown in Table 13-1.

PHYSIOLOGIC PROCESSES AND CONSEQUENCES

Physiologic Processes

Oral Intake

Normal intake requires appropriate ingestion of necessary foods to meet macronutrient (the kilocalorie sources of carbohydrates, fats, and proteins) and micronutrient (vitamins, minerals, phytochemicals, and water) needs. This involves informed food choices as well as efficient mastication and swallowing ability. For persons unable to ingest food orally, but who have an intact gastrointestinal tract, enteral nutrition may be provided through tube feeding. A common form of tube feeding is percutaneous endoscopic gastrostomy (PEG) feeding.

Digestion

Digestion is the process of mechanical and chemical breakdown of food matter and complex forms of macronutrients. Mechanical breakdown includes chewing as well as the mixing motions and peristaltic action of propelling food through the gastrointestinal tract. Efficient chemical breakdown of food matter through enzyme action is enhanced with thorough chewing because enzymes work on the surface of food particles. Chemical breakdown involves digestive enzymes; this begins in the oral cavity, where carbohydrates are metabolized into simple sugars. In the stomach, gastric enzymes begin to digest proteins into amino acids, and pancreatic enzymes finalize digestion in the small bowel with fats being converted into fatty acids. Bile, as produced in the liver and stored in the gallbladder, is involved in fat digestion as well through its emulsification and modification of dietary fats into absorbable forms. Damage to the pancreas, as found with alcohol abuse, can result in fat malabsorption and associated impaired absorption of fat-soluble vitamins, leading to deficiency of these vitamins. A healthy gallbladder is needed for optimal release of bile, which increases following ingestion of a fatty meal.

Absorption

Once food matter has been digested, the microscopic hair-like projections that line the intestinal tract (called villi, which contain capillaries) are able to absorb nutrients for transport through the vascular system. The upper portion of the small intestinal tract, the duodenum, is the primary site of absorption of trace minerals; the middle section, the jejunum, is the primary site of absorption of water-soluble vitamins and proteins; the lower section, the ileum, is the site of fat and fat-soluble vitamin absorption. Water is primarily absorbed in the colon. Malabsorption may occur without noticeable evidence, as is now recognized with uncontrolled celiac disease.[30] Confirmation of a diagnosis of celiac disease is based on the presence of specific antibodies as well as flattened villi.

Elimination

Large food particles and undigested fibers are not absorbed—they are eliminated through the colon. A healthy gastrointestinal tract with efficient peristaltic action is required for optimal elimination. Bulky stools, from adequate fiber intake, stimulate peristalsis. Elimination is enhanced with fiber intake; insoluble fiber adds bulk to the stool whereas soluble fiber softens stools by retaining moisture from adequate fluid intake. Exercise promotes the process of elimination.

Cellular Metabolism

Cellular metabolism includes the hormonal and enzymatic processes that occur within cell structures that allow various components (such as proteins, carbohydrates, or fats) to be produced or utilized for energy needs. Adequate intake of macro- and micronutrients is required for optimal cellular metabolism. Protein intake is essential for cellular ability to manufacture other forms of proteins, such as carrier proteins, and to enable tissue growth and repair. Adequate carbohydrate intake can provide the needed kilocalories to facilitate protein anabolism (the building process), and adequate fat intake with essential fatty acids is required for integrity of the phospholipid-based cell membranes. Carbohydrates are further required to provide glucose for the unique fuel needs of the brain and the rest of the neurologic system.

Because many cellular metabolic enzymes are composed of micronutrients, micronutrients assist in cellular metabolism. Zinc and magnesium are each known to be part of more than 200 different metabolic enzymes. Both zinc and folic acid are critical in the production of proteins and cellular structures, and without these micronutrients growth and tissue repair are severely impaired. Iron deficiency anemia contributes to impaired oxygenation because the iron in hemoglobin is responsible for the transportation of oxygen.

Consequences of Malnutrition

Protein is a component of every part of the body, ranging from its structural framework, such as skeletal muscle, to blood components, to carrier proteins that allow delivery of a vast array of micronutrients through the bloodstream to various tissues and organs. Protein deficiency has diverse consequences. The effects of protein malnutrition can be subtle or dramatic depending on the degree of deficiency (kwashiorkor is the severe form of protein malnutrition). At younger ages inadequate intake of protein and kilocalories (protein-calorie malnutrition [PCM], also known as marasmus) can lead to impaired growth and development, causing stunted growth; impaired cognition can develop if brain growth is diminished. At any age inadequate protein status will adversely impact the body's ability to repair or replace body tissues or produce other constituents such as immune factors.

Inadequate carbohydrate intake can alter cellular metabolism and result in the use of dietary protein as a fuel substrate, diminishing protein's intended function in cell growth and repair. Ultimately, if inadequate intake of carbohydrate continues there is a shift to use body lipids for fuel and a potential for excess ketone accumulation, especially if insulin availability is limited. Diabetic ketoacidosis results in lowered blood pH level; symptoms include nausea and vomiting and altered patterns of breathing.

Essential fatty acid deficiency affects all cellular membranes and is particularly a problem with premature infants who receive parenteral nutrition.[31] Docosahexaenoic acid (DHA), an omega-3 fatty acid, is now recognized as an essential fatty acid; deficiency or imbalance of omega-3 fatty acids and omega-6 fatty acids is related to impaired neurologic function. According to historical evidence, it is believed that a 1:1 ratio of omega-6 to omega-3 fatty acids is optimal. However, today's Western diet with its high intake of soybean oil has contributed to an altered ratio, ranging from 10:1 to 25:1. Deficiency of DHA can impair development of the brain and retina, and along with another omega-3 fatty acid, eicosapentaenoic acid (EPA), will adversely affect membrane receptor function and neurotransmitter production and utilization.[32] The chief source of DHA and EPA is marine oils, as found in fatty fish such as salmon, sardines, herring, mackerel, bluefish, and trout. Plant sources that provide the precursor for the marine form of DHA and EPA include canola oil, walnuts, and flaxseed.

Deficiency of vitamin C was one of the first recognized nutrient deficiency diseases, with the severe form of deficiency, scurvy, being a cause of death among early sea voyagers. British sailors were called "limey's" because their intake of citrus fruits while onboard sea vessels was found to prevent this condition. More recently, in the early twentieth century, when processed grains were becoming widespread in use, a mysterious grouping of ailments was found—initial dermatitis on sun-exposed areas along with diarrhea, dementia, and death. Once this condition, now known as pellagra, was determined to be from a B vitamin deficiency related to limited intake of whole grains, it became mandatory for processed white flour products to be enriched with vitamins B_1, B_2, and B_3, also known as thiamine, riboflavin, and niacin, respectively.

However, inadequate intake or absorption of micronutrients still exists today; emphasis on processed foods or exclusion of certain food groups, such as vegetables or dairy, as well as the increased prevalence of malabsorptive surgical weight loss procedures can result in deficiency conditions.[33,34]

Deficiency of B vitamins can also develop as a result of relentless vomiting, such as seen with hyperemesis of pregnancy.[35] Micronutrient deficiencies of fat-soluble vitamins occur with obesity because of their increased storage in adipose tissue, thereby lowering serum levels of these vitamins. This is true of both vitamin D and vitamin A.[36]

Some key micronutrient deficiency states include iron deficiency anemia, B vitamin deficiencies (e.g., Wernicke's encephalopathy and pellagra), scurvy from lack of vitamin C, night blindness progressing to total blindness from vitamin A deficiency, macular degeneration from lack of the phytochemical lutein and other carotenoids, and osteoporosis and hyperparathyroidism caused by vitamin D insufficiency. Other common issues of poor micronutrient status include impaired skin integrity resulting from vitamin C deficiency, poor wound healing associated with zinc deficiency, and a variety of anemias ranging from iron deficiency to copper deficiency, the latter often attributable to excessive zinc supplementation (see Table 13-2).

Malnutrition can also occur from excess macronutrient (kilocalorie) intake leading to weight gain. Consequences of obesity are related to chronic illnesses associated with metabolic syndrome (see Glucose Regulation concept). Excess intake of micronutrients is most likely to occur with high-dose vitamin and mineral supplements that has no bearing on food intake. The outcomes of excessive food or supplement intake on physiologic processes are numerous and complex, but some basic consequences can be expected.

ASSESSMENT

All nurses should know how to perform a basic assessment of nutritional status. Maintaining an awareness of risk factors for malnutrition helps to focus the interview and examination.

History

In the interview of the patient or family members it should be remembered that food has a strong emotional component and actual food or eating practices may not be revealed unless there is excellent interpersonal communication. This is especially true when interviewing parents if their child's growth and development is not within expected ranges. Generally, adults respond more openly to health provider concerns if they are aware of the rationale for the question. Mentioning some potential nutritional complications of a disease state or condition or asking about the individual's health concerns allows for focused interviewing, promotes discussion, and enables a fuller and more accurate assessment of needs.

The basic elements of a history—such as nutritional intake, diet restrictions, changes in appetite and intake, medical history, current medical conditions, current medications and treatments, allergies, family history, and social history—are essential to potentially identify risk factors associated with poor nutrition. In addition, it is important to consider the chief complaint/presenting symptoms because they might relate to nutrition and complete a symptom analysis. The most common presenting symptoms as related to nutrition

TABLE 13-2   COMMON VITAMIN AND MINERAL DEFICIENCIES AND TOXICITIES

NUTRIENT	CONSEQUENCES OF DEFICIENCIES	CONSEQUENCES OF TOXICITIES
Vitamin A	Night blindness	Loss of appetite, bone pain, hypercalcemia
Vitamin B_1 (thiamine)	Wernicke's encephalopathy with neurodegeneration	Toxicity rare
Vitamin B_3	Pellagra with 4 D's: dermatitis, diarrhea, dementia, death	Abnormal glucose metabolism, flushing, nausea and vomiting
Vitamin B_{12}	Pernicious anemia, psychiatric disorders	Toxicity unknown
Biotin	Hair loss	Toxicity unknown
Vitamin C	Bleeding tendency/scurvy	Inhibits zinc absorption, urinary stones
Vitamin D	Rickets/bone disease/muscle pain/falls	Hypercalcemia, renal stones, calcification of soft tissues
Copper	Anemia, skin lesions, neurologic disease, bone fragility	Found in Wilson's disease; neuron and liver cell damage
Iron	Anemia, fatigue, poor growth	Hemochromatosis (genetic) with liver, pancreatic, and cardiac damage
Magnesium	HTN, dysrhythmia, preeclampsia	Increased calcium excretion
Zinc	Dermatitis, impaired taste, impaired growth, low level of alkaline phosphatase enzyme	Copper deficiency, renal damage, nausea and vomiting, diarrhea

problems include the following: unplanned changes in weight; changes in appetite or intake; nausea and/or vomiting; difficulty chewing or swallowing; pain, especially abdominal discomfort; changes in bowel habits; or history of constipation or diarrhea.

Examination Findings

There are several techniques used to assess nutritional status including general observation, anthropometric measurements, and other various clinical findings from systems' assessment. Determining the body mass index (BMI) is an important initial step in assessing nutritional status and therefore determination of height and weight is required. The BMI formula using pounds and inches is:

$$\text{Weight} \div \text{Height} \div \text{Height} \times 703$$

General goals for BMI may be found in Table 13-3.

If BMI is within normal limits and weight has been stable, it is still important to have at least a brief assessment of oral intake to verify that macronutrients and micronutrients are being consumed in appropriate amounts. If there is any suspicion of poor nutritional status, lab work should be ordered by the attending provider to help assess protein status (albumin goal ≥3.5 mg/dl or pre-albumin goal ≥18 mg/dl) and to eliminate anemia from the diagnosis (hemoglobin/hematocrit ratio, mean corpuscular volume, and mean corpuscular height values in normal range).

Physical appearance and demeanor will give insight into health status. It is important to note skin integrity and turgor. The hair should be shiny and not brittle. The teeth should be free of cavities and the oral tissues moist, pink, and firm. The eyes should be bright and the sclera white. Optimal nutritional status is often observable.

The person who is well-groomed and providing past records indicates a well-organized individual, and one who cares about his or her health. Note the person's level of interest in the assessment/discussion of health, and if he or she is open to ideas and can state lifestyle changes that can be undertaken. To determine understanding of concepts discussed, use open-ended questions rather than questions that simply invoke a "yes" or "no" response. If there is a question regarding intellect, provide ample time for a response and encouragement because there may be a delayed processing time, but good intelligence.

Diagnostic Tests

Although most nurses are not able to directly order laboratory measurements, the nurse needs to be aware of important nutrition-related tests in order to alert the health care provider and request that laboratory assessments be undertaken when appropriate.

Protein Status

Measurement of albumin or pre-albumin level is the most common laboratory assessment performed, although this measurement alone is inadequate. Laboratory indices of inflammation, include an albumin/globulin ratio <1.0, an elevated erythrocyte sedimentation rate, or elevated C-reactive protein can indicate artificially low albumin levels. However, because inflammation adversely impacts nutritional well-being, measurements of albumin level are still helpful.

Glucose Metabolism

Determining hemoglobin A_{1c} level and/or testing fingerstick readings can provide insight into problems with glucose metabolism. Such testing is warranted if preexisting diabetes is present or if the patient is high risk, such as found in individuals who are obese, have a family history of diabetes, or have been diagnosed with other health conditions associated with metabolic syndrome (see Chapter 12). Interpretation of the A_{1c} reading with some conditions requires caution. This includes anemia and conditions of rapid turnover of red

TABLE 13-3   INTERPRETING BMI IN CHILDREN AND ADULTS

AGE GROUP AND APPROACH	BMI	INTERPRETATION
Children (percentile) BMI percentile for children: apply calculated BMI (weight in pounds/height in inches/height in inches × 703) to percentile growth chart (see www.cdc.gov/growthcharts/)	<5th	Underweight; may be acceptable if bone growth is adequate and child "follows the curve." Promote increased kilocalorie intake as needed if weight curve is declining
	5th to 85th	Optimal weight; still important to "follow the curve," and meet goals for bone growth
	85th to 95th	Overweight; goal to prevent obesity without causing risk to bone growth or emotional development
	≥95th	Childhood obesity; goal for young children is not to exceed percentile growth curve; promote physical activity and healthy eating to help "grow into weight"
Adults (calculated BMI) BMI calculated by weight in pounds/height in inches/height in inches × 703)	<19	Underweight; severe level <15 indicative of anorexia
	19-24.9	Optimal body weight composition. Elderly persons should strive for BMI >21
	25-29.9	Overweight; may be appropriate given health status
	30-34.9	Class I obesity; slow weight loss advised to promote permanent weight loss Not appropriate for elder population to lose weight[37-39]
	35-39.9	Class II obesity; slow weight loss advised May be a candidate for bariatric surgery if comorbidities present and not able to achieve long-term weight loss through diet and exercise
	≥40	Class III or "extreme" obesity (formerly known as morbid obesity) May be a candidate for bariatric surgery based on health status, age, and level of obesity and history of not being able to achieve long-term weight loss through diet and exercise

blood cells, as found with renal disease that can provide false low readings. However, renal disease can also provide falsely elevated levels of A_{1c} as a result of the test not being able to discriminate between other factors related to elevated levels. Finger-stick readings with self-monitoring of blood glucose level is optimal in these situations.

Fat Metabolism

For persons with preexisting cardiovascular disease, diabetes, or health conditions associated with metabolic syndrome, a lipid profile is generally warranted. This includes assessment of low-density lipoprotein (LDL) and high-density lipoprotein (HDL) cholesterol levels as well as measurement of triglycerides. Problems with fat metabolism, however, are found with pancreatitis and cystic fibrosis because of issues of digestion and absorption. In patients with cystic fibrosis or with other signs and symptoms of fat malabsorption, a fecal fat content can be ordered.

Electrolytes

Electrolytes should be assessed whenever concerns of dehydration or overhydration exist because even small deviations from the norm for potassium and sodium concentrations will increase risk of mortality as a result of altered physiologic processes. In conjunction with electrolytes, if dehydration is suspected, a blood urea nitrogen (BUN) to creatinine ratio that is elevated reinforces dehydration as the cause of either hypernatremia or hyperkalemia. Elevations of electrolyte

levels found with increased levels of chloride suggest diabetic ketoacidosis (DKA). Potassium levels should be periodically monitored when there is concern of hyperkalemia with CKD or hypokalemia with potassium-depleting diuretics. Hypokalemia may be due to hypomagnesemia. Hyponatremia may also be caused by excessive laxative use and the use of certain diuretics.

Other Nutrition-Related Labs

Tests to rule out anemia should be performed whenever there is a change in behavior/cognition or a change in skin integrity because lack of oxygenation from iron deficiency anemia will interfere with skin integrity whereas a vitamin B_{12} deficiency will affect neurologic functioning. If anemia is not related to these common causes, assessment of renal function with measurement of an estimated glomerular filtration rate (eGFR) is warranted because chronic kidney disease may be the cause. Anemia from copper deficiency should be ruled out if zinc supplements are consumed and signs and symptoms of copper deficiency are present, such as skin lesions.

With bone disease or muscle pain, calcium and vitamin D status should be obtained. Phosphorous levels (PO_4) should be monitored if there is advanced renal disease (stage 4 or 5 CKD with eGFR <30 ml/min/1.73m²). If liver disease is suspected an ammonia level (NH_3) can be ordered to eliminate toxin accumulation as the cause and to help determine dietary protein goals.

DXA Scans

A dual-energy x-ray absorptiometry (DXA) scan helps identify bone integrity. Bone loss may be related to poor nutrition, such as inadequate intake of calcium, vitamin D, and other micronutrients needed for bone health and strength. Bone loss may also be related to genetics, such as with uncontrolled celiac disease or vitamin D–resistant rickets, or be attributed to treatment regimens of medical conditions, such as the use of corticosteroids to suppress inflammation.

CLINICAL MANAGEMENT

Primary Prevention

Healthy Eating

A person who follows the *2010 Dietary Guidelines for Americans* and MyPlate (see ChooseMyPlate.gov), along with meeting the dietary reference intake (DRI) values as found on food labels generally can meet macro- and micronutrient needs and be said to have a healthy diet. Promotion of the inclusion of the minimum number of servings in MyPlate will meet the DRI micronutrient and macronutrient needs for general health needs. The *Dietary Guidelines* are aimed more at preventing chronic health diseases associated with excess intake of macronutrients, especially the solid type of fat known as saturated/trans fats or excess sugar or salt. Food labels with their DRI values reinforce the *Dietary Guidelines*. Food labels also state four marker nutrients: calcium, iron, vitamin A, and vitamin C. Generally if these micronutrients are included in adequate amounts from foods naturally high in them, the other needed micronutrients will also be obtained.

Physical Activity

Physical activity helps to prevent obesity. The general goals include 30 minutes of exercise, or equivalent physical activity, on most days of the week or ≥150 minutes weekly. Weight loss may require at least twice this amount of exercise. However, guidelines for exercise need to be individualized. A person who has sarcopenia or preexisting cardiovascular disease needs limited time intervals of exercise more frequently. This approach may also be most realistic for an individual who has never engaged in exercise.

Secondary Prevention (Screening)

Secondary prevention involves screening tests to detect disease. Screening for nutritional status in the general population is limited primarily to lipid screening, blood glucose screening, and BMI. The U.S. Preventive Services Task Force (USPSTF) recommends that lipids be assessed in men ≥35 years and women ≥45 years. Exceptions to this rule include lipid measurement in men ages 20 to 35 and women ages 20 to 45 when there is increased risk of coronary heart disease (CHD). Blood glucose screening is advised for persons with evidence of insulin resistance, such as central obesity found with metabolic syndrome (see Glucose Regulation concept).

For infants, routine screening that occurs at birth includes the following: glucose levels; at least 40 different genetically-linked metabolic disorders, including phenylketonuria and maple syrup urine disease, that are related to an inability to metabolize certain amino acids or to errors in fatty acid metabolism; carbohydrate disorders, including galactosemia; other congenital disorders that can affect nutritional status, including cystic fibrosis; and human immunodeficiency virus (HIV). The number of screenings varies from state to state.

Collaborative Interventions

There are several interventions to manage individuals who have nutritional-related health conditions. Interventions fall into the following major groups: dietary interventions, pharmacologic agents, and surgical interventions.

CLINICAL NURSING SKILLS FOR NUTRITION

- Assessment
- Tube feedings
  - Nasogastric tube
  - Gastrostomy tube
  - Jejunostomy tube
- Feeding-dependent patients
- Parenteral nutrition
- Medication administration

Dietary Interventions

Depending on kilocalorie needs or medical conditions such as hypoalbuminemia, hyperlipidemia, or hyperglycemia, the macronutrient quantities advised will vary. Micronutrient needs may be increased, such as potassium supplementation for persons prescribed potassium-depleting diuretics or vitamin D_3 supplementation for persons with chronic kidney disease (CKD). On the other hand, potassium or phosphorus could be restricted in persons with CKD.

Medical nutrition therapy (MNT) is provided by registered dietitians (RDs). These health professionals have the most knowledge about the macronutrient and micronutrient contents of foods; in addition, RDs can adjust a patient's food intake so that it not only is appropriate for health goals but also is a realistic and feasible dietary plan that addresses the multitude of lifestyle concerns related to family and work environments as well as usual food habits, finances, and food preparation abilities.

Nurses should be aware of basic therapeutic diets in order to help reinforce messages provided by RDs or to encourage referrals to an RD. Basic guidelines of limiting the intake of salt, sugar, and saturated fats; promoting consumption of fiber-containing foods; and moderating kilocalorie intake as found within the *Dietary Guidelines* are appropriate for the nurse to reinforce. Common institutional therapeutic diets include the No Added Salt diet (3 to 4 g of Na^+) used with hypertension and stable heart failure to the more restrictive 2 g of Na^+ diet for persons with severe heart failure and uncontrolled edema. Because sugar may be included within a diabetic diet as part of the total carbohydrate intake, the former No Concentrated Sweets diet is increasingly being replaced with a Consistent or Controlled Carbohydrate diet. A Renal diet typically implies restrictions in phosphorus, sodium, and potassium. In managing renal disease there may also be avoidance of excess protein intake for persons not on dialysis and fluid restrictions when urine output is impaired. The Therapeutic Lifestyle Changes (TLC) diet advised by the American Heart Association for persons with metabolic syndrome is not commonly offered within an institutional setting, but is aimed at a fat intake that is 35% of the total kilocalories, with an emphasis on monounsaturated fat sources such as olive, canola, and peanut oils as well as nuts and avocadoes. Saturated fat should be restricted to 7% of the total kilocalories and fiber intake increased, with the goal of low glycemic index meals to suppress the postprandial rise in glucose levels that may precede the diagnosis of diabetes.

Nurses also play a role in the administration of nutrition support via tube feedings. Tube feedings are indicated for an individual who is unable to eat or swallow but has an intact/functional gastrointestinal tract. Feeding tubes are inserted directly into the stomach or small intestine for the delivery of enteral feedings. A specific enteric feeding formula is determined by the RD based on patient need. The tube feeding is administered either by gravity or through a feeding pump.

Surgical Interventions

The most common surgical intervention affecting nutritional status is bariatric surgery; it is increasingly being used to control obesity and its associated manifestations of diabetes and hypertension. Generally, bariatric surgery has demonstrated good success when certain outcome measures are examined, such as weight loss, improved glucose level, and normalized blood pressure. However, weight gain can still occur after surgical interventions; also, other unintended complications can result in a variety of macro- and micronutrient deficiencies that are not easily managed either because of lack of adherence to dietary and supplement guidelines or because of limited knowledge of actual needs. There increasingly is a call to restrict the use of this procedure while investigations of both short-term and long-term health problems are resolved. This includes issues of correcting what appears to be Type 2 diabetes mellitus, while actually being the evolving autoimmune form Type 1[40] issues of prevention childhood obesity versus treatment with bariatric surgery,[41] especially in light of insufficient data regarding safety and effectiveness of long-term use of bariatric weight loss surgery.[42]

Nonmalabsorptive Bariatric Interventions

Forms of this type of bariatric surgery restrict the size of the stomach. This may be accomplished through the use of constricting bands that can later be adjusted or removed as needed. There are also surgical procedures that permanently remove portions of the stomach with the intent to limit volume of oral intake.

Malabsorptive Bariatric Procedures

These forms of bariatric surgery can significantly impact nutritional status because of reduced absorptive area and restrictions on the volume of food that can be ingested, at least initially. The most common form of malabsorptive bariatric surgical procedure is the Roux-en-Y gastric bypass. In this procedure most of the stomach and the proximal small intestine are bypassed with food entering a Y-shaped reconnection between the upper stomach and the distal portion of the duodenum or jejunum. The most malabsorptive procedure is the distal gastric bypass biliopancreatic diversion (DBP), which is often done in tandem with a duodenal switch (DS) in which the upper part of the stomach is surgically removed and the upper portion of the duodenum is reattached to the ileum, effectively bypassing most of the small intestine. This form of surgery has been associated with profound nutrient deficiencies along with the most weight loss of any bariatric procedure. See Table 13-2 for symptoms of common micronutrient deficiencies.

Pharmacologic Agents

In regard to pharmacologic agents for obesity management, research continues. There have been complications with previous forms of weight loss medications, and currently all of these medications have limitations on duration of use. There are a variety of pharmacologic agents that address blood pressure, lipid levels, and glucose levels along with other concerns such as altered thyroid function. Some nutritional issues include decreased absorption of fat-soluble vitamins because the medications interfere with fat absorption for weight loss purposes or lipid management, loss of B vitamins and magnesium[43] from proton pump inhibitors, and decreased absorption of B vitamins associated with antiseizure medications. Once a person is taking more than three medications, the potential implication to nutritional status is too complex to measure and is therefore unknown.

Parenteral nutrition is another type of pharmacologic agent used to provide either total or supplemental nutrition intravenously. Parenteral nutrition consists of a glucose-based intravenous solution (of various concentrations) and electrolytes, minerals, and amino acids. Fat emulsions (also known as lipids) may also be included or administered as a separate solution. Parenteral nutrition is usually indicated for individuals who are unable to process nutrients via the gastrointestinal tract for more than 4 to 5 days. Therapy can be short term or long term.

INTERRELATED CONCEPTS

Nutrition is interrelated with nearly all of the health and illness concepts as a preventive or disease management intervention. In addition, nutrition has an interrelated role with many body functions as presented in Figure 13-3. **Glucose regulation** is dependent on caloric intake and is critical to adequate metabolism of nutrients; in fact, glucose regulation can also be considered a subconcept of nutrition. For this reason, an overlap exists between these two concepts. Nutrition influences other metabolic processes such as **Immunity, Clotting,** and **Thermoregulation;** these all depend on adequate nutrients for optimal functioning. **Development** and **Culture** are also interrelated based on the influence of these concepts on dietary patterns and preferences.

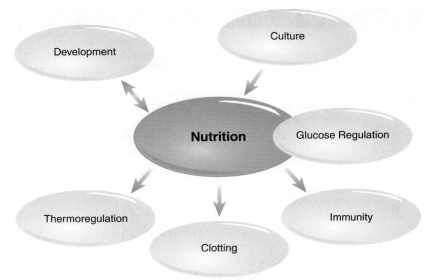

FIGURE 13-3 Nutrition and Interrelated Concepts.

MODEL CASE

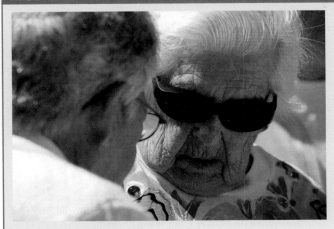

Mary Williams is a 73-year-old female who has stage 4 CKD (estimated glomerular filtration rate, eGFR, <30 mg/dl). She has a long history of morbid obesity (now defined as class III or extreme obesity) and uncontrolled diabetes, and now has heart failure as well. There is a family history of obesity with Mary's daughter having undergone bariatric surgery. Mary's obesity is related, in part, to her hyperphagia and craving for sweets. Having grown up on a working farm and tending to her horses, Mary has always consumed a relatively high caloric intake. After marriage she gained excess weight with pregnancies that was difficult to lose.

Mary currently resides in a long-term care center and is prescribed a No Added Salt diet to lessen the workload on the heart from potential fluid retention and a Controlled Carbohydrate diet to manage her diabetes. She has been having improved blood glucose levels since being changed to a basal/bolus insulin regimen with nursing staff providing mealtime insulin based on percentage of meal intake corresponding to an approximation of an insulin-to-carbohydrate ratio.

In the past, Mary had difficulty declining baked goods when they were offered at birthday parties and other social functions, although now that her health status is so tenuous, she has become overly restrictive with her sweets' intake in an attempt to protect her kidneys. She was advised by the facility dietitian to eat more sweets to help prevent excessive weight loss as a means to protect her kidneys, and to have her diabetes managed by additional bolus meal coverage insulin. Mary is skeptical, but somewhat relieved because her appetite and pleasure in eating other foods have diminished. She often has nausea, and many foods do not appeal to her. She has a long history of chronic anemia, now felt to be due to her CKD. Her potassium level has been elevated at 5.6 mEq/L, but by limiting her intake of high potassium foods, her level remains normal. In fact, she is now taking a potassium-depleting diuretic for her heart failure that caused her potassium level to decrease to 3.0 mEq/L, and Mary is pleased that she has been able to increase her potato intake.

Case Analysis

Mary is now realizing, unfortunately, the adverse effects of chronic obesity and uncontrolled diabetes as reflected in heart failure and chronic kidney disease. However, Mary has been successful in stabilizing renal function and avoiding dialysis by adhering to the following recommended treatment strategies: abiding by the medical intervention to promote heart function; using insulin to control blood glucose level; meeting dietary goals, including a maximum 1 g of protein/kg corrected body weight and consuming a moderate intake of sodium, potassium, and phosphorus; maintaining a stable weight; having a positive attitude. Her zealous avoidance of sweets resulted in weight loss, which has its pros and cons. One benefit of weight loss is reduced inflammation, which helps protect renal function; however, rapid weight loss increases Mary's risk of becoming frail because of sarcopenia and the increased workload on the kidneys, excreting the by-products of weight loss.

BOX 13-1 EXEMPLARS OF NUTRITION

Insufficient Nutrition*
- Starvation
- Protein-calorie malnutrition/Marasmus
- Eating disorders (anorexia nervosa, bulimia nervosa)
- Malabsorption syndromes
- Kwashiorkor
- Vitamin A deficiency
- B vitamin deficiencies
- Vitamin C deficiency
- Vitamin D deficiency
- Vitamin K deficiency
- Iron deficiency (anemia)
- Calcium deficiency (hypocalcemia)

Excess Nutrition
- Obesity
- Cardiovascular disease/hyperlipidemia
- Hypertension
- Type 2 diabetes mellitus
- Certain cancers

*Inadequate macronutrient or micronutrient intake or absorption.

EXEMPLARS

There are a large number of nutrition-related conditions. It is beyond the scope of this chapter to present all conditions, but some of the most common are presented in Box 13-1.

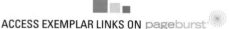

ACCESS EXEMPLAR LINKS ON pageburst

REFERENCES

1. Marzetti E, Privitera G, Simili V, et al: Multiple pathways to the same end: mechanisms of myonuclear apoptosis in sarcopenia of aging, *Sci World J* 10:340–349, 2010.
2. Narici MV, Maffulli N: Sarcopenia: characteristics, mechanisms and functional significance, *Br Med Bull* 95:139–159, 2010.
3. Barbarot S, Chantier E, Kuster A, et al: Symptomatic acquired zinc deficiency in at-risk premature infants: high dose preventive supplementation is necessary, *Pediatr Dermatol* 27(4):380–383, 2010.
4. Modi N, Uthaya S, Fell J, et al: A randomized, double-blind, controlled trial of the effect of prebiotic oligosaccharides on enteral tolerance in preterm infants, *Pediatr Res* 68(5):440–445, 2010.
5. Benelam B: Satiety and the anorexia of ageing, *Br J Commun Nurs* 14(8):332–335, 2009.
6. Cereda E, Pedrolli C, Zagami A, et al: Body mass index and mortality in institutionalized elderly, *J Am Med Dir Assoc* 12(3):174–178, 2011.
7. Berger MJ, Doherty TJ: Sarcopenia: prevalence, mechanisms, and functional consequences, *Interdiscip Top Gerontol* 37:94–114, 2010.
8. Ginde AA, Liu MC, Camargo CA Jr: Demographic differences and trends of vitamin D insufficiency in the US population, 1988-2004, *Arch Intern Med* 169(6):626–632, 2009.
9. Rovner AJ, O'Brien KO: Hypovitaminosis D among healthy children in the United States: a review of the current evidence, *Arch Pediatr Adolesc Med* 162(6):513–519, 2008.
10. Redmond N, Baer HJ, Hicks LS: Health behaviors and racial disparity in blood pressure control in the National Health and Nutrition Examination Survey, *Hypertension* 57(3):383–389, 2011.
11. Harper PS: The epidemiology of Huntington's disease, *Hum Genet* 89(4):365–376, 1992.
12. Marzetti E, Privitera G, Simili V, et al: The association between obesity and urban food environments, *J Urban Health* 87(5):771–781, 2010.
13. Esposito G, Imperato MR, Ieno L, et al: Hereditary fructose intolerance: functional study of two novel ALDOB natural variants and characterization of a partial gene deletion, *Hum Mutat* 31(12):1294–1303, 2010.
14. Dror DK, Allen LH: Effect of vitamin B_{12} deficiency on neurodevelopment in infants: current knowledge and possible mechanisms, *Nutr Rev* 66(5):250–255, 2008.
15. Honzik T, Adamovicova M, Smolka V, et al: Clinical presentation and metabolic consequences in 40 breastfed infants with nutritional vitamin B_{12} deficiency—what have we learned? *Eur J Paediatr Neurol* 14(6):488–495, 2010.
16. Mariani A, Chalies S, Jeziorski E, et al: Consequences of exclusive breast-feeding in vegan mother newborn—case report, *Arch Pediatr* 16(11):1461–1463, 2009.
17. Herrmann W, Obeid R, Schorr H, et al: Enhanced bone metabolism in vegetarians—the role of vitamin B_{12} deficiency, *Clin Chem Lab Med* 47(11):1381–1387, 2009.
18. Thacher TD, Abrams SA: Relationship of calcium absorption with 25(OH)D and calcium intake in children with rickets, *Nutr Rev* 68(11):682–688, 2010.
19. Krajcovicova-Kudlackova M, Babinska K, Valachovicova M: Health benefits and risks of plant proteins, *Bratisl Lek Listy* 106(6-7):231–234, 2005.
20. Karatzias T, Chouliara Z, Power K, et al: General psychopathology in anorexia nervosa: the role of psychosocial factors, *Clin Psychol Psychother* 17(6):519–527, 2010.
21. Swanson AM, Hughey LC: Acute inpatient presentation of scurvy, *Cutis* 86(4):205–207, 2010.
22. Andreu A, Moizé V, Rodríguez L, et al: Protein intake, body composition, and protein status following bariatric surgery, *Obes Surg* 20(11):1509–1515, 2010.
23. Sallé A, Demarsy D, Poirier AL, et al: Zinc deficiency: a frequent and underestimated complication after bariatric surgery, *Obes Surg* 20(12):1660–1670, 2010.
24. Rufenacht P, Mach-Pascual S, Iten A: Vitamin B_{12} deficiency: a challenging diagnosis and treatment, *Rev Med Suisse* 4(175):2212–2214, 2216–2217, 2008.
25. Naghshineh N, O'Brien Coon D, McTigue K, et al: Nutritional assessment of bariatric surgery patients presenting for plastic surgery: a prospective analysis, *Plast Reconstr Surg* 126(2):602–610, 2010.
26. Valentini L, Schaper L, Buning C, et al: Malnutrition and impaired muscle strength in patients with Crohn's disease and ulcerative colitis in remission, *Nutrition* 24(7-8):694–702, 2008.
27. Kuwabara A, Tanaka K, Tsugawa N, et al: High prevalence of vitamin K and D deficiency and decreased BMD in inflammatory bowel disease, *Osteoporos Int* 20(6):935–942, 2009.

28. Kazemi A, Frazier T, Cave M: Micronutrient-related neurologic complications following bariatric surgery, *Curr Gastroenterol Rep* 12(4):288–295, 2010.

29. Dumler F: Body composition modifications in patients under low protein diets, *J Ren Nutr* 21(1):76–81, 2011.

30. Volta U, Villanacci V: Celiac disease: diagnostic criteria in progress, *Cell Mol Immunol* 8(2):96–102, 2011.

31. Levant B, Zarcone TJ, Fowler SC: Developmental effects of dietary n-3 fatty acids on activity and response to novelty, *Physiol Behav* 101(1):176–183, 2010.

32. Simopoulos AP: Evolutionary aspects of diet: the omega-6/omega-3 ratio and the brain, *Mol Neurobiol* 44(2):203–215, 2011.

33. Singh S, Kumar A: Wernicke encephalopathy after obesity surgery: a systematic review, *Neurology* 68(11):807–811, 2007.

34. Ba F, Siddiqi ZA: Neurologic complications of bariatric surgery, *Rev Neurol Dis* 7(4):119–124, 2010.

35. Netravathi M, Sinha S, Taly AB, et al: Hyperemesis-gravidarum-induced Wernicke's encephalopathy: serial clinical, electrophysiological and MR imaging observations, *J Neurol Sci* 284(1-2):214–216, 2009.

36. McGill AT, Stewart JM, Lithander FE, et al: Relationships of low serum vitamin D_3 with anthropometry and markers of the metabolic syndrome and diabetes in overweight and obesity, *Nutr J* 7:4, 2008.

37. Rejeski WJ, Marsh AP, Chmelo E, et al: Obesity, intentional weight loss and physical disability in older adults, *Obes Rev* 11(9):671–685, 2010.

38. Zanni GR, Wick JY: Treating obesity in older adults: different risks, different goals, different strategies, *Consult Pharm* 26(3):142–148, 153–154, 2011.

39. Chapman IM: Weight loss in older persons, *Med Clin North Am* 95(3):579–593, 2011.

40. Deitel M: From bariatric to metabolic surgery in non-obese subjects: time for some caution, *Arq Bras Endocrinol Metabol* 53(2):246–251, 2009.

41. Whitlock EA, O'Connor EP, Williams SB, et al: Effectiveness of weight management programs in children and adolescents, *Evid Rep Technol Assess (Full Rep)* 170:1–308, 2008.

42. Colquitt JL, Picot J, Loveman E, et al: Surgery for obesity, *Cochrane Database Syst Rev*(2):CD003641, 2009.

43. Hoorn EJ, van der Hoek J, de Man RA, et al: A case series of proton pump inhibitor-induced hypomagnesemia, *Am J Kidney Dis* 56(1):112–116, 2010.

14

Elimination

Carolyn McKenzie

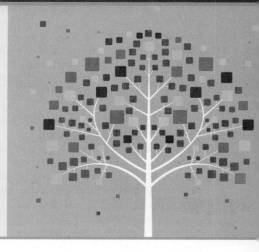

Elimination is a concept that has various applications across multiple disciplines including mathematics, economics, chemistry, and biology. From a biological perspective, elimination is a concept applicable to all living organisms—from the smallest of microbes, to plants, animals, and humans. This concept analysis will focus on elimination as a physiologic concept as it applies to humans. This analysis will include expected elimination patterns and problems associated with elimination.

DEFINITION(S)

Broadly speaking, the term elimination refers to the removal, clearance, or separation of matter. From a human physiologic perspective, the term elimination is defined as *the excretion of waste products.*[1] The human body eliminates various forms of waste through the skin, kidneys, lungs, and intestines. This concept analysis will focus on elimination of waste from the urinary system and the gastrointestinal system. Specific definitions for each follow. Bowel elimination is defined as *the passage of stool through the intestinal tract and dispelling the stool by means of intestinal smooth muscle contraction.*[1] Urinary elimination is defined as *the passage of urine through the urinary tract by means of the urinary sphincter and urethra.*[2,3] Other terms related to elimination include defecation (bowel) and micturition (urine). Bowel movements may be referred to as "stool" or "feces" and urination as "voiding." A variety of slang terms exist for both defecation and urination.

SCOPE AND CATEGORIES

As mentioned previously, the scope of this concept includes gastrointestinal and urinary elimination ranging from normal or expected function, to problems associated with elimination. The major categories representing problems associated with elimination include control, retention, and discomfort (Figure 14-1).

Control

The term continence refers to the purposeful control of urinary or fecal elimination. The ability to control is a normal and expected function associated with this concept. Incontinence refers to the loss of control of either urine or bowel elimination. With "control issues" both urinary and bowel incontinence may be exhibited by involuntary loss of stool or urine through normal routes. Control issues arise as a result of undeveloped elimination mechanisms, malfunctions in the mechanism of elimination, or alterations in cognition. Infants and toddlers lack control over the sphincters and muscles that control urination and bowel elimination. Voluntary sphincter and muscle control occurs as a normal process of development allowing the child to attain continence of both bladder and bowel elimination. Malfunctions in the elimination mechanism can result when injury or disease impacts neuromuscular integrity of the sphincters and muscles controlling elimination. Changes and/or loss of cognition can also result in the inability to control elimination.

Retention

Retention refers to keeping within the body materials normally excreted. Purposeful retention of urine and stool until an appropriate time for elimination is associated with control or continence (noted in the preceding paragraph). Retention represents an elimination associated with both urinary and bowel elimination. The mechanisms causing retention are usually associated with obstructions, inflammation, or ineffective neuromuscular activation within the bladder or the gastrointestinal tract. If untreated, both bowel and bladder retention can result in significant discomfort and potentially serious physiologic consequences that will be described in the sections that follow.

Discomfort

The process of elimination should be free of discomfort; in fact, when there is a significant urge, elimination often is associated with the relief of discomfort. Discomfort

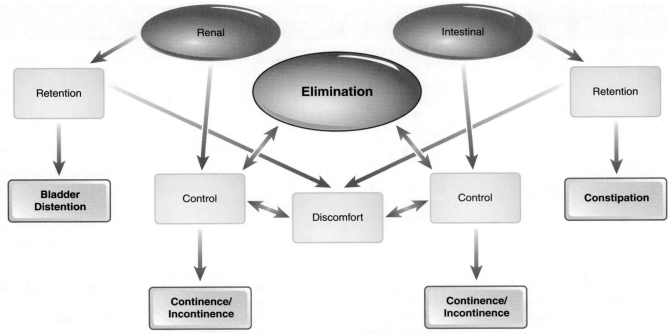

FIGURE 14-1 Scope and Categories of Elimination.

associated with urinary elimination can be associated with several underlying causes, but is most often associated with urinary tract infection. This is an important symptom signaling a need for medical treatment. Discomfort associated with bowel elimination can be associated with passage of hard stool, inflammation or injury to the anus, the presence of hemorrhoids (both internal and external), infection, or irritation of the intestinal lining attributable to frequent passage of stool. In children there can be telescoping of the bowel back into itself that can result in abdominal pain from obstruction and retention of stool.[4]

RISK FACTORS

Because elimination represents normal physiologic function, this concept applies to all individuals and problems with the elimination of urine and stool can affect any person regardless of age, gender, or race. General risk factors include conditions that result in neurologic impairment, altered mobility, cognitive impairment, and immunologic impairment or infection. Persons with trauma to the brain or spinal cord may experience bladder and bowel impairment attributable to interruption of bowel and bladder innervation by the spinal cord. If messages cannot be sent along the nervous system pathways, the anus and bladder are unable to function normally.

Many medical conditions can place an individual at risk for alterations in elimination, including cerebrovascular accidents (CVAs), spinal cord injury, diabetic neuropathy, dementia (including Alzheimer's disease), and acquired immunodeficiency syndrome (AIDS) or other autoimmune

diseases. Conditions specific to the gastrointestinal and urinary systems associated with risk include irritable bowel syndrome, Crohn's disease, urinary calculi, enlarged prostate, acute infection[5] chronic infections, and food allergies or intolerance, such as celiac disease.[6] Several congenital defects impair the elimination function such as defects of the spinal cord or brain, colon or rectal defects, and bladder defects.

Altered Urinary Elimination

Populations at risk for urinary incontinence include children younger than 3 years of age, the elderly, pregnant women, and women who are menopausal.[7] The prevalence of urinary incontinence ranges from 19% in women age 45 or younger up to 49% in women age 80 or older.[2] Because of the large numbers of women who have difficulty with urination, men may be somewhat overlooked when considering urination problems. Men are more likely to experience urination difficulties as they age because of changes (hyperplasia) in the prostate gland that may cause either urinary retention or increased urinary frequency because of incomplete emptying of the bladder. There are many reasons incontinence increases with age in both genders, such as pelvic floor muscle weakness for women and neurologic problems in men. Medications such as diuretics can also contribute to the involuntary loss of urine in both men and women.

Risk Factors for Altered Bowel Elimination

Bowel or fecal incontinence occurs in approximately 8% or 18 million Americans.[2] Bowel problems occur in men and women from both acute neurologic injury and progressive

TABLE 14-1 **CRITICAL ATTRIBUTES AND ANTECEDENTS ASSOCIATED WITH CONCEPT OF ELIMINATION**

CATEGORY	CRITICAL ATTRIBUTES	ANTECEDENTS
Bowel elimination (normal)	Presence of stool/feces Passage of stool Form of stool Color of stool Frequency of stool passage Retention of stool	Urge to defecate Possible intestinal cramping or feeling of fullness in rectum
Bladder elimination (normal)	Presence of urine Passage of urine Retention of urine Color of urine Frequency of urination Amount of urine	Urge to urinate Feeling of fullness or possible contraction of bladder

neurologic changes with advanced age. Excessive use of medications such as laxatives can contribute to incontinence issues in both genders. Persons at highest risk for incontinence are those with cognitive impairment, those who are exposed to radiation for treatment purposes, and those who take multiple medications, consume excessive amounts of caffeine, or have limited access to toilet facilities because of immobility or environmental or sociocultural factors.[8,9] Risk factors that place individuals at risk for stool retention include lack of adequate fluids, fiber, or exercise, as well as use of medications that dry the system, such as diuretics, narcotics, antidepressants, or anxiolytics. Pregnancy increases risk for stool retention because of the pressure of the fetus on the bowel.

PHYSIOLOGIC PROCESSES AND CONSEQUENCES

An overview of the normal physiologic process of elimination is presented followed by the problems and consequences of abnormal elimination patterns. Critical attributes and antecedents to bowel and bladder elimination can be found in Table 14-1.

Normal Urinary Elimination

In normal human urinary elimination there are specific structures involved. The kidneys, ureters, bladder, and urethra must all function adequately for normal urination to occur. The external urinary sphincter must be under the individual's control in order for continence to be successful. The main functional unit of the kidneys is the nephron, which consists of the glomerulus and the renal tubules including the loop of Henle. Various parts of the nephron are important in understanding the function, malfunction, and effects of medications on the urinary system. After the kidneys filter the blood using their functional semipermeable membrane called the glomerulus, urine begins forming. The urine contains the waste and toxins that have been removed from the blood. The rate of filtration is known as the glomerular filtration rate and is indicative of kidney

function. Some reabsorption of necessary elements occurs in the tubules. The loop of Henle conserves water and concentrates the urine.

The tubules have a role in the regulation of acid-base balance in the body by reacting to the stimulation of antidiuretic hormone, thereby allowing water reabsorption. The renal tubules are also affected by aldosterone, which stimulates the exchange of potassium and sodium to maintain electrolyte balance.

Urine then travels to the bladder and is stored as long as the sphincter that closes the bladder is functional and there are no obstructions from masses or strictures in the system. The bladder holds approximately 300 to 500 ml before the pressure increases enough to signal that elimination of the urine outside the body is required.

Normal Bowel Elimination

The intestinal tract is composed of the small and large intestines. The small intestine is primarily responsible for digestion and absorption of nutrients in food. Along the lining of the intestinal tract are villi that help propel the food as it is metabolized and formed into a waste product known as stool or fecal matter. The large intestine, which is 5 to 6 feet long and approximately 2 inches in diameter, has 4 parts: the cecum (and attached vermiform appendix), the colon, the rectum, and the anus. The function of the large intestine is to absorb water and electrolytes as the fecal matter moves through its walls. Mucus in the intestine helps lubricate the walls and aids in the expulsion of the stool. If there is excessive peristalsis and the stool moves through the large intestine quickly, less water is absorbed, resulting in a loose stool. If the peristalsis is reduced, feces pass through the large intestine slowly, resulting in greater absorption of water and a harder stool.

When the stool reaches the rectum, pressure stimulates the urge to defecate through stimulation of the intestinal smooth muscle and its stretch response. The urge to defecate can be suppressed until an appropriate environment is obtained. Repeated delay can cause difficulty in passage of the stool. The Valsalva maneuver can assist in passage of

TABLE 14-2	TYPES OF URINARY INCONTINENCE[8]
TYPE OF INCONTINENCE	**DESCRIPTION**
Stress	Leakage of small amounts of urine during physical movement (coughing, sneezing, exercising)
Urge	Leakage of large amounts of urine at unexpected times, including during sleep
Overactive bladder	Urinary frequency and urgency, with or without urge incontinence
Functional	Untimely urination because of physical disability, external obstacles, or cognitive problems that prevent person from reaching toilet
Overflow	Unexpected leakage of small amounts of urine because of full bladder
Mixed	Usually occurrence of stress and urge incontinence together
Transient	Leakage that occurs temporarily because of a situation that will pass (infection, taking a new medication, colds with coughing)

the stool; however, the Valsalva maneuver stimulates the vagus nerve, which can create problems such as bradycardia in some individuals and should be avoided if heart rhythm problems are present.[3]

Control Issues

Patterns of elimination change in the first few years in life. Infants and toddlers initially lack control, but control is attained during early childhood as a normal developmental milestone. Urinary and bowel control is expected among all adults; loss of control is considered an abnormal finding. Almost 25% of Americans may experience either fecal or urinary incontinence during their lifetime.[2] Individuals who are incontinent are at risk for skin breakdown (particularly if bedridden) and can potentially experience changes in daily activities, functional activities, and social relationships.

Urinary Incontinence

Urinary incontinence is a disruption in the storage or emptying of the bladder with involuntary release of urine. It is usually associated with dysfunction of the external and/or internal urinary sphincters, allowing urine to flow from the urethra. Factors affecting urinary incontinence may be psychological. Issues such as depression and anxiety may affect urinary elimination. Physical factors contributing to incontinence include cognitive impairments or recent surgical procedures affecting usual elimination. These are usually temporary issues that resolve once the causative factor is resolved. Types of urinary incontinence are listed in Table 14-2.[10]

Bowel Incontinence

Bowel incontinence is the involuntary passage of stool. Loss of sphincter control is the main problem that contributes to bowel incontinence. Loss of sphincter control can occur as a result of traumatic injury or pathologic changes to the rectum, or from neurologic injury. Bowel incontinence also can occur with diarrhea, particularly when it is associated with forceful intestinal peristalsis (cramping).

Retention Issues
Urinary Retention

Urinary retention occurs when the bladder continues to fill and the external sphincter does not allow the urine to be expelled from the bladder.[3] Retention is associated with significant discomfort caused by bladder distention. If left untreated, the pressure can lead to reflux (a backflow) of urine from the lower to upper urinary tract, causing dilation of the ureters and renal pelvis. The pressure can cause significant damage including pyelonephritis and renal atrophy. Chronic retention is associated with the persistent presence of urine left in the bladder after urination. This usually leads to chronic urinary tract infection attributable to the stasis of urine, or bladder dystonia.

There are several known causes of urinary retention including malfunction in nervous system innervation to the bladder, obstruction that causes the passage of urine to become blocked, or mechanical change in the shape of the bladder that causes retention, such as stretching with pocketing of urine.[11] For example, women may experience urinary retention if there is hard stool that presses against the bladder, or they may develop rectoceles or cystoceles that cause prolapse of the bladder and trapping of urine. Medications that may cause urinary retention include antidepressants, anticholinergics, and antihistamines.[11] Postoperatively, patients may have problems with urinary elimination as a result of the effects of anesthetics or the use of catheters during the surgical procedure. Psychosocial factors (such as fear or anxiety) may also affect the ability to successfully void.

Retention of Stool

Stool retention occurs when the person is unable to pass the stool successfully from the rectum. This condition is not normal for the young, but may be a common occurrence in people as they age as a result of the slowing of bodily functions. Stool retention in the young may occur as the "urge to defecate" is ignored and stool becomes hard to eliminate.

Postoperative stool retention may occur if the patient has received multiple doses of pain medications and anesthetics. Certain surgical procedures may also result in decreased peristalsis that contributes to further stool retention.

Stool retention usually results in constipation, defined as the difficult passage of hard, dry stool. When stool becomes lodged in the intestines or rectal vault, the condition may be referred to as a "bowel impaction." Liquid stool may pass around a hard, occlusive impaction, which can distract from the major problem—impacted stool. A consequence of ongoing retention of stool includes loss of appetite discomfort, and potentially fecal impaction.

Discomfort

The process of elimination should normally be free of pain or discomfort; in the case of significant urgency, the process of elimination can actually relieve discomfort.

Urinary Discomfort/Pain

The most common causes for urinary discomfort are associated with inflammation (often associated with infection) of the urinary tract or bladder distention associated with urinary retention. Pain associated with urinary tract infection is often described as a burning pain. Pain can also be associated with irritation when skin comes in contact with lesions on the genitalia, such as open herpes lesions.

Bowel Discomfort/Pain

Discomfort during the process of bowel elimination occurs occasionally with alterations in stool consistency; the passage of hard stool (with constipation) can create significant discomfort. Chronic conditions such as colitis or irritable bowel syndrome and excessive flatus or gas buildup in the bowel can also be very painful and unless dissipated or released they are very uncomfortable for the individual. An inflamed colon should be treated to alleviate discomfort. Bowel irritability that is characterized especially by constipation or diarrhea, cramping abdominal pain, and the passage of mucus in the stool can cause discomfort. Pain also can be associated with lesions such as an anal fissure or hemorrhoids. When these are present, an individual may avoid defecation because of the pain.

ASSESSMENT

Assessment of elimination includes taking a history, conducting a physical examination, and performing diagnostic testing when problems are identified.

History

Conducting a history is the first step to understanding problems associated with elimination. Common reported symptoms directly related to elimination include alterations in elimination patterns; changes in the appearance, frequency, or quality of stool or urine; or discomfort associated with elimination. It is also important to determine if there have been changes in diet or recent changes in health status (such as cognition, mobility, functional ability, or other medical conditions) and if there are new medications or changes in medications. Voluntary or involuntary (incontinence) emptying of the bowel or bladder must be assessed also to determine the impact of the condition on the individual.[3] Adults of all ages should be asked during routine assessment about urinary continence because it is an underreported phenomenon.[9]

Examination

Physical assessment incorporates four examination techniques: inspection, auscultation, palpation, and percussion.

Inspection

The abdomen is inspected for contour; abdominal or bladder distention is an abnormal finding. The genitalia are also inspected to examine the urinary meatus for evidence of redness, lesions, or discharge. Discharge from the urinary meatus is an abnormal finding and may suggest infection, especially if the patient reports pain with voiding. Inspection also involves observing the perianal area; the area should be free from redness or lesions; the presence of hemorrhoids or an anal fistula may be observed if the patient complains of pain with defecation. Inspection also includes looking at a stool or urine sample if available. Urine should be clear and yellow with mild odor. Very dark urine may be indicative of dehydration, may be a side effect of medication, or may indicate the presence of blood. Stool should be brown and formed. Stools that are black and tarry in appearance often signal gastrointestinal bleeding.

Auscultation

Auscultation is limited to the abdomen to listen to bowel sounds. Bowel sounds should be heard in all four quadrants. An absence of bowel sounds may be associated with paralytic ileus; hyperactive bowel sounds may be noted with gastrointestinal inflammation or with an intestinal obstruction.[12] Auscultation is not indicated in urinary assessment.

Palpation

Abdominal palpation is a physical examination technique for both urinary and bowel elimination. The abdomen should be soft and nontender with palpation over the entire abdomen and over the urinary bladder. Abdominal or urinary distention is considered an abnormal finding and may be associated with reduced peristalsis, or retention of stool or urine.

Rectal palpation is done to assess the rectal sphincter and to examine for the presence of masses, lesions, or impacted stool. Digital palpation is also part of the prostate examination. Although this is not directly an examination associated with elimination, prostate enlargement can result from a tumor (benign or malignant) or inflammation; both can contribute to urinary retention.

Percussion

Abdominal percussion may be performed to examine internal structures and may help to identify masses or excessive intestinal gas. Direct fist percussion over the costovertebral angle (over the flank area) should be painless; if sharp pain is produced it could signal the presence of a kidney infection.[12]

Diagnostic Tests

There are a number of diagnostic tests associated with elimination. In general, the diagnostic tests fall into one of three categories: laboratory, radiographic, and direct observation.

Laboratory Tests

Urinalysis. A urinalysis is one of the most common of all laboratory tests. It is useful for screening a number of conditions not associated with a problem in elimination and is obtained with either a sterile urine specimen or a clean-catch specimen. Bacteria indicate infection, whereas blood may indicate damage from infection or trauma to the urinary system. Urinary analysis that indicates the presence of bacteria or blood components in the urine may require further assessment of the urinary tract by a physician specialist in the field of urology.

Renal function tests. Laboratory tests assessing renal function include blood urea nitrogen (BUN), blood creatinine, and creatinine clearance tests. Creatinine and blood urea nitrogen are excreted entirely by the kidneys and therefore provide a measure of renal function.

Culture. Urine and stool cultures are relatively common laboratory tests. When a urinary tract infection is suspected, a urine culture determines the presence of and type of organism causing the urinary infection. Stool cultures are indicated when a parasitic infection is suspected.

Occult blood. When blood is suspected in stool, an occult blood test is indicated. It also represents a basic screening that should be performed as part of a rectal examination. The presence of blood in the stool could be related to a gastrointestinal bleed (inflammation, infection), hemorrhoids, or tumors.

Biopsy. A biopsy is a sample of tissue or cells that undergo pathologic evaluation. A biopsy can be taken from the rectum, colon, bladder, or kidney. Biopsies provide information associated with tumors or with general organ function.

Radiographic Tests and Scans

Numerous radiographic tests are used to assess elimination. Common radiographic tests include x-rays, computerized tomography (CT), magnetic resonance imaging (MRI), and ultrasound. These are used to detect a variety of problems, including the presence of an intestinal tumor, a congenital renal abnormality, or kidney stones. Angiography is used to assess renal blood flow and can detect renal artery stenosis.

Direct Observation Tests

The ability to directly observe internal organs can be accomplished with scopes. With regard to the concept of elimination, scopes can be used to visualize the colon *(colonoscopy),*[13] the sigmoid colon *(sigmoidoscopy),* the bladder *(cystoscopy),* or the urethra or ureters *(uroscopy).*

Other Diagnostic Tests

Several special tests are available to evaluate urinary elimination. These include bladder stress testing, uroflowmetry and other urine flow studies, and postvoid residual measurement through use of bladder scans or postvoid catheterization.

CLINICAL MANAGEMENT

Primary Prevention

The prevention of problems with elimination occurs with individual application of prevention measures based upon the person's normal bowel and bladder habits. By maintaining healthy bowel and bladder function with the intake of a healthy diet and adequate fluids, each person can promote the elimination of stool and produce the quality and quantity of urine that supports a healthy urinary system. Primary prevention through public education should occur regarding activities to promote bladder health, such as the following: encouraging adequate hydration, emptying the bladder with the first urge, maintaining normal body mass index (BMI), refraining from smoking, limiting intake of caffeinated beverages, and adhering to regular elimination habits and a consistent exercise program.

Environmental Factors

Avoidance of contaminated water and foods can assist in maintaining consistent bowel habits. Bacteria in water or food can cause diarrhea and colitis. Parasites can be present in water or food that is not properly prepared. Parasites not only can cause elimination problems but also can affect overall health. Laboratory testing can determine if parasites are present in the gastrointestinal system that may be causing problems with bowel elimination.

Maintaining Hydration

Water is a key element for prevention of bowel and urinary elimination problems. Water is absorbed by the stool to soften it and promote intestinal motility, which assists in the elimination of stool. Water serves the urinary system in that it increases volume, reduces bladder irritation, and helps eliminate toxins from the body. Fluids that may create difficulty in both bowel and bladder elimination include those with caffeine, which may cause an increase in frequency of elimination. Any substances that irritate the bowel or bladder will cause alterations in normal elimination patterns. Individuals can avoid problems by limiting the intake of fluids that contain caffeine, which may cause water to be withdrawn from the stool or cause irritation to the bladder.

Dietary Fiber

Fiber intake has been shown to assist in the prevention of stool retention, especially when implemented with adequate water intake and exercise.[8] Fiber creates enough friction along the bowel surface that it can assist in the production of a bowel movement. Adequate fluid intake with the fiber is imperative; at least six to eight glasses of decaffeinated fluids is recommended. Fiber should be slowly added to the diet to prevent abdominal discomfort and excessive gas formation in the intestine. The American Dietetic Association[14] recommends 14 g of fiber per 1000 kcal intake. The average is 25 g for adult women and 38 g for adult men.[14]

Maintenance of Regular Toileting Practices

Maintaining the individual's normal time of defecation is important in the regulation of bowel movements.[3] The use of familiar toileting facilities may also encourage defecation. Avoidance of foods that cause discomfort during digestion and absorption can help maintain normal bowel functioning. To prevent urinary incontinence or retention, there should be timely and complete emptying of the bladder. Women should not try to "hold" urine because this behavior encourages bacterial growth in the bladder and consequent urinary tract infection. Women who "over-toilet" themselves, however, may be avoiding the sensation of bladder fullness, which ultimately can cause more problems with urinary function.[9]

Secondary Prevention (Screening)

Two common screening tests associated with elimination are screening for occult blood and colonoscopy—both are considered effective for the detection of colon cancer. The U.S. Preventive Services Task Force (USPSTF) recommends occult blood testing, sigmoidoscopy, or colonoscopy for adults beginning at age 50 until 75 years of age.[15] These tests allow visualization of the colon and removal of precancerous lesions, averting the development of colon cancer. Screening for occult blood is performed annually or as a component of all digital rectal examinations. Screening associated with urinary elimination includes prostate cancer screening. The USPSTF does not condone routine screening for bladder cancer.[15]

Collaborative Interventions

Problems with elimination represent a wide range of conditions involving two major body systems—the gastrointestinal system and the urinary system. For the purposes of this chapter, common interventions are only briefly described; detailed information is available in various nursing textbooks.

Pharmacologic Agents

Antibiotics. Infections of the kidney and urinary tract are treated with antibiotics. Antibiotics are usually selected based on the provider's best judgment or based on the results of culture and sensitivity testing. Although a variety of agents are used, trimethoprim, trimethoprim with sulfamethoxazole, or nitrofurantoin are commonly prescribed for urinary tract infections; parenteral antibiotics are indicated for more severe infections such as pyelonephritis. Antibiotics may also be used prophylactically with urinary retention or recurrent urinary tract infection.

Antispasmodics. Anticholinergics are often used to relieve smooth muscle spasms in the bowel or bladder. Bladder spasms can occur as a consequence of neurologic injury. Anticholinergics can reduce bladder spasms, and can provide relief from urinary incontinence. Bowel spasms commonly occur with irritable bowel syndrome. Some antispasmodic medications (such as Imodium [loperamide]) are effective for the treatment of diarrhea because they cause a reduction in peristalsis and slow the passage of stool.

Agents to manage stool retention. Pharmacologic management to treat stool retention includes both prescribed and over-the-counter versions of laxatives, bulk-forming agents, bowel stimulants, lubricants, stool softeners, saline laxatives, and enemas. The drawback in using these medications is that the bowel can become dependent on laxatives and stimulants for the impulse to defecate. Medications for stool retention should be a last resort and discontinued as soon as the bowel elimination is achieved.[14]

Analgesics. Analgesics are indicated for relief of mild discomfort to severe pain for select urinary or bowel elimination conditions. Examples of conditions causing pain with elimination include kidney stones, cystitis, urinary tract infections, bladder spams, hemorrhoids, and rectal fissures.

Incontinence Management

Multidisciplinary management of the person with alterations in elimination must occur in order to successfully control the condition. The need for retraining the bowel and bladder is of paramount importance. Providing a regular toileting schedule, managing fluid intake, modifying the environment, avoiding indwelling catheters, providing high-quality skin care and assessment, and avoiding medications that contribute to incontinence are nursing actions that will promote urinary continence. Personal absorbent pads or bed-protecting pads may be used to catch episodes of incontinence in both mobile and immobile individuals. Biofeedback may be used to assist the person in gaining improved control over the muscles of elimination. Biofeedback involves placement of sensors onto the affected area of bowel so that the person can receive feedback regarding which muscles are being used to control bowel function.[16] Among those with dementia, toilet assistance (including timed voiding and prompted voiding) along with protective pads, and skin care are standard interventions.[17]

Invasive Procedures and Surgical Interventions Involving Urinary Elimination

A variety of surgical procedures are performed as treatment for urinary elimination problems. The benefits must outweigh the risks for utilization of these interventions because they can be invasive and sometimes lifestyle-altering procedures.

Procedures relieving urinary retention. The most common performed procedure to relieve urinary retention is urinary catheterization.[18] This can be done as-needed or an indwelling catheter can be inserted. Measures must be taken to prevent complications (such as infection) when urinary drainage systems are used for long period of time.[19]

Surgical intervention is often needed to treat other forms of obstructions, including surgery on the bladder, prostate, or ureters. Many procedures are conducted through a cystoscope. Stents, rigid tubes that provide an opening that is not normally present, may be used internally in the urethra and externally as part of anastomosis procedures performed for bladder cancer; stents maintain the patency of pathways for urinary elimination.

Renal calculi. Renal calculi (also known as kidney stones) often require surgical intervention if the stones are unable to pass through the urinary tract. A variety of surgical procedures are available to treat renal calculi, including *lithotripsy* (fragmentation of the stones through soundwave technology), *endourologic procedures* (insertion of a ureteroscope and crushing the stones with a surgical instrument called a lithotrite), or open procedures (*nephrolithotomy, pyelolithotomy, ureterolithotomy,* or *cystotomy*), where an incision is made and the stone is surgically removed.

Nephrectomy. At times surgical removal of the kidney is required, as with renal cancer. Other conditions such as polycystic kidney disease may require surgical intervention.

Prostate surgery. An enlarged prostate can cause significant urinary obstruction. A transurethral resection of the prostate (TURP) procedure may be indicated when other noninvasive treatment measures have failed.

Bladder surgeries. Surgical interventions of the bladder include a wide variety of procedures to treat many types of conditions such as prolapsed bladder or bladder cancer. Surgical treatment options include laser surgery, transurethral resection, and partial or total cystectomy. If the bladder is removed, urinary diversion is required.

Urinary diversion. Urinary diversion procedures involve diverting the ureters to a urinary stoma on the skin (usually on the abdomen). There are multiple types of diversion procedures that are described in greater detail in many nursing textbooks. Urinary diversion is required with a cystectomy and is also used in the treatment of other conditions such as bladder cancer, neurogenic bladder, or trauma to the bladder. Maintenance of skin integrity at the stoma site is of great importance. External urinary pouches are used in many cases to collect urine in these types of situations.

Invasive Procedures and Surgical Interventions Involving Bowel Elimination

Surgical procedures for bowel elimination problems are primarily associated with the colon, rectum, and anus and treat pathologic conditions or traumatic injury.

Colectomy. A colectomy (also referred to as a colon resection) involves removing a portion of the bowel. This may be done because of disease to a portion of the bowel (such as a cancerous tumor) or as treatment for traumatic injury. The two ends of the colon are reattached (anastomosed).

Colostomy/ileostomy. Diversion of the intestines (colon or small intestine) through a stoma on the skin is occasionally needed temporarily or permanently as a result of injured or diseased intestine, colon, or rectum. The use of external

devices (such as a colostomy pouch) is required for the collection of stool. Maintenance of skin integrity around the stoma is of utmost importance.

Rectal prolapse repair. Rectal prolapse is a condition that occurs when the rectum falls down into or through the anal opening. This is most common among young children and the elderly. Prolapse can occur from weak pelvic floor muscles or from excessive straining during bowel movements, as with chronic constipation. Surgical repair is indicated if prolapse occurs regularly or is associated with significant discomfort.

CLINICAL NURSING SKILLS FOR ELIMINATION

- Assessment
- Urinary catheterization
- Suprapubic catheter care
- Catheter irrigation
- Enema
- Nasogastric tube for gastric decompression
- Ostomy care
- Medication administration

Hemorrhoidectomy. This procedure involves the excision of internal or external hemorrhoids. Hemorrhoids may require surgical intervention if topical treatments and changes in diet do not eliminate their associated discomfort. Thus this procedure is usually only performed for patients with severe pain and multiple thrombosed hemorrhoids or when there is significant prolapse.

Fecal collection systems. A bag and tube system that uses a rigid tube inserted into the rectum is used to collect liquid stool in patients with incontinence who are not candidates for bowel retraining. These systems may also be used to relieve flatus.

INTERRELATED CONCEPTS

The concepts **Nutrition, Fluid and electrolyte balance, Mobility,** and **Cognition** are all interrelated and work together to ensure normal elimination. When any of these factors are depleted or impaired, problems with elimination may occur (see Figure 14-2).

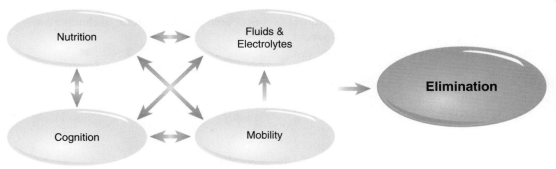

FIGURE 14-2 Elimination and Interrelated Concepts.

Nutrition. Mentioned previously, nutrition has a close interrelationship with bowel and urinary elimination. The types of foods and fluids ingested impact stool formation and urinary elimination.

Fluid and electrolyte balance. Inadequate fluids affect the urinary system and can contribute to the potential for infection. Inadequate fluids can also contribute to hard stool and constipation. Toxins cannot be eliminated from the body without adequate fluids. Elevated and reduced serum potassium and calcium levels impact neuromuscular transmission. Because peristaltic activity is dependent on smooth muscle action in the gastrointestinal track, altered electrolyte balances can negatively impact bowel elimination. Chronic elevations of serum calcium can lead to the formation of renal calculi thus negatively impacting urinary elimination.

Mobility. Lack of mobility can result in both urinary and bowel elimination problems. Mobility helps with stimulation of peristalsis. Immobility, particularly when an individual is in a supine position, can lead to ineffective bladder emptying.

Cognition. When a person has cognitive impairment, the potential for complications in both elimination mechanisms can result from the inability to obtain and maintain adequate food and fluid intake and can also lead to an inability to recognize cues for elimination—thus leading to incontinence.

MODEL CASE

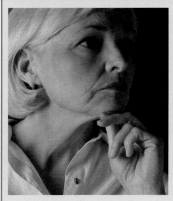

Ms. Andrea Doyle is a 61-year-old white female with a history of type 1 diabetes and has been bothered by osteoarthritis for the past couple of years. Her diabetes is well controlled with diet and insulin. Recently she began taking over-the-counter ibuprofen 400 mg twice a day to manage the arthritis.

For the past 6 weeks, Ms. Doyle has experienced abdominal pain and increased frequency of bowel movements. Her stools are loose and not formed; quite frequently they are a liquid consistency. Her life has been altered by the frequency of having to access a toilet because of the diarrhea. She had rectal bleeding and irritation from the frequent bowel movements and suffered from abdominal pain at night as well as during the day. She reported these symptoms to her primary care provider, who referred her to a gastroenterologist for evaluation.

An occult blood test showed blood in her stool. A stool culture was done to rule out parasitic infections; this was negative. Because it had been 9 years since her last colonoscopy, a colonoscopy was ordered to rule out pathology within the colon such as ulcerations or tumors. This screening test was also negative. The nurse practitioner suggested that Ms. Doyle change her arthritis medication from ibuprofen to celecoxib. Within 2 weeks Ms. Doyle has normally formed bowel movements and no abdominal pain.

Case Analysis
The symptoms described by Ms. Doyle are consistent with abnormal patterns of elimination. The diagnostic tests performed are routine given the symptoms and the time frame since the last screening tests. Nonsteroidal antiinflammatory drugs (NSAIDs) cause gastrointestinal distress, bleeding, and diarrhea, particularly in high doses and when not administered with food or milk. Celecoxib is a COX-2 inhibitor and is indicated for osteoarthritis, particularly when gastrointestinal inflammation is experienced with other NSAIDs.

EXEMPLARS

Exemplars of alterations in urinary elimination include conditions across the lifespan—ranging from bedwetting, which may occur as a child is learning to control bladder elimination, to incontinence, which may occur as a person ages and the muscles supporting the bladder become less efficient.

Bowel function also spans the lifecycle; a variety of issues may affect function as an infant, such as structural problems in the bowel (e.g., strictures and fissures), whereas functional issues such as constipation may occur as the person advances in age. Box 14-1 presents common exemplars of conditions associated with the concept of elimination.

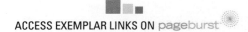

ACCESS EXEMPLAR LINKS ON pageburst

BOX 14-1 EXEMPLARS OF ELIMINATION

Control

Urinary
- Bedwetting
- Stress incontinence
- Urge incontinence

Bowel
- Diarrhea
- Fecal incontinence

Retention

Urinary
- Benign prostatic hypertrophy
- Prostate cancer
- Prostatitis
- Urethral stricture
- Bladder cancer
- Spinal cord injury

Bowel
- Constipation
- Fecal impaction
- Bowel obstruction
- Rectal cancer

Discomfort

Urinary
- Urinary tract infection
- Pyelonephritis
- Renal calculi
- Interstitial cystitis

Bowel
- Hemorrhoids
- Anal fissure
- Anorectal abscess
- Pilonidal cyst
- Constipation

REFERENCES

1. Venes D, editor: *Taber's cyclopedic medical dictionary*, ed 21, Philadelphia, 2010, FA Davis.
2. NIDDK (National Institute of Diabetes and Digestive and Kidney Diseases): *Fecal incontinence.* Accessed Feb 10, 2011, from http://digestive.niddk.nih.gov/ddiseases/pubs/fecalincontinence/.
3. Lewis S, Heitkemper M, Dirksen S, et al: *Medical-surgical nursing*, ed 8, St Louis, 2011, Mosby/Elsevier.
4. Hockenberry MJ, Wilson D: *Wong's essentials of pediatric nursing*, ed 8, St Louis, 2009, Mosby/Elsevier.
5. Mayo Clinic: *C. difficile.* Accessed Dec 27, 2010, from www.mayoclinic.com/health/cdifficile/DS00736.
6. National Digestive Diseases Clearinghouse: *Celiac disease.* Accessed Dec 27, 2010, from, http://digestive.niddk.nih.gov/ddiseases/pubs/celiac/index.htm#examples.
7. National Kidney and Urologic Diseases Information Clearinghouse (NIDDK, NIH): *Urinary incontinence in women.* Accessed Dec 27, 2010, from http://kidney.niddk.nih.gov/kudiseases/pubs/uiwomen/.
8. Wang K, Palmer MH: Women's toileting behavior related to urinary elimination: concept analysis, *J Adv Nurs* 66(8):1874–1884, 2010.
9. Palmer MH: Urinary incontinence. In Carreri-Kohlman V, Lindsey AM, West CM, editors: *Pathophysiological phenomena in nursing: human responses to illness*, ed 3, Philadelphia, 2003, Saunders http://digestive.niddk.nih.gov/ddiseases/pubs/diarrhea/2003.
10. *Crohn's disease.* Accessed Dec 27, 2010, from http://digestive.niddk.nih.gov/ddiseases/pubs/crohns/.
11. National Digestive Disease Information Clearinghouse NDDIC (NIDDK, NIH): *What I need to know about constipation.* Accessed Dec 27, 2010, from http://digestive.niddk.nih.gov/ddiseases/pubs/constipation_ez/.
12. Wilson S, Giddens J: *Health assessment for nursing practice*, ed 4, St Louis, 2009, Elsevier.
13. National Institute of Diabetes and Digestive and Kidney Diseases: *Colonoscopy.* Accessed Dec 27, 2010, from http://digestive.niddk.nih.gov/ddiseases/pubs/colonoscopy/.
14. *Fiber.* Accessed Dec 27, 2010, from www.eatright.org/About/Content.aspx?id=8355&;terms=daily+fiber+intake.
15. United States Preventive Services Task Force: www.uspreventiveservicestaskforce.org/recommendations.htm.
16. University of California, San Francisco: *Biofeedback.* Accessed Dec 27, 2010, from www.ucsfhealth.org/education/biofeedback_for_incontinence/index.html.
17. Hägglund D: A systematic literature review of incontinence care for persons with dementia: the research evidence, *J Clin Nurs* 19(3-4):303–312, 2010.
18. National Kidney and Urologic Disease Clearinghouse: *Urinary retention.* Accessed Dec 27, 2010, from http://kidney.niddk.nih.gov/kudiseases/pubs/UrinaryRetention/.
19. Newman DK: The indwelling catheter: principles for best practice, *J Wound Ostomy Continence Nurs* 34(6):655–663, 2007.

15

Perfusion

Susan F. Wilson

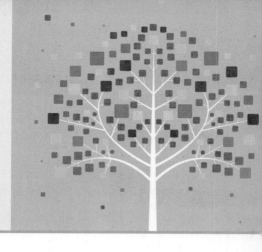

In order to survive, all cells need a consistent supply of blood to deliver oxygen and nutrients and to remove wastes. When the blood supply or perfusion is impaired, ischemia develops and can progress to necrosis, if prolonged. For this reason, perfusion is a critical concept for nurses to understand and incorporate into practice. The purpose of this concept analysis is to help the nurse acquire foundational knowledge about perfusion across the lifespan. In practice, nurses should be able to promote individual's healthy behaviors that optimize perfusion, identify individuals at risk of impaired perfusion, recognize when individuals are experiencing an impairment of perfusion, and respond with appropriate interventions.

DEFINITION(S)

For the purpose of this concept analysis, *tissue perfusion* refers to *the flow of blood through arteries and capillaries delivering nutrients and oxygen to cells and removing cellular waste products.* Perfusion is a normal physiologic process that requires the heart to generate sufficient cardiac output to transport blood through patent blood vessels for distribution in the tissues throughout the body. Thus maintaining cardiovascular health is essential to optimal perfusion. The extent of tissue damage from impaired perfusion depends on the size and location of the blood vessel and whether the blood supply is reduced or completely interrupted. When blood supply is available but decreased, the term *ischemia* is used. For example, when blood supply from coronary arteries to the myocardium is decreased but not absent, the term myocardial ischemia is used. The chest pain produced is called angina pectoris and the function of myocardial cells is reduced, but cells do not die. However, prolonged ischemia of tissue leads to necrosis, and eventually infarction if blood supply is not restored. Myocardial *infarction* indicates death of myocardial tissue with an inability to regenerate.

SCOPE AND CATEGORIES

The concept of perfusion and problems associated with impaired perfusion represent a wide range of physiologic processes and conditions. The scope of perfusion ranges from optimal perfusion to no perfusion (Figure 15-1).

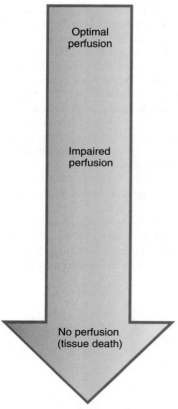

FIGURE 15-1 The Scope of Perfusion Ranges from Optimal, to Impaired, to a Total Lack of Perfusion.

Various degrees of reduced perfusion lie between the two ends of the spectrum. Two broad categories that describe the process and problems associated with perfusion are central perfusion (mechanisms for blood delivery) and local or tissue perfusion (actual amount of blood available to target tissues). Both of these categories are presented in Figure 15-2 and described further in the following sections.

Central Perfusion

Central perfusion is generated by cardiac output—the amount of blood pumped by the heart each minute. Cardiac output is an outcome of coordinated effects of electrical and mechanical factors that move blood through the heart into the peripheral vascular system. This central perfusion propels blood to all organs and their tissues from patent arteries through capillaries and returns the blood to the heart through patent veins. Although the mechanics of flow are the same to each target tissue, various factors can reduce cardiac output from the heart or cause systemic vasodilation or vasoconstriction to impair central perfusion. When central perfusion is impaired, clinical manifestations are systemic; in other words, the entire body is affected. Significant reduction of central perfusion results in shock, which occurs when blood supply to tissues is impaired because of inadequate cardiac output, significant blood loss, or vasodilation throughout the body.

Local/Tissue Perfusion

Tissue perfusion refers to the volume of blood that flows through target tissues. This perfusion is supplied by blood flowing from arteries to capillaries, which are surrounded by smooth muscles. The force of ventricular contractions creates a pressure, called capillary hydrostatic pressure, which pushes blood through capillaries into the interstitial spaces allowing delivery of oxygen, fluid, and nutrients to cells.

Different organs and tissues require different volumes of blood to maintain adequate function. Some organs such as the brain and intestines require much larger volumes of perfused blood compared to skeletal tissue, as an example. Inadequate tissue perfusion can result from poor central perfusion or from a mechanism within the organ itself, such as a blocked blood vessel leading to or from the tissue or from excessive edema within the tissue interfering with the cellular oxygen exchange.

RISK FACTORS

Adequate perfusion is required for life; therefore all individuals, regardless of age, gender, race, or socioeconomic status, are potentially at risk for impaired perfusion. Nurses need to recognize that some individuals are at greater risk for impairment. Some of these risk factors are controllable lifestyle behaviors, whereas others are not.

Populations at greatest risk of impaired perfusion are middle age and older adults, especially among males and African Americans. Also at risk are infants with congenital heart defects. Children and young adults commonly experience impaired perfusion as a result of trauma; this leads to central perfusion failure attributable to blood loss.

Adults in middle and old age are commonly affected by atherosclerosis involving the heart and peripheral vessels, myocardial disease, and other chronic conditions that negatively impact the cardiovascular system. Atherosclerosis is characterized by plaques of cholesterol and other lipids lining the inner layers of arteries, which results in obstructed blood flow. Older adults are at risk for impaired perfusion because of anatomic changes expected with advanced age such as fibrosis and sclerosis of the sinoatrial node and mitral and aortic valves.

A number of modifiable and nonmodifiable risk factors linked to impaired perfusion are presented in Table 15-1.

PHYSIOLOGIC PROCESSES AND CONSEQUENCES

Perfusion of blood begins when the heart is stimulated by an electrical impulse that originates in the sinoatrial (SA) node and travels to the atrioventricular (AV) node. From the AV node the impulse moves through a series of branches (bundle of His) and Purkinje fibers in the myocardium, which causes the ventricles to contract. The phase of the cardiac cycle when the ventricles contract is called systole. As the ventricles contract, they create a pressure that closes the mitral and tricuspid valves, preventing the backflow of blood into the atria. This ventricular pressure forces the aortic and pulmonic valves to open, resulting in ejection of blood into the aorta (from the left ventricle) and the pulmonary arteries (from the right ventricle). As blood is ejected, the ventricular pressure decreases, causing the aortic and pulmonic valves to close. The ventricles relax to fill with blood. The movement of blood from the atria to the ventricles is accomplished when the pressure of the blood in the atria becomes higher than the pressure in the ventricles. The higher atrial pressures passively open the mitral and tricuspid valves, allowing blood to fill the ventricles. The phase of the cardiac cycle when ventricles fill with blood is called diastole. Figure 15-3 shows the flow of blood through the right and left sides of the heart.

Pressure generated from the myocardial contraction supplies blood to the peripheral vascular system. Arteries, capillaries, and veins provide blood flow to and from tissues. The tough and tensile arteries and their smaller branches, the arterioles, are subjected to remarkable pressure from the cardiac output. They maintain blood pressure by constricting or dilating in response to stimuli. The more passive veins and their smaller branches, the venules, are less sturdy but more expansible, enabling them to act as a reservoir for extra blood, if needed, to decrease the workload on the heart. Pressure within the veins is low when compared with arterial circulation. The valves in each vein keep blood flowing in a forward direction toward the heart.

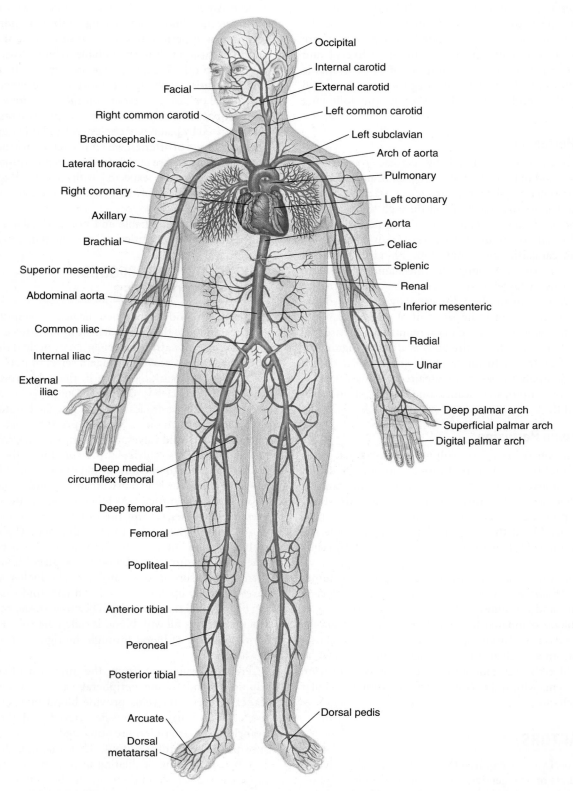

FIGURE 15-2 Arteries Supplying Central and Local Perfusion. (From Seidel et al: *Mosby's guide to physical examination,* St Louis, 2011, Mosby.)

TABLE 15-1	INDIVIDUAL RISK FACTORS FOR IMPAIRED PERFUSION
MODIFIABLE RISK FACTORS	**UNMODIFIABLE RICK FACTORS**
Smoking: nicotine vasoconstricts	Age: increases with age
Elevated serum lipids: contribute to atherosclerosis	Gender: men > women
Sedentary lifestyle: contributes to obesity	Genetics: family history
Obesity: increases risk for type 2 diabetes and atherosclerosis	
Diabetes mellitus: increases risk of atherosclerosis	
Hypertension: increases work of myocardium	

From Wilson S, Giddens J: *Health assessment for nursing practice,* ed 4, St Louis, 2009, Elsevier.

Consequences of Impaired Central Perfusion

Impairment of central perfusion occurs in conditions that decrease cardiac output or cause shock. Cardiac output is decreased when there is inadequate perfusion to the myocardium, inadequate impulse conduction through the heart, or malfunction of heart valves. First, any occlusion or constriction of coronary arteries that reduces blood flow to the myocardium can result in a myocardial infarction that decreases cardiac output. This impairment prevents the myocardium from performing the mechanical function of pumping blood to the body. Second, altered impulse conduction through the heart (from the SA node through the AV node to the right and left bundle branches and Purkinje fibers) interrupts the electrical function necessary for the myocardium to contract. Third, malfunction of heart valves, either stenosis or insufficiency, impairs flow of blood through the heart. Shock, the inability of central perfusion to supply blood to peripheral tissues, occurs when the heart is unable to act as a pump

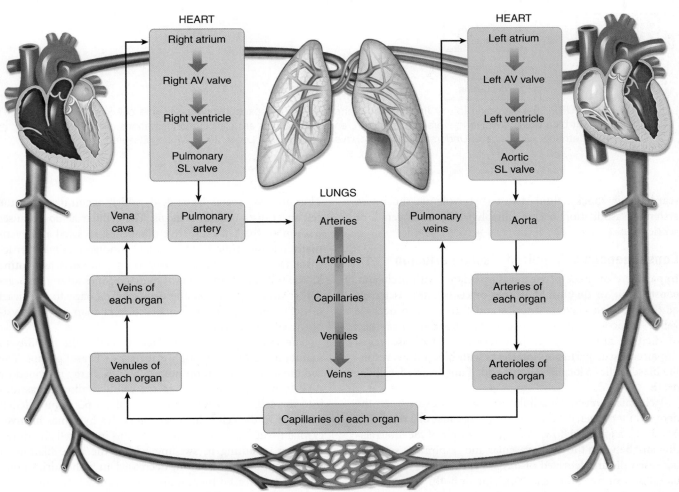

FIGURE 15-3 Diagram Showing Serially Connected Pulmonary and Systemic Circulatory Systems and How to Trace the Flow of Blood. Right heart chambers propel unoxygenated blood through the pulmonary circulation, and the left heart propels oxygenated blood through the systemic circulation. (From Huether S, McCance K: *Understanding pathophysiology,* ed 4, St Louis, 2008, Mosby/Elsevier.)

Reversible Cell Injury   Irreversible Injury (cell death)

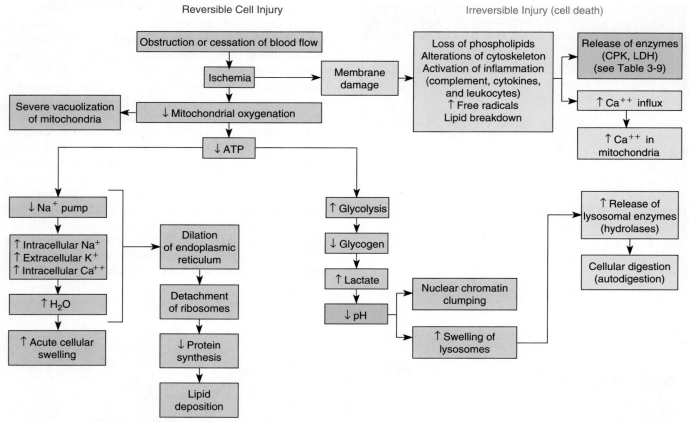

FIGURE 15-4 Hypoxic Injury Induced by Ischemia. Purple boxes involve reversible cell injury, light blue boxes involve irreversible cell death, and green boxes are clinical manifestations. (From Huether S, McCance K: *Understanding pathophysiology*, ed 4, St Louis, 2008, Mosby/Elsevier).

(cardiogenic shock), fluid is lost (hypovolemic shock), or systemic vasodilation occurs (anaphylactic, neurogenic, or septic shock).

Consequences of Impaired Tissue Perfusion

Impairment of tissue perfusion is associated with occlusion, constriction, or dilation of arteries or veins. Atherosclerosis or thrombi can occlude arteries and thrombi can occlude veins. Vasoconstriction can occur from frostbite. Examples of dilation are aneurysms in arteries and varicose veins. Impaired tissue perfusion interferes with blood flow, resulting in ischemia to localized tissue and, if uncorrected, cellular death.

Ischemia is *reversible* cellular injury that occurs when the demand for oxygen exceeds the supply because of a reduction or cessation of blood flow. This is an example of the interrelationship between the cardiovascular and respiratory systems, because cells are deprived of oxygen either from the lack of blood flow or from the lack of oxygen, or both.

Decreased oxygen to the mitochondria reduces adenosine triphosphate (ATP) production, which causes two problems. First, when oxygen is not available for the cells' usual oxidative metabolism, they are forced to use anaerobic metabolism, creating ATP from glycogen, to maintain cell function.

This process creates lactic acid, which accumulates in the cell and causes cellular acidosis. The cellular acidosis causes lysosomes, the cell's digestive organelles, to swell and eventually release acidic enzymes that autodigest cellular structures. Destruction of tissues releases enzymes such as creatine kinase (CK); measurement of these enzymes after a myocardial infarction indicates the degree of damage to the heart muscle.[1] Figure 15-4 presents a concept map of the physiologic effects of ischemia.

The second problem with lack of ATP is the inability to maintain the adenosinetriphosphatase (ATPase) pumps. The sodium-potassium pump normally uses energy provided by ATP to pump sodium out of the cell and allow potassium into the cell. When ATP is unavailable, a potassium deficit develops in the cell, which can cause dysrhythmias in myocardial tissue. Also, the sodium remains in the cell and draws in water, resulting in swelling within the cell, dilation of the endoplasmic reticulum, decreased mitochondrial function, and increased membrane permeability.[1] The increased membrane permeability allows calcium ions to enter the mitochondria, where they activate lipases and proteases and increase the production of free radicals.[2] The membrane damage initiates the inflammatory process, producing prostaglandins, thromboxanes, and cytokines. When ischemia persists, irreversible cell injury or cell death occurs from necrosis.

ASSESSMENT

Sources of data come from the patient as well as from physical assessment and laboratory findings. Assessment of perfusion involves recognizing indications of adequate and inadequate perfusion. The presence of central perfusion is noted by heart rate and blood pressure measurements within normal limits. Cerebral tissue perfusion is indicated by the patient's orientation to time, place, person, and situation; expected bilateral movement and sensation; clear speech; presence of carotid pulses; and absence of carotid bruit. Peripheral tissue perfusion is present when the patient's extremities are warm with color appropriate for race and the radial and dorsalis pedis pulse rates are between 60 and 100 beats per minute with regular rhythm, easily palpable upstroke, and smooth, rounded contour. Adequate peripheral tissue perfusion is also indicated when the capillary refill time is less than 2 seconds and the ankle-brachial index is greater than 0.9. Patients' reports of adequate perfusion include the presence of warm hands and feet and the absence of continuous pain in fingers and toes or leg pain when walking.[3]

History
Baseline History
When collecting subjective data from patients, nurses ask about lifestyle behaviors including diet, exercise, smoking, and alcohol consumption. A diet high in fat and carbohydrates together with minimal or infrequent exercise contributes to atherosclerosis and obesity. The nicotine present in cigarettes constricts blood vessels, contributing to hypertension and increasing the workload of the heart. Excessive alcohol intake is associated with dysrhythmias. Also, patients are asked if any chronic diseases, such as diabetes mellitus, renal failure, and hypertension, are present in either the patient or the patient's family. Nurses ask patients for a list of medications they take, both prescription and over-the-counter, including the reason for each medication and its efficacy. Patients are also asked about use of recreational or street drugs, such as cocaine because it is associated with myocardial infarction and stroke.[3]

Problem-Based History
When providing their history, patients may describe pain, shortness of breath (dyspnea), edema (swelling), and fainting (dizziness). When these symptoms are reported, the nurse follows up with a symptom analysis to obtain additional data, including the onset of the symptom; the location, duration, and severity of the symptom; a description of the symptom; factors that alleviate or aggravate the symptom; other associated symptoms; actions taken by the patient to relieve the symptom.[3]

Pain. A common symptom reported by patients with impaired tissue perfusion is pain. When there is inadequate perfusion to carry needed oxygen to meet tissue needs, patients experience ischemic pain. Ischemic pain occurs by the same process whether it is occurring in the coronary arteries of the heart or the femoral arteries of the legs.

Chest pain may be due to impaired blood flow to the myocardium or pulmonary emboli. Patients experience myocardial ischemia, also called stable angina, when there is an increased demand for oxygen on the heart. They often report a precipitating event such as physical exertion, exposure to cold temperatures, or emotional stress. Patients with angina pectoris describe their chest pain as a constricting or squeezing sensation that is relieved with rest and/or by taking one or more nitroglycerin tablets. By contrast, patients having acute coronary syndrome (unstable angina advancing to myocardial infarction) report severe chest pain that is not relieved by rest or nitroglycerin; shortness of breath; radiating pain to the jaw or arms; and nausea, vomiting, and diaphoresis. Although men and women may experience the same symptoms, some women report atypical chest pain, shortness of breath, and fatigue as their only indications of myocardial infarction. Patients experiencing pulmonary emboli report varied and nonspecific symptoms. Classic symptoms of chest pain and shortness of breath are reported only by about 20% of patients. The pain onset varies from gradual to sudden. Pleuritic chest pain also is reported at the onset of a pulmonary embolus.[4]

Pain in the legs attributable to impaired perfusion may be caused by peripheral arterial disease (PAD) or a deep vein thrombus. Patients with PAD may report pain when walking that is relieved with rest, called intermittent claudication. This pain indicates an inadequate supply of blood to transport needed oxygen to meet the demands of the leg muscles. As the arterial occlusion increases, patients may report "rest pain," which is leg pain while walking that is not relieved with rest. By contrast a venous thromboembolism causes pain because of pressure within the vein. Edema also develops from the obstruction of venous blood flow.

Dyspnea. Inadequate circulation of blood interferes with oxygen transport to tissues, making patients dyspneic or short of breath during activity. Thus this symptom may be reported by patients with primary perfusion problems, such as heart failure, or by those with primary gas exchange problems, such as chronic obstructive pulmonary disease. Patients may report having to sleep sitting up or using several pillows to prop up during the night. Lightheadedness may be reported attributable to inadequate oxygen transport to the brain. Nurses inquire about the duration of patients' shortness of breath as well as if the dyspnea occurs on inhalation or exhalation, or both. They ask what makes the dyspnea better and what makes it worse. Nurses ask if patients have any other symptoms occurring at the same time such as chest pain or swelling of the feet and ankles.[3] When an infant is being evaluated for heart disease, the mother or caretaker may report the infant needing to stop sucking "to catch his or her breath" or the infant exhibited a bluish color around the lips when sucking.[5]

Edema (swelling). Patients may report their socks leaving an indentation around their legs or edema in their feet that is worse at the end of the day. This edema reflects excessive fluid in the interstitial spaces, which indicates a fluid overload or an accumulation of fluids. The excessive fluid may occur from renal disease when blood cannot be filtered by the kidneys. Right-sided heart failure is another cause of peripheral edema that develops if the right ventricle is unable to eject its usual volume of blood. Reflux of blood occurs from the right ventricle into the right atrium, and then into the inferior and superior venae cavae. Because of the buildup of blood, the veins are unable to transport blood back to the right side of the heart, resulting in an accumulation of blood in the venous system that pushes fluid into the interstitial spaces, causing edema. Incompetent veins that develop from varicose veins may cause peripheral edema. Use Figure 15-2 to review the flow of blood from the venules of each organ to the right side of the heart.

Dizziness or fainting. Patients may report feeling dizzy. Using a symptom analysis, nurses collect more data to learn when this lightheadedness occurs as well as aggravating and relieving factors. If the dizziness occurs when the patient sits up suddenly, it is called orthostatic hypotension, which is defined as a 20 to 30 mm Hg drop in systolic blood pressure when a patient moves from a lying to a sitting or standing position. Nurses inquire about the duration of the dizziness. For many patients the dizziness subsides if they sit for a few seconds before standing. In contrast, dizziness unrelated to position changes may be caused by inadequate blood flow to the brain. The carotid arteries may be obstructed from atherosclerosis, preventing adequate blood flow to the brain.

Examination Findings
Central Perfusion

When assessing patients experiencing inadequate *central perfusion,* nurses may notice changes in vital signs such as hypotension or tachycardia. When assessing for orthostatic hypotension, blood pressure is measured in three positions: lying, sitting, and standing. Nurses compare these three blood pressure readings to confirm position changes as a contributing factor to the dizziness or fainting. Auscultation of the patient's heart may reveal S_1 and S_2 heart sounds as expected as well as S_3 or S_4 heart sounds or murmurs, indicating turbulent blood flow through the heart. There may be a change in mentation reflecting impaired blood flow to the brain, or shortness of breath can result from insufficient oxygenation of the blood or the accumulation of blood in the pulmonary capillaries. Additional findings may include changes in heart rhythm indicating altered cardiac electrical function; peripheral edema can develop from fluid retention or inadequate cardiac output. Patients may have a sympathetic nervous system response causing diaphoresis or anxiety.

Infants may have low weight and failure-to-thrive attributable to a weak suck and dyspnea while feeding. Children may not be as active and may squat on the playground to compensate for impaired perfusion. Characteristic heart murmurs are heard in infants with congenital heart disorders such as atrial septal defect, ventricular septal defect, and patent ductus arteriosus. Infants with coarctation of the aorta have high blood pressure and bounding pulses in the arms, but lower blood pressure, weak to absent pulses, and cool lower extremities.[6]

Tissue Perfusion

Manifestations of poor *tissue perfusion* are dependent upon the tissues involved. When assessing patients with impaired blood flow to the lower extremities, the nurse may notice less hair on the legs and pale skin on inspection. Palpation reveals cool skin, diminished to absent dorsalis pedal or posterior tibial pulses, and slowed capillary refill time. An ankle-brachial index (ABI) measurement of <0.9 indicates that the brachial blood pressure is stronger than the ankle blood pressure, confirming reduced perfusion to the lower extremities.

When ischemia involves the kidneys, for example in response to hemorrhagic shock, kidneys produce less urine because of lack of blood flow. The lack of perfusion stimulates the renin-angiotensin-aldosterone (RAA) system, resulting in a relative increase in blood pressure because of the effects both of angiotensin II (vasoconstricts blood vessels) and of increases in aldosterone secretion (retains sodium and then water, causing peripheral edema).

When ischemia involves the brain, manifestations produced depend on the extent of ischemia and the areas of the brain affected. For example, when mild atherosclerosis occludes the right carotid artery, patients experience a transient ischemic attack (TIA) that may involve left-sided weakness and difficulty speaking, conditions that usually resolve within 24 hours. In contrast, if blood supply to the right anterior cerebral artery is reduced or absent, patients will have a reduce level of consciousness and paralysis of the left leg.

Diagnostic Tests
Blood Tests

Enzymes and markers. Enzymes released from damaged cells and circulate in the blood can be measured to help confirm impaired perfusion.

- Creatine kinase (CK) is an enzyme present in myocardium (CK-MB), in muscle (CK-MM), and in brain (CK-BB) tissues. When enzymes are isolated, the level of CK-MB is elevated after a myocardial infarction.
- Lactate dehydrogenase (LDH) is an enzyme found in large amounts in the heart, liver, muscles, and erythrocytes. When enzymes are isolated, the level of LDH_1 isoenzyme is elevated after damage to the myocardium and erythrocytes.
- Natriuretic peptides include two hormones. Atrial natriuretic peptide (ANP) is a hormone secreted from right atrial cells when right atrial pressure increases; it is used to detect heart failure. Brain-type natriuretic peptide (BNP) is a hormone secreted from cardiac cells in increased amounts when pressures are high; it is used to detect heart failure.
- Troponin is a myocardial muscle protein released after myocardial injury. Increased blood levels of this protein are found in patients who have had a myocardial

infarction. Troponin also can be used to predict the likelihood of future cardiac events.[7]

- Homocysteine (Hcy) is an amino acid produced during protein metabolism. Elevated levels of Hcy can be hereditary or acquired from dietary deficiencies such as vitamin B_6, vitamin B_{12}, or folate. The link to perfusion is that elevated levels of Hcy have been identified as a predictor of coronary artery disease (CAD), cerebrovascular accident, peripheral arterial disease, and venous thrombosis.[8] Hcy promotes atherosclerosis by causing endothelial damage, promoting deposits of low-density lipoproteins, and promoting vascular smooth muscle growth.[7] Testing for Hcy has been recommended in those patients with a familial predisposition for early cardiovascular disease or history of cardiovascular disease in the absence of other common risk factors.[8]

- C-reactive protein (CRP) is a protein produced by the liver during acute inflammation and is emerging as an independent risk factor for CAD. Measurement of CRP using a high-sensitivity test (hsCRP) has been shown to predict the risk of future cardiac events in patients with unstable angina and myocardial infarction.[8]

Serum lipids. Serum lipids are measured to detect hyperlipidemia and include cholesterol lipoproteins (low-density lipoproteins [LDLs], high-density lipoproteins [HDLs], very-low-density lipoproteins [VLDLs], and triglycerides). These provide information about risk factors and possible presence of vessel disease.[7]

Electrocardiogram

An electrocardiogram (EKG) is performed by placing 12 leads on the patient's chest to record the electrical impulses through the heart. Six leads record electrical impulses in the frontal plane, whereas the remaining six leads record electrical impulses in the horizontal plane. The waveforms generated detect cardiac dysrhythmias by documenting on a screen or paper the electrical impulses generated by the heart during contraction and relaxation of atria and ventricles.[7] A 12-lead EKG is obtained to detect myocardial ischemia or infarction when patients complain of chest pain. An EKG also is used to continuously monitor the heart rhythm using one or more leads. Four leads are commonly used to monitor heart rhythm at the bedside.[9]

Cardiac Stress Tests

Exercise cardiac stress test. The exercise cardiac stress test (ECST) is one of the most common cardiac stress tests because it is relatively simple and noninvasive. Using a standardized protocol, the patient exercises on a treadmill with a progressive increase in speed and elevation. During the test, an EKG is recorded along with regular monitoring of heart rate and rhythm, blood pressure, and respiratory rate. If coronary artery disease is present, changes in electrical conduction or other symptoms such as chest pain may occur.

Pharmacologic stress test. Another common cardiac stress test involves the administration of certain pharmacologic agents which stimulate the physiologic effects of exercise. This is often done when patients are unable to perform the exercise stress test due to underlying conditions. Agents often administered include dobutamine and adenosine. EKG monitoring (or radionuclide imaging) is performed while the pharmacologic agents are given to detect problems with conduction, heart rate, or strength of contractions.

Radiographic Studies

Chest x-ray. Chest x-rays provide visualization of the lungs, ribs, clavicles, vertebrae, heart, and major thoracic vessels. For patients with impaired perfusion, x-rays are taken to visualize the size of the heart and lung fields.[8]

Ultrasound. Venous compression ultrasound is performed to determine if deep femoral, popliteal, and posterior tibial veins collapse with application of external pressure, which is normal. Veins with a deep vein thrombosis are unable to collapse. Duplex ultrasound is a combination of compression ultrasound and Doppler flow studies. Veins are examined for filling defects to help determine the location and extent of thrombus.[10]

Arteriogram. An arteriogram allows visualization of arteries by injecting radiopaque contrast into them so that the location and extent of occlusion can be identified. A cardiac catheterization is one type of arteriogram that allows visualization of coronary arteries and heart chambers. A catheter is passed into the heart through a peripheral vein or artery, depending on whether catheterization of the left or right side of the heart is being performed. Pressures are recorded through the catheter and radiographic contrast is injected to visualize the patency of coronary arteries.[7]

CLINICAL MANAGEMENT

Clinical management associated with the perfusion concept involves the prevention of illness and the early detection and appropriate management of cardiovascular problems. There are 24 objectives for heart disease and stroke in the *Healthy People 2020* document that reflect primary prevention, secondary prevention, and collaborative management strategies. (See *Healthy People 2020* at healthypeople.gov).

Primary Prevention

Primary prevention includes measures to promote health and prevent development of disease. There are several measures that prevent or diminish conditions that impair perfusion. Prevention measures are based on a heart-healthy lifestyle, which includes eating a healthy diet, exercising most days of the week, taking a daily low-dose aspirin, and not smoking. Recommendations by the American Heart Association[11] are presented in Box 15-2.

Secondary Prevention (Screening)

Secondary prevention includes screening and early diagnosis and prompt treatment of existing health problems. Its purpose is to shorten the duration and severity of consequences. Routine screening involves monitoring blood pressure and serum lipids.

BOX 15-1 *HEALTHY PEOPLE 2020* **OBJECTIVES FOR HEART DISEASE AND STROKE**

1. Increase overall cardiovascular health in the U.S. population.
2. Reduce coronary heart disease deaths.
3. Reduce stroke deaths.
4. Increase the proportion of adults who have had their blood pressure measured within the preceding 2 years and can state whether their blood pressure was normal or high.
5. Reduce the proportion of persons in the population (adults, adolescents, and children) with hypertension.
6. Increase the proportion of adults who have had their blood cholesterol checked within the preceding 5 years.
7. Reduce the proportion of adults with high total blood cholesterol levels.
8. Reduce the mean total blood cholesterol levels among adults.
9. Increase the proportion of adults with prehypertension who meet the recommended guidelines.
10. Increase the proportion of adults with hypertension who meet the recommended guidelines.
11. Increase the proportion of adults with hypertension who are taking the prescribed medications to lower their blood pressure.
12. Increase the proportion of adults with hypertension whose blood pressure is under control.
13. Increase the proportion of adults with elevated LDL cholesterol who have been advised by a health care provider regarding cholesterol lowering management including lifestyle changes and, if indicated, medication.
14. Increase the proportion of adults with elevated LDL cholesterol who adhere to the prescribed LDL cholesterol lowering management lifestyle changes and, if indicated, medication.
15. Increase aspirin use as recommended among adults with no history of cardiovascular disease.
16. Increase the proportion of adults ages 20 years and older who are aware of, and respond to, early warning symptoms and signs of a heart attack.
17. Increase the proportion of adults ages 20 years and older who are aware of and respond to early warning symptoms and signs of a stroke.
18. Increase the proportion of out-of-hospital cardiac arrests in which appropriate bystander and emergency medical services are administered.
19. Increase the proportion of eligible patients with heart attacks or strokes who receive timely artery-opening therapy as specified by current guideline.
20. Increase the proportion of adults with coronary heart disease or stroke who have their (LDL) cholesterol level at or below recommended levels.
21. Increase the proportion of adults with a history of cardiovascular disease who are using aspirin or antiplatelet therapy to prevent recurrent cardiovascular events.
22. Increase the proportion of adult heart attack survivors who are referred to a cardiac rehabilitation program at discharge.
23. Increase the proportion of adult stroke survivors who are referred to a stroke rehabilitation program at discharge.
24. Reduce hospitalizations of older adults with heart failure as the principal diagnosis.

LDL, Low-density lipoprotein.
From *Healthy People 2020;* accessed March 3, 2011, at www.healthypeople.gov/2020/topicsobjectives2020/default.aspx.

BOX 15-2 **AMERICAN HEART ASSOCIATION HEALTH PROMOTION RECOMMENDATIONS**

1. Eat a variety of fruits, vegetables, grains, legumes, fat-free or low-fat dairy products, fish, poultry, and lean meats:
   - Reduce sodium (salt) intake to less than 1500 a day.
   - Reduce saturated and trans fats to less than 10% of calories.
2. Participate in physical activity
   - Adults >20 yrs: at least 150 minutes/week of moderate intensity activity
   - Children 12-19 yrs: at least 60 minutes of moderate intensity activity every day
3. Refrain from smoking and have no exposure to environmental tobacco smoke.
4. Maintain blood pressure:
   - Adults over 20 years of age: <120/80 mm Hg
   - Children 8 to 19 years of age: <90th percentile
5. Maintain total cholesterol
   - Adults >20 years of age <200 mg/dL
   - Children 6-19 years of age <70 mg/dL
6. Maintain fasting blood glucose
   - Adults >20 years of age: less than 100 mg/dL
   - Children 12 to 19 years of age: less than 200 mg/dL
7. Achieve and maintain desirable weight
   - Adults >20 years of age: 25 kg/m².
   - Children 12-19 years of age: <85th percentile

Lloyd-Jones, DM et al: Defining and setting national goals for cardiovascular health promotion and disease reduction: the American Heart Association's strategic impact goal through 2020 and beyond. *Circulation* 2010, 121:586-613: originally published January 20, 2010. doi:10.1161/CIRCULATIONAHA.109.192703. Accessed September 19, 2011. Courtesy AHA.

Blood Pressure Screening

Blood pressure screening is a simple and cost-effective screening recommended across the lifespan. Beginning in infancy, blood pressure screening is recommended at every well-child visit, and at least annually. Among adults, the U.S. Preventive Services Task Force (USPSTF)[12] recommends screening for high blood pressure in adults ages 18 and older. For patients who have hypertension, the Joint National Committee on Prevention, Detection, Evaluation, and Treatment of High Blood Pressure[12] recommends screening every 2 years when blood pressures are less than 120/80 mm Hg. This same committee recommends screening every year when systolic blood pressures are 120 to 139 mm Hg or diastolic pressures are 80 to 90 mm Hg.

Lipid Screening

Recommendations for screening of lipids vary between men and women. The USPSTF strongly recommends screening men ages 35 and older for lipid disorders and screening men ages 20 to 35 if they are at increased risk for coronary artery disease. For women the USPSTF strongly recommends screening those ages 45 and older for lipid disorders if they are at increased risk for coronary heart disease. Among younger women, ages 20 to 45, The USPSTF recommends lipid screening if they are at increased risk for coronary heart disease.[12]

Collaborative Interventions

The management of individuals with impaired perfusion is highly dependent on the specific condition. The following sections describe common interventions implemented in the treatment of conditions resulting in impaired perfusion.

Nutrition Therapy

Nutrition therapy should meet the recommendations described under Primary Prevention, but the goal of the heart-healthy diet is tertiary prevention—to lower serum lipid levels and lose weight. For the reason, nutrition therapy is considered an intervention in both primary prevention and disease management.

Activity, Exercise, and Positioning

Activity and exercise are a regular part of any treatment regimen. Specifically it is included in the following applications:
- For the purpose of weight loss
- Cardiac rehabilitation after acute coronary syndrome[13]
- Progressive activity for patients with peripheral arterial disease
- Position lower extremities when seated or in bed
  - Dependent for arterial occlusion
  - Elevated for venous occlusion

Smoking Cessation

Smoking cessation is also considered both primary prevention and collaborative intervention for disease management. Refer to the Gas Exchange concept for interventions directed at smoking cessation.

Pharmacotherapy

- *Vasodilators* increase the diameter of blood vessels in a variety of ways that block normal mechanisms. For example, vasodilators can block the following: alpha-adrenergic receptors; calcium influx into vascular smooth muscle; formation of angiotensin II, which normally increases aldosterone concentration to retain sodium as well as vasoconstriction; or receptors that receive angiotensin II. Myocardial contractility is reduced for the purpose of lowering cardiac output by blocking calcium influx into the myocardium and blocking the beta-adrenergic receptors in the heart.[13] Vasodilators are used to treat hypertension as well as angina.

- *Vasopressors* decrease the diameter of blood vessels by stimulating the alpha-adrenergic or dopamine receptors to effect the normal mechanism of vasoconstriction.[13]
- *Diuretics* reduce blood volume by preventing the reabsorption of sodium in the kidneys, which increases urine output.
- *Antidysrhythmics* correct erratic electrical impulses to create regular cardiac rhythms. These agents act by blocking electrolytes that affect electrical conduction in the heart, such as sodium, potassium, and calcium, or by blocking beta-adrenergic receptors.[13]
- *Anticoagulants* prevent blood clotting at several locations in the clotting cascade to suppress the production of fibrin. They are most effective in preventing venous thrombosis.
- *Antiplatelet* agents prevent platelets from aggregating to form clots. They are most effective in preventing arterial thrombosis.
- *Thrombolytics* disrupt blood clots that are impairing perfusion by lysing fibrin.
- *Lipid-lowering agents* decrease the levels of lipids that contribute to atherosclerosis and result in blood vessel occlusion by reducing the synthesis of cholesterol.

Procedures and Surgical Interventions

There are many procedures and surgical interventions that improve electrical conduction in the heart as well as perfusion.

Pacemaker insertion. A pacemaker is an electronic device used to increase the heart rate in severe bradycardia by electronically stimulating the myocardium. The basic pacing circuit consists of a battery-operated pulse generator and one or more conducting leads that pace the atrium and one or both ventricles. Pacemakers can be external (temporary) or surgically implanted (permanent).[14]

Electrical cardioversion. The use of electric energy is an intervention to treat select abnormal cardiac rhythms. Cardiac defibrillation is used for emergency treatment during cardiac arrest when ventricular fibrillation or ventricular tachycardia is present. Synchronized cardioversion is a therapeutic procedure used to convert an abnormal rhythm, such as ventricular tachycardia with a pulse or atrial fibrillation, to a normal sinus rhythm. The procedure for cardioversion is the same as that for defibrillation with a few exceptions. If synchronized cardioversion is performed on a nonemergent basis, the patient is sedated before the procedure. The initial energy needed for synchronized cardioversion is less than the energy needed for defibrillation. Synchronized cardioversion starts at levels of 50 to 100 joules and is increased as needed.[14]

Intraaortic balloon pump. An intraaortic balloon pump (IABP) provides temporary circulatory assistance to the patient in the critical care unit who has a compromised heart. This pump reduces afterload to decrease the workload of the ventricles and augments the aortic diastolic pressure, resulting in improved coronary blood flow. Afterload is the force the ventricles must exert to open the pulmonic and aortic valves. The IABP consists of a sausage-shaped balloon that is inserted percutaneously or surgically into the femoral artery. The balloon is advanced toward the heart and positioned in the descending thoracic aorta just inferior to the left subclavian artery and superior to the renal arteries. A pneumatic device fills the balloon with helium at the start of diastole and deflates it just before the next systole. The EKG is the primary trigger used to initiate deflation on the upstroke of the R wave (of the QRS complex) and inflation on the T wave. IABP therapy is referred to as *counterpulsation* because the timing of the balloon is opposite that of ventricular contraction.[15]

Heart valve surgery. Heart valve surgery is a procedure to replace or repair one or more heart valves with a prosthetic valve. This surgery is indicated for patients with valves that have stenosis (do not open completely) or insufficiency (do not close completely). Valves may be mechanical or biological. Mechanical valves are constructed of metal alloys, pyrolytic carbon, and Dacron, while biological valves are constructed from bovine, porcine, or human (cadaver) cardiac tissue and usually contain some man-made materials.[16]

Cardiac transplant. A cardiac transplant is the transfer of a heart from one person after death to another person to treat a variety of terminal or end-stage heart conditions.[17]

Coronary artery bypass graft. Coronary revascularization is accomplished with a coronary artery bypass graft (CABG). This procedure surgically implants patent blood vessels to transport blood between the aorta and the myocardium distal to the obstructed coronary artery or arteries. The internal mammary artery, radial artery, and saphenous vein from the patient are used frequently as bypass grafts. CABG requires a sternotomy to gain access to the heart and cardiopulmonary bypass (CPB) to divert the patient's blood from the heart to the CPB machine. The CPB machine oxygenates the patient's blood and returns it to the patient, allowing the surgeon to operate on a nonbeating, bloodless heart while perfusion to organs is maintained.[18]

Peripheral artery revascularization. This procedure is accomplished using an autogenous vein or synthetic graft to bypass the lesion in the artery that is impairing perfusion. Femoropopliteal bypass is an example of this procedure in which a graft is attached to the femoral artery to divert blood around the occlusion and attached to the popliteal artery.[17] The femoral artery is clamped proximal to the insertion of the graft, allowing the surgeon to attach the graft to a bloodless artery.

Stent placement and angioplasty. Stents are inserted into arteries to hold them open. A stent is an expandable mesh-like structure designed to expand in the artery to maintain patency.[18] Cardiac catheterization and coronary angiography provide images of coronary circulation to identify lesions blocking coronary arteries. If appropriate, revascularization can be performed using balloon angioplasty. During this procedure, a catheter equipped with an inflatable balloon tip is inserted into the affected coronary artery. When the blockage is located, the catheter is passed through it, the balloon is inflated, and the blockage (atherosclerotic plaque) is compressed, which dilates the artery. Intracoronary stents are often inserted into the artery during an angioplasty to hold the artery open.

Endarterectomy. Endarterectomy is a surgical procedure in which the artery is opened to remove obstructing plaque that is impairing perfusion.[10] The carotid artery is a common site for this procedure, resulting in improved perfusion to the brain and thereby preventing an ischemic stroke.

CLINICAL NURSING SKILLS FOR PERFUSION

- Assessment
- Cardiac monitoring
- Hemodynamic monitoring
  - Continuous arterial blood pressure monitoring
  - Pulmonary artery pressure monitoring
- Circulatory assist devices
  - Intraaortic balloon pump
  - Ventricular assist device
- Medication administration

INTERRELATED CONCEPTS

Because all the cells in the body depend on perfusion to carry oxygen and nutrients to cells and remove wastes, this concept is interrelated to nearly all of the health and illness concepts within this textbook. Concepts that most closely interrelate with perfusion are **Pain, Clotting, Inflammation, Gas exchange, Elimination, Cognition, Mobility, Nutrition,** and **Patient education** (Figure 15-5).

Patients complain of pain when perfusion is impaired by clotting, whether it be in the coronary arteries, causing chest pain, or in the iliac or femoral arteries, causing leg pain when walking. Impaired tissue perfusion leading to ischemia creates lactic acid that contributes to pain.

Because impaired tissue perfusion to the legs causes pain during walking, peripheral arterial disease reduces the mobility of patients because of the pain they experience. Walking is a healthy lifestyle behavior to exercise the heart and improve central perfusion.

Inflammation occurs when there is tissue damage, which is linked to ischemia. Also it is the inflammation that develops after damage to the endothelium of arteries that initiates atherosclerosis.

Impaired perfusion results in impaired gas exchange because the blood carries oxygen from alveoli to cells and carbon dioxide away from cells to alveoli for exhalation.

Elimination from the kidneys is an indirect indicator of cardiac output because blood flows from the heart through the aorta to the renal arteries and through nephrons that produce urine.

Cognition is altered when perfusion to the brain is impaired. The neurons require a consistent supply of oxygen and glucose to maintain function.

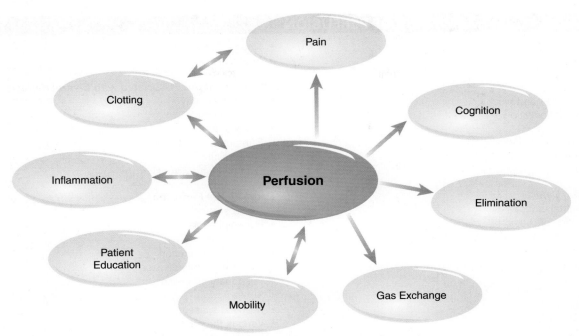

FIGURE 15-5 Perfusion and Interrelated Concepts.

MODEL CASE

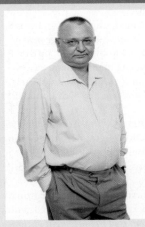

George Jones is a 63-year-old male who went to the emergency department with chest pain. He had experienced this chest pain for 30 minutes and it was not relieved after taking four nitroglycerin tablets 5 minutes apart. He reports the pain feels "like an elephant is sitting on my chest." He is diaphoretic and appears anxious. His vital signs are temperature 99° F, blood pressure 100/68 mm Hg, heart rate 110 beats/ min, and respiratory rate 24 breaths/min. Mr. Jones is obese and has type 2 diabetes mellitus, hyperlipidemia, and hypertension. He quit smoking last year after a 40-year history of one pack of cigarettes a day. His troponin level is elevated and the EKG shows ST segment elevation. The nurse administers oxygen and draws blood for arterial blood gas analysis. Mr. Jones is told he will have a cardiac catheterization to locate the blockage, determine its severity, and evaluate left ventricular function.

The cardiac catheterization revealed a 90% blockage in one coronary artery. The cardiologist performed a balloon angioplasty and placed a stent in Mr. Jones' blocked coronary artery to reestablish perfusion. Mr. Jones was admitted to the cardiovascular surgery unit, and was ambulating within 24 hours after stent placement. The nurse's goals for Mr. Jones' plan of care are to maintain effective cardiac output, control pain, relieve anxiety, and balance physical activity with energy-conserving activities. The nurse also played a significant role in Mr. Jones' therapy by teaching him and his family about lifestyle changes, including diet and exercise, and the purpose of his prescribed medications, including adverse effects and the importance of following the medication regimen. Mr. Jones is referred for cardiac rehabilitation after discharge.

Case Analysis

This case exemplifies an impairment of local perfusion of the heart that could have developed into central impairment if Mr. Jones had not been treated. He had several risk factors, including obesity, that contributed to type 2 diabetes. The hyperlipidemia and diabetes mellitus contributed to the blockage of his coronary artery and his hypertension, which increased the workload of his heart. Mr. Jones' manifestations were consistent with impaired tissue perfusion to the myocardium. The stent reestablished perfusion to the myocardium. Mr. Jones' recovery and prevention of further cardiovascular disease will be improved by his lifestyle changes.

■■■ BOX 15-3 EXEMPLARS OF PERFUSION

Central Perfusion
Cardiac Dysrhythmias
- Atrial fibrillation
- Asystole
- Third-degree heart block
- Ventricular fibrillation

Valvular Heart Disease
- Aortic stenosis or insufficiency
- Mitral valve prolapse

Congenital Defects
- Atrial septal defect (ASD)
- Coarctation of the aorta
- Tetralogy of Fallot
- Ventricular septal defect (VSD)

Shock
- Anaphylactic shock
- Cardiogenic shock
- Hemorrhagic shock
- Neurogenic shock
- Septic shock

Other Conditions Associated with Central Perfusion
- Cardiomyopathy
- Cor pulmonale
- Endocarditis
- Ruptured arterial aneurysm (leading to shock)
- Heart failure
- Pulmonary hypertension

Local/Tissue Perfusion
- Atherosclerosis
- Hyperlipidemia
- Hypertension
- Myocardial infarction
- Peripheral artery disease
- Pulmonary embolism
- Stroke
- Raynaud's disease
- Venous thrombosis

EXEMPLARS

There are multiple known conditions that contribute to impaired perfusion, far more than are described in this text. Box 15-2 lists common conditions associated with impaired perfusion across the lifespan; further details about these conditions can be found in pathophysiology, medical-surgical, and pediatric nursing textbooks.

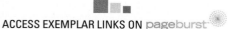

ACCESS EXEMPLAR LINKS ON pageburst

REFERENCES

1. Wilson S, Giddens J: *Health assessment for nursing practice*, ed 4, St Louis, 2009, Mosby/Elsevier.
2. Porth C: *Essentials of pathophysiology*, ed 3, Philadelphia, 2011, Wolters Kluwer/Lippincott Williams & Wilkins.
3. McCance K, Grey T: Altered cellular and tissue biology. In Huether S, McCance K, editors: *Understanding pathophysiology*, ed 4, St Louis, 2008, Mosby/Elsevier, pp 62–95.
4. Malone M, et al: Nursing management: lower respiratory problems. In Lewis S, editor: *Medical-surgical nursing: assessment and management of clinical problems*, ed 8, St Louis, 2011, Mosby/Elsevier, pp 545–586.
5. Hueckel R, Wilson D: The child with disturbance of oxygen and carbon dioxide exchange. In Hockenberry M, Wilson D, editors: *Wong's nursing care of infants and children*, ed 8, St Louis, 2007, Mosby/Elsevier, pp 1273–1313.
6. O'Brien P, Baker A: The child with cardiovascular dysfunction. In Hockenberry M, Wilson D, editors: *Wong's nursing care of infants and children*, ed 8, St Louis, 2007, Mosby/Elsevier, pp 1436–1502.
7. Pagana K, Pagana T: *Mosby's diagnostic and laboratory test reference*, ed 10, St Louis, 2011, Mosby/Elsevier.
8. DiSabatino A, Bucher L, et al: Nursing assessment: cardiovascular system. In Lewis S, editor: *Medical-surgical nursing: assessment and management of clinical problems*, ed 8, St Louis, 2011, Mosby/Elsevier, pp 715–737.
9. Bucher L, et al: Nursing management: dysrhythmias. In Lewis S, editor: *Medical-surgical nursing: assessment and management of clinical problems*, ed 8, St Louis, 2011, Mosby/Elsevier, pp 818–840.
10. Wipke-Tevis D, Rich K, et al: Nursing management: vascular disorders. In Lewis S, editor: *Medical-surgical nursing: assessment and management of clinical problems*, ed 8, St Louis, 2011, Mosby/Elsevier, pp 866–896.
11. American Heart Association: *Getting healthy*. Accessed Jan 25, 2011, at www.heart.org/HEARTORG/GettingHealthy/Getting Healthy_UCM_001078_SubHomePage.jsp.
12. www.uspreventionservicestaskforce.org. Accessed March 5, 2011.
13. Bucher L, Castellucci D, et al: Nursing management: coronary artery disease and acute coronary syndrome. In Lewis S, editor: *Medical-surgical nursing: assessment and management of clinical problems*, ed 8, St Louis, 2011, Mosby/Elsevier, pp 760–796.
14. Lehne R: *Pharmacology for nursing care*, ed 7, Philadelphia, 2010, Saunders/Elsevier.
15. Bucher L, et al: Nursing management: dysrhythmias. In Lewis S, editor: *Medical-surgical nursing: assessment and management of clinical problems*, ed 8, St Louis, 2011, Mosby/Elsevier, pp 818–840.
16. Bucher L, Seckel M, et al: Nursing management: critical care. In Lewis S, editor: *Medical-surgical nursing: assessment and management of clinical problems*, ed 8, St Louis, 2011, Mosby/Elsevier, pp 1681–1716.
17. Kupper N, Mitchell D, et al: Nursing management: inflammatory and structural heart disorders. In Lewis S, editor: *Medical-surgical nursing: assessment and management of clinical problems*, ed 8, St Louis, 2011, Mosby/Elsevier, pp 841–865.
18. Bouffard L, et al: Nursing management: heart failure. In Lewis S, editor: *Medical-surgical nursing: assessment and management of clinical problems*, ed 8, St Louis, 2011, Mosby/Elsevier, pp 797–817.

Gas Exchange

Susan F. Wilson

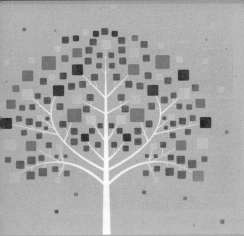

All cells depend on a consistent supply of oxygen and removal of waste in order to survive. A reduction or lack of oxygen and/or a buildup of waste leads to demise. For this reason, gas exchange is a critical concept for nurses to understand and incorporate into practice. The purpose of this concept analysis is to help nurses acquire foundational knowledge about gas exchange across the lifespan. In practice, nurses should be able to promote individual's healthy behaviors that optimize gas exchange, identify individuals at risk of impaired gas exchange, recognize when individuals are experiencing an impairment in gas exchange, and respond with appropriate interventions.

DEFINITION(S)

For the purposes of this concept analysis, **Gas Exchange** is defined as *the process by which oxygen is transported to cells and carbon dioxide is transported from cells.* This normal physiologic process requires interaction among the neurologic, respiratory, and cardiovascular systems. The brainstem houses the pons and medulla oblongata that drive inspiration and expiration. The lungs deliver oxygen to the pulmonary capillaries where it is carried by hemoglobin to cells. After cellular metabolism, carbon dioxide is carried in hemoglobin to the lungs where it is exhaled. Figure 16-1 shows the process of gas exchange. Thus adequate functioning of these systems is essential for optimal gas exchange. When delivery of oxygen is impaired, tissues become ischemic and lactic acidosis contributes to cellular death. Likewise, if elimination of carbon dioxide is impaired, respiratory acidosis may cause disorientation, tremors, seizures, and coma.[1,2]

Several other terms are important as they relate to this concept. *Ischemia* is insufficient flow of oxygenated blood to tissues that may result in hypoxia and subsequent cell injury or death. *Hypoxia* is insufficient oxygen reaching cells, whereas *anoxia* is the total lack of oxygen in body tissues. *Hypoxemia* is reduced oxygenation of arterial blood.

SCOPE AND CATEGORIES

The concept of gas exchange and problems associated with impaired gas exchange represent a variety of physiologic processes. Three broad categories that describe these processes are ventilation, transport, and perfusion. Ventilation is the inhalation of oxygen and exhalation of carbon dioxide. Oxygen diffuses from the alveoli to the erythrocytes in the pulmonary capillary to be perfused (transported) to cells. Carbon dioxide moves from cells to the erythrocytes for perfusion (transport) back to the alveoli to be exhaled.

Ventilation

Ventilation is the process of inhaling oxygen into the lungs and exhaling carbon dioxide from the lungs. Ventilation may be impaired by the unavailability of oxygen, such as at high altitudes, as well as by any disorder affecting the nasopharynx and lungs. Clinical manifestations depend on the area affected, but patients must work harder to breathe or must change the route air enter the lungs. For example, when patients have narrowed bronchi because of asthma, they use accessory muscles to move air into the lungs until the bronchi are dilated again. The accessory muscles include the trapezius and sternocleidomastoid; these muscles contract during inspiration to help patients inhale when they are experiencing airway obstruction or constriction. Likewise, when patients have edema of the sinuses, they are unable to breathe through the nose; instead, these patients breathe through the mouth until the edema subsides.

Transport

Transport refers to the availability and ability of hemoglobin to carry oxygen from alveoli to cells for metabolism and to carry carbon dioxide produced by cellular metabolism from cells to alveoli to be eliminated. Transport is impaired when the amount of hemoglobin is low, which occurs when patients have anemia for any reason.

Anemia is defined as an abnormally low number of circulating red blood cells (RBCs), low level of hemoglobin, or both.[2] Causes of anemia can be classified in three ways: decreased production of RBCs, increased loss of RBCs, or premature destruction of RBCs. Production of red blood cells is reduced when nutrients needed to form them are deficient, such as iron, vitamin B_{12}, and folate. Another cause is a reduction in the amount of erythropoietin, which normally stimulates the bone marrow to produce red blood cells. Chronic renal failure is a common cause of decreased erythropoietin production. Anemia of chronic disease is associated with decreased RBC production and may include chronic inflammatory, autoimmune, infectious, and malignant disorders. Older adults experience a reduction in RBC mass, which increases their risk of anemia. Blood loss from acute or chronic causes reduces the number of red blood cells, thus making hemoglobin unavailable to carry oxygen. An example of an acute cause is hemorrhage. Conditions such as peptic ulcers or colon cancer, however, are associated with chronic slow blood loss. Finally, destruction of red blood cells occurs in hemolytic anemias when the spleen destroys these cells prematurely, such as sickle cell crisis.

Perfusion

Perfusion, as it relates to the concept of gas exchange, refers to the ability of blood to transport oxygen-containing hemoglobin to cells and return carbon dioxide–containing hemoglobin to the alveoli. Perfusion can be impaired by a decreased cardiac output as well as by thrombi, emboli, vessel narrowing, vasoconstriction, or blood loss. When perfusion is impaired, oxygen does not reach cells, resulting in ischemia and perhaps necrosis if not resolved. Likewise, the carbon dioxide transport from the cells to the alveoli is impaired and may lead to respiratory acidosis.

RISK FACTORS

Because adequate gas exchange is required for life, all individuals—regardless of age, gender, race, or socioeconomic status—potentially are at risk for gas exchange impairment. Nurses need to recognize, however, that some individuals are at greater risk for impairment. Some of these risk factors are controllable due to lifestyle behaviors, whereas others are not.

Populations at Risk

Populations at greatest risk are infants, young children, and older adults. Infants are at risk because they have fetal hemoglobin. Fetal hemoglobin (HbF) is present for the first 5 months of life and results in shortened survival of red blood cells, causing physiologic anemia by age 2 to 3 months. Contributing to anemia at about 6 months is the lower level of hemoglobin caused by gradually diminishing maternal iron stores.[3] Infants and young children are at risk for impaired gas exchange because they have less alveolar surface area for gas exchange as well as narrow branching of peripheral

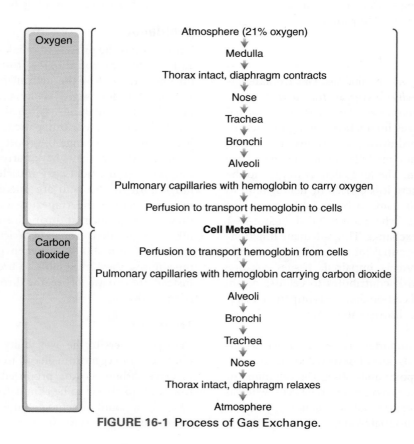

FIGURE 16-1 Process of Gas Exchange.

airways that are easily obstructed by mucus, edema, or foreign objects.[4]

Older adults are at risk for impaired gas exchange because of anatomic and physiologic changes that are expected with advanced age. The chest wall becomes stiffer with loss of elastic recoil. Respiratory muscles become weaker, reducing the effectiveness of coughing, normally a protective mechanism to prevent aspiration. Additional expected changes are dilation of alveoli, decreased surface area for gas diffusion, and decreased pulmonary capillary network. Finally, the ability to initiate an immune response to infection is decreased in older adults.[1]

Individual Risk Factors

A number of personal risk factors are linked to impairment in gas exchange. Nonmodifiable risk factors include age (as described under Populations at Risk), air pollution, and allergies. *Tobacco use* is the single most preventable cause of death and disease in the United States and is the most significant risk factor for impaired gas exchange. Boxes 16-1 and 16-2 present data about those who use tobacco. Risk for aspiration is increased during an altered state of consciousness such as from a chemical alteration (e.g., alcoholism, drug overdose, anesthesia) or from a neurologic disorder (e.g., head injury, seizure, stroke). *Altered oropharyngeal flora* increases the number of microorganisms that can be aspirated. Patients requiring *tracheal intubation* are at risk because of altered oropharyngeal flora as well as the bypassing of protective mechanisms for the alveoli. *Bed rest and prolonged immobility* reduce thoracic expansion, which can increase the risk for atelectasis and pneumonia. *Chronic disease*, such as cystic fibrosis, chronic obstructive pulmonary disease (COPD), or heart failure, increases risk because of mucus and fluid accumulation in the airways and alveoli. *Immunosuppression* alters the body's natural ability to fight infection, whether it is from a systemic disorder (such as aplastic anemia), a cancer (such as leukemia), or a treatment regimen (such as cancer chemotherapy).

PHYSIOLOGIC PROCESSES AND CONSEQUENCES

Breathing is involuntary because changes in ventilation rate and volume are stimulated and regulated automatically by the nervous system to maintain arterial blood gases within normal ranges.[1] Chemoreceptors in the medulla sense carbon dioxide levels, and when carbon dioxide concentration is elevated, these receptors transmit impulses to the diaphragm and intercostal muscles to contract. As the diaphragm contracts, negative pressure pulls in 21% oxygen from the atmosphere. The nose warms and humidifies the air and it flows to

---

BOX 16-1 USE OF TOBACCO PRODUCTS BY ADULTS, ADOLESCENTS, AND CHILDREN

Adults

20.6% of adults ages 18 years and older were current cigarette smokers in 2008 (age adjusted to the year 2000 standard population).

2.3% of adults ages 18 years and older were current users of snuff or chewing tobacco products in 2005 (age adjusted to the year 2000 standard population).

2.2% of adults ages 18 years and older were current cigar smokers in 2005 (age adjusted to the year 2000 standard population).

Adolescents

26.0% of adolescents in grades 9 through 12 used cigarettes, chewing tobacco, snuff, or cigars in the past 30 days in 2009.

19.5% of adolescents in grades 9 through 12 smoked cigarettes in the past 30 days in 2009.

8.9% of adolescents in grades 9 through 12 used smokeless (chewing tobacco or snuff) tobacco products in the past 30 days in 2009.

14.0% of adolescents in grades 9 through 12 smoked cigars in the past 30 days in 2009.

Children and Adolescents

7.7% of children and adolescents ages 12 to 17 years who had not previously used tobacco products in their lifetime first used tobacco products in the past 12 months in 2008.

From *Healthy People 2020*. Accessed Feb 15, 2011, at www.healthypeople.gov/hp2020/Objectives/TopicAreas.aspx.

BOX 16-2 CHARACTERISTICS OF SMOKERS

By Gender

23.5% men
17.9% women

By Age

21.8% ages 18–24 years
24.0% ages 25–44 years
21.9% ages 45–64 years
9.5% ages 65 years and older

By Race/Ethnicity

23.3% of American Indians/Alaska natives
21.3% of blacks (non-Hispanic)
14.5% of Hispanics
22.1% of whites (non-Hispanic)

By Education

49.1% adults with a General Educational Development (GED) diploma
33.6% of adults with 9–11 years of education
11.1% of adults with an undergraduate college degree
5.6% of adults with a graduate college degree

By Poverty Status

31.1% of adults who live below the poverty level
19.4% of adults who live at or above the poverty level

From Centers for Disease Control and Prevention. Accessed Feb 15, 2011, at www.cdc.gov/tobacco/data_statistics/fact_sheets/adult_data/cig_smoking/index.htm.

alveoli through patent airways (trachea and bronchi). Alveolar walls are lined with single layer of epithelial cells, called type I alveolar cells, that provide structure. In between these type I cells are thicker type II alveolar cells that produce surfactant—a lipoprotein that coats the inner surface of alveoli to keep them open. Tiny pores called pores of Kohn allow some air to pass from one alveolus to another, permitting collateral ventilation and even distribution among alveoli. The high pressure of oxygen causes it to diffuse from the alveoli into the pulmonary capillaries. These capillaries are separated from the alveoli by a single layer of flat epithelial cells. In the pulmonary capillaries oxygen attaches to hemoglobin and is carried as oxyhemoglobin (HbO_2). Hemoglobin saturation is measured by the saturation of arterial hemoglobin (represented SaO_2). At the cellular level oxygen is released from hemoglobin, called hemoglobin desaturation. Oxygen dissolved in plasma is measured by the partial pressure of oxygen in the artery or PaO_2. Dissolved oxygen diffuses into the interstitial space and then diffuses into cells to be used in metabolic processes.[1,2]

Carbon dioxide, a by-product of cellular metabolism, is transported to the atmosphere in the reverse order of oxygen and lowers the arterial carbon dioxide level. Carbon dioxide dissolved in plasma is measured by the partial pressure of carbon dioxide in the artery or $PaCO_2$. The lower $PaCO_2$ value turns off signals from the medulla until the carbon dioxide level rises again to repeat the gas exchange process.

Consequences

Gas exchange is compromised when there is impairment of ventilation, altered transport of oxygen, or inadequate perfusion.

Impaired ventilation may occur in the following conditions:

- Inadequate muscle or nerve function to move air into the lungs, such as cervical spinal cord injury
- Narrowed airways from bronchoconstriction (such as in asthma) or from obstruction (such as in chronic bronchitis or cystic fibrosis)
- Poor gas diffusion in the alveoli, such as in pulmonary edema, acute respiratory distress syndrome, or pneumonia

Altered transport of oxygen occurs when sufficient red blood cells are not available to carry oxygen, such as in anemia.

Inadequate perfusion develops when cardiac output is reduced, such as in myocardial infarction. Perfusion is also impaired when peripheral blood vessels are constricted or obstructed and unable to carry blood, such as in peripheral arterial disease.

The term "gas exchange" can be misinterpreted because the word "exchange" can mean "swap, substitute or trade." However, as described by Dalton's law of partial pressures, the pressure exerted by each gas is independent of the pressure exerted by other gases. Oxygen diffuses from the alveoli to the pulmonary capillary because the pressure of oxygen in the alveoli is higher than the pressure of oxygen in the capillaries. Gases diffuse from areas of high concentration to areas of low concentration. Gases exchange back and forth between the atmosphere and the blood and between the respiratory and cardiovascular systems.[1,2] Believing that oxygen diffuses based on the diffusion of carbon dioxide is incorrect. These two gases are independent; they do not exchange with each other.

ASSESSMENT

Nurses gather data from the patient's history, physical examination, and the patient's diagnostic test results. Assessment of gas exchange involves recognizing indications of adequate and inadequate ventilation, transport, and perfusion. Adequate ventilation is apparent when the following occur:

- Breathing is quiet and effortless at a rate appropriate for age.
- Oxygen saturation (SaO_2) is between 95% and 100%.
- Skin, nail beds, and lips are appropriate colors for the patient's race.
- Thorax is symmetric with equal thoracic expansion bilaterally.
- Spinous processes are in alignment; scapulae are bilaterally symmetric.
- Anteroposterior (AP) diameter of the chest is about a 1:2 ratio of AP to lateral diameter.
- Trachea is midline.
- Breath sounds are clear bilaterally.[5]

History
Baseline History
When collecting subjective data from patients, nurses ask about lifestyle behaviors including diet, exercise, and smoking habits. Nurses ask about patients' work and home environments to identify potential respiratory irritants. Also, patients are asked about any chronic diseases as well as allergies that may affect the respiratory system. Nurses ask patients about medications they take, both prescription and over-the-counter, and the reason each medication is taken as well as its efficacy.[5]

Problem-Based History
There are several symptoms often reported by individuals experiencing gas exchange impairment including cough, shortness of breath, and chest pain. When a symptom is reported, a symptom analysis is conducted.

Cough. When a cough is reported or observed, ask if the cough causes fatigue or interferes with sleep. Also ask if the cough is productive or nonproductive. Inquire about the color and consistency of productive coughs. Question the patient about factors that alleviate or aggravate the cough as well as any self-treatment measures taken to relieve the cough. Also ask about other symptoms that accompany the cough, such as fever or shortness of breath.

Shortness of breath. Patients may report having to sleep sitting up or using several pillows to prop themselves up during the night. Lightheadedness may be reported as a result of inadequate oxygen transport to the brain. Inquire about what precipitated the shortness of breath and if it occurs during inhalation or exhalation, or both. The patient should be asked what factors alleviate or aggravate the dyspnea and also if there are other symptoms such as cough, chest pain, or swelling of the feet and ankles.[5]

Chest pain with breathing. Ask when the chest pain occurs, what activity is associated with the pain, and how long the pain lasts. Inquire if the onset of chest pain was gradual or sudden, and ask for a description of the pain, such as sharp or dull, pain radiation, and severity.

Examination Findings

Vital Signs

Inadequate gas exchange is noticed by changes in vital signs such as respiratory rate, oxygen saturation (SaO_2), heart rate, and temperature. Changes in respiratory rate to tachypnea may be due to increased work of breathing. The SaO_2 value may drop below 95% when oxygen is not being transported by erythrocytes to cells. Tachycardia may occur either from anxiety caused by not being able to breathe well or from anemia. Temperature may be elevated because of an infection, such as pneumonia or respiratory syncytial virus (RSV).

Inspection

If a patient is having difficulty breathing, the nurse may notice the patient assuming a position to ease the work of breathing (such as sitting leaning forward). Patients with impaired gas exchange often appear anxious because of the sensation of not getting enough air or a feeling of suffocation. Low oxygen saturation may impair mentation as a result of lack of adequate oxygen supply to the brain. Patients may use accessory muscles on inspiration to help get air into the lungs. They may use pursed-lip breathing on exhalation to keep airways open longer. The skin and lips may appear pale because of anemia or hypoxemia. A late sign of hypoxemia is cyanosis. Clubbing of nails develops in patients with chronic hypoxic disorders such as cystic fibrosis or chronic obstructive pulmonary disease. The thorax may be asymmetric with unequal thoracic expansion unilaterally attributable to pneumothorax. Scoliosis is a curvature of vertebrae that creates asymmetric expansion of the thorax as well as malalignment of spinous processes and scapulae. When patients develop a barrel chest from air trapped in alveoli from emphysema, their ratio of anteroposterior to lateral diameter changes from a normal ratio of 1:2 to a ratio of 1:1 respectively. The trachea shifts from midline away from the lung that is experiencing a tension pneumothorax.[5]

Additional assessment findings commonly noted in infants and young children with inadequate gas exchange are flaring of the nares, chest wall retractions on inspiration, grunting on inspiration, cyanosis around the lips when sucking, and the need to stop during feeding to breathe.[4]

Auscultation

During auscultation, narrowed bronchi may produce expiratory and/or inspiratory wheezing or stridor. Mucus or secretions in the bronchi may create rhonchi and fluid in alveoli may generate crackles.[5]

Diagnostic Tests

There are a number of diagnostic tests associated with gas exchange that are used to assess for impairment.

Laboratory Tests

Arterial blood gases (ABGs). ABGs reveal measurements of pH and oxygen, carbon dioxide, and bicarbonate concentrations in arterial blood. They are used to detect respiratory acidosis and alkalosis. Respiratory acidosis develops during hypoventilation when carbon dioxide is retained, such as in patients with chronic obstructive pulmonary disease. Respiratory alkalosis develops during hyperventilation when excessive carbon dioxide is exhaled, such as during anxiety or hysteria.

- The pH is inversely proportional to the actual hydrogen ion concentration. Normal values are between 7.35 and 7.45. The pH values below 7.35 indicate acidosis and above 7.45 indicate alkalosis.[6]
- SaO_2 is an abbreviation for "saturation of arterial oxygen" and represents the percentage of arterial hemoglobin that is saturated with oxygen. This value accounts for about 97% of arterial oxygen. The normal value for adults is 95% to 100% and for newborns 40% to 90%.[6]
- PaO_2 is an abbreviation for the "partial pressure of arterial oxygen" and represents the pressure of oxygen dissolved in arterial blood. This value accounts for about 3% of oxygen. The normal value for adults is 80 to 100 mm Hg and for newborns is 60 to 70 mm Hg.[6]
- $PaCO_2$ is an abbreviation for the "partial pressure of arterial carbon dioxide" and represents the pressure of carbon dioxide dissolved in arterial blood. The $PaCO_2$ is a measurement of ventilation capability. Normal values for adults are 35 to 45 mm Hg and for children less than 2 years 26 to 41 mm Hg.[6]
- HCO_3 is an abbreviation for bicarbonate and represents most of the carbon dioxide in the blood. Serum bicarbonate level is regulated by the kidneys. Normal values are 22 to 26 mEq/L. There is a direct proportional relationship between HCO_3 concentration and pH; thus when HCO_3 concentration is above normal, the pH increases, indicating alkalosis. When the HCO_3 concentration is below normal, the pH decreases, indicating acidosis. The kidneys compensate for primary respiratory acid-base alterations. For example, in respiratory acidosis, the kidneys compensate by retaining HCO_3 in an attempt to regain acid-base balance. However in respiratory alkalosis, the kidneys compensate by excreting HCO_3 in an attempt to regain acid-base balance.[6]

Complete blood count (CBC). The CBC is obtained from venous blood and includes measurements of red blood cell count (RBC), hemoglobin (Hb), hematocrit (Hct), and white blood cell count (WBC).

- Red blood cell (RBC) count determines the oxygen-carrying capacity of the blood. Each RBC carries hemoglobin that transports oxygen to tissues and carbon dioxide from tissues. Patients who have anemia have decreased numbers of RBCs, which reduces the patient's oxygen-carrying ability.

- Hemoglobin (Hb) level reflects the number of RBCs in the venous blood and determines the oxygen and carbon dioxide transport capability.
- Hematocrit (Hct) measures the percentage of venous blood volume that is composed of red blood cells. The Hct closely reflects the hemoglobin and RBC values.
- White blood cell (WBC) count measures the number of leukocytes in venous blood. The WBC differential measures the percentage of each leukocyte (e.g., neutrophils, eosinophils, basophils, or monocytes) contained within the total number of WBCs. Elevations in total WBC count occur when there is inflammation and often that inflammation is due to infection. Decreases in WBC count occur with certain cancers as well as an adverse effect of chemical or radiation therapy to treat cancer. Patients with low WBC counts are at risk for newly acquired infection because the immune system is unable to respond optimally.[6] The WBC differential is helpful in suggesting a generalized cause of the abnormal value. For example, elevated neutrophils indicate an acute inflammation, whereas increased monocytes indicate a chronic infection. Eosinophils are elevated during allergies.

Sputum examination. Studying sputum specimens can help diagnosis respiratory disorders. Culture and sensitivity are performed on a single specimen to detect bacteria and determine which antibiotic is most effective. Gram stain of sputum distinguishes gram-positive from gram-negative bacteria. Testing a series of three early-morning sputum samples for acid-fast bacillus is diagnostic for tuberculosis. A single sputum specimen for cytologic examination is performed to detect a pulmonary malignancy.[7]

Skin tests. Mantoux screens for tuberculosis. A positive reaction to the skin test indicates patients have developed antibodies to *Mycobacterium tuberculosis*. Allergies detected by skin tests may indicate causes of bronchoconstriction. The sweat chloride test screens for cystic fibrosis, which produces high levels of chloride in the sweat.

Pathologic analysis. Tissue from the lungs or bronchus may be taken for pathologic analysis, particularly if a malignant tumor is suspected.

Radiologic Studies

Chest x-ray. Chest x-ray films are very useful in detecting impaired ventilation because they provide visualization of the lungs, ribs, clavicles, vertebrae, heart, and major thoracic vessels. They are useful in identifying foreign bodies, infiltrations in pneumonia, tubercles in tuberculosis, tumors in cancer, or edema. In patients with COPD, chest x-rays show the flat diaphragm and barrel chest configuration of ribs and vertebrae. Also, chest x-rays can identify pleural effusion, pneumothorax, hemothorax, or empyema.[7]

Computed tomography. Computed tomography (CT) scans of the chest produce three-dimensional images of the lungs and are useful in detecting pulmonary densities, space-occupying tumors, and pulmonary emboli.[7]

Ventilation-perfusion scans. Ventilation-perfusion scans ($\dot{V}/\dot{Q}$) use radioactive particles to diagnosis disorders involving both perfusion and ventilation. Radioactive particles are injected into peripheral veins to detect impaired perfusion to the lungs. Also, inhaled radioactive particles are used to detect impaired lung function. This scan is used to diagnose pulmonary emboli.[7]

Positron emission tomography. Positron emission tomography (PET) scans use intravenous injection of radioactive chemical compounds to distinguish benign from malignant pulmonary nodules.[7]

Pulmonary Function Studies

Pulmonary function tests assess the presence and severity of diseases in large and small airways. A spirometer measures the volume of air moving in and out of the lungs and then calculates the lung capacities.[7] One example of its use is for patients with asthma. Because their bronchoconstriction worsens, they exhale less air. This finding is reported as decreased forced expiratory volume.

Pulmonary function tests are also used to distinguish between obstructive and restrictive pulmonary diseases. Because air trapping increases for patients with obstructive lung disease such as cystic fibrosis or chronic obstructive pulmonary disease, more air remains in their lungs, which is reflected as an increase in reserve volume. Obstructive lung diseases impair patient's ability to get air **out of** the lungs. By contrast, patients may develop restrictive lung diseases from intrapulmonary or extrapulmonary causes. Intrapulmonary causes include pulmonary fibrosis or empyema. Extrapulmonary causes include chest wall trauma or cervical spinal cord injury. Restrictive lung diseases impair the patient's ability to get air **into** the lungs as reflected in a decreased tidal volume.

Endoscopy Examination

Bronchoscopy is an endoscopic examination in which a flexible fiberoptic bronchoscope is extended through the bronchi for the purpose of diagnosis, specimen collection, or tissue biopsy.[7]

CLINICAL MANAGEMENT

Clinical management related to gas exchange includes health promotion and the management of emerging or present conditions that compromise gas exchange. The ultimate goal is to optimize gas exchange.

Primary Prevention

Primary prevention includes measures to promote health and prevent development of disease. There are several measures that prevent conditions that impair gas exchange.

Infection Control

One of the simplest primary prevention measures is infection control. Proper hand hygiene helps to prevent respiratory tract infections. All individuals should be taught the importance of hand hygiene and proper hand washing technique; in addition, individuals should be instructed to clean surfaces that are frequently touched, such as doorknobs and countertops. Coughing or sneezing into a tissue or into the elbow or sleeve reduces the particles delivered into the air. Avoiding large groups of people reduces the airborne transmission of microorganisms.

Smoking Cessation

Smoking cessation is important for both primary prevention, discussed here, as well as an intervention to treat disease. *Healthy People 2020* goals related to tobacco use include reducing tobacco use by adolescents and adults; decreasing the initiation of tobacco use by children, adolescents, and young adults; and increasing smoking cessation attempts by adults, including pregnant women.[8]

Nicotine in tobacco products is the psychoactive drug that produces dependence, the most common form of chemical dependence in the United States. The American Lung Association and American Cancer Society have resources to help patients stop smoking.[9,10] Quitting smoking is difficult and may require multiple attempts. Smokers often report lack of success in smoking cessation because of stress, weight gain, and withdrawal symptoms. Those symptoms include irritability, anxiety, difficulty concentrating, and increased appetite.

People who are successful at smoking cessation greatly reduce their risk for disease and premature death. In addition to nicotine, cigarette smoke contains at least 250 chemicals known to be toxic or carcinogenic.[11] Health benefits of smoking cessation include lowering the risk for lung and other cancers and reducing the risk for coronary heart disease, stroke, peripheral vascular disease, and chronic obstructive pulmonary disease. When women in their reproductive years quit smoking, they reduce the risk for infertility. Smoking cessation in women who are pregnant reduces the risk of delivering a low birth weight baby.[11]

Immunizations

Immunizations prevent infection by bacteria or viruses, such as diphtheria, *Haemophilus influenzae* type b (Hib), H1N1 flu, influenza, measles, pneumococcal pneumonia, pertussis, and rubella. Schedules for these immunizations from infancy to adulthood are found on the CDC website.[12]

Preventing Postoperative Pulmonary Complications

After a surgical procedure, patients are encouraged to deep breathe and cough at least every 2 hours and/or use an incentive spirometer to prevent pneumonia and atelectasis. This device encourages deep breathing for patients and measures the air inhaled as an outcome indicator that is useful for nursing assessment.

Preventing deep vein thrombosis is essential for all patients who are less active than usual so that pulmonary emboli are prevented. This includes patients after a surgical procedure or those whose disease process prevents them from ambulating as much as usual. One intervention is to subcutaneously administer an anticoagulant to reduce clotting of platelets. Another intervention is to apply elastic stockings to the legs or use intermittent compression devices to the lower legs to prevent venous stasis. A third intervention is to encourage ambulation as soon as possible.

Secondary Prevention (Screening)

Secondary prevention includes screening and early diagnosis and prompt treatment of existing health problems. Its purpose is to shorten the duration and severity of consequences. There are few routine screenings for problems associated with gas exchange. A Mantoux skin test may be administered to individuals who have exposure risks to tuberculosis.

Collaborative Interventions
Smoking Cessation

Although smoking cessation is typically considered primary prevention (to prevent respiratory illness), it is also considered an important intervention strategy among individuals who have a disease process because smoking exacerbates respiratory and cardiovascular disease.

Pharmacotherapy

Pharmacotherapy plays a very important role in managing individuals with impaired gas exchange. Agents can be used to open upper and lower airways to improve gas exchange by dilating airways, reducing edema, increasing a cough's effectiveness, and killing or limiting the growth of microorganisms. Depending on the pharmacologic agent, these drugs are administered through a number of routes including oral, intravenous, or inhalation through inhalers or nebulizer (aerosol). Descriptions of general classifications of agents are presented next; consult a pharmacology textbook for further information about specific agents.

Drugs that affect upper airways

- Antihistamines relieve symptoms of sneezing, rhinorrhea, and nasal itching experienced in allergic rhinitis. They are more effective when taken prophylactically. Antihistamines block the histamine$_1$ (H$_1$) receptors to cause vasoconstriction and decreased capillary permeability of small arterioles and venules.[13]
- Decongestants relieve congestion in passageways and sinuses. Intranasal glucocorticoids exert an antiinflammatory effect to prevent or suppress major symptoms of allergic rhinitis such as congestion, rhinorrhea, sneezing, nasal itching, and erythema. Sympathomimetics act as decongestants by activating the alpha$_1$-adrenergic receptors on nasal blood vessels to cause vasoconstriction that shrinks edematous membranes, thereby reducing nasal drainage.[13]

Lower airway bronchodilators

- Glucocorticoids reduce bronchial hyperreactivity that occurs in asthma by suppressing inflammation. Specifically, they decrease synthesis and release of inflammatory mediators such as leukotrienes, histamine, and prostaglandins; decrease infiltration of inflammatory cells such as eosinophils and leukocytes; and decrease edema of airway mucosa. They may be given by inhalation, orally, or intravenously.

- Sympathomimetic agents are beta$_2$ agonists that act on these receptors to relax the bronchial smooth muscle of the lung to relieve bronchospasm. These agents stimulate the normal sympathetic nervous system to open airways.[13]
- Anticholinergics improve lung function by blocking muscarinic receptors in the bronchi, causing bronchodilation. These agents block the normal parasympathetic nervous system so it cannot stimulate constriction of airways.[13]

Agents to help cough up mucus. Mucolytics react directly with the mucus to make it more liquid. They are delivered by inhalation. Expectorants cause the cough to be more productive by stimulating the flow of respiratory tract secretions.

Agents to suppress cough. Coughing is a protective mechanism and is useful to expectorate sputum. However, when coughing is chronic and nonproductive, it may prevent sleep or tire the patient, making cough suppression therapeutic. Most antitussives act within the central nervous system.

Antimicrobials. Respiratory tract infections are treated with antimicrobials to kill or limit growth of microorganisms.

Agents to aid smoking cessation. Five products available as first-line treatment for smoking cessation are used as nicotine replacement therapy (NRT). They are available in gum, lozenge, patch, inhaler, or nasal spray form. NRT allows smokers to substitute a drug source of nicotine for the nicotine in cigarettes and gradually withdraw the replacement nicotine to wean the smoker off nicotine completely.[13]

Oxygen Therapy

Delivery of humidified oxygen is a cornerstone of gas exchange intervention. Nurses collaborate with respiratory therapists to supply patients with oxygen and teach them how to use oxygen at home when applicable. Oxygen therapy is provided through a variety of delivery mechanisms when patients require more than 21% oxygen. A nasal cannula is used to deliver 24% oxygen (at flow rates of 1 L/min) to 44% oxygen (at flow rates of 4 L/min) through plastic nasal prongs. This is a safe and simple method that is used for long-term therapy. The cannula allows patients to eat, talk, and cough while wearing this device. Patients whose pulmonary disease causes retention of carbon dioxide, such as those with chronic obstructive pulmonary disease (COPD), should not use oxygen levels greater than 3 L/min.[14] Their bodies have adjusted to chronically high levels of carbon dioxide (hypercapnea) so that carbon dioxide no longer acts as the stimulant to breathe. For these patients, low blood oxygen levels become the stimulant to initiate breathing. Thus giving these patients oxygen >3 L/min can eliminate their stimulus to breathe, causing hypoventilation and, if prolonged, death.

Another oxygen delivery device is a simple face mask that covers the patient's nose and mouth. This mask delivers between 35% and 50% humidified oxygen at flow rates of 6 to 12 L/min and is used for short-term therapy because of its uncomfortable fit.[14]

Partial or nonrebreathing masks are used for short-term therapy when patients need higher levels of humidified oxygen between 60% and 90% at flow rates of 10 to 15 L/min. Oxygen flows into a reservoir bag and mask during inhalation. To attain these high levels of oxygen, the mask must fit snugly over the nose and mouth and may be uncomfortable.[14]

Venturi masks can deliver precise, high flow rates of humidified oxygen. These lightweight, cone-shaped devices are fitted to the face and are able to deliver 24%, 28%, 31%, 35%, 40%, and 50% oxygen. These masks are used to deliver low, constant oxygen concentrations to patients with COPD.[14]

Oxygen delivery devices such as a tracheostomy collar are available to provide humidified oxygen to patients with tracheostomy tubes.

Airway Management and Breathing Support

Patients with an acute disorder causing impaired gas exchange may need airway support. Before arrival of the emergency team, the nurse may insert an oropharyngeal airway to maintain the patient's breathing. Patients may require intubation using an endotracheal tube or tracheostomy tube. Humidified oxygen is delivered to the trachea and bronchi. When breathing support is needed, the patient's respiratory rate and volume are controlled by a ventilator.

Chest Physiotherapy and Postural Drainage

Chest physiotherapy and postural drainage are performed for the purpose of loosening and moving secretions into large airways where they can be expectorated. Chest physiotherapy includes percussion (cupping and clapping) and vibration to loosen secretions. Postural drainage involves positioning the patient in specific positions (e.g., head down, on left and right sides, and supine and prone) to use the benefit of gravity to remove secretions after they are loosened from specific segments of the lungs. Patients with cystic fibrosis use this procedure frequently to help remove the thick secretions formed by their disorder.

Invasive Procedures

There are a number of therapeutic interventions that are invasive. The nurse generalist does not perform these interventions, but provides care for patients during and after the procedures.

Chest tubes. Chest tubes are placed in the pleura to remove air (pneumothorax) and/or blood (hemothorax) from the pleural space so that the lungs can be reexpanded after thoracic surgery or trauma. Nurses monitor the amount and appearance of drainage from chest tubes and change the dressing around these tubes as ordered.

Thoracentesis. Thoracentesis is a procedure to relieve a pleural effusion by inserting a needle into the pleural space to remove fluid. Nurses assist physicians with this procedure and monitor the patient's vital signs, lung sounds, and pain level afterward.

Bronchoscopy. Bronchoscopy is a procedure that can be diagnostic or therapeutic. The procedure involves insertion of a bronchoscope through the trachea into bronchi. The diagnostic effect is directly visualizing the airway or taking tissue samples for biopsy. The therapeutic effects can include removing foreign objects and suctioning mucous plugs from airways or lavaging airways. Airway patency can also be accomplished using laser therapy, electrocautery, cryotherapy, and stents placed through a bronchoscope.[7]

Nutrition Therapy

Nutrition therapy is needed to provide energy for the increased work of breathing and support the immune system. High-protein, high-calorie, nutritious foods and drinks meet the needs of these patients. Small meals are advised for patients who become dyspneic while eating. For the patients with a productive cough, offer oral care before meals to reduce any lingering taste of sputum.[14]

Positioning

Two positions are important interventions for patients with impaired gas exchange. The first position is *sitting up*. Patients with acute or chronic impaired gas exchange breath more easily in high Fowler's position, Fowler's position, or semi-Fowler's position. These positions use gravity to move the diaphragm away from the lungs to reduce the work of breathing. Orthopnea refers to an abnormal condition in which a person must sit or stand to breathe comfortably. Patients with chronic pulmonary disease may use a tripod position or prefer sleeping while leaning forward over a table.

The second position is *lying horizontally*, which helps patients who are hypoxemic and have acute lung disease. The distribution of pulmonary capillary blood flow is affected by gravity in different body positions. The greatest volume of pulmonary blood flow occurs in the gravity-dependent areas of the lung. Thus the areas of the lung that are most dependent become the best ventilated and perfused.[1] Even though thoracic expansion of the dependent lung is reduced somewhat by the mattress, the gravity-dependent lung still has better ventilation and perfusion than the other lung. This principle can be seen in Figure 16-2 and applied to patients who have one lung affected more than the other. If the right lung is affected, the patient experiences the best ventilation and perfusion when lying on the left side. The patient will be turned routinely to prevent pressure ulcers, but may perhaps spend

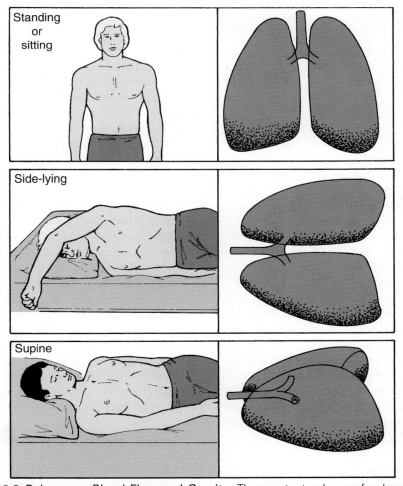

FIGURE 16-2 Pulmonary Blood Flow and Gravity. The greatest volume of pulmonary blood flow normally will occur in the gravity-dependent areas of the lung. Body position has a significant effect on the distribution of pulmonary blood flow. (From Huether S, McCance K: *Understanding pathophysiology,* ed 4, p 707, St Louis, 2008, Mosby.)

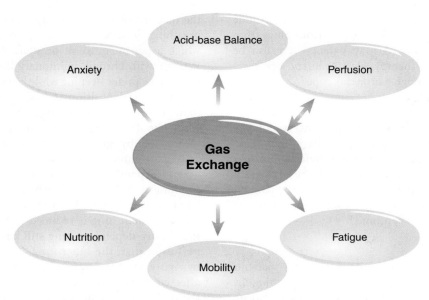

FIGURE 16-3 Gas Exchange and Interrelated Concepts.

CLINICAL NURSING SKILLS FOR GAS EXCHANGE

- Assessment
- Oxygen administration
- Positioning
- Peak expiratory flow rate
- Nebulizers
- Chest physiotherapy
- Airway suctioning
- Endotracheal tube and tracheostomy care
- Chest tube
- Mechanical ventilation
- Medication administration

more time in the position that provides the best ventilation and perfusion until recovery. The "good lung down" is a way to remember this position.[15]

Other Interventions

Alternate activity with rest periods; for example, if the patient becomes dyspneic after a bath or shower, allow a rest period before a meal or exercise. Many patients with COPD perceive they can breathe easier when there is an increase in air circulation, which they accomplish by using an electric fan.

Patient's coping may be improved by encouraging them to express their feelings about their impaired gas exchange and how it has changed their lives. Nurses may be able to help patients locate needed resources.

INTERRELATED CONCEPTS

Gas exchange is interrelated to nearly all of the health and illness concepts within this textbook because all cells in the body depend on gas exchange and removal of gases. Concepts that most closely interrelate with gas exchange are **Anxiety, Acid-base balance, Perfusion, Nutrition, Mobility,** and **Fatigue.** Figure 16-3 illustrates the interrelationship of these concepts.

Acid-base balance is affected by gas exchange in several ways. Diseases that retain carbon dioxide, such as COPD, create increased levels of carbonic acid, which causes respiratory acidosis. Conversely, when excessive carbon dioxide is exhaled such as during an anxiety attack, less carbonic acid is formed, causing a respiratory alkalosis. Finally, hypoxia attributable to inadequate perfusion, such as from a myocardial infarction, causes lactic acid formation that causes metabolic acidosis.

Mobility may be reduced when patients with impaired gas exchange become dyspneic when walking or climbing stairs. Fatigue is related to gas exchange in two different ways. When anemia is a cause of impaired gas exchange, the fatigue may be a manifestation of the anemia. However, when the patient must use accessory muscles and work hard to breathe, such as those with emphysema, they exert significant energy to breath, which contributes to fatigue.

Nutrition is a concern for patients who expend more than usual energy to breathe, such as those with emphysema and cystic fibrosis. They required high-calorie, high-protein, and nutritious foods in small servings so they do not tire while eating. Patients with anemia need food high in iron to maintain or increase their hemoglobin levels.

EXEMPLARS

There are multiple conditions that contribute to impaired gas exchange, more than are described in this text. Box 16-3 lists common conditions associated with impaired gas exchange across the lifespan; further details about these conditions can be found in medical-surgical and pediatric nursing textbooks.

MODEL CASE

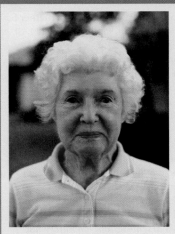

Martha Moore is an 87-year-old woman with a history of osteoporosis and hypertension. She had an exploratory laparotomy for a small-bowel obstruction 2 days ago. Before assessing this patient, the nurse noticed Mrs. Moore's hemoglobin level was 9 g and her SaO_2 was 90%. During this morning's assessment Martha reports her cough kept her awake last night. Vital signs reveal temperature 101° F, blood pressure 150/78 mm Hg, heart rate 100 beats/min, respiratory rate 24 breaths/min. On auscultation the nurse hears crackles in both lungs. The patient reports a sharp pain in her chest when she took the deep breath. After the deep breath for auscultation, the patient has a productive cough and the nurse notices the sputum is green with rust-colored tinting. Martha reports she tries not to cough because it causes abdominal pain at her incision site.

The nurse recognizes that Mrs. Moore has symptoms suggesting pneumonia as a postoperative complication. The nurse knows Mrs. Moore needs to deep breathe, increase activity as tolerated, and increase fluid intake. The nurse works with Mrs. Moore to implement the plan of care. The nurse asks Mrs. Moore to use the incentive spirometer now and notices she is moving only 800 ml of air. The nurse emphasizes the importance of using the incentive spirometer about 10 times every hour while awake to help get air into Mrs. Moore's lungs. Together they agree on a goal of moving 1500 ml. The nurse also talks with Mrs. Moore about giving her pain medication to relieve the abdominal pain. To further reduce pain when coughing, the nurse recommends that Mrs. Moore hold a pillow over her incision when she coughs to splint the incision site. After receipt of pain medication, Mrs. Moore is assisted to sit on the side of the bed and walk to a chair to eat the clear liquid breakfast. The nurse encourages Mrs. Moore to drink all of the liquids to help liquefy her secretions. When the surgeon makes rounds, the nurse reports the findings from Mrs. Moore's assessment and the plan of care initiated. The surgeon orders a chest x-ray, aspirin as needed for fever, an antibiotic, and iron tablets. After a bath, a nap, pain medication, and use of incentive spirometry with coughing, Mrs. Moore is assisted to walk in the hall. Before discharge, Mrs. Moore is taught about ways to treat her anemia with foods rich in iron and with the daily iron tablet. The outcome of this plan of care is that by discharge Mrs. Moore will be able to move at least 1500 ml on the spirometer, have clear breath sounds bilaterally, have a SaO_2 greater than 95%, be afebrile, and be able to state the plan to treat her anemia.

Case Analysis

This case clearly exemplifies impairment in gas exchange in a number of ways. Mrs. Moore has several classic risk factors including her age, a recent surgical procedure, and hesitancy to cough for fear of abdominal pain. The clinical presentation of Mrs. Moore's signs and symptoms is consistent with two types of gas exchange impairments: bacterial pneumonia, a very common exemplar of impaired gas exchange representing impairment of ventilation, and anemia, which impairs the oxygen-carrying capacity of the blood.

▪▪▪ BOX 16-3   EXEMPLARS OF GAS EXCHANGE

Impairment of Ventilation
- Acute respiratory failure
- Adult respiratory distress syndrome
- Airway obstruction
- Asthma
- Atelectasis
- Chronic obstructive pulmonary disease
- Cystic fibrosis
- Infant respiratory distress syndrome
- Lung cancer
- Pleural effusion
- Pneumonia
- Pneumothorax
- Respiratory syncytial virus (RSV)
- Tuberculosis
- Trauma and flail chest

Impairment in Perfusion
- Aneurysm
- Heart failure
- Peripheral artery disease
- Pulmonary emboli
- Shock

Impairment in Transportation
- Aplastic anemia
- Folic acid deficiency anemia
- Iron deficiency anemia
- Hemolytic anemia
- Megaloblastic anemia
- Pernicious anemia
- Thalassemia

Some disorders impairing ventilation are acute, from which patients recover completely. These disorders include acute respiratory failure, influenza, pneumonia, pulmonary edema, and respiratory syncytial virus (RSV). Other disorders requiring lifestyle changes are chronic, such as cystic fibrosis and chronic bronchitis and emphysema, called chronic obstructive pulmonary disease when they occur together. Asthma is a chronic disorder that has remissions and exacerbations. The prognosis of lung cancer is variable depending on the type of lung cancer and its degree of progression when detected. Tuberculosis can easily be detected and treated, but treatment requires a minimum of 6 months of antibiotic therapy. When drug therapy is successfully completed, the bacteria lie dormant in the lung for the rest of the patient's life and can be reactivated if the patient's immune system is compromised in any way.

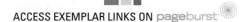

ACCESS EXEMPLAR LINKS ON pageburst

REFERENCES

1. Brashers V: Alterations of pulmonary function. In Huether S, McCance K, editors: *Understanding pathophysiology*, ed 4, St Louis, 2008, Mosby/Elsevier, pp 714–747.
2. Porth C: *Essentials of pathophysiology*, ed 3, Philadelphia, 2011, Wolters Kluwer/Lippincott Williams & Wilkins.
3. Wilson D: Health promotion of the infant and family. In Hockenberry M, Wilson F, editors: *Wong's nursing care of infants and children*, ed 8, St Louis, 2007, Mosby/Elsevier, pp 499–606.
4. Hueckel R, Wilson D: The child with disturbance of oxygen and carbon dioxide exchange. In Hockenberry M, Wilson D, editors: *Wong's nursing care of infants and children*, ed 8, St Louis, 2007, Mosby/Elsevier, pp 1273–1386.
5. Wilson S, Giddens J: *Health assessment for nursing practice*, ed 4, St Louis, 2009, Mosby/Elsevier.
6. Pagana K, Pagana T: *Mosby's diagnostic and laboratory test reference*, ed 10, St Louis, 2011, Mosby/Elsevier.
7. Norris C, et al: Nursing assessment respiratory system. In Lewis S, editor: *Medical-surgical nursing: assessment and management of clinical problems*, ed 8, St Louis, 2011, Mosby/Elsevier, pp 496–518.
8. *Healthy People 2020 goals for tobacco use:* Accessed Feb 12, 2011, at www.healthypeople.gov/2020/topicsobjectives2020/default.aspx.
9. American Lung Association: *Stop smoking.* Accessed Jan 15, 2011, at www.lungusa.org/stop-smoking.
10. American Cancer Society: *Stay healthy, guide to quitting smoking.* Accessed Jan 15, 2011, at www.cancer.org/Healthy/StayAwayfromTobacco/GuidetoQuittingSmoking.
11. www.cdc.gov/tobacco/data_statistics/fact_sheets/cessation/quitting/#dependence. Accessed Feb 16, 2011.
12. www.cdc.gov/vaccines/recs/schedules/adult-schedule.htm#hcp immunizations.
13. Lehne R: *Pharmacology for nursing care*, ed 7, Philadelphia, 2010, Saunders/Elsevier.
14. Kaufman J: Nursing management: obstructive pulmonary disease. In Lewis S et al: *Medical-surgical nursing: assessment and management of clinical problems*, ed 8, St Louis, 2011, Mosby/Elsevier, pp 587–640.
15. Yeaw E: How position affects oxygenation. Good lung down? *Am J Nurs* 92(4):27–29, 1992.

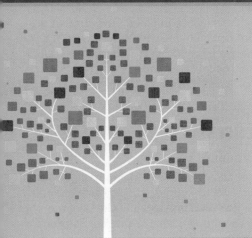

All cells depend on a consistent supply of blood. When injury occurs to veins and arteries, the clotting process is initiated to stop the blood loss. This represents an important physiologic protective mechanism allowing the body to maintain homeostasis when injury occurs. However, excessive clotting can impair perfusion, whereas inadequate clotting increases blood loss. For this reason, clotting is a critical concept for nurses to understand and incorporate into practice. The purpose of this concept analysis is to help nurses acquire knowledge about clotting across the lifespan. In practice, nurses should be able to promote healthy behaviors that optimize clotting, identify individuals at risk of impaired clotting, recognize when individuals are experiencing impaired clotting, and respond with appropriate interventions.

DEFINITION(S)

For the purposes of this concept analysis, clotting is defined as *a physiologic process in which blood is converted from a liquid to a semisolid gel.* This is a normal and expected physiologic event. Although clotting can occur within an intact blood vessel, the process usually starts when veins or arteries are injured.[1] Multiple coagulation factors interact in a sequence with fibrin and platelets to form a blood clot. The result of the clotting process is hemostasis, the stoppage of blood flow.

The clotting process can become impaired in two ways. First, when clotting factors are not available, patients experience excessive bleeding. Alternatively, if blood clots form when they are not physiologically indicated, then a *thrombus* (blood clot) may obstruct a blood vessel and interfere with blood flow. Effects of impaired clotting vary depending upon the extent of impairment and the anatomic location.

SCOPE AND CATEGORIES

The concept of clotting and problems associated with impaired clotting represent a variety of physiologic processes. The scope of the concept represents a continuum—ranging from excessive clotting beyond physiologic need on one end of the spectrum, to impaired clotting resulting in bleeding on the other. Expected physiologic clotting processes fall in the middle of this continuum. Two categories are related to the anatomic location of the impairment, whether it is local or systemic. Figure 17-1 depicts this scope and categories.

RISK FACTORS

Impaired clotting affects all individuals regardless of age, gender, race, or socioeconomic status. Common risk factors are described in the following sections.

Age

Older adults have increased risk for clotting because of expected physiologic changes that occur with advanced age such as increased platelet adhesiveness,[2] which promotes blood stasis.

Genetics

Several genetic disorders are associated with hematologic conditions. The classic example is hemophilia, a recessive genetic disorder caused by the inability to produce adequate clotting factor needed for blood coagulation. Certain types of thrombocytopenia are also inherited diseases.

Immobility

Immobility contributes to blood clot formation by slowing the return of venous blood to the heart. Slow blood flow results in stasis, a risk factor for thrombi formation. Immobility may occur as a result of paralysis or an unconscious or impaired cognitive state, or from bed rest needed to recover from an illness or surgery. Individuals who are confined to a sitting position for long periods (such as long flights) are also susceptible to the formation of venous clots.

Smoking

Smoking is a known risk factor that contributes to hypercoagulability of the blood—a contributing factor to clot formation.

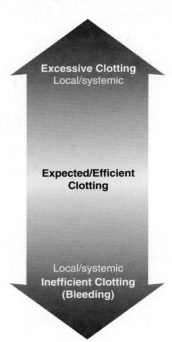

FIGURE 17-1 Scope and Categories of Clotting Concept.

Underlying Medical Conditions Leading to Bleeding

Thrombocytopenia

Thrombocytopenia is a condition manifested by a reduction in the number of platelets. A severe decrease in the amount of circulating platelets makes one susceptible to uncontrolled bleeding with injury, or even spontaneous bleeding. Thrombocytopenia may be caused by inherited disorders, acquired disorders, or medical treatment that results in bone marrow suppression. Chemotherapy and radiation therapy are examples of treatments that often cause bone marrow depression, which can lead to a reduction in the number of platelets. Some conditions, such as leukemia, affect the bone marrow directly by decreasing platelet production.

Hemophilia

Hemophilia is caused by genetic disorders that are associated with defective or deficient coagulation factors. Thus individuals with hemophilia are at risk for excessive bleeding.

Underlying Medical Conditions Leading to Excessive Clotting

Polycythemia

Polycythemia is a condition associated with the production and presence of too many red blood cells (RBCs). When this occurs, the increased number of RBCs makes the blood more viscous, thus increasing the risk of thrombi formation. A chromosomal mutation is one cause of polycythemia. A second cause is a compensatory mechanism for chronic hypoxemia that increases the number of erythrocytes to improve oxygen transport. A malignant or benign tumor can also cause polycythemia by increasing erythropoietin production, which stimulates production of more erythrocytes.

Atrial Fibrillation

Atrial fibrillation produces inefficient blood flow through in the atria that results in stasis of blood within the atrium. The stasis allows for formation of clots that may become emboli and enter the cerebral circulation, causing a stroke (also known as "brain attack" and "cerebral vascular accident").[3]

PHYSIOLOGIC PROCESSES AND CONSEQUENCES

Normal Clotting Process

The homeostatic process is a protective mechanism to prevent excessive bleeding when vascular injury occurs. In a normal clotting process, the damaged vessel, platelets, and clotting factors work together to stop bleeding. The first response is vasoconstriction to reduce blood loss. The second response is formation of a platelet plug, which develops in 3 to 7 minutes. Next, clotting factors are activated either from the intrinsic or from the extrinsic pathway and proceed in a coagulation cascade to the common final pathway. At the end of this pathway thrombin stimulates fibrinogen to form insoluble fibrin that stabilizes the clot.[4] Figure 17-2 illustrates the coagulation cascade.

Pathophysiologic Process of Excessive Clotting/Thrombi

Normal homeostatic processes can become impaired when excessive clotting factors lead to thrombus formation. A thrombus can form in arteries or veins.

Arterial Thrombosis

Arterial thrombi are associated with conditions that increase platelet counts or RBC production or that create turbulent blood flow with platelet adhesion. Another source of thrombi is atherosclerosis, which begins with injury to the endothelium. Hypertension causes endothelial injury from the increased pressure of blood in the arteries creating a shearing force. Other causes of endothelial injury include exogenous chemical agents such as toxins from cigarette smoke and endogenous agents such as cholesterol.

When a thrombus blocks an artery, it interrupts the flow of oxygenated blood to the tissue, leading to ischemia. If left untreated, this results in cell death; however, if adequate collateral circulation exists, it can compensate for the reduced blood flow and avert cell death. The pathologic consequence of such an event is determined by the location (coronary artery, cerebral artery, femoral artery) and size of the affected artery. The larger the artery impacted, the larger amount of tissue affected.

Venous Thrombosis

Venous thrombosis is the formation of a blood clot in a vein—usually in association with inflammation within the vein. Superficial and deep veins may be affected. Three factors associated with the formation of venous thrombosis are hypercoagulability of the blood, injury to the vessel wall endothelium, and stasis of blood flow.[2] These three factors are commonly known as Virchow's triad (Figure 17-3). Hypercoagulability develops because of an imbalance between clotting mechanisms and

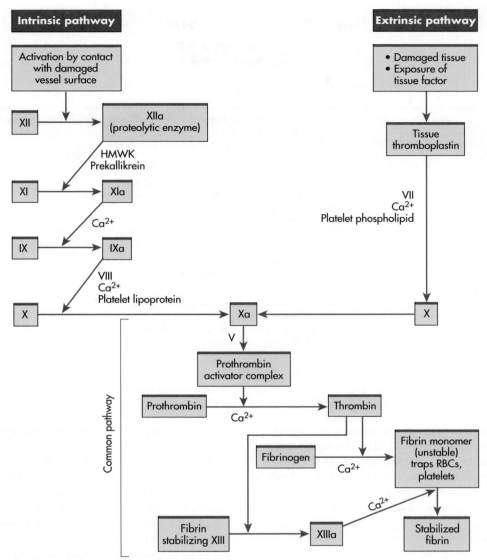

FIGURE 17-2 Coagulation Cascade. Coagulation cascade showing steps in the intrinsic and extrinsic pathways. (From Lewis S, et al: *Medical-surgical nursing: assessment and management of clinical problems,* ed 8, St Louis, 2011, Mosby/Elsevier.)

coagulation or because of an increase in fibrin production. Endothelial damage leads to release of clotting factors or activation of platelets. Stasis of venous blood occurs when there is dysfunction of venous valves, inactivity of extremity muscles, or change in unidirectional venous blood flow.[5]

A thrombus that detaches becomes an embolus and can lodge in pulmonary vessels, creating a pulmonary embolus.

Pathophysiologic Process of Inadequate Clotting/Bleeding

Bleeding occurs after injury to arteries and veins, but also can occur spontaneously when the factors needed for clotting are absent. These clotting factors include platelets and clotting factors II (prothrombin), VII, VIII, IX, and X. The extent of bleeding can be as minor as bruising or as significant as hemorrhage. Disorders that cause bleeding include thrombocytopenia, liver diseases, hemophilia A, hemophilia B, and

von Willebrand's disease. Thrombocytopenia is defined as a platelet count below 150,000/mm³, although the decrease is not considered significant unless the platelet count falls below 100,000/mm³. Risk for hemorrhage after minor trauma increases when the platelet count falls below 50,000/mm³ and may result in the formation of petechiae, purpura, or ecchymosis. Spontaneous bleeding without trauma, such as a spontaneous nosebleed, occurs when the platelet count ranges from 10,000/mm³ to 15,000/mm³. Liver disease, such as cirrhosis, impairs the liver's synthesis of clotting factors, including factors II, VII, IX, and X. Reduction in the amounts of these clotting factors prevents formation of clots after trauma or hemorrhage. Hemophilia A and hemophilia B are similar in that they are both recessive sex-linked genetic disorders in males whose affected clotting factor is defective or deficient. The difference is the affected clotting factor. In hemophilia A it is factor VIII, whereas in hemophilia B it is factor IX. By

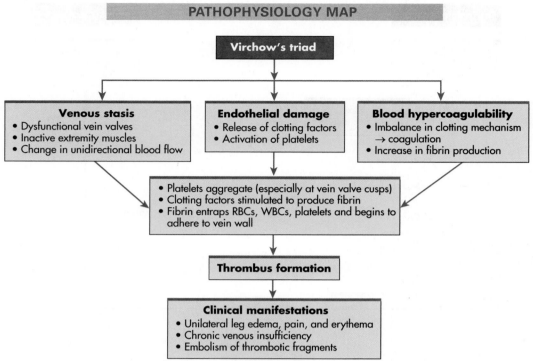

FIGURE 17-3 **Virchow's Triad.** Virchow's triad showing the pathophysiology of venous thromboembolism. (From Lewis S, et al: *Medical-surgical nursing: assessment and management of clinical problems*, ed 8, St Louis, 2011, Mosby/Elsevier.)

contrast, von Willebrand's disease is a bleeding disorder that is an autosomal dominant genetic disorder affecting both genders; affected individuals have a deficiency in von Willebrand factor coagulation protein and factor VIII as well as a platelet dysfunction. Absence of these clotting factors results in spontaneous bleeding, including nosebleeds and hematuria.[5]

ASSESSMENT

Nurses gather data from the patient's history, physical assessment, and diagnostic test results. Assessment of clotting involves recognizing indications of adequate and inadequate blood clotting. Adequate clotting is apparent when the patient forms a blood clot after endothelial damage. Peripheral pulses are present, and the skin is warm and dry without discolorations or edema. Also, blood pressure and heart rate are at expected rates for the patient's age.

History
Baseline History
Baseline history includes current and past medical conditions. Nurses inquire about patients' chronic diseases. As mentioned previously, many medical conditions are associated with bleeding or clotting disorders. Common conditions associated with clotting disorders are listed in Box 17-2 at the end of the chapter.

Also included in the baseline history are medications the patient is currently taking because many medications affect clotting.[6] Aspirin is taken daily by many people to reduce the potential for clot formation because of its antiplatelet effects.

Warfarin (Coumadin) is a prescription drug taken to prevent blood clotting by interfering with the four vitamin K–dependent clotting factors (II, VII, IX, X). Nurses also ask about herbal and dietary supplements that may affect clotting. These supplements include bilberry, black cohosh, chamomile, chondroitin sulfate, feverfew, garlic, ginger, ginkgo biloba, ginseng, goldenseal, omega-3 fatty acids, melatonin, niacin, soy, and turmeric.[7]

Lifestyle behaviors are also important to assess as part of the history. Questions include exercise habits, including the kind of exercise and how often it is performed and for what length of time, because exercise increases blood flow. Nurses ask patients about smoking habits because nicotine causes vasoconstriction and is a toxin that damages the endothelium, contributing to atherosclerosis.

Bleeding Problems
Adults may report bleeding from gums when brushing teeth, from the rectum after defecation, or after a minor trauma. Patients may report fatigue or dyspnea from anemia caused by blood loss. When applicable, women are asked if the amount of blood lost during menses has increased. Patients may describe bleeding that takes longer than usual to stop. Patients with prolonged bleeding may report blood loss from anywhere in the body including nosebleeds; new bruises; black, tarry stools; blood in emesis, sputum, or urine; or bleeding from the mouth. Indications of intracranial bleeding may include a headache, changes in vision, sudden difficulty talking, or weakness of one arm or leg.

In children with hemophilia, the parents may report bleeding after minor trauma such as from a circumcision, during loss of deciduous teeth, or after a slight fall. Bleeding into a joint (hemarthrosis) may produce complaints of stiffness, tingling, or ache of knees, elbows, and ankles. Reports of hematuria are not uncommon.[8]

Clotting

Symptoms associated with a thrombus vary depending upon location. A venous thrombus impairs venous return and creates an inflammatory response. Symptoms include pain, edema, and redness in the affected extremity. In most cases, venous thrombosis is reported in the lower extremities. In contrast, a thrombus in an artery interrupts blood flow to the tissue and creates an ischemic response. Hallmark symptoms reported by patients experiencing arterial ischemia include pain (often severe) and abnormal sensations (paresthesia).

Examination Findings
Bleeding

When assessing patients with *prolonged bleeding*, nurses may notice petechiae, ecchymosis, and purpura during inspection of the skin that indicate localized bleeding in the subcutaneous tissue. For patients with hemophilia, subcutaneous and intramuscular hemorrhages are common. Hemarthrosis results in warmth, redness, edema, and severe pain of affected joints followed by decreased joint range of motion.[8] Bleeding into the brain produces varying manifestations of stroke depending on the amount of blood released and the area of the brain affected. When bleeding is excessive, changes to vital signs—specifically increased heart rate and decreased blood pressure—may be noted.

Clotting

When assessing patients with a thrombosis, nurses find different manifestations depending on whether arteries or veins are affected. Clots within veins frequently develop in lower extremities, where they impair perfusion and cause pain, redness, and edema with an increased circumference of the affected extremity. The patient may have a palpable firm vein that is tender to touch. When venous thrombi become emboli, the emboli flow superiorly in the inferior vena cava and lodge in pulmonary capillaries. Manifestations produced from pulmonary emboli vary by location affected and size of the emboli; however, the classic triad includes dyspnea, chest pain, and hemoptysis.[9]

As mentioned previously, an arterial thrombus in lower extremities impairs perfusion. Accompanying the common reported symptoms of *pain* and *paresthesia,* other clinical manifestations include *pulselessness, pallor,* and *poikilothermia (cool skin* temperature over the affected area). These are often referred to as "the five P's." Blood clots that travel as emboli through the carotid circulation can impair perfusion to the brain, producing manifestations of a brain attack that vary by location affected and size of the emboli.

Diagnostic Tests
Laboratory Tests

Prothrombin time (PT). PT measures the adequacy of the extrinsic system and common pathways in the clotting mechanism, which include clotting factors I (fibrinogen),

II (prothrombin), V, VII, and X. When these clotting factors are found in decreased amounts, the PT is prolonged, meaning more time is needed for blood to clot. PT results are reported in seconds along with a control value. The patient's value should be approximately equal to the control. A normal finding is 11.0 to 12.5 seconds. The PT is used to monitor the therapeutic ranges of anticoagulants such as warfarin (Coumadin) and these therapeutic values are 1.5 to 2.5 times normal.[10]

International normalized ratio (INR). INR was established by the World Health Organization to measure clotting using a standardized international sensitivity index. Using this index standardizes the INR results regardless of the reagents or methods used to analyze the blood. The INR is used to monitor the effectiveness of anticoagulant therapy such as warfarin (Coumadin) that is given to inhibit the formation of blood clots.[10]

Partial thromboplastin time (PTT). PTT measures the intrinsic system and common pathway of clot formation, which includes factors I (fibrinogen), II (prothrombin), V, VIII, IX, X, XI, and XII. Factors II, VII, IX, and X are vitamin K–dependent factors. When there are reduced amounts of these clotting factors, the PTT is prolonged, meaning more time is needed for blood to clot. Like the PT values, the PTT results are reported in seconds along with a control value. The patient's normal value should be approximately equal to the control. A normal finding is 60 to 70 seconds. Activators were added to PTT reagents to shorten normal clotting time and provide a narrow normal range. This shortened time is called activated PTT or APTT, with a normal value of 30 to 40 seconds. The PTT is used to monitor the therapeutic ranges of patients taking anticoagulants such as heparin and these therapeutic values are 1.5 to 2.5 times normal.[10]

Fibrinogen. Fibrinogen (or clotting factor I) is part of the common pathway in the coagulation system. It is converted to fibrin by the action of thrombin during the coagulation process. Reduced fibrinogen level occurs in patients with liver disease, malnutrition states, and consumptive coagulopathies such as disseminated intravascular coagulation (DIC). Normal values for adults range from 200 to 400 mg/dl and for newborns 125 to 300 mg/dl.[10]

Platelet count. This is the number of platelets (thrombocytes) per cubic millimeter of blood. This test is performed on patients with suspected bleeding disorders or clotting disorders. Normal values are as follows: adults and children, 150,000 to 400,000 per mm^3; premature infants, 100,000 to 300,000 per mm^3; newborns, 150,000 to 300,000 per mm^3; infants, 200,000 to 475,000 per mm^3.[10]

D-Dimer. The D-dimer test assesses the activity of both thrombin, used to form blood clots, and plasmin, used to break down blood clots. While plasmin breaks down fibrin clots, fibrin degradation products and D-dimer are produced. The D-dimer assay provides a highly specific measurement of the amount of fibrin degradation that occurs as the clot is dissolved. Normal plasma does not have detectable amounts of fragment D-dimer. This test is used to confirm a diagnosis of disseminated intravascular coagulation (DIC).[10]

RBC count, hemoglobin, and hematocrit. These measures are used to diagnose the presence of polycythemia. Individuals with polycythemia have elevated levels of hemoglobin, hematocrit, and RBCs with microcytosis.

Bone marrow examination. An examination of the bone marrow may be done to assess for evidence of hyper- or hypoproduction of platelets and RBCs. This test may be indicated for polycythemia or thrombocytopenia.

Radiologic Tests

Noninvasive venous studies. Ultrasound is used as a non-invasive approach for evaluation for venous thrombosis.

Arteriograms. Arteriograms allow visualization of arteries by injecting radiopaque contrast into them so that the location and extent of occlusion or dilation can be identified.[10]

Venograms. Venograms of the lower extremities allow visualization of veins by injecting radiopaque contrast into them so that the location and extent of thrombi can be identified.[10]

CLINICAL MANAGEMENT

Clinical management related to clotting includes health promotion and the management of emerging or present conditions that compromise clotting. The ultimate goal is to optimize the clotting process. The *Healthy People 2020 Goals for Bleeding and Clotting* are summarized in Box 17-1 and link to all phases of care.[11]

Primary Prevention

Primary prevention includes measures to promote health and prevent disease. For problems associated with excessive bleeding, the only true primary prevention measure is genetic counseling. Genetic counseling is advised for couples who have a family history of bleeding disorders and want to start a family. Genetic counseling will assist couples to comprehend the medical facts, understand risks and options, and make an informed decision. Measures to prevent bleeding as a complication of a disease process or medical treatments for other conditions are discussed under the collaborative care section.

For this concept, most primary prevention measures relate to prevention of blood clots. Strategies for prevention include minimizing the risks for blood stasis, increased blood viscosity, and vessel injury. Patients at risk for venous stasis or those with clotting disorders are encouraged to enhance blood flow by performing leg exercises, engaging in regular walking, or wearing compression stockings. High-risk patients (such as those following knee or hip replacement surgery) are administered anticoagulant therapy as a prophylactic measure. These agents will be discussed further in sections that follow. Women with an increased risk for clots may be advised to avoid taking birth control pills because of their adverse effect on clotting. Teaching patients about the importance of smoking cessation is a priority because nicotine both causes vasoconstriction, that contributes to stasis of blood flow, and damages the endothelium, contributing to atherosclerosis. Maintaining adequate hydration reduces the potential for increased blood viscosity.

Secondary Prevention (Screening)

Secondary prevention includes screening and early diagnosis and prompt treatment of existing health problems. There are no routine screening tests indicated for the general public related to this concept.

Collaborative Interventions for Bleeding Disorders
Prevention of Bleeding

Prevention and control of bleeding are the cornerstones for management of individuals with bleeding disorders. Patients must learn to recognize signs and symptoms of bleeding and to notify the health care provider when indications of bleeding occur. They also must be taught strategies to minimize risk for trauma. Patients with bleeding disorders or individuals who are taking anticoagulants are taught to avoid taking drugs that contribute to bleeding such as any drugs containing aspirin. They are encouraged to avoid situations that could cause injury resulting in bleeding, such as participation in contact sports. Nurses may teach strategies designed to avoid bleeding. For example, patients learn to use a soft bristle toothbrush to avoid bleeding from gums while brushing teeth. They use an electric razor rather than a blade razor to avoid nicks to the skin. Patients are encouraged to avoid blowing their nose forcefully to reduce the likelihood of nosebleeds. They should avoid getting tattoos and body piercings. Women who are menstruating should count the number of pads or tampons they use daily and notify the health care provider if that number increases. Patients should understand the importance of notifying health care personnel before seemingly benign invasive procedures such as teeth cleaning, manicure, or pedicure.[12]

Medications given by injection should be avoided if possible to prevent the needle stick that causes bleeding. When an injection is unavoidable, nurses use the smallest size needle possible.[12] Additionally, nurses monitor laboratory tests such

---

BOX 17-1   *HEALTHY PEOPLE 2020* OBJECTIVES FOR BLEEDING AND CLOTTING

1. Increase the proportion of persons with bleeding disorders who receive recommended vaccinations.
2. Reduce the number of persons who develop venous thromboembolism.
3. Reduce the number of adults who develop venous thromboembolism during hospitalization.
4. Increase the proportion of providers who refer women with symptoms suggestive of inherited bleeding disorders for diagnosis and treatment.
5. Increase the proportion of women with von Willebrand's disease (vWD) who are timely and accurately diagnosed.
6. Reduce the proportion of persons with hemophilia who develop reduced joint mobility because of bleeding into joints.

From www.healthypeople.gov/2020/topicsobjectives2020/default. aspx; accessed Feb 12, 2011.

as INR to assess risk and to provide direction in medication management.

Management of Bleeding Episodes

During episodes of active bleeding, the obvious goal is to control hemorrhage. Direct pressure over bleeding sites is indicated. The use of topical agents (such as Gelfoam or fibrin foam) might also help to slow the bleeding. Ice applications are also indicated for topical bleeding or bleeding within a joint space. Pharmacologic agents (discussed next) and the provision of supportive care, such as volume replacement and oxygen support, may be needed to prevent the progression of bleeding to the point of hemodynamic instability.

Pharmacotherapy

Clotting factor replacement or stimulating agents. There are several agents used to replace factor VII and factor IX—the deficient clotting factors associated with hemophilia. Desmopressin acetate is a synthetic vasopressin agent that stimulates release of factor VIII and von Willebrand factor. This agent is useful for milder forms of hemophilia.[12]

Platelet replacement agents. Several pharmacologic agents are used to increase the number of platelets. Platelet growth factor agents (such as oprelvekin, romiplostim, and eltrombopag) stimulate bone marrow production of platelets. A transfusion of platelets is also a way to increase a patient's platelet volume, but this is generally performed to treat life-threatening hemorrhage.

Collaborative Interventions for Clotting Disorders

Because there are several conditions that can lead to clotting, collaborative interventions are dependent on the underlying cause.

Pharmacotherapy

Several groups of drugs are used to treat individuals with clotting disorders and to prevent the formation of clots among high-risk individuals.

Anticoagulants. Two common anticoagulant agents used to prevent the formation of blood clots include warfarin and heparin. Warfarin (Coumadin) acts by decreasing the production of four vitamin K–dependent clotting factors: II (prothrombin), VII, IX, and X. Coumadin is the only oral anticoagulant currently available.[13] Heparin acts by inactivating clotting factors, primarily thrombin and factor Xa. Low-molecular-weight (LMW) heparin drugs, such as enoxaparin (Lovenox) or dalteparin (Fragmin), are the most commonly used agents in this category.

Antiplatelets. Agents such as aspirin or clopidogrel (Plavix) act as antiplatelets by preventing platelet aggregation.

Direct thrombin inhibitors. These synthetic agents are direct, reversible inhibitors that bind to free and bound thrombin. By inhibiting thrombin, these agents prevent the conversion of fibrinogen to fibrin and the activation of factor XIII. Examples of this category of agents are hirudins, synthetic thrombin inhibitors, and factor Xa inhibitors.[13]

Thrombolytic agents. Agents to dissolve blood clots are thrombolytic agents such as streptokinase, alteplase (a tissue plasminogen activator [t-PA]), tenecteplase, and reteplase. These agents act by digesting fibrin in clots and breaking down plasmin and other clotting factors. All of these agents have risks of serious bleeding.[13]

Invasive Procedures

Phlebotomy. Phlebotomy, or the removal of blood, is a common treatment to prevent clots for individuals with polycythemia. The goal of this treatment is to reduce blood volume, blood viscosity, and bone marrow activity. Phlebotomy may be needed as often as every 2 to 3 months.

Thrombectomy. A thrombectomy is the removal of a thrombus from a vessel. This can be accomplished through a catheter placed percutaneously or as an open surgical procedure (e.g., direct arteriotomy or venous thrombectomy) in which the vessel is opened to remove the thrombus.

Filters. Filter devices are used to prevent pulmonary embolism for individuals with clotting disorders who are unable to take anticoagulant agents or have a history of pulmonary emboli. Filters (also known as vena cava interruption devices) are inserted percutaneously through the right femoral vein or right internal veins and floated into the vena cava, where they block blood clots from reaching the pulmonary capillaries.

Nutrition Therapy

Warfarin (Coumadin) is an anticoagulant that acts by interfering with vitamin K–dependent clotting factors (VII, IX, X, and II [prothrombin]). The dosage of this drug is adjusted regularly to maintain the INR between 2 and 3. Patients taking warfarin should keep their vitamin K intake consistent to maintain the therapeutic effects of the drug. If the dietary intake of vitamin K increases, then the dose of warfarin must be increased as well and vice versa. Sources of vitamin K include green, leafy vegetables such as spinach or kale, mayonnaise, canola oil, and soybean oil.[13]

Positioning

Positioning affects blood flow and comfort. Patients with a deep venous thrombosis (DVT) (also known as venous thromboembolism [VTE]) in a lower extremity are taught to elevate the affected leg when lying or sitting to facilitate venous return to the heart. By contrast, patients with an arterial thrombus of a lower extremity are taught to position the affected leg in a dependent position to use gravity to improve perfusion to the feet. During the acute phase after a brain attack, patients are positioned with the head of the bed elevated at least 30 degrees to facilitate venous blood flow from the brain to help prevent cerebral edema. Positioning for all patients prescribed bed rest includes preventing pressure ulcers by repositioning patients as needed to maintain perfusion in dependent areas. Bed rest patients wear sequential compression devices (SCDs) to stimulate venous return to the heart.

MODEL CASE

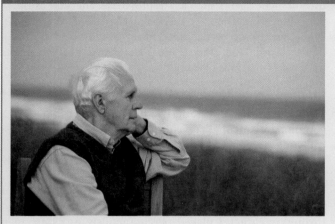

Arthur Rosen is a 78-year-old widower who lives alone. He has a history of atrial fibrillation and has a prescription for warfarin 5 mg once a day. Arthur finished his Coumadin prescription 3 weeks ago and did not have an opportunity to obtain the refill. He was admitted to the hospital for treatment of an ischemic stroke attributable to cerebral emboli. His manifestations were paralysis and anesthesia of the left leg. During the morning assessment the nurse notices Arthur's left thigh is red and edematous. Arthur tells the nurse his left upper leg feels achy. The circumference of the right leg is 51 cm, whereas the

circumference of the left leg is 53 cm. Arthur has no feeling in his left leg. His vital signs reveal temperature 98° F, blood pressure 140/72 mm Hg, heart rate 86 beats/min, respiratory rate 18 breaths/min. Based on these recent changes, the nurse suspects a deep vein thrombosis (DVT) and notifies the physician of these changes. An ultrasound of the extremity is performed and confirms a DVT. Arthur is prescribed immediate full bed rest and a new order for intravenous heparin is started until his INR is ≧2.0 for 24 hours. Also the nurse notifies the physical therapist of the suspected DVT so that therapy can be rescheduled. The nurse elevates Arthur's left leg on two pillows and does not perform the passive range-of-motion exercises of the lower extremities she had earlier planned.

Case Analysis

This case exemplifies impairment of clotting in several ways. Arthur had a history of atrial fibrillation. This disorder causes stasis of blood in the left atrium, which can cause clot development. These clots can dislodge, allowing emboli to travel to the cerebral circulation. The emboli lodged in the right anterior cerebral artery, impairing blood flow to the right frontal and parietal lobes. This lack of perfusion caused the paralysis and anesthesia of the left leg. Arthur's therapy is bed rest with limited mobility until he becomes stronger. Immobility is a risk factor for the development of thrombi, particularly in the lower extremity.

INTERRELATED CONCEPTS

Concepts that interrelate with clotting are **Perfusion, Gas exchange, Intracranial regulation, Mobility, Pain,** and **Patient education.** Figure 17-4 illustrates the interrelationship of these concepts.

Perfusion is impaired when blood clots slow or stop blood flow as well as when the absence of clotting results in hemorrhage.

Gas exchange is impaired when pulmonary emboli reduce pulmonary capillary blood available to carry oxygen from alveoli to cells.

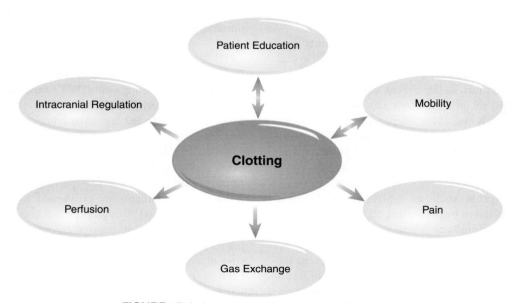

FIGURE 17-4 Clotting and Interrelated Concepts.

Intracranial regulation is affected either by blood clots or by hemorrhage, which produce disorders such as brain attack or communicating hydrocephalus.

Mobility is reduced due to illness or recovery from surgery. This immobility increases the risk for deep vein thrombosis (DVT). Treatment for DVT is bed rest, which further impairs mobility.

Pain is experienced from an arterial thrombus or constriction impairing perfusion to a lower extremity as well as by hemorrhage in a joint space.

Patient education is needed to help patients manage their bleeding or clotting disorders. Individuals with clotting disorders require patient education; likewise inadequate education can lead to complications.

EXEMPLARS

There are multiple conditions that contribute to impaired clotting, more than are described in this text. Box 17-2 lists common conditions associated with impaired clotting across the lifespan; further details about these conditions can be found in medical-surgical and pediatric nursing textbooks. Some disorders are acute whereas others are chronic. The acute disorders include disseminated intravascular coagulation (DIC) and deep vein thrombosis. Disorders that usually are chronic are polycythemia, thrombolytic and hemorrhagic strokes, immune thrombocytopenic purpura (ITP), and hemophilia.

BOX 17-2   EXEMPLARS OF CLOTTING

Clotting Disorders

Local
- Arterial thrombi
- Venous thrombosis

Systemic
- Disseminated intravascular coagulation
- Polycythemia

Bleeding Disorders
- Bone marrow depression
- Disseminated intravascular coagulation
- Heparin-induced thrombocytopenia
- Hemophilia A and B
- Immune thrombocytopenia purpura (ITP)
- Leukemia
- Thrombocytopenia
- von Willebrand's disease

ACCESS EXEMPLAR LINKS ON pageburst

REFERENCES

1. Porth C: *Essentials of pathophysiology*, ed 3, Philadelphia, 2011, Wolters Kluwer/Lippincott Williams & Wilkins.
2. Rote N, McCance K: Structure and function of the hematologic system. In Huether S, McCance K, editors: *Understanding pathophysiology*, ed 4, St Louis, 2008, Mosby/Elsevier, pp 481–507.
3. Centers for Disease Control and Prevention: *ICD-9-CM Coordination and Maintenance Committee Meeting, April 1-2, 2004* Accessed Jan 18, 2011, at www.cdc.gov/nchs/data/icd9/agendaapril04%20revised.pdf.
4. Lungstrom N, Emerson R: Alterations in hemostasis and blood coagulation. In Copstead L, Banasik J, editors: *Pathophysiology*, ed 3, St Louis, 2005, Mosby/Elsevier, pp 363–381.
5. Rote N, McCance K, Mansen T: Alteration of hematologic function. In Huether S, McCance K, editors: *Understanding pathophysiology*, ed 4, St Louis, 2008, Mosby/Elsevier, pp 508–549.
6. Wilson S, Giddens J: *Health assessment for nursing practice*, ed 4, St Louis, 2009, Mosby/Elsevier.
7. Wipke-Tevis D, Rich K: Nursing assessment: vascular disorders. In Lewis S, et al editors: *Medical-surgical nursing: assessment and management of clinical problems*, ed 8, St Louis, 2011, Mosby/Elsevier, pp 866–896.
8. Bryant R: The child with hematologic or immunologic dysfunction. In Hockenberry M, Wilson D, editors: *Wong's nursing care of infants and children*, ed 8, St Louis, 2007, Mosby/Elsevier, pp 1503–1557.
9. Malone M: Nursing management: lower respiratory problems. In Lewis S, et al: *Medical-surgical nursing: assessment and management of clinical problems*, ed 8, St Louis, 2011, Mosby/Elsevier, pp 545–586.
10. Pagana K, Pagana T: *Mosby's diagnostic and laboratory test reference*, ed 10, St Louis, 2011, Mosby/Elsevier.
11. *Healthy People 2020 goals for bleeding and clotting:* Accessed Feb 12, 2011, at www.healthypeople.gov/2020/topicsobjectives 2020/default.aspx.
12. Rome SI: Nursing assessment: hematologic problems. In Lewis S, et al: *Medical-surgical nursing: assessment and management of clinical problems*, ed 8, St Louis, 2011, Mosby/Elsevier, pp 661–713.
13. Lehne R: *Pharmacology for nursing care*, ed 7, Philadelphia, 2010, Saunders/Elsevier.

18

Reproduction

Jan Lamarche Zdanuk

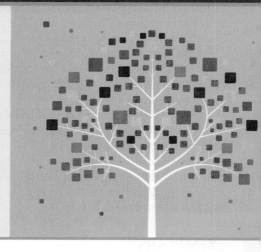

The creation of all life occurs as a result of reproduction. As a foundational concept in the biological sciences, reproduction has been studied extensively. Two main types of reproduction described are sexual and asexual reproduction. With asexual reproduction an organism can create genetic copies of itself. Viruses, bacteria, fungi, and some plants reproduce through such a process. Sexual reproduction is a biological process in which a combination of genetic material from two sources is needed. Mammals, fish, reptiles, and most plants reproduce through this process. The purpose of this concept analysis is to present the concept of reproduction as it applies to humans and in the context of nursing. Because human reproduction involves male and female sexual interaction, the scope of this concept includes both genders, although the majority of discussion focuses on the female.

DEFINITION(S)

There are multiple definitions of human reproduction in the literature. However, the foundational principle of human reproduction is that it is the process by which human beings produce a new individual. Sexual intercourse between a man and a woman may result in the conception of a child. The sex glands or gonads (ovaries in the female and testes in the male) produce the germ cells (oocytes and spermatozoa) that unite and grow into a new individual.

During intercourse, the interaction between the male and female reproductive systems results in fertilization of the woman's ovum by the man's sperm. When the germ cells unite, a process known as fertilization begins. Fertilization of the ovum may also be achieved outside the uterus without sexual intercourse in a process called artificial insemination. Childbirth will follow a typical gestation period of 40 weeks. For the purpose of this concept analysis, reproduction is defined as *the total process by which organisms produce offspring*. In humans the concept is referred to as human reproduction.[1]

SCOPE AND CATEGORIES

The scope of this concept ranges from normal reproductive health—including contraception, unplanned pregnancy, and planned pregnancy—to problems associated with human reproduction.

Normal Reproductive Health
Contraception

Contraception is the intentional prevention of pregnancy during sexual intercourse.[2] The effectiveness of contraception varies and depends on both the method and user characteristics. For example, oral contraceptive pills (OCPs) are 99% effective in preventing pregnancy if taken as directed. Because ovulation is prevented, pregnancy cannot occur. To achieve this level of effectiveness, the user must remember to take the OCPs each day at the same time. Other methods of contraception include natural family planning, spermicides, injectable and implantable progestins, coitus interruptus, sterilization, and barrier methods such as male and female condoms, diaphragms, cervical caps, sponges, vaginal contraceptive rings, transdermal patches, and intrauterine devices.

Conception and Pregnancy

Pregnancy is a normal physiologic process that occurs without incident in the large majority of cases. The fertility rate varies by age and global location. It is important to note that the U.S. teen pregnancy rate of 72 pregnancies per 1000 women ages 15 to 19 (in 2006) continues to be one of the highest in the developed world; it is more than twice as high as rates in Canada (28 per 1000 women ages 15 to 19 in 2006) and Sweden (31 per 1000 women ages 15 to 19 in 2006). Each year, almost 750,000 U.S. women ages 15 to 19 become pregnant.[3] As stated earlier in this concept, pregnancy begins with the fertilization of an ovum by a sperm—also known as conception. A normal pregnancy without complications typically involves a 40-week gestation period and results in a live birth. Further discussion about the process of pregnancy will be detailed later in this concept.

Pregnancy is usually a planned and/or expected event among couples who engage in consensual intercourse without contraceptive measures. Unplanned pregnancy occurs when contraceptive efforts fail, when consensual sexual intercourse occurs without contraceptive measures and with no specific intent to create a pregnancy, when couples engage in sexual intercourse and lack education regarding conception and pregnancy, and when intercourse is not consensual.

Problems Associated with Reproduction

There are several categories of problems associated with reproduction, including conception challenges and problems or complications maintaining or carrying a pregnancy through full-term birth.

Infertility

There are a number of problems that lead to infertility, and contributing factors can originate in both males and females. These include genetic problems (such as *Turner's syndrome* or *Klinefelter's syndrome*). Ovarian factors affecting female fertility include developmental anomalies, primary or secondary anovulation, pituitary or hypothalamic hormone disorder, adrenal gland disorder, congenital adrenal hyperplasia, disruption of hypothalamic-pituitary-ovarian axis, amenorrhea after discontinuing oral contraceptive pills, premature ovarian failure, and increased prolactin levels. Uterine, tubal, and peritoneal factors affecting female fertility include developmental anomalies, reduced tubal motility, tubal inflammation, tubal adhesions, endometrial and myometrial tumors, uterine adhesions, endometriosis, chronic cervicitis, and inadequate cervical mucus. Other factors affecting female fertility include nutritional deficiencies such as anemia, obesity, thyroid dysfunction, and idiopathic conditions.[4]

Structural or hormonal disorders affecting male fertility include undescended testes, hypospadias, varicocele, obstructive lesions of the vas deferens or epididymis, low testosterone levels, hypopituitarism, endocrine disorders, testicular damage caused by mumps, or retrograde ejaculation. Other factors affecting male fertility include sexually transmitted infections; exposure to environmental hazards such as radiation or toxic substances; exposure of the scrotum to high temperatures; nutritional deficiencies; obesity; presence of antisperm antibodies; substance abuse; changes in sperm caused by cigarette smoking, heroin, marijuana, amyl nitrate, butyl nitrate, ethyl chloride, or methaqualone; decrease in libido attributable to heroin, methadone, selective serotonin reuptake inhibitors, or barbiturates; or impotence caused by alcohol, antihypertensive medications, and idiopathic conditions.[4] Patients with infertility are usually referred to a reproductive endocrinologist or obstetrician who specializes in infertility.

Maintaining a Pregnancy

There are a multitude of reproduction problems characterized by failure to maintain a pregnancy. These problems are related to maternal/fetal complications and are categorized by trimester. First trimester complications may include hyperemesis gravidarum, maternal/fetal infections such as rubella or toxoplasmosis, ectopic pregnancy, trauma, or spontaneous abortion (miscarriage). Spontaneous abortion in the first trimester usually results from chromosomal abnormalities.

Complications of pregnancy that become evident during the second and third trimesters include fetal congenital and chromosomal anomalies, maternal systemic conditions (such as gestational diabetes, gestational hypertension), and infections. Many other complications can occur later in pregnancy such as preterm labor, premature rupture of the membranes, placenta previa, abruptio placentae, trauma, fetal distress, and intrauterine fetal death.[5] Patients experiencing problems maintaining a pregnancy are usually referred to a perinatologist or maternal fetal medicine specialist.

RISK FACTORS

Populations at Risk

Human reproduction is inefficient with as many as 30% of pregnancies resulting in spontaneous losses.[6] In spite of predictions to reach a human population of 7 billion in 2011 and 9 billion by 2050, 15% of couples worldwide are childless because of infertility.[6,7] Risk factors affecting successful human reproduction and fertility transcend all races and nations, with third-world developing countries largely being affected the greatest because of poverty. About 97% of the global growth in the next 40 years will be in Asia, Africa, Latin America, and the Caribbean. The high fertility rates in the developing world will fuel the majority of reproductive growth, especially in Africa where women give birth six or seven times, as compared to two times in the United States and one or two times in Canada. Projections for the most populous nation in 2050 will be India at 1.7 billion, overtaking China, which is forecast to reach 1.4 billion. The United States is anticipated to reach a population of 439 million.[8]

The adolescent population worldwide is a reproductive high-risk group. Women younger than 15 years have a 60% higher death rate than those older than 20 years.[9] Adolescent pregnancy concerns and complications include impaired nutrition, anemia, infections, depression, social isolation, preeclampsia, protracted labor, cephalopelvic disproportion, premature delivery, and cesarean section.[10] The impact on the woman is lifelong and includes the risks of higher dropout rates, completing school later or not at all; lower income; and dependence on government assistance and living in poverty.

The teen birth rate in the United States is at the lowest level in 70 years but higher than many other developed countries.[11] There are differences between ethnicities with the 2009 birth rate for U.S. Hispanics at 70:1000; Blacks 50:1000; and Whites 26:1000. Western Europe and other countries are considerably lower. In the United Kingdom the teen birth rate is approximately 24:1000; Ireland 16:1000; Canada 13:1000; Sweden 8:1000; France 7:1000; Italy and Japan 5:1000; and the Netherlands 4:1000. The disparity has been in existence for decades and may be due to differences in approaches to birth control.[11]

Individual Risk Factors

There are numerous risk factors for women and men affecting reproductive health and pregnancy outcomes. These can be categorized into biophysical, psychosocial, sociodemographic, and environmental factors. Some of the risk factors for human reproduction fit into multiple categories.[9]

Biophysical Factors

Genetic concerns encompass defective genes, inherited disorders, chromosome anomalies, multiple gestation, large fetal size, and ABO incompatibilities. Nutritional concerns include malnutrition, fad diets, young age, inadequate or excessive weight gain, and anemia. Medical and obstetric disorders encompass complications of past or current pregnancies, obstetric illnesses, and previous pregnancy losses.[9,10]

Changes in fertility and sexual functioning do occur in males as they grow older. There is no maximum age at which a man cannot father a child, as evidenced by men in their sixties or older conceiving with younger women. With age, male testes become smaller and softer. Sperm shape, quality, quantity, and motility decline. There is also an increased risk of genetic defects in the sperm.[12]

Psychosocial Factors

Psychosocial factors include smoking, excessive caffeine intake, alcohol and drug abuse, psychologic status including impaired mental health, addictive lifestyles, spousal abuse, and noncompliance with cultural norms.[9,10]

Sociodemographic Factors

Sociodemographic factors include low income, inadequate prenatal care, age at both ends of the reproductive years (<16 and >35 years), parity, marital status, geographic location (urban versus rural), and ethnicity.[10,13] It is beyond the scope of this concept analysis to discuss every ethnic group worldwide. However, there are a disproportionate number of non-White women who die of pregnancy-related causes annually compared to Caucasian women (a 3:1 ratio). African-American newborns have the highest rate of prematurity, low birth weight, and infant mortality.[9]

Environmental Factors

Environmental factors affecting reproductive health and pregnancy outcomes include industrial pollution, tobacco, radiation, chemical exposure, bacterial and viral infections, drugs (over-the-counter [OTC], therapeutic, and illicit), and stress.[9,10]

PHYSIOLOGIC PROCESSES AND CONSEQUENCES

Expected Physiologic Process of Pregnancy

In order for normal human reproduction to occur, there are several complex developmental and physiologic events that must occur sequentially. A new individual begins with a sperm from a male and an oocyte from a female. The sperm and oocytes are produced in the reproductive system and are called gametes. They provide a mechanism that mixes genetic material from past generations to form a new individual. The sequential process of human reproduction includes gametogenesis, ovulation, fertilization, cleavage, implantation, and embryo and fetus.[14,15]

Gametogenesis

The formation and development of germ cells is called gametogenesis.[9] Gametogenesis begins in utero at 5 weeks' gestation when germ cells migrate to the gonadal ridge from the yolk sac. The gamete has a diploid number of 46 chromosomes. For survival, the number of chromosomes must remain constant. A specialized form of cell division called meiosis produces cells with a haploid number of 23 chromosomes. Two sequential meiotic cell divisions occur during gametogenesis. Homologous chromosomes pair during prophase and separate during anaphase. The first meiotic division is a reduction division in which each new cell forms a secondary oocyte or spermatocyte retaining the haploid number of chromosomes. In the second meiotic division, each chromosome divides to form two chromatids that are drawn to a different pole of the cell. The daughter cells that are produced contain a haploid number of chromosomes representative of each pair.[15]

The process of egg formation (ovum) begins during fetal life in a female and is known as oogenesis. The ovaries at birth contain all the cells that may undergo meiosis during a woman's reproductive stage of life. Only 400 to 500 ova out of 2 million oocytes will mature during a woman's reproductive years. Primary oocytes begin their first meiotic division before birth but remain suspended in prophase until puberty. At puberty, monthly cycles begin and usually one oocyte matures and completes the first meiotic division. The second meiotic division begins at ovulation but progresses only to metaphase when division is arrested. If the zona pellucida (inner layer) is penetrated by a sperm, the second meiotic division is completed.[15]

Ovulation

The results of a series of events occurring in the ovary cause an expulsion of the oocyte from the ovarian follicle known as ovulation. The ovarian cycle is driven by multiple important hormones: (1) gonadotropic hormone, (2) follicle-stimulating hormone (FSH), and (3) luteinizing hormone (LH). The cilia in the tubes are stimulated by high (4) estrogen levels, which propel the ovum toward the uterus. The zona pellucida (inner layer) and corona radiata (outer layer) form protective layers around the ovum. If an ovum is not fertilized within 24 hours of ovulation by a sperm, it is usually reabsorbed in a woman's body.[15]

Fertilization

With the process of fertilization, embryonic development begins. Fertilization usually occurs in the lower third of the fallopian tube (Figure 18-1). A sperm penetrates the

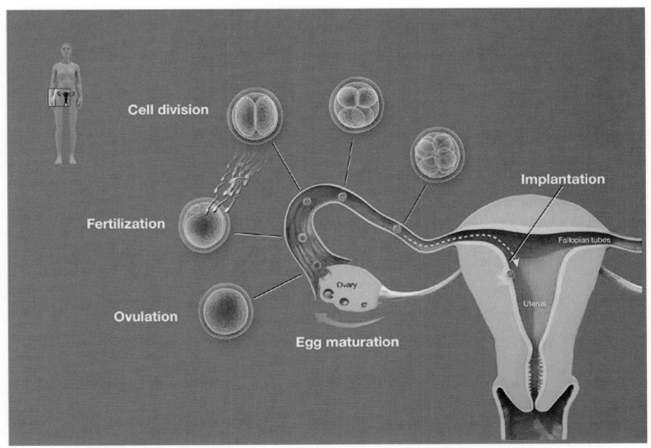

FIGURE 18-1 Human Fertilization. (From Nobel Committee for Physiology or Medicine: *Fertilization process in humans,* 2010. Accessed at http://nobelprize.org/nobel_prizes/medicine/laureates/2010/adv.pdf.)

ovum membrane and the sperm and ovum are enclosed in a process called the cortical reaction. The ovum nucleus becomes the female pronucleus and the second meiotic division is completed. The head of the sperm enlarges to form the male pronucleus and the tail degenerates. Fertilization results in a new cell called the zygote, which bears the diploid number of chromosomes. One half of the zygote genetic material was obtained from the maternal gamete and one half was obtained from the paternal gamete.[15]

Remember that the primary spermatocyte contained two sex chromosomes, one X and one Y; the primary oocyte contained two sex chromosomes, both X chromosomes. During the first reduction division, two secondary spermatocytes were produced—one X and one Y, establishing X and Y cell lines. The X-bearing cell line was established during oogenesis. Female gametes will all be X bearing and male gametes will be either X or Y bearing. A female develops through the fertilization of the ovum by an X-bearing sperm, producing an XX zygote; a male is produced through the fertilization of a Y-bearing sperm, producing an XY zygote. Therefore at fertilization, chromosomal gender is established.[9]

Cleavage

With the zygote enclosed in the zona pellucida, cleavage occurs in the fallopian tube. Although there is an increase in the number of cells, there is no increase in mass. Approximately 30 hours after fertilization, the zygote divides and two blastomeres are produced. The conceptus journeys down the reproductive tract while rapidly dividing. About 3 days after fertilization, a cell mass of 12 to 16 blastomeres known as the morula enters the woman's uterus.[15]

Implantation

A cavity is formed within the morula 4 days after fertilization. It becomes a blastocyst and floats freely within the uterus for 2 days. Spaces form between the central cells of the morula and fluid passes through the zona, collecting in these spaces. The cells then separate into an outer layer know as a trophoblast and an inner layer known as an embryoblast. The blastocyst receives nourishment from the endometrial glands in the uterus including carbohydrates, pyrimidines, purines, and amino acids by active and passive transport. While the blastocyst implants into the endometrium at 6 days following fertilization, the zona pellucida lyses and degenerates (Figure 18-2). By 9.5 days following ovulation, the blastocyst

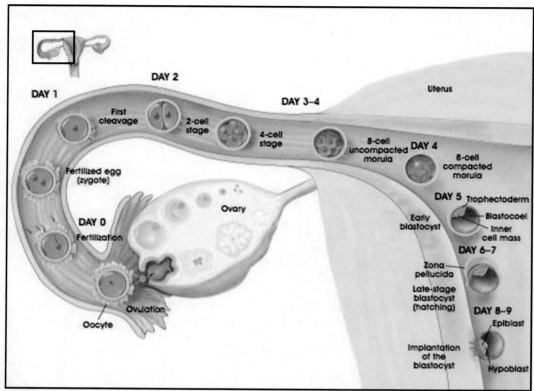

FIGURE 18-2 Blastocyst Implantation. (From National Institutes of Health: *Blastocyst implantation picture, 2010.* Accessed Nov 15, 2010, from www.stemcells.nih.gov.)

is completely imbedded into the decidua. The idea that the human implantation window is narrow has been challenged. Evidence obtained from in vitro fertilization programs suggests that the window for implantation may be 2 or even 3 days later than expected but the issue is still being studied.[15]

Embryo and Fetus

Stages of development include ovum, embryonic, and fetal. The beginning of the fourth week to the end of the eighth week comprise the embryonic period. Teratogenicity is a major concern because all external and internal structures are developing in the embryonic period. A pregnant woman should avoid exposure to all potential toxins during pregnancy especially alcohol, tobacco, radiation, and infections during embryonic development. At the end of this period, the embryo has human features. The fetal period follows from the ninth week until birth. The normal human fetus grows about 1.5% per day. Pregnancy normally lasts 9 calendar months, 280 days, 40 weeks, or 10 lunar months. Conception normally occurs 2 weeks after the first day of the last menstrual period (LMP); therefore the length of the pregnancy is computed from the first day of the LMP.[9] The process of human development is presented in Figure 18-3.

Consequences

The majority of the risk factors affecting reproductive health have been discussed in the previous sections. The physiologic processes affecting fertility in the female are often caused by damage to the fallopian tubes, which obstructs potential contact between the egg and sperm. Male infertility is often caused by impaired sperm quality, quantity, and motility. The inability to conceive a child is a reproductive dilemma that affects more than 15% of all couples worldwide.

ASSESSMENT

The assessment of human reproduction involves history, examination, and diagnostic testing. Nurses should have a basic understanding of the elements of an assessment; they should also be able to recognize abnormal findings and understand common diagnostic tests related to normal reproduction.

History

Elements of a history that reflect reproductive health include the following: normal sexual history; absence of previous or current neoplasms, polyps, or fibroid tumors; absence of alterations in pelvic support, including uterine displacement, uterine prolapse, cystocele, or rectocele; absence of urinary incontinence or genital fistulas; normal Pap history; and normal menstrual history. Additional pertinent history includes rubella and hepatitis B immune status, mental health, dietary history (with normal calcium and folic acid intake), absence of eating disorders,

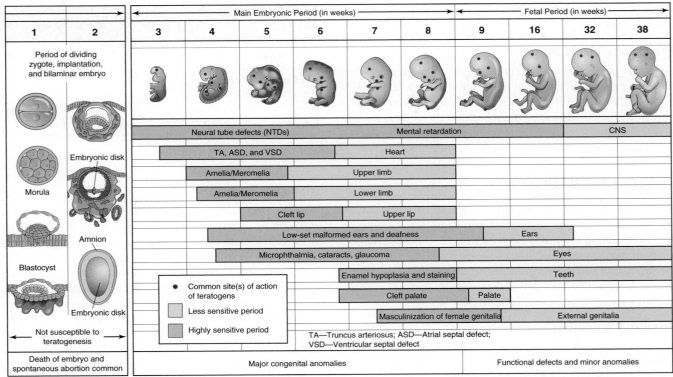

Main Embryonic Period (in weeks) — Fetal Period (in weeks)

Period of dividing zygote, implantation, and bilaminar embryo

Morula
Embryonic disk
Amnion
Blastocyst
Embryonic disk

Not susceptible to teratogenesis

Death of embryo and spontaneous abortion common

Neural tube defects (NTDs) — Mental retardation — CNS

TA, ASD, and VSD — Heart

Amelia/Meromelia — Upper limb

Amelia/Meromelia — Lower limb

Cleft lip — Upper lip

Low-set malformed ears and deafness — Ears

Microphthalmia, cataracts, glaucoma — Eyes

Enamel hypoplasia and staining — Teeth

Cleft palate — Palate

Masculinization of female genitalia — External genitalia

• Common site(s) of action of teratogens
☐ Less sensitive period
☐ Highly sensitive period

TA—Truncus arteriosus; ASD—Atrial septal defect;
VSD—Ventricular septal defect

Major congenital anomalies — Functional defects and minor anomalies

FIGURE 18-3 Critical Periods in Human Development. (From Lowdermilk DL, Perry SE, Cashion K, et al, editors: *Maternity & women's health care,* ed 10, p 276, St Louis, 2011 Elsevier/Mosby.)

limited alcohol and caffeine intake, negative illicit drug use, being within ideal child-bearing age, and no known genetic or inherited familial disorders. Positive findings that are not expected would alert the nurse that additional testing, screening, or monitoring may be needed. If pregnant, changes may include amenorrhea, fatigue, nausea, and vomiting for 4 to 12 weeks due to increasing levels of human chorionic gonadotropin (hCG). Increased levels of estrogen and progesterone can cause breast enlargement, fullness, tenderness, and heightened sensitivity, as well as increased urinary frequency.

Examination

Common elements of a physical exam history that reflect reproductive health include the following: normal temperature, pulse rate, respiratory rate, and blood pressure; weight appropriate for height; benign physical findings, especially in the heart, lungs, breasts, abdomen, pelvis, adnexa, and genitourinary, rectal, and lymph systems.

Changes observed by the woman's health care provider include softening and compression of the lower uterine segment (Hegar's sign), softening of the cervical tip (Goodell's sign), positive urine or serum pregnancy test after 4 weeks, visualization of the fetus by real-time ultrasound at 5 weeks, a violet blue vaginal mucosa and cervix at 6 weeks (Chadwick's sign), fetal heart tones at 6 weeks by ultrasound, fetal heart tones at 8 weeks by Doppler, Braxton Hicks contractions starting at 16 weeks, passive movements of the fetus

at 16 weeks (ballottement), and palpable fetal movements at 19 weeks.

Diagnostic Tests

Some of the routine laboratory testing that may be done prenatally includes the following: urine or serum pregnancy test, complete blood count (CBC), blood type and Rh factor, rubella titer, tuberculosis (TB) skin test, urinalysis (UA), urine culture, renal function test, Pap smear, glucose tolerance test, and tests for *Neisseria gonorrhoeae, Chlamydia,* hepatitis B, human papillomavirus (HPV), group B *Streptococcus,* rapid plasma reagin, and HIV.

Depending on the woman and her fetus, more monitoring or testing may be needed. A maternal assay to detect trisomy 21 (Down syndrome) is available from 11 to 14 weeks' gestation. Measurement of level of maternal serum alpha-fetoprotein (MSAFP) may be offered to detect neural tube defects from 14 to 34 weeks' gestation. Maternal level of alpha-fetoprotein usually correlates with week of gestation. Elevated AFP levels have been associated with neural tube defects.

Obtaining amniotic fluid (amniocentesis) to examine fetal cells for genetic disorders, neural tube defects, fetal hemolytic disease, or fetal lung maturity may be needed. If the testing reveals abnormal or positive findings, treatment and further monitoring may be necessary to ensure the health of the woman and her fetus. Perinatologists and maternal fetal medicine specialists may be consulted for assistance with managing high-risk pregnancies through tertiary centers.

Pregnancy Monitoring

During the first and second trimesters, the woman is usually seen once a month. The third trimester starting at 28 weeks begins with visits every 2 weeks. At 36 weeks, the visits are weekly until birth. The individual needs of the child-bearing family are considered and the pregnant woman may need less or more frequent visits depending on her health status.[10,11]

CLINICAL MANAGEMENT

The health management related to reproduction includes utilizing interventions to prevent problems and optimize health, screening for problems, and providing collaborative interventions if problems arise. The levels of care related to the concept of human reproductive health are discussed next; for the pregnant female, prenatal care is the cornerstone to nursing care.

Primary Prevention

Primary prevention refers to health promotion activities that further health and well-being.[16] An example of primary prevention would be teaching a group of high school students about reproductive health. Topics to discuss may include abstinence; the importance of safe sex; contraceptive options; tobacco, alcohol, and drug cessation; avoidance of environmental toxins; folic acid supplementation; and the need for preconception counseling and prenatal care throughout pregnancy.[10]

Nurses should be instrumental in providing anticipatory guidance to adolescents by providing instruction in human sexuality and maternal and newborn care, offering parenting classes, and promoting healthy lifestyles through education about proper nutrition and exercise. Education provided during teachable moments—at the right place and time—can change the course of a woman's life.

Secondary Prevention (Screening)

Secondary prevention refers to early detection of disease and disease sequelae associated with reproduction.[16] An example of secondary prevention relating to reproductive health would be continuing prenatal care in the second trimester of pregnancy. The purpose of prenatal care would be to determine the gestational age of the fetus, identify risk for and minimize reproductive complications, define the health status of the fetus and the mother, provide education and counseling, and perform the normal screening done at prenatal clinic visits.[10] Screening includes CBC, blood type and Rh, rubella titer, TB skin test, UA, urine culture, renal function test, Pap smear, glucose tolerance test, and tests for *Neisseria gonorroheae*, *Chlamydia*, HPV, rapid plasma reagin and HIV.

Collaborative Interventions

This level of prevention focuses on the management of problems; it refers to assessing, treating, and minimizing illness as a result of disease.[16]

CLINICAL NURSING SKILLS FOR REPRODUCTION

- Assessment
- Prenatal care
- Fetal monitoring
- Breastfeeding
- Contraception education
- Medication administration

High Risk Pregnancy

Women experiencing a high-risk pregnancy are often referred to a perinatologist. Factors related to high risk child-bearing are categorized as biophysical, psychosocial, sociodemographic, and environmental. *Biophysical factors* include genetics, nutritional status, and obstetric-related illnesses. *Psychosocial factors* include effects of nicotine, caffeine, alcohol, and drugs on the developing fetus and maternal psychologic status. *Sociodemographic factors* include low income, lack of prenatal care, pregnant adolescents or older mothers, parity, marital status, residence, and ethnicity. *Environmental factors* related to high-risk pregnancy may include infections, radiation exposure, chemical exposures such as lead or mercury, therapeutic and/or illicit drugs, cigarette smoke, industrial pollutants, poor diet, and stress.

Collaborative interventions for the management of high risk pregnancy include ongoing assessment of maternal and fetal well-being that includes maternal weight, blood pressure, and presence of protein in the urine. Ongoing fetal assessment may include ultrasound to assess fetal growth and fetal monitoring for heart rate.

Assisted Reproductive Technologies

The inability to conceive a child is a reproductive dilemma that affects more than 15% of all couples worldwide. Couples who are unable to conceive naturally may consult specialists and seek assisted reproductive technology (ART) procedures such as in vitro fertilization–embryo transfer (IVF-ET), gamete intrafallopian transfer (GIFT), zygote intrafallopian transfer (ZIFT), therapeutic donor insemination (TDI), or intracytoplasmic sperm injection (ICSI).[9]

Abortion

Abortion is termination of pregnancy before 20 weeks' gestation. Indications may include (1) a woman's request, (2) genetic disorders of a fetus, (3) incest or rape, and (4) preserving the health of a woman. The most common planned clinic abortion procedure is called vacuum aspiration. It is used up to 16 weeks after a woman's last menstrual period. Another type of abortion procedure performed in a hospital is called dilation, curettage, and evacuation. This is usually performed later than 16 weeks after a woman's last menstrual period.[17]

MODEL CASE

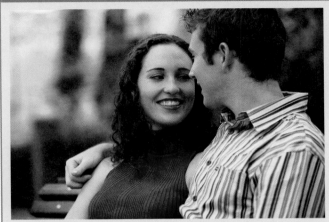

Katherine Cordova is a 28-year-old female, gravida 0, para 0, who presents with her male partner to the community women's clinic for a preconceptional counseling appointment. Katherine received an email from her health insurer about a new program offered at the clinic, designed to guide health promotion and disease prevention in support of *Healthy People 2020* initiatives.[21] The components of the program address preconception education, risk assessment, and intervention in order to improve maternal, infant, and child health.[18]

The couple has been together for 2 years and is contemplating starting a family. Both Katherine and her partner are social drinkers and smoke cigarettes. They are weight appropriate for height, exercise three times a week, and do not use drugs or take medications. Katherine and her partner are advised to stop all alcohol and tobacco use. She stopped her birth control pills the month before her appointment at the woman's clinic.

Katherine is prescribed prenatal vitamins that include folic acid 400 micrograms daily. They are counseled to continue exercising and structure their diets around fruits, green leafy vegetables, and whole grains. A risk factor assessment including rubella and hepatitis B immune status is positive for immunization. There is no past history of herbal or nonprescription drug use, current or chronic illnesses. Katherine and her partner are both college educated, employed full time, have health insurance, and are homeowners. There are no apparent financial concerns. There are no known environmental home or workplace safety concerns. They have supportive, extended families nearby and there is no history of domestic violence.

Two months after the couple attended their preconception counseling appointment, Katherine becomes pregnant. The couple has stopped drinking alcohol and smoking cigarettes, and also has avoided exposure to secondhand smoke. Katherine calls the clinic to schedule her first prenatal appointment.

Case Analysis

This case study illustrates an example of a visionary couple who seek anticipatory guidance to improve reproductive health and pregnancy outcomes before starting a family. They are counseled on primary prevention measures to reduce problems associated with conception and pregnancy, and Katherine is taking measures to access prenatal care throughout her pregnancy.

INTERRELATED CONCEPTS

Figure 18-4 shows the interrelationships of major concepts that influence or are impacted by the process of human reproduction. Reproduction and **Sexuality** are obviously closely related. The effect of proper **Nutrition** and **Glucose regulation** on human reproduction and pregnancy outcomes has been prevalent in the literature. In the 1950s, studies concluded that prenatal folic acid supplementation prevented pregnancy-induced megaloblastic anemia. In the 1990s, further research studies confirmed that periconceptual folic acid supplementation and folic acid food fortification prevented the occurrence of neural tube defects.[19]

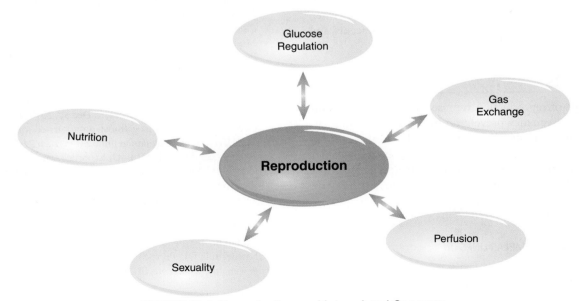

FIGURE 18-4 Reproduction and Interrelated Concepts.

BOX 18-1   EXEMPLARS OF REPRODUCTION

Normal Reproductive Health
Contraception
- Hormonal contraception
- Intrauterine device
- Cervical cap
- Contraceptive sponge
- Condoms and spermicides

Pregnancy
- Planned, uncomplicated pregnancies
- Unplanned, uncomplicated pregnancies

Problems Associated with Reproduction
Conception
- Infertility

Gestational Conditions
- Gestational diabetes
- Gestational hypertension
- Iron deficiency anemia

- Preeclampsia
- Eclampsia
- HELLP syndrome
- Hyperemesis gravidarum
- Miscarriage
- Premature dilation of the cervix
- Ectopic pregnancy
- Abruptio placentae
- DIC*
- Sexually transmitted infections
- Preterm labor
- Dystocia
- Prolapsed umbilical cord

Fetal Complications/Genetic Congenital Defects
- Neural tube defects (spina bifida)
- Intrauterine growth restriction
- Impaired fetal brain development
- Fetal alcohol syndrome
- Premature delivery

*DIC, Disseminated intravascular coagulation; HELLP syndrome, syndrome of hemolysis, elevated liver enzymes, and low platelet count.

Adequate **Perfusion** of maternal blood to the growing fetus is absolutely essential, as is adequate **Gas exchange.** A female who smokes tobacco may reduce oxygenation to her developing fetus and can lead to a number of complications. Smoking cessation has been recognized as the most important preventable risk factor for improving reproductive and pregnancy outcomes worldwide.[20]

Understanding the interrelationships of these major concepts helps nurses recognize risk factors and their potential effect on the human reproductive process and pregnancy outcomes. These are important steps in providing anticipatory guidance, clinical judgment, and screening when planning for reproductive health needs of adolescents and child-bearing families.

EXEMPLARS

The concept of reproduction represents many clinical situations, from pregnancy prevention to conception and pregnancy. A comprehensive discussion related to all these factors is beyond the scope of this concept, and is best left to other textbooks devoted to sexual and reproductive health. Box 18-1 presents common exemplars related to reproductive conditions seen in clinical practice.

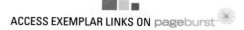

ACCESS EXEMPLAR LINKS ON pageburst

REFERENCES

1. *Pearson Education Dictionary, 2010:* Retrieved April 23, 2011, from www.ldoceonline.com/Biologytopic/reproduction.
2. Stewart F, Trussell J, Van Look P: Emergency contraception. In Hatcher R, Trussell J, Nelson A et al, editors: *Contraceptive technology,* New York, 2007, Ardent Media.
3. Kost K, Henshaw S, Carlin L: *U.S. teenage pregnancies, births and abortions: national and state trends and trends by race and ethnicity, 2010.* Retrieved May 31, 2011, from www.guttmacher.org/pubs/USTPtrends.pdf.
4. Gingrich PM: Infertility. In Lowdermilk DL, Perry SE, Cashion K, et al, editors: *Maternity & women's health care,* St Louis, 2012, Elsevier/Mosby.
5. Moore MC: Maternal and fetal nutrition. In Lowdermilk DL, Perry SE, Cashion K, et al, editors: *Maternity & women's health care,* St Louis, 2012, Mosby/Elsevier.
6. Dey SK: How we are born, *J Clin Invest* 120(4):952–955, 2010.
7. U.S. Census Bureau International Data Base: *World's 50 most populous countries: 2010.* Accessed Dec 31, 2010, at www.infoplease.com/world/statistics/most-populous-countries.html.
8. CNN Tech: *World population projected to reach 7 billion in 2011* 2009. Accessed Dec 31, 2010, at http://articles.cnn.com/2009-08-12/tech/world.population_1_fertility-rates-world-population-data-sheet-population-reference-bureau?_s=PM TECH.
9. Perry SE: Conception and fetal development. In Lowdermilk DL, Perry SE, Cashion K, et al, editors: *Maternity & women's health care,* St Louis, 2012, Mosby/Elsevier.
10. Lamarche Zdanuk J: Assessment and health promotion. In Lowdermilk DL, Perry SE, Cashion K, et al, editors: *Maternity & women's health care,* St Louis, 2011, Mosby/Elsevier.

11. Strobbe M: *U.S. teen birth rate still far higher than W. Europe, Washington Post.* Accessed Dec 31, 2010, at www.washingtonpost.com/wp-dyn/content/article/2010/12/30/AR2010123002716_pf.html.

12. American Society for Reproductive Medicine: *Age and fertility, a guide for patients, 2003.* Accessed Dec 1, 2010, at www.reproductivefacts.org/uploadedFiles/ASRM_Content/Resources/Patient_Resources/Fact_Sheets_and_Info_Booklets/agefertility.pdf.

13. Gillem-Goldstein J: Methods for assessment for pregnancy at risk. In DeCherney A, Nathan L, editors: *Current obstetric and gynecologic diagnosis and treatment*, New York, 2003, Lange Medical Books/McGraw-Hill.

14. Lewis R: *Human genetics: concepts and applications*, Boston, 2008, McGraw-Hill.

15. Reece EA, Hobbins JC: *Handbook of clinical obstetrics: the fetus and mother*, Malden, Mass, 2007, Blackwell.

16. Baldwin JH, O'Neil MC: Health promotion and wellness. In Saucier Lundy K, Janes S, editors: *Community health nursing, caring for the public's health*, Boston, 2009, Jones and Bartlett.

17. *In clinic abortion procedures, 2011.* Retrieved May 31, 2011, from www.plannedparenthood.org/health-topics/abortion/in-clinic-abortion-procedures-4359.asp.

18. *Healthy People 2020: Healthy people in healthy communities, 2010.* Accessed Dec 31, 2010, at www.healthypeople.gov.

19. Tsunenobu T, Picciano MF: Folate and human reproduction, *Am J Clin Nutr* 83(5):993–1016, 2006.

20. Cnattingius S: The epidemiology of smoking during pregnancy: smoking prevalence, maternal characteristics, and pregnancy outcomes, *Nicotine Tob Res* 6(suppl 2):S125–S140, 2004. Retrieved Dec 15, 2010, from doi: 10.1080/14622200410001669187.

Sexuality

Barbara H.M. Pascoe

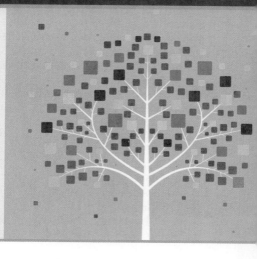

Perhaps the most difficult of the health and illness concepts to describe is human sexuality. Nurses are likely to find discussion related to estimated date of delivery or menstrual irregularities very straightforward; however, when the conversation turns to one regarding sexual health, nurses may find themselves at a loss. To foster optimal sexual health, it is essential that nurses, as well as other health care professionals, become cognizant of sexual health implications and develop a comfort level in evaluating, educating, and providing treatment related to sexuality. Ideally, this work is performed within the context of normal growth and development and well-being across the lifespan. As nurses, it is important to take into account individual behaviors that may increase risk and consider the impact of illness or disability on sexual health. Professionals working in health care settings must develop an understanding of the sexual behaviors of the populations they serve.[1]

DEFINITION(S)

For the purposes of this concept analysis, the World Health Organization (WHO) definition of sexuality is used: "*…a state of physical, emotional, mental and social well-being related to sexuality; it is not merely the absence of disease, dysfunction or infirmity. Sexual health requires a positive and respectful approach to sexuality and sexual responses, as well as the possibility of having pleasurable and safe sexual experiences, free of coercion, discrimination and violence.*"[2] To fully understand the broader concept of sexuality, it is also necessary to become familiar with the terms used when discussing this topic. These include *sex, sexual acts, sexual and gender identity,* and *sexual orientation and behavior* (Box 19-1). In 2001 the Surgeon General of the United States issued a "Call to Action" to promote sexual health and responsible sexual behavior. This document addressed the significant public health challenges related to sexual behavior in America and proposed strategies for initiating dialogue on issues of sexuality and sexual health.[3] Since that time, sexual health has emerged as a concept that addresses clinical issues as diverse

as teen pregnancy, sexual dysfunction (SD), and sexually transmitted infections (STIs).[4]

As we explore the historical context of sexuality in America, we can credit Alfred Kinsey and his colleagues at Indiana University for the first qualitative research on human sexual behavior.[5] Kinsey's work was born from the frustration of working with college students who sought answers to questions about their own sexual behavior; but at the time, no one professional was able to provide answers. In the 1940s and 1950s it was extremely difficult for any adult to glean factual information regarding sexuality without the shroud of moral, philosophic, or social interpretation.[5] In his research, Kinsey conducted confidential interviews with more than 20,000 subjects, followed by the publication of reports related to human male and female sexual behavior.[6,7] This groundbreaking work opened the door for other researchers to further explore human sexuality.

From 1957 through the 1990s, William Masters and Virginia Johnson pioneered their study of the human sexual response.[8] Unlike Kinsey, whose work was based upon interviews only, Masters and Johnson carried the research related to human sexuality one step further, by recording biological data related directly to the human sexual response during intercourse and self-stimulation. This work resulted in the development of the four-stage model of the *human sexual response cycle.*[8] Masters and Johnson utilized this model to develop a treatment program for a variety of sexual dysfunctions (i.e., premature ejaculation, impotence, vaginismus).[9]

In spite of the decades-long quest for knowledge and understanding, it appears there is still much to learn about human sexuality. Over the past 20 years we have seen unparalleled societal changes that alter the landscape of sexual health. These changes include access to the Internet for sexual information, the development of pharmaceuticals to treat erectile dysfunction, changes in behavior that have increased the transmission of herpetic viruses, and the launch of a vaccine to treat cancers associated with these viruses.[4] In 2010, the Center for Sexual Health Promotion conducted the National Survey of Sexual Health and Behavior (NSSHB) among a

> ### BOX 19-1 DEFINITIONS RELATED TO THE CONCEPT OF SEXUALITY
>
> - **Sex:** One of four primary drives that also includes thirst, hunger, and avoidance of pain.
> - **Sexual Acts:** Occur when behaviors include genitalia and erogenous zones.
> - **Sexuality:** Is the result of biological, psychologic, social, and experiential factors that mold an individual's sexual development, self-concept, body image, and behavior. Sexuality depends on four interrelated psychosexual factors.
>   1. **Sexual Identity:** Whether one is male or female based on biological sexual characteristics
>   2. **Gender Identity:** How one views one's gender as masculine or feminine, socially derived from experiences with the family, friends, and society
>   3. **Sexual Orientation:** How one views one's self in terms of being emotionally, romantically, sexually, or affectionately attracted to an individual of a particular gender
>   4. **Sexual Behavior:** How one responds to sexual impulses and desires

From Shives L: Basic concepts of psychiatric mental health nursing, Philadelphia, 2008, p 466, Wolters Kluwer/Lippincott Williams & Wilkins.

sample of almost 6000 participants. The results of this work will enable nursing, medical, and public health professionals to provide meaningful sexual health education, offer appropriate treatment and risk prevention options, and spearhead public health initiatives related to contemporary sexuality.[4]

SCOPE AND CATEGORIES

The concept of sexuality ranges in scope from positive sexual identity and function to dysfunction or impairment. The concept categories of sexuality encompass the lifespan of all human beings.

Infancy and Childhood

We evidence the first glimmer of the development of sexual identity as we watch excited new parents dress their baby daughters in pink and their infant sons in blue. The combination of *biological, societal, cultural,* and *familial* influences interact to form a child's developing sexuality and gender expectations as shown in Figure 19-1.[10]

Adolescent Sexuality

It is not until a child approaches adolescence and develops secondary sex characteristics that issues may arise around a sense of gender identity and related concepts, and behaviors and attitudes about one's self and others in the context of the adolescent's society.[10] Although today's adolescents are being raised during a period of relative conservatism, the sexual

behavior of these teens continues to be a topic of significant importance to parents, schools, health care professionals, and public health officials.[11] Data from the most recent national survey of 14 to 17 year olds indicate that sexual behavior changes significantly during as little as a 1-year period during this timeframe.[11] By the age of 17, both males and females have achieved physical sexual maturity and partnered sexual behavior is reported in 49% of teen males and 40% of adolescent females.[11,12] Sexual challenges for adolescents can include unwanted pregnancy, sexually transmitted infections (STIs), and issues related to gender identity.[10]

Adult Female Sexuality

Societal change since the time of Kinsey's work had the most significant impact on female sexuality that has occurred in centuries. During the 1960s medical advances provided women (primarily married women) access to oral contraceptives and the subsequent reduction of unwanted pregnancy.[13] The women's rights, civil rights, and gay rights movements, in conjunction with the sexual revolution, finally allowed women many of the sexual freedoms long experienced only by men.[13] It was during the 1980s, amidst the emergence of the human immunodeficiency virus (HIV) epidemic, that U.S. health officials became concerned about how little was actually known regarding female sexuality. The National Health and Social Life Survey (NHSLS), conducted in 1992, released data confirming that the sexual behavior of women had changed markedly since the time of Kinsey, with increased dialogue regarding the full range of sexual behaviors—vaginal intercourse, oral sex, anal sex, and masturbation—as well as expanded opportunities for same-sex marriage and civil unions.[13] As expected, women between the ages of 18 and 29 report the highest frequency of partnered sexual activity, followed by women between the ages of 30 and 39 years.[13] Just over 50% of women between 18 and 49 years of age reported masturbating in the prior 90-day period.[13] Sexual behaviors of any cohort of women vary widely depending upon culture, religion, and personal differences. For many women, child-bearing age is a time when they first seek care related to their sexual needs (e.g., contraception, preconception care, screening, concerns regarding sexually transmitted diseases, or prenatal care).[11]

Much of the focus in the past had been on younger adults, although recent evidence has shown that more women may

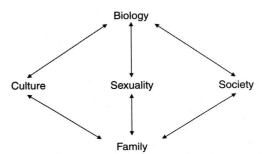

FIGURE 19-1 Factors Influencing the Development of Sexuality. (From Brown RT, Brown JD: *Primary care clinic office practice adolescent sexuality,* Vol 33, p 374, Philadelphia, 2006, Saunders/Elsevier.)

experience a greater proportion of their "sexual lives" after menopause.[13] The perimenopausal period is defined as that time in a woman's life that ultimately leads to the cessation of menses and ovulatory function.[12,14] This transition, approximately 4 years in length, is marked by menstrual irregularity accompanied by vasomotor symptoms.[14] Once a woman completes a consecutive period of 12 months without menses she is considered "menopausal."[14] Many women believe that these physiologic changes during the middle years contribute to decreased sexual interest; however, these commonly held beliefs are more closely related to cultural myths and negative societal messages.[12] Female sexuality at this age, a "multidimensional phenomenon," consists of not only sexual desire and response but also presentation and view of oneself as a woman.[14] Women who perceive themselves as being less attractive as they age find it more difficult to incorporate sexuality into their lifestyle.[12] There is a significant lack of research regarding the perimenopausal/menopausal period and the effect upon sexuality. Although sexual disturbances have been reported in 5% to 85% of women during this transition, this is a meaningless statistic because there is no consistent definition for sexual health during the climacteric.[14] Alterations in hormone levels, urogenital aging, and pain during intercourse, attributable to changes in the vaginal mucosa, may all contribute to decreased sexual activity during the menopausal transition.[14]

Adult Male Sexuality

Recent studies have shown that there are significant differences in how the adult male determines that he has experienced "good sex" compared to the adult female.[15] Data reveal that less than 30% of women are orgasmic at any sexual encounter, in contrast to 80% of men.[15] Oddly enough, reports of satisfaction were similar. Libido in adult women has long been considered to be less than that of men, necessitating a longer period of foreplay than required by the adult male.[15] The results from the NSSHB indicate that the age cohorts of sexually active men closely mirror those of women, with partnered sexual intercourse being the highest in the 20- to 30-year age group (80% of men).[16] Masturbation is a frequent and common practice among men, reported by 95.5% of adult males between the ages of 25 and 39 and 60% of men through the age of 59.[16] Only when health declines is there a drop in this activity. Anal intercourse with other men was the least commonly reported of all sexual activities.[16]

As men age, they take longer to achieve an erection and reach orgasm.[12] This naturally occurring process makes sexual activity difficult for many men and so frustrating for others that they lose interest in their partners entirely. Of particular concern is the decrease in condom use as men age, with less than 20% of men older than 50 years of age reporting condom use with sexual activity.[17] This is not necessarily the result of a lack of activity but, rather, ignorance and unawareness about the risk of contracting STIs.[17] Other poorly understood influences contribute to male sexuality and subsequent behavior, including cultural upbringing, societal factors, and personal beliefs.[18] Poor sexual performance (impotence) continues to be one of men's greatest concerns.[18] This may explain why fear of interference with sexual arousal has been cited as another reason for lack of condom use.[19] Herein lies an opportunity for the nurse to offer education regarding appropriate condom use and screening for STIs.

Elder Sexuality

As previously mentioned, sexual health is a basic human right important to all individuals, regardless of their age. Health care providers should become attentive to the sexual needs of older adults, which may be easier said than done. Even the latest of studies report that little is known about how older adults experience their sexual lives; however, we know that 20% to 30% of both women and men remain sexually active well into their eighties.[20] Scientific data confirm that as men and women age, hormone levels diminish, resulting in decreased libido and a decline in sexual capability.[15] Population-based surveys confirm that both advanced age and poor health have a negative effect on sexuality.[15,20]

Women are living longer than men and experience good health for a greater period of their golden years.[20] As a result they spend a larger portion of their lives as sexually active adults. Unfortunately, it is a reality that older women are less "pursued" and consequently have fewer opportunities to develop healthy sexual relationships.[12] The most commonly cited reasons for postmenopausal women to be sexually inactive are poor relationships, partner unavailability, or partner illness and incapacitation.[12,15,20] For many aging couples, having a positive and loving relationship may be more important than the sexual act itself.[15]

RISK FACTORS

It is important for the nurse to be aware that some groups of patients will have more problems related to the concept of sexual health than others.

Adolescents

Perhaps the most significant of these groups is teens, in particular adolescent girls, because of the risk for unplanned pregnancy. Worldwide, teen pregnancy rates are used as a measure of adolescent sexual and reproductive health.[21] The majority of teen pregnancies are unintended and reflect the extent to which adolescent girls have the capacity to control their sexual health.[21] In the United States alone, 1 million adolescent females (4 out of 10) become pregnant each year, resulting in approximately 450,000 births annually.[12] Pregnancy in the teenage girl under the age of 16 introduces a tremendous physical burden during an already stressful period of growth and development.[12] The adolescent parent usually lacks the financial resources to support a pregnancy and may or may not have their own parents' help, support, or involvement. A teenage mom may not have the emotional maturity to understand the importance of receiving consistent prenatal care or avoiding exposure to teratogens during her pregnancy.[12] Just as adolescent girls are at increased risk for unintended pregnancy, they are also vulnerable to contracting a variety of STIs. Teens who experience their first sexual encounter before the age of 13 years or have more than six partners are at increased risk for both pregnancy and infection.[10]

Minorities

Minority teens are the most vulnerable population for early child-bearing. In the 13- to 17-year-old age group, Hispanic and African-American girls experience double the rate of pregnancy than do Caucasian adolescents.[22] Unintended pregnancy is not the only sexual concern of minorities. Major disparities continue to exist between African-American and Hispanic individuals and their Caucasian counterparts for a variety of sexually transmitted diseases, in particular HIV (human immunodeficiency virus).[19,23] Sexual health researchers have found that the explanatory factors for these rates of infection are actually not related to race or ethnicity, but rather to social concerns such as poverty, racism, migration, and stigma.[23,24] These important data provide a baseline for nurses to develop appropriate sexual and other health care initiatives.

Intellectual and Developmental Disabilities (IDDs)

It may be difficult to argue that no population faces the sort of sexual (and reproductive) restraints as the disabled. Individuals with IDDs are entitled to move towards both sexual and social maturity in the same manner as the rest of the population.[25] Historically these patients were often institutionalized, sterilized, and portrayed as sexually threatening by their families, health care providers, and society in general.[25] At a time when these individuals have moved into mainstream society, it is important that they are able to learn about healthy sexuality and be given the opportunity to develop both friendships and appropriate relationships with the opposite gender.[25] If sexual health is not promoted within this population then unhealthy forms of sexuality and sexual abuse of these individuals are likely to occur.[25] Nurses should be educated to recognize such abuse and address sexual concerns with these patients and their families.

Newly Unpartnered

A rather unique population at increased risk for negative sequelae are those adults who have recently separated from their long-term partners because of death or divorce and are now exposed to an entirely new sexual paradigm. These adults may begin dating and suddenly have several new and unknown sexual partners.[12] Depending upon their age, HIV, AIDS (acquired immunodeficiency syndrome), and other STIs may not have been of concern when these adults were initially partnered. Although HIV/AIDS infections in the United States are now considered to be chronic conditions, all parties who have intercourse must be cognizant of their risk for exposure to this and other diseases and receive appropriate health education.[12]

Individual Risk Factors

Although sexual activity is considered a normative process, some individuals inadvertently place themselves at increased risk for sexual health problems. These individuals are primarily those who engage in sexual activity with multiple and casual partners and/or refrain from "safe sex" practices.[12] According to the most recent surveys these individuals are comprised of minorities, young people (in particular gay, lesbian, and bisexual youths), and men who have sex with men regardless of race.[10,19,24]

High-risk sexual behaviors that place African-American youths at risk include an increased likelihood that they will be sexually active (45.7%), more varied sexual experiences, and intercourse with greater than four sexual partners during their teen years.[26] Hispanic and Caucasian youths may have lower rates of risk because of lower levels of reported sexual activity (35.9% and 31.3%, respectively); however, they are less likely to use a condom than their African-American peers (53.5%, 56.8%, and 67.1%, respectively).[26] In comparison to their heterosexual counterparts, gay, lesbian, and bisexual youths have been found to engage in more high-risk sexual practices.[10] Young women who primarily have sex with women also report that they are likely to engage in sexual activity with men who are homosexual, bisexual, or injection drug users.[10] Adolescent boys who participate in sexual activity with bisexual men are at significantly increased risk for possible transmission of HIV and AIDS.[10] New cases of HIV diagnosis are increasing among men who have sex with men (particularly those of racial minorities) perhaps because of the "glamorization" of anal intercourse, misperceptions that partners are at low risk, and the belief that medical advances in the treatment of AIDS have eliminated the need for appropriate protection during sexual activity.[10,28]

Of secondary importance is the influence of nonsexual high-risk behavior such as the use of alcohol, marijuana, or other illicit substances. Prior research has shown that when these substances are ingested close to the time of sexual activity, the rate of sexual risk-taking increases.[27,28] The abuse of alcohol or drugs most often results in impaired judgment and consequently less thoughtfulness related to the sexual act.[12]

PHYSIOLOGIC PROCESSES AND CONSEQUENCES

The four-stage sexual response model, first proposed by Masters and Johnson,[8] presents the classic physiologic phases of sexual response for men and women. The four stages include excitement phase, plateau phase, orgasmic phase, and resolution phase; these stages are presented in Table 19-1. Although this model is useful for understanding sexual response from a physiologic perspective, there are other things to consider.

Positive Sexual Attitudes and Behaviors

How do we best define positive sexual attitudes and behaviors? This question has plagued many researchers and if glossy magazine covers are any indication, the general public as well. In the past clinical research has focused primarily on sexual psychopathologies and dysfunction.[29] Practitioners often equate positive sexual functioning with Masters and Johnson's sexual response cycle, rather than considering the psychologic and emotional components of what truly makes an optimal sexual encounter.[29] More recent research has provided nurses, physicians, and therapists with knowledge regarding the prominent components or building blocks of optimal sexuality.

The most predominant component is that of *being present*— in the moment and fully attentive.[29] Participants describe this as "utter immersion and intensely focused attention" where they are fully embodied in the experience and able to allow

TABLE 19-1	FOUR-STAGE MODEL OF THE HUMAN SEXUAL RESPONSE CYCLE	
REACTIONS COMMON TO BOTH GENDERS	**FEMALE REACTIONS**	**MALE REACTIONS**
Excitement Phase Heart rate and blood pressure increase. Nipples become erect. Myotonia begins.	Clitoris increases in diameter and swells. External genitalia become congested and darken. Vaginal lubrication occurs; upper two thirds of vagina lengthen and extend. Cervix and uterus pull upward. Breast size increases.	Erection of penis begins; penis increases in length and diameter. Scrotal skin becomes congested and thickens. Testes begin to increase in size and elevate toward body.
Plateau Phase Heart rate and blood pressure continue to increase. Respirations increase. Myotonia becomes pronounced; grimacing occurs.	Clitoral head retracts under clitoral hood. Lower one third of vagina becomes engorged. Skin color changes occur: red flush may be observed across breasts, abdomen, or other surfaces.	Head of penis may enlarge slightly. Scrotum continues to grow tense and thicken. Testes continue to elevate and enlarge. Preorgasmic emission of two or three drops of fluid appears on head of penis.
Orgasmic Phase Heart rate, blood pressure, and respiration increase to maximum levels. Involuntary muscle spasms occur. External rectal sphincter contracts.	Strong rhythmic contractions are felt in clitoris, vagina, and uterus. Sensations of warmth spread through pelvic area.	Testes elevate to maximum level. Point of "inevitability" occurs just before ejaculation and an awareness of fluid in urethra. Rhythmic contractions occur in penis. Ejaculation of semen occurs.
Resolution Phase Heart rate, blood pressure, and respirations return to normal. Nipple erection subsides. Myotonia subsides.	Engorgement in external genitalia and vagina resolves. Uterus descends to normal position. Cervix dips into seminal pool. Breast size decreases. Skin flush disappears.	Fifty percent of erection is lost immediately with ejaculation; penis gradually returns to normal size. Testes and scrotum return to normal size. Refractory period (time needed for erection to occur again) varies according to age and general physical condition.

From Lowdermilk DL, Perry SE, Cashion K, et al, editors: *Maternity & women's health care,* ed 10, St Louis, 2011, Mosby/Elsevier.

thinking to stop and arousal take over.[29] For most of the participants interviewed, being present was inextricably linked with a second component of *authenticity,* described as "feeling free to be themselves with their partner."[29] A third theme that emerged was that of *intense emotional connection,* described as heightened intimacy during the sexual encounter. Many couples felt that intimacy needed to be present both inside and outside of the bedroom, whereas others pointed out that "great sex" also occurred in new relationships, with friends or "play partners."[29] Another building block of optimal sexuality is *sexual and erotic intimacy,* described as a deep sense of caring for one another regardless of the length of the relationship.[29] Most of the surveyed participants identified excellent *communication* as crucial to the success of any sexual encounter.[29] This includes not only verbal communication but also empathy and making one's needs known through touch. Last, but certainly not the least important, ultimate sexual pleasure appears to include *transcendence,* a combination of heightened mental, emotional, physical, relational, and spiritual states of mind.[29] This picture of "great sex" that is painted by these six attributes is certainly different than that touted from the news-stands. These findings illustrate that optimal sexuality is not necessarily about technique or skill, but rather about attitude, positive behaviors, and healthy relationships.

Consequences

From both a physiologic and psychologic standpoint, it is important for nurses to understand the consequences of poor functioning of this concept. The former Surgeon General of the United States, M. J. Elders, reported that 30% of health care costs are directly related to sexuality.[1] Sex should be viewed as necessary for a "lifetime of pleasure" and not just for procreation once or twice in a lifetime. Let us now consider what happens to the human condition when sexual health is not present.

Gender Identity

As part of normal growth and development, all adolescents must work to understand both their identity and their sexuality.[10] Gender identity is defined as "a personal and culturally defined construct based upon one's perception of being male or female."[28] Perhaps the most complex task of adolescence is this formulation of a sexual identity. Transgender youths are those whose gender identity is in direct contrast to their biologic sexual assignment; for example, someone who has been born a female yet feels that she has a male gender identity.[28] In the past, one's sexual orientation was either heterosexual or homosexual; however, more recent studies suggest that gender identity development may occur along a continuum. Terminology such as *bisexual* or *questioning* may more accurately describe the journey that adolescents experience in order to determine their sexual orientation.[28] LGBTQ (lesbian, gay, bisexual, transgender, and questioning) youths face a more challenging period of development because they must reconcile themselves as having a "minority" sexual orientation.[10,28] Studies have shown that LGBTQ adolescents encounter health risks at a much higher rate than their heterosexual peer group.[10,28] These youths are more likely to engage in unsafe sexual practices and experience higher rates of mental health illness (anxiety, depression, adjustment disorders), and they are at an increased risk for both suicidal ideation and actual suicide attempts.[10,25,28] Researchers have speculated that the reasons for this are twofold: the added developmental task of not conforming and victimization by their peer group.[28]

Sexual Dysfunction

"What is sexual dysfunction (SD)?" This negative consequence of human sexuality is "any disturbance to the psycho-physiological changes that occur during *sexual response* or any changes in the level of *desire*."[30] Such changes to the sexual response cycle are likely to result in "marked distress and interpersonal difficulty."[30] It appears that SD is very common among the general population, with rates varying from 19% to 50%.[31] Upon further investigation, researchers suggest that this issue is more prevalent among women, with 40% to 45% of women reporting SD at some point in time, compared to 20% to 30% of men.[30,31] In women this is most often evidenced by either decreased (or absent) desire or the inability to reach orgasm.[30] To assist clinicians in both diagnosis and treatment, the American Psychological Association has developed categories to describe disorders related to each stage of the sexual response cycle. Sexual arousal in both men and women may be diminished by biological factors such as hormones or illness (e.g., hypertension, diabetes, or cancer); however, psychologic factors, such as anxiety, mood disorders, or stress, appear to play a more significant role in sexual health.[30-32] In many patients the best predictor of sexual health is emotional well-being as opposed to the impairment of the physiologic aspects of arousal.[30] Positive sexual functioning contributes to both a healthy sense of self and a general feeling of happiness.[18,29] When SD occurs, both men and women are at risk for developing anxiety, stress, depression, and avoidance of their normal patterns of sexual behavior. The quality of one's sex life remains a major quality of life indicator with a direct impact on one's interpersonal relationships.[29,31] Nurses must remain cognizant that sexual dysfunction, regardless of the cause, is likely to result in a number of negative consequences.[31]

ASSESSMENT

Despite the importance of sexual health and the high prevalence of sexual problems in the general population, questions related to sexual health are infrequently raised by clinicians during routine examinations.[33] Patients report a high level of embarrassment discussing such concerns with their health care providers, with only one in five self-reporting their sexual issues.[33] Nurses' attitudes do not differ in this respect. Recent studies indicate that nurses are hesitant to engage their patients in discussions related to sexual problems for a number of reasons: invasion of privacy, fear of creating increased anxiety, and a belief that sexuality is never as important as other immediate problems.[34] Within the hospital setting, 70% of nursing staff report that a heavy workload and lack of time prevent them from completing a thorough sexual assessment.[34] If the patient presents with an illness likely to impact sexual function (e.g., cancer of the breast, cervix, or prostate), then there is a greater chance that the nurse will include sexual health as part of the assessment.[35] Regardless of the practitioner's level of discomfort, a complete sexual assessment is essential in order to provide optimal nursing care across the lifespan.

History

Any health assessment, whether in the hospital or an outpatient setting, generally begins with an interview often referred to as the patient's history. This interview should always be conducted in a private and comfortable setting. The nurse will begin by introducing himself/herself and query the patient regarding how he/she would like to be addressed; for example, an 18 year old may prefer to be addressed in a different manner than a patient in their sixties. This is an ideal opportunity to evaluate the communication variations that occur while working with patients from different cultures. Questions should be posed in a nonjudgmental manner and the patient must be assured that all answers will be kept strictly confidential. Patients may be hesitant to ask questions regarding sexual functioning, for fear of appearing ignorant. The nurse's responsibility is to put the patient at ease, utilizing receptive body language and asking open-ended questions to garner information.

The history includes information from the following categories: biographic data, reason for seeking care, history of present illness, past health, family history, review of systems, and functional assessment.[12] It is during the review of systems that the nurse will inquire about sexual health and sexual activity. A careful sexual history should include questions related to usual sexual patterns, number of partners (both same sex and opposite sex), frequency of sexual activity, level of satisfaction, sexual knowledge, and any perceived problems.[12,36] Box 19-2 presents history information to include in a history to assess for high-risk behaviors. This is an ideal time for the nurse to encourage the patient to ask questions about sexuality or sexual functioning that may be causing distress.[36] If the patient is an adolescent, excuse the parent in order to allow the teen to discuss his or her sexual concerns without fear of repercussions. Adolescents may express concerns regarding their altered appearance, voice changes, and impulse control.[36] All patients should be screened for possible abuse. Questions to illicit this information might include asking whether the patient has ever been physically

BOX 19-2   ASSESSING STI AND HIV RISK BEHAVIORS

Sexual Risk
- Are you sexually active now?
- If no, have you had sex in the past?
- Have you ever had an oral, vaginal, or anal sexual experience with another person?
- With how many different people have you had a sexual experience? 1? 2? 3? 4 to 10? More than 10?
- Have your partners been men or women, or both?
- Have you ever thought that a sex partner put you at risk for AIDS* or an STI (IF drug user, bisexual)?
- Have you ever had an STI (herpes, gonorrhea, genital warts, *Chlamydia*)?
- Have you ever had sex against your will?
- How do you protect yourself from HIV and STIs?
- Do you use male condoms? Female condoms? Other barriers?

Drug Use—Related Risk
- Have you ever injected drugs using shared equipment, including street drugs, steroids?

- Have you ever had sex with a person who uses and shares?
- Have you ever had sex while stoned, high, or drunk, so that you cannot remember the details?
- Have you ever exchanged sex for drugs, money, or shelter?

Blood-Related Risks
- Have you ever had a blood transfusion?
- Have you ever had sex with a person who had a blood transfusion?
- Have you ever had sex with a person with hemophilia?
- Have you ever received donor semen, egg, or transplanted organ or tissue?
- Have you ever shared equipment for tattoo and/or body piercing?

Other
- Have you ever had a test for HIV?
- Have you ever worried about AIDS and would like to talk with someone about it?

*AIDS, Acquired immunodeficiency syndrome; HIV, human immunodeficiency virus; IV, intravenous; STI, sexually transmitted infection.
Adapted from Hatcher R, Trussell J, Nelson A, et al, editors: *Contraceptive technology*, ed 19, New York, 2007, Ardent Media; Lowdermilk DL, Perry SE, Cashion K, et al, editors: *Maternity & women's health care*, ed 10, St Louis, 2011, Elsevier/Mosby.

or emotionally abused, has been forced to have sex against one's will, or has a history of childhood sexual abuse.[12]

Examination

Once the history is completed, the patient is ready for the physical examination. The patient is instructed to undress and provided with an examination gown. If the patient is elderly or has a disability he or she may require assistance with disrobing and assistance onto the examination table.

Female Examination

A complete pelvic examination is completed for females. The woman should be assisted into a lithotomy position with her feet supported by knee or heel stirrups. Adolescents and women who have anxiety at the thought of an impending pelvic exam should be encouraged to perform slow deep-breathing exercises.[12] The gynecologic examination includes external inspection, external palpation, internal examination, collection of specimens, vaginal examination, bimanual palpation, and sometimes rectovaginal palpation. Findings might include the following: healed scars from childbirth or trauma, hymenal tags, bulges (cystoceles or rectoceles), thinning of the vaginal wall, fistulas, masses, lesions, and inflammation. This is an excellent time to provide the woman with an opportunity to learn the skills necessary to perform a regular vulvar self-examination and Kegel exercises.[12]

Male Examination

The male examination includes examination of the genitalia and the digital rectal examination (DRE). The practitioner should begin by examining both the penis and the testicles. The scrotum is palpated very gently and may reveal such findings as hydrocele, hernia, masses, nodules, or inflammation.[37] The penis is also evaluated and may manifest ulcerations, nodules, and discharge.[37] This might be an opportune time to instruct the patient on the technique used to perform a testicular self-exam so that the patient may self-discover an abnormality in his testicles (often an indication of testicular cancer).[37] Every man older than age 40 should also undergo a DRE to screen for cancer of the prostate.[37] This may well be the most embarrassing, but essential, procedure for the male patient because it allows the practitioner to assess the size, shape, and texture of the prostate as well as any tenderness or presence of nodules.[37]

Diagnostic Tests

A thorough assessment of sexual health includes laboratory and diagnostic procedures. Women who have been sexually active for 3 years or who are 21 years of age are advised to have an annual Papanicolaou (Pap) test in order to screen for cervical cancer.[12] A prostate-specific antigen (PSA) test is recommended annually for men at increased risk for prostate cancer.[37] This includes men with a family history of prostate cancer or men of African-American descent.[37] Tests for specific STIs are ordered at the discretion of the provider; however, all sexually active men and women should have a VDRL (Venereal Disease Research Laboratory) and an RPR (rapid plasma reagin) performed.[12,38] This is of particular importance before initiating sexual intercourse with a new partner.[38] Patients who present with STI symptomatology will have much more thorough testing ordered dependent upon their clinical presentation.[39] A patient presenting with a vaginal infection might be screened for trichomoniasis, candidiasis, and vaginosis whereas a patient with genital warts will only receive testing for human papillomavirus (HPV).[39] Tests for HIV are usually ordered for patients that belong to high-risk populations, including men who have sex with men and all pregnant women.[12,39] All adults should be screened at least once in order to determine a baseline for HIV status.[38]

CLINICAL MANAGEMENT

Healthy People 2020 is a national campaign designed to improve the health of all Americans.[40] Eight specific objectives, selected from 42 topic areas, relate specifically to sexuality and reproduction and provide the basis for many of the prevention and screening guidelines.[40] These objectives include, but are not limited to, the following: the reduction of all STIs, an increase in the number of adolescents who abstain from sexual intercourse or use protection if sexually active, an improvement in annual screening rates, an increase in the number of adolescents who receive formal instruction in reproductive health topics, and the reduction of pregnancy rates among female adolescents.[40]

Primary Prevention

Primary prevention strategies are those implemented in order to avoid the development of disease. These strategies may be population based or initiated at the level of the individual. Disease processes associated with human sexuality include STIs, HIV, and cervical cancer; however, prevention strategies must also address concerns related to unintended pregnancy.

When used correctly, the (male) condom continues to be the single most effective method for preventing sexually transmitted diseases as well as being a very highly effective contraceptive agent.[16,19] Condoms are consistently used by 80% of teenage males and 69% of adolescent females, clearly indicating that this has become normative behavior for many youth.[11,19] Along with consistent condom use, access to quality reproductive health education and increased oral contraceptive use have resulted in decreasing trends in teen pregnancy rates over the past decade.[21]

Although we have seen success related to primary prevention techniques within the adolescent population cohort, condom use has been found to decline with age; it is less common in more established relationships and for women using other methods of contraception.[16,19] When surveyed, only 25% of adult men and 21% of women have reported using a condom within the last 12 months.[19] As previously noted, this is an opportunity for both primary care practitioners and public health professionals to provide education directed at adults.[20]

Other primary prevention measures are those "individual activities" aimed at deterring infection. This would include knowing one's partner, reducing the number of partners, avoiding partners who themselves have had many sexual encounters, eliminating casual sexual encounters, and avoiding unsafe sexual practices.[4,12] By educating patients towards behavior change, nurses may be able to reduce high-risk behaviors and consequently lessen the risk of contracting STIs. Of significance in the realm of primary prevention is the recent introduction of a vaccine to prevent cervical cancers associated with the sexually transmitted human papillomavirus (HPV).[4] This vaccine has been successfully marketed amidst concern that its use would have a negative effect on sexual behavior. The American College of Obstetrics and Gynecology has recommended that girls should receive either one of the two FDA-approved vaccines (Cervarix and Gardasil) before becoming sexually active.[12,41] Ideally, the vaccine should be routinely administered at the age of 11 or 12; however, it can be given up until the age of 26 regardless of sexual activity.[41]

Secondary Prevention (Screening)

In contrast to primary prevention strategies, secondary prevention attempts to diagnose an existing disease in its earliest stages. This is often referred to as screening with a goal of reducing morbidity and mortality and preserving quality of life.

Human Papillomavirus (HPV)

Although we now have the ability to vaccinate young women in order to protect them from the sequelae of HPV infection, it should be noted that the vaccine only protects against 70% of HPV-related cancers and 90% of HPV cases of genital warts.[12] The vaccine is a tremendous preventive tool; however, it does not replace necessary screening for cervical cancers. Cervical cytologic screening guidelines remain unchanged and should be followed regardless of vaccination status.[41] Screening begins no later than age 21 and is recommended annually for women younger than 30.[41] By the age of 30 and after at least three normal surveys, screening may be reduced to every 2 to 3 years.[12]

HIV Screening

The Centers for Disease Control and Prevention recommends HIV testing for all patients ages 13 to 64 years in all health care settings (e.g., urgent-care centers, inpatient services, substance abuse clinics, and primary care settings).[42] The exception would be patient populations with a prevalence rate of less than 0.1%.[42] Of particular importance are patients who present with tuberculosis, patients seeking treatment for other STIs, pregnant women, and newborns.[42] Patients at increased risk of contracting HIV should be screened annually.[42] This includes injection drug users and their partners, persons who have sex for money or drugs, men who have sex with men, and heterosexual persons who have sex with more than one partner.[42] Any patients presenting with an opportunistic-like illness or symptoms of AIDS should be tested for HIV.[42] Screening should always be performed with informed consent and is always voluntary.[42] Should a patient decline testing, it must be noted in his or her medical record.[42]

Other Sexually Transmitted Infections

The CDC strongly recommends the screening of asymptomatic women who are at high risk and for whom STIs would otherwise go undetected.[39] This includes, but is not limited to, women who have *Chlamydia,* gonorrhea, syphilis, the herpes simplex virus, hepatitis, and bacterial vaginal infections.[12,39] Early screening will guide the clinician to select the appropriate treatment modality and improve outcomes.

Effective screening will also reduce transmission of STIs, because education can be provided in order to reduce risk among a patient's sexual partners.

Collaborative Interventions
Disorders of Male Sexual Function

Erectile dysfunction (ED), more commonly known as impotence, is the inability for a man to either achieve or maintain an erection for a sufficient length of time to complete the sexual act.[37] Phosphodiesterase type 5 inhibitors are commonly prescribed pharmacologic agents for the treatment of ED. Other treatment modalities for ED include surgery (penile implants or transurethral resection of the prostate) and the use of negative-pressure vacuum devices.[37]

Ejaculation problems include both premature ejaculation and inability to ejaculate under any circumstances.[37] Premature ejaculation occurs when a man has no ability to control the ejaculatory reflex and reaches orgasm much sooner than desired.[37] Behavioral therapies and sexual counseling have proven to be very successful in addressing the psychologic component of these disorders.[37]

Relief of Menopausal Symptoms

Sexuality is a lifelong healthy behavior that does not necessarily end with the transition to menopause. There are women that accept child-bearing as a necessary responsibility of marriage and find that entering the climacteric gives them permission to forego sexual activity entirely.[12] For other women, lack of lubrication is frequently cited as the cause for sexual problems when they reach middle age.[12,14] A number of water-soluble lubricants (e.g., K-Y Intrigue, FemGlide) are now readily available and provide much relief for the pain that occurs during intercourse because of vaginal dryness.[12] Other treatment options available to the menopausal woman include hormone replacement therapy, herbal therapy, homeopathic remedies, and acupuncture.[12] Nurses have the ability to provide accurate information to patients regarding the physiology of menopause and its effect on sexuality.[12] The nurse should be seen as supportive of healthy sexual function and may refer women or couples for sexual counseling if problems continue.[12]

Management of Pelvic Organ Prolapse

Symptoms of sexual dysfunction and altered body image often coexist with prolapse of the female reproductive organs (uterus, cystocele, rectocele).[12,43] Approximately 50% of women experience some degree of prolapse by the time they reach the age of 40.[43] For this cohort of women, intercourse may be painful or embarrassing and associated with fecal or urinary incontinence.[43] Conservative management includes lifestyle changes—such as losing weight, avoiding constipation, reducing high-impact exercise (e.g., running)—and pelvic muscle floor training (Kegel exercises).[12,43] Mechanical devices such as vaginal pessaries are a safe, simple, and inexpensive option for many women. For patients with a greater degree of uterine prolapse and little success with other options, surgery may be necessary; however, there is a 30% chance of the surgery failing because of recurrent uterine prolapse.[43] Nursing care requires a great deal of sensitivity because many women are very embarrassed by their condition and have many concerns about resuming sexual activity postoperatively.[12]

Treatment of STIs

Preventing infection remains the most effective way of reducing the adverse consequences of STIs, in particular those that are not readily curable.[12] In cases where prevention has been unsuccessful, prompt diagnosis and treatment are essential. Nurses are often able to reassure the patient enough to open dialogue regarding possible exposure, testing, and treatment options.[12] For all sexually transmitted diseases, CDC guidelines should be strictly followed.[44] These are available by searching www.cdc.gov.[44]

INTERRELATED CONCEPTS

The concept of sexual health represents the "integration of somatic, emotional, intellectual and social aspects of sexual being in ways that are enriching and enhance personality, communication and love."[2] **Sexuality** and interrelated concepts are presented in Figure 19-2. This model illustrates some concepts that may be impacted by normative sexual functioning and/or have an impact on sexuality.

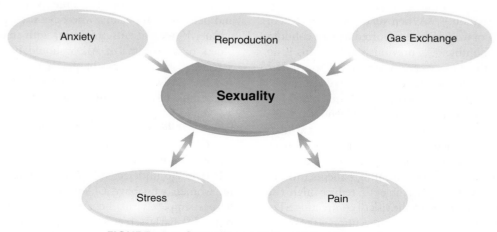

FIGURE 19-2 Sexuality and Interrelated Concepts.

Reproduction. The most obvious overlap between concepts is that of sexuality and reproduction. An example is the decision to use contraception before sexual activity or undergoing an abortion after intercourse when an unplanned pregnancy occurs. Even the woman who intentionally becomes pregnant may find that her sexual relationship with her partner is altered as a result of her advancing pregnancy. Emotional distress may be experienced by those who are unable to conceive a baby. This may lead to feelings of guilt, failure, anger, and sadness. A nurse can assist by discussing alternatives for conceiving such as in vitro fertilization (IVF). Adoption may be another alternative to be considered and discussed. Once a need has been identified, referrals to various health care specialists and agencies are often facilitated by the nurse.

Pain. One physiologic barriers to healthy sexual functioning is pain. For the patient who has pain as a result of intercourse, the use of lubricants should be encouraged. If the person has chronic pain, then sexual activity should be planned for a time when pain medication has been taken and has begun to take effect.[37]

Gas exchange. The patient who has poor gas exchange may encounter challenges with sexual activity associated with hypoxia. The patient should be instructed to utilize oxygen during intercourse and assume activity at a time of day when he or she is most well rested.[37]

Anxiety. A patient who has lost a body part because of cancer or trauma may be anxious about the resumption of sexual activity because of an altered sense of self. The nurse should encourage the patient to share his or her concerns with his or her partner before engaging in sexual activity.[37] A healthy sense of self contributes to sexual health and vice versa.

Stress. If a patient is undergoing extreme stress from other life issues (e.g., work, children, parents) this may have a negative impact on sexual functioning. The nurse can assist the person to identify stressors and provide the patient with techniques to reduce stress (e.g., exercise or support groups).[37]

EXEMPLARS

Any number of exemplars could be chosen to effectively illustrate the concept of human sexuality. Those presented in Box 19-3 address a continuum of concerns that have a significant impact upon a person's sexual health and well-being across the lifespan.

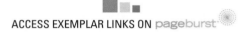

ACCESS EXEMPLAR LINKS ON pageburst

MODEL CASE

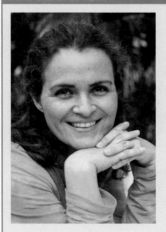

Anna Garner is a 44-year-old married White female with an appointment to see her nurse practitioner (NP) for her annual examination. As part of her annual physical, Anna will be having a pelvic examination including a Papanicolau test in order to screen for cervical cancer. Anna has three teenage daughters, all born by spontaneous vaginal delivery. Several years ago Anna returned to work full time at a rather sedentary job. Anna has found her weight to be increasing over these past few years and is now carrying 164 pounds on her 5 foot, 1 inch frame. Over the years Anna and her NP have developed a trusting and therapeutic relationship. As part of the history-taking process the NP asks Anna if she has ever been "hit, slapped, or forced to have sex against her wishes." Anna states that she has not; however, she hesitates in her response. The NP senses that she may need to elicit further information from Anna without making her feel uncomfortable. She queries Anna to see if there have been any changes in the past year related to the sexual relationship that she has with her partner. Anna appears somewhat embarrassed; but, with some encouragement, she goes on to explain that in the past she and her husband have always enjoyed intercourse two to three times a week and that this is a very important part of their marriage. Anna states that for the last 9 to 10 months she has begun to "lose urine" during intercourse. Sometimes this occurs during foreplay and on other occasions it will happen during orgasm. Anna reports that she often interrupts their sexual activity to go to the bathroom. Recently she is finding excuses to avoid sex altogether and is concerned that she is driving her husband away. The NP explains to Anna that this condition is referred to as "stress or coital incontinence" and may be the result of childbearing, aging, and her recent weight gain. Education is provided regarding the necessity for urodynamic evaluation and the possible treatment modalities available. These may include the use of pessaries, a medication regimen, pelvic floor rehabilitation, or even surgery. Anna is instructed on how to perform Kegel exercises during her pelvic examination. The NP reassures Anna that although this condition is neither uncommon nor life threatening, if left untreated it may result in other unanticipated symptomatology including depression, loss of self-esteem, altered body image, worsening of incontinence, reduced social interaction, and decreased sexual interest and activity. Anna is very reassured by this education and agrees to the treatment plan.

▪▪▪ BOX 19-3 EXEMPLARS OF SEXUALITY

Sexually Transmitted Infections
Protozoa
- Trichomoniasis

Parasites
- Pediculosis
- Scabies

Viruses
- Cytomegalovirus
- Hepatitis A and hepatitis B
- Herpes simplex virus 1 and 2 (HSV)
- HIV
- Human papillomavirus (HPV)

Bacteria
- Chancroid
- *Chlamydia*
- Genital mycoplasmas
- Gonorrhea
- Group B *Streptococcus*
- Syphilis

Intimate Partner Violence
- Genital trauma
- Rape-trauma syndrome

- Sexual harassment
- Sexual assault

Sexual Dysfunction and Alteration
- Anorgasmia
- Coital incontinence
- Decreased libido
- Dyspareunia
- Erectile dysfunction
- Impotence
- Premature ejaculation
- Menopause
- Vaginismus

Sexuality and Pregnancy
- Anticipated body changes
- Bleeding
- Changing attitudes towards sexual activity
- Decreased libido
- Fatigue, nausea
- History of miscarriage
- History of premature births
- Multiple pregnancy
- Placenta previa

REFERENCES

1. Elders MJ: Sex for health and pleasure throughout a lifetime, *J Sex Med* 7(suppl 5), 2010.
2. World Health Organization: *Defining sexual health; report of a technical consultation on sexual health, Jan 28-31, 2001*, Geneva, Switzerland, 2006, Author.
3. Office of the Surgeon General: *The Surgeon General's call to action to promote sexual health and responsible sexual behavior*, Rockville, Md, 2001, Author.
4. Herbenick D, Reece M, Schick V, et al: Sexual behavior in the United States: results from a national probability sample of men and women ages 14-94, *J Sex Med* 7(suppl 5), 2010.
5. Goldstein I: Looking at sexual behavior 60 years after Kinsey, *J Sex Med* 7(suppl 5), 2010.
6. Kinsey AC, Pomeroy WB, Martin CE: *Sexual behavior in the human male*, Philadelphia, 1948, WB Saunders.
7. Kinsey AC, Pomeroy WB, Martin CE, et al: *Sexual behavior in the human female*, Philadelphia, 1953, Saunders.
8. Masters WH, Johnson VE: *Human sexual response*, Boston, 1966, Little, Brown.
9. Masters WH, Johnson VE: *Human sexual inadequacy*, Boston, 1970, Little, Brown.
10. Brown RT, Brown JD: Adolescent sexuality, *Prim Care Clin Office Pract* 33, 2006.
11. Fortenberry JD, Schick V, Herbenick D, et al: Sexual behaviors and condom use at last vaginal intercourse: a national sample of adolescents ages 14 to 17 years, *J Sex Med* 7 (suppl 5), 2010.
12. Lowdermilk DL, Perry SE, Cashion K, et al, editors: *Maternity & women's health care*, ed 10, St Louis, 2011, Mosby/Elsevier.
13. Herbenick D, Reece M, Schick V, et al: Sexual behaviors, relationships, and perceived health status among adult women in the United States: results from a national probability sample, *J Sex Med* 7(suppl 5), 2010.
14. Berg J: Dimensions of sexuality in the perimenopausal transition: a model for practice, *JOGNN*, July/August 2001.
15. Freedman M: Partnership issues and sexuality, *Clin Obstet Gynecol* 52(4), 2009.
16. Reece M, Herbenick D, Schick V, et al: Sexual behaviors, relationships, and perceived health status among adult men in the United States: results from a national probability sample, *J Sex Med* 7(suppl 5), 2010.
17. Barclay LB: Commentary on the national survey of sexual health and behavior, *J Sex Med* 7(suppl 5), 2010.
18. Kelly D: Male sexuality in theory and practice, *Nurs Clin North Am* 39, 2004.
19. Sanders SA, Reece M, Herbenick D, et al: Condom use during most recent vaginal intercourse event among a probability sample of adults in the United States, *J Sex Med* 7(suppl 5), 2010.
20. Schick V, Herbenick D, Reece M, et al: Sexual behaviors, condom use, and sexual health of Americans over 50: implications for sexual health promotion for older adults, *J Sex Med* 7 (suppl 5), 2010.
21. McKay A, Barrett M: Trends in teen pregnancy rates from 1996-2006: a comparison of Canada, Sweden, U.S.A. and England/Wales, *Can J Hum Sex* 19(1–2), 2010.
22. Talashek ML, Alba ML, Patel A: Untangling the health disparities of teen pregnancy, *J Spec Pediatr Nurs* 11(1), 2006.
23. Dodge B, Reece M, Herbenick D, et al: Sexual health among U.S. black and Hispanic men and women: a nationally representative study, *J Sex Med* 7(suppl 5), 2010.

24. Fenton KA: Time for change: rethinking and reframing sexual health in the United States, *J Sex Med* 7(suppl 5), 2010.

25. Ailey SH, Marks BA, Crisp C, et al: Promoting sexuality across the lifespan for individuals with intellectual and developmental disabilities, *Nurs Clin North Am* 38, 2003.

26. Lederman RP, Chan W, Roberts-Gray C: Sexual attitudes and intentions of youth aged 12-14 years: survey comparisons of parent-teen prevention and control groups, *Behav Med* 29(Winter), 2004.

27. Herbenick D, Reece M, Schick V, et al: An event-level analysis of the sexual characteristics and composition among adults ages 18 to 59: results from a national probability sample in the United States, *J Sex Med* 7(suppl 5), 2010.

28. Dowshein N, Garofalo R: Optimizing primary care for LGBTQ youth, *Contemp Pediatr* 26(10), 2009.

29. Kleinplatz PJ, Menard AD: Building blocks toward optimal sexuality: constructing a conceptual model, *The Family Journal: Counseling and Therapy for Couples and Families*, Jan 2007.

30. Sobczak JA: Female sexual dysfunction: knowledge development and practice implications, *Perspect Psychiatr Care* 45(3), 2009.

31. Zakhari R: Female sexual dysfunction: a primary care perspective, *J Am Acad Nurse Pract* 21, 2009.

32. Forrest KA: Men's reproductive and sexual health, *J Am College Health* 49(6), 2001.

33. Shifren JL, Johannes CB, Monz BU, et al: Help-seeking behavior of women with self-reported distressing sexual problems, *J Women's Health* 18(4), 2008.

34. Magnan MA, Reynolds KE, Galvin EA: Barriers to addressing patient sexuality in nursing practice, *MEDSURG Nurs* 14(5), 2005.

35. Shell JA: Including sexuality in your nursing practice, *Nurs Clin North Am* 42, 2007.

36. Carpenito-Moyet LJ: *Handbook of nursing diagnosis*, ed 12, Philadelphia, 2008, Wolters Kluwer/Lippincott Williams & Wilkins.

37. Smeltzer SC, Bare BG: *Brunner & Suddarth's textbook of medical-surgical nursing*, ed 10, Philadelphia, 2004, Lippincott Williams & Wilkins.

38. U.S. Department of Health and Human Services: *Screening tests and immunization guidelines for men*. Available at www.womenshealth.gov (updated March 18, 2010).

39. Centers for Disease Control and Prevention (CDC): Sexually transmitted diseases treatment guidelines, *Morbid Mortal Wkly Rep (MMWR)* 51(RR-6), May 10, 2002.

40. Office of Population Affairs: *Reproductive health and Healthy People 2020*. Available at www.healthypeople.gov (updated Dec 2010).

41. American College of Obstetrics and Gynecology (ACOG): Committee Opinion #344: human papillomavirus vaccination, *Obstet Gynecol*, Sept 2006.

42. Centers for Disease Control and Prevention (CDC): Revised recommendations for HIV testing of adults, adolescents and pregnant women in health-care settings, *Morbid Mortal Wkly Rep (MMWR)* 55(RR-14), Sept 22, 2006.

43. Richardson K, Hagen S, Glazener C, et al: The role of nurses in the management of women with pelvic organ prolapse, *Br J Nurs* 18(5), 2009.

44. Centers for Disease Control and Prevention (CDC): Sexually transmitted diseases treatment guidelines, 2010, *Morbid Mortal Wkly Rep (MMWR)* 59(RR-12), Dec 17, 2010.

20

Immunity

Carolyn E. Sabo

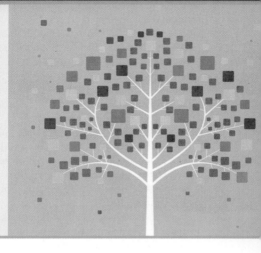

The ability of the human body to sustain health within the environment requires multiple protective mechanisms. One of the most complex protective mechanisms is the immune response. When immune processes are functioning optimally, the body has the ability to mount an efficient defense in response to the invasion of foreign substances. Such a response is critical to maintaining health. It is reasonable then to conclude that multiple health problems occur in the absence of a normal immune response. Although this concept analysis will describe the concept of immunity from the perspective of both normal and abnormal functioning, the primary focus will be on that of abnormal function because of the multitude of health-related problems that result.

DEFINITION(S)

Immunity is commonly defined as a physiologic process that provides an individual with protection or defense from disease. It is a characteristic that allows one to be insusceptible or resistant to a particular disease or condition and is derived from the Latin word "immunis" meaning exempt.[1,2] Immunity is accomplished through the actions of the immune system, which is a bodywide, complex, interrelated group of cells, tissues, and organs that work within a dynamic communication network to protect the body from attacks by foreign antigens, typically proteins. These foreign antigens may include microorganisms (bacteria, viruses, parasites, or fungi), but may also be proteins found in pollens; foods; bee, snake, or spider venom; vaccines; transfusions; and transplanted tissues.[3,4] This definition represents the perspective of normal function. As noted earlier, this concept includes abnormal function leading to health problems. For the purpose of this concept analysis, a broader definition of immunity is used: *the normal physiologic response to microorganisms and proteins as well as conditions associated with an inadequate or excessive immune response.*

There are additional terms that are used to differentiate type of immunity protection. *Innate immunity* (also referred to as

natural or native) is the immunity present at birth; it provides nonspecific response not considered antigen specific. *Acquired immunity* refers to immunity protection that is gained after birth either actively or passively. *Active acquired immunity* develops after the introduction of a foreign antigen resulting in the formation of antibodies or sensitized T lymphocytes. For example, active immunity may be obtained artificially through the immune response to an immunization or it may be obtained naturally through the immune response to exposure to infectious pathogens such as varicella-zoster virus. *Passive acquired immunity* occurs by the introduction of preformed antibodies—either from an artificial route, such as a transfusion of immunoglobulin (Ig), or from a natural route, such as from a mother to her fetus through placental blood transference or through colostrum transfer during breastfeeding.[1,4-6]

SCOPE AND CATEGORIES

The complexity of immunity often makes it a difficult topic to fully understand from a traditional presentation. From a conceptual perspective, it is useful to think about what this concept represents from a very broad view and considering the context of patient-related issues. Such a perspective may make the pathologic details described later easier to understand. The scope of immunity and related immunity problems are described as optimal and abnormal responses, with the two opposite ends of the abnormal function being suppressed immune response and exaggerated immune response (Figure 20-1).[7-9]

Optimal Immune Response

An optimal immune response involves the three primary protective functions:

1. Protects the body from invasion of microorganisms and other antigens.
2. Removes dead or damaged tissue and cells.
3. Recognizes and removes cell mutations that have demonstrated abnormal cell growth and development.

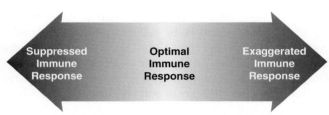

FIGURE 20-1 Scope of Immunity Concept.

To accomplish these functions the immune system reacts with three lines of defense. The first line of defense is the skin boundary surfaces including mucous membranes, enzymes, natural microbial flora, and complement proteins. The second line of defense is accomplished by the activities of phagocytes, natural killer T lymphocytes, granulocytes, and macrophages providing innate, nonspecific immunity. Finally, the third line of defense comes from antibodies derived from B lymphocytes and the T lymphocytes resulting from learned or acquired specific immunity.[8-10] These components of the immune system will be further discussed throughout this concept.

Suppressed Immune Response

To the far left of the immune response spectrum is a hypo- or suppressed immune response. Individuals who have suppressed immune responses are referred to as immunocompromised or are considered to be in a state of immunodeficiency. *Primary immunodeficiency* occurs as a result of improperly developed cells or an absence of cells required to execute the immune response. *Secondary immunodeficiency* is a loss of immune functioning (in a person with previously normal immune function) as a result of an illness or treatment. Individuals with suppressed immune responses are unable to provide an adequate immune defense against the invasion of microorganisms or foreign proteins. As a result, they are at significant risk for infection, or if immunosuppression occurs over time, they are at risk for cancer because of the loss or removal of mutating cells.[8-10]

Exaggerated Immune Response

To the far right of the immune response spectrum (Figure 20-1) is a hyperimmune or exaggerated immune response. Considering the list of normal protective functions, this is a situation in which there is an overreaction of the immune response. Although initially this may seem like a positive outcome with better protective mechanisms, an exaggerated immune response is actually very problematic.

Hyperimmune or exaggerated immune responses range among allergic reactions, cytotoxic reactions, and autoimmune reactions. A critical component of the immune system is its ability to differentiate between "self" and "non-self." This capability is accomplished by the presence of unique proteins on the surface of every cell that distinguish each individual as "self" and are as unique to each individual as fingerprints. When this recognition fails, the immune system may begin attacking host cells in an exaggerated immune response. This process leads to the development of autoimmune diseases

and disorders (e.g., rheumatoid arthritis or systemic lupus erythematosus).[8-10] This autoimmune process is discussed in greater detail in the sections that follow.

RISK FACTORS

Populations at Risk

People from all age, socioeconomic, and racial/ethnic groups can potentially have impaired immune systems. However, some population groups and individuals are at greater risk than others. Risk factors for insufficient and exaggerated immune function are presented separately in the sections that follow.

Suppressed Immune Response
Age

In the very young, the immune system is immature with inadequate lymphocyte function, particularly T lymphocyte deficiency. Newborn T lymphocyte responses are functional at birth, but B lymphocyte response and antibody production are significantly diminished. In the last trimester of development the fetus is able to initiate an antibody response with immunoglobulin M (IgM) (though antibody production remains low), whereas IgG and IgA responses are underdeveloped.[9] Newborns rely on immune protection received from placental blood transfer with the mother and from the high levels of immunoglobulin found in colostrum during breastfeeding. Over the next few months, maternal antibodies are slowly destroyed with the rate of catabolism exceeding the rate of newborn immunoglobulin production.[11] This mild hypogammaglobulinemia contributes to the increased risk of infection in the newborn.

In the elderly, loss of immune effectiveness occurs in part because of the physiologic aging and shrinking of the thymus gland, leaving it at about 15% of its maximum size by middle age and decreasing the ability of T lymphocytes to mature in the gland over time.[11] Research has also demonstrated that elderly people have fewer T lymphocytes, produce fewer immunoglobulins, experience a delayed and diminished hypersensitivity response, and demonstrate an increase in autoantibodies.[8,9] B lymphocyte function is diminished secondary to a decrease in circulating memory cells that evolve after about 60 years of age. These changes in B and T lymphocyte function leave the elderly immunocompromised and more susceptible to infection and cancers.[11]

Nonimmunized State

Individuals who are not immunized are susceptible to a number of infections including rubella, measles, mumps, tetanus, diphtheria, hepatitis, and others. Many of these diseases can be fatal to the very young, the elderly, or those who are immunocompromised as a result of disease processes or their treatment and other environmental factors.

Environmental Factors

Environmental factors such as poor nutrition, exposure to pollutants (including tobacco smoke) or heavy metals, and other stressors may depress immune functioning.[12-15] Unsafe sanitary conditions, food and water contamination, and poor hand hygiene also contribute to disease transmission and are particularly dangerous to the very young or elderly and those with some other chronic illnesses. Some of these situations are easily remedied by the individual, whereas others require more of a community-focused attention to solving the problem.

Chronic Illnesses

Depressed immune function can develop as a result of chronic illness or treatments for medical conditions. In addition to primary immunodeficiency conditions that directly impair the immune system (such as human immunodeficiency virus [HIV]), many chronic conditions (such as diabetes mellitus, chronic obstructive pulmonary disease, malnutrition, and cancer) also lead to reductions in immune function as a secondary consequence to the disease or its treatment. The Centers for Disease Control and Prevention (CDC) has issued recommendations for cancer patients, cancer survivors, and caregivers concerning the link between cancer and influenza. Although currently living with cancer or being a cancer survivor does not increase the chance of contracting influenza, these people are at increased risk for complications from influenza, including hospitalization and death.[16]

Medical Treatments

Medical treatments may be implemented specifically to inhibit an optimal immune response or they may lead to immunosuppression as a consequence of the treatment. For instance, in the case of tissue graft or tissue transplantation, immunosuppression is necessary to keep the body from rejecting the graft because it is recognized as foreign or not a part of the self. Conversely, pharmacologic treatments for autoimmune hypersensitivity reactions, such as systemic lupus erythematosus, or cancers include treatment regimens that inhibit the immune response. The stress associated with many medical treatments, both psychologic and physical, places an added burden on the immune system and may leave the individual vulnerable to illness. Research has demonstrated that achieving the daily recommended doses of vitamins and minerals contributes to a properly functioning immune system. New research is addressing the role of vitamins A and D in protecting and supporting the immune response. In addition to their usefulness in the daily diet for health maintenance,[8,9] supplementation with these vitamins may be a valuable contribution to many medical treatment regimens.

Genetics

An individual's genetic base, overall health, and history of exposure to potential antigens influence immune functioning.[17] A number of genetic diseases may lead to depressed or absent functioning of parts or all of the immune system. As a group, complement deficiencies are comparatively rare and their prevalence varies depending on the specific deficiency and the age of a person. Another immune deficiency, common variable immunodeficiency, is one of the most prevalent primary immunodeficiency diseases with an estimated 1 case per 30,000 population.[13] Allergies to food or environmental stimuli and type 1 diabetes mellitus are also considered a type of immune dysfunction. The incidence of those diseases is widespread in both children and adults of all ethnic origins, with variations depending on geography and ethnicity. An increase in the incidence of autoimmune diseases such as fibromyalgia, multiple sclerosis, and asthma is also being seen in children and adults.[13,18]

High-Risk Behaviors and Substance Abuse

A number of high-risk behaviors have been associated with the development of a dysfunctional immune system. Transmission of human immunodeficiency virus (HIV) and hepatitis virus may be directly related to high-risk sexual behaviors and sharing needles among intravenous drug abusers. According to Waldschmidt and colleagues,[19] excessive alcohol consumption leads to compromised immunity (innate and acquired), dysfunction of components of the immune system, and increased risk of infection.

Pregnancy

Immunity is influenced by pregnancy, creating a situation where the mother is immunocompromised. The developing fetus exists in what has been termed a "privileged" immunity environment where fetal antigens from the father do not stimulate an immune response and rejection of the graft created by the fetus-placenta connection and the mother.[4] New research has demonstrated that the placental barrier between mother and fetus is open to communication between mother and fetal cells. It has been found that fetal cells may remain in the mother's tissues for long periods of time, creating a situation termed *microchimerism* or a mixing of cells of different origins. A microchimerism may also be created in the fetus and research is investigating the role that this may play in the development of autoimmune diseases.[9]

Exaggerated Immune Response
Gender, Race, Ethnicity

Some hypersensitivity disorders have higher incidence and prevalence by virtue of gender, race, or ethnicity. For example, systemic lupus erythematosus occurs more often in women than men by a 10:1 ratio and African Americans are eight times more likely to contract the disease than Caucasians/non-Hispanics.[9]

Genetics

Genetics is often responsible for the formation of an exaggerated immune response. An exaggerated reaction may be minor and serve more as an annoyance, such as seen with some environmental or food allergies, or may lead to destruction of normal tissue, loss of organ function, or death. In some cases, the genetic basis for the development of hyperimmune disorders requires that the gene or chromosome be carried by both parents (or sometimes only one parent), and some disorders require an environmental or physiologic trigger (e.g., hormonal changes seen in puberty) in addition to the predisposition to a hyperimmune disorder created by genetics.

Environmental or Medication Exposure

Environmental or medication exposure to a foreign antigen may elicit an exaggerated immune response. Foods, drugs, pollens, dust, molds, bee venom, vaccines, or serum may all evoke hypersensitivity reactions (types I, II, or III), and some may evoke more than one type of hypersensitivity.[6,8,9] Generally, these hypersensitivity reactions do not occur on first exposure to the foreign antigen but rather on reexposure. However, genetic predisposition, exposure by the mother during fetal development, or other contributing factors may cause an exaggerated response on first presentation of the pathogen. In many cases, individuals who manifest an allergic type of exaggerated response to one type of pathogen (e.g., pollen) will demonstrate a similar reaction to other antigens in the same or similar class.

Medication exposure may act similarly to environmental exposure in inducing an exaggerated response. Some individuals report an allergic type of exaggerated reaction on first exposure to some medications (e.g., penicillin). The inactive substances contained in medication preparations may also evoke an exaggerated response, even though the active portion of the medication is nonallergenic. In this case, changing from one brand of the medication to another may solve the problem. In some individuals, a previously expressed exaggerated immune response may be amplified further in the presence of specific medications. For example, cancer treatment that includes the use of monoclonal antibodies has triggered exaggerated hypersensitivity reactions in some patients although a more mild reaction to the same pathogen was experienced in the past. It is critical that information on any reaction to medications or any known allergies be elicited before first administration of a medication.

PHYSIOLOGIC PROCESSES AND CONSEQUENCES

Recognition of the "self" and recognition of foreign proteins are the hallmarks of a properly functioning immune system. The individual must be able to differentiate between host and foreign proteins in order to respond appropriately. With the invasion of foreign proteins, a protective response is needed; failure to respond appropriately (immunosuppression or immunodeficiency) results in infections. Likewise, the body must maintain the ability to recognize host proteins and not initiate an immune response. When this recognition fails, the immune system launches an attack on host cells (hyperimmune response).

Normal Physiologic Immune Functioning
Major Histocompatibility Complex Proteins

Surface proteins called major histocompatibility complex (MHC) proteins are divided into two classes, with class I being found on all cells and class II on specialized cells.[4] Major histocompatibility complex proteins function, in part, to differentiate cells of the self/host from foreign proteins. Substances that are "non-self" are capable of initiating an immune response. A foreign antigen may be a whole cell, a virus, a bacterium, a MHC marker protein, or a small portion of a larger foreign protein. Epitopes are the markers on foreign antigens that cause the immune response in individuals.[3,4] The MHC provides what has been termed a "scaffold" that presents the foreign antigen to the immune cells. The empty MHC scaffold, also termed a self-marker scaffold, of a foreign cell from a donor organ may be introduced into the host during a transplant. These MHC self-marker scaffolds are the individual's tissue type or human leukocyte antigen (HLA).[3,4]

Organs Comprising the Immune System

Organs of the immune system are spread throughout the body. They are termed lymphoid organs and include the bone marrow, thymus gland, spleen, tonsils, adenoids, and appendix. From these organs, the lymphocytes are formed, grow, mature, and are released into the body. The body's lymphatic system provides the network by which organs of the immune system are connected. The blood also provides a connection among the organs and provides the route for lymphocyte movement throughout the body.

Origin of Cells in an Immune Response

A variety of components work together to provide an immune response. All cells in the immune system are derived from stem cells in the bone marrow and begin as either myeloid progenitor or lymphoid progenitor cells. Myeloid progenitors include neutrophils, monocytes (which become macrophages in body tissues), eosinophils, basophils, and mast cells. Lymphoid progenitor cells include B lymphocytes (which become plasma or memory B cells), mature T lymphocytes, and natural killer cells.

B and T lymphocytes. During fetal development, B and T lymphocytes are produced in large numbers. All immune cells begin as immature stem cells in the bone marrow and grow into specific immune cell types such as B or T lymphocytes and phagocytes. Preprocessing and maturation of the B lymphocytes occur in the liver during mid-fetal life and in the bone marrow during late-fetal life and after birth. Maturation of T lymphocytes occurs in the thymus gland. This process is called generation of clonal diversity. As a person is challenged by the presence of foreign antigens during life, *specificity* of lymphocytes to a specific antigen emerges, a process termed clonal selection.[8,9] On reexposure to the same antigen, the person will have a more rapid and efficient immune response, indicating a *memory* capacity for the immune system.

Antibody production. Antibodies are secreted by B lymphocytes. Antibodies or immunoglobulins (Ig) are formed after a B lymphocyte encounters and engulfs an antigen and then interacts with helper T lymphocytes; the B lymphocyte then begins producing identical copies of a specific antibody. The antibody consists of two identical heavy chains and two identical light chains that form a "Y" shape, or variable region, on top of what is termed the constant region. The Y shape variable arms are matched to an invading antigen and the constant version links the antibody to other components in the immune response. This region is identical in all antibodies of the same class. Researchers have identified nine classes of antibodies or immunoglobulins (four forms of IgG, two forms of IgA, and one form each of IgE, IgM, and IgD). Immunoglobulins are found in various concentrations at different sites around the body.[4,8,9]

- IgG: primary immunoglobulin in the blood (80% to 85% of circulating immunoglobulins); may enter tissue spaces; selectively crosses the placenta; coats antigen for more effective and efficient presentation for an immune response; binds to macrophages and neutrophils for increased phagocytosis
- IgD: found within the cell membrane of B lymphocytes
- IgE: responsible for allergy symptoms and increases in the presence of parasitic worms; normally found in trace amounts
- IgA: protects entrances to the body; found in high concentrations in body fluids (tears, saliva, secretions of the respiratory and gastrointestinal [GI] tracts)
- IgM: remains in the blood and efficiently kills bacteria; largest of the immunoglobulins; first antibody produced with an initial (primary) immune response

Phagocytes. Phagocytes are found throughout the body and are usually responsible for recognizing and ingesting foreign antigens as they enter the body. Macrophages and neutrophils are the primary phagocytic cells responsible for this first line of defense during an immune response. Because macrophages are the primary defensive cells against antigen entry to the body, when awaiting the need for phagocytic activity, large numbers of macrophages are stored in connective tissue, the spleen and liver, and the lining of the gastrointestinal and respiratory tracts. Neutrophils remain circulating in the blood.[3,4,8,9]

Phagocytosis is the process of ingesting cellular material and involves the ability of phagocytes to be selective in recognizing cells that must be ingested and discarded. Healthy cells of the self tend to be smooth and covered with a smooth protein coat that normally functioning phagocytes tend to ignore. Antibody-antigen complexes have rougher surfaces and are particularly susceptible to phagocytic functioning. Although both neutrophils and macrophages are phagocytes, in an immune response the macrophages are more effective than neutrophils.[8]

Complement system. The complement system works to enhance the immune response and to help rid the body of antibody-antigen complexes. The complement system is comprised of 25 major proteins that circulate in an inactive form in the blood and are engaged in a cascade of interactions when the first protein molecule (C1) encounters an antigen-antibody complex. The complement cascade is also responsible for the dilation and ultimate leaking of fluid from the vascular system, leading to the redness and swelling during the inflammatory process that are associated with an immune response.[3,4,8,9]

Lymphocyte Function in an Immune Response

A general overview of immune system development and maturation leading to an immune response to a foreign antigen is presented in Figure 20-2.

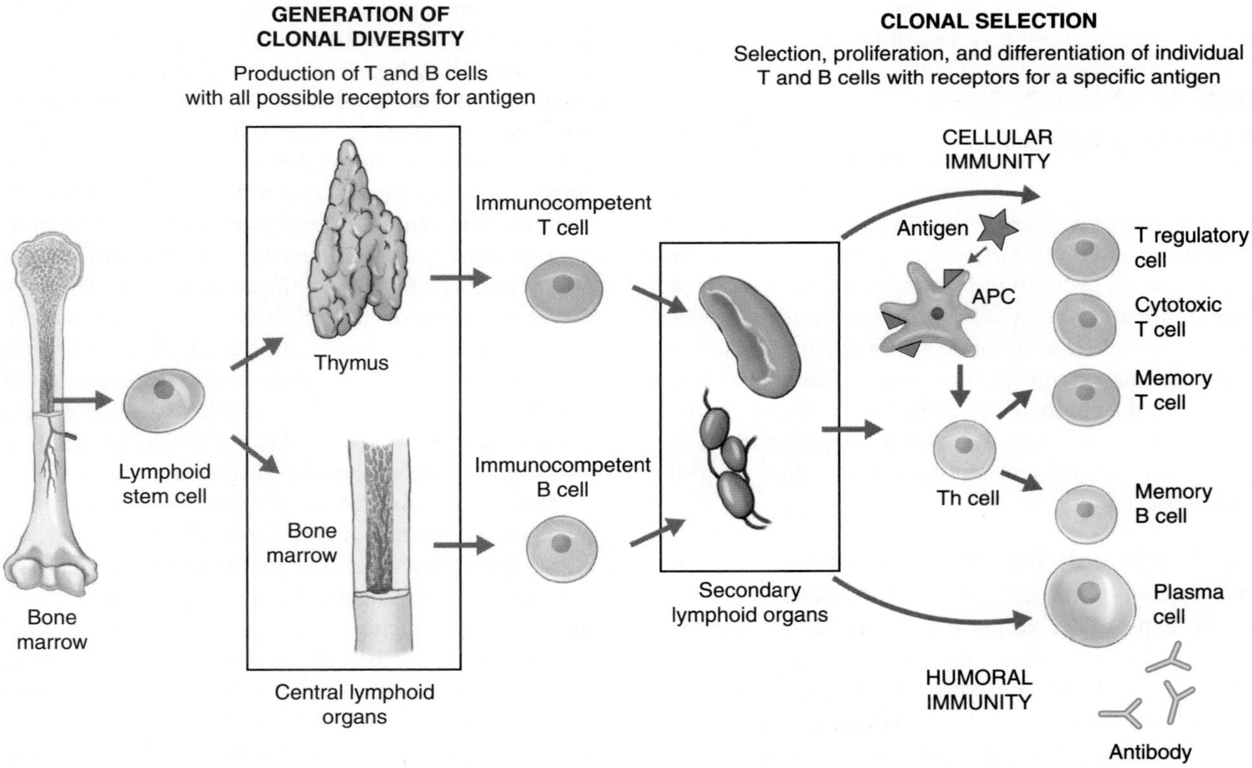

FIGURE 20-2 Overview of Immune Response. (From McCance KL, Huether SE: *Pathophysiology: the biologic basis for disease in adults and children,* ed 6, St Louis, 2010, Mosby/Elsevier.)

B lymphocyte response. McCance and colleagues[9] differentiate immunoglobulins as all molecules that have specificity to an antigen and an antibody as one particular set of immunoglobulins with specificity against a known antigen. Immunoglobulin, or antibody, is a glycoprotein produced by B lymphocyte plasma cells in response to the presentation of an antigen. Plasma cells are B lymphocytes that have differentiated into plasma cells and memory cells from exposure to an antigen. The major classes of immunoglobulins and areas of focus in an immune response have been previously identified. Immunoglobulins are primarily responsible for the body's response to invading bacteria and viruses and provide the humoral immunity component of an immune response.

T lymphocyte response. T lymphocytes undergo differentiation on exposure to a foreign antigen, developing into subtypes of cells that may directly attack the antigen or stimulate the activation of other leukocytes. Cytotoxic T lymphocytes attack and kill antigens directly with preference for viruses or mutated cells that have become cancerous. This type of innate immunity is termed cellular or cell-mediated immunity.[3,4,8,9]

Several types of T lymphocytes (or T cells) may be classified into three primary groups: helper T cells, cytotoxic T cells, and suppressor T cells. Helper T cells (CD4 cells) comprise approximately 75% of all T lymphocytes. They help in the functions of the immune system by regulating most of the system's functions via the protein mediators, lymphokines. They help direct and encourage other T cells and also help to activate B lymphocytes. Cytotoxic T cells, also termed killer cells, directly kill foreign antigens and may kill cells of the self. Suppressor T cells suppress the function of both helper and cytotoxic T cells in order to prevent hyperimmune responses.[8]

Complement system response. The 25 primary proteins of the complement system contribute to an immune response by amplifying and increasing the efficiency and efficacy of the other components of the immune system. The complement system also contributes to the inflammatory response, which will be discussed in Concept 21. The primary activities resulting from activation of the complement cascade include increasing bacterial susceptibility to phagocytosis, lysing some types of bacteria and foreign antigens, producing chemotactic substances, increasing vascular permeability, and increasing smooth muscle contraction.[20]

Dendritic Cell Function in an Immune Response

Dendritic cells were discovered about 35 years ago and have come to be recognized as potent cells in asserting control from initiation to termination of the immune response. Dendritic cells have a "sentinel" function throughout the body as they look for foreign antigens and alert lymphocytes to the presence of injury or infection. They are also considered *antigen presenting cells;* they bind to antigens and then process and present them to both B and T lymphocytes in an immune response. They have been found to directly activate helper and killer T cells and present cancer cells to cytotoxic T cells, which respond by killing mutant cells.[21-25]

Suppressed Immune Response

An inadequately functioning immune system leaves the individual immunocompromised. When an individual is immunocompromised, all body systems may be affected. An individual may be immunocompromised because of a dysfunctional immune system or may be induced to an immunocompromised status by medication or treatment for other diseases.

Consequences

A depressed immune system may be created with medication in order to avoid rejection of transplanted tissue or it may be induced as a result of treatment for various types of cancer. In the treatment of some types of leukemia, destruction of the bone marrow is necessary before healthy stem cells may be reintroduced and a healthy immune system regrows. Throughout the treatment process, the immune system is partially destroyed, leaving the individual immunocompromised. Conversely, some cancers such as multiple myeloma, Hodgkin's disease, and non-Hodgkin's lymphomas may directly lead to immune system dysfunction and immunocompromise. Cancer, particularly in the elderly, has been associated with an immunocompromised state and a diminished ability to recognize and destroy mutant cells.

Primary immunodeficiency (PI) is a situation wherein the entire immune defense system is inadequate and the individual is missing some, if not all, of the components necessary for a complete immune response. The National Institutes of Health (NIH) has identified more than 70 different types of immunodeficiencies.[26-28] Ten warning signs of primary immunodeficiency were also identified by the NIH with PI suspected if two or more of the signs are evident.[29] The 10 warning signs include the following: 4 or more new ear infections within 1 year; 2 or more serious sinus infections within 1 year; 2 or more months taking antibiotics with little effect; 2 or more pneumonias within 1 year; failure of an infant to gain weight or grow normally; recurrent, deep skin or organ abscesses; persistent thrush in mouth or fungal infection on skin; need for intravenous antibiotics to clear infections; 2 or more deep-seated infections including septicemia; and a family history of primary immunodeficiency. Common variable immunodeficiency is one of the most prevalent PI diseases and is manifest with a defect in antibody formation following a defect in B lymphocytes that interferes with the ability of the cells to differentiate into plasma (antibody-producing) cells.[15]

A number of other health problems develop for the immunocompromised individual. Some problems include an increase in the incidence of infection by bacteria and viruses, the development of superinfections such as methicillin-resistant *Staphylococcus aureus* (MRSA) or *Clostridium difficile* (*C. difficile* or *C. diff.*), or the development of treatment-resistant fungal infections secondary to antibiotic treatment for primary bacterial infections.[30-33]

Exaggerated Immune Response

An exaggerated immune response will generally be classified as one of four classes of hypersensitivity disorders: type I, IgE-mediated or atopic ("allergic"); type II, tissue-specific or

TABLE 20-1   IMMUNOLOGIC MECHANISMS OF TISSUE DESTRUCTION

TYPE	NAME	RATE OF DEVELOPMENT	CLASS OF ANTIBODY INVOLVED	PRINCIPAL EFFECTOR CELLS INVOLVED	COMPLEMENT PARTICIPATION	EXAMPLES OF DISORDERS
I	IgE-mediated reaction*	Immediate	IgE	Mast cells	No	Seasonal allergic rhinitis
II	Tissue-specific reaction	Immediate	IgG IgM	Macrophages in tissues	Frequently	Autoimmune thrombocytopenic purpura, Graves' disease, autoimmune hemolytic anemia
III	Immune complex–mediated reaction	Immediate	IgG IgM	Neutrophils	Yes	Systemic lupus erythematosus
IV	Cell-mediated reaction	Delayed	None	Lymphocytes, macrophages	No	Contact sensitivity to poison ivy and metals (jewelry)

*Ig, Immunoglobulin.

From McCance KL, Huether SE: *Pathophysiology: the biologic basis for disease in adults and children,* ed 6, St Louis, 2010, Mosby/Elsevier.

cytotoxic; type III, immune complex–mediated; and type IV, cell-mediated or delayed hypersensitivity. Copstead and Banasik define hypersensitivity as "a normal immune response that is inappropriately triggered or excessive, or produces undesirable effects on the body."[34] The pathology associated with hypersensitivity reactions is summarized in Table 20-1.

Hypersensitivity Reactions

Exaggerated immune responses may be localized or they may affect all body systems. A bee sting may cause a localized type I allergic reaction or it may cause a systemic anaphylactic reaction. Systemic anaphylactic reactions caused by a number of foreign antigens are also considered type I hypersensitivity reactions. Type II tissue-specific reactions may lead to myasthenia gravis, hyperacute graft rejection with transplanted tissues, or autoimmune-based hemolytic anemia. Type III immune complex–mediated responses are the basis for rheumatoid arthritis or systemic lupus erythematosus (SLE). Type IV cell-mediated responses are seen with delayed transplant grant rejection or poison ivy allergic responses.[9,10,18,35]

Consequences

Multisystem or singular bodywide system disease may result from an initiating hypersensitivity response. Cardiovascular diseases may emerge as a consequence of autoimmune disorders such as Graves' disease or SLE. Renal failure may result from chronic glomerulonephritis or polycystic kidney disease. HIV disease weakens the immune system and a variety of opportunistic diseases and infections will ultimately result.[36]

Autoimmune disorders occur when the immune system attacks and destroys healthy cells of the self following a breakdown of what has been termed "self tolerance." With more than 80 autoimmune disorders already identified, an individual may have more than 1 autoimmune disorder simultaneously.[37] This type of immune disorder is associated with three potential outcomes: destruction of one or more types of body tissues, abnormal organ growth, or changes in organ function. The degree of destruction and functional loss varies dramatically and depends on the type of immune disorder, age, overall physical and nutritional health, and treatment options. Some of the more commonly occurring autoimmune diseases include rheumatoid arthritis, systemic lupus erythematosus, muscular sclerosis, Graves' disease, and diabetes mellitus. Genetic predisposition is an important factor in the development of autoimmune diseases with manifestation of the disease often associated with some type of environmental trigger such as bacterial or viral infections or physiologic or environmental stressors.[8,9,34]

ASSESSMENT

Assessment of immune disorders and dysfunction begins with a thorough health history and physical examination. Basic laboratory and diagnostic testing procedures are followed with more specific tests depending on the individual's history and current presenting symptoms. Genetic testing may also be important to confirm a diagnosis, to determine appropriate counseling concerning the person's prognosis, or to make reproduction recommendations.

History

The health history is useful to determine a patient's risk for an altered immune response and to determine if symptoms are described that link to problems with the immune system. The history should include current and past medical problems including treatments, especially the presence of conditions associated with immune problems (see Box 20-1). The patient should be asked about allergies to substances including the response that occurs with exposure. Also included are current medications taken by the patient and the vaccination history. It is also important to ask questions related to general health status including energy levels, nutritional status including normal dietary intake, and recent changes in weight and wound healing. Associated health topics of concern include health problems during pregnancy, conditions causing significant or consistent psychologic stress, exposure to environmental agents or stressors, physical trauma, and a history of exposure to microorganisms that may cause immunosuppression (Epstein-Barr virus, human immunodeficiency virus, cytomegalovirus, herpes simplex virus type 6, or hepatitis B virus among others).

Examination Findings

Examination findings indicative of immune status are presented from the perspective of normal (optimal) immune functioning, suppressed immune functioning, and exaggerated immune functioning.

Clinical Findings Indicative of Optimal Immune Functioning

Clinical indicators of optimal immune functioning reveal an individual who generally appears well and is well nourished. Vital signs are within normal parameters for age; lymph nodes should be soft, movable, and nontender (although lymph nodes are often not palpable among older adults). Wounds that may be present are healing within a timeframe normal for the type of wound.

Clinical Findings Indicative of Suppressed Immune Functioning

Clinical indicators of suppressed immune functioning may be mild or widespread, and may be indicative of impending immune system failure. Vital signs may or may not be within normal parameters for age depending on the amount of suppression and the degree to which the host is immunocompromised. The individual will generally not appear to be well nourished, may present with weight loss or wasting syndrome, and may complain of generalized fatigue or malaise. Impaired wound healing is present and with sufficient immune system suppression opportunistic infections and diseases may also be present. As a result of inflammation and infection within the central nervous system, psychologic evaluation should be included because it may disclose a change in cognitive functioning or depression. The presence of seizure activity or changes in motor behavior should also be determined. Should the individual present with clinical manifestations indicating significant immunocompromise, a more thorough evaluation for the presence of clinical manifestations related to specific opportunistic infections and diseases would be appropriate.

Clinical Findings Indicative of Exaggerated Immune Functioning

Clinical findings associated with an allergic response may vary from typical mild symptoms (sneezing, watery eyes, and nasal congestion) to severe responses (rashes, swelling, and shock syndrome). They may produce a minor decrease in quality of life or be life threatening.

Clinical manifestations of autoimmune disorders are often vague and less obvious while often affecting multiple organ systems. Symptoms may become apparent when systems become impacted. For example, cardiovascular symptoms may include pericarditis, congestive heart failure, pulmonary or peripheral edema, and anemia. Renal symptoms will range from no symptoms to glomerulonephritis and from acute to chronic renal failure and end-stage renal disease. Musculoskeletal manifestations can include joint pain or the inability to control movements, including walking, as seen with multiple sclerosis. Some autoimmune disorders have classic findings. For example, a subtle butterfly rash across the nose and cheeks is a common finding associated with systemic lupus erythematosus.

Laboratory and Diagnostic Testing
Primary Testing

Laboratory and diagnostic testing begins with basic blood tests to determine red blood cell and white blood cell counts with differential evaluation. A fluorescent antinuclear antibody (FANA) test is standard in the evaluation of potential autoimmune diseases. Screening tests—C-reactive protein (CRP) and erythrocyte sedimentation rate (ESR)—may also be completed. CRP is used to determine inflammation in the body and not to diagnose a specific immune dysfunction. It may also be used to follow the progress of and response to treatment for diseases such as rheumatoid arthritis, systemic lupus erythematosus, and other autoimmune disorders. An ESR is useful in monitoring inflammatory or cancerous diseases, rheumatoid arthritis and other autoimmune diseases, and tuberculosis.[38-40]

Allergy Testing

Allergy testing is often important in diagnosis and it may necessitate a skin test, an allergen-specific immunoglobulin (IgE) blood test, or both. Skin testing helps determine allergens to which the individual is sensitive and the IgE blood test measures the amount of IgE in the blood— higher levels are associated with a more severe allergic response. Circulating blood levels of immunoglobulin M and A (IgM and IgA) may also be measured.

Advanced or Disease-Specific Testing

More specific blood testing includes cytogenic analysis to detect chromosomal instability, indicative of chromosomal disorders, DNA analysis to detect genetic mutations, and enzyme-linked immunosorbent assay (ELISA) to determine blood levels of IgG subclasses and diagnose IgG deficiency. T lymphocyte levels and proliferative response to antigen introduction testing aids in determining T cell capacity in an immune response and provides another avenue for information. Rheumatoid factor (RF) is a blood test to determine the presence of antibodies against immunoglobulins and is evaluated in combination with other blood tests on the immune system.[2,41] The ELISA and confirmatory Western blot tests are done to confirm the presence of antibodies to HIV infection. The TORCH antibody panel looks for the presence of antibodies to cytomegalovirus, herpes simplex, rubella, and toxoplasmosis.[41] Complement system testing is done to determine the presence of deficiencies or abnormalities in complement proteins, addressing both quality and activity of the proteins. Deficiencies contribute to increased incidence and severity of infections and autoimmune dysfunction.

Test of Organ Function

Tests of organ function are often performed to aid in assessing specific organ function or to monitor the effectiveness of treatment regimens. These tests include hemoglobin A_{1c} levels in diabetes mellitus management, hepatic function tests, or thyroid screening panels. In most cases, serial laboratory testing is recommended to assess both progression of disease and effectiveness of treatment strategies.

CLINICAL MANAGEMENT

The clinical management of individuals with immunosuppression or hyperimmune conditions varies widely depending on the type of condition, severity, and attribute variables such as age, health status, and underlying medical conditions. Such variables must be considered when making clinical management decisions.

Primary Prevention

The cornerstone of primary prevention for immune system disorders is based on recommended vaccinations across the lifespan. The Centers for Disease Control and Prevention's (CDC) Advisory Committee on Immunization Practices (ACIP) has established recommended vaccination schedules for children (birth to 6 years), adolescents (7 to 18 years), a "catch-up" schedule (4 months to 18 years), and adults (over 18 years). An additional schedule for teens and adolescents (beginning with the child's 11- to 12-year checkup or as soon thereafter as possible) was also established and is particularly targeting teens and college students. All of the schedules and updates can be accessed at www.cdc.gov/vaccines/recs/schedules/child-schedule.htm.

Primary prevention also includes reduction of modifiable risk factors noted earlier in this concept analysis. This includes avoiding high-risk behaviors, minimizing exposure to environmental triggers, eating a proper diet, and engaging in regular exercise. Research has demonstrated that achieving the daily recommended doses of vitamins and minerals contributes to a properly functioning immune system. New research is addressing the role of vitamins A and D in protecting and supporting the immune response and may serve a valuable contribution to many medical treatment regimens in addition to their usefulness in one's daily diet for health maintenance.[8,9]

Secondary Prevention (Screening)

Secondary prevention focuses on screenings for the presence or emergence of immune system disorders. There are few screenings specifically directed at immune system dysfunction for the general public. However, some screenings (such as HIV screening) are recommended for high-risk groups.

MODEL CASE

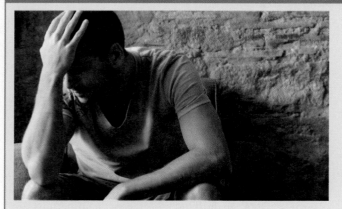

Jonathan Eckert is a 22-year-old white male who has been involved in a number of high-risk sexual behaviors. Three months ago he developed a 4-day course of fever and chills, malaise, lethargy, night sweats, diarrhea, and anorexia. He believed he had acquired the flu (influenza) and self-medicated with acetaminophen, vitamin C, and increased fluid intake. He became increasingly concerned about his health because he had friends who were infected with human immunodeficiency virus (HIV), so he contacted his primary care provider to obtain a blood screening test for HIV and hepatitides B and C.

His screening test for hepatitides B and C was negative and the HIV screening tests—ELISA and confirmatory Western blot—both returned positive for HIV infection. Additional laboratory testing was done to assess his red blood cell (RBC) count, white blood cell (WBC) count with differential, and CD4 and CD8 lymphocyte counts (lymphocyte immunophenotyping). All of his blood tests were within the normal range. A skin test for tuberculosis (TB) returned negative and a chest x-ray was unremarkable.

Jonathan has developed an infection with HIV and is currently asymptomatic. His immune system has responded to the pathogen invasion by producing antibodies to the virus and cytotoxic T lymphocytes are also responding to the viral infection. At this time, he is not a candidate for highly active antiretroviral therapy (HAART); however, he must continue to monitor his immune functioning. He was given information on, and demonstrated understanding of, the need to maintain a healthy lifestyle with appropriate nutrition, physical activity, stress management, avoidance of cigarettes and other forms of tobacco, maintenance of appropriate vaccinations including an annual influenza vaccination, and adherence to safer sexual practices to avoid reinfection with a potentially more virulent strain of the virus and transmission of the virus to others. He was given information on community support groups and a referral to a care provider specializing in HIV/AIDS care.

Collaborative Interventions

Collaborative treatment strategies vary depending on whether the immune dysfunction is one of deficiency or an exaggerated response. Thus interventions may range from supporting an inadequate immune response or diminishing the consequences of an exaggerated response. An overview of selected clinical management strategies for the treatment of immune system diseases or dysfunction is found in Table 20-2.

INTERRELATED CONCEPTS

The concept of **Immunity** is closely related to the concepts of **Inflammation** and **Infection.** There exists overlap among the concepts in the areas of pathology, laboratory and diagnostic tests, clinical manifestations, nursing interventions, and clinical outcomes. A discussion of the concepts inflammation and infection is found in Concepts 21 and 22, respectively. **Tissue integrity** is also closely aligned to immunity because a defect in tissue integrity will cause the body to invoke an immune response and may lead to both inflammation and infection. **Stress** has been discussed as a pathologic influence that both may initiate an immune response and may lead to immune dysfunction. Both inadequate nutrition and extreme or prolonged fatigue are stressors to the body, either of which may cause the individual to become immunocompromised, or cause the individual to have an exaggerated preexisting immune response. These concepts were previously discussed as methods by which an individual may become immunocompromised.

TABLE 20-2   INTERVENTIONS IN THE CLINICAL MANAGEMENT OF IMMUNE DYSFUNCTION

MANAGEMENT OF CLINICAL MANIFESTATIONS	CLINICAL OUTCOMES
Suppressed Immune Response	
Infection	
• Clinical management of infection and opportunistic diseases is typically an important part of clinical care; interventions and clinical outcomes are discussed in Concept 22: Infection	• Normal GI transit time • Resolution of infection • Adequate hydration • Adequate nutrition
Gastrointestinal Dysfunction	• Resolution of skin rash
• Pharmacologic treatment of diarrhea, candidiasis, and fluid and electrolyte loss	• Restoration of adequate nutrition, body weight, and BMI
Skin Disorders	
• Pharmacologic treatment of skin rash	
Nutrition	
• Multiple vitamin and mineral supplements • Dietary supplements such as Ensure or equivalent • Evaluation of weight and BMI*	
Exaggerated Immune Response	
Anaphylaxis	
• Support of airway, breathing, and circulation: subcutaneous epinephrine if type 1 reaction; other bronchodilators; intubation and ventilator support, circulatory volume expanders, and vasopressors to maintain blood pressure and circulating volume • Pharmacotherapy: epinephrine and bronchodilators as described above • Education: avoiding contact with pathogen initiating anaphylactic response; proper use of an EpiPen for self-administration of epinephrine	• Adequate ventilation • Restoration of blood pressure and pulse to prereaction normal levels • Adequate urine output indicating adequate circulatory volume • Modulation of hypersensitivity responses • Management of pain experience • Maintenance of joint and muscle mobility; self-care for ADLs‡ where possible; restoration or maintenance of adequate levels of physical activity
Immunosuppression	
• Pharmacotherapy: corticosteroids, chemotherapeutic agents, NSAIDs,† immunomodulators	
Pain Management	
• Pharmacotherapy: NSAIDs, corticosteroids • Hypothermia or hyperthermia treatments as appropriate • Maintenance of mobility and physical activity	

*BMI = Body mass index.
†NSAIDs = Nonsteroidal antiinflammatory drugs.
‡ADLs = Activities of daily living.

EXEMPLARS

Examples of diseases that may develop with immune system diseases represent cases of just B or T lymphocyte dysfunction, hypersensitivity reactions, complement dysfunction, or dysfunction of more than one component. Many examples have been introduced throughout this unit. Box 20-1 provides a brief overview of some of the more common diseases that may lead to immunocompromise.

When considering an immune response, it is most important to remember that the response is a complex interaction between a foreign antigen and a wide variety of differing cells and is also dependent on genetic, environmental, and overall health parameters that are unique to each individual. The presence and progress of immune responses and the development of immunocompromise is unique to each individual and requires a thorough review of health history, presenting symptoms, and laboratory and diagnostic data when determining nursing care strategies.

BOX 20-1 EXEMPLARS OF IMMUNITY

Suppressed Immune Response
- Classic complement pathway deficiency
- Deficiencies of immunoglobulin A, G, D, or M
- DiGeorge syndrome
- Hodgkin's and non-Hodgkin's lymphoma
- Human immunodeficiency virus (HIV)
- Plasma cell disorders
- Primary immunodeficiency
- Severe combined immunodeficiency

Exaggerated Immune Response

Allergic Responses
- Allergic reaction
- Allergic rhinitis

Autoimmune Responses
- Anaphylaxis
- Autoimmune thrombocytopenic purpura
- Crohn's disease
- Diabetes mellitus (type 1, insulin-dependent)
- Glomerulonephritis
- Graves' disease
- Multiple sclerosis
- Myasthenia gravis
- Rheumatoid arthritis
- Systemic lupus erythematosus
- Ulcerative colitis

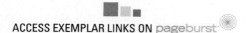

ACCESS EXEMPLAR LINKS ON pageburst

REFERENCES

1. Mosby: *Dictionary of medicine, nursing, and health professions*, ed 8, St Louis, 2009, Mosby/Elsevier.
2. Taber: *Cyclopedic medical dictionary*, ed 21, Philadelphia, 2009, FA Davis.
3. National Institutes of Health: *Immune system*, 2008. at www.niaid.ni.gov/topics/immuneSystem/pages/whatisimmunesystem.aspx. Accessed Sept 20, 2010.
4. National Cancer Institute: *Understanding the immune system*, 2006. at http://cancer.gov/cancertopics/understandingcancer. Accessed Sept 20, 2010.
5. Centers for Disease Control and Prevention: *Immunity types*, 2009. at www.cdc.gov/vaccines/vacgen/immunity-types.htm. Accessed Sept 15, 2010.
6. National Institutes of Health: *U.S. National Library of Medicine: Immune response*, 2010. at www.nlm.nih.gov/medlineplus/ency/article/000821.htm. Accessed Sept 15, 2010.
7. University of Hartford: *Immune System*, 2001. at http://whaweb.hartford.edu/BUGL/immune.htm. Accessed Sept 15, 2010.
8. Hall JE: *Textbook of medical physiology*, ed 12, Philadelphia, 2011, Saunders/Elsevier.
9. McCance KL, Huether SE: *Pathophysiology: the biologic basis for disease in adults and children*, ed 6, St Louis, 2010, Mosby/Elsevier.
10. National Institutes of Health: *National Institute of Allergy and Infectious Diseases: Immune system, disorders of the immune system*, 2008. at www.niaid.nih.gov/topics/immuneSystem/Pages/disorders.aspx. Accessed Sept 20, 2010.
11. National Institutes of Health: *U.S. National Library of Medicine: Aging changes in immunity*, 2008. at www.nlm.nih.gov/medlineplus/ency/article/004008.htm. Accessed Sept 15, 2010.
12. Burns CE, Dunn AM, Brady MA, et al: *Pediatric primary care*, ed 4, St Louis, 2009, Saunders/Elsevier.
13. Arizona Center for Advanced Medicine: *Immune system dysfunction*, 2009. at http://arizonaadvancedmedicine.com/articles/immune_system_dysfunction.html. Accessed Nov 30, 2010.
14. Chaganti RK, Schwartz RA: *Complement deficiencies*, 2009. at http://emedicine.medscape.com/article/135478. Accessed Nov 30, 2010.
15. Park CL: *Common variable immunodeficiency*, 2010. at http://emedicine.medscape.com/article/885935. Accessed Nov 30, 2010.
16. Centers for Disease Control and Prevention: *Cancer, the flu, and you*, 2010. at www.cdc.gov/cancer/flu. Accessed Nov 15, 2010.
17. Nolan D, Gaudieri S, Mallal S: Host genetics and viral infections: immunology taught by viruses, virology taught by the immune system, *Cur Opin Immunol* 18, 2006.
18. Winfield JB: *Fibromyalgia*, 2010. at www.emedicine.medscape.com/article/329838-overview. Accessed Nov 1, 2010.
19. Waldschmidt TJ, Cook RT, Kovacs EJ: Alcohol and inflammation and immune responses: summary of the 2006 Alcohol and Immunology Research Interest Group (AIRIG) meeting, *Alcohol* 42, 2007.
20. Fix D: *Components and functions of the complement system*, 2010. at www.cehs.siu.edu/fix/medmicro/cment.htm. Accessed Nov 30, 2010.
21. Steinman R: *Introduction to dendritic cells*, 2009. at www.lab.rockefeller.edu/steinman. Accessed Nov 30, 2010.
22. Steinman R: *Dendritic cells initiate the immune response*, 2009. at www.lab.rockefeller.edu/steinman/dendritic_intro/immune Response. Accessed Nov 30, 2010.

23. Steinman R: *Dendritic cells and immune tolerance*, 2009. at www.lab.rockefeller.edu/steinman/dendritic_intro/immuneTol erance. Accessed Nov 30, 2010.

24. Leon B, Ardavin C: Monocyte-derived dendritic cells in innate and adaptive immunity, *Immunol Cell Biol* 86, 2008.

25. Maason F, Mount AM, Wilson NS, et al: Dendritic cells: driving the differentiation programme of T cells in viral infections, *Immun Cell Biol* 86, 2008.

26. National Institutes of Health: *National Institute of Child Health & Human Development: Primary immunodeficiency*, 2008, at www.nichd, nih.gov/publications/pubs/primary_immuno.cfm. Accessed Sept 15, 2010.

27. National Institutes of Health: *U.S. National Library of Medicine: Immune system and disorders*, 2010, at www.nlm.nih.gov/ medlineplus/immunesystemanddisorders.html. Accessed Dec 9, 2010.

28. National Institutes of Health: *U.S. National Library of Medicine: Immunodeficiency disorders*, 2010, at www.lm.jih.gov/medl ineplus/ency/article/000818.htm. Accessed Sept 15, 2010.

29. National Primary Immunodeficiency Resource Center: *10 Warning signs of primary immunodeficiency*, 2009, at http:// info4pi.org/aboutPI/index.cfm?section=aboutPI&content= warningsigns. Accessed Dec 9, 2010.

30. Mayo Clinic: *MRSA infection*, 2010. at www.mayoclinic.com/ health/mrsa/DS00735. Accessed Oct 12, 2010.

31. Davis C: *MRSA infection*, 2008, at www.emedicinehealth.com/ script/main/art.asp?articlekey=86302&. Accessed Oct 12, 2010.

32. Mayo Clinic: *C. difficile*, 2010, at www.mayoclinic.com/health/ c-difficile/DS00736. Accessed Dec 12, 2010.

33. Centers for Disease Control and Prevention: *Clostridium difficile infection*, 2010, at www.cdc.gov/HAi/organisms/cdiff/ Cdiff_infect.html. Accessed Dec 12, 2010.

34. Copstead LC, Banasik JL: *Pathophysiology*, ed 4, St Louis, 2010, Saunders/Elsevier.

35. Heib V, Becker M, Taube C, et al: Advances in the understanding of mast cell function, *Br J Haematol* 142, 2008.

36. Iwami S, Miura T, Nakaoka S, et al: Immune impairment in HIV infection: existence of frisky and immunodeficiency thresholds, *J Theoret Biol* 260, 2009.

37. National Institutes of Health: *U.S. National Library of Medicine: Autoimmune disorders*, 2009, at www.nlm.jih.gov/medline plus/ency/article/000816.htm. Accessed Sept 15, 2010.

38. Shiel WC: *Antinuclear antibody test (ANA)*, 2010, at www. medicinenet.com/script/main/art.asp?articlekey-7083. Accessed Dec 12, 2010.

39. National Institutes of Health: *U.S. National Library of Medicine: ESR*, 2009, at www.nlm.nih.gov/medlineplus/ency/article/ 003638.htm. Accessed Dec 12, 2010.

40. National Institutes of Health: *U.S. National Library of Medicine: C-reactive protein*, 2009, at www.nlm.nih.gov/medlineplus/ ency/article/003356.htm. Accessed Dec 12, 2010.

41. Pagana KD, Pagana TJ: *Diagnostic and laboratory test reference*, ed 8, St Louis, 2010, Mosby/Elsevier.

Inflammation

Carolyn E. Sabo

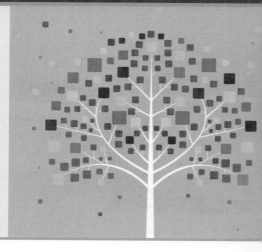

Inflammation is a normal and expected physiologic response to cellular injury. The response is protective in that it provides an opportunity for the body to heal and repair the injury. This biophysical concept is foundational to patient care across the lifespan.

DEFINITION(S)

The term inflammation is derived from the Latin "inflammare"—to set on fire. As a concept, inflammation is defined as *an immunologic defense against tissue injury, infection, or allergy*. It is a protective process initiated to minimize or remove the pathologic agent or stimuli triggering the inflammation and to promote healing. Although inflammation is always present with infection, inflammation often occurs in the absence of infection. Inflammation is the body's physiologic response to injury—not the agent causing the injury as is seen with infection. The inflammatory process is very similar regardless of the cause of cellular injury; however, there is variability in the degree of response depending on the severity and scope of injury and the physiologic capacity of the affected individual.[1-7]

The inflammatory process produces four potential outcomes.[6-9]

1. The first outcome is divided into two parts. First, a period of acute inflammation ensues, which is the initial response to tissue damage. This response is nonspecific and focuses on eradicating dead tissue, promoting an immune response, and protecting against infection. A period of restitution follows wherein the damaged tissue is replaced by identical functioning tissue created by removing the injurious agent/pathogen and allowing cells to regenerate. This is the optimal and desirable outcome of an inflammatory response.
2. A second outcome is fibrous repair of the damaged tissue and the formation of scar tissue. In this scenario, the damaged cells are unable to repair with functioning cells and nonspecialized fibrous tissue is produced. This outcome is most commonly seen in the presence of substantial tissue damage.
3. The third outcome is the development of chronic inflammation. The pathologic agent remains active despite an initial inflammatory and immune response. Tissue destruction continues and is associated with repeated attempts at immune system resolution with consequent continued production of fibrous scar tissue rather than newly generated functioning tissue. This outcome is associated with increased incidence of morbidity and mortality.
4. The fourth potential outcome is initial death of tissue and ultimately death of the host.

SCOPE AND CATEGORIES

The categories of inflammation can be classified as acute, chronic, or repair/restorative. An initial injury leading to an inflammatory response may be from various sources, including mechanical trauma (e.g., laceration, splinter, crushing); thermal, electrical, or chemical injury; radiation damage; or biological assault (viral, bacterial, or fungal infections). The role of an acute inflammatory response is to eradicate the harmful stimuli from the body and initiate repair. Chronic inflammation may be a complication of the inflammatory process, not allowing for repair, or it may be a consequence of disease, as seen in rheumatoid arthritis.[1-11]

Acute Inflammation

Acute inflammation is the immediate response to tissue injury and is short in duration (minutes to days). It is characterized by five cardinal signs: redness (rubor), swelling (fumor), heat (calsor), pain (dolor), and loss of function (functio laesa). It is also associated with three physiologic changes: increased blood flow (hyperemia); increased vascular permeability; and migration of leukocytes from the blood to the tissues (diapedesis or extravasation).[9,10,12-14] Immediately after an injury, exudate moves from the vascular system to the area of injury. Exudate carries proteins, fluid, lymphocytes, monocytes, macrophages, granulocytes, and complement proteins. The various cells in the exudate work to eradicate the pathologic organism, remove tissue debris, secrete cytokines, and initiate healing. In an acute inflammatory response, neutrophils will appear first in the greatest numbers and are followed by macrophages. A subclass of cytokines, the leukotrienes or interleukins, is important in modulating activity to ensure that the immune response does not become excessive and destroy healthy tissue surrounding the site of injury. The different components of the immune response are mediated by different chemical signals that promote selective aspects of the immune response, are overlapping in areas of control, and serve to ensure that both the immune and the inflammatory responses cease when the invading pathogen has been eradicated and repair is initiated.[9,12,14,15] The physiologic processes will be described in more detail later in this concept.

Chronic Inflammation

Inflammation that continues for weeks to years after initial injury is termed chronic; tissue is repeatedly being destroyed and repaired, thus impairing healing. The response is out of proportion to the stimulus or is directed against an inappropriate target. Localized chronic inflammation will result in the formation of a granuloma—an accumulation of macrophages, fibroblasts, and collagen—as seen with untreated *Mycobacterium tuberculosis*. Systemic chronic inflammation may result from many diseases or may be the consequence of disease processes, including autoimmune diseases such as the inflammatory bowel diseases ulcerative colitis (UC) and Crohn's disease.[4] The pathologic processes associated with chronic inflammation will be explained in more detail later in this concept.

RISK FACTORS

Populations at Risk

Individuals of all ages, genders, ethnic and socioeconomic groups, geographic location, and prior health history are susceptible to an acute or chronic inflammatory process. Age plays a role in the development of more severe inflammatory responses. For the very young, an immature immune system may provide a foundation for a more severe inflammatory response because the immune system is unable to control a minor pathogen and infection may be severe. For the elderly, the immune system becomes less able to respond to foreign pathogens, resulting in a stronger inflammatory response than might have been encountered earlier in life. Those who are uninsured or underinsured are at increased risk because they may not have access to sufficient or early health care intervention and a comparatively simple inflammatory response to injury may escalate to one with more severe injury or to a chronic inflammatory state.

Individual Risk Factors

Individual risk factors for an inflammatory response include the presence of autoimmune diseases and allergies, exposure to pathogens with or without resultant infection, and being very young or elderly with a compromised immune system. Genetics plays a role in the emergence of chronic inflammatory processes because many autoimmune diseases have a genetic basis for predisposition and involve an inflammatory response. Certain chronic disease processes such as atherosclerosis, rheumatoid arthritis, diabetes mellitus, and cancer may lead to or be the result of chronic inflammation. Research is also underway evaluating the role of obesity and vitamin D and magnesium deficiency in the development of chronic inflammation.[2-4,16-21]

Any process that weakens the immune system increases the potential for what might have been a mild inflammatory response to develop into an acute severe inflammation or chronic inflammatory process.[22,23] The absence of effective hand hygiene procedures, the sharing of personal hygiene or grooming material and equipment, poor sanitation, poor nutrition, and living or congregating in tight spaces with large numbers of people increase the risk for infection and accompanying inflammation. Within the health care system, the absence of effective use of Standard Precautions increases the individual's risk for infection and an inflammatory response. Environmental factors, such as pollution and smoking or exposure to repeated trauma, also increase the risk of stimulating an inflammatory response.

PHYSIOLOGIC PROCESSES AND CONSEQUENCES

The functioning of the immune system and the primary activities of an immune response, both acute and chronic, were presented in Concept 20: Immunity. An inflammatory response is often directly linked to the activities of the immune system, demonstrating an overlap and interplay of physiologic processes between the two systems (immune and inflammatory) providing protection to the host. It has also been noted that an inflammatory process has two primary functions directed at a positive outcome for the individual: (1) restitution of normal functioning cells following injury or (2) fibrous repair when functional cells cannot be restored. Negative consequences of an inflammatory response are also possible and may include an overly severe immune response to stimuli resulting in additional tissue damage or an inadequate response leading to infection or chronic inflammation and illness.

Inflammation is a process involving white blood cells (WBCs) and a number of different chemicals that serve to protect the body against invading pathogens or cellular/tissue trauma. White blood cells are attracted to an area of inflammation by chemotaxis. Chemotaxis is a complex process involving more than a dozen different chemicals whose release is initiated by stimuli that may generally be placed into four categories: (1) bacterial or viral exotoxins; (2) degenerative by-products of inflammation; (3) products of complement system activation; and (4) reactive products of plasma clotting in the inflamed area.

Pro-inflammatory hormones are mediating factors in the inflammatory response and are critical to the effective implementation of the response. There are three major hormone groups: prostaglandins, cytokines, and histamines. In general, the pro-inflammatory hormones increase blood flow to the injured area, increase vascular membrane permeability, activate various components of an immune response including the

TABLE 21-1　**EFFECTS OF PRO-INFLAMMATORY MEDIATORS**

PRO-INFLAMMATORY FACTOR	SOURCE	EFFECT ON INFLAMMATORY RESPONSE
Prostaglandins Leukotrienes	Phospholipids from mast cell and other cell membranes; derived from arachidonic acid in cell membrane	Mediate late stages of acute inflammatory response Increase vasodilation Increase vascular permeability Active in anaphylactic hypersensitivity reactions
Bradykinins	Plasma protein Kinins	Increase vascular permeability Increase vasodilation Responsible for pain production
Complement proteins	Macrophages Liver endothelium	Primarily from proteins C3a, C4a, and C5a: initiate chemotaxis of neutrophils and macrophages Activate mast cells and basophils to release histamine, heparin, and other chemicals Result in increased blood flow, increased vascular permeability, and leaking of plasma proteins to extracellular fluid
Histamine Serotonin	Mast cells Basophils	Mediates early acute inflammatory response Increases vasodilation Increases vascular permeability
Interleukin-1 (IL-1)	Macrophages Neutrophils B lymphocytes Dendritic cells Other antigen-presenting cells (APCs)	Promotes T lymphocyte proliferation and differentiation Promotes release of acute-phase inflammatory proteins Promotes neutrophil adhesion to endothelial cell walls Promotes development of fever
Interleukin-8 (IL-8)	T lymphocytes Monocytes (blood) Macrophages (tissue)	Chemotaxic factor for neutrophils Chemotaxic factor for T lymphocytes
Interleukin-17 (IL-17)	Helper T lymphocytes (Th17 cells)	Increases chemotaxis of neutrophils Increases chemotaxis of macrophages Increases epithelial cell chemokine production
Platelet-activating factor	Platelets	Promotes secretion of chemical mediators Promotes vasodilation and increased permeability Activates neutrophils
Transforming growth factor-beta (TGF-β)	T lymphocytes Activated macrophages Fibroblasts	Inhibits T and B lymphocyte activity Chemotaxic factor for macrophages Increases macrophage IL-1 production Inhibits macrophages
Tumor necrosis factor-alpha (TNF-α)	Activated macrocytes Selected lymphocytes	Promotes cellular proliferation Increases phagocytosis Increases leukocytosis Induces fever Promotes neutrophil adhesion to endothelial cell walls Toxic to some tumor cells

Adapted from Taber: *Cyclopedic medical dictionary*, ed 21, p 1189, Philadelphia, 2009, FA Davis; Hall JE: *Textbook of medical physiology*, ed 12, Philadelphia, 2011, Saunders/Elsevier; McCance KL, Huether SE, Brashers VL et al: *Pathophysiology: the biologic basis for disease in adults and children*, ed 6, p 229, St Louis, 2010, Mosby/Elsevier; Copstead LC, Banasik JL: *Pathophysiology*, ed 4, p 196, St Louis, 2010, Saunders/Elsevier.

complement system of proteins, attract leukocytes to the area of injury, promote angiogenesis, stimulate growth of connective tissue, and cause fever.[1,12] Specific actions of selected pro-inflammatory, mediating hormones are found in Table 21-1.

Acute Inflammation

The pathologic processes associated with acute inflammation are complex, yet sequential, as shown in Figure 21-1. They involve a constant interaction with various components of the immune system and are regulated by feedback systems. The primary steps in an acute inflammatory response have the following sequence:

- Injury to or death of tissue and release of chemical mediators
- Vasodilation and increased blood flow to the small vessels surrounding the area of injury

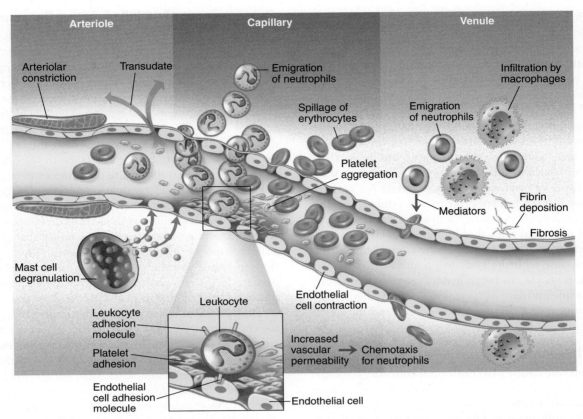

FIGURE 21-1 Acute Inflammation Response. (From McCance KL, Huether SE, Brashers VL et al: *Pathophysiology: the biologic basis for disease in adults and children*, ed 6, Fig. 6-3, p 188, St Louis, 2010, Mosby/Elsevier.)

- Swelling and partial retraction or separation of activated endothelial cells
- Increased vascular permeability and leakage of water, salts, fibrinogen (later becoming fibrin), and other small plasma proteins into the surrounding tissue
- "Walling off" of the area from surrounding tissues to delay the spread of the pathogen and toxic products from the pathogen
- Margination and emigration of polymorphonucleocytes, monocytes, lymphocytes, and macrophages (later) to the endothelial cell walls and out of the vascular system to the area of injury; margination of endothelial cell walls by neutrophils is possible because of the increased level of cellular adhesiveness created by activation of the endothelial cell
- Exudates exiting the vascular system fill spaces left by damaged, necrotic tissue
- Movement of glucose and oxygen to the area in support of removal of necrotic tissue and cellular repair
- Release of nitric oxide and prostacyclin, endothelin, thromboxane A$_2$, angiotensin II, growth factor, and chemokines from activated endothelial cells

Neutrophils are of significant importance in an acute inflammatory response. Movement of neutrophils is mediated by several chemotaxic factors that arise from the area of tissue damage. The chemotaxic factors bind to the surface of the neutrophils and cause them to release additional factors, resulting in pathogen breakdown from lysosomal cytoplasmic enzymes. The neutrophils are also directly involved in phagocytosis after they bind to antibodies already connected to the antigen. In preparation for the neutrophil, opsonization has occurred with either the antibody or the complement proteins; then neutrophil lysosomal granules can be released to begin phagocytosis. It should be noted that during the process of phagocytosis, reactive oxygen species (ROS) are created by the neutrophils and macrophages. The ROS binds with the lysosomes to help kill the invading pathogen.[10,24]

Neutrophil blood counts increase fourfold to fivefold within a few hours after the onset of acute severe inflammation, making more neutrophils available to continue the inflammatory response. Neutrophils comprise the primary WBC component of exudate created during an acute inflammatory response to bacterial invasion. Band cells, or immature neutrophils, may also be present in the blood to achieve the increased numbers of neutrophils required of the severe response. The bone marrow will also significantly increase production of both granulocytes and monocytes; however, it takes 3 to 4 days before these cells are mature and ready to leave the bone marrow.[2]

Lymphocytes are most prominent in inflammatory responses to viral antigens. They are also important in combination with monocytes and macrophages in situations of chronic inflammation. Eosinophils are most evident in inflammatory responses to parasitic infections and in association with allergic hypersensitivity immune reactions. Mast cells and basophils release histamine, which contributes to the increased vascular permeability seen in an inflammatory response.[9,15]

An acute inflammatory response may last minutes to days with the majority of activity taking place in the first 12 to 24 hours after tissue injury. The response may be localized or systemic. Localized inflammatory responses begin when damaged tissue or invading organisms activate the immune system. Complement system proteins and cytokines begin a cascading sequence of events that lead to the classic signs and symptoms associated with the immune response. Autoimmune reactions may cause systemic activation of the inflammatory response with the body being attacked by its own cells. In most people, the inflammatory response may last up to 5 days while invading pathogens are destroyed, phagocytosis of antigens and necrotic tissue occurs, and fibroblasts begin the process of tissue healing.

Chronic Inflammation

Macrophages are critical in a chronic inflammatory response. They release tissue thromboplastin to facilitate hemostasis and to promote fibroblast activity. They are instrumental in removing necrotic tissue and foreign pathogen material from the area of injury (debridement), allowing for repair and healing. Macrophages and lymphocytes will comprise the majority of the WBCs found in the exudate during a chronic inflammatory response. Unfortunately, when inflammation is chronic, healing processes may be interrupted by reinjury or renewed inflammation and immune system activity with the inflammatory cycle being reactivated.

Chronic inflammation may also be subclinical, manifesting with elevated levels of nonspecific blood markers such as C-reactive protein (CRP) or an increased erythrocyte sedimentation rate (ESR) with no obvious overt symptoms. A white blood cell scan (WBC scan), or inflammatory scan, may be required to identify areas of inflammation. Low-grade chronic inflammation has been associated with systemic manifestations including body aches and pains, frequent infections, diarrhea, dry eyes, and shortness of breath.[16,17,25,26]

Regardless of whether the inflammation is acute or chronic a number of systemic manifestations result. Localized symptoms discussed earlier in this concept analysis will depend on the degree of injury and the resistance of the host to injury. Systemic responses include neutrophilia, fever, malaise, loss of appetite, and muscle catabolism. The liver will respond by releasing a number of proteins, called acute-phase proteins, which include complement system proteins, clotting factors, and protease inhibitors. The acute-phase proteins also stimulate an increase in the level of fibrinogen, promoting hemostasis. C-Reactive protein and serum amyloid are also released by the liver. The CRP assists in opsonization of the foreign pathogen to facilitate phagocytosis.[2-4]

Consequences of an Inflammatory Response

As a collaborative function in an immune response, inflammation will help to attract lymphocytes, complement proteins, cytokines, cells to promote hemostasis, and phagocytes to the site of the immune response, which fosters resolution of the pathologic invasion, moderation of the immune response, and promotion of repair and healing. Activity from selective pro-inflammatory mediators (bradykinins) will cause stimulation of pain signals alerting the brain to danger and allowing for action to be taken to remove the host from danger or alert the host to the presence of trauma. Spinal cord injuries are an example of one type of trauma where the inflammatory response may cause significant additional tissue damage if swelling to the damaged region is not controlled. The physiologic response to injury that an inflammatory response provides, in this case with increased blood flow, increased vascular permeability, and the movement of exudate to the damaged tissue, may cause additional compression-based trauma to an already damaged spinal cord.

Excessive stimulation of the inflammatory response and the development of chronic inflammation may also be a consequence of hypersensitivity reactions by the immune system, including allergies and autoimmune diseases such as asthma, rheumatoid arthritis, multiple sclerosis, and systemic lupus erythematosus. In these diseases, an initial immune response and resultant inflammatory response trigger a sequence of cyclic physiologic responses that result in a pathologic disease process.

Systemic pathology may also result from an inflammatory response. Wisse[27] studied the metabolic effects of obesity and identified the potential role of inflammation within fat cells as a basis in generating metabolic syndrome. The role of cytokines secreted by adipose tissue in modulating an immune response and promoting a chronic inflammatory condition was discussed. Research on the role of reducing inflammation by altering selected dietary fatty acid intake and thus reducing the amount of arachidonic acid levels in cell membranes is ongoing. Because arachidonic acids play a role in the production of pro-inflammatory molecules, altering the level of this acid may influence the severity of an inflammatory response.[28] Multisystem organ failure associated with sepsis or septic shock invokes both a strong immune and a strong inflammatory response. One of the negative consequences of inflammatory activity in the presence of shock is that inflammatory mediators instigate activation of coagulation inhibitors of fibrinolysis and may cause diffuse endovascular injury, organ dysfunction, or death. Widespread inflammation may also lead to hypovolemia, pleural effusion, respiratory distress, renal failure, and death.[29-31]

Chronic inflammation has been linked to a number of systemic diseases or diseases with systemic consequences if the affected individual is compromised. In 2003, the American Heart Association (AHA) and the Centers for Disease Control and Prevention (CDC) published a joint scientific statement presenting findings suggesting the important role that inflammation plays in the development of atherosclerosis. More recent studies have discussed the role of inflammation in coronary artery calcification, a critical component in the development of coronary atherosclerosis. Silverstein discussed the relationship between chronic renal disease, the pro-inflammatory state that exists in individuals with this disease, and the need to mediate the inflammatory process to prevent consequential tissue damage.[32-34] Research is ongoing on the relationship between inflammation and blood-brain barrier dysfunction with suggestions that inflammatory challenges that occur during brain development may have consequences later in life for a variety of neurologic disorders. Similarly, inter-relationships among autoimmune diseases such as asthma and diabetes mellitus, cancer, and inflammation have been studied for years and are no longer considered theoretical.[2-4,35-40]

ASSESSMENT

As with any other pathologic process, the basis and extent of disease must be assessed in order to guide appropriate treatment interventions to either eradicate or manage inflammation, whether it is acute or chronic. Assessment of an individual for the presence of inflammation includes asking appropriate questions to elicit a history and conducting a physical examination. In addition, laboratory and diagnostic testing aids in the diagnosis. Common clinical findings associated with inflammation are featured in Table 21-2.

History

The history should be focused on determining the nature of the inflammatory trigger (e.g., recent injury, exposure to allergens, exposure to infectious agents) and the patient's physiologic ability to respond, or more specifically the risk for an ineffective inflammatory response. The nurse should also inquire about the presence of symptoms commonly associated with inflammation including swelling, pain, and fatigue. It is also important to determine the duration of the inflammatory process and the treatment measures, if any, that have already been initiated.

Examination Data

There are several classic findings associated with inflammation. Obvious trauma or minor wounds will likely appear red, be warm to the touch, and be associated with some degree of pain. Swelling may be present with or without an open wound, such as would be seen with a strained or sprained joint. Drainage or pus may be evident from a laceration or other injury where the skin or mucosal surface has been broken. Anytime an infection is evident, some degree of inflammation will also be present. Inflammation associated with an immune response, but without external trauma, will present with some combination of swelling, pain, fever, and decreased or absent functioning of the tissue or organ. Severe inflammation may be associated with shock syndrome or multiorgan failure, significant hyperthermia, seizure, coma, or death.

Laboratory and Diagnostic Data

Laboratory testing and diagnostic data collection will be determined by the clinical presentation of the individual, evidence of obvious trauma, likelihood of exposure to infection-causing pathogens, and health history particularly as related to immune dysfunction or deficiency or a history of any chronic illnesses.

Blood Tests

Blood testing for white blood cell counts with differential is helpful in determining if neutrophil, lymphocyte, or macrophage cell counts are elevated, indicating bacterial or viral infection and acute or chronic inflammation. C-Reactive protein (CRP) and erythrocyte sedimentation rate (ESR) blood testing are nonspecific tests that will confirm the presence of inflammation, though not the location or cause. Various serologic tests for viruses or antibodies against pathogens, such as hepatitis, human immunodeficiency virus (HIV), Epstein-Barr, severe acute respiratory syndrome (SARS), herpes simplex, syphilis, methicillin-resistant *Staphylococcus aureus* (MRSA), *Clostridium difficile (C. diff.)*, and *Helicobacter pylori*, among many others, will be helpful in determining the cause of inflammation and guide treatment regimens to eradicate or control infection and minimize damage from inflammation.[26]

Radiographic and Other Testing

Computer-assisted tomography (CT), magnetic resonance imaging (MRI), proton emission tomography (PET) scans, or a colonoscopy is useful in determining the location and extent of inflammation within the body.

CLINICAL MANAGEMENT

Primary Prevention

Preventing inflammation is directed at reducing risk for injury and infection. Although many injuries occur as a result of accidents with an associated inflammatory response being unavoidable, some precautions can be taken. Following appropriate hand hygiene precautions can significantly decrease the risk of pathogen transmission among people, thus reducing the potential for an inflammatory response. Similarly, keeping wounds clean and covered will help accelerate the healing process, potentially decreasing the total or length of an inflammatory response. Using designated safety equipment when involved in sports or other physical activity can also minimize the incidence of injury. Additionally, being aware of food and water safety standards and any issues that

TABLE 21-2	CLINICAL MANIFESTATIONS OF INFLAMMATION
LOCAL MANIFESTIONS	**SYSTEMIC MANIFESTATIONS**
Swelling	Fever
Pain	Leukocytosis
Heat	Increase in plasma proteins
Redness	Malaise
Exudate	Fatigue
Serous exudate	
Fibrinous exudate	
Purulent exudate	
Hemorrhagic exudate	

may arise from contamination can prevent the transmission of pathogens and avoid potential inflammation associated with an immune response.

Secondary Prevention (Screening)

There are no routine screening procedures for inflammation, making primary prevention strategies critical in reducing the incidence and severity of inflammatory responses.

Collaborative Interventions

The clinical management of inflammation is directed at mediating the inflammatory process to promote repair and healing and avoid an excessive inflammatory response that may lead to further tissue injury. Some general guidelines to treatment can be made depending on the cause of the inflammation. If inflammation is due to infection, the underlying cause of the infection must be eradicated. If inflammation is due to a hypersensitivity type immune response, such as allergies, asthma, or autoimmune diseases, management of inflammation must be combined with management of the immune response and the pathologic consequence of immune dysfunction (e.g., diabetes mellitus, inflammatory bowel syndrome, rheumatoid arthritis, or muscular sclerosis). If inflammation is due to an uncomplicated strain or sprain, the standard treatment regimen of *rest*, *ice*, *compression*, and *elevation* (RICE) combined with nonsteroidal antiinflammatory drugs (NSAIDs) will help with both management of pain and moderation of the inflammatory response.

Chronic inflammatory responses to disease require careful monitoring to prevent or slow the process of tissue damage that may result in organ failure. Treatment of the underlying cause of the disease, support for ongoing tissue function, and prevention of organ or limb dysfunction or deformity are all important areas of clinical management. Sometimes treatment is aimed at finding alternative routes to achieve physiologic outcomes, such as providing insulin to the individual with type 1 diabetes mellitus, replacing endogenous insulin that is no longer being manufactured in the pancreas.

Rest, Ice, Compression, Elevation (RICE)

RICE represents a set of activities directed at minimizing the swelling associated with a sprain or strain. As described previously, swelling of the tissues immediately surrounding an area of injury is a part of the normal inflammatory response. By minimizing swelling, the injured tissue and surrounding tissue will be protected from additional damage resulting from the swelling itself. The first 24 to 48 hours after the injury is the critical period when RICE measures will be most beneficial. Typically, icing of the sprain or strain for 20 minutes at a time every 2 to 3 hours is indicated and leaving the ice in place for a longer period of time may cause additional tissue damage. Compression of the damaged area also helps to minimize swelling; but, the compression wrap must be snug yet not so tight to impede circulation (be alert to fingers or toes becoming cool, tingling, or turning blue in color). Whenever possible, elevation of the injured area above the level of the heart is useful in helping to minimize swelling.[41]

Immobilization Devices

Immobilization devices such as splints or slings contribute to the ability to rest the injured area. Wheelchairs, walkers, or crutches may also be useful in minimizing weight bearing to an injured extremity. If bed rest is indicated, leg exercises or pneumatic compression devices should be considered to protect against thrombus formation in the legs.

Pharmacologic Agents

Pharmacologic intervention options are diverse and depend on the cause of inflammation. Three major goals of treatment include reducing inflammation, managing fever, and providing pain relief. For this reason, many pharmacologic agents prescribed for the treatment of inflammation have one or more of these properties.

Steroidal agents. Glucocorticoids (e.g., prednisone) are steroids used to suppress the immune system and thus suppress an inflammatory response. They are particularly effective in reducing the swelling and pain that accompanies inflammation. Steroids such as prednisone are used in a wide range of inflammatory conditions—from swelling secondary to trauma to inflammation found in allergies and autoimmune diseases such as rheumatoid arthritis or systemic lupus erythematosus.[42]

Nonsteroidal antiinflammatory agents. Nonsteroidal antiinflammatory drugs (NSAIDs), such as ibuprofen or naproxen, are important in the management of pain, fever, and inflammation. These medications may be found as over-the-counter products or they may be combined with narcotics (e.g., hydrocodone or oxycodone) and require a prescription. Significant inflammation may require the use of cyclooxygenase (COX) inhibitors. COX-1 is produced by all tissues and promotes a number of protective functions. COX-2 is produced primarily at sites of tissue injury and acts to mediate inflammation and to sensitize receptors to painful stimuli. It is also found in the brain, where it helps to mediate fever and assist the brain in pain perception. Inhibition of COX-2 is important in treating an inflammatory response because the medication triggers processes that lead to suppression of inflammation, control of pain, and reduction of fever. First-generation NSAIDs inhibited both COX-1 and COX-2 and newer generation NSAIDs (e.g., celecoxib) are able to inhibit COX-2 only.[42]

Recombinant DNA and monoclonal antibodies. Recombinant DNA and monoclonal antibody development has produced an entirely new line of pharmacologic treatment for inflammation. Interleukin-1 (IL-1) antagonists inactivate IL-1 receptors whereas tumor necrosis factor-alpha (TNF-α) inhibitors prevent it from producing its inflammatory actions, but leave the individual more susceptible to infection. Recombinant protein C helps the body dissolve microvascular clots formed during inflammation, and although infliximab (Remicade) is a TNF inhibitor, it has been key to more recent treatments of lymphoma, rheumatoid arthritis, and inflammatory bowel diseases.[42]

Antipyretics. Fever is a common physiologic response to an inflammation. For this reason, antipyretics are often

MODEL CASE

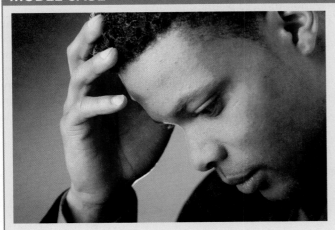

Chris Shomni is a 25-year-old male in a stressful, professional position. He was recently diagnosed with ulcerative colitis (UC) after developing abdominal pain and cramping and bloody diarrhea intermittently (though more frequently recently) over the last several weeks. He has lost 10 pounds in the last 4 weeks and has complained of nausea and fatigue. A colonoscopy demonstrated the presence of significant inflammation and ulcers in the colon and rectum. No strictures, perforations, or areas of paralysis of the colon were noted. Biopsy and further evaluation of the colonoscopy confirmed the presence of UC and ruled out Crohn's disease. He has no family history of inflammatory bowel disease. Assessment of the skin revealed the presence of erythema nodosum lesions, which are characteristic of UC. Laboratory testing further identified the presence of lowered red blood cell (RBC) and hemoglobin levels, elevated platelet count, and normal white blood cell (WBC) count. Serum total protein and albumin levels were low.

Diagnosis of UC was made with complications of anemia and hypoalbuminemia. Mr. Shomni was also demonstrating impaired nutrition as a result of impaired nutrient absorption and diarrhea and anemia secondary to inflammation of the bowel and loss of fluid, protein, and RBCs. Pain from inflammation and abdominal cramping was present, but not significant, and he was at risk for fluid volume deficiency. It was determined that the bowel needed to be rested, that bowel resection surgery was not indicated at this time, and that inflammation must be reduced. Mr. Shomni was admitted to the hospital to begin treatment for inflammation, rest the bowel, reduce his diarrhea, and balance his fluid and electrolyte levels.

Overall goals of treatment for Chris include controlling colon inflammation, ensuring adequate nutrition and hydration, and relieving pain and diarrhea. With control of inflammation and diarrhea, it is expected that the anemia and hypoalbuminemia will resolve. Pharmacologic intervention included aminosalicylates containing 5-aminosalicylic acid (5-ASA) to control inflammation. Corticosteroids to reduce inflammation will only be used if Chris has an exacerbation of his UC and his disease becomes severe and nonresponsive to 5-ASA. If Mr. Shomni does not respond sufficiently to the 5-ASA or corticosteroids, the use of immunomodulators such as 6-mercaptopurine (6-MP) or monoclonal antibodies such as infliximab (Remicade) may have to be introduced in the future. With chronic inflammatory bowel disease, at some point in his life Mr. Shomni may need to have surgery for a colostomy or ileostomy because tissue damage to the intestinal tract may be so severe that it no longer functions.

Chris was discharged after 3 days with new medications and instructions to avoid enteric and time-released medications, an understanding of dietary changes to limit high-fiber food intake, strategies for stress reduction, and actions to be taken should early signs and symptoms of an inflamed or infected bowel be evident.

Case Analysis

Inflammatory bowel disease encompasses two primary inflammatory processes: ulcerative colitis and Crohn's disease. Ulcerative colitis (UC) is a chronic inflammatory disease with symptoms that may range from mild to severe. Chris Shomni's case provides a classic example of chronic inflammation with symptoms including abdominal pain and cramping, bloody diarrhea, weight loss, nausea, and fatigue. Clinical symptoms included significant inflammation and ulcers in the colon and rectum evident during his colonoscopy and erythema nodosum lesions on his skin. Primary treatment regimens were directed at reducing and controlling Mr. Shomni's colon inflammation, relieving pain and diarrhea, and enhancing his nutrition and hydration status.

administered for fever management. Antipyretic agents, such as acetaminophen, aspirin, and nonsteroidal antiinflammatory drugs (NSAIDs), described previously, reduce fever by inhibiting cyclooxygenase. These are often administered in combination with opioid analgesic agents.

Analgesics. Nonopioid analgesic agents, such as acetaminophen or aspirin, are the most common type of analgesic used for pain relief caused by inflammation. NSAIDs are also considered analgesics because a reduction in inflammation tends to also relieve associated pain. Opioid analgesic agents are used when inflammatory pain is severe.

Antimicrobials. Antibiotics, antivirals, and other antimicrobials are important in treating the underlying cause of infection leading to inflammation. Antimicrobials

encompass a wide variety of medications that are required to treat diseases associated with immune and inflammatory responses. These are discussed further in Concept 22: Infection.

INTERRELATED CONCEPTS

Several concepts featured in this textbook are interrelated to inflammation (Figure 21-2).

Immunity and **Infection** are probably the most closely related concepts. Many of the pathophysiologic processes associated with inflammation are also found in both immunity and infection with pathology from one process overlapping those of the other two processes or with one process triggering another. This can be seen with hypersensitivity reactions of the immune system triggering an inflammatory response or infection stimulating an inflammatory response.

Tissue integrity is at risk in an inflammatory response as is impaired mobility and pain associated with an initial injury and with the consequences (swelling) of an inflammatory response.

Thermoregulation may be influenced by inflammation depending on the severity of the response to tissue injury.

Adequate **Gas exchange** is at risk in the presence of inflammation-induced pleural effusion.

Hemostasis alterations in the form of microvascular **Clotting** may also be a consequence of inflammation, particularly if it is chronic.

Both **Fatigue** and **Stress** are often associated with injury and recovery from an acute inflammatory response and may be an even greater consequence of chronic inflammation from an autoimmune hypersensitivity reaction.

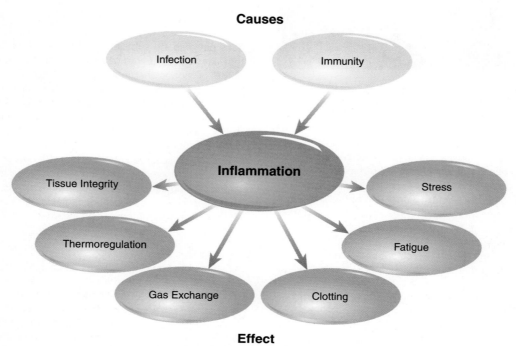

FIGURE 21-2 Inflammation and Interrelated Concepts.

■■■ BOX 21-1   EXEMPLARS OF INFLAMMATION

Acute Inflammation
- Acute infection
- Bronchitis
- Bursitis
- Cellulitis
- Gastroenteritis
- Joint sprain or strain
- Nephritis
- Rheumatic fever
- Sinusitis
- Tendonitis
- Tonsillitis

Chronic Inflammation
- Atherosclerosis
- Chronic infection
- Chronic obstructive pulmonary disease
- Cirrhosis

- Diverticulitis
- Fibromyalgia
- Gingivitis
- Myocarditis
- Osteoarthritis
- Psoriasis
- Ulcerative colitis
- Vasculitis

Autoimmune-Based Inflammation
- Asthma
- Crohn's disease
- Goodpasture's syndrome
- Multiple sclerosis
- Myasthenia gravis
- Rheumatoid arthritis
- Systemic lupus erythematosus

EXEMPLARS

Exemplars for the concept of inflammation are presented in Box 21-1. These examples are divided into diseases or conditions that represent acute inflammation, chronic inflammation, or inflammation based on the presence of an autoimmune hypersensitivity response. It should be noted that overlap often occurs between acute and chronic inflammation with chronic inflammatory conditions having acute exacerbations and acute inflammatory responses developing into chronic conditions. Thus some artificial division among the three types of inflammation is unavoidable.

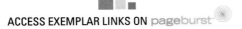

ACCESS EXEMPLAR LINKS ON pageburst

REFERENCES

1. Taber: *Cyclopedic medical dictionary*, ed 21, Philadelphia, 2009, FA Davis.
2. Hall JE: *Textbook of medical physiology*, ed 12, Philadelphia, 2011, Saunders/Elsevier.
3. McCance KL, Huether SE, Brashers VL, et al: *Pathophysiology: the biologic basis for disease in adults and children*, ed 6, St Louis, 2010, Mosby/Elsevier.
4. Copstead LC, Banasik JL: *Pathophysiology*, ed 4, St Louis, 2010, Saunders/Elsevier.
5. Kimball J: *Inflammation*, 2010. at http://users.rcn.com/jkimball. ma.ultranet/BiologyPages/I/Inflammation.html. Accessed Oct 27, 2010.
6. Cleveland Clinic: *Inflammation: what you need to know*, 2006. at http://my.clevelandclinic.org/symptoms/inflammation/hic_inflammation_what_you_need_to_know.aspx. Accessed Oct 27, 2010.
7. Mosby: *Dictionary of medicine, nursing, and health professions*, ed 8, St Louis, 2009, Mosby/Elsevier.
8. Kessler J: *Inflammation, repair, and cellular growth*, n.d., at www.uvm.edu/~jkessler/PATH301/301infla.htm. Accessed Sept 24, 2010.
9. Kahn MA, Solomon LW: *Acute inflammation, wound healing & repair I*, 2007. at www.ocw.tufts.edu/data/51/551512.pdf. Accessed Sept 24, 2010.
10. State University of New York at Stony Brook: *Inflammation* n.d. at www.path.sunysb.edu/coursemat/hbp310inflam.htm. Accessed Sept 24, 2010.
11. National Institutes of Health, National Library of Medicine: *Inflammation*, 2010. at http://ghr.nlm.nih.gov/glossary=inflammation. Accessed Sept 20, 2010.
12. Women-to-Women: *The biology behind inflammation—proinflammatory hormones*, 2010. at www.womentowomen.com/inflammationproinflammatoryhormones.aspx. Accessed Sept 27, 2010.
13. Krakauer T, Buckley MJ, Fisher D: Proinflammatory mediators of toxic shock and their correlation to lethality, *Media Inflam*, article ID517594, 2010.
14. Mamet J, Baron A, Lazdunski M, et al: Proinflammatory mediators, stimulators of sensory neuron excitability via the expression of acid-sensing ion channels, *J Neurosci* 22, 2002.
15. Humpath.com: *Acute inflammation* n.d. at www.humpath.com/Acute-inflammation. Accessed Sept 24, 2010.
16. Pick M: *What is chronic inflammation*, 2010. at www.womentowomen.com/inflammation/whatischronicinflammation.aspx. Accessed Sept 27, 2010.
17. Pick M: *C-reactive protein (CPR and hs-CRP)—are you on fire?* 2010. at www.womentowomen.com/understandyourbody/tests/crp.aspx. Accessed Sept 27, 2010.
18. Pick M: *Inflammation—the key to chronic disease?* 2010. at www.womentowomen.com/inflammation/default.aspx. Accessed Sept 27, 2010.
19. Challem J: *The dangers of inflammation*, 2005. at www.functionalingredientsmag.com/content/print.aspx?topic=the-dangers-of-inflammation. Accessed Dec 15, 2010.
20. Nielsen FH: Magnesium, inflammation, and obesity in chronic disease, *Nutr Rev* 68, 2010.
21. Ferrante AW: Obesity-induced inflammation: a metabolic dialogue in the language of inflammation, *J Int Med* 262, 2007.
22. Lopes-Virella MF, Carter RE, Gilbert GE, et al: Risk factors related to inflammation and endothelial dysfunction in the DDCT/EDIC cohort and their relationship with nephropathy and macrovascular complications, *Diabet Care* 31, 2008.
23. Chung HY, Cesari M, Anton S, et al: Molecular inflammation: underpinnings of aging and age-related diseases, *Ageing Res Rev* 8, 2009.
24. Kimball J: *Reactive oxygen species (ROS)*, 2010. at http://users.rcn.com/jkimball.ma.ultranet/BiologyPages/R/ROS.html. Accessed Dec 5, 2010.
25. Aronson D, Avizohar O, Levy Y, et al: Factor analysis of risk variables associated with low-grade inflammation, *Atherosclerosis* 200(1):206–212, 2008.
26. Pagana KD, Pagana TJ: *Diagnostic and laboratory test reference*, ed 8, St Louis, 2010, Mosby/Elsevier.
27. Wisse BE: The inflammatory syndrome: the role of adipose tissue cytokines in metabolic disorders linked to obesity, *J Am Soc Nephrol* 15, 2004.
28. Clifton P: Dietary fatty acids and inflammation, *Nutr Dietet* 22, 2009.
29. Al-Khafaji AH, Sharma S, Eschun G: *Multisystem organ failure of sepsis*, 2010. at http://emedicine.medscape.com/article/169640-print. Accessed Nov 27, 2010.
30. Dellinger RP, Cinel I, Sharma S, et al: *Septic shock*, 2010. at http://emedicine.medscape.com/article/168402-print. Accessed Nov 27, 2010.
31. Rubins J: *Pleural effusion*, 2010, at http://emedicine.medscape.com/article/299959-print. Accessed Nov 27, 2010.
32. Pearson TA, Mensah GA, Hong Y, Smith S: AHA Conference Proceedings. CDC/AHA Workshop on Markers of Inflammation and Cardiovascular Disease: Application to Clinical and Public Health Practice: overview, *Circulation* 110:e543–e544, 2004.
33. Li JJ, Zhu CG, Yu B, et al: The role of inflammation in coronary artery calcification, *Ageing Res Rev* 6, 2007.
34. Silverstein DM: Inflammation in chronic kidney disease: role of the progression of renal and cardiovascular disease, *Pediatr Nephrol* 24, 2009.
35. Stolp HB, Dziegielewska KM: Review: role of developmental inflammation and blood-brain barrier dysfunction in neurodevelopmental and neurodegenerative diseases, *Neuropathol Appl Neurobiol* 35, 2009.
36. Ferguson LR: Chronic inflammation and mutagenesis, *Mutat Res* 690, 2010.
37. Buck I, Morceau F, Grigorakaki C, et al: Linking anemia to inflammation and cancer: the crucial role of TNF, *Biochem Pharmacol* 77, 2009.

38. Murdoch JR, Lloyd CM: Chronic inflammation and asthma, *Mutat Res* 690, 2010.

39. Garcia C, Feve B, Ferre P, et al: Diabetes and inflammation: fundamental aspects and clinical implications, *Diabet Metab* 36(5):327–338, 2010.

40. Jacobs M, van Greevenbroek MMJ, van der Kallen CJH, et al: Low-grade inflammation can partly explain the association between the metabolic syndrome and either coronary artery disease or severity of peripheral arterial disease: the CODAM study, *Eur J Clin Invest* 39, 2009.

41. Quinn E: *RICE—rest, ice, compression and elevation soft tissue injury first aid* at http://sportsmedicine.about.com/cs/rehab/a/rice.htm. Accessed Feb 14, 2010.

42. Lehne RA: *Pharmacology for nursing care*, ed 7, St Louis, 2010, Saunders/Elsevier.

Infection

Carolyn E. Sabo

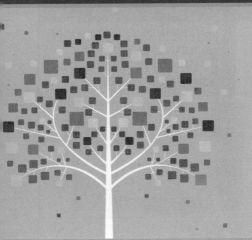

Microorganisms are found throughout the environment. As a consequence, humans are constantly exposed to a multitude of microorganisms at any moment. Although many microorganisms do not pose a health threat to humans, some microorganisms cause human disease and are known as pathogens. Our bodies are constantly confronted with pathogens in the forms of bacteria, viruses, parasites, or fungi. These pathogens are routinely found on the skin; the mucous membranes; the linings of the respiratory, gastrointestinal, and urinary tracts; and the mouth and eyes.[1] Typically, an individual's immune system is able to rid the body of the pathogens without developing an infection. An infection occurs when a susceptible host is invaded by a pathogen that multiplies and causes disease. This concept presentation will provide an overview of the infection concept, including identifying individuals most at risk, recognizing signs and symptoms of infection, and understanding ways to treat or manage an infection.

DEFINITION(S)

For the purposes of this concept analysis, infection is defined as *the invasion and multiplication of microorganisms in body tissues, which may be clinically unapparent or result in local cellular injury due to competitive metabolism, toxins, intracellular replication, or antigen-antibody response.* Several additional terms are important to understand that are used in this concept analysis. Terms used to describe the classification of organisms causing infection include *bacterial, viral, fungal,* and *protozoal.* These will be described further in the next section. Terms are also used to describe the trajectory of infection. When an infection occurs, it may be *acute* (resolving in a few days or weeks) or *chronic* (an infection that typically lasts longer than 12 weeks and in some cases is noncurable). Terms are also used to describe the extent of spread in the body. A *localized* infection is limited to a specific body area. Disseminated is a term used to describe a spread of infection from an initial site to other areas of the body. The term

systemic is used to describe an infection that affects the body as a whole, or has spread throughout the body. A common type of systemic infection known as sepsis is defined as the presence of pathogens in the blood or other tissues throughout the body.

Two additional terms that are significant to the concept of infection are epidemic and pandemic. The term *epidemic* is used to describe a situation in which there are more cases of an infectious disease than is normal for the population or geographic area. A *pandemic* is a worldwide epidemic of a disease.[2] The global nature of our modern world presents challenges because people with asymptomatic infections can travel from home to virtually anyplace in the world in less than 24 hours. Professional conferences, worldwide sporting events, and gatherings for various types of entertainment can bring people together from all over the world. They are often transported to and from the events in confined airplanes and participate in events in close proximity of others. Exposure to infection leads to the spread of disease before returning to their homes. As a result, infection management initiatives at times are implemented on a global basis, particularly in the event of a pandemic.

SCOPE AND CATEGORIES

Infections may be categorized in several ways, including on the basis of the multiple variables involved such as mode of transmission, trajectory of illness, and body systems affected. The most common way to categorize and discuss infections is based on the classification of the causative microorganism.

The most common microorganisms initiating an infection are bacteria, viruses, fungi, and parasites or protozoa. Table 22-1 identifies common pathogens for each of these microorganism categories. When considering an infection, leukocytes found in the blood and tissue-derived leukocytes are primarily responsible for protecting the body. Whether the invading organism is a bacterium, virus, parasite, or fungus will influence how the immune system will respond. B lymphocytes

TABLE 22-1	COMMON PATHOGENS		
BACTERIA	**VIRUS**	**FUNGUS**	**PARASITE OR PROTOZOA**
Methicillin-resistant *Staphylococcus aureus* (MRSA)	Human immunodeficiency virus (HIV)	Tinea pedis	Giardiasis
Clostridium difficile (C. diff.)	Hepatitis A, B, C, or E virus	Candidiasis	Trichinosis
Vancomycin-resistant *Enterococci* (VRE)	Human papillomavirus (HPV)	Histoplasmosis	Toxoplasmosis
Streptococcus pyogenes (group A)	Ebola virus	Lobomycosis	Malaria
Corynebacterium diphtheria	Hanta virus	Cryptococcosis	Ascariasis
Escherichia coli	SARS-associated coronavirus	Aspergillosis	Pediculosis
Mycobacterium tuberculosis	Respiratory syncytial virus	Coccidioidomycosis	Cryptosporidiosis
Pseudomonas aeruginosa			*Pneumocystis jirovecii* pneumonia
Neisseria gonorrhoeae			
Clostridium tetani			

and T lymphocytes take "leadership" roles depending on whether it is a bacterial or viral invasion, the complement system is always present to enhance the immune response, and dendritic cells will help to modulate the immune response.[3-8]

Bacterial Infections

Bacteria, the pleural form of bacterium, are one-celled organisms without a true nucleus or cellular organelles. They synthesize deoxyribonucleic acid (DNA), ribonucleic acid (RNA), and proteins and can reproduce independently, but require a host for a suitable environment for multiplication. Bacteria cause cellular injury by releasing toxins that are either exotoxins (enzymes released by gram-positive bacteria into the host) or endotoxins (part of the bacterial cell wall of gram-negative bacteria that can cause damage to the host even if the bacteria are dead). Diseases caused by bacterial invasion depend on the type of bacterial pathogen and the area of the body that is primarily invaded.[9]

Viral Infections

A virus is defined as a pathogen with a nucleic acid within a protein shell requiring invasion of a host for replication. An invading virus may immediately cause disease or may remain relatively dormant for years. The virus causes cellular injury by blocking its genetically prescribed protein synthesis processes and using the cell's metabolic processes for the reproduction of the virus. Diseases develop as a result of interference of normal cellular functioning of the host, with destruction of the virus by the immune system also requiring death of the host cell.[9]

Fungal Infections

A fungus may be defined as a microorganism belonging to the kingdom Fungi, which includes yeasts, molds, and mushrooms. They may grow as single cells (yeasts) or as multicellular filamentous colonies (molds or mushrooms). In an otherwise healthy individual, fungi do not cause disease and are contained by the body's natural flora. Fungi causing disease are termed fungi imperfecti, and in the immunocompromised individual they can result in infections that lead to death.[9] Other fungal infections such as tinea pedis (athlete's foot) or ringworm may also develop in the individual with a competent immune system.

Protozoa/Parasitic Infections

Protozoa include a subcategory termed parasitic protozoa and, with few exceptions, generally infect individuals with compromised immune responses. They are typically found in dead material in water and soil and are spread by the fecal-oral route by ingesting food or water that is contaminated with the parasitic spores or cysts. Disease may develop in an otherwise healthy individual when the spores invade organs and stimulate an immune response, interfering with normal functioning of the organ system.[9]

Other Types of Infections

Sometimes an infection will develop that begins as one type and after an additional pathogen is introduced a secondary infection occurs. Fungal infections may develop when treatment for a bacterial infection decimates the body's natural flora or bacterial infections may arise while a debilitated body is treated for a viral infection. When considering bacterial infections, some bacteria are always pathogenic, are never part of the normal flora, but may cause subclinical infection (*Mycobacterium tuberculosis*); some bacteria are part of the normal flora but can become pathogenic (*Escherichia coli*); some are part of the normal flora but can cause infection if they reach deep tissues, perhaps by surgery (*Staphylococcus epidermidis*); and some bacteria are part of the normal flora and become pathogenic when the individual is immunocompromised (*Acinetobacter*).[9,10]

McCance and colleagues[11] noted an increase in morbidity and mortality secondary to infections in part attributable to the emergence of previously unknown infections and the reemergence of infections that were considered controlled in various parts of the world. As these infections manifest, globalization of travel and increased ease of introducing new infections into a geographic area have contributed to changes in morbidity and mortality.

Health care–acquired and community-acquired infections are emerging as significant public health concerns. Although methicillin-resistant *Staphylococcus aureus* (MRSA) and

Clostridium difficile (C. diff.) are debilitating health care–acquired diseases, community-acquired MRSA is even more prevalent in some areas. Hospitals and other health care centers have been proactive in providing alcohol-based solutions for hand hygiene in both patient care rooms and public areas, but this same attention to infection prevention has not translated nearly as extensively to sporting arenas, areas where children gather for sporting and other group events, restaurants, food stores and other shopping facilities, movie theaters, and other group activity locales.

RISK FACTORS

Populations at Risk

Infectious diseases may cause health concerns for all individuals regardless of age, ethnicity, gender, socioeconomic status, geographic location, or prior health history. That said, there are risk factors linked to some population groups based on age, socioeconomic status, and geographic location. Of the 10 leading causes of infant deaths, bacterial sepsis ranked number 7 and disorders related to short gestation and low birth weight ranked number 2. Because an infant's immune system is immature and compromised at birth, any additional stress such as low birth weight further places the infant at risk for infection.[12,13]

The growing population of individuals of low socioeconomic status has increased the risk of infection for several reasons. Those who are uninsured or underinsured may be at risk for the consequences of absent or insufficient preventive health care. For example, if the cost of vaccinations is too expensive or the ability to access clinics where free vaccinations may be provided is not available, both children and adults can be at risk for acquiring infections from which they should be protected. Further, this same population may not have the resources available to travel for preventive health care screenings or treatments for infection, to purchase medicines, or to buy food and food supplements that may contribute to health maintenance, disease prevention, and more rapid recovery from infections and other illnesses. Meanwhile, the prevalence of some diseases and infections is increasing in specific age or ethnic groups (human immunodeficiency virus [HIV]) or in geographic locations worldwide (cholera and malaria), all of which influence the prevalence of infection in the United States.

Individual Risk Factors

Individual risk factors for infection are influenced by a number of variables. The immune status of the host is one very important risk factor as is the type and dose of exposure to microorganisms.

Compromised Host Because of Immunodeficiency

Individual risk factors for infection include being very young or elderly because these individuals have immune systems that are immature or becoming less responsive and efficient with age. Those who are immunocompromised are also at increased risk for infection. Immunocompromised immune systems may develop as a result of genetic factors (primary immunodeficiency), malnutrition, preexisting infection with other pathogens (e.g., HIV or Epstein-Barr virus), acute or chronic psychologic or environmental stress, use of medications to prevent rejection of transplanted organs, and the presence of or treatment for cancer. These processes associated with immunocompromise were previously discussed in the Immunity concept.

Compromised Host Because of Chronic Disease

Chronic illness and associated treatments increase the risk for infection. In the United States, infections in adults including chronic lower respiratory tract diseases, influenza and pneumonia, nephritis, septicemia, and chronic liver disease accounted for 5 of the top 15 leading causes of death in 2007.[14] Diseases such as diabetes mellitus, inflammatory disorders, cancers, and hepatic or respiratory disorders challenge the immune system and increase individual vulnerability to infection. Pathologic changes within these body systems may alter the structural integrity of the system and create an environment conducive to infection while treatment regimens are imposed that may also increase the risk of infection. Treatment strategies requiring the introduction of invasive lines (parenteral or other catheters), immunosuppressive medications (corticosteroids), antibiotics or antivirals, surgery, or intubation and mechanical ventilation all expose the body to avenues of entry for pathogenic organisms. In association with chronic illness–derived immunosuppression, required treatment regimens may only serve to enhance the risk of individual infection.

Environmental Conditions

Exposure to unsafe sanitation conditions may also make an individual vulnerable to a multitude of pathogens. These pathogens may directly cause infection or challenge the immune system and increase the potential for infection upon future introduction of other microorganisms. Crowded living conditions increase the likelihood of the spread of disease and may also contribute to less than optimal sanitary conditions, all of which increase the potential for infection. Other environmental factors influence the individual's susceptibility to infection and include the presence or absence of clean food and water, conditions involving food preparation, and sufficiency of air ventilation.

PHYSIOLOGIC PROCESSES AND CONSEQUENCES

Pathogens may be highly virulent and able to cause disease when small numbers invade the body. Other pathogens are weakly virulent and able to cause disease only when an excess number invade the body or the host body is already weakened by disease, malnutrition, excessive fatigue, or other stresses. Opportunistic infections, such as seen in human immunodeficiency virus (HIV) infection, cause disease when the host immune system is severely compromised.

The transmission of an infection from one person to another is a major public health concern. Some diseases are communicable before symptoms are evident in the carrier (herpes simplex virus, varicella-zoster virus, human papillomavirus, influenza, or poliomyelitis), whereas others remain communicable after initial symptoms have subsided (human immunodeficiency virus, Epstein-Barr virus). Some infections remain dormant within the host and may resurface as the same or as a different disease; an example is the varicella-zoster virus (VZV)—it first presents as chickenpox and later may manifest as shingles.[15] The "iceberg" concept of infectious disease has also emerged. This concept postulates that there are three levels of infection: the vast majority of a population may, at any given time, carry an infection wherein they are asymptomatic or undiagnosed. This group is thought to be the largest section of individuals, the part of the iceberg that is underwater. A smaller population group presents with an infection that manifests as less severe, symptomatic disease; the smallest group presents with classical, clinical symptoms of disease, and are those at the very tip of the iceberg. Epidemiology is important in the study of infection because it is concerned with the manner in which a disease spreads through groups or a population and the application of this information to the control of health problems.[9,10,15]

Infection Process

The process of infection requires the following six elements, all of which must be present for the infection to develop: (1) pathogen, (2) susceptible host, (3) reservoir, (4) portal of exit (from the reservoir), (5) mode of transmission, and (6) portal of entry (to the susceptible host) (see Figure 22-1). The reservoir is anywhere the pathogen may live and

multiply, either in the body or on objects contaminated with the organism (door handles, stagnant water, health care equipment). Portals of exit for a pathogen include urine or feces, saliva, blood, skin, or the gastrointestinal tract. Portals of entry include broken skin, intimate sexual contact, mouth, gastrointestinal tract, and contaminated food or water. The spread of infection is dependent on a reliable mode of transmission. Following basic hand hygiene principles and adhering to Standard Precautions are the most effective methods of blocking transmission of infection in community and health care settings. The Centers for Disease Control and Prevention (CDC) has published guidelines for infection control and hand hygiene within health care settings as well as guidelines related to health care–associated infections.[16-22] The guidelines are updated periodically and serve as excellent resources for ensuring adherence to infection control principles.

Pathogen Invasion

When a pathogen invades the body a number of immune system responses are initiated to minimize tissue and organ damage. B lymphocytes are activated to differentiate into plasma cells for the production of antibodies and memory cells in preparation for a future reexposure. T lymphocytes directly kill the invading organism, secreting lymphokines that attract and stimulate the activity of macrophages. Macrophages and monocytes initiate phagocytosis. The complement system is activated to enhance the entire immune response. Some tissue damage will occur as a result of endotoxins released by the pathogen that kill host cells, neurotoxins that affect nerve impulse transmission, or enterotoxins that damage cells of the gastrointestinal tract. Clinical manifestations associated

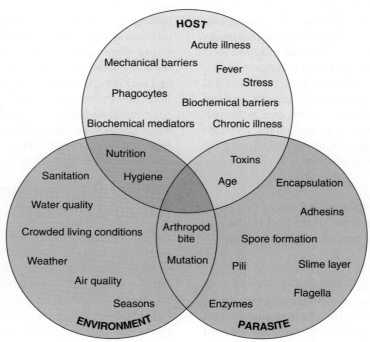

FIGURE 22-1 Process of Infection: Interactions of Host, Microorganisms, and the Environment. (From Copstead LC, Banasik JL: *Pathophysiology,* ed 4, Fig. 8-4, p 167, St Louis, 2010, Saunders/Elsevier.)

with the release of endotoxins may be mild (fever, chills, weakness, and malaise) or severe (shock syndrome or disseminated intravascular coagulation [DIC]). Some injuries leading to infection will also manifest with swelling and tenderness at the site, drainage from a wound, or red streaks on the skin leading away from the injury. These common, mild manifestations are indicative of an inflammatory response.[1]

Infections remain a significant cause of morbidity and mortality as a result of the emergence of antibiotic-resistant bacteria, the development of infections that have become resistant to multiple antibiotics, and the occurrence of both infections that had previously been controlled and newly discovered infections. Some bacteria are becoming smarter, with the ability to produce toxins and extracellular enzymes that destroy phagocytic cells, coat part of an antibody to prevent its activation of the complement system, or degrade and suppress an immune response.[11] Exotoxins released by bacteria may act locally at the site of infection or enter the blood and produce symptoms throughout the body. Symptoms associated with release of exotoxins from various pathogens include profuse diarrhea (cholera), spastic paralysis (tetanus), phagocyte death (gangrene), and prevention of nerve impulse transmission (botulism). As discussed next, severe exotoxin release may cause septic shock syndrome, which if not controlled rapidly can lead to death.

PHYSIOLOGIC PROCESSES AND CONSEQUENCES

Infections that are severe, poorly responsive to therapy, or initially untreated may challenge the body's restorative and compensatory responses, leading to the development of septic shock syndrome and multisystem failure. Symptoms of failure may include hypotension, tachycardia, tachypnea, oliguria or anuria, hypoxia, hypercapnia, seizures, or coma. The pathologic processes leading from uncontrolled infection or septicemia to multisystem failure and the symptoms just identified involve a complex interaction among a number of body systems. A bacterial infection will be described as the foundation for this potential progression.

Unresponsive or Untreated Infection

When a bacterial pathogen invades the body and initiates an immune response, lymphocytes (to produce antibodies), the complement system, and phagocytes will respond aggressively. Following invasion, bacteria will cause cellular injury by the release of either exotoxins or endotoxins, or both, into the host and initiate an inflammatory response. Exotoxins released during bacterial growth damage host cells as do endotoxins released after bacterial cell death. In some cases, a combination of the relative virulence of the bacteria and the immunocompromised status of the host may allow for the bacterial infection to overwhelm the immune system and cause significant host damage before the mounting of an effective defense against the bacteria. When this happens, the host will initiate compensatory actions to support vital functions, but these actions will eventually fail without supportive treatments, leading to death of the host.

Vascular, renal, and nervous system compensation. An inflammatory response to the invading bacteria will initiate the host defense mechanisms. This response will trigger a complement system response and all of the activities inherent in that type of response. Vascular permeability will be increased and allow for the shift of fluid from the intravascular compartment to the extravascular/extracellular spaces in the tissues, leading to hypovolemia and hypotension. The nervous system will attempt to compensate for the hypotension with peripheral vascular constriction and shunting of blood from nonessential to essential organs such as the brain, heart, and lungs. Acute systemic hypoperfusion may ensue and result in increased heart rate and cardiac contractility in an effort to maintain the cardiac output. In this early period, inadequate tissue perfusion may have caused organ damage despite a hyperdynamic cardiovascular state.

The renal system will initially attempt to compensate by creating a vasodilatory response of the glomeruli in an attempt to maintain an internal degree of pressure to continue filtration. Continued hypoperfusion of the kidneys leads to decreased urine output to retain cardiovascular volume, resulting in oliguria or anuria. Peripheral vasoconstriction may lead to increased cardiac ventricular preload. Should the myocardium be compromised, an increase in ventricular afterload may challenge the pulmonary vascular system with excess fluid that the ventricles cannot eject.

Respiratory compensation. The respiratory system will attempt to compensate for inadequate tissue perfusion (oxygenation) or hypoxemia by increasing the rate of respiration. This process may well be hampered by cardiovascular decompensation, leading to decreased cardiac output and resultant fluid accumulation and pulmonary edema. Inadequate tissue perfusion (hypoxia) and hypercapnia will result, leading to central nervous system decompensation as evidenced by an early change in mental status progressing to seizures, stupor, and coma.

Multisystem failure. Without effective treatment, the bacterial invasion leads to the development of septic shock syndrome with multiorgan failure. Eventually the consequences of inadequate tissue perfusion, overextended compensatory mechanisms, and host cell damage will result in irreversible organ failure and death of the host.[11,23] Figure 22-2 provides an overview of the primary pathologic processes and consequences of a bacterial infection leading to septic shock syndrome.

ASSESSMENT

History

A thorough health history includes questions to help the nurse understand an individual's risk potential for infection, recognize symptoms associated with infection, and appreciate factors associated with a presenting infection. Questions to gain information about an individual's risk for infection include those about the incidence of injury, known exposure to pathogens, and a history of prior infections. Current or immediate past treatment for cancer,

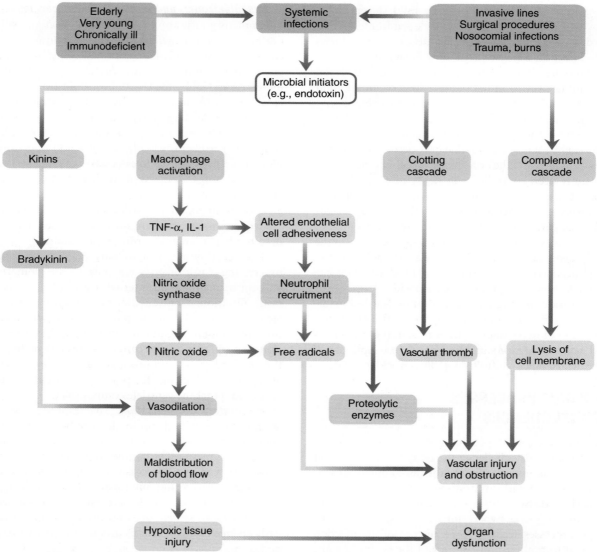

FIGURE 22-2 Pathophysiologic Process of Septic Shock. (From Copstead LC, Banasik JL: *Pathophysiology*, ed 4, p 501, St Louis, 2010, Saunders/Elsevier.)

recent surgical procedures, the presence of autoimmune or immunodeficiency disease, and use of immunosuppressant medication regimens must also be assessed. Travel should also be evaluated, particularly outside of the United States or to underdeveloped areas of the world that may expose the individual to pathogens in air, food, and water or to pathogens that are generally not found in the United States, such as smallpox. Other avenues of inquiry may include assessing incidences of interaction with larger groups of people, such as recent exposure to sports teams or attending entertainment or sporting events where the close proximity of others may facilitate the transmission of infectious pathogens.

Symptoms of infection are those verbalized by the patient and are often caused by the inflammatory response to infection, such as pain, swelling, or redness (see the Inflammation concept); other clinical manifestations may be those associated with the effect of the infectious process itself on the body system. Specific symptoms are often influenced by the affected organ, such as a cough with an infection of the respiratory system. Some symptoms are a result of generalized stress to the host, such as fatigue or malaise.

Examination Findings

Physical examination findings of particular importance in assessing for the presence of infection include fever, swelling, chills, malaise, redness or drainage in or around a wound, pain, and respiratory congestion.[11,23-26] In general, clinical manifestations associated with infection parallel those of inflammation. Should infection with *Clostridium difficile* (*C. diff.*) or parasites be suspected, the presence of watery diarrhea, loss of appetite, nausea, and abdominal pain or tenderness should also be evaluated because these symptoms may be indicative of infection with these pathogens.[14]

Laboratory and Diagnostic Tests

Laboratory and diagnostic studies are foundational to the diagnostic process for infections. Laboratory studies may be done on any type of body fluid or tissue and can prove the presence of infection. Radiographic diagnostic tests provide additional information to understand the location and extent of infections.

Complete Blood Count

The complete blood count with a white blood cell (WBC) differential count is one of the most critical laboratory tests to evaluate the presence of infection. Elevated levels of B and T lymphocytes, neutrophils, and monocytes are indicative of infection, particularly a bacterial or viral infection. Neutrophil counts are significantly elevated with bacterial infections and may lead to an increase in the number of band cells (immature neutrophils) when an infection is acute. Parasitic infections may result in an increase in the number of basophils and eosinophils; however, these two WBCs are not elevated in the presence of bacterial or viral infections.

Culture and Sensitivity

A culture and sensitivity (C&S) test is done to identify the invading pathogen and to determine the antimicrobial most likely to be effective in treatment. This test can be done on any body fluid, tissue, or exudates and is critical in the management of infections. Some of the most common specimens for C&S are obtained from the genitourinary tract (urine culture), respiratory tract (sputum culture), oropharynx (throat culture), blood, wounds, and spinal fluid. Specimens may also be obtained from within the body during invasive procedures or surgeries or from invasive equipment such as intravenous lines, feeding tubes, endotracheal tubes, and indwelling urinary catheters. Nurses are often responsible for the collection of specimens for C&S and it is critical that correct collection procedures are followed to avoid sample contamination leading to incorrect pathogen identification. Details of collection procedures are typically outlined in textbooks about laboratory and diagnostic procedures.

Other Laboratory Tests

There are several other blood and body fluid screening tests used to determine the presence of or evaluate an infection. These include C-reactive protein (CRP), erythrocyte sedimentation rate (ESR), and various serologic tests for the detection of a virus or antibodies against pathogens such as hepatitis, HIV, Epstein-Barr virus, severe acute respiratory syndrome (SARS), herpes simplex virus, syphilis, MRSA, *C. difficile,* and *Helicobacter pylori,* among many others.[27]

Radiographic Tests

Radiographic tests typically do not lead to an affirmative diagnosis of infection by themselves, because this requires confirmation through pathologic analysis (gained through laboratory testing). Radiographic tests are useful in visualizing certain body tissues to gain insight to the possibility of an infection (if not yet diagnosed) and/or the extent and scope of some confirmed infections. Chest x-rays, computer-assisted tomography (CAT) scans, magnetic resonance imaging (MRI) scans, positron emission tomography (PET) scans, and indium (indium-111) scans are examples of radiographic testing procedures that are useful in identifying areas of infection and inflammation within the body.

CLINICAL MANAGEMENT

Success in the prevention and treatment of infections has progressed dramatically over the past century with the introduction of antibiotics, the modernization of sanitation practices, the development of public health initiatives, and the spread of immunization programs. Morbidity and mortality rates for polio, influenza, pneumonia, and many other infections have decreased substantially with some infections being nearly eradicated worldwide. In the United States, smallpox vaccinations are no longer recommended and poliomyelitis is nearly eradicated with widespread vaccination protocols. Progress is being made in the development of vaccines for other diseases such as HIV, and a combined vaccination for smallpox and anthrax is being investigated.[2,11,28-31]

Success gained in the prevention and treatment of infections must also be tempered by the following facts: some community- or hospital-acquired bacterial infections are now difficult to treat because of emerging antibiotic resistance (e.g., methicillin-resistant *Staphylococcus aureus* [MRSA] and vancomycin-resistant *Enterococci* [VRE]); the prevalence of hospital-acquired infections is increasing in the form of both MRSA and *Clostridium difficile;* tuberculosis remains one of the world's leading causes of death; and foodborne and waterborne bacteria (*Salmonella* and *Campylobacter*) continue to cause debilitating diarrheal disease around the world. Following Alexander Fleming's discovery of penicillin in 1928, 70 years of using more and more potent antimicrobials has resulting in bacteria and viruses that are resistant to even the most potent weapons in our arsenal. The National Institute of Allergy and Infectious Diseases (NIAID) issued a statement of concern about the increasingly difficult process of disease management given the microbial resistance that has emerged against some of the most powerful antimicrobials. The NIAID particularly expressed concern related to treating staphylococcal infection, tuberculosis, influenza, gonorrhea, *Candida* infection, and malaria.[11,14,32-35] Continued research to find more powerful antimicrobials, while teaching the population about the consequences of overuse or inappropriate use of antimicrobials, will challenge health care providers and researchers for years to come.

Primary Prevention

Primary prevention involves all measures to prevent infections and begins with the administration of vaccinations. Worldwide, health care organizations have demonstrated various levels of success in providing vaccinations to their population in an effort to eradicate some of the more devastating infectious diseases such as polio and smallpox. Standard vaccinations in the U.S. arsenal to control the spread of disease through prevention of initial infection include those for human papillomavirus (HPV); hepatitis A and hepatitis B; varicella; measles, mumps, and rubella (MMR); influenza (annual); pneumococcus; tetanus, diphtheria, pertussis (Td/Tdap); and polio.

Infection control has been defined by the World Health Organization as measures aimed at the protection of those who might be vulnerable to acquiring an infection, including both individuals residing in the community and persons receiving care for health care problems within a wide variety of settings. The basic tenant of infection control is identified as *hygiene* and encompasses such topics as patient safety, infection control and prevention in health care, injection safety, and food safety.[36]

The following are some recommendations for infection control proposed by the CDC: keep hands clean by washing thoroughly with soap and water (for at least 30 seconds) or using an alcohol-based hand rub (for at least 15 seconds); keep cuts and scrapes clean and covered with a bandage until healed; avoid contact with other people's wounds and bandages; and refrain from sharing personal items such as towels or razors. In athletic settings, participants should shower immediately after participation and before using whirlpools. Uniforms should be washed and dried after each use. In health care settings, prevention of infection requires following accepted principles of hand hygiene, Standard Precautions, and contact precautions. Visitors should follow hand hygiene principles and avoid touching the dressings, catheters, or wound sites of an infected person.[37-39]

Hand hygiene is a critical component to the prevention of infection and the spread of disease. The CDC has an entire section on its website that addresses the issues of hand hygiene as a method of saving lives. Topics include the correct method for washing hands, situations that warrant hand washing, the use and limitations of hand sanitizers, and numerous publications and educational materials that are available. Further information is on the CDC website at www.cdc.gov/handwashing.

Secondary Prevention (Screening)

Secondary prevention through disease screening is less effective in controlling infection. Health care standards of care are strongly directed at prevention of infection, but should infection occur, therapy options become important in treating the infection without the misuse or overuse of antimicrobials.

The areas of screening most strongly supported are those for the identification of sexually transmitted diseases such as bacterial infections (*Chlamydia trachomatis, Neisseria gonorrhoeae,* or group B *Streptococci*), viral pathogens (human immunodeficiency virus, herpes simplex virus, hepatitis virus, or human papillomavirus [HPV]), fungal pathogens (*Candida albicans),* or protozoa (*Giardia lamblia*). Pap smears for sexually active women can be used as screening tools not only for cancer cells but also for the presence of HPV as well.

Collaborative Interventions

Management of infections requires both treatment of the infectious process itself and support for the affected body systems. The goal of treatment is to eradicate the infection,

---

CLINICAL NURSING SKILLS FOR INFECTION

- Hand hygiene
- Personal protective equipment
  - Gloves
  - Mask
  - Protective eyewear
  - Gown
  - Cap
- Isolation precautions
- Sterility
- Collecting specimens for culture
- Medication administration

---

prevent secondary infections, and limit damage to the body. Many interventions are related to supporting affected body systems. The following infection control measures are critical for a rapid recovery and are universal in that they apply to infection treatment regardless of the system involved: know and follow the principles of effective hand hygiene; clean and disinfect environmental surfaces; avoid close contact with infected individuals or crowded conditions in which bacterial or viral infections may be easily disseminated.[16-18]

Antimicrobials

Interventions in the treatment of various infections begin with the use of antibiotics, antivirals, and other antimicrobials. The laboratory and diagnostic testing identified previously helps to direct the health care provider to the appropriate antimicrobial. Instructing the infected individual to complete the full course of antimicrobial therapy helps to avoid a secondary infection, or reemergence of infection because of inadequate initial treatment.

Antibiotic agents. There are several classifications of antibiotics, based on bacterial spectrum and activity (bactericidal or bacteriostatic). Spectrum refers to the number of organisms affected by the antibiotic (i.e., broad-spectrum or narrow-spectrum antibiotic). Activity refers to the way in which the antibiotic kills bacteria. Bactericidal agents attack and kill the bacteria directly whereas bacteriostatic agents interfere with replication of the pathogen. The common classifications of antibiotics are presented in Table 22-2. Antibiotics within a structural class generally have similar patterns of effectiveness, toxicity, and allergic potential.

Antiviral agents. Like antibiotics, antiviral agents either kill viruses or suppress their replication, preventing their ability to multiply and reproduce. These agents are primarily used to minimize the severity of illness by limiting the viral spread. Common classifications of antiviral agents are presented in Table 22-2.

Antifungal agents. Antifungal agents kill fungal organisms. Because there are various types of fungi that cause infection, multiple classifications of antifungal agents are available and include polyenes, imidazoles, triazoles, thiazoles, allylamines, and echinocandins.

TABLE 22-2   CLASSIFICATION OF ANTIBIOTIC AND ANTIVIRAL AGENTS

ANTIBIOTICS	ANTIVIRAL AGENTS
Penicillin	Adamantane
Cephalosporins	Antiviral chemokine receptor
First generation	agonist
Second generation	Antiviral interferon
Third generation	Neuraminidase inhibitors
Fourth generation	Nonnucleoside reverse transcrip-
Fluoroquinolones	tase inhibitors (NNRTIs)
Tetracyclines	Nucleoside reverse transcriptase
Macrolides	inhibitors (NRTIs)
Aminoglycosides	Protease inhibitors
	Purine nucleosides

Nutrition and Fluids

Replacement of fluids and electrolytes (oral or parenteral) is critical in the presence of fever, vomiting, or diarrhea. Adequate rest and nutrition provide the body with energy needed for optimal functioning of the immune system and resolution of infection. Allowing time for rest and ensuring adequate fluids and nutritional intake are equally important.

INTERRELATED CONCEPTS

The concept of infection is closely aligned with several concepts featured in this textbook. These interrelated concepts are presented in Figure 22-3.

Immunity and **Inflammation.** The immune system is critical in providing a sentry level of alert for early identification

MODEL CASE

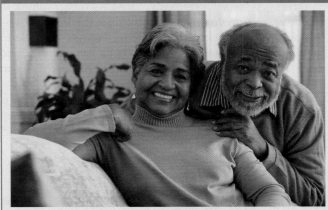

Mrs. Bovier is a 72-year-old woman who recently spent 5 days in the hospital for pneumonia where she received intravenous antibiotics and respiratory therapy. She was discharged 1 week ago and has been at home with her elderly husband, who assists in her care. She has arthritis and typically is not very physically active.

Mrs. Bovier returned to her primary care provider for a checkup and complained of increasing difficulty breathing, headache, and coughing up yellowish colored sputum. On examination she was found to have a low-grade fever, chest auscultation revealed areas of atelectasis, oxygen saturation (PaO_2) was 91%, and she was diaphoretic. A sputum specimen was obtained for culture and sensitivity that later revealed the presence of MRSA. Chest x-ray confirmed pulmonary congestion and atelectasis. Laboratory analysis showed an elevated white blood cell (WBC) count, the presence of band cells (immature neutrophils), and an elevated erythrocyte sedimentation rate (ESR).

Mrs. Bovier was again hospitalized because of the severity of her respiratory distress, the need for intravenous antibiotics to manage the MRSA pulmonary infection and pulmonary therapy to assist in resolving her pulmonary congestion, and the need for contact isolation because of her recurrent pneumonia and MRSA infection. Mrs. Bovier's age and lack of physical activity are complications that may influence MRSA treatment, requiring a more watchful course of initial therapy.

Hospital care for Mrs. Bovier included instruction in methods to improve the productivity of her cough, humidified oxygen to assist with loosening secretions while improving ventilation, and respiratory therapy to help with expectoration and to facilitate lung expansion and air exchange. She received intravenous vancomycin, mucolytic agents, a bronchodilator, and expectorants to treat her pulmonary disease and assist in breathing.

On discharge Mrs. Bovier received instructions in the proper technique for effective hand hygiene; the importance of avoiding large crowds of people as well as areas where people are smoking, to diminish her exposure to irritating respiratory stimuli; and the need to increase her physical activity, including frequent ambulation in her home, to help stimulate deep breathing and avoid peripheral vascular clot formation. She demonstrated understanding of her medication regimens and the need to maintain adequate food and fluid intake to support her immune system and provide energy while healing. The need for rest to promote healing was also emphasized. Finally, Mrs. Bovier was instructed on warning signs of recurring pulmonary disease or dysfunction.

Case Analysis

Health care–acquired MRSA is the most severe form of MRSA, with life-threatening infections such as bacteremia, surgical site infections, pneumonia, septic arthritis, toxic shock syndrome, and endocarditis as consequences. People at risk for acquiring MRSA infections include patients and visitors of patients in health care settings.

Mrs. Bovier met a number of the criteria that put her at risk for the development of MRSA. She was elderly, had been hospitalized with pneumonia (foreign pathogen), and had received intravenous antibiotics (invasive port of entry for MRSA). When she sought follow-up care to her hospitalization for pneumonia, she was found to have pulmonary congestion, hypoxemia, and fever. Diagnostic data revealed atelectasis on chest x-ray, an elevated white blood cell count, and immature neutrophils indicating the presence of a bacterial infection. These are classic clinical findings associated with infection. Diagnosis and treatment measures were consistent with the standards of care.

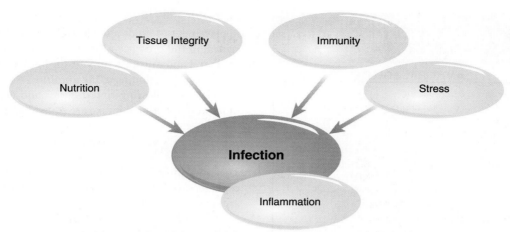

FIGURE 22-3 Infection and Interrelated Concepts.

of pathogen entry into the body. The immune system is the first line of defense against infection and the body's primary method of response to an invading organism. Inflammation is part of the body's response to a foreign antigen with many of the symptoms of infection being those of the body's inflammatory response (redness, swelling, pain).

Tissue integrity. Tissue integrity is critical to avoiding infection with the skin being the largest component of the immune system. Intact tissues are less vulnerable to pathogen entry and form natural barriers to infection.

Stress. As noted previously, stress—whether physical, emotional, or environmental—challenges the immune system and makes it more vulnerable to damage, less able to respond effectively and efficiently to pathogen invasion, and more difficult for the body to respond to treatment for an infection.

Nutrition. Maintaining adequate nutrition and rest is also necessary for the body to respond to active infection treatment regimens and support the work of an immune response.

■ ■■ BOX 22-1   EXEMPLARS OF INFECTION

Neurologic
- Encephalitis
- Meningitis

Respiratory
- Pneumonia
- Respiratory syncytial virus

Cardiovascular
- Endocarditis
- Myocarditis

Eyes
- Conjunctivitis

Ears
- Otitis media

Skin
- Cellulitis
- Methicillin-resistant *Staphylococcus aureus* (MRSA)
- Pressure ulcers
- Surgical wounds

Gastrointestinal
- *Clostridium difficile (C. diff.)*
- Gastroenteritis
- Hepatitis
- Tapeworm

Genitourinary
- Cystitis
- Pyelonephritis
- Urinary tract infection

Reproductive
- *Candida albicans*
- *Chlamydia trachomatis*
- Group B *Streptococci*
- Herpes simplex virus
- Human papillomavirus
- *Neisseria gonorrhoeae*

Systemic
- Human immunodeficiency virus
- Measles
- Mumps
- Sepsis

EXEMPLARS

Table 22-1 identifies examples of common infections that may be reviewed. A variety of infections have been presented as recurring, emerging, resistant, and global infections. Infections that were once under control or eradicated in various geographic areas are now reestablishing themselves within the United States and worldwide. Box 22-1 presents some of the more commonly occurring infections by body systems. Some infections have been present for a long time and have become resistant to our most effective antimicrobials. Research agendas are constantly focused on developing new generations of antibiotic classes or categories because antimicrobial resistance has made treatment of many infectious pathogens increasingly difficult. The global nature of our modern world makes prevention of infection a priority and transmission of infections to previously uninfected populations far more important than ever before. Finally, understanding the interrelationships between immunity and infection is critical for assessment, diagnosis, and treatment of people with infections.

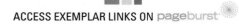

ACCESS EXEMPLAR LINKS ON pageburst

REFERENCES

1. Hall JC: *Textbook of medical physiology*, Philadelphia, 2011, Elsevier/Saunders.
2. Ross AL, Brave A, Scarlatti G, et al: Progress towards development of an HIV vaccine: report of the AIDS Vaccine 2009 Conference, *Lancet Infect Dis* 10(5):305–316, 2010.
3. National Institutes of Health: *Immune system*, 2008, at www.niaid.ni.gov/topics/immuneSystem/pages/whatisimmunesystem.aspx. Accessed Sept 20, 2010.
4. Steinman R: *Introduction to dendritic cells*, 2009, at www.lab.rockefeller.edu/steinman. Accessed Nov 30, 2010.
5. Steinman R: *Dendritic cells initiate the immune response*, 2009. at www.lab.rockefeller.edu/steinman/dendritic_intro/immune Response. Accessed Nov 30, 2010.
6. Steinman R: *Dendritic cells and immune tolerance*, 2009. at www.lab.rockefeller.edu/steinman/dendritic_intro/immuneTolerance. Accessed Nov 30, 2010.
7. Leon B, Ardavin C: Monocyte-derived dendritic cells in innate and adaptive immunity, *Immun Cell Biol 86*, 2008.
8. Maason F, Mount AM, Wilson NS, et al: Dendritic cells: driving the differentiation programme of T cells in viral infections, *Immun Cell Biol 86*, 2008.
9. Taber: *Cyclopedic medical dictionary*, ed 21, Philadelphia, 2009, FA Davis.
10. Pallen M: *Principles of pathogenesis: bacterial infection*, n.d. at www.infection.bham.ac.uk/Teaching/pathogenesis.ppt#1. Accessed Oct 6, 2010.
11. McCance KL, Huether SE, Brashers VL, et al: *Pathophysiology: the biologic basis for disease in adults and children*, St Louis, Mo, 2010, Mosby/Elsevier.
12. Xu J, Kochanek KD, Murphy SL, et al: Deaths: final data for 2007, *CDC Natl Vital Stat Rep* 58, 2010.
13. National Institutes of Health, U.S. National Library of Medicine: *Aging changes in immunity*, 2008, at www.nlm.nih.gov/medlineplus/ency/article/004008.htm. Accessed Sept 15, 2010.
14. Centers for Disease Control and Prevention: *Information for healthcare providers*, 2005, at www.cdc.gov/ncidod/dhqp/id_CdiffFAQ_HCP.html. Accessed Sept 15, 2010.
15. Ehrlich SD: *Varicella-zoster virus*, 2009, at www.umm.edu/altmed/articles/varicella-zoster-000080.htm. Accessed Oct 20, 2010.
16. Rutala WA, Weber DJ: *HICPAC: Guideline for disinfection and sterilization in healthcare facilities*, 2008, at www.cdc.gov/hicpac/pdf/guidelines/Disinfection_Nov_2008. Accessed Dec 20, 2010.
17. Centers for Disease Control and Prevention: *Guideline for hand hygiene in health-care settings, Morbid Mortal Wkly Rep*, 2002, at www.cdc.gov/mmwr/PDF/rr/rr5116.pdf. Accessed Dec 20, 2010.
18. Centers for Disease Control and Prevention: *Guideline for isolation precautions: preventing transmission of infectious agents in healthcare settings 2007*, 2007, at http://cdc.gov//ncidod/dhqp/pdf/isolation2007.pdf. Accessed Dec 20, 2010.
19. Centers for Disease Control and Prevention: *Type of health-care-associated infections*, 2010, at http://cdc.gov/HAI/infection Types.html. Accessed Dec 20, 2010.
20. Centers for Disease Control and Prevention: *Preventing healthcare-associated infections*, 2010, at http://cdc.gov/HAI/prevent/prevention.html. Accessed Dec 20, 2010.
21. Centers for Disease Control and Prevention: *Monitoring healthcare-associated infections*, 2010, at http://cdc.gov/HAI/surveillance/monitorHAI.html. Accessed Dec 20, 2010.
22. Centers for Disease Control and Prevention: *First state-specific healthcare-associated infections summary data report CDC's national healthcare safety network (NHSN) January-June, 2009 Q and A, 2010*, at http://cdc.gov/HAI/surveillance/QA_state Summary.html. Accessed Dec 20, 2010.
23. Copstead LC, Banasik JL: *Pathophysiology*, ed 4, St Louis, 2010, Saunders/Elsevier.
24. Centers for Disease Control and Prevention: *About MRSA*, 2008, at www.cdc.gov/mrsa/mrsa_initiative/skin_infection/index.html. Accessed Sept 15, 2010.
25. Jernigan J, Kallen A: *Methicillin-resistant Staphylococcus aureus (MRSA) infections, 2010, Presentation at the Nevada State Health Division Conference on "MRSA, Healthcare-associated Infections,"* Las Vegas, Nev, Nov 16, 2010.
26. McKenna M: *SUPERBUG: the fatal menace of MRSA*, New York, 2010, Free Press SimonSchuster.
27. Pagana KD, Pagana TJ: *Diagnostic and laboratory rest reference*, ed 8, St Louis, 2010, Elsevier/Mosby.
28. Merkel TJ, Perera PY, Kelly VK, et al: Development of a highly efficacious vaccinia-based dual vaccine against smallpox and anthrax, two important bioterror entities, *Proc Natl Acad Sci U S A* 107(42):18091–18096, 2010.
29. Centers for Disease Control and Prevention: *Smallpox disease overview*, 2007, at www.bt.cdc.gov/agent/smallpox/overview/disease-facts.asp. Accessed Nov 15, 2010.
30. Centers for Disease Control and Prevention: *Questions and answers about smallpox disease*, 2009, at www.bt.cdc.gov/agent/smallpox/faq/smallpox_disease.asp. Accessed Nov 15, 2010.
31. Centers for Disease Control and Prevention: *Polio disease—questions and answers*, 2007, at www.cdc.gov/vaccines/vpd-vac/polio/dis-faqs.htm. Accessed Nov 15, 2010.
32. National Institutes of Health, National Institute of Allergy and Infectious Diseases: *Bacterial infections*, 2010. at www.niaid, nih.gov/topics/bacterialinfections/pages/default.aspx. Accessed Sept 15, 2010.

33. National Institutes of Health, National Institute of Allergy and Infectious Diseases: *Bacterial infections, research activities*, 2007, at www.niaid.nih.gov/topics/bacterialinfections/research/Pages/activities.aspx. Accessed Sept 15, 2010.

34. Centers for Disease Control and Prevention: *MRSA infections*, 2010, at www.cdc.gov/mrsa/index.html. Accessed Sept 15, 2010.

35. National Institutes of Health, National Institute of Allergy and Infectious Diseases: *Antimicrobial (drug) resistance*, 2009, at http://niaid.nih.gov/topics/antimicrobialResistance/Understanding/Pages/healthissue.aspx. Accessed Sept 15, 2010.

36. World Health Organization: *Infection control*, 2010, at www.who.int/topics/infection_control/ed. Accessed Feb 21, 2011.

37. Centers for Disease Control and Prevention: *Personal prevention of MRSA skin infections*, 2010, at www.cdc.gov/mrsa/prevent/personal.html. Accessed Nov 26, 2010.

38. Centers for Disease Control and Prevention: *Prevention of MRSA infections in healthcare settings*, 2010, at www.cdc.gov/mrsa/prevent/healthcare.html. Accessed Nov 26, 2010.

39. Centers for Disease Control and Prevention: *Prevention of MRSA infections in athletic facilities*, 2010, at www.cdc.gov/mrsa/prevent/athletic.html. Accessed Nov 26, 2010.

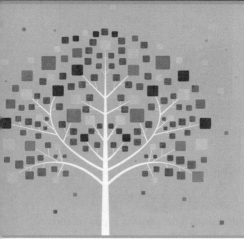

The 10-month-old child taking his first steps, the 6-year-old girl riding a bicycle, the high school jock "dunking" the basketball, the newly married couple dancing at their wedding, the 40-year-old neighbor walking his dog, and the 76-year-old grandmother knitting a scarf are all examples of mobility accomplished through functions of the musculoskeletal and nervous systems. As a basic physiologic process, mobility is required for optimal health. Changes in mobility can significantly impact biophysical health, psychosocial health, and functional status. Nurses should be familiar with interventions to promote optimal mobility, prevent situations leading to immobility, and minimize complications when immobility occurs.

DEFINITION(S)

Mobility refers to purposeful physical movement, including gross simple movements, fine complex movements, and coordination. Mobility is dependent upon the synchronized efforts of the musculoskeletal and nervous systems as well as adequate oxygenation, perfusion, and cognition. More specifically, mobility requires adequate energy, adequate muscle strength, underlying skeletal stability, joint function, and neuromuscular coordination to carry out the desired movement. For the purposes of this concept analysis, mobility is defined as a *"state or quality of being mobile or movable."*[1,p1479] There are many variations on the term mobility seen throughout the literature worth mentioning. The term *immobility* refers to an inability to move. *Impaired physical mobility* describes a state in which a person has a limitation in physical movement, but is not immobile;[2] *impaired bed mobility* refers to the inability to change positions in bed independently. Although immobility is typically considered a negative state, there are times that immobility or immobilization is therapeutic. For example, the immobilization of a shoulder if it has been dislocated provides desired rest, recovery, and comfort.

The term *deconditioned* is used to describe a loss of physical fitness. This applies not only to an athlete who fails to maintain an optimal level of training but also to an individual who fails to maintain optimal physical activity. In the context of health care, this term applies to patients who experience extended immobility (following prolonged bed rest, as an example) resulting in an overall deconditioned state of the musculoskeletal and cardiopulmonary systems. This is particularly a problem among older adults. A term with similar meaning in the nursing literature is *disuse syndrome.*[2]

SCOPE AND CATEGORIES

Scope

The scope of mobility as a concept ranges on a continuum from complete immobility to partial mobility (also referred to as impaired mobility) to full mobility (Figure 23-1). Mobility can be considered on a micro or macro perspective. Mobility and immobility may refer to a particular part of the body (an arm or leg as an example), or it can refer to the entire body. Thus mobility and immobility are not mutually exclusive; a patient with an immobilized extremity can be mobile, for example. Also, because mobility is on a continuum, a change in mobility may be temporary.

Categories

The primary categories of immobility are best described based on causative factors. Obvious categories are neurologic disorders (including the brain, the spinal cord, and the peripheral nerves), musculoskeletal disorders (bones, joints, muscles), or a combination of both (neuromuscular conditions). Mobility can also be negatively impacted by several other physiologic conditions (particularly cardiovascular and pulmonary conditions leading to fatigue) in the absence of neuromuscular dysfunction (Figure 23-2).

RISK FACTORS

Populations at Risk

All individuals are potentially at risk for altered mobility regardless of age, ethnicity, race, or socioeconomic status. Because of the effects of aging the population group at greatest risk for impaired mobility is older adults. These changes predispose

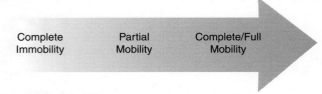

FIGURE 23-1 Scope of Mobility as a Concept.

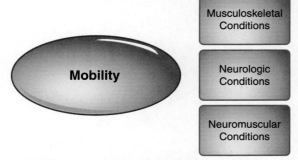

FIGURE 23-2 Categories of Mobility Concept.

older individuals to a greater incidence of falls and greater challenges regaining full mobility following a period of impaired mobility. An estimated 90% of hip fractures are a result of falling; 76% of hip fractures occur among elderly women.[3]

Individual risk factors for changes in mobility are often attributed to acute and chronic conditions, chronic pain, and injury/trauma. Specifically, individuals with orthopedic injury, congenital deformities, neurologic disorders, strokes, head injury, spinal injury, nutritional deficiencies, and cardiopulmonary conditions are particularly susceptible. Side effects and adverse effects of many medications (such as corticosteroids and chemotherapy) and medical treatments can also affect mobility.

PHYSIOLOGIC PROCESSES AND CONSEQUENCES

Physiology of Mobility

Optimal mobility relies on bones, joints, articular cartilage, tendons and ligaments, skeletal muscle, and the mechanics of muscle contraction.

Bones

The skeleton has three overarching roles as related to mobility: acts as the structural foundation for the body and as leverage to move body parts, supports and protects tissues and internal organs, and provides attachment sites for muscles and ligaments. Bones also serve as a storage center for calcium and as a production center for red blood cells within the bone marrow.[4] The human body has 206 bones divided into 2 groups: the axial skeleton (bones that comprise the skull, thorax, and spinal column) and the appendicular skeleton (bones that comprise the upper and lower extremities).

All structures designed for use over time require ongoing maintenance and intermittent repair. The same is true for the skeletal system. Remodeling is a term that describes an ongoing maintenance of bone tissue through a process where new bone tissue replaces existing bone tissue in bone-remodeling units.[5] The remodeling process also provides the mechanism to repair injured bones (for example, a fracture). Remodeling requires adequate nutrition, hormonal regulation, and blood supply. The severity of the bone injury and the availability of remodeling elements influence the rate or speed that injured bone heals.

Joints

Bones come together at joints. Joints provide stability to bones and allow skeletal movement. Mobility is impacted by the degree of joint freedom; joints allow for skeletal positioning to carry out the desired action. The various types of movement provided by joints include flexion, extension, rotation, adduction, abduction, supination, and pronation. Some of the most common problems associated with mobility arise as a result of joint pain and/or changes in joint function.

Three classifications of joints (based on stability and movement) include synarthrosis joints (nonmovable), amphiarthrosis joints (slightly movable), and diarthrosis joints (freely movable).[5] Joints are also classified by structure. Fibrous joints serve to hold bones together in place with connective tissue. For example, the tibia and fibula are held together by a fibrous ligament. Cartilaginous joints feature cartilage material that holds the joint together and provides some movement. For example, ribs are attached and held to the sternum by cartilaginous material, allowing movement for the process of breathing, yet providing chest stability required for the breathing process. Joints that allow the most movement are also the most complex. Synovial joints have multiple elements including a joint capsule, synovial membrane, joint cavity, synovial fluid, and articular cartilage. Articular cartilage acts as a cushion by distributing joint loads over a wide area, thereby reducing prolonged compression of articulating bones within the joint. Without cartilage, significant friction and pain result from joint movement.

Muscles

Skeletal muscle differs from other types of muscle in the body in many ways, but one of the most important differences is that it is under voluntary control.[4] Optimal skeletal muscle function depends on the following five factors: nerve impulses reaching the muscle, muscle fibers response to nerve stimulus, proprioception, mechanical load, and joint mobility. Impairment of any one of these factors negatively impacts purposeful movement.

Nerve impulses reach skeletal muscle from the spinal cord and peripheral nerves via motor neurons. The motor neurons innervate a group of muscle fibers known as the motor or muscle unit. There are many different types of muscle fibers within a muscle unit depending on the function and type of responsiveness required. Muscles that maintain body posture do not have the same need for quick responsiveness as do the ocular muscles, as an example, but are less sensitive to fatigue.

Muscle movement occurs in response to nerve stimulation of the muscle fibers triggering muscle contraction. On a cellular level, the functional units of muscle contraction are myofibrils. Movement occurs in a reciprocal fashion among muscle groups. If one group contracts, another group must relax. As an example, flexion of the elbow to move the forearm up requires contraction of the biceps muscles and relaxation of the triceps muscles; likewise, flexion of the elbow joint requires contraction of the triceps muscles and relaxation of the biceps muscles. If both are contracted at the same time, no movement occurs.

Proprioception is the mechanism that provides a sense of position and movement; this process allows for accuracy in the degree of movement with muscle contraction. Mechanical load of movement is associated with having adequate strength within the muscle group to carry out the desired task. For example, most humans would struggle to pick up a 250-pound object and walk 50 feet with it. However, such a feat is entirely possible for individuals who are well conditioned for this.

Age-Related Differences

Significant changes to the musculoskeletal system occur throughout infancy and childhood as a function of growth and development. The appendicular skeleton (extremities) grows faster than the axial skeleton (head, thorax, and spine)—partly because the appendicular skeleton is disproportionately shorter than the axial skeleton. Throughout infancy, childhood, and adolescence bones change in composition, grow in length and diameter, and undergo changes in rotation and alignment. Similarly, the size and composition of muscles undergo changes as a result of physical growth and development throughout childhood, and are a major factor in weight gain during adolescence.[5,6]

A number of musculoskeletal changes occur with aging. In the spinal column, a thinning of vertebral disks, shortening of the spinal column, and onset of kyphosis with spinal column compression occurs. Bone density decreases and becomes brittle (particularly in females), leaving older adults more susceptible to fracture. Cartilage becomes rigid and fragile and there is a loss of resilience and elasticity of ligaments. Muscle mass and tone reduce significantly in late adult years. Cumulatively, these changes result in mobility impairment attributable to reduced range of motion and pain in joints, reduced muscle strength, and increased risk for bone fracture.[3]

Physiologic Consequences of Immobility

Attaining and/or maintaining mobility is paramount to health. The human body was designed to move; thus when movement is limited, consequences occur. A state of immobility has a significant impact on the entire body; literally all body systems are potentially negatively impacted.

Cardiovascular Complications

Cardiovascular complications occur both with central and with peripheral perfusion. A lack of physical activity results in reduced cardiac capacity. According to one study a 15% reduction in muscle mass will occur after 12 weeks of complete immobility.[7] This translates to reduced force of cardiac contraction and a reduction in cardiac output. The loss of endurance and the deconditioned state present challenges when the resumption of physical activity is desired.

Problems also occur within the vascular system. Decreased efficiency of orthostatic neurovascular reflexes and diminished vasopressor mechanism cause orthostatic hypotension intolerance when an individual attempts to attain an upright position because of blood pooling in the extremities.[5] Adequate perfusion and venous return depend on skeletal muscle contraction, and frequent changes in body position. Because muscular contraction (particularly in the legs) facilitates venous return, venous stasis occurs during periods of inactivity. Slowed blood flow provides an opportunity for the formation of blood clots. Deep vein thrombosis is a relatively common complication associated with immobility.

Respiratory Complications

Physical activity is associated with full lung expansion, particularly among those engaging in exercise. Immobility contributes to reduced lung expansion and eventually leads to atelectasis (an airless state of the alveoli), and reduced capacity for gas exchange. Pooling of respiratory secretions, coupled with a reduced cough effort, places the immobilized patient at risk for stasis pneumonia.

Musculoskeletal Complications

Muscle tone, joint movement, and maintenance of bone density require active skeletal contraction and weight bearing. Skeletal muscle adapts to nonuse by reducing mass. Thus prolonged immobility leads to significant reductions in muscle mass and atrophy; in fact, an average loss of 25% muscle mass occurs with permanent immobility.[7] The lack of activity leads to contracture in the joint, primarily as a result of muscle shortening. Muscle atrophy and joint contraction are particularly concerning because together these negatively affect functional ability.[8]

The lack of weight bearing leads to bone demineralization and calcium loss from the skeletal system. The degree of bone demineralization and calcium depletion is related to the severity and duration of immobility as well as the degree of weight-bearing ability. Over time, osteoporosis can develop in response to immobility.

Integument System

Sustained pressure on the skin reduces perfusion to the tissues. A reduced flow of oxygenated blood causes hypoxemia of the tissues and increases the risk for skin breakdown. Individuals who lack the ability to move in bed (impaired bed mobility) have increased risk not only because of pressure but also because of shearing forces that often accompany certain positions or occur during transfers. These problems are further exacerbated if the patient has a poor nutritional status and is incontinent. Development of pressure ulcers commonly results.

Gastrointestinal Complications

Constipation is a frequently reported complication of immobility for several reasons. First, not being able to assume an optimal upright position makes having a bowel movement more challenging; for many people, relying on the assistance of others to have a bowel movement is embarrassing and may lead to reluctance in acting on the urge. From a physiologic standpoint, the gastrointestinal tract slows during states of immobility, resulting in reduced peristaltic motility. Constipation, reduced appetite, and anorexia negatively impact nutritional status.

Urinary Complications

Immobility leads to three common problems that occur within the urinary system: renal calculi, urinary stasis, and infection. Renal calculi result from stasis of urine in the renal pelvis and because of increased circulating serum calcium levels (as a result of bone reabsorption mentioned earlier). The bladder loses tone, making it difficult to completely empty the bladder, particularly in a lying position for voiding. This often results in urinary tract infection because the presence of urinary stasis provides an optimal environment for the growth of bacteria.

Psychologic Effects

Acute and chronic psychologic conditions that result from immobility include boredom, depression, feelings of helplessness/hopelessness, grieving, anxiety, anger, disturbed body image, and decreased verbal and nonverbal communication. Individuals who are unable to work or are even unable to meet basic activities of daily living often experience a loss of self-worth or value associated with the role change. Social isolation and mood disturbances are common.

Psychologic effects of immobility are especially concerning among children. For children, physical activity is integral to daily activity. Not only is it essential for physical growth and development, but also it is central to expression, communication, and making sense of the world around them. Immobilization can interfere with intellectual and psychomotor function. Emotional responses range from anger and aggressive behavior to passive quiet demeanor and withdrawal. Developmental regression is common. Children often become less communicative and may experience depression; in some cases, hallucinations occur.[6]

ASSESSMENT

History

The history, as it related to the concept of mobility, includes general health information (past health history, medications, surgery/treatments) and social history (lifestyle, employment, family assessment, activities of daily living) as a starting point.[9] Additionally, the history includes an investigation of specific symptom's experienced by the patient. Areas of questions specific for mobility include:

- Presence of pain with movement
- Recent changes in mobility or problems with balance
- Presence of fatigue
- Recent falls
- Recent changes in ability to complete activity of daily living

Examination Findings

Objective data regarding the assessment of the musculoskeletal system include an assessment of gait and body posture; joints; size, symmetry, and strength of muscles; and range-of-motion of joints.[9] Pediatric assessment also involves observation of motor activities as related to developmental milestones.[6]

Expected findings include erect posture and symmetry of extremities. Gait should be smooth, coordinated, and balanced. The spine should be straight with expected curvatures. Muscles and joints should be assessed for size, symmetry, strength, range of motion, and stability. Comparisons are made between right and left sides.[9] Assessment of muscle strength is done utilizing a muscle strength scale (0 = no detection of muscular contraction; 5 = full muscle strength). Findings considered abnormal include observed deformity of bone or joint, edema, ecchymosis, localized warmth and redness, a loss of function, numbness, guarding (due to pain), and limitations in movement or mobility. Further information related to conducting an assessment of the musculoskeletal system can be found in physical assessment textbooks.

Diagnostic Tests

There are many diagnostic tests used to evaluate musculoskeletal disorders. These are briefly described next.

Radiographic Diagnostics

- The x-ray evaluates the integrity of bones and joints and is the most common radiographic test used to diagnose fractures.
- Computed tomography (CT) scan identifies soft tissue and bony abnormalities and evaluates musculoskeletal trauma.
- Magnetic resonance imaging (MRI) uses radiowaves and magnetic fields to provide an image of soft tissue. This is used most efficiently to evaluate soft tissues, such as a vertebral disk, tumor, ligaments, and cartilage.[10]
- Myelogram is a radiographic study of the spinal cord and nerve root using a contrast dye. This is particularly useful in the evaluation of individuals with back pain.
- Arthrography (arthrogram) is a visualization of a joint by injection of a radiopaque substance into the joint cavity, allowing for the evaluation of bones, cartilage, and ligaments. This is most commonly performed on the knee and shoulder joints, but also can be done on hips, ankles, and wrists.[10]
- Bone mineral density (BMD) is a diagnostic test used to determine the core mineral content and the density of bone. This test is used for the diagnosis of osteoporosis and osteopenia.
- Bone scan evaluates the bone uptake of a radionuclide material; the uptake is related to the metabolism of the

bone. The primary indication of this test is to detect metastatic cancer in the bone,[10] but it is also used to evaluate avascular necrosis or unexplained bone pain.

Other Diagnostic Tests

- Arthroscopy is a procedure that allows direct visualization of the interior of a joint through an endoscope. This procedure is most commonly performed on the knee, but can be done on other joints as well.
- Electromyography (EMG) is an evaluation of electrical activity generated within the muscle. This is used to determine the quality of neuromuscular innervation.
- Laboratory tests can be used to provide various types of information about the functional state of muscles, bones, or joints. Types of tests include blood tests (such as alkaline phosphatase, calcium, phosphorus, uric acid, creatine kinase, blood urea nitrogen [BUN], creatinine, and myoglobinuria), analysis of joint fluids, and pathologic analysis of biopsied tissue (such as a muscle biopsy or bone biopsy).

CLINICAL MANAGEMENT

Primary Prevention

Regular physical activity is associated with multiple health benefits and is foundational to primary prevention measures.[11,12] Prevention of problems associated with mobility is relatively simple—that is, maintaining the highest level of regular physical activity possible along with optimal nutrition, keeping an ideal body weight, and getting adequate rest. Taking measures to prevent injury and trauma are also considered primary prevention strategies.

Nutrition, as a primary prevention strategy, links to musculoskeletal development. During infancy, childhood, and adolescence, adequate protein and calcium in the diet is critical for the musculoskeletal development described previously. Adequate calcium intake is also necessary to prevent osteoporosis among older individuals. Maintaining a healthy body weight prevents excessive joint strain and is associated with fewer problems with back pain. Falls represent one of the most common mobility problems among older adults; thus fall prevention is an important aspect of primary prevention. Strategies include participating in regular physical activity (to maintain muscle strength and balance), making the environment safer (e.g., avoiding hazards, using hand rails, wearing sturdy shoes with nonslip soles, having adequate lighting), and optimizing vision.[3]

Secondary Prevention (Screening)

The primary areas to highlight related to mobility and screening are osteoporosis, mobility screening, and fall risk assessment. For osteoporosis screening, the United States Preventive Services Task Force (USPSTF) recommends screening of women age 65 years and older as well as younger women who have increased fracture risk; dual-energy x-ray absorptiometry of the hip and spine is the recommended method to measure bone density. There is no recommendation for the

screening interval.[13] Further, the USPSTF concludes evidence is insufficient to recommend screening for men.[13]

There are a large number of mobility and fall risk assessment screening tools available. In a review of the literature, Scott and colleagues reviewed 38 different fall and mobility assessment tests for use among older adults and concluded most are reliable. However, they were unable to conclude if one screening test was better than another because of the wide range of settings for use.[14] One of the most common screening tests is the Timed Get-Up-and-Go test that measures mobility in people who are able to walk on their own (assistive devices allowed).[15] Another common screening is the Performance-Oriented Mobility Assessment (POMA) test,[16] which aids in the identification of gait and balance impairments.

Collaborative Interventions

Numerous interventions for the care of individuals with limitations in mobility exist and are usually presented based on the underlying medical condition or diagnosis. Interventions specific for a health condition associated with changes or loss in mobility often overlap. From a conceptual perspective, a general discussion of interventions delivered by various members of the health care team that directly impact mobility is presented based on the following categories: care of the immobilized patient, exercise therapy, pharmacologic agents, surgical interventions, immobilization, and assistive devices.

Care of Immobilized Patient

Many nursing interventions are incorporated into care for the immobilized patient, regardless of the underlying condition. First, the patient should be positioned with appropriate *body alignment*. This is important to prevent injury to extremities and joints and is critical to prevent pulmonary complications. For example, pillows are commonly used to support the body alignment of a patient placed in a Sims position. The patient should be *repositioned* at least once every 2 hours. The patient dependent on caregivers for positioning is at significant risk for skin breakdown because of prolonged pressure over bony prominences. Thus *skin care* is a priority for immobilized patients; the skin should be kept clean, dry, and protected to prevent skin breakdown. The skin is regularly monitored and examined for evidence of adequate circulation.

Because immobilized patients are at risk for stasis pneumonia, coughing and deep breathing is part of the standard treatment plan. Patients with adequate cognition are encouraged to use an incentive spirometer every hour to maintain ventilator capacity. Rotational bed therapy has been shown to reduce the incidence of pneumonia among patients receiving mechanical ventilation in intensive care settings.[17]

Bed exercises should be encouraged to the extent possible to minimize atrophy and maintain joint movement. Many types of exercise can be done including flexion and extension of the foot to promote venous blood return and prevent venous stasis.[18] If a patient has a trapeze bar over the bed, pull-up exercise should be encouraged if he or she is able. Range-of-motion (ROM) exercise is critical to promote circulation and to minimize complications to the joints.[18,19] Active ROM is performed by the patient; assisted ROM is a patient doing most of the exercise, but under the guidance/assistance of a health professional. Passive ROM involves the nurse taking each affected joint through the full range of motion. It is important not to force the joints past the point of resistance. If tolerated, patients should be encouraged to stand at the side of the bed to promote weight bearing. Doing this a few times a day for a few minutes helps to reduce bone demineralization.

Exercise Therapy

Exercise therapy is a cornerstone intervention in the management of individuals with impairments in mobility. Several forms of exercise therapy exist including Exercise Therapy: Ambulation, Exercise Therapy: Joint Mobility, Exercise Therapy: Stretching and Exercise Therapy: Balance. Exercise therapy is performed by nurses or physical therapists in acute care, community-based, and home care settings. The goal of exercise therapy is rehabilitative or preventive and is often done in multiple combinations. There are many examples of exercise therapy such as ROM exercises mentioned earlier, water exercise, and gait training. Specific exercise therapy interventions are created based upon patient needs in collaboration with physicians, nurses, physical therapists, and occupational therapists.

Pharmacologic Agents

Many of the drugs used to treat mobility problems are for the relief of pain or inflammation, or to treat underlying conditions. It is beyond the scope of this concept to describe each drug separately, but general categories are briefly presented.

Antiinflammatory agents. Inflammation is a common primary or secondary finding among conditions leading to changes in mobility, from an underlying autoimmune condition to a traumatic injury. Antiinflammatory agents, such as corticosteroids and nonsteroidal antiinflammatory drugs (NSAIDs), are by far the most common used. Another group of agents used to reduce inflammation are the immunomodulators. These function to weaken or modulate the activity of the immune system, thereby decreasing the inflammatory response.

Analgesics and muscle relaxants. Although a reduction in inflammation provides some relief of discomfort associated with inflammation, analgesic agents are an important component of drug therapy. Agents that are specific for analgesia include opioids (such as morphine), NSAIDs, and aspirin, among many others. Although not considered analgesics, muscle relaxants provide relief from discomfort by eliminating muscle spasms.

Supplements. In addition to adequate dietary intake, nutritional supplementation with vitamin D and calcium is a useful prevention and treatment measure for osteoporosis, particularly for postmenopausal women. Bisphosphonates are antiresorptive agents that slow or stop the reabsorption of calcium from the bone, resulting in maintained or increased bone density and strength. These agents are used to treat osteoporosis.

Surgical Interventions

Many conditions that impact mobility are treated with surgical intervention. Surgical intervention can be either curative or palliative, depending on the underlying cause.[18] Examples of surgical interventions related to mobility/immobility include arthroscopic procedures, open and/or closed reduction of a fracture with or without external and/or internal fixation, amputation, synovectomy, osteotomy, debridement, arthroplasty, arthrodesis, diskectomy, and spinal fusion. Specific details about these procedures can be found in medical-surgical textbooks.

Immobilization

Following an injury or surgery, immobilization of a joint or bone is often necessary to provide stability and hold the appendage in place so that healing can occur. Following a fracture, as an example, bone remodeling takes several weeks before the fracture is stable. Immobilization is necessary to enhance the healing process, protect the bone from further injury, and provide comfort to the patient. Common examples of immobile devices include casts, splints, abductor pillows, shoulder restraints, braces, and traction. Assessment to verify adequate perfusion (presence of pulse and/or rapid capillary refill in nail beds), movement, and sensation is critical. Another indication for immobilization is to prevent injury. For example, spinal immobilization is routinely applied to all patients with suspected spinal injury in the prehospital setting by strapping the patient on a backboard and using a cervical collar to prevent head rotation.[20]

Assistive Devices

Assistive devices are objects to provide assistance with a task. Many types of assistive devices are commonly used in patient care including assistive devices for mobility/ambulation and assistive devices for activities of daily living (ADLs). Common mobility/ambulation assistive devices include canes, crutches, walkers, wheelchairs, and prostheses.[21] Patients must be taught to use these devices correctly to avoid injury.

CLINICAL NURSING SKILLS FOR MOBILITY

- Assessment
- Patient transfers
- Positioning
- Range-of-motion exercises
- Continuous passive motion
- Sequential compression device and elastic stockings
- Ambulation
- Assistive devices
  - Cane
  - Crutches
  - Walker
  - Wheelchair
- Traction
- Heat and cold therapy
- Immobilization devices
- Medication administration

Causes

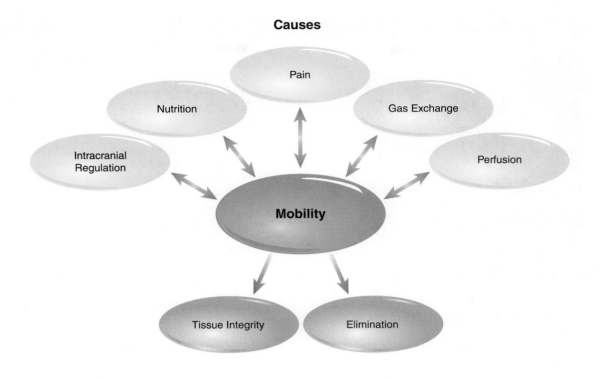

Effect

FIGURE 23-3 Mobility and Interrelated Concepts.

INTERRELATED CONCEPTS

Mobility links to numerous concepts featured in this textbook. Those considered most important are shown in Figure 23-3 and discussed further.

Gas exchange. Individuals who have inadequate gas exchange may become immobile because of excessive fatigue. Immobile patients are at risk of developing complications associated with gas exchange, such as stasis pneumonia.

Intracranial regulation. Individuals who have intracranial regulation problems may become immobile as a result of unsteadiness and imbalance.

Nutrition. Individuals who are immobile may be unable to purchase, prepare, and/or consume adequate nutrition; likewise, individuals with inadequate nutrition may have decreased mobility because of excessive fatigue.

Pain. Either acute or chronic pain may interfere with mobility; likewise, some conditions associated with immobility cause pain.

Perfusion. Individuals who have perfusion problems are less able to be mobile because of reduced oxygenated blood reaching peripheral tissues. Among individuals who are immobile, perfusion is less effective because of reduced venous return.

Tissue integrity. Individuals who are immobile may have diminished tissue integrity or be at risk of experiencing such problems, such as skin breakdown.

Elimination. Individuals who are immobile may have changes to their pattern of elimination or be at risk of experiencing problems such as constipation or urinary retention.

EXEMPLARS

Many clinical exemplars related to mobility and impaired mobility exist. Box 23-1 presents some of the most common causes across the lifespan based on the following categories: trauma and injury, congenital defects, skeletal disease, neuromuscular dysfunction, muscle, and joint and connective tissue. There are certainly far more conditions than listed. Specific information about these exemplars is readily available in medical-surgical, pediatric, and gerontologic textbooks.

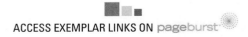

ACCESS EXEMPLAR LINKS ON pageburst

MODEL CASE

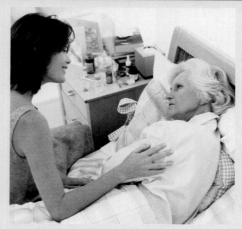

Mrs. Lydia Martin, an 81-year-old widow, lives alone in her single-story home. She prides herself in being fully independent. During the middle of the night, Mrs. Martin fell in her home while walking to the bathroom. She was unable to get up, so she crawled to the telephone and dialed 911. She was transported to the emergency department and underwent diagnostic tests including hip and femur x-ray and computerized tomography, which confirmed a left femoral neck fracture. Her past medical history reveals anxiety, osteoporosis, arthritis, and cataracts.

Mrs. Martin underwent an open reduction internal fixation (ORIF) surgical procedure. Following surgery, she had a compression dressing with ice to the left hip, a Foley catheter, antiembolism stockings, a sequential compression device, and an order to use the incentive spirometer every hour while awake. Her medications included hydrocodone bitartrate 7.5 mg/acetaminophen 750 mg (Vicodin ES) 2 tabs orally every 4 hours, as needed for pain po and enoxaparin (Lovenox) 40 mg daily subcutaneously.

On post-op day 1, the physical therapist began to work with Mrs. Martin; the goal of the session was to get her out of bed to a chair. During the attempted transfer, Mrs. Martin's surgical site was painful and her Foley catheter was pulled, causing pelvic pain. She screamed in pain and refused to continue the process. Mrs. Martin was anxious and fearful of pain; she also became worried that she would never walk again and would end up in a nursing home. She was unwilling to move and declined physical therapy the next 3 days. Mrs. Martin became constipated and lost her appetite. She also developed a stage 2 pressure ulcer over her sacrum. Eventually, on post-op day 4 Mrs. Martin agreed to work with the physical therapist. By this time she experienced significant weakness and fatigue and was unable to move independently. Mrs. Martin was later transferred to a rehabilitation center to continue regaining her mobility.

Case Analysis

This case exemplifies the concept of mobility in many ways. Mrs. Martin's age and injury were significant risk factors for a fall and hip fracture. Following surgery, she was immobile for several days because of pain and experienced several consequences of immobility including constipation, loss of appetite, poor nutrition, and impaired skin integrity. Mrs. Martin's fear of not being able to return home is substantiated in the literature; it is estimated that up to 25% of older adults who lived independently before a hip fracture spend up to 1 year in a nursing facility to recover and 20% die within 1 year.[22,23]

■■■ BOX 23-1   EXEMPLARS OF MOBILITY

Trauma and Injury
- Amputation
- Fractures
- Joint dislocation
- Spinal cord injury
- Sprains

Congenital Defects
- Clubfoot
- Developmental hip dysplasia
- Metatarsus adductus
- Spina bifida
- Syndactyly

Skeletal Disease
- Bone tumors
  - Fibrosarcoma
  - Myelogenic tumors
  - Osteosarcoma
- Metabolic bone disorders
- Osteochondroses

- Osteomyelitis
- Osteoporosis
- Osteogenesis imperfecta
- Rickets
- Spine
  - Herniated disk
  - Low back pain (acute/chronic)
  - Scoliosis
  - Spinal stenosis

Neuromuscular Dysfunction
- Amyotrophic lateral sclerosis
- Cerebral palsy
- Guillain-Barré syndrome
- Huntington's disease
- Multiple sclerosis
- Muscular dystrophy
- Myasthenia gravis
- Parkinson's disease
- Spinal muscular atrophy
- Stroke

Muscle
- Disuse atrophy
- Fibromyalgia
- Myotonia
- Myositis
- Rhabdomyoma
- Rhabomyosarcoma

Joint and Connective Tissue
- Ankylosing spondylitis
- Gout
- Systemic lupus erythematosus
- Systemic sclerosis
- Tendonitis

Arthritis
- Juvenile rheumatoid arthritis
- Psoriatic arthritis
- Osteoarthritis
- Rheumatoid arthritis

REFERENCES

1. Taber: *Cyclopedic medical dictionary*, Philadelphia, 2009, FA Davis.
2. Ackley BJ, Ladwig GB: *Nursing diagnosis handbook*, ed 9, St Louis, 2010, Mosby.
3. National Center for Injury Prevention and Control, Centers for Disease Control and Prevention: *Preventing falls among seniors.* Available at www.cdc.gov/ncipc/duip/spotlite/falls.htm.
4. Copstead LC: *Pathophysiolgy*, ed 4, St Louis, 2010, Saunders.
5. McCance KL, Huether SE: *Pathophysiology: the biologic basis for disease in adults and children*, ed 10, St Louis, 2010, Elsevier/Mosby.
6. Hockenberry MJ, Wilson D: *Wong's essentials of pediatric nursing*, ed 8, St Louis, 2009, Mosby/Elsevier.
7. Hill J: Cardiac plasticity: mechanisms of disease, *N Engl J Med* 358:1370–1380, 2008.
8. Kasper CE: Skeletal muscle atrophy. In Carrieri-Kohlman V, Lindsey AM, West CM, editors: *Pathophysiological phenomena in nursing*, St Louis, 2003, Saunders.
9. Wilson S, Giddens J: *Health assessment for nursing practice*, ed 4, St Louis, 2009, Mosby/Elsevier.
10. Pagana KD, Pagana TJ: *Mosby's diagnostic and laboratory test reference*, ed 10, St Louis, 2011, Mosby/Elsevier.
11. U.S. Department of Health and Human Services: *Healthy People 2020*, Nov 2010. Available at www.healthypeople.gov/2020/default.aspx.
12. Pender N, Murdaugh C, Parsons MA: *Health promotion in nursing practice*, ed 6, Upper Saddle River, NJ, 2011, Pearson.
13. United States Preventive Services Task Force: Accessed at www.uspreventiveservicestaskforce.org/recommendations.htm.
14. Scott V, Votova K, Scanlan A, et al: Multifactorial and functional mobility assessment tools for fall risk among older adults in community, home-support, long-term and acute care settings, *Age Aging* 36(2):130–139, 2007.
15. Wall JC, Bell BS, Campbell S, et al: The timed get-up-and-go test revisited: measurement of component tasks, *J Rehabil Res Dev* 37(1):109–111, 2000.
16. Tinetti ME: Performance-oriented assessment of mobility problems in elderly patients, *JAGS* 34:119–126, 1986.
17. Goldhill DR, Imhoff M, McLean B, et al: Rotational bed therapy to prevent and treat respiratory complications: a review and meta-analysis, *Am J Crit Care* 16(1):50–61, 2007.
18. Lewis SL: *Medical-surgical nursing—assessment and management of clinical problems*, ed 8, St Louis, 2011, Elsevier/Mosby.
19. The Arthritis Foundation: *Range-of-motion exercises,* 2004. Retrieved May 1, 2011, from Practical Help from the Arthritis Foundation: www.arthritis.org.
20. Peery CA, Brice J, White WD: Prehospital spinal immobilization and the backboard quality assessment study, *Prehosp Emerg Care* 11(3):293–297, 2007.
21. Kedlaya D: *Assistive devices to improve independence,* 2008. Retrieved May 5, 2011, from Medscape Reference, http://emedicine.medscape.com/article/325247-overview.
22. Magaziner J, Hawkes W, Hebel JR, et al: Recovery from hip fracture in eight areas of function, *J Gerontol Med Sci* 55A(9): M498–507, 2000.
23. Leibson CL, Toteson ANA, Gabriel SE, et al: Mortality, disability, and nursing home use for persons with and without hip fracture: a population-based study, *J Am Geriatr Soc* 50:1644–1650, 2002.

24

Tissue Integrity

Debra Hagler

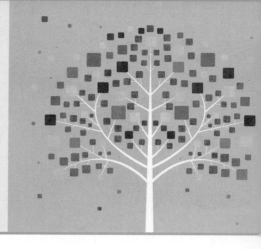

The skin is the largest organ of the body and supports several functions critical for life including management of temperature, conservation of fluid, and protection from infection.[1] Maintenance of skin and tissue integrity is a fundamental component of nursing care. Not only do nurses play a pivotal role in maintaining skin and tissue integrity, but they also contribute independently and collaboratively to the care management when that integrity is disrupted.

DEFINITION(S)

Tissues are organized groups of cells with common functions. Of the four types of tissues— muscle, neural, connective, and epithelial—the concept of tissue integrity is most closely aligned with epithelial tissue. The term *impaired skin integrity* is specifically focused on damage to the epidermal and dermal layers of epithelial tissue, but deep damage to skin integrity is often associated with disruption of other underlying tissues as well. For the purposes of this concept, tissue integrity is defined as *the state of structurally intact and physiologically functioning epithelial tissues such as the integument (including the skin and subcutaneous tissue) and mucous membranes.* The term *impaired tissue integrity* reflects varying levels of damage to one or more of those groups of cells.[2,3]

SCOPE AND CATEGORIES

The scope of the concept tissue integrity ranges from an intact state serving as the body's protective barrier to some level of disrupted or impaired tissue integrity. Disrupted skin integrity ranges from superficial or partial-thickness injury of the epidermis to deep or full-thickness injury of the dermis and deeper tissues (Figure 24-1). Six major categories of impaired skin integrity include trauma/injury; loss of perfusion; immunologic reaction; infections and infestations; thermal or radiation injury; and lesions. Within each of these categories, partial- or full-thickness injury can occur.

Trauma/Injury

Tissue trauma or injury includes intentional and unintentional damage that can range from a superficial abrasion or scrape to a deep wound penetrating the skin and subcutaneous layers, with possible extension to muscle, internal organs, and bone. In areas where there is little or no subcutaneous tissue (such as the back of the hand, top of the foot, or the skull), a relatively minor blunt or penetrating injury may extend directly through the skin layers to the muscle or bone. A surgical incision is an example of an intentional injury to the skin, inflicted to reach deeper structures for a therapeutic purpose.

Loss of Perfusion

All tissue requires a continuous supply of oxygenated blood. The skin is relatively tolerant of poor circulation compared to other organs, and in times of shock even survives a temporary shunting of oxygenated blood away from the skin to protect the perfusion of other organs such as the heart and brain. However, prolonged poor perfusion or a short period of no perfusion can lead to tissue necrosis. Examples of impaired tissue integrity resulting from a chronic state of poor perfusion include ulcerations or necrosis and loss of toes related to diabetes and/or peripheral arterial disease. Examples of short-term or temporary disruption of perfusion to tissue caused by unrelieved pressure are dermal or pressure ulcers. Dermal ulcers are also described as bedsores, pressure sores, and pressure ulcers. Dermal ulcer is a more general term than pressure ulcer; dermal tissue damage may be caused by a number of factors, including excessive pressure on tissue, but the damage seen in a dermal ulcer is not necessarily caused by pressure.[2]

Immunologic Reaction

The skin is a visible indicator of an allergic response to a foreign substance, and the presence of redness, rash, or hives is a common way that allergies are first noted. Common substances that lead to skin irritation and/or local allergic

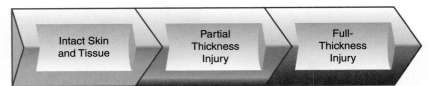

FIGURE 24-1 Scope of Concept. Tissue integrity ranges from intact skin, to partial-thickness injury, to full-thickness injury.

response are soaps, detergents, cleaning products, fragrances, and metals such as nickel, silver, and copper.[4] In addition, many common skin disruptions are thought to be chronic immune responses to unknown antigens. As an example, psoriasis is a recurrent inflammatory disease that affects 2% of the population in the United States.[5] In rare cases, a hypersensitivity response to a medication can cause extensive tissue sloughing. Severe hypersensitivity disorders such as Stevens-Johnson syndrome or toxic epidermal necrolysis involve large areas of epidermal tissue sloughing with high risk for life-threatening fluid loss, body heat loss, and widespread infection.[1]

Infections and Infestations

Skin and mucous membrane infections can be the result of bacteria, fungi, or viruses. Live arthropods can cause tissue disruption by burrowing under the skin or attaching to skin structures such as hair shafts.

Bacterial Infection

Bacteria are normally present on the skin and generally cause no harm, but pathogenic bacteria can cause superficial or deep infection. A small abrasion or lesion can provide a portal for opportunistic or pathogenic infectious organisms to infect deeper tissues. Superficial skin infections involve only the dermis, but deeper bacterial infection causes cellulitis, an inflammation of the subcutaneous and potentially muscle tissues. Impetigo, caused by staphylococci or beta-hemolytic streptococci, is the most common superficial bacterial infection, and spreads easily among small children on contact. A common bacterial infection of the skin seen in adolescents is acne vulgaris.[6]

Fungal Infections

The fungi that cause superficial fungal infections live on the dead skin cells of the epidermis. *Candida albicans* and other *Candida* species thrive in warm, moist areas of the skin and mucous membranes, particularly the mouth, the vagina, and the skin folds. In the absence of normal flora's bacterial protection on the skin or mucous membranes, *Candida* can grow more readily. It is common for a person to experience a fungal infection with *Candida* after a course of antibiotics for a bacterial infection decreases the normal protective flora and allows the *Candida* to flourish. Tinea refers to a group of diseases caused by a fungus that vary in skin sites and the types of fungal species, such as tinea capitis on the head and tinea pedis (athlete's foot) on the feet.[4]

Viral Infections

There are several viruses known to cause a disruption in skin integrity. A common form of skin virus is the verruca, or wart. Although warts most commonly occur on the skin of the hands and feet, they also can be found on the genitalia. Herpes simplex virus (HSV) can infect the skin and mucous membranes; HSV type 1 (HSV-1) is found on the face and mouth, whereas HSV-2 is found on genital mucosa.[4]

Infestations

The skin can be infested with live arthropods such as mites and lice. Mites such as scabies burrow into the epidermis and lay eggs. Mites are transmitted person-to-person or through infested sheets or clothing, where they can live for up to 2 days. Lice most commonly infect the body, head, or pubic hair. Lice lay eggs along the hair shafts and are transmitted by personal contact, clothing and bedding, and shared hair care items or hats.

Thermal or Radiation Injury

Thermal and radiation injuries to the skin range from the common sunburn to extensive scald burns and radiation burns. Sunburn appears after the epidermis is exposed to excessive ultraviolet radiation (UVR), and appears as redness and inflammation, and may extend to blistering with chills, fever, and pain, followed by peeling skin. Radiation therapy, used to treat some forms of cancer, requires careful monitoring and skin care to prevent burns. Burns resulting from a scald with hot liquids or contact with flame/heated items cause a series of chemical and mechanical events at the tissue level. The initial tissue response to burns is inflammation and vasoconstriction; edema at the site of a burn can last for several days. Later, fibroblasts produce the proteins collagen and elastin, which restore some structure and elasticity to the wound. Macrophages attack bacteria and foreign substances to clean the wound. New vascular networks form and new epithelial cells grow and cover the open area from the wound edges to the center as the wound begins to contract.[4]

Lesions

Lesions can range from benign skin growths and vascular lesions to invasive malignant tumors. The most common types of skin cancers, named for the type of cell that has become malignant, are melanoma, basal cell, and squamous.[7] Even benign skin growths may cause concern if they cause pressure on or displacement of other structures or change the person's appearance in a distressing way.

RISK FACTORS

All individuals are potentially at risk for impaired tissue integrity, regardless of age, gender, race, or ethnicity. However, there are factors that place some populations at greater risk for tissue disruption.

Populations at Risk

Infants and Children

Some risk factors for skin disruptions are related to age or developmental level. For example, diaper rash is a common rash among infants and toddlers; likewise, this age group is also at risk for injuries to the skin secondary to uncertain mobilization, the affinity for grasping and placing various objects in their mouth, and the inability to protect themselves from environmental dangers. Communicable skin infections such as impetigo are more commonly transmitted where there is frequent skin-to-skin contact, such as in child-care centers or schools when children play together. School-age children may experience frequent minor tissue injuries such as abrasions, bruises, and lacerations that occur during active play.

Older Adults

Changes related to the aging process increase the risk of impaired skin integrity. These changes include a loss of lean muscle mass; decreases in skin thickness, strength, moisture, and elasticity; decreased arterial and venous blood flow; and a diminished perception of pain and pressure that may prevent early recognition of tissue injury.[8] Skin changes often associated with aging are a result of sun and environmental damage over a long period of time, leading to a wrinkled and leathery appearance. In addition, hair and nail growth slow with aging and a decrease in sebaceous gland activity can result in rough, dry, and itchy skin.[4]

Personal Risk Factors

There are a number of risk factors that increase risk for impaired skin integrity. Health conditions associated with poor peripheral perfusion, malnutrition, obesity, fluid deficit or excess, impaired physical mobility, and immunosuppression increase the risk of tissue disruption. In addition, exposure to chemical irritants, radiation, excessively hot or cold temperatures, and mechanical damage may cause a loss of tissue integrity. Individuals who have undergone medical treatments, surgical procedures, or invasive procedures also have disruptions to skin integrity.

Skin Cancer Risk

Basal cell skin cancer usually occurs in areas that have been exposed to the sun, such as the face, and is the most common skin cancer in light-skinned persons. Squamous cell skin cancer is usually found in areas less exposed to the sun, such as the legs or feet, and is the most common type of skin cancer in dark-skinned persons. Melanoma is a virulent and potentially life-threatening form of skin cancer that has a good prognosis if detected early. Melanoma, which begins in

---

BOX 24-1   COMMON CONDITIONS ASSOCIATED WITH DERMAL ULCER DEVELOPMENT

- Peripheral vascular disease
- Myocardial infarction
- Stroke
- Multiple trauma
- Musculoskeletal disorders/fractures/contractures
- Gastrointestinal bleed
- Spinal cord injury (e.g., decreased sensory perception, muscle spasms)
- Neurologic disorders (e.g., Guillain-Barré syndrome, multiple sclerosis)
- Unstable and/or chronic medical conditions (e.g., diabetes, renal disease, cancer, chronic obstructive pulmonary disease, congestive heart failure)
- Preterm neonates
- Dementia
- Recent surgical patient (This risk may be related to length of time on operating room/procedure table, hypotension, or type of procedure.[12])

From Institute for Clinical Systems Improvement (ICSI): *Pressure ulcer prevention and treatment: health care protocol,* Bloomington, Minn, 2010, Author.

---

the pigment cells or melanocytes, can grow on any skin surface, and is found most commonly in men on the head, neck, and torso. In women, melanoma is more commonly found on the torso or the lower legs. Although rare in people with dark skin, when it does develop, melanoma is found under the nails and on the palms and soles. Fair-skinned men and women older than 65 years, persons with atypical moles, and those with more than 50 moles are at substantially increased risk for melanoma. Other risk factors for skin cancer include family history and a considerable history of sun exposure and sunburns.[9]

Dermal Ulcer Risk

In 2007, about 1 of every 100 residents of nursing homes was reported to have 1 or more pressure ulcers. The *Healthy People 2020* initiative has established an objective of reducing the prevalence of pressure ulcers by 10% from the 2007 rate.[10] Recognition of risk factors is critical for meeting this goal. Risk factors include those with impaired cognition or sensory perception, immobility, friction and shearing, poor nutrition, impaired perfusion or oxygenation, impaired sensation, and incontinence/moisture. Certain medical conditions (many of which are associated with these risk factors) also are associated with increased risk (Box 24-1).

PHYSIOLOGIC PROCESSES AND CONSEQUENCES

Physiologic Processes

Epithelial cells join to cover nearly every internal and external surface of the body, providing protection from the external environment, absorption of needed substances, secretion

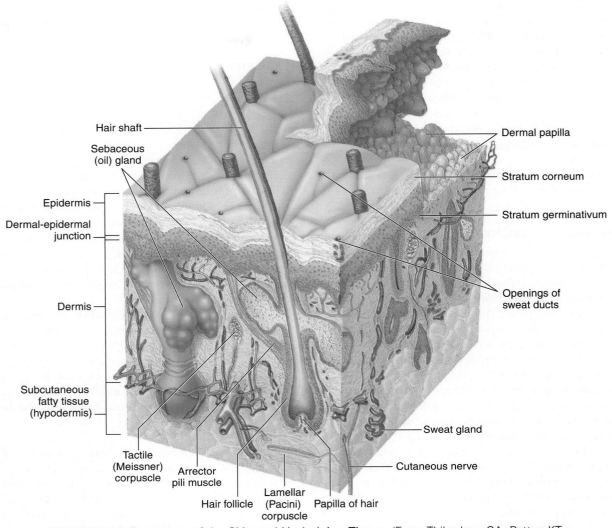

FIGURE 24-2 Structures of the Skin and Underlying Tissue. (From Thibodeau GA, Patton KT: *Anatomy and physiology*, ed 5, St Louis, 2003, Mosby.)

Labels: Hair shaft, Sebaceous (oil) gland, Epidermis, Dermal-epidermal junction, Dermis, Subcutaneous fatty tissue (hypodermis), Tactile (Meissner) corpuscle, Arrector pili muscle, Hair follicle, Lamellar (Pacini) corpuscle, Papilla of hair, Dermal papilla, Stratum corneum, Stratum germinativum, Openings of sweat ducts, Sweat gland, Cutaneous nerve

into body cavities, and excretion of wastes from the body. The skin, as an external surface, protects other body tissues and organs from mechanical trauma, fluid loss, chemical disruption, and infectious organisms. The nerves in the skin layer provide a safety mechanism as sensations of pain, temperature, and touch inform a person about the environment and reveal the need to take actions that prevent or limit damage to the skin and deeper structures. The integument is made up of the two layers commonly known as skin, the epidermis and the dermis, and the underlying subcutaneous or fat tissue (Figure 24-2). Sweat glands and the small muscles in the dermal layer that control piloerection (goosebumps) help to maintain body temperature in a fairly narrow range despite widely varying air temperatures. Subcutaneous tissue, under the dermal layer, contains fat cells that assist in temperature regulation as well as additional sweat glands.

Mucous membranes are those epithelial tissues, located continuously with the skin, that line the eyelids, nose and mouth, ears, genital area, urethra, and anus. Some, but not all, mucous membranes secrete thick, slippery mucus that helps protect the body from infection.[4]

Expected Physiologic Process for Wound Healing

Tissue injuries and wounds heal by processes of primary, secondary, or tertiary intention. Primary intention healing occurs when wound margins are well approximated, as in a sutured surgical incision or a simple laceration, and takes place more rapidly than the other types of healing. Secondary intention healing processes occur when wounds such as ulcerations have edges that do not approximate; repairing the larger wound surface area takes longer because it requires generating granulation tissue to fill the gap. Tertiary intention healing processes occur when a wound is sutured closed only after a long period of healing, and results in more scarring than wounds closed with primary intention. Tertiary closure takes place when a wound closure is delayed until resolution of infection or wound contamination; then the clean and partially healed wound is sutured to facilitate continued wound healing.

There are three phases of wound healing: inflammatory, granulation, and maturation. The inflammatory phase lasts 3 to 5 days while blood clots form at the site of injury and platelets release growth factors to begin the healing process. A matrix of cells and debris forms at the site and is later removed by macrophages. During the granulation phase, new vessels and collagen structures are formed, resulting in a very vascular pink wound. White blood cells continue to remove debris while epithelium begins to grow from the edges toward the center of the wound.

The maturation phase, which may continue for months or years, involves collagen fiber remodeling and contraction of the scar.[11,12]

Consequences of Impaired Skin Integrity

When tissue integrity is impaired, a number of body functions are affected, including thermoregulation, elimination, fluid and electrolyte balance, protection from infection, safety, comfort/pain, and body image. The skin normally regulates body temperature within a narrow range through the constriction or relaxation of piloerector muscles, vasodilation and vasoconstriction of vessels in the dermis, and the production of sweat. In the absence of skin integrity, such as in an overwhelming burn surface, the ability to regulate body heat and prevent excess fluid loss is impaired, requiring external maintenance of temperature and massive fluid replacement. Whether the skin is disrupted by a small abrasion or a massive wound, that loss of the skin as a barrier means that underlying structures are no longer protected from the environment's infectious and chemical dangers. Even a small open wound provides a portal that could lead to an overwhelming infection if the person is immunocompromised or the infectious agent is particularly virulent. Loss of deep skin structures such as nerve endings prevents normal sensation that provides cues about the environment and helps promote safety in active movement. Because the skin has many sensory nerve endings, particularly over the hands and face, injuries and lesions of the skin can be painful. The skin's ready visibility as the external surface of the body means that, unlike some other health conditions which can be hidden from casual view, skin conditions are often visible to others. Skin conditions may affect body image and even cause psychologic distress because they may alter the person's mental model of how he or she appears.[2]

ASSESSMENT

The assessment of skin involves taking a history, conducting an examination of the skin, and performing diagnostic testing.

History

The history should begin with questions related to overall health including past and current conditions, current medications taken, known allergies, and family history.

Medications may cause rashes through an allergic reaction, a side effect of the medication, or by inducing hypersensitivity to sunlight. Box 24-2 lists specific information about tissue integrity to discuss during the health history.

Examination
Inspection

Examination of the skin starts with inspection, which includes color and presence of lesions. Normal adult skin is a consistent color, ranging for individuals from light pink, to olive tones, to deep brown, with relatively darker shades in areas of sun exposure. Oral and eye mucosa may appear pale pink to darker pink, red, or brown. Skin findings may vary by natural skin color; for example, cyanosis may appear as a blue-gray color in light-skinned persons, whereas it appears as an ashen gray color in dark-skinned persons and is particularly visible in the nail beds and mucosa. The more visible areas for identifying generalized changes in skin color for a dark-skinned person are those areas with the least pigmentation, particularly the subglossal mucosa, the buccal mucosa, the palpebral conjunctiva, and the sclera.[13]

There are a wide range of types of skin lesions, including both normal variations and lesions that indicate possible disease. A bright light, a ruler, and a magnifying glass are helpful tools for skin inspection. Describe the lesions' location, size, shape, color, elevation, consistency, and pattern. Describe the grouping of multiple lesions in rings, lines, or diffusely scattered arrangements and the color, odor, and consistency of any exudates.[14]

Palpation

The skin should be smooth and intact with an even surface, and minimal perspiration or oiliness except after exercise or heat exposure. There should not be dryness, peeling, or cracking, although there may be calluses over the hands, feet, elbows, and knees. Skin folds should not be excessively moist or macerated. Skin mobility and turgor are assessed by picking up and slightly pinching the skin on the forearm or under the clavicle. The skin should move easily when lifted and should return to place immediately when released.

BOX 24-2   HEALTH HISTORY RELATED TO TISSUE INTEGRITY

- Previous history of skin disease (allergies, hives, psoriasis, eczema)
- Change in pigmentation
- Change in mole (size or color)
- Excessive dryness or moisture
- Pruritus
- Excessive bruising
- Rash or lesion
- Medications
- Hair loss
- Change in nails
- Environmental or occupational hazards
- Self-care behaviors

From Jarvis CL: *Physical examination and health assessment*, ed 5, Philadelphia, 2008, Saunders.

Age Variations

Infants have thinner, more permeable skin and less subcutaneous fat than older children and adults. This leads to a higher potential for fluid loss and challenges in regulating temperature for maintaining warmth. Adolescents experience increased sebum and sweat production, which commonly results in acne on the face and neck.

Skin thins through the aging process and subcutaneous fat is lost over the hands, feet, and lower arms and legs. Older adults may appear to have skin hanging loosely over other tissues. Checking for skin turgor using the older adult's hand may give a false impression of dehydration. The loss of subcutaneous tissue in the hands causes an appearance of skin tenting even when hydration is normal. Therefore check the skin turgor in the forearm or under the clavicle instead. Skin tears may occur with minimal contact or pressure as a result of the thin, fragile texture.

Assessment of Dermal Ulcers

Dermal ulcers are assessed for size and depth, as well as for level of tissue injury. If a wound is covered with eschar, a dry scab covering, it is not possible to determine the stage of the wound. The eschar may have to be removed through pharmacologic, mechanical, or surgical debridement to allow for accurate assessment and to promote healing. Pressure ulcers are classified by four stages, presented in Box 24-3.

BOX 24-3   STAGES OF PRESSURE ULCERS

Suspected Deep Tissue Injury: Localized area of discolored (purple or maroon) intact skin or blood-filled blister due to underlying soft tissue damage resulting from pressure or shear. May be difficult to detect among individuals with dark skin tone. May include a thick blister over a dark wound bed; wound may become covered with eschar.

I. Nonblanchable erythema of intact skin usually over bony prominence; darkly pigmented skin may not have visible blanching

II. Partial-thickness skin loss involving epidermis or dermis presenting as a shallow open ulcer with a red-pink wound bed, without slough; may also present as an intact or open/ruptured serum-filled blister

III. Full-thickness skin loss involving damage or necrosis of subcutaneous tissue that may extend to, but not through, underlying fascia; may include undermining and tunneling

IV. Full-thickness skin loss with extensive destruction, tissue necrosis, or damage to muscle, bone, or supporting structures

Non Stageable: Full thickness tissue loss in which base of ulcer is covered by slough (yellow, tan, gray green or brown) and/or eschar (tan, brown, or black). True depth of the wound cannot be determined until the slough and/or eschar is removed to expose the base of the wound.

From National Pressure Ulcer Advisory Panel: *Pressure ulcer stages revised by NPUAP,* 2007. Available at www.npuap.org/pr2.htm.

Diagnostic Tests

There are only a few common diagnostic tests linked to the concept of skin integrity.

- *Woods lamp:* Use of a Woods lamp (black light) or immunofluorescence is an enhanced method of inspection involving magnification and special lighting. It is used to identify the presence of infectious organisms and proteins associated with specific skin conditions.

- *Tissue biopsy:* Various types of biopsies—such as punch, incision, excision, and shave—are conducted for pathologic evaluation of tissue when skin lesions are suspected to be malignant. The type and depth of biopsy are based on the lesion and the location.

- *Wound cultures:* Cultures identify the organisms causing infection. Because some bacteria are present on healthy skin, normal skin flora may be identified in wound cultures along with any pathogenic bacteria.

- *Patch testing:* This is a test used to identify specific allergens causing dermatitis. One or many potential allergens can be tested simultaneously by applying a small amount of the substance to a marked area of the skin, usually on the back.[15]

CLINICAL MANAGEMENT

Primary Prevention

Primary prevention measures guard against development of disease. Primary measures to prevent disruption to skin integrity include basic hygiene measures, nutrition, and protection from excessive sun exposure and other environmental hazards.

General Skin Hygiene

Basic skin hygiene prevents many common skin irritations and infections. Infants and toddlers may need frequent cleansing of hands and face to remove food residue and frequent perineal care to prevent irritation from urine and stool. During adolescence, sebaceous and sweat glands become more active; therefore more frequent bathing becomes necessary to reduce body odors and oils. In older adults, sebaceous and sweat glands become less active again and skin loses some of its moisture and elasticity. Older adults may find that a complete daily bath with soap can cause excessively dry skin, and may prefer to bathe less frequently and use a gentle moisturizing cleanser.

Hygiene practices are often linked to cultural norms and rituals. Although in North America it is common to bathe or shower daily and to use deodorant, people of a variety of cultures may prefer to bathe less frequently or not bathe when they are ill or after childbirth.[16]

Nutrition

Adequate protein, calories, minerals, vitamins, and hydration are needed for maintenance of healthy skin. In the chronic absence of adequate nutrition, skin becomes dry and flaky, hair appears dull, and subcutaneous fat disappears. Even a short period of poor nutrition, such as before and after abdominal surgery when eating is not possible, can damage tissue integrity and delay wound healing.[12]

BOX 24-4   RECOMMENDATIONS FOR PROTECTION FROM SUN EXPOSURE

- Avoid outdoor activities during the middle of the day. The sun's rays are the strongest between 10 AM and 4 PM. When you must be outdoors, seek shade when you can.
- Protect yourself from the sun's rays reflected by sand, water, snow, ice, and pavement. The sun's rays can go through light clothing, windshields, windows, and clouds.
- Wear long sleeves and long pants. Tightly woven fabrics are best.
- Wear a hat with a wide brim all around that shades your face, neck, and ears. Keep in mind that baseball caps and some sun visors protect only parts of your skin.
- Wear sunglasses that absorb UV radiation to protect the skin around your eyes.

- Use sunscreen lotions with a sun protection factor (SPF) of at least 15. (Some doctors will suggest using a lotion with an SPF of at least 30.) Apply the product's recommended amount to uncovered skin 30 minutes before going outside, and apply again every 2 hours or after swimming or sweating.
- Sunscreen lotions may help prevent some skin cancers. It is important to use a broad-spectrum sunscreen lotion that filters both *UVB* and *UVA radiation*. But you still need to avoid the sun during the middle of the day and wear clothing to protect your skin.

From National Cancer Institute: *What you need to know about melanoma and other skin cancers*, 2010, NIH Pub No. 10-7625.

Sun Exposure

Box 24-4 lists National Cancer Institute[7] recommendations for skin cancer prevention through protection from sun exposure. Population-based interventions designed to increase sun-protective behaviors in recreational settings include offering culturally relevant educational materials and reminders at the entrances to the setting; providing sun-safety training for, and role modeling by, lifeguards, aquatic instructors, recreation staff, parents, and children; increasing the availability of shaded areas; and having sunscreen readily available.[17]

Burn Prevention

Smoke alarms should be installed and maintained to help prevent burns in the home setting. Hot-water temperature should be set at a maximum of 120° F to avoid scald burns. Infants and toddlers are at particular risk for burns. Parents should be advised not to carry their infant and hot liquids or foods at the same time. Milk and formula should not be heated in the microwave because it can heat unevenly and scald the infant's mouth. Young children should be kept away from hot oven doors, irons, wall heaters and grills, electrical cords, and cups or dishes of hot food. Older children should be taught stovetop and microwave oven safety.[18]

Dermal Ulcer Prevention

Prevention of pressure ulcers requires initial assessment and daily reevaluation and documentation for inpatients at risk of pressure ulcer development, using a tool such as the *Braden Scale for Predicting Pressure Sore Risk*.[19] The Braden scale consists of six subscales based on common causes of dermal ulcers: sensory perception, moisture, activity, mobility, nutrition, and friction and shear. Adults scoring less than 18 of 23 possible points on the Braden scale are considered at risk for dermal ulcers. The scale is often completed as part of a health care facility admission assessment and may be repeated daily in acute care facilities, depending on the initial risk level. Those persons found to be at higher risk should have more intensive preventive measures instituted to maintain tissue integrity and protect from further tissue damage.[8] Those at risk in home settings can be taught to assess their own skin

and to have family or caregivers assist in monitoring the skin. Prevention interventions include minimizing or eliminating friction and shear (such as sliding on sheets), minimizing pressure through frequent repositioning and use of pressure-relieving devices, managing moisture on skin surfaces, and maintaining adequate nutrition and hydration.[20]

Secondary Prevention (Screening)

Malignant melanoma is a particularly virulent type of skin cancer, but early detection and treatment improves the outcome. Use the mnemonic ABCDEF to remember the early signs of melanoma during a skin assessment, and teach the mnemonic to patients to guide their own comprehensive monthly skin self-assessments.[7]

- **A**symmetry: The shape of one half does not match the other half.
- **B**order that is irregular: The edges are often ragged, notched, or blurred in outline. The pigment may spread into the surrounding skin.
- **C**olor that is uneven: Shades of black, brown, and tan may be present. Areas of white, gray, red, pink, or blue may also be seen.
- **D**iameter: There is a change in size, usually an increase. Melanomas can be tiny, but most are larger than the size of a pea (larger than 6 millimeters or about ¼ inch).
- **E**volving: The mole has changed over the past few weeks or months.

Collaborative Interventions
Pharmacotherapy

Medications for skin disorders include topical and oral or parenteral antibiotics, steroids, topical moisturizers, and anticancer agents or immunosuppressive chemotherapy.

Antibiotics. When a specific organism is identified through culture, topical or parenteral antibiotics may be prescribed. Common fungal infections such as athlete's foot may be treated with over-the-counter antifungal creams or sprays. When arthropod infestations appear in the skin, an antibiotic is commonly administered in a shampoo or lotion form applied to the affected area.

Steroids. Topical steroids are often used to treat allergic dermatitis and the irritating symptom of pruritus (itching). Oral or parenteral steroids may be used when urticaria (hives) manifest on the skin, indicating a systemic allergic reaction.

Emollients. Lotions, creams, and ointments may be used to retain moisture in the skin or as a base for other medications. Gels and powders are used when there already is excessive moisture present.

Chemotherapy agents. When skin lesions are malignant, cancer chemotherapy and systemic adjunct therapy may be used.[15]

Wound Care

Cleansing. The goal of wound cleansing is to promote wound healing by removing debris and excessive exudates. Shallow wounds that appear healthy are generally cleaned with mild soap and water, and deeper but healthy wounds are cleaned gently with normal saline. Harsh solutions such as diluted bleach, acetic acid, or hydrogen peroxide can break down the cell walls of the newly formed tissues, so those solutions are reserved for use in heavily contaminated wounds.

Dressings. Wounds may be mechanically protected to promote healing in a moist but not soggy environment using a simple adhesive bandage or more complex dressings. Dry dressings are used to absorb excessive exudates whereas moist dressings are used to maintain a slightly damp environment to promote tissue repair. Nonadherent dressings are useful when the wound drainage is slight and may dry between dressing changes, causing the dressing to stick to the fragile wound surface wound and then disrupt the wound during dressing removal. Occlusive and semiocclusive dressings are used for clean wounds that have minimal drainage but need to be protected from environmental pathogens, such as a central intravenous catheter puncture site. Hydrocolloid, hydrogel, and alginate dressings are used to absorb exudates while maintaining a therapeutically moist wound surface to promote healing. Vacuum-assisted closure systems are special dressings for complex wounds attached to a device that maintains negative pressure at the wound surface, aiding in removal of large amounts of exudates.[12]

The Institute for Clinical Systems Improvement[21] suggests that multiple aspects of care be integrated when treating a person with a pressure ulcer (see Box 24-5).

Phototherapy

Some skin disorders such as psoriasis and atopic dermatitis respond to controlled phototherapy with UV light. Protection from excessive UV exposure is important to prevent tissue damage.

Surgical Treatment

Excisions—knife or laser. Surgical removal is indicated for benign lesions such as deep plantar surface warts unresponsive to other therapy and malignant lesions such as squamous, basal cell, and melanoma skin cancers. Surgical excision of primary melanoma includes not only removal of the lesion but also removal of an additional margin around

---

> **BOX 24-5   CARE REQUIRED FOR A PERSON WITH A PRESSURE ULCER**
>
> - Establishing the treatment goal
> - Moist wound healing
> - Cleansing the wound
> - Choosing appropriate topical wound care products
> - Wound debridement
> - Consideration of adjunct therapy (negative-pressure wound therapy, electrical stimulation)
> - Pain management
> - Management of nutrition (specific nutrient goals, vitamin and mineral supplement)
> - Surgical consultation
> - Patient and staff education
> - Discharge plan or transfer of care
> - Documentation of all items in patient's medical record

From Institute for Clinical Systems Improvement (ICSI): *Pressure ulcer prevention and treatment: health care protocol,* Bloomington, Minn, 2010, Author.

the lesion to ensure eradication of malignant cells. For example, a 4-mm lesion would be removed along with an additional 2-cm margin around the lesion, which means that the resulting wound would be 4.4 cm in diameter, much larger than the size of the original lesion.[22]

Debridement. Wounds covered with a dry, leathery eschar surface may not be able to heal until the eschar is removed. Surgical debridement enables a rapid removal of the eschar and debris, whereas debridement using topical collagenase or wet to dry dressings is done slowly over a longer period of time. Collagenase ointment breaks down the peptide bonds in necrotic ulcer or burn wound tissues without damaging the healthy tissue.[23]

Skin grafts. When there is extensive damage associated with large or deep burns, wound excision and skin grafting are required to cover and heal the burn wounds. Grafts may be taken from other areas of the person's skin, from living or nonliving donors, or as porcine grafts. In addition to grafts, skin substitutes and bioengineered skin coverings are available.[12]

Nutrition

Tissue maintenance and repair is dependent on adequate nutrition. Protein and vitamins A and C are particularly critical for wound healing because they are required for collagen synthesis. In the absence of adequate nutrition, delayed wound healing and infection are likely outcomes. Early provision of enteral or parenteral nutrition is important to consider for patients at risk of prolonged inadequate nutrition.[12]

> **CLINICAL NURSING SKILLS FOR TISSUE INTEGRITY**
>
> - Assessment
> - Skin hygiene
> - Wound care
> - Medication administration

Causes

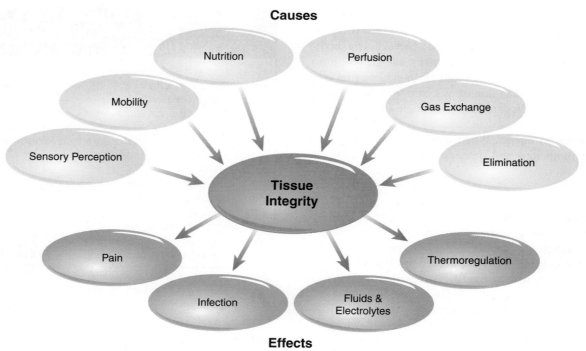

Effects

FIGURE 24-3 Tissue Integrity and Interrelated Concepts. This is a cause-and-effect model showing the concepts that impact tissue integrity, and those concepts that are negatively impacted when tissue integrity is disrupted.

MODEL CASE

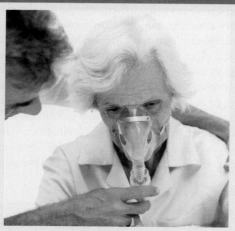

Mrs. Ramona Garcia, a 76-year-old female, is admitted to a medical respiratory unit with pneumonia after 4 days of difficulty breathing, fever, and a productive cough with purulent sputum. She reports that she has been sleeping sitting upright in a chair for the past week because it was too difficult to breathe lying down. When Mrs. Garcia's breathing is comfortable enough for her to be turned briefly for a full skin assessment, the nurse notes a 4-cm red area on the buttock over the left ischial tuberosity that does not blanch to pressure.

Recognizing the reddened area as a stage I dermal ulcer likely related to the prolonged pressure from sitting, the nurse collaborates with the patient, family, and health team on a plan for prevention of further tissue breakdown including frequent movement and positioning, adequate nutrition, hygiene for prevention of moisture collection from sweat or urine that might lead to skin maceration, and use of pressure-relieving devices.

Case Analysis

Mrs. Garcia has a serious medical problem that has kept her in a sitting position struggling for airflow over several days. Continuously sitting up to improve her air exchange has prevented her from relieving the pressure on her ischium, which she would normally have done by changing her position when she noticed discomfort. Poor perfusion from the near constant pressure on her ischium and a low capillary oxygen level from her respiratory illness have begun to cause damage at the tissue level. Mrs. Garcia's nurse identifies a reddened area of skin that does not blanch to touch as a stage I dermal ulcer and realizes that any further injury to the area could result in deep tissue damage and an open wound. In order to promote tissue healing and prevent further injury, the nurse begins tissue integrity interventions promptly and recognizes that helping Mrs. Garcia maintain comfortable air exchange will encourage her to position herself off of the dermal ulcer.

INTERRELATED CONCEPTS

Concepts related to tissue integrity include **Perfusion, Gas exchange, Nutrition, Mobility, Sensory perception, Elimination, Pain, Fluid and electrolyte balance, Thermoregulation,** and **Infection.** Adequate perfusion with oxygen- and nutrient-enriched blood promotes tissue integrity; in the absence of oxygen or sufficient nutrition the tissues can be suffocated and/or starved, leading to atrophy or necrosis. Adequate sensory perception and mobility provide the stimulus and action needed to prevent prolonged pressure from limiting the perfusion to a specific tissue area.

In the presence of tissue integrity, the skin functions to maintain fluid and electrolyte balance and thermoregulation. Production of sweat, which includes both water and electrolytes, serves to cool the excessive body temperatures that could lead to organ damage and to remove wastes. The skin and mucous membranes provide a barrier to most organisms and many toxic substances in the environment. The nerves of the skin provide feedback about temperature and pressure that serve as a safety mechanism for the person negotiating the environment. Unrelieved pressure on a body tissue eventually causes injury. Urinary or bowel incontinence can also contribute to impairment of tissue integrity through skin contact with caustic excretions. Finally, a loss of tissue integrity often results in pain because the skin is laden with sensory nerve endings reactive to the irritation of the local damage. These interrelationships are depicted in Figure 24-3.

EXEMPLARS

There are a large number of clinical exemplars related to skin integrity. Box 24-6 presents common clinical conditions associated with tissue integrity impairment by categories noted earlier: trauma/injury, loss of perfusion, immunologic conditions, infections, thermal/radiation, and lesions.

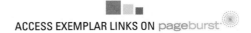

ACCESS EXEMPLAR LINKS ON pageburst

BOX 24-6 EXEMPLARS OF TISSUE INTEGRITY

Trauma/Injury
- Abrasion
- Blister
- Chemical irritant
- Ecchymosis
- Hematoma
- Laceration
- Surgical incision

Loss of Perfusion
- Dermal ulcer
- Diabetic foot ulcer

Immunologic Disorders
- Atopic dermatitis
- Psoriasis
- Scleroderma
- Stevens-Johnson syndrome
- Systemic lupus erythematosus
- Toxic epidermal necrolysis

Infection
Bacterial
- Cellulitis
- Impetigo

Fungal
- Tinea capitis
- Tinea cruris
- Tinea pedis (athlete's foot)
- Vaginitis

Viral
- HSV-1 (oropharyngeal)
- HSV-2 (genital)
- Verruca (warts)

Infestations
- Lice
- Scabies

Thermal/Radiation
- Burns
- Frostbite
- Radiation burns
- Sunburn

Lesions
- Basal cell carcinoma
- Benign tumors
- Malignant melanoma
- Squamous cell carcinoma

REFERENCES

1. Huether SE, McCance KL: *Pathophysiology: the biologic basis for disease in adults and children*, ed 6, St Louis, 2010, Elsevier.
2. Carpenito-Moyet LJ: *Nursing diagnosis: application to clinical practice*, ed 13, Philadelphia, 2010, Wolters Kluwer.
3. Venes D, editor: *Taber's cyclopedic medical dictionary*, Philadelphia, 2009, FA Davis.
4. Porth CM, Matfin G: *Pathophysiology: concepts of altered health states*, ed 8, Philadelphia, 2009, Wolters Kluwer.
5. Camisa C: *Handbook of psoriasis*, Malden, Mass, 2004, Blackwell.
6. Pickering LK, Baker CJ, Kimberlin DW, et al: *Red Book: 2009 report of the Committee on Infectious Diseases*, ed 28, Elk Grove Village, Ill, 2009, American Academy of Pediatrics.
7. National Cancer Institute: *What you need to know about melanoma and other skin cancers*, 2010, NIH Pub No. 10–7625.
8. Berman A, Kozier B, Erb G, et al: *Kozier & Erb's fundamentals of nursing: concepts, process, and practice*, New York, 2008, Pearson.
9. U.S. Preventive Services Task Force (USPSTS): Screening for skin cancer: USPSTS recommendation statement, *Ann Intern Med* 150:188, 2009.
10. U.S. Department of Health and Human Services: *Healthy People 2020: the road ahead, 2010,* at http://healthypeople.gov/2020/default.aspx. Accessed Jan 22, 2011.
11. Zaiontz RG, Lewis SL, et al: Inflammation and wound healing. In Lewis SL, Heitkemper M, Dirksen S, editors: *Medical-surgical nursing: assessment and management of clinical problems*, ed 8, St Louis, 2011, Mosby.
12. Barbul A, Efron DT: Wound healing. In Brunicardi FC, editor: *Schwartz's principles of surgery*, New York, 2010, McGraw-Hill.
13. Jarvis CL: *Physical examination and health assessment*, Philadelphia, 2008, Saunders.
14. Wilson S, Giddens J: *Health assessment for nursing practice*, St Louis, 2009, Mosby.
15. Sinni-McKeehen B: Nursing assessment: integumentary system; Nursing management: integumentary system. In Lewis SL, Heitkemper M, Dirksen S et al, editors: *Medical-surgical nursing: assessment and management of clinical problems*, ed 8, St Louis, 2011, Mosby/Elsevier.
16. Potter PA, Perry AG, Stockert P, et al: *Basic nursing*, ed 7, St Louis, 2011, Mosby/Elsevier.
17. Guide to Community Preventive Services: *Preventing skin cancer: education and policy approaches in outdoor recreation settings*, 2010, at www.thecommunityguide.org/cancer/skin/education-policy/outdoorrecreation.html. Accessed Jan 22, 2011.
18. Gardner HG: American Academy of Pediatrics Committee on Injury, Violence, and Poison Prevention: Office-based counseling for unintentional injury prevention, *Pediatrics* 119(1):202–206, 2007.
19. Bergstrom N, Braden BJ, Laguzza A, et al: The Braden scale for predicting pressure sore risk, *Nurs Res* 36(4), 1987.
20. Ayello EA, Sibbald RG, et al: Preventing pressure ulcers and skin tears. In Capezuti E, Zwicker D, Mezey M et al, editors: *Evidence-based geriatric nursing protocols for best practice*, ed 3, New York, 2008, Springer.
21. Institute for Clinical Systems Improvement (ICSI): *Pressure ulcer prevention and treatment: health care protocol*, Bloomington, Minn, 2010, Author.
22. American Society of Plastic Surgeons: *Evidence-based clinical practice guideline: treatment of cutaneous melanoma*, Arlington Heights, Ill, 2007, Author.
23. Ramundo J, Grey M: Collagenase for enzymatic debridement: a systematic review, *J Wound Ostomy Continence Nurs* 36(6):S4, 2009.

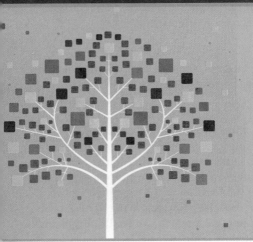

Sensory Perception

Louise Fleming

Sensory perception represents a complex physiologic process that allows humans to interact efficiently within the environment. These senses provide the basis for social interactions, communication, and learning. Sensory perception also provides a level of protection through detection and reaction to dangers within the environment. Impairment in any of the five senses can lead to significant challenges that can negatively impact development, health, and well-being with consequences that are potentially significant. This concept presentation provides an overview of the concept, including recognizing who is most at risk for impairment in sensory perception, and possible treatment when impairment occurs.

DEFINITION(S)

To describe the concept of sensory perceptual processes and alterations in these processes, it is important first to define both sensation and perception and then to understand how they relate to one another. Sensation is the ability to perceive stimulation through one's sensory organs such as the nose, ears, and eyes. This stimulation can be internal, from within the body, or external, from outside the body, and includes feelings of pain, temperature, and light. External stimuli are commonly received and processed through the five senses: vision, hearing, taste, smell, and touch. Examples of external stimulation are a loud noise or distinct smell such as garlic or vanilla. Perception is defined as the process by which we receive, organize, and interpret sensation. Sensory perception can then be defined as the ability to receive sensory input and, through various physiologic processes in the body, translate the stimulus or data into meaningful information.[1] For the purposes of this concept analysis, the definition of sensory perception is *the ability to receive sensory input and, through various physiologic processes in the body, translate the stimulus or data into meaningful information.*

SCOPE AND CATEGORIES

Populations at Risk

Both sensation and perception occur within various parts of body systems and through a complex interaction of both sensory receptors and the nervous system. For persons to interact fully with the environment in which they live, it is important that these systems are as functional as possible. The major categories that form this concept link to the five senses:
- Vision
- Hearing
- Taste
- Smell
- Touch

Within each of these categories, the level of function ranges from optimal functioning to impairment. For the purposes of this concept, impairment of sensory perception includes altered function or perceptual ability—but does not include psychiatric applications such as auditory, visual, or tactile hallucinations or psychosis. The *physiologic* processes of these systems and the consequences of impairment are presented later in this concept.

RISK FACTORS

Populations at Risk

All human populations, regardless of age, gender, ethnicity, or socioeconomic status, are at risk for disturbances in sensation and perception. However, there are certain populations associated with increased risk. The population at the highest risk is the elderly population as a result of changes in sensory perceptual functioning associated with the aging process.

Elderly Population

There are many studies that illustrate a link between a decline in sensory/perceptual functions and the aging process.

Research has been done examining all five senses, with the majority of the studies focused on decreased vision and hearing abilities in the elderly population. The National Social Life, Health, and Aging Project (NSHAP) began a major research study in 2005 exploring the health and social factors, related to aging, of older Americans. This was the first national study attempting to provide a comprehensive assessment of sensory function among older adults. The study examined more than 3000 people ages 57 to 85, and the data showed decline among all five senses within the elderly population.[2]

Vision

According to the Centers for Disease Control and Prevention,[3] as of 2004 blindness or low vision affected more than 3 million Americans ages 40 years and older, and this number is predicted to double by 2030 because of the increasing epidemics of diabetes and other chronic diseases and also because of our rapidly aging population. Low vision is defined as best-corrected visual acuity of less than 20/40 in the better seeing eye, and blindness is considered corrected visual acuity of 20/200 in the better seeing eye.[4] The primary reasons for visual problems in older adults include not only age-related systemic diseases such as type 2 diabetes and hypertension that can cause visual problems, but also primary eye disorders that typically affect the older population such as cataracts, glaucoma, and macular degeneration.[5] In addition, as one enters middle age, there is a natural decrease in the ability to focus on near objects as a result of the reduced elasticity of the lens, called presbyopia.[6]

Hearing

Hearing loss is a common condition among older adults and is present in about one third of people more than 60 years of age and half of people more than 85 years of age.[7] Age-related hearing loss, called presbycusis, is typically sensorineural (caused by pathologic changes in the inner ear or in the nerve pathways from the inner ear to the brain) and refers to a decrease in the ability to hear and process sound that is associated with aging and cannot be explained by the patient's genetic history, other diseases, or injury to the auditory system.[8]

Olfactory and Gustatory

As we age, the olfactory epithelium decreases as a result of cell death. In addition, there are also a decreased number of nasal cilia receptors available to assist in sending olfactory signals to the brain. The loss of smell typically begins around age 60, with increasing loss into the seventies and eighties. Not only is the ability to smell decreased with aging, but also the ability to distinguish between various smells is greatly affected.[9] A recent study of more than 90 people age 45 to 84 years showed olfactory impairment in almost 25% of the subjects and impairment increased with age in both genders.[10]

It is somewhat unknown as to why one's sense of taste tends to decline with age. It is thought to be related to both the decrease in olfaction and also the potential chewing problems and tooth loss.[11] Furthermore, decreased levels of certain hormones, such as testosterone, in the elderly population can contribute to a decrease in cell growth, including taste cells located in taste buds. The decrease in the number of taste cells thus leads to a decrease in the sense of taste.[9]

Tactile Perception

As part of the aging process, there is evidence that tactile thresholds (perceptibility to the sense of touch) tend to increase. An example of this would be a delay in the process of sensing a wrinkled sheet under the back or a slight prick from a small needle, thus resulting in potential injuries. In addition, certain tests that measure the ability to accurately assess tactile sensation tend to show a decline in function that corresponds with aging—a decline of 1% per year between the ages of 20 and 80.[12] Sensation at the fingertips and toes tends to decline faster, especially when studying the ability to accurately assess heat and cold, which can lead to problems with burns and potential frostbite in the elderly population.[9] A study conducted in 2010[13] found that when evaluating sensation thresholds of older (mean age 93) and younger subjects (mean age 28), to match the performance of the younger subjects, the older subjects required two to more than five times the tactile stimulation required by the younger group.

Individual Risk Factors

Significant individual risk factors include medications, medical conditions, lifestyle choices, and occupation.

Adverse Reactions and Side Effects of Medications

Changes in sensory perception function are a common side effect or adverse effect of many medications, particularly when taken for a long time, such as with chronic illness (Table 25-1). Visual disturbances are among the most common

TABLE 25-1	COMMON MEDICATIONS THAT CAN AFFECT SENSATION AND PERCEPTION
DRUG CLASSIFICATION	**POSSIBLE SIDE EFFECTS**
Antihistamines (loratadine, diphenhydramine)	Blurred vision, dry mouth
Antihypertensives (beta blockers, calcium channel blockers, ACE* inhibitors)	Blurred vision
Miotic eye drops (pilocarpine, carbachol)	Changes in vision, increase in near-sightedness, blurred vision
Antiseizure drugs (topiramate, acetazolamide)	Numbness in hands and feet, dry mouth, tinnitus (ringing in ears), blurred vision, eye pain, metallic taste
Diuretics (furosemide)	Hearing loss, tinnitus
Chemotherapeutic drugs	Alterations in taste and smell
Antibiotics	Alterations in taste and smell, ototoxicity

*ACE, Angiotensin-converting enzyme.

undesirable side effects associated with medication therapy. Examples include blurred vision, papillary constriction, retinal toxicity, halo effects, and dry eyes.[9] Ototoxicity, as an adverse medication effect, can result in permanent or temporary inner ear problems that can affect not only hearing, but also balance and possibly speech. This represents one of the main preventable causes of deafness.[14]

Many drugs also affect both taste and smell. In fact, medications (especially chemotherapy agents) are the most common cause of taste disturbances.[15] It is often reported that up to half of all cancer patients experience changes in their taste and/or smell perception.[16] A 2007 study[17] showed that more than 80% of those surveyed who were undergoing chemotherapy for advanced cancer experienced chemosensory abnormalities and 50% of those reported disturbances in both taste and smell. In addition, when alterations in taste and smell were considered severe, they were associated with poor nutrient intakes, food enjoyment, and quality of life.[17] Other drugs that cause taste disturbances include antimicrobial drugs, antivirals, antihypertensives, calcium channel blockers, and diuretics. If it is possible for the medication to be discontinued, the person's sense of smell and taste is often restored; however, some medications do induce long-term changes in taste and smell, and occasionally produce permanent sensory loss.[18]

Paresthesia, a feeling of numbness/tingling typically in the hands and feet, can also be caused by various medications including select antineoplastic agents. Certain anticonvulsants can cause paresthesia in the hands, feet, face, and lips, which do not tend to improve until the medication is discontinued.

Complications from Medical Conditions

Visual disturbances secondary to other medical conditions are not uncommon. Brain tumors, cancers, head injuries, infectious diseases, stroke, and some cardiovascular diseases, such as hypertension, can affect vision.[9] These same conditions are also risk factors for producing auditory problems.

Sinus and upper respiratory tract infections, seasonal allergies, and also dental problems can alter both the sense of smell and the sense of taste. In addition, nasal polyps and exposure to certain environmental chemicals can cause disturbances in both smell and taste.

Cerebrovascular accidents (CVAs) or strokes can affect many aspects of sensation and perception in the body. Alterations in taste sensation, balance issues, and visual disturbances can result from CVAs depending on the area of the brain affected. Another type of neurologic disturbance that can affect perception, especially when looking at alterations in touch, is autism. Children and adults with autism report sensory disturbances such as insensitivity to pain as well as unusual sensory responses to visual, auditory, tactile, and olfactory stimulation. According to Leekam and colleagues,[19] studies have shown that although many children with developmental delays have problems with sensory and perception, these problems tend to be more prevalent in children with autism.

Lifestyle Choices and Occupation

Certain lifestyle choices can increase the risk of sensory and perceptual alterations. Smoking creates an increased risk for alterations in both smell and taste primarily because it damages the taste receptors on the tongue and sensory receptors in the nose. A 2008 study showed that when a smoker who experiences a decreased sense of smell and taste stops smoking, both senses are typically returned to their proper level of functioning.[20]

Individuals exposed to loud noise at work or for recreation have risk for hearing deficit. This loss can be spontaneous or occur over time, typically when decibels are greater than 85. This occurs because such loud vibrations damage the small hairlike cells in the inner ear, and once such damage has occurred, it is typically irreversible.[21] In addition, those persons who work where flying debris is commonly present, such as miners and steel workers, and those who work with certain chemicals are at high risk for eye injuries, especially when not wearing protective equipment.

PHYSIOLOGIC PROCESSES AND CONSEQUENCES

Vision

Vision requires functioning of the visual system, which includes the eyes, surrounding optic muscles, and cranial nerves II (optic), III (oculomotor), IV (trochlear), V (trigeminal), and VI (abducens). The eyelid, conjunctiva, lacrimal gland, and eye muscles all compose the external eye, which helps to regulate and control the visual input as well as protect the eye, aid with tear production, and move the eye when desired. The internal eye consists of three separate layers including the outer sclera and cornea; the middle layer that houses the choroid, ciliary body, and iris; and the innermost layer, which is the retina.[22] The iris allows light to enter the eye and regulates the amount of light entering the eye at any given time. The lens bends entering light rays so that they can properly fall on the retina. The ciliary body, which consists of ciliary muscles, is fed by the choroid, a highly vascular structure (Figure 25-1).

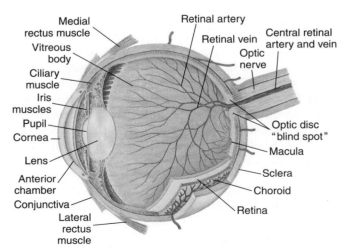

FIGURE 25-1 Structures of the Eye. (From Seidel H, Ball J, Dains J et al: *Mosby's guide to physical examination*, St Louis, 2011, Mosby.)

TABLE 25-2	CRANIAL NERVES AND FUNCTION
CRANIAL NERVE	**FUNCTION**
I: Olfactory	Smell reception and interpretation
II: Optic	Visual acuity and visual fields
III: Oculomotor	Raising eyelids, extraocular movements, papillary constriction
IV: Trochlear	Downward and inward eye movement
V: Trigeminal	Jaw opening and closing; sensation to eye, forehead, nose, mouth, teeth, ear, and face
VI: Abducens	Eye movement laterally
VII: Facial	Controls most facial expressions; taste with anterior two thirds of tongue; excretion of tears and saliva
VIII: Acoustic	Hearing and equilibrium
IX: Glossopharyngeal	Swallowing and speaking; sensation of nasopharynx, gag reflex, and taste to posterior third of tongue; secretion of salivary glands and carotid reflex; certain speech sounds and swallowing
X: Vagus	Sensation behind ear and portion of external ear canal; secretion of digestive enzymes, peristalsis; carotid reflex; heart, lungs, and digestive processes
XI: Spinal accessory	Turn head and shrug shoulders
XII: Hypoglossal	Tongue movement, speech, and swallowing

Modified from Seidel H, Ball J, Dains J, et al: *Mosby's guide to physical examination*, St Louis, 2006, p 764, Elsevier.

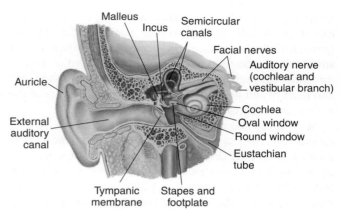

FIGURE 25-2 Structures of the Ear. (From Seidel H, Ball J, Dains J, et al: *Mosby's guide to physical examination*, St Louis, 2011, Mosby.)

The innermost area of the eye is the retina, which transforms light impulses into electrical impulses that are transmitted to the optic nerve. The optic nerve, in turn, communicates with the brain to produce vision.[22] Cranial nerves II through VI all have important roles in eye function (Table 25-2).

Poor vision and blindness can lead to many adverse physical and psychosocial effects. Some of these include depression, anxiety, and loss of self-worth. In addition, as will be discussed later in this concept, visual disturbances can lead to difficulty in instituting and maintaining meaningful interpersonal relationships and establishing vocations. Among children, poor vision contributes to developmental delay and may lead to learning challenges in school. There are also countless safety risks associated with blindness and low vision. Some include injury from falls, cooking fires, and travelling.

Hearing

Hearing, which involves the body's auditory system, is composed of the peripheral and central auditory systems. The peripheral system involves the external, middle, and inner ear and is concerned with hearing and processing sound. The external ear includes the auricle and external auditory canal and functions primarily to collect and transmit sound

to the tympanic membrane and to protect the inner ear[3] (Figure 25-2).

The middle ear is an air-filled space that is located in the temporal bone. It connects to the throat/nasopharynx by the eustachian tube, whose primary function is to equalize air pressure on both sides of the eardrum. The eustachian tube opens to allow airflow when chewing and swallowing. Vibrations of the tympanic membrane (or eardrum), which separates the external ear from the middle ear, cause the auditory ossicles to move and transmit sound waves to the oval window. Once these vibrations reach the oval window, they have been greatly amplified in comparison to when they first came in contact with the eardrum. The inner ear consists of a bony labyrinth surrounding a membrane. Within this structure is the cochlea, closely connected to hearing ability, and the vestibular system, which helps control balance.[23]

Sound waves stimulate this series of actions, and once these waves reach the inner ear, the hairlike cells of the cochlea pick up the vibrations. These cochlear cells initiate nerve impulses that are carried by nerve fibers to cranial nerve VIII (vestibulocochlear) and then to the brain, where the cerebellum receives the signals and helps to maintain a sense of balance.

Hearing loss can be devastating, because it will initially decrease the ability to communicate, maintain relationships, work, and learn. Children with hearing loss, especially if undetected for long periods of time, are at risk for developmental delays and often experience frustration and isolation. As with vision impairment, hearing loss also can lead to injury.

Taste

A person's gustatory system, or sense of taste, involves various cranial nerves and is directly related to the ability of the mouth and tongue to swallow and chew. Taste signals from taste buds located on the tongue are transmitted to the nucleus of the solitary tract (NST) in the medulla of the brain and then sent to other areas within the brain. Senses of smell converge here along with visceral sensory fibers from the esophagus, stomach, intestines, and the liver, which allow taste and odor signals to initiate digestive activity.[9]

Loss of taste often results in a decreased appetite, which can lead to weight loss and malnutrition. In addition, there can be serious health dangers associated with decreased taste such as food poisoning from ingesting spoiled foods and eating foods that can burn the tongue and esophagus. Finally, the satisfaction of eating food is closely related to the taste preferences of a person, which would be lost.

Smell

Sense of smell is controlled primarily by cranial nerve I (olfactory) and is critical in the desire to eat and maintain a healthy nutritional state.[9] Smell depends on sensory receptors in the nose that respond to airborne chemicals. These airborne chemicals bond to the cilia receptors in the nose, which trigger a series of reactions that eventually lead to signals travelling along the olfactory nerve to the brain. The brain then processes this information and makes a determination as to the type of smell.[24]

Any loss of smell can have a negative effect on a person's quality of life. The sense of smell is often closely related to taste, because these senses work together as part of the chemosensory system. Thus, because decreased taste can result in nutritional problems, so can a decreased sense of smell. Decreased sense of smell is also associated with health risks. Sense of smell is often an early warning sign of danger from the environment such as fire, gas leaks, spoiled food, or dangerous chemicals.

Touch

Sense of touch, or the somatosensory system, is controlled by a large network of touch receptors and nerve endings in the skin. These receptors transmit the senses of pain, temperature, pressure, itching, and others to the brain for processing.

Clearly, there are major health risks associated with an impaired somatosensory system. These would include the decreased ability to sense pain, potentially leading to injury and possible infection of wounds associated with injury. In addition, decreased sensitivity to heat and cold could lead to burns and hypothermia. Being able to stand erect and steady is closely related to peripheral sensation.[12]

ASSESSMENT

An assessment includes conducting a history and examination as well as diagnostic testing when sensory perceptual conditions are suspected. Some conditions, such as autism, can initially manifest with sensory perceptual disturbances. Often these disturbances can lead to other issues such as social isolation, withdrawal, behavioral problems, and developmental delays, especially in children.

History and Physical Examination

When performing any type of physical assessment, it is necessary to first complete a thorough history of the patient, including past medical, surgical, family, and social history. For infants, it is important to ask about prenatal and maternal history. Because of the potential for adverse effects with medications, it is also important to gain a list of all medications (prescription and over-the-counter) used by the patient. Health history questions should also specifically ask about sensory perceptual symptoms/problems for each of the categorical areas. In addition, a detailed physical examination related to the patient complaint is crucial. Common symptoms that suggest impairments are described for each category.

Vision

When assessing vision, some important questions that should be asked include whether the patient has experienced any changes in vision, such as blurred vision, difficulty seeing close up and/or far away, peripheral visual changes, and eye pain. In an infant/toddler, it is crucial to ask caregivers if tracking of the eyes has been observed when the child is watching movement and to ensure that the eyes have been observed moving in synchrony.

Examination of the eyes starts by inspecting external eye structures, including the eyebrows, eyelashes, and eyelids, paying attention to symmetry, size, and extension. In addition, the nurse should palpate both the eyelid and the eye and inspect the conjunctiva, the thin membrane that covers the inner eyelid and sclera, closely for redness and irritation. The sclera should be predominantly white and the lens should be transparent.

One of the most obvious tests to conduct initially when evaluating the visual system is to test for visual acuity. Visual acuity refers to the clarity of vision and is basically a measure of how well a person sees. This is typically done using the Snellen eye chart. Visual acuity is then recorded as a fraction in which the numerator shows the distance that the patient was from the chart, typically 20 feet, and the denominator represents the distance that the average eye can read that same line of the chart.[22] For example, 20/60 means a patient can see clearly at 20 feet what the average eye sees at 60 feet.

Movement of the eyes is typically controlled by cranial nerves III, IV, and VI and by six extraocular muscles. The ability to produce eye movement is typically tested by having the patient follow a finger, keeping the head stationary, as it moves through the six cardinal fields of gaze.[22] A person's inability to follow through all the fields can indicate a host of visual disorders. Nystagmus, a rapid, involuntary movement of the eye, can often be detected during this part of the visual assessment.

Evaluating the interior of the eye allows for visualization of the optic disc, arteries, veins, and retina. This is done using an ophthalmoscope, and often following dilation of the pupils, although this is not always necessary. Some unexpected findings would include hemorrhages, optic disc swelling (referred to as papilledema), or cotton wool spots, which are poorly defined yellow areas on the retina, and often are related to damage of the nerve fibers.[22] Finally, checking for papillary response to light should be evaluated in both the adult and the pediatric population.

Hearing

Difficulty hearing, tinnitus, and ear pain are common complaints that prompt a patient to have the auditory system evaluated by a health care professional. For the pediatric population, frequent problems with otitis media are common and can include symptoms such as ear drainage, pain, and fever.

Inspection of the outer portion of the ear, or auricle/pinna, includes noting the symmetry, size, shape, and possible discharge. The evaluation of the inner ear is done using an otoscope. The nurse should look for cerumen, or earwax, noting its color and odor if present.[22] The tympanic membrane (see Figure 25-2) should be translucent with a pearly, gray color. Some abnormal findings would include a bulging or retracted tympanic membrane (or eardrum) and/or perforations of the tympanic membrane. Evaluating hearing can be accomplished using several methods. Assessing the patient's ability to hear during general conversation is the most common approach. If hearing deficit is suspected, further diagnostic studies are indicated.

Taste

The most common complaint associated with the sense of taste is lack of one. Most patients who think they have a taste disorder actually have a problem with smell.[31] One of the most important tasks during a health history assessment of a patient experiencing alteration in taste is obtaining a complete list of current medications, because many medications contribute to this loss.

Taste is typically assessed by an inspection of the tongue and oral cavity, looking for any abnormalities such as an atrophied tongue or a tongue that does not appear red and moist.[22] Overgrowth of yeast or ulcerations or nodules should be noted. However, often patients with taste disturbances have normal appearing, well-functioning tongues.

Smell

Assessing the sense of smell is first done by obtaining a detailed history, including medications the patient is taking, and assessing for recent upper respiratory tract complaints such as sinus infections, allergies, and nasal polyps, which often prompt a patient to seek medical attention. Proper inspection of the nose, looking for abnormalities such as nasal discharge or blockages, and evaluation of the color and size of the nose are vital when evaluating the olfactory system. If discharge is observed, the nurse should note the color, consistency, odor, and amount. Nasal breathing is assessed by pinching one naris, or nostril, and asking the patient to breathe in and out with his or her mouth closed, alternating nostrils. Breathing should be quiet and effortless.[22]

Touch

Touch and balance are largely regulated by the body's neurologic system. Alterations in perception can often manifest as balance disturbances. Balance is routinely tested by the Romberg test, which involves asking patients to stand with their feet together and arms at their sides with their eyes first open, and then to shut their eyes. Some slight swaying is normal, but the patient should be able to stand still for the most part. The nurse should observe the patient's gait for abnormal findings such as shuffling, staggering, and asymmetric stride.

Evaluating sensory function is accomplished by having the patient identify stimuli affecting the major peripheral nerves including the hands, arms, feet, legs, and abdomen. Cranial nerve VII, the trigeminal nerve, is most closely associated with sensory function. The patient should be able to correctly identify if a stimulus feels sharp or dull and the location of the sensation. In addition, the patient should be able to properly differentiate temperature (hot/cold), the location of the stimulus, and the correct side of the body that is being stimulated.[22] Monofilament testing is a relatively inexpensive and easy-to-use test for assessing peripheral neuropathies that cause decreased sensation to the extremities, and is often used when testing neuropathy in persons with diabetes. Monofilaments are single-fiber nylon threads that are placed on the patient's skin, typically on the feet. An abnormal finding is that the patient will not be able to detect the presence of the filament.[26]

Diagnostic Tests

After a basic history and a physical assessment are completed, occasionally further diagnostic testing is warranted. These are described by sensory classification.

Vision

Some common visual diagnostic tests include evaluating peripheral vision by testing visual fields with automated perimetry. A patient looks straight ahead into a device with a concave dome, while small flashes of light are shown sporadically in all visual fields. The patient then pushes a button every time he or she sees a light. Decreased visual field acuity could be indicative of glaucoma, optic nerve damage, and other visual problems. Another example would include noncontact tonometry, or the puff-of-air test. This involves an eye's resistance to a puff of air from a small hand-held jet, which calculates a range of intraocular pressure (IOP). Elevations in IOP can be indicative of glaucoma. Radiographic examinations of the brain may be indicated if a tumor is suspected of causing visual disturbances.

Hearing

If hearing loss is suspected in an initial examination, a referral to a certified audiologist is often done. There are several ways audiologists can test hearing. One is a pure-tone air conduction hearing test, which determines the faintest tones a person can hear at selected frequencies ranging from low to high. Typically earphones are worn so that information can be obtained for each ear separately.[27] Pure-tone tests are often conducted on school-age children every few years and are used for adults when hearing difficulties are reported.[27] Other common screening methods used often with infants are otoacoustic emissions (OAEs) and auditory brainstem response (ABR). OAEs are sounds from the inner ear after the cochlea has been stimulated by a sound, and this is measured by using a small probe in the ear canal. Those with hearing loss do not produce such sounds.

The ABR test is performed by placing electrodes on the head and recording brain wave activity in response to sounds.[27]

CLINICAL MANAGMENT

Primary Prevention

Many measures exist to prevent injury and disease to the eyes, ears, mouth, and the nose. Basic measures to protect the eyes and ears include the use of protective devices; patient education related to these practices is essential. Safety goggles are recommended for selected sporting activities and work activities in which small particles (such as sawdust, wood chips, metal pieces, vegetation debris) are present in the air. According to *Healthy People 2020,* more than 2000 workers in the United States receive medical treatment each year because of eye injuries that occur on the job.[28] The use of ear plugs or other ear protection is also a requirement in many work settings involving loud machinery and is suggested for other activities such as attending loud concerts. Wearing helmets when riding a bicycle, skiing, or participating in contact sports can prevent brain injury—another cause of sensory disturbances.

Primary prevention extends beyond wearing protective devices. Infants receive silver nitrate ointment in their eyes to help reduce the chances of the mother passing on certain sexually transmitted diseases. Regular oral hygiene prevents diseases to the mouth, reducing risks for changes in taste or smell. Proactive management of many chronic conditions can prevent complications that negatively affect the sensory organs such as diabetes and heart disease, as already discussed.

Secondary Prevention (Screening)

Screening tests are common for vision and hearing. There are no routine screenings to evaluate the sense of smell or taste.

Vision

Vision screens are recommended across the lifespan. Starting in the newborn period, a pediatric eye evaluation is recommended. Certain children, such as those who are born premature or with family histories of vision problems, should be referred to pediatric ophthalmologists shortly after birth. According to the American Academy of Pediatrics,[29] eye evaluations in pediatrician's offices for children up to age 3 years should occur with at least all well-child checkups and include history, assessment, external inspection of the eyes and lids, ocular motility assessment, pupil examination, and red reflex examination. After age 3, the evaluation should also include age-appropriate visual acuity measurement and an attempt at ophthalmoscopy. Any abnormal findings would warrant a referral to a pediatric ophthalmologist.

For adults, the American Optometric Association (AOA) recommends that adults up to age 40 receive an eye exam at least every 2 years.[30] The same recommendation is true for middle-age adults, those up to age 60; however, special attention should be paid to people with chronic conditions such as diabetes, heart disease, and hypertension because visual problems can occur among these patients. In addition, this is the time frame when presbyopia often begins to develop.

For older adults, those more than 60 years of age, yearly eye exams are recommended to screen for simple vision loss related to aging as well as age-related eye disorders such as glaucoma and macular degenerative disease.[30] This population is more likely not only to have chronic conditions, but also to have eye-specific problems such as cataracts, macular degenerative disease, glaucoma, and retinal detachment. Eye examination with dilation and careful inspection can often diagnose these problems, but tonometry is necessary when considering glaucoma, a disease in which fluid pressure in the eye is consistently elevated, causing damage to the optic nerve and leading to loss of vision. Tonometry involves the use of a covered probe to gently touch the corneal surface several times to record the average intraocular pressure. The cornea is anesthetized first with eye drops before the pressures are measured. Normal intraocular pressure is 10 to 22 mm Hg, and pressures greater than 22 mm Hg are considered abnormal. Those with ongoing pressures greater than 27 mm Hg are at a higher risk of glaucoma.[23]

Hearing

Hearing tests are often done within 48 hours of birth in the hospital setting. The two common screening methods used with infants are otoacoustic emissions (OAEs) and auditory brainstem response (ABR), which have already been discussed. Outer and inner ear inspection, with the use of an otoscope, is typically done with each well-child visit; however, for adults, otoscopic inspection is usually completed only when the patient reports a hearing problem.

Collaborative Interventions

Vision

For many visual problems, especially those associated with decreased visual acuity, corrective lenses (glasses and contact lenses) are a relatively easy and inexpensive treatment.

Surgery. There are a number of surgical procedures performed to treat conditions of the eye. Laser-assisted in situ keratomileusis (LASIK) is a surgical procedure that involves cutting a small flap in the cornea and then retracting the flap. Pulses from a computer-controlled laser then remove small parts of the cornea, permanently reshaping its surface. The reshaped cornea can better focus light onto the eye and onto the retina, allowing for improved vision.[31] The most common treatment for cataracts is surgery, which is also an option for macular degenerative disease. In addition to surgery, those with macular degeneration also have the option of injectable drug treatments and photodynamic therapy.[32] Microsurgical procedures and laser procedures are also available to treat many visual disorders and are being done more frequently.[33]

Pharmacotherapy. Certain visual disorders can be initially treated with beta-adrenergic eye drops, which decrease production of aqueous humor. Other types of eye drops prescribed include prostaglandin analogs, adrenergic agonists, and carbonic anhydrase inhibitors. In addition, oral forms of carbonic anhydrase inhibitors can also be prescribed. In addition to surgery, those with macular degeneration also have the option of injectable drug treatments and photodynamic therapy.[32] Other common forms of ophthalmic pharmacotherapy include antibiotic, steroidal, and analgesic agents.

Hearing

Surgery. For recurrent otitis media in children, surgical intervention may become necessary. The decision to perform surgery should be based on the response to medical treatment first, an evaluation of possible hearing loss, and the appearance of the tympanic membrane (or eardrum) itself. A myringotomy is performed to correct recurrent otitis media; in this surgical procedure a small incision is made in the tympanic membrane, fluid is removed, and a small tube is inserted. This surgery is typically done as an outpatient procedure with the patient being administered a general anesthetic.[34]

Cochlear implants are devices that are surgically implanted to provide direct electrical stimulation to the auditory nerve. Both children and adults with profound hearing loss, typically not helped by hearing aids, may have success with these implants. Although a cochlear implant will not restore hearing, it may allow for the perception of sound.[35]

Adaptive Methods

Adaptive methods provide additional options for hearing and vision problems and include braille, guide dogs, sign language, closed caption television, and assistive listening. As previously mentioned, if a person is experiencing sensory loss from medication therapy, it is likely that discontinuing the therapy will result in the loss being restored.

CLINICAL NURSING SKILLS FOR SENSORY PERCEPTION

- Assessment
- Eye irrigation
- Ear irrigation
- Administering eye and ear medications

INTERRELATED CONCEPTS

As previously mentioned, the concept of sensory perception is interrelated with several other health and illness concepts discussed in this textbook (Figure 25-3).

Intracranial regulation. The brain is an amazing organ with more than 100 billion cells that regulate sensory input and output. Any disturbance of these vital processes will disrupt many other human functions. For example, a brain tumor that affects intracranial regulation can disrupt neurologic function and interfere with all five senses. Depending on the location and size of the tumor, symptoms such as blurred or double vision, tinnitus, and loss of taste and smell can occur.

Pain. Pain is a sensation that most people do not want to experience; however, sometimes pain is necessary to provide the brain with the signals needed to cause action to remove the pain source. An example of the interrelatedness of pain and sensation and perception would be a patient with diabetes who is experiencing peripheral neuropathy and steps on a nail, but cannot properly feel the pain because of the nerve damage to the foot. Without the pain, the patient might not realize that he or she has a wound and would not seek treatment, leading to a possible infection that would be difficult to treat. In addition, problems such as uveitis, inflammation of the inner eye, or ear infections can cause pain.

Interpersonal relationships. Vision- and hearing-impaired persons often must use adaptive measures in order to communicate effectively, and this can present challenges when having and maintaining interpersonal relationships. For example, only a minority of people in the United States are able to use and understand sign language, which creates a clear communication barrier for those in society who are hearing impaired. This barrier also can create challenges to many other aspects of life such as one's occupation and

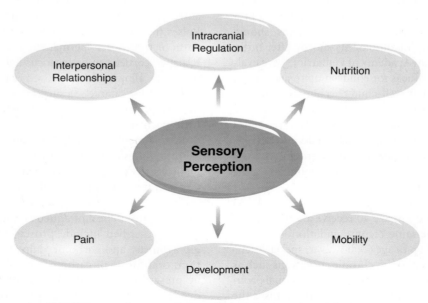

FIGURE 25-3 Sensory Perception and Interrelated Concepts.

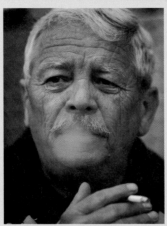

Mr. Robert Holton is a retired 74-year-old male who spent his entire working career as a self-employed carpenter. He has a 22-year history of type 2 diabetes; he also has hypertension and emphysema. He is an active smoker (52-pack year smoking history), although he has attempted to stop smoking on several occasions. He wears a hearing aid in each ear because of hearing loss as a result of working around machinery for several years.

Robert presents for a routine 3-month visit with the nurse practitioner accompanied by his wife. Mrs. Holton reports that Robert's feet smell very bad, but he does not seem to notice the odor. The nurse practitioner removes Robert's shoes and socks; a large infected foot ulcer is observed on the bottom of the foot. Robert is surprised that he was unaware of the wound. When asked about other changes, Robert does not respond. Mrs. Holton reports that he recently failed his visual acuity test for driver's license renewal, and now must depend on her for transportation. She adds that he has become increasingly withdrawn over the last 6 months, and does little to communicate with her or others and is not interested in leaving the house. She asks the nurse practitioner if he is depressed.

Case Analysis

This case illustrates many aspects of this concept. Mr. Holton is an older adult with diabetes, a chronic condition known to lead to changes in vision (attributable to diabetic retinopathy) and peripheral sensation (attributable to peripheral neuropathy). Along with the natural changes associated with aging, Mr. Holton's smoking history has contributed to his reduced sense of smell. The loss of tactile and olfactory sensation contributed to his lack of awareness of a diabetic foot ulcer that had developed. Mr. Holton's hearing loss can be attributed to his age and past work history with machinery. A common response to hearing and vision loss is social isolation—particularly when independence is lost—such as with the loss of his driver's license.

developing meaningful relationships with others who are not hearing impaired.

Mobility. Certain disorders, especially neurologic disorders, have the potential to alter sensation and perception in many ways. For example, when a person has suffered a neurologic impairment, such as a cerebrovascular accident (CVA), often mobility is limited, and potentially the ability to see and speak is altered, affecting communication. Another common manifestation may be paralysis and paresthesia of an arm or leg. This results in a person having difficulty in ambulating and lifting, greatly affecting mobility.

Nutrition. The inability to taste and smell reduces the desire to eat, because these senses have a vital role in initiating the digestive process. This often leads to inadequate nutrition, which would negatively affect both children and adults; however, children experiencing poor nutrition can have delayed physical and mental development.[6] For example, patients undergoing chemotherapy often experience taste disturbances that decrease their desire for food, leading to nutritional deficiencies.

EXEMPLARS

There are multiple exemplars of sensory perception. Box 25-1 presents common exemplars that represent disorders that affect a person's sensory perceptual functioning. When looking at gustatory, olfactory, and somatosensory disorders, what is listed in the box is more typically a systemic disorder, not one that specifically targets the sensory perceptual system itself. For example, sinus infections often cause loss of smell because of the swelling of the nasal membranes, but they certainly cause other more systemic symptoms such as fever, sore throat, and headaches. A decreased ability to detect odors is called hyposmia and complete loss of the ability to detect odors is anosmia. Similarly, a reduced ability to taste is called hypogeusia and complete lack of ability to taste is ageusia. Dysgeusia is a condition in which a foul, salty, or metallic taste persists in the mouth.[25]

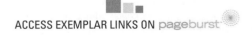

ACCESS EXEMPLAR LINKS ON pageburst

■■■ BOX 25-1   EXEMPLARS OF SENSORY PERCEPTION

Visual Exemplars
- Premature retinopathy
- Amblyopia
- Presbyopia
- Cataracts
- Retinal detachment
- Macular degenerative disease
- Glaucoma
- Traumatic injury

Auditory Exemplars
Sensorineural Hearing Loss
- Genetic
- Ototoxic drugs
- Trauma
- Exposure to loud noise

Conductive Hearing Loss
- Otitis media
- Allergies
- Perforated eardrum
- Earwax
- Presence of foreign body
- Tumors
- Traumatic injury

Gustatory Exemplars
- Radiation to head and neck
- Head injury
- Surgeries to ear, nose, and throat
- Dental problems
- Brain tumor

Olfactory Exemplars
- Sinus infections
- Nasal polyps
- Brain injury
- Dental problems
- Parkinson's disease
- Alzheimer's disease
- Brain tumor

Somatosensory Exemplars
- Peripheral neuropathy
- Peripheral artery disease
- Stroke
- Third-degree burns
- Spinal cord injury

REFERENCES

1. Day A: Sensation, perception, and cognition. In Daniels R, editor: *Nursing fundamentals: caring and clinical decision making,* Florence, Ky, 2008, Delmar Cengage Learning.
2. Schumm L, McClintock M, Williams S, et al: Assessment of sensory function in the national social life, health, and aging project, *J Gerontol B Psychol Sci Soc Sci* 64:i76, 2009.
3. Centers for Disease Control and Prevention: *Vision health initiative fast facts,* 2009, at www.cdc.gov/visionhealth/basic_information/fast_facts.htm. Accessed Nov 28, 2010.
4. Eye Diseases Prevalence Research Group: Causes and prevalence of visual impairment among adults in the United States, *Arch Ophthalmol* 122:477, 2004.
5. Sharts-Hopko N: Lifestyle strategies for the prevention of vision loss, *Holist Nurs Pract* 24:284, 2010.
6. Schiffman S: Sensory impairment: taste and smell impairments with aging. In Wales C, Ritchie C, editors: *Handbook of clinical nutrition and aging,* ed 2, Totowa, NJ, 2009, Humana Press.
7. National Institute on Deafness and other Communication Disorders: *Hearing loss and older adults,* 2010, at www.nidcd.nih.gov/health/hearing/older.htm. Accessed Dec 1, 2010.
8. Bance M: Hearing and aging, *CMAJ* 176:925, 2007.
9. Schiffman S: Critical illness and changes in sensory perception, *Proc Nutr Soc* 66:331, 2007.
10. Murphy C, Schubert C, Cruickshanks K, et al: Prevalence of olfactory impairment in older adults, *JAMA* 288:2307, 2007.
11. Boyce J, Shone G: Effects of ageing on smell and taste, *Postgrad Med J* 82:239, 2006.
12. Wickremaratchi M, Llewelyn J: Effects of ageing on touch, *Postgrad Med J* 82:301, 2005.
13. Craig J, Rhodes R, Busey T, et al: Aging and tactile temporal order, *Attention Percept Psychophys* 72:226, 2010.
14. Yorgason J, Fayad J, Kalinec F: Understanding drug ototoxicity: molecular insights for prevention and clinical management, *Expert Opin Drug Saf* 5:383, 2006.
15. Madnani N, Khan K: Doc, I can't taste my food! *Indian J Dermatol Venerol Leprol* 76:296, 2010.
16. Ripamonti C, Fulfaro F: Taste alterations in cancer patients, *J Pain Symptom Manag* 16:349, 1998.
17. Hutton J, Baracos V, Wismer W: Chemosensory dysfunction is a primary factor in the evolution of declining nutritional status and quality of life in patients with advanced cancer, *J Pain Symptom Manag* 33:156, 2007.
18. Doty R, Bromley S: Effects of drugs on olfaction and taste, *Otolaryngol Clin N Am* 37:1229, 2004.
19. Leekam S, Nieto C, Libby S, et al: Describing the sensory abnormalities of children and adults with autism, *J Autism Dev Disord* 37:894, 2007.
20. Vennemann M, Hummel T, Berger K: The association between smoking and smell and taste impairment in the general population, *J Neurol* 255:1121, 2008.
21. National Institute on Deafness and other Communication Disorders: *Noise induced hearing loss,* 2008, at www.nidcd.nih.gov/health/hearing/noise.asp. Accessed Dec 3, 2010.
22. Seidel H, Ball J, Dains J, et al: *Mosby's guide to physical examination,* St Louis, 2006, Elsevier.
23. Smith S, Neely S: Visual and auditory systems. In Lewis S, Heitkemper M, Dirksen S, et al: *Medical-surgical nursing: assessment and management of clinical problems,* St Louis, 2007, Mosby/Elsevier.

24. National Institute on Deafness and Other Communication Disorders: *Smell disorders*, 2010, at www.nidcd.nih.gov/health/smelltaste/smell.html. Accessed Nov 20, 2010.

25. National Institute on Deafness and Other Communication Disorders: *Taste disorders*, 2010, at www.nidcd.nih.gov/health/smelltaste/taste.html. Accessed Dec 1, 2010.

26. Dros J, Wewerinke A, Bindels P, et al: Accuracy of the monofilament testing to diagnose peripheral neuropathy: a systematic review, *Ann Fam Med* 7:556, 2009.

27. American Speech Language Hearing Association: *Hearing screening and testing*, 2011, at www.asha.org/public/hearing/Hearing-Testing/. Accessed Dec 1, 2010.

28. HealthyPeople.gov: *Vision*, 2010, at http://healthypeople.gov/2020/topicsobjectives2020/overview.aspx?topicid=42. Accessed March 3, 2011.

29. American Academy of Pediatrics: Eye examination in infants, children, and young adults by pediatricians, *Pediatrics* 111:902, 2003.

30. American Optometric Association: *Comprehensive eye and vision examination*, 2011, at www.aoa.org/x4725. Accessed Nov 20, 2010.

31. U.S. Department of Health and Human Services: *Lasik*, 2009, at www.fda.gov/MedicalDevices/ProductsandMedicalProcedures/SurgeryandLifeSupport/LASIK/default.htm. Accessed Dec 1, 2010.

32. Mayo Clinic Staff: *Cataracts*, 2010, at www.mayoclinic.com/health/cataracts/DS00050. Accessed Jan 4, 2011.

33. Dahl A: *Glaucoma*, 2011, at www.medicinenet.com/glaucoma/article.htm. Accessed Jan 3, 2011.

34. Cunha J: *Ear tubes*, 2011, at www.medicinenet.com/ear_tubes/article.htm. Accessed March 3, 2011.

35. American Speech Language Hearing Association: *Cochlear implants*, 2011, at www.asha.org/public/hearing/Hearing-Testing/. Accessed Dec 1, 2010.

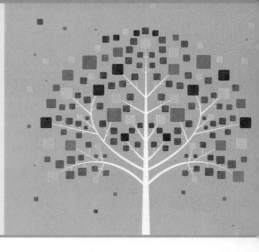

Pain

Chris Pasero and Jan Belden

ain is one of the most common reasons people seek health care. The field of pain management has experienced rapid growth in technology and research over the past several years. Although progress has been made, pain continues to be undertreated in all care settings. As the only health care professionals who provide 24-hour presence 7 days a week, nurses play an important role in the management of pain and can be instrumental in ensuring their patients receive the best possible pain relief available.

DEFINITION(S)

The American Pain Society (APS) defines pain as "an unpleasant sensory and emotional experience associated with actual or potential tissue damage, or described in terms of such damage."[1, p1] This definition describes pain as a complex phenomenon with multiple components that impact a person's psychosocial and physical functioning. The accepted clinical definition of pain, which was proposed by Margo McCaffery in 1968, is accepted worldwide and reinforces that pain is a highly personal and subjective experience: "Pain is whatever the experiencing person says it is, existing whenever he says it does."[2, p8] This is why all accepted guidelines consider the patient's report to be the most reliable indicator of pain.[3]

SCOPE AND CATEGORIES

In general discussion, pain is usually described as being *acute* or *chronic (persistent)*.[4] Acute pain and chronic pain differ from one another primarily in their duration. For example, tissue damage as a result of surgery, trauma, or burns produces acute pain, which is expected to be relatively short-lived and to diminish with normal healing. Chronic pain may result from underlying medical conditions, such as cancer pain from tumor growth or osteoarthritis pain from joint degeneration, and can persist throughout a person's lifespan. Patients may experience both acute and chronic pain as part of their disease process. For example, some patients with cancer have continuous chronic pain and also experience acute

exacerbations of pain periodically or are exposed to repetitive painful procedures related to cancer treatment.

Pain is most often classified by its inferred pathology as being either *nociceptive pain* or *neuropathic pain*.[4] Nociceptive pain refers to the normal functioning of physiologic systems that leads to the perception of noxious stimuli (tissue injury) as being painful. Simply stated, nociception means "normal" pain transmission.[4] Pain from surgery, trauma, burns, and tumor growth are examples of nociceptive pain. Patients often describe this type of pain as "aching," "cramping," or "throbbing."

Neuropathic pain results from the abnormal processing of sensory input by the nervous system as a result of damage to the brain, spinal cord, or peripheral nerves.[4] Simply stated, neuropathic pain is pathologic. Examples of neuropathic pain include postherpetic neuralgia, diabetic neuropathy, phantom pain, and poststroke pain syndrome. Patients with neuropathic pain use very distinctive words to describe their pain, such as "burning," "sharp," and "shooting."

Some patients have a combination of nociceptive and neuropathic pain. For example, a patient may have nociceptive pain as a result of tumor growth and if the tumor is pressing against a nerve plexus the patient may also report radiating sharp and shooting neuropathic pain. Sickle cell pain is usually a combination of both nociceptive pain from the clumping of sickled cells, and resulting perfusion deficits, and neuropathic pain from nerve ischemia.

Some painful conditions and syndromes are not easily categorized and thought to be unique with multiple underlying and poorly understood mechanisms. These are referred to as *mixed pain syndromes* and include fibromyalgia and some low back and myofascial pain.

RISK FACTORS
Populations at Risk

With rare exception, everyone experiences pain at some point during the course of a lifetime. However, some individuals are at higher risk for pain than others. Although not all older adults experience pain, the incidence of pain increases with age, placing this population at higher risk for pain than younger individuals.[5,6] Pain has been shown to be very common in the older adult in the inpatient acute care setting[7,8] and in the outpatient setting, such as in nursing homes.[9] This is in large part because older adults suffer many of the conditions associated with pain, including musculoskeletal disorders, such as degenerative spine conditions and arthritis.[5] They are frequent recipients of surgical procedures[7,10] and at increased risk of injury from falls and trauma, all of which can result in pain.[8] Some pain syndromes, such as postherpetic neuralgia, poststroke pain, and diabetic neuropathy, are more prevalent in the older population.[11] Cancer is more common in older adults than in younger adults, and as many as 80% of cancer patients experience pain as a consequence of the disease process as well as its treatment.[5]

The older adult is at high risk for undertreatment of pain as well. Many are reluctant or unable to report their pain because of illness or cognitive impairment.[6] Research shows that clinicians fail to provide adequate analgesia based on the misconception that analgesics are not needed or fears that analgesics may cause adverse effects, such as confusion and respiratory depression.[7,8,12,13]

At the other end of the age spectrum, neonates are also at risk for pain, primarily from procedures. Healthy neonates may experience painful heelsticks, venipuncture, and circumcision.[14] Critically ill infants are at very high risk for pain. One study showed that 151 sick neonates were exposed to a mean number of 14 painful procedures per day, including endotracheal intubation and suctioning, insertion of chest tubes, and arterial and venous punctures, during the first 2 weeks after admission to a tertiary neonatal intensive care unit (NICU).[15]

Similar to critically ill infants, critically ill children, adolescents, and adults experience a significant amount of pain from underlying painful pathologic conditions and the repetitive painful procedures to which they are exposed during the course of care.[12,16] Research has shown that the single most painful procedure in the ICU is turning,[17,18] which underscores the high prevalence of pain in the critical care setting.

Regardless of age, anyone who cannot report pain using the customary pain assessment methods and tools, such as the 0 to 10 Numeric Rating Scale or Faces Pain Scale-Revised, is at risk for undertreatment of pain. These individuals are referred to as *nonverbal* and include infants, toddlers, the cognitively impaired, and anesthetized, critically ill, comatose, and imminently dying patients.[3]

PHYSIOLOGIC PROCESSES AND CONSEQUENCES OF PAIN

Pain triggers a number of physiologic stress responses in the human body. Unrelieved pain can prolong the stress response and produce a cascade of harmful effects in all body systems (Figure 26-1). The stress response causes the endocrine system to release excessive amounts of hormones, such as cortisol, catecholamines, and glucagon. Insulin and testosterone levels decrease.[19] Increased endocrine activity in turn initiates

a number of metabolic processes, in particular accelerated carbohydrate, protein, and fat destruction (catabolism), which can result in weight loss, tachycardia, increased respiratory rate, shock, and even death.[20] The immune system is also affected by pain as demonstrated by research showing a link between unrelieved pain and a higher incidence of nosocomial infections[21] and increased tumor growth.[22,23]

Effects on the cardiovascular system are dramatic and include increased postoperative blood loss[24] and hypercoagulation,[20,25] which can lead to myocardial infarction and stroke. Unrelieved pain impacts the respiratory system, causing small tidal volumes and decreases in functional lung capacity, which can lead to pneumonia, atelectasis, and an increased need for mechanical ventilation.[20,26,27]

ASSESSMENT

The gold standard of pain assessment is the patient's report of the pain experience.[1-3] A thorough pain assessment is obtained by asking the patient a number of questions and serves as the foundation for effective pain management. It is used to establish the initial treatment plan and determine when changes are needed.[3] The following are components of a comprehensive pain assessment:

- **Location(s) of pain:** Ask the patient to point to the area(s) of pain on the body.
- **Intensity:** Ask the patient to rate the intensity of pain using a reliable and valid pain assessment tool. A number of scales in several language translations have been evaluated and made available for use in clinical practice and for educational purposes.[3] The following scales are most commonly used:
  - *Numeric Rating Scale (NRS):* The NRS is most often presented as a horizontal 0 to 10 point scale, with word anchors of "no pain" at one end of the scale, "moderate pain" in the middle of the scale, and "worst possible pain" at the end of the scale.
  - *Faces Pain Scale-Revised (FPS-R):* The FPS-R has six faces to make it consistent with other scales using the 0 to 10 metric. The faces range from a neutral facial expression to one of intense pain and are numbered 0, 2, 4, 6, 8, and 10. Patients are asked to choose the face that best describes their pain. The FPS-R is valid and reliable for use in children and adults, including cognitively intact and impaired elders.[28] Although young children may be able to select a face on a faces scale, they are unable to optimally quantify pain (identify a number) until approximately 8 years of age.[29]
  - *Wong-Baker FACES Pain Rating Scale:* The FACES scale consists of six cartoon faces with word descriptors, ranging from a smiling face on the left for "no pain (or hurt)" to a frowning, tearful face on the right for "worst pain (or hurt)." The faces are most commonly numbered using a 0, 2, 4, 6, 8, 10 metric; however 0 to 5 can also be used. Patients are asked to choose the face that best describes their pain. The FACES scale is used in adults and children as young as 3 years old.

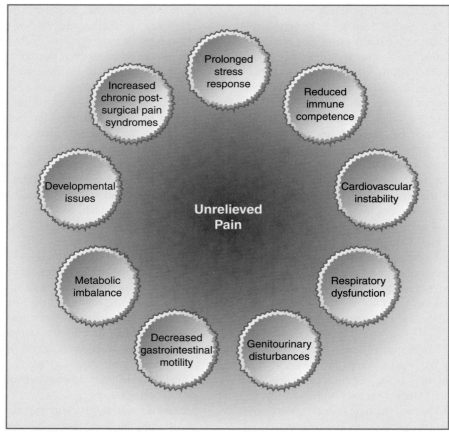

FIGURE 26-1 Overview of the Harmful Effects of Unrelieved Pain. This figure depicts some of the adverse effects of unrelieved pain on multiple domains. (Adapted from Pasero C, McCaffery M, editors: *Pain assessment and pharmacologic management,* St Louis, 2011, Mosby/Elsevier.)

- *Verbal Descriptor Scales:* A Verbal Descriptor Scale (VDS) uses a series of different words or phrases to describe the intensity of pain, such as *"no pain, mild pain, moderate pain, severe pain, very severe pain,* and *worst possible pain."* The patient is asked to select the phrase that best describes his or her pain intensity. The scale can be presented horizontally or vertically and can be helpful for patients with difficulty using a numeric scale.[30]
- **Quality:** Ask the patient to describe how the pain feels. Descriptors such as "burning" or "shooting" may identify the presence of neuropathic pain.
- **Onset and duration:** Ask when the pain started and whether it is constant or intermittent.
- **Alleviating and relieving factors:** Ask the patient what makes the pain better and what makes it worse. The answers help to determine which pain medications and nonpharmacologic interventions are effective and which are not.
- **Effect of pain on function and quality of life:** Ask the patient to describe medication side effects (e.g., constipation, nausea, sedation) and difficulty sleeping or eating. Assess for comorbidities, such as anxiety and depression.

It is particularly important to ask patients with chronic pain about how pain has affected their lives; what could they do before the pain began that they can no longer do, or what do they want to do but cannot do because of the pain?
- **Comfort-function (pain) goal:** Discuss the expectation of functional goal achievement. For example, tell surgical patients that they will need to deep breathe, cough, turn, and ambulate or participate in physical therapy after surgery. Patients with chronic pain can be asked to identify their unique functional or quality-of-life goals, such as being able to work, walk the dog, or garden. Ask the patient to identify (using a 0 to 10 scale) a level of pain that will allow accomplishment of the identified functional or quality-of-life goals with reasonable ease. A realistic goal for most patients is 2 or 3, and pain intensity ratings that are consistently above the goal warrant further evaluation and consideration of an intervention and possible adjustment of the treatment plan.[3]
- **Other information:** The patient's culture, past pain experiences, and pertinent medical history such as comorbidities, laboratory tests, and diagnostic studies are considered when establishing a treatment plan.[12]

BOX 26-1 PASERO OPIOID-INDUCED SEDATION SCALE (POSS) WITH INTERVENTIONS*

S = Sleep, easy to arouse
Acceptable; no action necessary; may increase opioid dose if needed

1 = Awake and alert
Acceptable; no action necessary; may increase opioid dose if needed

2 = Slightly drowsy, easily aroused
Acceptable; no action necessary; may increase opioid dose if needed

3 = Frequently drowsy, arousable, drifts off to sleep during conversation
Unacceptable; monitor respiratory status and sedation level closely until sedation level is stable at less than 3 and respiratory status is satisfactory; decrease opioid dose 25% to 50%[†] or notify primary[‡] or anesthesia provider for orders; consider administering a nonsedating, opioid-sparing non-opioid, such as acetaminophen or a NSAID, if not contraindicated; ask patient to take deep breaths every 15 to 30 minutes.

4 = Somnolent, minimal or no response to verbal and physical stimulation
Unacceptable; stop opioid; consider administering naloxone[§,¶]; call Rapid Response Team (Code Blue); stay with patient, stimulate, and support respiration as indicated by patient status; notify primary[‡] or anesthesia provider; monitor respiratory status and sedation level closely until sedation level is stable at less than 3 and respiratory status is satisfactory.

Copyright 1994, Chris Pasero. Used with permission.
*Appropriate action is given in italics at each level of sedation.
[†]Opioid analgesic orders or a hospital protocol should include the expectation that a nurse will decrease the opioid dose if a patient is excessively sedated.
[‡]For example, the physician, nurse practitioner, advance practice nurse, or physician assistant responsible for the pain management prescription.
[§]For adults experiencing respiratory depression mix 0.4 mg of naloxone and 10 ml of normal saline in a syringe and administer this dilute solution very slowly (0.5 ml over 2 minutes) while observing the patient's response (titrate to effect).
[¶]Hospital protocols should include the expectation that a nurse will administer naloxone to any patient suspected of having life-threatening opioid-induced sedation and respiratory depression.

Breakthrough Pain

An important part of the pain assessment is to determine whether the patient is experiencing *breakthrough pain* and if its treatment is effective. Breakthrough pain (also called *pain flare*) is a transitory exacerbation of pain in a patient who has relatively stable and adequately controlled baseline pain.[12] When breakthrough pain is brief and precipitated by a voluntary action, such as movement, it is referred to as *incident pain*. Another type of breakthrough pain called *idiopathic pain* is not associated with any known cause and often lasts longer than incident pain. Episodes of pain that occur before the next analgesic dose is due are called *end-of-dose failure pain*. A fast-onset, short-acting formulation of a first-line analgesic, such as morphine, oxycodone, hydromorphone, or fentanyl, is used to manage breakthrough pain. Analgesic doses or the frequency of their administration is adjusted as needed to minimize the occurrence of breakthrough pain.[12]

Reassessment

Following initiation of the pain management plan, pain is reassessed and documented on a regular basis as a way to evaluate the effectiveness of the treatments. At a minimum, pain should be reassessed with each new report of pain and before and after the administration of analgesics.[31] The frequency of reassessment depends on the stability of the patient's pain and is guided by institutional policy. For example, in the acute care hospital setting, reassessment may be necessary as often as every 10 minutes when pain is unstable during the titration phase (gradual increases in dose to establish analgesia) and every 8 hours in patients with stable pain.

Findings that warrant further evaluation or notification of the prescriber include pain ratings that continue to be higher than the patient's comfort-function goal, a change in the location or quality of pain, and the development of medication-induced side effects that do not respond to treatment.

Nurse monitoring of side effects is essential to ensure patient safety during analgesic administration. Life-threatening opioid-induced respiratory depression is the most serious of the opioid side effects; however, nurses can be key to preventing this complication by performing systematic assessments of their patients' sedation levels (Box 26-1).[12,32,33] Less opioid is required to produce sedation than to produce respiratory depression, a characteristic that makes sedation a particularly sensitive indicator of impending respiratory depression. Gradual increases in sedation level warrant prompt reduction of opioid dose and increased frequency of nurse monitoring until the patient demonstrates an acceptable level of sedation.[12,32]

Challenges in Assessment

Many patients are unable to provide a report of their pain because they are cognitively impaired or too young (infants and small children) to use customary self-report pain assessment tools. Other patients who present challenges in pain assessment are the critically ill (intubated, unresponsive) and those who are receiving neuromuscular blocking agents or are sedated from anesthetics and other drugs given during surgery. All of these patients are collectively referred to as "nonverbal" patients.[34]

When patients are unable to report pain using traditional methods, an alternative approach based on the Hierarchy of

---

BOX 26-2   HIERARCHY OF IMPORTANCE OF PAIN MEASURES*

1. Attempt to obtain the patient's self-report, the single most reliable indicator of pain. Do not assume a patient cannot provide a report of pain; many cognitively impaired patients are able to use a self-report tool, such as the Faces Pain Scale-Revised (FPS-R) or Verbal Descriptor Scale (VDS).

2. Consider the patient's condition or exposure to a procedure that is thought to be painful. If appropriate, assume pain is present (APP) and document APP when approved by institution policy and procedure.

3. Observe behavioral signs (e.g., facial expressions, crying, restlessness, and changes in activity). There are many behavioral pain assessment tools available that will yield a pain behavior score and may help to determine if pain is present. However, it is important to remember that a behavioral score is not the same as a pain intensity score. Pain intensity is unknown if the patient is unable to provide it.

A surrogate who knows the patient well (e.g., parent, spouse, or caregiver) may be able to provide information about underlying painful pathology or behaviors that may indicate pain.

4. Evaluate physiologic indicators with the understanding that they are the least sensitive indicators of pain and may signal the existence of conditions other than pain or a lack of it (e.g., hypovolemia, blood loss). Patients may have normal or below normal vital signs in the presence of severe pain. The absence of an elevated blood pressure or heart rate does not mean the absence of pain.

5. Conduct an analgesic trial to confirm the presence of pain and to establish a basis for developing a treatment plan if pain is thought to be present. An analgesic trial involves the administration of a low dose of nonopioid or opioid and observing patient response. The initial low dose may not be enough to illicit a change in behavior and should be increased if the previous dose was tolerated, or another analgesic may be added. If behaviors continue despite optimal analgesic doses, other possible causes should be investigated. In patients who are completely unresponsive, no change in behavior will be evident and the optimized analgesic dose should be continued.

Copyright 1999, Margo McCaffery, Chris Pasero. Used with permission.
*Shows the recommended framework for pain assessment in nonverbal patients.[3,34,35]

Importance of Pain Measures is recommended.[3,34,35] The key components of the Hierarchy are to (1) attempt to obtain self-report; (2) consider underlying pathology or conditions and procedures that might be painful (e.g., surgery); (3) observe behaviors; (4) evaluate physiologic indicators; and (5) conduct an analgesic trial (Box 26-2 for detailed information on each component).

CLINICAL MANAGEMENT

For most of the health and illness concepts presented in this text, clinical management includes all phases of health promotion including primary and secondary prevention. However, for the concept of pain, the relevant focus of clinical management involves interventions to treat pain.

Collaborative Interventions
Pharmacologic Strategies

Pain is a complex phenomenon involving multiple underlying mechanisms. This mandates the use of more than one analgesic, sometimes provided by more than one route of administration, to manage it. Guidelines recommend the use of multimodal analgesia for all types of pain.[1,12,36,37] A multimodal regimen combines drugs with different underlying mechanisms. This allows lower doses of each of the drugs in the treatment plan, which reduces the potential for each to produce adverse effects.[12,36] Furthermore, multimodal analgesia can result in comparable or greater pain relief than can be achieved with any single analgesic.[12]

Multimodal analgesia is discussed most often in the context of nociceptive-type pain treatment (e.g., postoperative pain); however, neuropathic pain is a multifaceted phenomenon with many underlying mechanisms, which underscores the importance of using a multimodal approach to manage this type of pain as well.[37] The use of multimodal analgesia should be the rule, rather than the exception, in pain treatment.

Analgesics. There are three major analgesic groups:
- Nonopioid analgesics
- Opioid analgesics
- Adjuvant analgesics

Figure 26-2 shows the first-line analgesics in each group.

Nonopioid analgesics are appropriate alone for mild to some moderate nociceptive-type pain and are added to opioid analgesics as part of a multimodal analgesic regimen for more severe nociceptive pain.[12,38] For example, unless contraindicated, all surgical patients should routinely be given acetaminophen and an NSAID in scheduled doses throughout the postoperative course. Opioid analgesics are added to the treatment plan to manage moderate to severe postoperative pain. A local anesthetic is sometimes administered epidurally or by continuous peripheral nerve block. An anticonvulsant may be added to the treatment plan as well to control severe pain or prevent a chronic postsurgical pain syndrome, such as postthoracotomy or postmastectomy pain.[39]

Anticonvulsants and antidepressants are first-line analgesics for neuropathic pain.[37] These analgesics require a period of several days to weeks of dose titration to determine efficacy and safety and to achieve adequate pain control. Lidocaine patch 5% is used for well-localized peripheral neuropathic types of pain, such as postherpetic neuralgia (shingles-related pain). Long-term opioid therapy can be effective for some individuals with neuropathic pain as well.[12] It is not unusual to find a multimodal pain treatment regimen for a person with neuropathic pain that includes an antidepressant, anticonvulsant, local anesthetic, and an opioid.

Routes of administration. A variety of routes of administration are used to deliver analgesics. A principle of pain management is to use the oral route of administration whenever

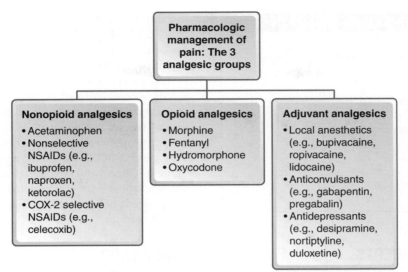

FIGURE 26-2 Pharmacologic Management of Pain. This figure shows the three analgesic groups and examples of first-line options within each group.

feasible.[12] All of the first-line analgesics used to manage pain are available in short-acting and long-acting formulations. For patients who have continuous pain, a long-acting analgesic, such as modified-release oral morphine, oxycodone, or hydromorphone, or transdermal fentanyl, is used to treat the persistent baseline pain. A fast-onset, short-acting analgesic (usually the same drug as the long-acting) is used to treat breakthrough pain if it occurs.[12]

When the oral route is not possible, such as in patients who cannot swallow or are NPO or nauseated, other routes of administration are used, including intravenous (IV), subcutaneous, transdermal, and rectal. Opioids are often given by IV patient-controlled analgesia (PCA), whereby patients manage their own pain by pressing a button attached to an infusion pump to deliver a preset bolus dose of pain medication. The concept of PCA recognizes that only the patient can feel the pain and only the patient knows how much analgesic will relieve it.[12] Patients who use PCA must be able to understand the relationships between pain, pushing the PCA button, and pain relief. They must also be able to cognitively and physically use the PCA equipment.[12] Some of the methods used to manage pain are accomplished via catheter techniques such as intraspinal analgesia and continuous peripheral nerve block infusions with or without PCA capability. Nurses play a key and extensive role in the successful management of these therapies, and the American Society for Pain Management Nursing (ASPMN.org) provides guidelines for care.[40]

Nonpharmacologic Strategies

Nonpharmacologic strategies encompass a wide variety of nondrug treatments that may contribute to comfort and pain relief. These include the body-based (physical) modalities, such as massage, acupuncture, and application of heat and cold, and the mind-body methods, such as guided imagery, relaxation breathing, and meditation. There are also biologically-based therapies that involve the use of herbs and vitamins, and energy therapies such as reiki and tai chi.[41]

Nonpharmacologic methods may be effective alone for mild to some moderate-intensity pain and are used to complement, but not replace, pharmacologic therapies for more severe pain.[42] The effectiveness of nonpharmacologic methods can be unpredictable, and although not all have been shown to relieve pain, they offer many benefits to patients with pain.[41,42] For example, research has shown that nonpharmacologic methods can facilitate relaxation and reduce anxiety and stress.[43-45] Many patients find the use of nonpharmacologic methods helps them cope better with their pain and feel greater control over the pain experience.[44] These effects may ultimately contribute to improvements in overall quality of life.

Research shows that individuals with pain are interested in self-management of their health care and want to use alternative strategies.[41] Nurses play a key role in introducing and educating patients about nonpharmacologic techniques and are often involved in providing or facilitating their use.[46] The following list provides examples of nonpharmacologic measures that are noninvasive and relatively easy to incorporate into daily clinical practice. They can be used individually or in combination with other nondrug therapies.

- Proper body alignment achieved through proper *positioning* and regular repositioning can help prevent or relieve pain. Pillows can be used to maintain the position and support the patient's back and extremities.[46]
- Thermal measures such as the *application of localized, superficial heat and cooling* may relieve pain and provide comfort by decreasing sensitivity to pain and muscle spasms and alleviating joint and muscle aches. The two measures are often used interchangeably.[43]
- *Mind-body therapies* are designed to enhance the mind's capacity to affect bodily function and symptoms[41,46,47] and include music therapy, distraction techniques, meditation, prayer, hypnosis, guided imagery, relaxation techniques, and pet therapy, among many others.[43,44]

CLINICAL NURSING SKILLS FOR PAIN

- Pain assessment
- Nonpharmacologic pain management
  - Massage
  - Splinting
  - Relaxation and guided imagery
  - Distraction
- Pharmacologic pain management
  - Oral medications
  - Intravenous medications
  - Epidural analgesia
  - Patient-controlled analgesia
  - Local anesthesia

INTERRELATED CONCEPTS

The two types of pain, nociceptive pain (from tissue damage) and neuropathic pain (from nerve damage), share common effects when left untreated or inadequately managed. Figure 26-3 demonstrates that some of the most disturbing effects of unrelieved pain are seen in the musculoskeletal system with impaired muscle function (**Mobility**), **Fatigue,** and immobility. Inadequately managed pain in the postoperative setting limits the patient's ability to ambulate and participate in important physical therapy activities,[48] prolongs recovery,[49,50] and is associated with a higher incidence of complications including long-term disability.[7,12,51] In the outpatient setting, individuals with poorly managed chronic pain report inability to complete even the simplest of activities of daily living (**Functional ability**), which can result in loss of independence and greater reliance on family, friends, and the health care system.[52,53]

The adverse effects of unrelieved pain on quality of life are numerous and can be particularly devastating because they affect both the person with pain and the person's family and friends. Patients with poorly managed chronic pain frequently report sleep disturbances,[54] are more likely to rate their general health as poor,[55] and describe having suicidal thoughts (**Mood and affect**).[20] Research has even shown that severe chronic pain is associated with increased mortality, independent of sociodemographic factors, such as income, age, and gender.[56]

EXEMPLARS

As mentioned previously, most individuals experience pain across the lifespan and in many different ways. Thus there are multiple situations encountered by the nurse that will require pain assessment and interventions. A discussion of each situation is beyond the scope of this concept analysis; however, Box 26-3 presents the most common pain conditions in the context of the major categories of pain.

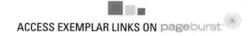

ACCESS EXEMPLAR LINKS ON pageburst

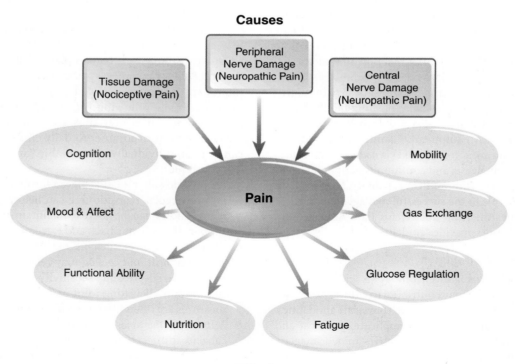

FIGURE 26-3 Interrelated Concepts: Causes and Effects of Pain.

MODEL CASE

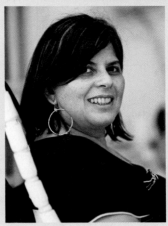

Jenny Alvers is a 38-year-old otherwise healthy female who has been admitted directly to the ICU after an automobile accident and emergency abdominal surgery. In addition to surgery, she has deep face, neck, and chest lacerations and contusions. Jenny is on a ventilator and somewhat disoriented and restless with elevated blood pressure and heart rate. She is unable to provide a report of pain but, based on her pathologic condition, the nurse assumes that Jenny has pain and consults with the surgeon about orders for a continuous IV opioid infusion. Knowing that Jenny will be subjected to painful procedures such as endotracheal suctioning and wound care during her stay in the ICU, the nurse also requests supplemental IV opioid doses to administer prophylactically. Jenny's sister reported that Jenny has no allergies but experienced severe nausea when she was given IV morphine following an appendectomy 3 years ago. The surgeon prescribes an IV infusion of hydromorphone at a dosage appropriate for an adult with moderate to severe pain and supplemental IV hydromorphone bolus doses every hour as needed. Scheduled doses of IV acetaminophen and IV ibuprofen are also ordered.

The nurse suspects that Jenny's restlessness could be related to unrelieved pain and therefore administers an IV hydromorphone loading dose before initiating the infusion. Infusions of IV ibuprofen followed by IV acetaminophen are also administered. An aqua pad circulating cool water is placed over Jenny's chest to provide additional analgesia. The nurse reduces the external stimuli in the room as much as possible and provides Jenny with calm reassurance and orientation while caring for her. Within 45 minutes of these interventions, Jenny is no longer restless, her vital signs are within normal limits and stable, and she appears to be resting comfortably.

Case Analysis

Pain assessment in Jenny is a challenge because she is unable to report pain using customary assessment tools. According to the Hierarchy of Pain Measures, when self-report of pain cannot be obtained, clinicians should assume pain is present based on the existence of painful pathology. Behaviors, if present, may also be observed as possible indicators of pain. The nurse correctly suspected that Jenny's restlessness might be due to unrelieved pain and administered analgesia promptly. It is important to note that elevated vital signs, which often accompany restlessness, are not reliable measures of pain, but they are sometimes used to further support the assumption that acute pain may be present. When Jenny recovers enough to provide a report of pain, self-report tools such as the NRS or FPS-R will be introduced and used to assess her pain.

The type of pain is used to determine the appropriate treatment approach. Jenny has experienced surgery as well as significant trauma-related tissue damage, both of which yield nociceptive pain. The first-line analgesics for moderate to severe nociceptive pain include opioids and nonopioids, such as acetaminophen and NSAIDs. Because Jenny is on a ventilator, the analgesics are administered by the IV route. Fortunately, there are several opioid and some nonopioid analgesics available in IV formulation. Administration of a loading dose (IV bolus in this case) before initiation of the maintenance analgesic (IV infusion) is recommended to establish rapid analgesia. When Jenny is able to take oral fluids, analgesics will be given orally.

■■■ BOX 26-3 EXEMPLARS OF PAIN

Nociceptive Pain
Somatic Pain
- Ankylosing spondylitis
- Cancer pain (tumor growth) and pain associated with bony metastases
- Labor pain (cervical changes and uterine contractions)
- Osteoarthritis pain
- Osteoporosis pain
- Pain of Ehlers-Danlos syndrome
- Rheumatoid arthritis pain
- Surgical trauma
- Wound and burn pain

Visceral Pain
- Crohn's disease
- Irritable bowel syndrome
- Organ-involved cancer pain
- Pancreatitis
- Ulcerative colitis

Neuropathic Pain
Centrally-Generated Pain
- Complex regional pain syndrome
- Pain following spinal cord injury
- Phantom pain as a result of peripheral nerve damage
- Poststroke pain

Peripherally-Generated Pain
- Alcohol-nutritional neuropathy
- Diabetic neuropathy
- Nerve root compression, nerve entrapment
- Pain of Guillain-Barré syndrome
- Postherpetic neuralgia
- Some types of neck, shoulder, and back pain
- Trigeminal neuralgia

Continued

> ### ■■■ BOX 26-3   EXEMPLARS OF PAIN—cont'd
>
> **Mixed Pain**
> - Fibromyalgia
> - Myofascial pain
> - Pain associated with human immunodeficiency virus (HIV)
>
> - Pain associated with Lyme disease
> - Some headaches
> - Some types of neck, shoulder, and back pain

REFERENCES

1. American Pain Society (APS): *Principles of analgesic use in the treatment of acute and cancer pain*, ed 6, Glenview, Ill, 2008, Author.
2. McCaffery M: *Nursing practice theories related to cognition, bodily pain, and man-environment interactions*, Los Angeles, 1968, University of California.
3. McCaffery M, Herr K, Pasero C: Assessment. In Pasero C, McCaffery M, editors: *Pain assessment and pharmacologic management*, St Louis, 2011, Mosby/Elsevier, pp 13–176.
4. Pasero C, Portenoy RK: Neurophysiology of pain and analgesia and the pathophysiology of neuropathic pain. In Pasero C, McCaffery M, editors: *Pain assessment and pharmacologic management*, St Louis, 2011, Mosby/Elsevier, pp 1–12.
5. American Geriatrics Society (AGS): Pharmacological management of persistent pain in older persons, *J Am Geriatr Soc* 57:1331–1346, 2009.
6. Herr K: Pain in older adult: an imperative across all health care settings, *Pain Manag Nurs* 11(2):S1–S10, 2010.
7. Pasero C: Postoperative pain management in the older adult. In Gibson SJ, Weiner DK, editors: *Pain in older persons*, Seattle, 2005, International Association for the Study of Pain (IASP), pp 377–401.
8. Titler MG, Herr K, Schilling ML, et al: Acute pain treatment for older adults hospitalized with hip fracture: current nursing practices and perceived barriers, *Appl Nurs Res* 16(4):211–227, 2003.
9. Takai Y, Yamamoto-Mitani N, Okamoto Y, et al: Literature review of pain prevalence among older residents of nursing homes, *Pain Manag Nurs* 11(4):209–223, 2010.
10. Cook DJ, Rooke GA: Priorities in perioperative geriatrics, *Anesth Analg* 96:1823–1836, 2003.
11. American Geriatrics Society (AGS): The management of persistent pain in older persons, *J Am Geriatr Soc* 50(1):S205–S224, 2002.
12. Pasero C, Quinn TE, Portenoy RK, et al: Opioid analgesics. In Pasero C, McCaffery M, editors: *Pain assessment and pharmacologic management*, St Louis, 2011, Mosby/Elsevier, pp 277–622.
13. Ardery G, Herr K, Hannon BJ, et al: Lack of opioid administration in older hip fracture patients, *Geriatr Nurs* 24(6):353–359, 2003.
14. Pasero C: Pain relief for neonates, *Am J Nurs* 104(5):44–47, 2004.
15. Simons SH, van Dijk M, Anand KS, et al: Do we still hurt babies? A prospective study of procedural pain and analgesia in neonates, *Arch Pediatr Adolesc Med* 157(11):1058–1064, 2003.
16. Puntillo KA, Pasero C, Li D, et al: Evaluation of pain in the ICU patient, *Chest* 135(4):1069–1074, 2009.
17. Puntillo KA, White C, Morris AB, et al: Patients' perceptions and responses to procedural pain: results from Thunder Project II, *Am J Crit Care* 10(4):238–251, 2001.
18. Stanik-Hutt JA, Soeken KL, Belcher AE, et al: Pain experiences of traumatically injured patients in a critical care setting, *Am J Crit Care* 10(4):252–259, 2001.
19. Beilin B, Shavit Y, Trabekin E, et al: The effects of postoperative pain management on immune response to surgery, *Anesth Analg* 97:822–827, 2003.
20. Pasero C, Paice JA, McCaffery M: Basic mechanisms underlying the causes and effects of pain. In McCaffery M, Pasero C, editors: *Pain: clinical manual*, ed 2, St Louis, 1999, Mosby, pp 15–34.
21. Weatherston KB, Franck LS, Klein NJ: Are there opportunities to decrease nosocomial infection by choice of analgesic regimen? *Arch Pediatr Adolesc Med* 157:1108–1114, 2003.
22. Page GG: Analgesia administration attenuates surgery-induced tumor promotion, *Reg Anesth Pain Med* 27(2):197–199, 2002.
23. Page GG: Acute pain and immune impairment, *Pain Clin Updates* 12(1):1–4, 2005.
24. Guay J: Postoperative pain significantly influences postoperative blood loss in patients undergoing total knee replacement, *Pain Med* 7(6):476–482, 2006.
25. Kehlet H, Wilmore DW: Multimodal strategies to improve surgical outcome, *Am J Surg* 183:630–641, 2002.
26. Erb J, Orr E, Mercer D, et al: Interactions between pulmonary performance and movement-evoked pain in the immediate postsurgical period: implications for perioperative research and treatment, *Reg Anesth Pain Med* 33(4):312–319, 2008.
27. Shea RA, Brooks JA, Dayhoff NE, et al: Pain intensity and postoperative pulmonary complications among the elderly after abdominal surgery, *Heart Lung* 31:440–449, 2002.
28. Ware L, Epps DE, Herr K, et al: Evaluation of the revised faces pain scale, verbal descriptor scale, numeric rating scale and Iowa pain thermometer in older minority adults, *Pain Manag Nurs* 71:117–125, 2006.
29. Spagrud LJ, Piira T, Von Baeyer CL: Children's self-report of pain intensity. The faces pain scale—revised, *Am J Nurs* 103(12):62–64, 2003.
30. Herr KA, Spratt KF, Mobily PR, et al: Pain intensity assessment in older adults: use of experimental pain to compare psychometric properties and usability of selected pain scales with younger adults, *Clin J Pain* 20:207–219, 2004.
31. Miaskowski C, Cleary J, Burney R, et al: *Guideline for the management of cancer pain in adults and children*, Glenview, Ill, 2005, American Pain Society.
32. Pasero C: Assessment of sedation during opioid administration for pain management, *J PeriAnesth Nurs* 24(3):186–190, 2009.
33. Nisbet AT, Mooney-Cotter F: Selected scales for reporting opioid-induced sedation, *Pain Manag Nurs* 10(3):154–164, 2009.
34. Herr K, Coyne PJ, Key T, et al: Pain assessment in the nonverbal patient: position statement with clinical practice recommendations, *Pain Manag Nurs* 7(2):44–52, 2006.
35. Pasero C: Challenges in pain assessment, *J PeriAnesth Nurs* 24(1):50–54, 2009.
36. Ashburn MA, Caplan RA, Carr DB, et al: Practice guidelines for acute pain management in the perioperative setting. An updated report by the American Society of Anesthesiologists task force on acute pain management, *Anesthesiology* 100(6):1573–1581, 2004.

37. Dworkin RH, O'Connor AB, Backonja M, et al: Pharmacologic management of neuropathic pain: evidence-based recommendations, *Pain* 132(3):237–251, 2007.

38. Pasero C, Portenoy RK, McCaffery M: Nonopioid analgesics. In Pasero C, McCaffery M, editors: *Pain assessment and pharmacologic management*, St Louis, 2011, Mosby/Elsevier, pp 177–276.

39. Pasero C, Polomano RC, Portenoy RK: Adjuvant analgesics. In Pasero C, McCaffery M, editors: *Pain assessment and pharmacologic management*, St Louis, 2011, Mosby/Elsevier, pp 623–818.

40. Pasero C, Eksterowicz N, Primeau M, et al: Registered nurse management and monitoring of analgesia by catheter techniques, *Pain Manag Nurs* 8(2):48–54, 2007.

41. Bruckenthal P: Integrating nonpharmacologic and alternative strategies into a comprehensive management approach for older adults with pain, *Pain Manag Nurs* 11(2):S23–S31, 2010.

42. McCaffery M: What is the role of nondrug methods in the nursing care of patients with acute pain? *Pain Manag Nurs* 3(3):77–80, 2002.

43. McCaffery M, Pasero C: Practical nondrug approaches to pain. In McCaffery M, Pasero C, editors: *Pain: clinical manual*, ed 2, St Louis, 1999, Mosby, pp 399–427.

44. Kwekkeboom KL, Cherwin CH, Lee JW, et al: Mind-body treatments for the pain-fatigue-sleep disturbance symptom cluster in persons with cancer, *J Pain Symptom Manag* 39:126, 2010.

45. Allred KD, Byers J, Sole ML: The effect of music on postoperative pain and anxiety, *Pain Manag Nurs* 11:15, 2010.

46. Gatlin CG, Schulmeister L: When medication is not enough: nonpharmacologic management of pain, *Clin J Oncol Nurs* 11:699, 2007.

47. National Center for Complementary and Alternative Medicine (NCCAM): *What is CAM?* at http://nccam.nih.gov/health/whatiscam/overview.htm. Accessed Dec 20, 2010.

48. Morrison RS, Magaziner J, McLaughlin MA, et al: The impact of post-operative pain on outcomes following hip fracture, *Pain* 103:303–311, 2003.

49. Kehlet H, Wilmore DW: Evidence-based surgical care and the evolution of fast-track surgery, *Ann Surg* 248(2):189–198, 2008.

50. Pavlin DJ, Chen C, Penaloza DA, et al: Pain as a factor complicating recovery and discharge after ambulatory surgery, *Anesth Analg* 95(3):627–634, 2002.

51. Pavlin DJ, Chen C, Penaloza DA, et al: A survey of pain and other symptoms that affect the recovery process after discharge from an ambulatory surgery unit, *J Clin Anesth* 16(3):200–206, 2004.

52. Rudy TE, Lieber SJ: Functional assessment of older adults with chronic pain. In Gibson SJ, Weiner DK, editors: *Pain in older persons*, Seattle, 2005, International Association for the Study of Pain (IASP), pp 153–173.

53. Simmonds MJ, Novey D, Sandoval R: The differential influence of pain and fatigue on physical performance and health status in ambulatory patients with human immunodeficiency virus, *Clin J Pain* 21(3):200–206, 2005.

54. Turk DC, Cohen MJM: Sleep as a marker in the effective management of chronic osteoarthritis pain with opioid analgesics, *Semin Arthritis Rheum* 39(6):477–490, 2010.

55. Mantyselka PT, Turunen JHO, Ahonen RS, et al: Chronic pain and poor self-rated health, *JAMA* 290(18):2435–2442, 2003.

56. Torrance N, Elliott AM, Lee AJ, et al: Severe chronic pain is associated with increased 10 year mortality. A cohort record linkage study, *Eur J Pain* 14:380–386, 2010.

27

Stress

Lynne Buchanan

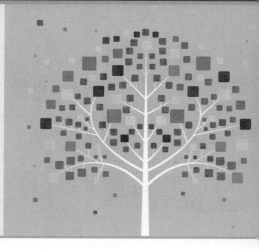

tress is a common topic in society and is a frequently used term. We have all used the word to express pressure or emotional strain. Although in early representations stress was often viewed as unhealthy, contemporary views use stress to understand the individual's perceptions of the requirements of an event, demand, or stressor as well as the individual's pattern of response. Stress is unhealthy when an individual cannot adapt and exhausts resources. The classic interpretation is that stress is a multidimensional concept that is interrelated with other concepts including cognitive appraisal, coping, and adaptation.[1]

The word stress has existed since the fourteenth century with a meaning of hardship, adversity, or affliction. Over the years, stress has been described from three perspectives—stimulus, response, and interaction. A stimulus perspective focuses on demands or events in the environment, such as a natural disaster or terrorist attack. In contrast, stress from a response perspective is interactional—between individual and environment—with cognitive appraisal determining a series of reactions. In the early 1950s, Hans Selye proposed a reaction theory that stated stress is the sum of all the effects of factors that act on the body with both pleasant and unpleasant stressors being equally important.[2] Though early experiments supported various species responded in a stereotypical reaction to events such as infection, trauma, nervous strain, heat, cold, or fatigue in a response termed the general adaptation syndrome, continuing work demonstrated no uniform response to all stimuli. Other theorists later proposed stress as a mediator between life events and adaptation but were criticized because of the assumption that all life events were negative.[3] Lazarus[4] proposed a cognitive appraisal approach, and the current concept of stress developed from this view. The contemporary view is that stress is a concept with psychologic, physiologic, and behavioral components; stress is interactional between the individual and the environment and is influenced by personal appraisal; and stress has defined end points and measurable outcomes.

DEFINITION(S)

A general definition is that stress is a pattern of physiologic and psychologic responses determined through cognitive appraisal.[1] To add focus for practice and research, experts suggested that stress be treated as an organizing concept for understanding a wide range of phenomena important in human adaption, health, and disease.[4] According to this viewpoint, stress is a complex blend of variables with multiple subparts and processes. Therefore the meaning of the concept for each discipline is delineated so that stress does not come to represent anything and everything that is perceived and adapted to.

Stress has been proposed in the nursing literature as a pattern of physiologic and psychologic responses to perceptions of extraordinary physical, environmental, or psychosocial demands.[5] This definition was then revised so that it applied to stress experienced with ordinary events during daily living—stress is a pattern of physiologic and psychologic responses to perceptions of demand or threat determined by cognitive appraisal, adaptation, and coping.[5] Stress is also defined as interactional, viewed as the state of affairs arising when persons relate to situations in certain ways.[1,4] In general, a person experiences stress when a demand exceeds coping abilities, resulting in reactions such as disturbances of cognition, emotion, and behavior that adversely affect well-being.[6] For the purposes of this concept analysis, stress is defined as *an event or demand made on the individual/family that causes the individual/family to appraise the event/demand for scope and meaning and to determine whether resources for management are exceeded and whether the event/demand is neutral (no stress), challenging, or threatening. It is the appraisal that determines the end result (outcome) of health, disability, or dysfunction.* The manifestations of stress are not always physically visible; they are complex and their purpose is to protect equilibrium and productivity. However, if stress is prolonged or severe, it can have unhealthy consequences, especially when exceeding the person's resources and ability to cope.[7,8]

SCOPE AND CATEGORIES

Stress is a set of responses (cognitive, emotional, and behavioral) to single or multiple events or demands that are sometimes called stressors. The response to the event or demand is determined by the interaction between the person and environment and the process of cognitive appraisal. The full scope of the experience is no stress (neutral), challenging, or threatening. A no stress experience is perceived by the individual to be neutral or easily managed through existing resources and does not disturb equilibrium. A challenging experience is perceived by the individual to be manageable but requires mobilization of resources—in other words, it is an event that can be positively addressed; it does not tax resources, harm the individual, or disturb the body's ability to maintain equilibrium and homeostasis. A threatening experience is perceived as taxing and exceeds existing resources and personal capabilities, causes disruption of equilibrium and homeostasis, and, if severe and/or chronic, impacts health and well-being.

Figure 27-1 illustrates an organizing framework for the concept of stress that nurses can use in their practice. In the framework there are factors that exist before or concomitant with the event or demand that are called antecedents. These include individual characteristics, family and community, and environment. The framework assumes the individual, who has unique characteristics, is interacting with family, community, and environment. Every individual is presumed to experience the scope of stress each day. The personal appraisal and reappraisal assist the individual to focus the scope of the experience and determine the magnitude as no stress, challenge, or threat. Developmental level, cognitive functioning, coping, adaptation, and capacity to respond interact when information is processed and these factors assist in the formation of meaning and response. It is the secondary appraisal or exploration of deeper meaning that shapes the full meaning of the event or demand. Psychologic and physiologic responses occur. The alarm response has specific sympathetic nervous system effects. If the responses become severe, prolonged, and chronic, there is a high potential for disability and dysfunction, which may manifest as visible signs and symptoms in the individual, family, or community. The far right box of Figure 27-1 depicts clinical management. Health promotion and protection, early diagnosis and treatment and disability limitation, and restoration and

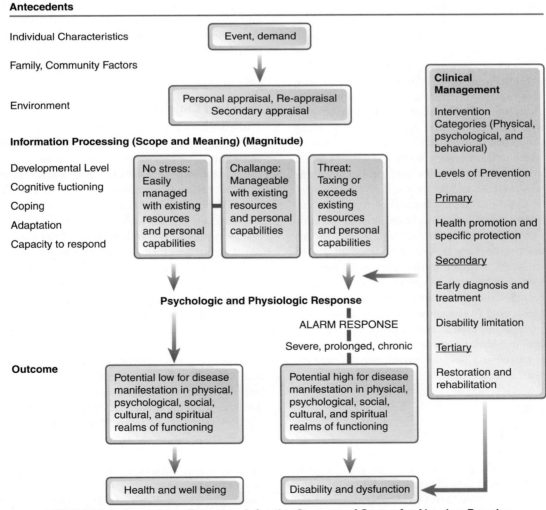

FIGURE 27-1 Organizing Framework for the Concept of Stress for Nursing Practice.

rehabilitation interventions can impact the trajectory and determine the course and severity of disability and dysfunction. It should be noted that primary prevention should be a goal of intervention by nurses in order to prevent the occurrence of disability and dysfunction, and thereby maintain health and well-being.

A health care–related example to illustrate the organizing framework in Figure 27-1 is that of an individual who is newly diagnosed with diabetes and must learn new behaviors including how to manage insulin injections. The psychologic and physiologic stress-related responses that are initiated are determined by personal appraisal of the event and the demands placed on the individual and family. The scope of the experience is evaluated as no stress, challenge, or threat. If the capacity for dealing with new demands is reached, the response may impact health and well-being. This is especially true if threat and alarm responses are severe, prolonged, or chronic. This same event may also exceed the family's coping and adaptation ability, reaching capacity to deal with the demands. Caregiver strain is more likely to occur in a family if they reside in a community setting that lacks adequate resources to manage the demands. The individual and family may isolate themselves for protection and energy conservation. The outcome is determined by the interaction of all of the following factors: the current level of functioning of the individual and family (antecedents), the information processing (for scope and meaning), and the psychologic and physiologic responses. According to the practice framework in Figure 27-1, the nurse is involved through clinical management after the assessment and diagnosis, and implements appropriate interventions aimed at reinforcing personal capabilities. The emphasis of clinical management in the illustration is on health promotion and protection whenever possible, which in this example might include education about disease and management principles, proper immunizations, nutrition, exercise, and lifestyle.

The stress concept also has a temporal component, representing short periods of time in seconds and minutes or longer periods of time spanning hours, days, and years. An example of a short-term event that must be handled is pain and anxiety from a small cut that needs suturing. An example of a long-term event that must be responded to is chronic illness with pain and other symptoms where the individual and family may become overwhelmed and experience taxing of resources. The number of events occurring within a time frame is also important because a high number over a short time may represent a negative experience if resources are taxed and capacity is reached.

RISK FACTORS

Populations at Risk

Individuals among all population groups experience risk from stress throughout the lifespan. According to the National Health Interview Survey, 75% of the general population experience at least some stress every 2 weeks.[9] Serious psychologic distress is prevalent in our society, and *Healthy People 2020*

has set a goal to improve mental health both through preventive measures and by ensuring access to appropriate, quality mental health services.[10]

Some specific populations at risk for negative consequences associated with stress are children and older adults, those with life-threatening acute and chronic diseases, and caregivers and family members dealing with acute and chronic diseases. Older adults may experience a decline in resources and capacity over time, making them at risk for stress consequences including depression and suicide. Caregiver family members of the older person with Alzheimer's disease, for example, may have chronic stress and immune system alterations.[11,12]

Infants, toddlers, and children have not had time to develop abilities and resources to cope with chronic or high-level stressors and depend on others for support, health, and well-being. Children with chronic stress have been shown to have developmental growth problems and failure-to-thrive.

Adults with chronic or severe stress who experience prolonged threat and chronic stress response may develop visceral fat, inflammation, and hormonal and metabolic changes contributing to heart disease.[13] Adults who experience prolonged psychologic stress are susceptible to diseases and conditions because of the negative impact of stress on the immune system; studies have shown this population to be more likely to have upper respiratory tract or viral infections, impaired wound healing, and faster cancer tumor growth rates.[13]

Impaired Cognition

There are a variety of factors that place an individual at risk for negative outcomes from stress. Individuals with impaired cognition are at risk for poor outcome because of the inability to adequately appraise and process information related to stress and the environment.[14-17] An appraisal is a necessary subpart because it assists with determining scope (no stress, challenge, or threat) and through reappraisal and secondary appraisal leads to full meaning of the event. The human cognitive architecture consists of two parts: working memory associated with consciousness and long-term memory. Researchers who study cognition claim that humans are conscious of and monitor events within the contents of their working memory.[14] All other cognitive functioning is hidden until it is transferred into the working memory. Information processing allows full meaning of the scope of the event/demand and requires working and long-term memory. Any factor that impacts cognition and working and long-term memory will affect cognitive appraisal and outcome. An example is an older adult with cognition impairment and memory problems or a person of any age with a brain injury impacting cognition or memory.

In a classic study, investigators found that the working memory in an adult is only able to hold seven items or elements of information at a time.[15] Therefore adults who overload their working memory will also be at greater risk for disability or dysfunction outcome because they may not be able to learn as well, may not be able to focus on the right things, or may have narrowed their focus so much they miss important cues. An example is a young or middle-age adult who experiences a high number of stressful life events and stressors in a short period of time with few coping resources and support systems.

Developmental Level and Age

In Figure 27-1 the subparts of developmental level and age are also important factors because nervous system development and experiences that form memory and capacity take time. On one end of life continuum are infants and children who have less experience, minimal developed ability, and reduced capacity for managing stress. On the other end of the spectrum are older adults with diseases affecting memory, cognition, and appraisal. In short, any health condition or situation that affects consciousness, memory, personal appraisal, information processing, and the ability to accurately interpret events places an individual at risk for disability and dysfunction. The nurse should consider not only physical diseases, such as dementia and brain injury, but also situations of serious psychologic distress, such as inadequate coping ability, impaired mental health, developmental delay, or a high number of unanticipated events occurring over a short period of time.

Socioeconomic and Cultural Factors

Other individual risk factors that should be mentioned are culture and socioeconomic level. A person from a foreign country who does not speak the native language may misinterpret events or make an inaccurate appraisal. A person of lower socioeconomic status who is illiterate cannot accurately interpret and respond to events that require reading. A homeless person or recently unemployed person may lack resources to pay for shelter, food, and health care services such as counseling or medications and be in such a poor state of health he or she cannot adequately process information. An individual who is exposed to toxic wastes in his or her residence could have developmental delays or alterations in nervous system function. Individuals living within communities with no preparedness plans may be at risk for poor outcome if subjected to a terrorist attack, mass shooting, or tornado, for example.

PHYSIOLOGIC PROCESSES AND CONSEQUENCES

Stress and response is a universal phenomenon that all people of all ages experience daily. If people have the ability and resources to deal with daily stress, the experience does not negatively impact health outcomes. However, stress that is severe, prolonged, and chronic with inadequate coping and resources has a high probability to result in disability and dysfunction.

Physiology of the Stress Response

When an individual is faced with stress (event or demand), he or she appraises the event/demand as no stress or challenging (perceived ability and resources to cope, does not exceed capacity) or as threatening. A perceived demand or event initiates a response in the central nervous system and endocrine system. It includes limbic system sympathetic nervous system (SNS) response. There is a point when the individual perceives the full meaning of the event as nontaxing to resources and not exceeding capacity for management. If capacity is reached and the event or demand exceeds a certain threshold, then health and well-being are impacted. For the person who appraises threat, if the event or demand is severe or chronic, the responses reach a point where damage begins to occur in the body, causing disease. A person in chronic stress has heightened responses and can exhaust the ability of the body to maintain homeostasis, at which point physical and/or psychologic and social manifestations occur.

A simplified schematic of the SNS response is shown in Figure 27-2, which illustrates the general response. The piece of the schematic that occurs in the mind is not shown in Figure 27-2, and the mind and body are interactive in determining the eventual body and behavioral responses. Although not visible, an assumption is that a taxing and threatening situation that is chronic and prolonged heightens the responses and over time causes adverse health consequences. One of the links between the psychologic, cognitive, and physical systems and disease manifestations is through the impact on the immune system.[11,12,16,17]

An assumption of Figure 27-2 is that all events and demands are consciously or subconsciously responded to and are appraised as stressors. A stressor activates the limbic system and the hypothalamus secretes corticotropin-releasing hormone (CRH). The limbic system activates the SNS (norepinephrine and epinephrine), the pituitary gland, and the adrenal glands. This assists to direct energy for adaptation to the central nervous system and the body. Perceived events or demands cause an anticipatory response beginning in the limbic system. The limbic system is responsible for emotions and cognition. The limbic system directs the endocrine response by stimulating neural pathways for sensory information and directs the central SNS response by directly stimulating the locus ceruleus to release norepinephrine. Effects of norepinephrine are arousal, vigilance, anxiety, and labile emotions.[17] The anterior and posterior pituitary gland is also stimulated. The anterior pituitary releases several hormones including endorphins, adrenocorticotropic hormone (ACTH), prolactin, and growth hormone. Cortisol is released along with a myriad of responses that affect organs such as the liver, heart, lungs, and immune system.

Pathophysiologic Consequences

Some examples of diseases linked with untreated or prolonged stress are coronary heart disease, hypertension, stroke, dysrhythmia disorders, obesity, tension headache, backache, autoimmune disease, infection, ulcers, bowel problems, urinary problems, eczema, acne, diabetes, menstrual cycle disorders, fatigue, depression, and insomnia.[17,18] Research is ongoing about the exact mechanisms of disease causation

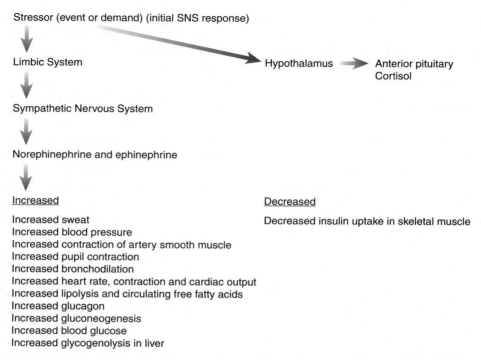

Stressor (event or demand) (initial SNS response)

Limbic System

Sympathetic Nervous System

Norephinephrine and ephinephrine

Hypothalamus → Anterior pituitary
Cortisol

Increased

Increased sweat
Increased blood pressure
Increased contraction of artery smooth muscle
Increased pupil contraction
Increased bronchodilation
Increased heart rate, contraction and cardiac output
Increased lipolysis and circulating free fatty acids
Increased glucagon
Increased gluconeogenesis
Increased blood glucose
Increased glycogenolysis in liver

Decreased

Decreased insulin uptake in skeletal muscle

FIGURE 27-2 Physiology of Alarm Response Sympathetic Nervous System Effects.

in chronic stress. There are theories proposing the harmful effects of prolonged inflammatory responses, inhibitory effects on the immune system, and effects on target organs including the cardiovascular system, where a relationship has been found between mental or emotional stress and myocardial ischemia, left ventricular dysfunction, and ventricular dysrhythmia.[17,18] If left untreated, chronic stress can result in exhaustion, adrenal cortex depletion, and even death.[7,8]

ASSESSMENT

Stress is observable by nurses in the clinical setting and can be evaluated using assessment tools that capture the physical, cognitive, psychologic/emotional, and behavioral signs and symptoms. Signs and symptoms can manifest in a variety of ways and may vary in their seriousness. Nurses should recognize individuals who are experiencing a challenging or threatening stress response and serious psychologic distress so that appropriate interventions can be initiated.

History

When conducting a history, the nurse queries about the past and current state of health (past medical history, current conditions, current medications), family history, psychosocial history, and stress symptoms associated with body systems. Past or current conditions that may be associated with stress include ulcers, stroke, hypertension, and heart disease. Anxiety, anger, depression, and irritability may become significant if they lead to thoughts of blame, revenge, or even suicide. Symptoms that could be associated with stress include unexplained abdominal pain, headaches, insomnia, lack of concentration, excessive sweating, skin eruptions, hair loss, hyperventilation, palpitations, tightening of the chest, and anxiety. Nurses should ask about the individual's perception of the event or demands and link the perception to physiologic responses.

The information is used to develop a clinical management plan to reduce stress and induce relaxation as well as to determine the reason the person sought an appraisal of the threat. Simply asking the patient if he or she feels threatened by this demand or event and how long he or she has felt this way could illicit accurate information as a basis for further therapeutic communication. The communication is used to collect additional information to formulate the nursing diagnosis and evidence-based clinical management plan.

Examination

Because of the physiologic response to stress noted in the previous section, examination findings are associated with the sympathetic nervous system response. In an acute phase these signs may include elevated heart rate, elevated blood pressure, increased respiratory rate and depth, and dilated pupils. Such findings may not be as evident when stress is chronic.

A priority of the physical exam should be assessment of common signs and symptoms and the association between symptoms and disease/dysfunction. An example is when an individual describes tension headaches from muscle contraction response and inability to perform activities of daily living. The nurse should also assess for other findings that support the stress response such as excess tension in other muscles, excessive sweating, rapid heartbeat, irregular rhythms, and hyperventilation. The clinical manifestations are not specific to the stress response, but become more obvious when considered with subjective data.

TABLE 27-1	EVIDENCE-BASED PRACTICES FOR CLINICAL MANAGEMENT OF STRESS		
TYPE OF STRESS INTERVENTION CATEGORIES	**SIGNS AND SYMPTOMS**	**EXAMPLES OF INTERVENTION**	**OUTCOMES**
Psychologic and emotional	Anxiety, anger, depression, irritability, frustration, overreaction, memory loss, lack of concentration	Cognitive behavioral skills training Meditation Stress inoculation Time management	Reduced anxiety and anger Reduced depression Reduced strain
Physiologic	Muscle tension, headache, stomachache, acid reflux, tachycardia, hyperventilation, elevated BP*	Biofeedback Muscle relaxation Therapeutic touch/massage Exercise	Reduced somatization Reduced forehead muscle tension (EMG)* Reduced BP Reduced level 0 to 10 scale Reduction in number and severity of stress signs and symptoms
Behavioral	Smoking, overeating, substance abuse	Health education Smoking cessation Counseling	Healthier lifestyle Improved health status

*BP, Blood pressure; EMG, electromyogram.

CLINICAL MANAGEMENT

As shown in Figure 27-1, the health outcome can be either health and well-being or disability and dysfunction. The clinical management of stress is an important component because it is a determinant of outcome. Clinical management is guided by the signs and symptoms in the history and physical exam and is used to determine type of stress and intervention category. The levels of prevention (primary, secondary, and tertiary) and examples of settings and intervention strategies are shown in Table 27-2.

Primary Prevention

Primary prevention refers to activities that prevent or decrease the probability of occurrence of an injury, physical or mental illness, or health-threatening situation in an individual or family, or an event or illness in the population by combating harmful forces and by strengthening the capacity of individuals to withstand these forces.[5,19,20] Primary care settings focused on wellness and prevention of stress-related disease and disability include the workplace, schools, senior centers, community wellness centers, primary health care clinics, and medical homes (residences in which multiple health care providers work collaboratively to provide a health care provider for every individual). In 2007, about 27% of individuals were receiving care through medical homes and this number is expected to grow.[21]

Primary prevention strategies can also be aimed at specific groups who are high risk. For example, four intervention strategies for individuals at risk for heart disease are using positive self-talk, employing emergency stress stoppers, finding sources of pleasure, and performing daily relaxation training.[22-24]

Research has shown that a positive attitude, such as feeling optimistic, contributes to health and well-being and that developing a positive attitude and learning skills to cope with stress are foundations of primary prevention.[24,25] Unhealthy traits such as chronic anxiety, worry, and negativism are linked with poor outcome.[23] Stress prevention management also involves counseling, education, and implementation of techniques to manage problem-oriented and emotion-oriented stress. To prevent physical symptoms, relaxation and deep breathing are effective and individuals can learn to prevent the stress response through cognitive behavioral strategies.[25,26]

Secondary Prevention (Screening)

Secondary prevention refers to screening and detection, allowing for prompt interventions. This enables the individual to return to maximum potential and normal function as quickly as possible. Most of the interventions shown in Table 27-1 are appropriate and can be chosen by the nurse after the assessment phase.

As shown in Table 27-2, secondary prevention settings may overlap with primary care settings and include clinics, schools, senior centers, health fairs, and hospitals. Screening for stress-related diseases and commonly affected organ systems should be targeted to high-risk populations.

A number of easy-to-use stress screening tools are available for secondary prevention to detect stress levels. Stress checklists can be administered as part of a health visit or in other settings such as those previously listed. The checklists measure a number of physical signs and symptoms (tenseness of muscles, tenseness of facial expression, headache, body ache, rapid heartbeat, irregular heartbeat, gastric distress, nausea, sleep problems), psychologic/emotional symptoms (anger, irritability, forgetfulness, lack of focus, depression, sadness, anxiety, crying, and anger), and behavioral responses (eating problems, weight gain or loss, illicit drug use, crying outbursts, and social withdrawal).[24-27] A response rating scale from 0 (no stress) to 10 (highest stress) is simple but yields good results and is a suitable starting point for the novice nurse.

Other tools, although more sophisticated, are simple to use and easy to administer and have good reliability and validity to rate daily symptoms of stress, daily hassles, or life events. The *Holmes Life Events Scale* is an example of a tool that measures life events and can be administered and scored by novice nurses. It has been extensively used and is still current.[3] Other tools measure thoughts, feelings, and actions or coping skills in response to stressful situations and are considered a reflection of ability to handle stress levels. One tool used widely to assess stress and actions/coping skills is *The Ways of Coping Checklist, Revised*.[1,4,27] It assesses both positive and negative methods of coping with stressful situations including problem-focus, seeking social support, blaming self, blaming others, wishful thinking, and avoidance. There

are a variety of other general self-report stress and coping tools for secondary prevention of stress that are comprehensive and psychometrically robust. More information can be found in the Coping concept.

Collaborative Interventions

Tertiary prevention refers to restoring the person to optimal function. It includes prompt treatment, follow-up, rehabilitation, and education. Clinical management first focuses on identifying the best practice interventions that will provide immediate alleviation of stress. The latter part of clinical management has a broader goal to seek the root causes of stress and to booster resources and coping ability; goals include not only alleviating the stress response but also preventing it. Table 27-1 shows examples of evidence-based practices for clinical management of stress for immediate initiation of relaxation responses. These are based on the stress intervention category.

Psychologic/emotional stress—which has signs and symptoms including anxiety, anger, depression, irritability, frustration, overreaction, and inability to concentrate—is best treated using cognitive behavioral skills training, meditation, stress inoculation, and time management. Outcomes should be measured after implementation of the intervention. Physiologic stress with signs and symptoms of muscle tension often responds well to biofeedback, yielding outcomes such as decreased somatization, muscle tension, and blood pressure as well as a reduction in the number and severity of stress signs and symptoms. In behavioral-expressed stress in which overeating, smoking, and substance abuse are evident, health education and counseling are used to achieve health and well-being and improve health status outcomes of weight loss, smoking cessation, and sobriety, respectively.

Clinical management requires nurses to use basic clinical judgment and diagnostic reasoning skills. The data gathered in the assessment phase are the foundation for decision making and conclusions and direct the clinical management. For example, one conclusion (nursing diagnosis) that might be supported in an individual with many life demands and events over a short period of time is stress overload. Stress overload is defined as excessive amounts and types of demands that require action.[19] The defining characteristics of stress overload are anger, impatience, feelings of pressure or tension, inability to function or make decisions, physical symptoms, and a psychologic distress rating of 7 or more on a 10-point scale. The interventions are to mobilize support, reduce stress through relaxation, and initiate cognitive behavioral therapy.[20]

Common collaborative treatments include medications (prescribed by a physician, physician assistant, or nurse practitioner) and counseling (provided by nurses, pharmacists, and psychologists), all with a focus on rehabilitation. As shown in Table 27-2, settings for tertiary level care sometimes overlap with primary and secondary level care centers, including clinics, hospitals, and rehabilitation centers. However, these services are increasingly being provided by skilled

TABLE 27-2	LEVELS OF PREVENTION, SETTINGS AND INTERVENTION STRATEGIES
LEVEL OF PREVENTION	**SETTINGS AND INTERVENTION STRATEGIES**
Primary Health promotion and protection	Settings: Workplace, schools, senior centers, community wellness centers, primary health care clinics, medical homes Individual interventions: Stress management techniques, stress reduction techniques, stress inoculation, counseling, health education, behavioral lifestyle change to wellness focus Family interventions: Family enhancement, social support enhancement, social network building Community interventions: Wellness programs
Secondary Early diagnosis and treatment Disability limitation	Settings: Primary care clinics, schools, senior centers, health fairs, hospital settings Individual: Screenings for stress-related diseases Family: Disease screenings Community: Disability limitation programs, exercise programs
Tertiary Restoration and rehabilitation	Settings: Clinics, hospitals, community rehabilitation centers Individual: Pulmonary and cardiac rehabilitation programs focused on stress management Family: Family rehabilitation programs Community: Community rehabilitation programs

teams working collaboratively in the community where the focus is not only on rehabilitation but also on the family and support networks. Common collaborative treatments are medications and counseling. The nurse is an integral member of the team because he or she provides education about medication use and supports counseling interventions.

Medication Treatment

The nurse is a member of the collaborative team and supports the prescriptive authority component through education and counseling. Some examples of medication categories used for stress management are drugs that act on the central and peripheral nervous systems, including anxiolytics and hypnotics, antidepressants, psychotherapeutics, muscle relaxants, narcotics, and antimigraine agents.[28] Selective serotonin reuptake inhibitors (SSRIs) are commonly used and are also safe for the elderly population. Tricyclic antidepressants (TCAs) are not well tolerated in older adults but can be used in young and middle-age adults. The nurse's role is safe medication administration using evidence-based guidelines that include education about side effects and drug interactions.

Counseling

Counseling generally consists of group and individual psychotherapy. Counseling recommendations are made in a collaborative manner involving the nurse, physician, and psychologist or psychiatrist. Nurses who are trained in special counseling techniques such as cognitive behavioral therapy are qualified to treat mild stress but need to have protocols for referral to more qualified individuals such as psychiatric mental health advanced practice nurses, psychologists, and psychiatrists.

Nurses working in tertiary care centers need to have a basic understanding of counseling principles for stress management because they will encounter individuals and families in stress situations. For the patient who is not experiencing an acute episode or who has symptoms of stress that can be treated at the bedside in the hospital and clinic, the guidelines in Table 27-2 can be used to decide which type of intervention to provide. For example, there is evidence to support that psychologic/emotional stress is best managed by cognitive behavioral skills training, meditation, stress inoculation, and time management; physiologic stress is optimally managed by biofeedback, muscle relaxation, touch, massage, and exercise; and stress that fits the behavioral category is best managed by health education and counseling.[22-26] There is also evidence that counseling, education, and medications combined in a multicomponent program are helpful for some patients. A good example of the use of multicomponent therapy is for individuals under stress who use tobacco for relaxation. Studies show that the smoking cessation rate doubled when both medications and intense counseling were used as compared to either intervention alone.[29]

INTERRELATED CONCEPTS

Three of the most common interrelated concepts with stress are adaptation, **Cognition,** and **Coping** (Figure 27-3). These are discussed throughout this concept and are also presented in the following text.

Adaptation is closely related to stress and is used to explain the ability and capacity that are present when faced with demands of living. Adaptation is defined as decrement in components of response patterns to perceived physical, environmental, and psychosocial demands of living.[5] Capacity is part of adaptation and is a measure of ability and functioning within one's defined roles. Capacity has a maximum amount that can be obtained. When reached, the individual and/or family can no longer adapt or function at an adequate level. Individuals and families who reach maximum capacity are at risk for disability and dysfunction. In adaptation, the ability to adapt positively to change is indicative of health. Illness occurs when the individual cannot adapt or adapts in ways that are unhealthy (for example, by smoking or using drugs).

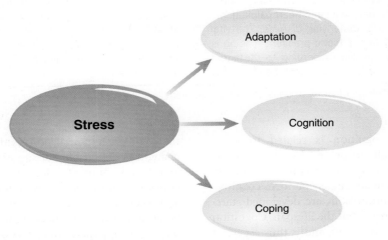

FIGURE 27-3 Stress and Interrelated Concepts.

MODEL CASE

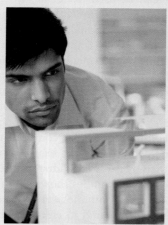

Jufar Hai is a 21-year-old male and a second-generation American whose grandparents and parents were immigrants from the Middle East. Neither of his grandparents spoke English. His father learned English as a teenager. Jufar is currently attending a state college; his parents pay for his tuition and Jufar pays for his books and room and board.

Jufar started smoking at age 14 because it was culturally acceptable. He finds smoking helps to relieve stress and makes him feel relaxed. He eats a lot of fast food because it is cheap and he does not have time to cook for himself since he is also working two part-time jobs. Jufar says his goal is to get an advanced degree in a science field and take care of his parents and grandparents. He also hopes to own his own home in the next 5 years and has a separate savings account for this purpose. He follows the religious practices of Islam and views himself as a practicing Muslim.

Assessing and Managing the Problem

Jufar presents to the student health clinic with a chief complaint of "stomach pains and a pounding heart." He has health insurance through his employer. Jufar has no chronic conditions and takes no medications. He states that he visits a physician only when he is ill.

The nurse practitioner conducts a comprehensive history and assessment. While conducting the history, she learns that Jufar was told by his parents 3 weeks ago that they expect him to marry his father's best friend's daughter, whom he has never met. Jufar feels anxious about this because the girl is from a prominent family in the Muslim community. He states: "I cannot stand all of this pressure anymore and feel stressed out all of the time. I feel like I have a huge weight on my shoulders to meet everyone's expectations. I am having trouble eating, my stomach hurts and I am nauseous. I am not sleeping well either." Although Jufar's most prominent physical symptoms were stomach pain and heart palpitations, the nurse finds no evidence of underlying disease. The vital signs are all normal except Jufar's blood pressure reading is slightly elevated at 128/80 mm Hg. According to the latest practice guidelines, this blood pressure measurement may place Jufar at risk for pre-hypertension, which requires lifestyle intervention.

There is information to support further assessment to determine behavioral risk factors including stress in Jufar's life, which may account for the symptoms. The *Holmes Life Events Scale* and *The Ways of Coping Checklist, Revised,* reveal many life events and a score that places Jufar at risk for disease. Jufar uses several negative coping skills, including smoking, avoidance, and risk-taking behavior. On the 0 to 10 scale, Jufar scores 8.

When Jufar states that he smokes in order to relax, the nurse asks Jufar if he wants to quit in the next 30 days. He states he is too stressed at this time to take on another task in his life but will think about it. Jufar is taught by the nurse to use progressive muscle relaxation, music, and daily exercise for managing his stress. The nurse tells Jufar that she will check the blood pressure measurement the next time he comes to the clinic but that she would like him monitor his blood pressure at home and shows him how to use an automatic cuff. He is given a referral for health education classes for stress management, a brochure about quitting smoking, and a community center phone number that conducts smoking cessation classes and counseling.

Case Analysis

Jufar has multiple demands in his life and it is clear that he has reached his capacity for meeting them. To gain more information the nurse administered a stress rating tool. The nurse recognized some of the defining characteristics of stress overload in this case. Jufar's self-rating of stress was high. The nurse recognized many stress symptoms that were of concern: physical (heart palpitations, stomach pain), psychologic (anxiety), and behavioral (not eating and sleeping well, using smoking to relax). The nurse concluded that Jafar had stress overload and taught him some basic stress management techniques to manage acute symptoms and also instituted a referral for counseling for smoking cessation, crisis intervention, emotional support, and family and support system enhancement. He was scheduled for a follow-up visit in 3 months. His blood pressure was to be monitored at home and he was to be closely watched for the next few months to see if his blood pressure decreased to normal levels. If he is unable to reduce his stress level or slightly high blood pressure, and if his heart palpitations and stomach pain return, a comprehensive lifestyle management plan would be started and medications may also be prescribed. Depending on the findings, referrals for professional counseling from a psychologist could also be implemented.

Cognition. Functional cognition is related to stress because it is the mental faculty or process by which knowledge is acquired and gained through perception, reasoning, and intuition and is needed to adequately perform cognitive appraisal of an event. Cognition skills are developed starting at birth and continue throughout the lifespan. Cognition is essential for information processing and is thus a part of the mediation of reactions. Cognition is a functional part of the cognitive appraisal process that reflects the unique and changing relationships taking place between the individual and the environment. Adequate cognition and cognitive processes that are intact allow cognitive appraisal, reappraisal, and secondary appraisal. Cognitive appraisal is only able to be accomplished if a person can think and process information. Reappraisal (the process of sorting out the impact of newly acquired information) and secondary appraisal

BOX 27-1   EXEMPLARS OF STRESS

Physiologic
Acute, Life-Threatening Conditions
- Acute renal failure
- Myocardial infarction
- Respiratory failure
- Sepsis
- Trauma
- Acute pain

Chronic, debilitating disease
- Cancer
- Chronic obstructive pulmonary disease
- Chronic kidney disease
- Dementia
- Diabetes
- Heart failure
- Liver failure
- Obesity
- Chronic pain

Psychologic/Emotional
- Death/end of life (of family member, close friend, or pet)
- Divorce
- Loss of job
- Loss of home
- Change in personal finances

Behavioral
- Alcohol addiction
- Drug addiction
- Gambling addiction
- Substance abuse
- Tobacco addiction

(a judgment of what might be done) also require intact cognition. In the conceptualization of stress, fully functional cognition is required for the full realm of cognitive appraisal to occur and is thus important to formulating meaning of events and responses.

Coping. Coping is also a related concept in stress. It is typically associated with success at adaptation and is usually a process rather than an outcome.[1] In the Figure 27-1 framework, coping is seen as a determinant of magnitude of response. If there is effective coping, the outcome is health and well-being. Coping, like stress, can be measured but many times is presumed to be present when an individual and family are healthy and functional. A closely related concept to stress and coping is vulnerability. Vulnerability is conceptualized as the degree of coping resources. Higher coping resources and ability to use them is associated with decreased vulnerability. Ineffective coping is defined as the inability to form a valid appraisal of stress, to make adequate choices of practice responses, and to use available resources.[19,27] The defining characteristics of ineffective coping are abuse of chemicals, change in communication patterns, decreased use of social support, destructive behavior, fatigue, high illness rate, inability to meet basic needs and role expectations, inadequate problem solving, lack of goals, inability to attend to information, poor concentration, risk-taking behavior, sleep disturbances, maladaptive coping style, and inability to cope.[19]

EXEMPLARS

Clinical examples of physical, psychologic, emotional, and behavioral demands and events that lead to the stress response are shown in Box 27-1. Nurses should note that not everything a person experiences leads to a threat and stress response that impacts health. Health is impacted when a person relates to the demand or event in a certain way and feels threatened. These individuals are most vulnerable because of poor coping ability and lack of resources. The examples in the box are events that formulate a perception of demand, and when events exceed coping abilities, reactions are initiated that disturb cognition, emotions, and behaviors to an extent that adversely affect well-being. An additional factor to consider is the severity and duration of events/demands and whether they are acute or chronic. Also a very high number of demands or events for which one is ill-prepared that occur over a short time can be perceived as threatening, adversely affecting well-being.

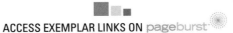

ACCESS EXEMPLAR LINKS ON pageburst

REFERENCES

1. Lazarus RS, Folkman S: *Stress, appraisal and coping*, New York, 1984, Springer.
2. Selye H: The general adaptation syndrome and the diseases of adaptation, *J Clin Endocrinol Metab* 6:117, 1946.
3. Holmes TH, Rahe RH: Social readjustment rating scale, *J Psychosomat Res* 11:213–218, 1967.
4. Lazarus RS, Lazarus BN: *Passion and reason: making sense of our emotions*, New York, 1994, Oxford University Press.
5. Mitchell P, Buchanan L: Physiologic adaptations during psychoemotional stress. In Underhill S, et al editors: *Cardiac nursing*, ed 2, Philadelphia, 1989, Lippincott Williams & Wilkins, p 165.
6. Forshee BA, Clayton MF, McCance KL: Stress and disease. In McCance K, Huether S, Brashers V, et al editors: *Pathophysiology: the biologic basis for disease in adults and children*, ed 6, St Louis, 2010, Mosby, p 336.
7. Selye H: Stress syndrome, *Am J Nurs* 65(3):97–99, 1965.
8. Selye H: Confusion and controversy in the stress field, *J Human Stress* 1:37–44, 1975.
9. Accessed at www.cdc.gov/niosh/docs/99-101.
10. Accessed at www.healthypeople.gov/2020/topicsobjectives2020/overview.aspx?topicid=28.

11. Kiecolt-Glaser J, et al: Chronic stress and immune function in family caregivers of Alzheimers disease victims, *Psychosomat Med* 45(5):523, 1987.

12. Antoni MH: The influence of biobehavioral factors on tumor biology: pathways and mechanisms, *Nat Rev Cancer* 6(3):240–248, 2006.

13. Sher L: Effects of psychological factors on the development of cardiovascular pathology role of the immune system and infection, *Med Hypotheses* 53(2):112–113, 1999.

14. Sweller J, van Merrienboer J, Paas F: Cognitive architecture and instructional design, *Educ Psychol Rev* 10(3):251–296, 1998.

15. Miller GA: The magical number seven, plus or minus two: some limits on our capacity for processing information, *Psychol Rev* 63:81–97, 1956.

16. Miller R: The aging immune system. Primer and perspective, *Science* 273:70–74, 1996.

17. McCance K, Huether S, Brashers V, et al: *Pathophysiology: the biologic basis for disease in adults and children*, ed 6, St Louis, 2010, Mosby.

18. Sharma R, Coats AJ, Anker SD: The role of inflammatory mediators in chronic heart failure: cytokines, nitric oxide, and endothelin A, *Int J Cardiol* 72(2):175–186, 2000.

19. Ackley BJ, Ladwig GB: *Nursing diagnosis handbook. An evidence-based guide to planning care*, ed 8, St Louis, 2006, Mosby/Elsevier.

20. Murray RB, Zentner JP, Yakimo R: Health promotion concepts and theories. In Beckmann Murray R, et al editors: *Health promotion strategies through the lifespan*, Upper Saddle River, NJ, 2009, Pearson Education, p 42.

21. Goroll AH, Berenson RA, Schoenbaum SC, et al: Fundamental reform of payment of adult primary care: comprehensive payment for comprehensive care, *J Gen Int Med* 22(3):410–415, 2007. doi: 10.1007/s11606-006-0083-2. PMID 17356977.

22. Greiner P, Edelman CL: Health defined: objectives for promotion and prevention. In Edelman CL, Mandle C, editors: *Health promotion throughout the life span*, ed 6, St Louis, 2006, Mosby/Elsevier.

23. Caplan RP: Stress, anxiety, and depression in hospital consultants, general practitioners, and senior health service managers, *BMJ* 309(6964):1261–1264, 1994.

24. Carrington P, Collings GH Jr, Benson H, et al: The use of meditation-relaxation techniques for the management of stress in a working population, *J Occup Med* 22(4):221–231, 1980.

25. Sims J: The evaluation of stress management strategies in general practice: an evidence led approach, *Br J Gen Pract* (422)577–581, 1997.

26. Bruning NS, Frew DR: Effects of exercise, relaxation, and management skills training on physiological stress indicators: a field experiment, *J Appl Psychol* 72(4):515–521, 1987.

27. Pearlin LI, Schooler C: The structure of coping, *J Health Soc Behav* 19(1):2–21, 1978.

28. Karch AM: *Focus on nursing pharmacology*, ed 5, Philadelphia, 2011, Wolters Kluwer/Lippincott Williams & Wilkins, pp 299–512.

29. Fiore MC, Jaen CR, Baker TB, et al: Treating tobacco use and dependence: 2008 update, *Clinical practice guideline*, Rockville, Md, May 2008, U.S. Department of Health and Human Services, U.S. Public Health Service.

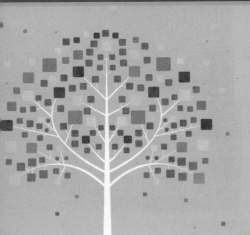

Coping

Jean Giddens and Kelley Edds

When an individual experiences physiologic or psychologic stress, a response is needed to adapt or modify the impact of the stressor. Considering the large number and variety of stressors humans experience throughout the lifespan, it is clear that a wide variety of responses occur; some responses are helpful and some are not. Coping is a multifaceted concept involving human cognition, individual perception, and behavior. In nursing, understanding the concept of coping as a relationship between the person and environment is an important component of care delivery.

DEFINITION(S)

The definition of coping in nursing has not yet reached a consensus. Research in the area of coping has studied this concept from a number of perspectives. One of the classic definitions of coping is from Lazarus and Folkman[1] and is described as *an ever changing process involving both cognitive means and behavioral actions, in order to manage internal or external situations that are perceived as difficult and/or beyond the individual's current resources.* This definition encompasses the relationship of the person and the environment. When the internal or external demands of the environment surpass current resources, the individual will attempt to maintain equilibrium by utilizing coping strategies. Ray and colleagues[2] defined coping as *being action oriented toward a goal of changing a situation;* in other words, the conscious or unconscious behaviors of an individual to avoid harm and restore balance. Keil further defines coping as *abstract thoughts based on past experiences to reduce stress.*[3]

It is apparent from the varying definitions that coping represents continual changes in behavior and cognition, in order to modify or adapt the person-environmental relationship to reduce stress. This adaptation or modification is behavior driven and can be conscious or unconscious.

Coping is based on individual perception, relationship to the environment, and evaluation of the environment as well as availability of resources. Furthermore, an individual's control over internal and external demands has an impact on coping and change.

SCOPE AND CATEGORIES

Scope

The scope of coping as a concept ranges from effective (or adaptive) coping responses to ineffective (or maladaptive) coping responses that result from constructive or destructive coping mechanisms (Figure 28-1). Coping mechanisms are stress management efforts. Constructive mechanisms occur when an individual treats the stressor as a warning and elects to resolve the problem.[4] Destructive mechanisms occur when an individual addresses the anxiety or the feeling associated with the stressor without resolving the problem—this is also seen as evasion. This continuum is not necessarily one or the other; some coping strategies may be partially effective or partially ineffective. Ineffective coping refers to the inability to assess the stressor and/or respond appropriately. When coping is ineffective, many problems can result, depending on the seriousness of the stressor event.

The scope of coping is also viewed from the perspective of an individual, family, or community. Individual coping links to the coping capacity of an individual/patient. Family coping refers the coping ability of family members when faced with challenges with one or more family members. On a community level, coping refers to the adaptive patterns and problem-solving capacity of a community when faced with challenges.[5] This concept analysis will focus primarily on individual coping.

Categories

Coping can be divided into two main categories: problem-focused and emotion-focused coping. Problem-focused

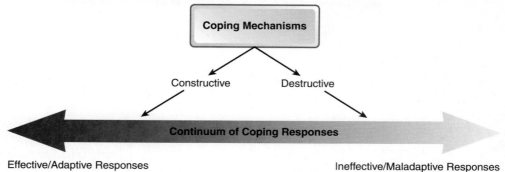

FIGURE 28-1 Scope of Coping.

coping involves the cognitive process of evaluating the situation and taking an action to manage the situation. Problem-focused coping can be carried out as aggressive efforts or rational efforts to change the situation or stressor.[6] Emotion-focused coping is more indirect and emphasizes regulation of the emotional response that occurs in a given situation. Forms of emotion-focused coping can include isolation or withdrawal from seeking social support or it can involve use of drugs or alcohol as a means to escape the threat.[6] Research has shown that although both problem-focused coping and emotion-focused coping occur together, strategies that incorporate problem-focused coping strategies are much more effective.[3] Inherent in these categories is the assumption that the individual is able to cognitively appraise the situation and current resources and decide on a course of action that will produce change.[6,7] It is important to note that types of coping can change depending on the perceived outcomes of the stressor and the perceived availability of resources.[6] For example, when a role is threatened, the individual utilizes more of a problem-focused direct coping plan to relieve or eliminate the stressor.

RISK FACTORS

All individuals use a variety of coping mechanism throughout life regardless of age, race, or gender. Although most individuals have effective coping mechanisms, there are risk factors associated with ineffective coping capacity. These depend on how the individual perceives the stressful event and the ability to identify and use resources. Any perceived threat to self or a loved one's well-being can be judged not only as a stressor but also as a situation in which one has little control. The ability to determine what resources are available and how those resources can be utilized is essential for coping. Therefore risk factors for poor coping link to one or more of the following:

- Inability to accurately assess the stressor
- Denial or avoidance of the stressor
- An actual or perceived lack of control over the situation
- An actual or perceived lack of support
- No experience or poor past experiences handling stressful situations

Impaired Cognition

Limited cognitive functioning is a key risk factor for poor coping. How well an individual appraises the stressful event(s) and utilizes available resources is central to positive outcomes. Individuals with poor cognition may also have limited experience managing stressful events, and thus may not take any action—either purposefully or as a form of denial.[8]

Limited Psychosocial Resources

Most researchers agree that personality variables impact the perception of the stressor or stressful event, although there is controversy as to how personality plays a role in coping.[9,10] Individuals who have poor self-esteem or those who feel depressed and lack motivation to respond to stressors are at risk for poor coping. Hardiness is the individual's sense of control over the stressful events, coupled with a commitment and challenge toward life events. Individuals who have a high degree of hardiness or resilience are generally better able to cope than those who have poor self-esteem.[11] Those with limited physical or financial resources are also at greater risk for poor coping because they may be less able to access appropriate interventions.

Age
Children

Research on children's perception of stressful events is based upon age and developmental stages as well as the child's level of self-efficacy and self-control.[12] Self-efficacy and self-control are challenged by chaos and loss of autonomy.[13] Harsh experiences in childhood, including dysfunctional family dynamics, can lead to poor coping skills later in life. Studies have reported that younger children who are unexpectedly admitted to the hospital are usually at higher risk for poor coping. Also, children whose parents experience extreme amounts of stress also have shown result in poor coping behaviors.[14]

Adolescents

There is a well-established relationship between adolescent coping and high-risk behaviors. Adolescents who have poor or insufficient coping are at risk for drug use, high-risk sexual behaviors, psychologic distress, and suicide. It is assumed that improving adolescent coping skills will result in changes in perception and reaction to stressors in different, more positive ways.[15] There has actually been relatively little research related to the measurement of coping among adolescents; therefore this is an area that requires additional exploration to further understand this concept.[15]

Older Adults

Older adults have unique risks for impaired coping compared to other age groups. Although they may have some advantage in coping experiences, many older adults may lack social supports or resources, may have less resilience because of health conditions, and may suffer from altered perceptions of stress events, particularly if cognitive function is impaired. There is a tendency for older adults with Alzheimer's disease to select escape mechanisms and emotional strategies as opposed to actually solving the underlying problem.[16] This underscores the importance of cognitive skills for adequate coping.

Changes in Health or Chronic Health Conditions

Individuals confronted with serious health issues are also vulnerable to poor coping styles. Franks and Roesch reported that individuals in a chronic state of disease who view their disease in a positive manner were more likely to use coping strategies.[17] However, individuals who viewed their disease negatively engaged in denial. Roesch and Weiner also reported that individuals who perceived their disease as uncontrollable were prone to denial and avoidance.[18]

EXPECTED COPING RESPONSES AND CONSEQUENCES

Responding to a Stressor

Effective coping involves two phases: primary appraisal and secondary appraisal. *Primary appraisal* is the initial assessment of the stressor to determine if the stressor is to be considered a threat. The individual evaluates the potential for harm to self or to a loved one's well-being, self-esteem, or personal values and may determine how much personal control can be exercised over the situation. The second phase of coping is *secondary appraisal*. Here, the individual evaluates the resources available to overcome, eliminate, or reduce the stressor.

It should be obvious then, that primary and secondary appraisal requires cognitive skill so that the stressor is accurately assessed and appropriate resources are identified. However, even with full cognitive capacity there can be wide variability in *how a stressor is perceived* and the *access, recognition, and application* of appropriate resources.

Multiple variables influence perspectives for primary and secondary appraisals. Key elements include level of education, past life experiences, current coping style, values, expectations, beliefs, self-efficacy, and worldviews. An individual's world is heavily influenced by his or her culture. A situation itself may or may not be perceived as stressful, depending upon one's culture, and the response to an event is often culturally based—such as religious beliefs, social values, beliefs concerning the meaning or purpose an event, and the individual's beliefs concerning his or her own purpose in life.

Cultural beliefs such as shame, discrimination, gender constraints, help-seeking activities, and stigma may affect how the individual copes in a situation.[19,20]

Consequences of Poor Coping

Consequences of poor coping can result in multiple issues, particularly for the individual already in a stressful state. Specific consequences are difficult to describe because these are highly variable, depending on the type and number of stressors involved, the way the stressors are perceived, the length of time the stressor occurs, the type of coping mechanism (if any) implemented (and degree of effectiveness), and the resilience of the individual. In other words, two individuals faced with the same stressor often have very different outcomes because of the variables described. The consequences of poor coping can be physical, psychosocial, or both. Examples include a decline in physical health status; the development of mental health problems (such as depression and anxiety); a reduction in functional ability; a change in social status, financial status, or relationships; and alterations in family dynamics. The concept *stress* (Concept 27) details the physiologic and psychosocial consequences of unresolved stress.

The type of coping strategy or resource one uses can have an effect on the outcome. Maladaptive coping responses often lead to physical health problems. The use of alcohol or drugs to escape the stressor can lead to self-injury or long-term consequences such as addiction. Likewise, failure to adequately respond to a stressor can result in health consequences as a result of the stressor itself. An individual who uses avoidance or denial will have far less favorable outcomes associated with the stressful event.[6] Levine found that although denial in cardiac patients led to fewer hospital episodes they were also found to be less likely to follow discharge instructions, such as adding an exercise regimen. As a result these patients had more rehospitalizations 1 year following the cardiac event.[21] Avoidance, as a coping tool, can be somewhat useful in situations that are perceived as short term and uncontrollable.[22] However, avoiding the stressful event or feelings surrounding the stressful event can lead to increased emotional distress, longer recovery times, less effective problem solving, and maladaptive responses.

ASSESSMENT

Nurses learn about an individual's perceived stressors and coping responses through a detailed history and examination. It is important to remember that coping is a way to manage a stressor. The assessment of coping should be kept separate from the outcome of the stressors itself. The individual may use maladaptive coping strategies to deal with the stressor, but this may or may not impact the outcome. Furthermore, the individual's background and culture may affect how the individual copes. Nurses should focus on the efficacy of the coping strategy, as opposed to the final outcome of the given stressor, to be effective in helping the individual. This information will guide the nurse in how to proceed with improving the individual's coping ability.

History

If an individual is experiencing a significant stressor, the history should provide data so the nurse can determine the individual's appraisal stage and determine coping strategies being used. Knowing if the individual has used or is using problem-based or emotional-based coping strategies is also important to determine.

Perception of Threat

The assessment of the individual and how he or she will cope with a stressor may be a very delicate matter, depending upon the given situation, the perceived threat, and the amount of control the individual has over the stressor. The nurse needs to understand the individual's perception of the event. This may be accomplished by asking the question, "What is the meaning of this event for you?" Recall, that the meaning or perception is developed from several factors including past experiences, internal needs, external needs, ability to acknowledge the problem, cognitive ability, values, expectations, culture, social supports, and perceived control over the situation. The nurse may want to also explore these areas with the individual in order to obtain a sense of how successfully the individual has coped in the past and if there are pertinent cultural beliefs that should be taken into consideration. This information will allow for the nurse to better understand the individual's coping ability as well as to aid the individual in finding more efficient ways to cope with the present stressor.

Past Coping Patterns

It is important to understand patterns of how the individual has coped in the past. Did this person turn to alcohol use or seek a support person for help? It is also helpful to gain insight into the strengths and/or weaknesses of the individual's coping patterns. Did the alcohol use help the person relax to better deal with the stressors or did the alcohol use become an additional problem? Did the person become withdrawn and isolative? Did the individual seek assistance from a support person? It is important to emphasize that the individual is to be the primary source of this information. No one else can describe that individual's comprehensive internal perception attached to the given stressor or the effectiveness of past coping strategies.

Medical and Social History

As part of the interview, the nurse will want to understand the stressor event in the context of the individual's current and past health and social history. The health history will help the nurse understand other health-related issues that can impact coping responses. Past social history may include questions concerning the individual's childhood caregivers, family history, and the family's coping strategies, as well as questions assessing how the individual navigated through difficult situations as a teenager. Relevant personal history also includes highest education level achieved, current and past occupations, social patterns, daily activities, sleeping patterns, eating patterns, and drug/alcohol use. The history also includes biographical data such as ethnicity, marital status and number of children, current living arrangements, and religious preference.

Examination

Observation of behavior is the key element associated with an examination of coping. This includes how the individual functions in the presence of the stressor and how the individual reacts when speaking of the stressor.[23] Because both primary and secondary appraisal require adequate cognitive functioning, a mental status assessment is essential. General observations such as personal appearance, grooming, facial expressions, and affect will aid the nurse in determining the extent to which the individual is reacting to the stressor, the individual's current cognitive ability, and the individual's current coping ability.[24] Assessment of the individual's thought process through conversation is essential. This information may reveal coexisting mental health concerns such as mood disorders, anxiety, or impaired thinking.

Evidence of poor coping behaviors includes anger, anxiousness, sadness, or hopelessness. Evidence of adequate coping behavior includes insight and engagement with the primary appraisal and the development of a coping plan. Willingness to use coping strategies or problem-solving techniques is also consistent with positive coping. For example, perhaps the individual makes a written list of the pros and cons of the situation, in order to determine if a threat actually exists, and then proceeds to make a list of support resources available to him/her.

The actual measurement of coping is very difficult because of the complexity of this concept. Many coping measurement instruments have been developed to quantify and measure coping. Several have been developed for specific age groups or situations. Box 28-1 presents examples of coping measurement instruments.

CLINICAL MANAGEMENT

The clinical management of coping can be very complex and challenging. The nurse is expected to understand that the construct of coping is very personal and involves both

---

BOX 28-1 COPING MEASUREMENT INSTRUMENTS

- The Miller Behavioral Style Scale
- The Mainz Coping Inventory
- The Billings and Moos Coping Measures
- The Ways of Coping Questionnaire (WCQ)
- The Coping Strategy Indicator (CSI)
- The Life Events and Coping Inventory (LECI) (children)
- The Adolescent Coping Orientation for Problem Experiences Inventory (A-COPE) (adolescents)
- The Life Situations Inventory (LSI) (middle and older adult)
- The Stress and Coping Process Questionnaire (SCPQ)
- The Coping Inventory for Stressful Situations (CISS)

internal and external needs. Once the nurse is aware of the individual's perception of the stressor, past coping experiences, and also perceived control and support, the nurse will be in a better position to guide the individual toward a positive coping experience.

Primary Prevention

Primary prevention strategies for coping are nonspecific and link to general strategies that optimize wellness. Maintaining good health and proper nutrition, exercising regularly, sustaining positive personal relationships and social support networks, and preserving positive self-esteem are all common mechanisms related to positive coping. Community-based support programs for situational stressors are described further in the Stress concept.

Collaborative Interventions

Clinical management of an individual with ineffective coping is directed toward the reduction of perceived threats and the reinforcement of perceived control over the stressor. Mentioned previously, there are two general types of coping patterns and strategies: problem-focused coping and emotion-focused coping.

Problem-focused coping strategies are most commonly applied when stressors can be modified, changed, or controlled. These are strategies that attempt to find solutions or improvements to the underlying stressor. Examples of problem-focused coping strategies are a newly diagnosed patient attending a patient education seminar to learn about optimal disease management or a caregiver gaining support through the access of community resources.

Emotion-focused coping strategies address the feelings one has as a result of the stressor. These strategies do not work toward a solution to the problem, but can help create a feeling of well-being; examples include performing physical activity to relieve stress associated with an overwhelming work schedule or attending a support group to discuss one's feelings.

In many cases a combination of problem-focused and emotion-focused coping strategies is utilized. It is important to emphasize that not all coping strategies are effective in all situations. Coping flexibility refers to the ability to change and adapt coping strategies over time based on changes in stressors and personal conditions.

Attempting to guide an individual towards enhanced coping abilities can be extremely challenging, because there are numerous variables to consider. Once those variables have been identified, the nurse can more efficiently help the patient choose a clinical management strategy that will best support the individual's needs. Specific strategies include education, planning, accessing resources, and cognitive restructuring.

Education

Education regarding the situation and alternative coping measures is a powerful tool to increase self-efficacy and control. The cancer patient who is educated about treatment alternatives and is given a choice of treatment will feel more in control of the situation. From here, the nurse can help the individual select emotion-focused coping strategies. When emotion-focused and problem-focused coping strategies are combined, there is a greater sense of positive coping.

Developing an Action Plan

Another way to increase control and self-efficacy is to develop an action plan or coping plan with the individual. The nurse can assist the patient to consider various coping methods in various situations and develop an individualized plan. For example, the nurse might help the cancer patient identify several relaxation techniques or perhaps create a list of activities to complete when he or she is feeling better. The nurse may also help the individual to develop a list of things to accomplish while undergoing treatment, such as reading a book or learning to use a computer program—something that is interesting but not physically taxing.

Accessing Resources

Another important strategy is to identify and access supportive resources that can help the individual. Such resources can range from a support group to a mentor, or to a clinical service. Resources may also be beneficial for the individual to discuss problem-solving concerns or decision-making ideas.

Cognitive Restructuring

Another potential strategy involves a cognitive restructuring of the stressor. Here the individual is encouraged to look at the stressor from other perspectives. This is referred to as positive reappraisal—that is, seeing the stressor from a more positive viewpoint.[8] When using this strategy, the nurse must understand and take into account the individual's worldview, which originates from the individual's values, beliefs, and culture. Positive appraisal has shown to increase the individual's strategies for coping, sense of control, and perception of the stressor.[25] This change in the perception of the stressor can lead to changes in emotions, as well as behaviors toward the stressor, and can increase the individual's ability to cope. For example, an individual suffering from panic attacks attributable to an upcoming surgery may be asked to identify what aspect of the surgery he or she finds upsetting. The perception is likely negative; as an example, a patient may fear not waking up from surgery. In this situation the nurse could provide education to the patient about the surgery and the strengths of the surgeon, as well as the success rate of the procedure. The nurse has added doubt to the perception of, "I won't wake up from the surgery." The individual can then begin to turn the negative thinking into a more positive pattern of thought. This increased understanding can provide the patient with a greater sense of control and a much more positive perception of the upcoming surgery.

INTERRELATED CONCEPTS

The concept of coping is multifaceted and involves links to several interrelated concepts featured in this textbook.

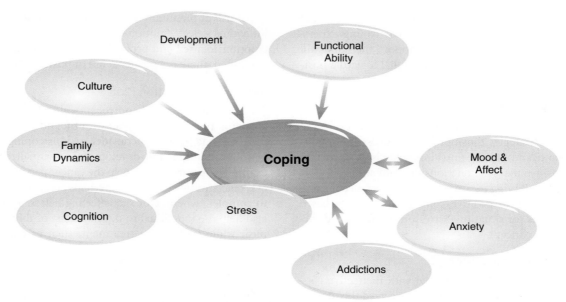

FIGURE 28-2 Coping and Interrelated Concepts.

MODEL CASE

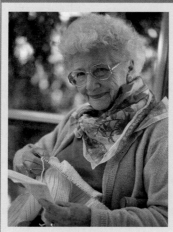

Mrs. Joyce Foster is a 68-year-old female who has recently undergone treatment for lung cancer. She became a widow 2 years ago following the sudden and unexpected death of her husband of 46 years. She has a close circle of friends in her quilting group and she has a very close relationship with her two sons and their families; these relationships have helped Joyce cope with her cancer diagnosis. A nurse at the cancer clinic has also provided Joyce with information about cancer treatment and ways to minimize the negative side effects of chemotherapy. Joyce looks forward to completing her treatments and getting on with life. She has set a goal to complete two quilts in the next 3 months to donate to a group children's home in her community.

Case Analysis

Mrs. Foster has a stressor (new diagnosis of cancer). Based on her actions she is practicing problem-focused and emotional-focused coping strategies that seem to be successful. She has accurately interpreted the threat, as evidenced by compliance with therapy, and she is using available resources to cope with the stressor. There is evidence that she has good coping abilities.

Stress is highly interrelated because coping is a stress response—coping either is a positive response or is a cause of stress if it is maladaptive. Although stress is usually viewed as a negative event, it can also be perceived as a positive attribute with individual control. The terms stress and coping can be viewed as having an equal, but different effect upon an individual. Stress can be viewed as a situation requiring coping or it can result from negative coping methods. Thus coping is how the individual views and addresses the stressor.

A second obvious interrelated concept is the health and illness concept **Cognition.** Adequate cognitive skills are essential for primary and secondary appraisal. Individuals with poor appraisal capabilities may fail to recognize or accurately perceive situations requiring attention, thereby exacerbating the situation. Additional concepts also impact one's appraisal, including the attribute concepts **Culture** and **Development. Functional ability** and **Family dynamics** are additional concepts that link to coping strategies and can also be a reason for poor coping. The concepts **Addiction, Anxiety,** and **Mood and affect** are interrelated because they can result from maladaptive coping, and they can also escalate poor coping strategies. These interrelated concepts are presented in Figure 28-2.

EXEMPLARS

As mentioned previously, coping ranges in scope from positive to maladaptive responses. There are many examples of positive coping behaviors and many examples of maladaptive behaviors. Although it is beyond the scope of this concept to list all examples, Box 28-2 presents common examples of

CONTRARY CASE

Carlie Wendell is a 10-year-old female who has recently been diagnosed with diabetes. She has no history of any major illnesses. Carlie lives with her single mother and four younger siblings in a small apartment. Her mother is unemployed and the family has very limited resources. When the nurse meets with Carlie and her mother, Carlie is crying. She has been told by her mother that she is sick because she eats too much candy and that she will have to have shots every day. The nurse observes that Carlie is angry, isolative, and tearful. Carlie's mother is present, but not engaged in the discussion. She tells the nurse she can't afford the medications needed to take care of Carlie's problem.

Case Analysis

Like the model case, the patient is upset with the diagnosis. However, this case reveals the patient's coping ability to be negative. Her primary appraisal is that the disease is a threat. However, unlike the model case, this patient's secondary appraisal reflects that she has fewer resources available. This child lacks an understanding of her condition and does not have the capacity to draw on coping resources. The mother may lack an understanding of access to resources that may help Carlie.

BOX 28-2 EXEMPLARS OF COPING

Exemplars of Positive Coping Behaviors
- Art therapy
- Counseling
- Diversional activities
  - Reading
  - Games
  - Television
  - Movies
  - Outings
- Education classes
- Imagery
- Journaling
- Massage
- Meditation
- Music therapy
- Physical activity
- Relaxation techniques
- Therapeutic communication
  - Active listening
  - Empathy
- Spiritual resources
- Social interactions
  - Family
  - Friends
  - Support groups

Exemplars of Maladaptive Coping Behaviors
- Alcohol abuse
- Anxiety
- Bullying
- Denial
- Dependency
- Developmental delay
- Drug abuse
- Emotional outbursts
- Excessive eating
- Impaired functional status
- Nonadherence to treatment plan
- Social isolation/withdrawal
- Violence towards others
- Violence towards self (suicide)

---

both types of responses. Positive coping strategies represent both cognitive and emotional responses.

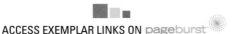

ACCESS EXEMPLAR LINKS ON pageburst

REFERENCES

1. Lazarus RS, Folkman S: *Stress, appraisal, and coping,* New York, 1984, Springer.
2. Ray C, Lindop J, Gibson S: The concept of coping, *Psychol Med* 12(2):385–395, 1982.
3. Keil RMK: Coping and stress: a conceptual analysis, *J Adv Nurs* 45(6):659–665, 2004.
4. Stuart G: Stuart stress adaptation model of psychiatric nursing care. In Stuart GW, editor: *Principles and practice of psychiatric nursing,* ed 9, St Louis, 2009, Elsevier/Mosby.
5. Ackley BJ, Ladwig GB: *Nursing diagnosis handbook: an evidence-based guide to planning care,* ed 8, St Louis, 2006, Mosby/Elsevier.
6. Folkman S, Lazarus R, Dunkel-Schetter C, et al: Dynamics of a stressful encounter: cognitive appraisal, coping, and encounter outcomes, *J Personality Soc Psychol* 50(5):992–1003, 1986.
7. Clarke M: Stress and coping: constructs for nursing, *J Adv Nurs* 9(1):3–13, 1984.
8. Folkman S, Moskowitz J: Coping: pitfalls and promise, *Psychology* 55(1):745, 2004.
9. Heth J, Somer E: Characterising stress tolerance: controllability awareness and its relationship to perceived stress and reported health, *Personality Individ Diff* 33:883–895, 2002.
10. Tyson P, Pongruengphant R, Aggarwal B: Coping with organizational stress among hospital nurses in Southern Ontario, *Int J Nurs Stud* 39(4):453–459, 2002.
11. Taylor S, Stanton A: Coping resources, coping processes, and mental health, *Clin Psychol* 3(1):377, 2007.

12. Zeitlin S, Williamson G: *Coping in young children: early intervention practices to enhance adaptive behavior and resilience,* Baltimore, Md, 1994, Paul H. Brookes Publishing.

13. Skinner E, Wellborn J: Children's coping in the academic domain, *Int J Behav Dev* 13:157–176, 1997.

14. Small L: Early predictors of poor coping outcomes in children following intensive care hospitalization and stressful medical encounters, *Pediatr Nurs* 28(4):393–401, 2002.

15. Garcia C: Conceptualization and measurement of coping during adolescence: a review of the literature, *J Nurs Schol* 42(2):166–185, 2010.

16. Nery de Souza-Talarioc J, Correâ Chaves E, Nitrini R, et al: Stress and coping in older people with Alzheimer's disease, *J Clin Nurs* 18:457–465, 2008.

17. Franks H, Roesch S: Appraisals and coping in people living with cancer: a meta-analysis, *Psycho-oncol* 15(12):1027–1037, 2006.

18. Roesch S, Weiner B: A meta-analytic review of coping with illness: do causal attributions matter? *J Psychosomat Res* 50(4):205–219, 2001.

19. Boss P: *Loss, trauma, and resilience: therapeutic work with ambiguous loss,* New York, 2006, WW Norton & Co.

20. Norris F, Alegria M: Mental health care for ethnic minority individuals and communities in the aftermath of disasters and mass violence, *CNS Spectrums* 10(2):132–140, 2005.

21. Levine J, Warrenburg S, Kerns R, et al: The role of denial in recovery from coronary heart disease, *Psychosomat Med* 49(2):109, 1987.

22. Suls J, Fletcher B: The relative efficacy of avoidant and non-avoidant coping strategies: a meta-analysis, *Health Psychol* 4(3):249–288, 1985.

23. Edelman C, Mandle C: *Health promotion throughout the life span,* St Louis, 2010, Mosby/Elsevier.

24. Folkman S, Moskowitz J: Positive affect and the other side of coping, *Am Psychol* 55(6):647, 2000.

25. Moskowitz J, Folkman S, Collette L, et al: Coping and mood during AIDS-related caregiving and bereavement, *Ann Behav Med* 18(1):49–57, 1996.

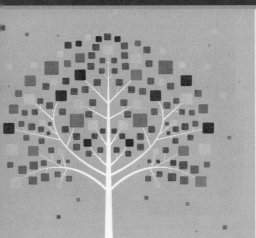

Mood and Affect

Robert Elgie

Mood and affect is a psychosocial concept that underlies all other concepts in the significant impact it has on health outcomes. The purpose of this concept analysis is to enable the generalist practice nurse to recognize the signs and symptoms of affective instability so that these patients can be managed safely and referred to advanced practitioners for evaluation and treatment of any possible mood spectrum disorders.

DEFINITION(S)

The term *mood* is defined as the way a person feels, and the term *affect* is defined as the observable response a person has to his or her own feelings.[1] The *mood spectrum* is a continuum, or spectrum, of all possible moods that any person may experience. *Mood spectrum disorders* disrupt the individual's ability to function normally and individuals with mood spectrum disorders are at increased risk for many problems such as health status impairment, addiction, and potential for violence.[2] Mood spectrum disorders must be diagnosed by physicians or other qualified advanced practitioners trained in making medical/psychiatric diagnoses; that is to say the diagnosis of mood spectrum disorders is not within the scope of practice of the generalist nurse.

However, because mood is a subjective experience and affect is an objective reflection of mood, the evaluation of mood is often done in terms of affect, and generalist practice nurses are qualified and expected to assess affect. In particular, nurses must be able to recognize unstable affective states known as *affective instability*. Signs of affective instability, such as crying, rage, euphoria, and blunting, indicate the need for further assessment because such individuals may have a mood disorder;[3] this important nurse responsibility will be discussed in more detail in the Assessment section of this concept analysis.

Several additional terms form a foundation for understanding this concept; the application of these terms will also be discussed in the Assessment. The term *euthymia* is used to describe normal, healthy fluctuations in mood. The term *functional status* describes the individual's ability to perform activities of daily living (ADLs) and to realistically solve problems of daily living.[4]

It is important for nurses to have a sufficient understanding of medical/psychiatric diagnostic models to facilitate collaborative care. For example, *depression* and *mania* are medical/psychiatric diagnostic terms used to indicate the extreme poles of the mood spectrum disorders.[5] Conceptually, *depression* is characterized by such overwhelming sadness and despair that one feels drained of energy. An individual suffering from *depression* may feel so sad and empty that he or she becomes incapacitated by a loss of the will to live and suicidal thoughts may prevail.

Caution should be exercised in the use of the word *depression* to avoid misunderstandings for a couple of reasons. First, the word *depression* is commonly misused to describe normal euthymic sadness when there is little or no loss of functional status. Second, *depression* is a medical/psychiatric diagnostic term and the clinical psychiatric use of the word *depression* has a variety of diagnostic applications. For clarity in this concept the undiagnosed mood state characterized by sadness, despair, and loss of functional status will be referred to as *melancholy*.

The term *mania* is used as a defining characteristic of some medical/psychiatric bipolar diagnoses that nurses are not qualified to make; however, like recognizing affective instability, nurses are qualified and expected to recognize *mania*. Individuals with *mania* are recognizable in the nursing paradigm by the presence of euphoric or agitated affective states, and they often suffer from varying degrees of *perceptual disturbances* (hallucinations) as well. Racing thoughts, grandiose delusions, difficulty concentrating, impulsivity, and lack of insight are not uncommon. Consequently, individuals with mania experience impaired functional status, and behavior associated with mania may be reckless and dangerous.

Another term used as a defining characteristic for some medical/psychiatric diagnoses is the term *hypomania*. Nurses are expected to be able to recognize *hypomania* as an affective state. *Hypomanic* affective states are expansive or agitated and possibly euphoric, but to a less severe degree than in *mania* and with less impairment. Although the individual with *hypomania* experiences racing thoughts and agitation or euphoria, perceptual disturbances are much less likely in *hypomania*. To facilitate the assessment of affective instability in the generalist nurse conceptual paradigm, the presence of perceptual disturbances will be used to distinguish *mania* from *hypomania* in this analysis.

SCOPE AND CATEGORIES

There is considerable evidence to support a conceptual model of mood and affect in a single spectrum of possible affective states.[3,6-8] The left sidebar of Figure 29-1 illustrates the full range of this spectrum from extreme melancholy to extreme mania in language consistent with the current generalist nurse paradigm and scope of practice to be used in this analysis. The narrow band of euthymia is located in the middle of the spectrum and in Figure 29-1 the green curve illustrates normal euthymic mood cycling. The amplitude and frequency of euthymic mood cycles may be normally regular or irregular and vary from one person to another.

Conceptually, mood spectrum disorders occur when the mood cycles downward from the euthymic range into affective states seen as melancholy, or when the mood cycles upward from the euthymic range into hypomania or severe mania. As the mood cycles further out of euthymia in either direction the functional status decreases proportionately. Initially, functional status may suffer from symptoms that are less severe, such as persistent tardiness attributable to oversleeping, or irritability and lethargy. Loss of appetite and interest in normal activities is common. In more extreme mood states such as mania or severe melancholy the individual may be completely disabled and experience symptoms of acute confusion such as hallucinations and/or delusions.

RISK FACTORS

As mentioned earlier in this concept, fluctuations within the euthymic range occur normally and even daily among all populations and across the lifespan. However, although anyone may experience mood spectrum disorders, there are known risk factors. The most recent, broad-based assessment of mood spectrum disorders in the United States was the National Comorbidity Survey Replication (NCS-R) study conducted from 2001 to 2003; this study was based on 9282 interviews.[9]

According to the NCS-R, the 12-month prevalence of clinically significant depression in the general population was

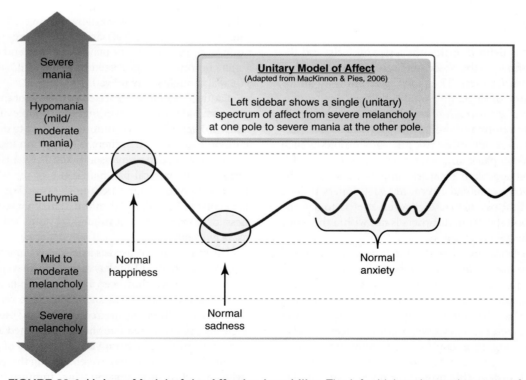

FIGURE 29-1 Unitary Model of the Affective Instability. The left sidebar shows the scope of affect in the generalist nurse paradigm from severe melancholy at one pole to severe mania at the other pole. The green line depicts normal mood as it cycles within the euthymic range from happiness to sadness and back to happiness. (Adapted from MacKinnon DF, Pies R: Affective instability as rapid cycling: theoretical and clinical implications for borderline personality and bipolar spectrum disorders, *Bipolar Disord* 8:1-14, 2006.)

6.6%, and the lifetime prevalence was 16.2%. Individual risk factors for depression are stress, early trauma, neglect, abuse, family history, comorbid medical and psychiatric disorders, and personality disorders. The rate of depression among women is two to three times higher than that in men and the first episode of depression for either gender usually occurs during adolescence or early adulthood. The incidence of depression peaks bimodally, occurring with the highest frequency during the late twenties/early thirties and again during the late sixties. Comorbid anxiety or substance-related disorders prevail in 75% to 80% of those with depression and 22% of adults report comorbid substance dependence.[10] Among those who reported no psychologic distress only 7% reported substance dependence.[10]

PHYSIOLOGIC PROCESSES AND CONSEQUENCES

Various neuroimaging studies of mood spectrum disorders demonstrate reduced blood flow and abnormal phosphorous metabolism in the cerebral cortex and especially the prefrontal cortex.[6] The activity of various neurotransmitters is also disturbed in mood spectrum disorders, particularly the levels of dopamine, norepinephrine, and serotonin. This is why medical interventions are aimed at restoring neurotransmitter balance.

Interpersonal relationships and productivity may be greatly limited by functional status impairment during mood spectrum disorders. Psychosocial variables such as negative life events, personality traits, and individual cognitive styles are associated with mood spectrum disorders.[6] There are a variety of psychotherapeutic approaches to addressing psychosocial variables that may cause or result from mood spectrum disorders; some of the more common approaches will be discussed in the Collaborative Care section of this concept.

Patients with mood spectrum disorders are high users of medical care and the incidence of mood spectrum disorders is increased in general medical care patients.[9] The most ominous consequence, of course, is the increased potential for suicide. Probably because of increased energy levels, patients on the manic or hypomanic pole of the mood spectrum are at a higher risk for suicide than those with low energy at the melancholic pole. Rates of suicidal ideation and attempts among individuals with manic and hypomanic mood states range between 35% and 50%.[11] A study of more than 25,000 patients found that patients with *undiagnosed* mania or hypomania were four times more likely to attempt suicide than those who were diagnosed.[12] This is an extremely important point that emphasizes recognition and exploration of affective instability with prompt referral to appropriate advanced practice services. It should be noted that energy and cognition in individuals at the melancholic pole may cycle unpredictably toward mania with a corresponding increase in risk for suicide attributable at least in part to the increase of energy and ability to plan. Clear data on the prevalence of shifting from melancholy toward mania are not available but for safety reasons nurses should be aware of this possibility and assess accordingly.

ASSESSMENT

Remembering that generalist practice nurses are not qualified to diagnose mood spectrum disorders, they should be able to recognize affective instability as an outward manifestation of a *possible* mood spectrum disorder. Affective instability may present as any combination of agitation, sadness, elation, or blunting. Blunting is particularly difficult to recognize because it may not by noticeable immediately; blunting is an absence or diminished presence of any affect and this should be considered a sign of affective instability. Speech may be monotone during blunting and responses may be unusually brief. Blunting must not be overlooked because it may mask dangerously unstable affect.

The combined interaction between mood, energy, and cognition results in what we call affect;[3] therefore the recognition of affective instability is facilitated by an analysis of mood, energy, and cognition. The defining characteristics for the mood and affect concept in this analysis are derived from the diverse presentations of affective instability that result from the various problematic ways that mood, energy, and cognition interact. The defining characteristics are (1) *persistent* mood disturbance, (2) functional impairment, and (3) disturbed vegetative functioning (sleep, appetite, and energy). To facilitate assessment, each of these characteristics will be discussed individually.

Persistent Mood Disturbance

To be clear, the assessment of mood by nurses does not mean the diagnosis of mood spectrum disorders, but rather the assessment of how the individual feels. Therefore the assessment of mood should be based on the patient's report. Occasionally, nurses will infer mood from affect but this can be misleading because affect is not always congruous with mood. For example, individuals may laugh and cry simultaneously. In any case, persistent mood disturbance may include sadness, melancholy, irritability, lack of interest in normal activities (anhedonia), euphoria, elation, rage, or the lack of any ability to feel emotions at all. Moods should fluctuate normally in the full range of euthymia, but moods should not fluctuate so rapidly or to such extremes or for so long that functional status is disrupted.

The important point that underlies this defining characteristic is the idea of persistence. Anyone will normally experience sadness, irritability, and even euphoria or rage occasionally. But daily, persistent melancholic feelings for longer than 2 weeks or persistent manic feelings for more than 4 days endorse a nursing assessment of persistent affective instability.[13] To illustrate useful reasoning in the recognition of persistent mania and hypomania by nurses, the fieldworkers who administered the face-to-face questionnaires during the NCS-R study were trained to ask the following:

Some people have periods lasting several days or longer when they feel much more excited and full of energy than usual. Their minds go too fast. They talk a lot. They are very restless or unable to sit still and they sometimes do things that are unusual for them, such as driving too fast or spending too much money. Have you ever had a period like this lasting several days or longer? …Or have you ever had a period lasting several days or longer when most of the time you were so irritable that you started arguments, shouted at people, or hit people?[14,p2]

Functional Impairment

A useful way to assess functional impairment is to think of it as the inability to realistically solve ordinary problems of daily living.[4] Functional status may also be known as *functional ability,* although *functional ability* refers more specifically to the *capacity* of an individual to perform ADLs whereas functional *status* refers to the individual's actual performance of the ADLs, which may not utilize his or her total functional capacity.[4] Functional impairment is closely linked to disturbed vegetative functioning.

Disturbed Vegetative Functioning

Vegetative functioning refers to the individual's appetite, sleep, and energy level. Some clinicians may evaluate sexual energy or changes in sexual desire (libido) as a separate measure of vegetative functioning. During a melancholic period the patient typically exhibits reduced energy level, increased sleep, decreased appetite, and decreased interest in sex. Atypically, individuals with melancholy may overeat, may become more sexual, or may be too agitated to sleep—this is known as mixed state depression in the medical/psychiatric paradigm.[15]

Mental Status Assessment

The mental status assessment is well within the nursing scope of practice and important in analyzing the defining characteristics for the mood and affect concept. In all areas of nursing, the ability to assess mental status efficiently and accurately is so important that it may be referred to as the sixth vital sign.[16] In the same way that a nurse should generally be aware of any patient's pulse rate and character, respiratory rate and character, blood pressure, temperature, and pain, the nurse should also know the following mental status items: *general appearance, motor activity, mood, affect, speech,* and *alertness and orientation.*

The assessment and continuous monitoring of mental status enables the nurse to accurately assess *cognitive status* and *functional status.* There are instruments such as the Mini-Mental State Exam, the Neecham Confusion Scale, or the Confusion Assessment Method Instrument and others that permit the nurse to quantifiably measure mental status for particular situations such as monitoring changes during or between shifts, day to day, or over the long term.[17] However, although these instruments can be very useful, they are not replacements for the *continuous* monitoring and documentation of the patient's mental status that makes it a sixth vital sign.

A complete discussion of the mental status examination is beyond the scope of this concept presentation, but sources are readily available that provide details of this part of the assessment. It is helpful to remember that the assessment of information processing lies at the heart of the mental status assessment. That is to say, assessing the patient's ability to process information is the purpose of the mental status assessment. Specifically, the patient's appearance; motor functioning; speech and speech content; cognitive processes such as perception, judgment, insight, and memory; alertness and orientation combine to form a clinical impression of the patient's total information processing ability, and thereby form a basis for clinical management.

CLINICAL MANAGEMENT

An effective and easy-to-remember way for nurses to translate data from the mental status assessment to clinical management is by analyzing it in the context of affect and the three main components of affect: (1) mood, (2) energy, and (3) cognition. Figure 29-2 illustrates these components and the normal cycling of euthymia into an unstable melancholy and then back into euthymia. Note that during the unstable period illustrated in Figure 29-2 the individual displays a melancholic mood (green line) with reduced energy (red line) but increased cognition (blue line). Behaviorally, this individual would struggle with persistent sadness and low energy but agitated thoughts that disturbed his or her sleep. For individuals with affective instability, one or more of the three affective components will cycle out of euthymia in either direction, causing a variety of behavioral responses. By studying Figure 29-2 one can picture different affective (behavioral) manifestations. What makes the assessment of disorders associated with affective instability so challenging is that each affective component may cycle at different rates and extremes. Different combinations of affective components will have quite different manifestations. Also, when components occur simultaneously at the extremes then the disabling effects are increased.

Primary Prevention

Primary prevention measures for mood spectrum disorders are not well established and efforts toward prevention focus on societal egalitarian interventions such as reduction in poverty, racism, violence, and stress.[2] According to systematic reviews,[2] programs that target prevention of mood disorders have been shown to reduce the severity of symptoms, but these programs tend to be early interventions rather than true prevention programs. Similar systematic reviews of universal prevention programs showed them to be ineffective.

Secondary Prevention (Screening)

Secondary prevention or screening efforts are aimed at early detection of mood spectrum disorders with hopes of preventing serious consequences, and there is compelling evidence to support mood disorder screening.[2] The U.S. Preventive Services Task Force (USPSTF) recommends the routine screening of adults for mood disorders in primary care.[18] The USPSTF further recommends that primary care

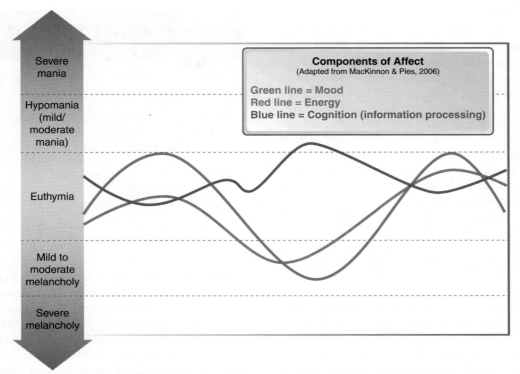

FIGURE 29-2 Components of Affect. Green line = mood; red line = energy; blue line = cognition. (Adapted from MacKinnon DF, Pies R: Affective instability as rapid cycling: theoretical and clinical implications for borderline personality and bipolar spectrum disorders, *Bipolar Disord* 8:1-14, 2006.)

physicians "remain alert"[19,p1001] for mood spectrum disorders in children and adolescents and that systems should be established to handle the diagnosis, treatment, and follow-up care for individuals who screen positive for mood spectrum disorders. According to the USPSTF, the following two questions may be as effective as longer screening measures: (1) "Over the past two weeks, have you ever felt down, depressed, or hopeless?" (2) "Have you felt little interest or pleasure in doing things?"[19,p1002]

Screening instruments do not diagnose mood spectrum disorders; instead they measure the severity of associated symptoms.[19] By measuring the severity of symptoms associated with mood spectrum disorders, screening instruments assist clinicians to assess acuity and treatment effectiveness. There are numerous screening instruments validated for use at different times in the lifespan and appropriate for varying levels of cognition.[19] Whatever instrument is used, it is important to realize that simple screening questions only detect about half of patients with mood spectrum disorders.[20] For this reason it is recommended that nurses do not completely rely on screening instruments, but use their assessment skills to detect affective instability followed by an assessment of functional status and potential for violence when indicated. It is noteworthy that diminished functional status may appear vaguely as somatic symptoms and vegetative complaints such as fatigue, sleep disturbance, pain, altered interest in sexual activity, or other persistent vague complaints.[19]

Collaborative Care

Individuals suffering from mood spectrum disorders are known to be lethargic in seeking treatment. Because the generalist nurse is quite likely to be the first clinician to detect the possibility of a mood spectrum disorder, it is imperative that the nurse is also able to discuss with the patient treatment options and reasonable expectations for treatment outcomes. In this way, the nurse may exert a substantial influence in convincing the patient to seek care. This influence is done most effectively with communication techniques called *motivational interviewing*.[21] Although additional training is helpful, motivational interviewing techniques lie within the generalist nurse scope of practice and the effectiveness of motivational interviewing for mood spectrum disorders and suicidal ideation has been established.[21] Motivational interviewing was first developed to motivate individuals suffering from addictions to pursue change, and so it will be further discussed in the addiction concept of this text (see the Addiction concept).

In addition to motivational interviewing, collaborative care for mood spectrum disorders consists of psychotherapy and/or pharmacotherapy and/or brain and vagus nerve stimulation therapies (e.g., electroconvulsive therapy [ECT]). Collaborative care also includes managing emergent situations (potential for suicide and/or other violence) among individuals suffering from affective instability. Each of these areas of interventions is discussed next. The nursing role in collaborative care may include case management activities when functional status impairment persists.

Psychotherapy Options

There are many different types of psychotherapy, and no particular therapy has been found to be more effective than any other.[22] Compared to pharmacotherapy, there are fewer well-designed clinical trials of psychotherapy "because of the lack of a 'placebo therapy' condition."[22,p6] However, there is sufficient evidence, including randomized controlled trials, to conclude that long-term outcomes of pharmacotherapy versus psychotherapy are similar.[22] Relapse rates appear to be lower in psychotherapy following termination of treatment.[23] Psychotherapy has been found to take about 8 weeks for a 50% remission rate, 26 weeks for a 75% remission rate, and 52 weeks for an 80% remission rate.[23]

Because a person's thoughts and beliefs have been found to affect mood, cognitive therapy attempts to change thoughts and beliefs as needed to be more adaptive and healthy. In comparison, behavioral therapy is aimed at changing patterns of behavior that are repeated over time with the same negative results. Cognitive and behavioral therapy is a combined approach that has been found to be effective in numerous applications that share the characteristic of repetitive dysfunctional patterns.[23] Interpersonal therapy focuses on communication patterns and the way the patient relates to others. Grief issues respond well to interpersonal therapy, and the patient is provided the opportunity to learn ways to express such uncomfortable feelings. Variations of this modality have been demonstrated to be effective in managing bipolar spectrum disorders.[23] Family-focused therapy includes family members in a therapeutic process aimed at problem solving and managing conflict in ways that produce positive outcomes. All these therapeutic approaches are known to adapt well to the treatment of mood disorders in children and adolescents.[23]

Play therapy is an approach for children in which toys and games are used to establish rapport so that the child may better express himself/herself. Toys and games may also be used for children who lack the cognitive abilities of expression. Sand tray therapy is a variant of play therapy wherein the child is encouraged to playfully make patterns in the sand. Other therapeutic modalities include light therapy, art therapy, and animal-assisted therapies, each with its own applications. Light therapy is used to treat seasonal affect disorder (SAD), a mood disorder that tends to occur during the winter months when there is less light. For some individuals, decreasing light is associated with melancholy. Animal therapies are often used in the recovery from psychologic trauma, and art therapies may help with psychologic self-healing.[23]

Pharmacotherapy for Mood Spectrum Disorders

The main drug categories used in the treatment of mood spectrum disorders are antidepressants and mood stabilizers; antianxiety agents (anxiolytics) are also used (Table 29-1). Generally speaking, antidepressants are prescribed to treat patients diagnosed with depression and mood stabilizers are used to treat diagnoses associated with mania and hypomania such as the various bipolar diagnoses.[5]

TABLE 29-1	PHARMACOTHERAPY FOR MOOD SPECTRUM DISORDERS	
ANTIDEPRESSANTS	**MOOD STABILIZERS**
Selective serotonin reuptake inhibitors (SSRIs)	Lithium
Serotonin-norepinephrine reuptake inhibitors (SNRIs)	Antiepileptic drugs (AEDs)
Tricyclic antidepressants (TCAs)	Second-generation antipsychotic medications
Norepinephrine-dopamine reuptake inhibiters (NDRIs)	
Monoamine oxidase inhibitors (MAOIs)	

Antidepressants. There are five subcategories of antidepressants: the selective serotonin reuptake inhibitors (SSRIs), the norepinephrine-dopamine reuptake inhibiters (NDRIs), the tricyclic antidepressants (TCAs), the serotonin-norepinephrine reuptake inhibitors (SNRIs), and the monoamine oxidase inhibitors (MAOIs). There are many factors affecting the choice of antidepressant medications, with remission or partial remission dependent on the particular neurochemical imbalance. The current first-line choice for the treatment of depression is the SSRI category because positive response rates are excellent and this category has the best rate of compliance as a result of its lower incidence of adverse effects.[22] SSRIs may be prescribed by primary care providers. If depression is complicated by anxiety, the anxiety may dissipate once the antidepressant medication takes effect, but this will take at least 3 weeks. During this period anxiety may temporarily be treated with an anxiolytic, but persistent agitation may be treated with a mood stabilizer. Individual responses to any pharmacotherapy are highly variable. To achieve a positive response the dose must often be increased after the initial 3 weeks; therefore it is not unusual for it to take 4 to 6 weeks to achieve a positive response.

The dual-action antidepressants known as SNRIs affect serotonin and norepinephrine levels, and these are also used in some cases of depression that do not respond to treatment, known as refractory depression.[22] For many years the TCA antidepressants were the standard choice in the treatment of depression and they are still used occasionally; however, because of their multiple adverse effects TCAs are rarely or never used as first-line choices.[22] Overdose of TCA medications is lethally dangerous, so compliance and risk for suicide must be carefully evaluated before initiating medications from this category.

The MAOI antidepressants have also been demonstrated to be effective in the treatment of refractory depression but they are never used as first-line treatment because of concerns about potentially fatal interactions (hypertensive crisis) between MAOI medications and foods containing tyramine. Tyramine occurs widely in foods, especially "spoiled" (fermented) or pickled foods. Foods to be avoided include many meats, chocolate, alcoholic beverages, cheese, tofu, beans, pineapples, plums, raspberries, figs, and nuts.

It is not unusual for patients to experience some mild side effects when SSRI medications are initiated or when the dosage is increased.[24] These side effects should subside within a couple of weeks and include insomnia, abdominal discomfort, and mild headaches. However, there is some potential for any antidepressant medication, including the safer SSRI category, to produce a dangerous condition known as *serotonin toxicity*.[24] Serotonin toxicity may occur abruptly, and initial presentation includes tachycardia, shivering, diaphoresis, dilated pupils, myoclonus (intermittent tremor or twitching), and hyperreflexia. Hyperthermia is common during serotonin toxicity, and temperatures may reach as dangerously high as 106° F (41° C). Serotonin toxicity is treated with serotonin blockade drugs such as chlorpromazine or cyproheptadine.

Patients should be instructed not to abruptly discontinue antidepressant medications, because this may result in anticholinergic rebound symptoms known as SSRI withdrawal syndrome (also known as SSRI discontinuation syndrome). In SSRI withdrawal syndrome the individual experiences flulike symptoms such as headache, diarrhea, nausea, vomiting, chills, dizziness, fatigue, insomnia, agitation, impaired concentration, and vivid dreams. Symptoms last from 1 to 7 weeks, and may be dangerous if there is an increased presence of suicidal ideation.

Mood stabilizers. The mood stabilizers are either lithium or antiepileptic drugs (AEDs); numerous antipsychotic medications also have been approved as mood stabilizers. Lithium and antiepileptic drugs (AEDs) have been the two main types of pharmacologic agents used as mood stabilizers for many years, and in recent years increasing numbers of later generation antipsychotic drugs have been approved and used for this purpose. Lithium was discovered in 1817. The first paper discussing its use for treatment of mania was published in 1949 and the FDA approved it for use in 1970. Its presumed action is through the regulation of the neurotransmitter glutamate. Kidney and thyroid function should be established before initiation of lithium therapy and it is important to note that lithium has a very narrow therapeutic blood range of between 0.8 and 1.4 mEq/L. The toxic range begins at 1.5 mEq/L and may even overlap the therapeutic range, making dosage calculations difficult.

Patients taking lithium should be taught to recognize early signs of lithium toxicity, including diarrhea, vomiting, drowsiness, muscular weakness, and lack of coordination. Severe symptoms include ataxia (failure or irregularity of muscle action), giddiness, tinnitus (ringing in the ears), blurred vision, and a large output of dilute urine. Long-term side effects include thirst, frequent urination, tremors, diarrhea, weight gain, and edema. The cause of weight gain is not definitely known, and it may even be due to an increased consumption of caloric beverages for thirst.[24] Patients taking lithium should be instructed to maintain a steady fluid and electrolyte balance through dietary sources because lithium is lost during perspiration, affecting its narrow therapeutic range. Lithium should not be taken by pregnant or breastfeeding women.

Three AED medications are used as mood stabilizers. They are carbamazepine, valproic acid/valproate, and lamotrigine. These three AEDs are similarly effective at inducing remission, but risk is substantial.[25] The prescribing specialist must carefully evaluate advantages and disadvantages of each medication. Some antipsychotic medications approved as mood stabilizers may provide better control of mania and a faster time to remission compared with valproic acid during treatment for manic or mixed episodes of bipolar disorder.[25]

Brain Stimulation Therapy

The brain stimulation therapies are used primarily for treatment-resistant mood disorders[23] that have failed to respond to other therapies. During electroconvulsive therapy (ECT), the patient is sedated with a general anesthetic and a seizure lasting less than 1 minute is induced with electricity through electrodes placed at precise locations. It is not known exactly how brain stimulation works to relieve depression, but a general course of treatment is three sessions per week for 4 weeks. Common side effects include headaches, nausea, muscle aches, and occasional loss of memory. Magnetic pulses may be used instead of electricity in a brain stimulation therapy called repetitive transcranial magnetic stimulation.[23] Nursing management of patients who undergo brain stimulation therapies is identical to preoperative and postoperative nursing care of patients who are administered a general anesthetic. Nurses should perform teaching before the procedure so the patient will know what to expect. After the procedure nurses should monitor the airway and mental status and assist the patient by orienting him or her to person, place, time, and situation as in any postoperative procedure.

Managing the Potential for Suicide and Other Violent Potential

The generalist nurse who suspects the possibility of a mood spectrum disorder should first assess for emergency situations. It should be considered an emergency when patients are at risk for suicide or violence; these patients should not be left alone. Any patient who presents with decreased functional status and affective instability should be evaluated for suicidal ideation. If there is any doubt regarding the severity of affective instability, functional status, or suicidal ideation the nurse should order continuous observation and refer the patient for an immediate, full evaluation.

Figure 29-3 demonstrates affective states associated with varying levels of suicide risk and potential for violence. In this figure the individual reflects a persistently low mood as depicted by the green line. On the left side of the figure cognition and energy are dropping, so despite the low mood he or she will tend to lack the energy and cognitive ability necessary to plan and carry out a suicidal act.

Comparatively, in the center of Figure 29-3 the individual's energy and cognition begin to cycle upward, increasing the risk of suicide. *This condition may sometimes occur on initiation of antidepressant medications.* On the far right side of the figure the mood is very low whereas energy and cognition are very high. The individual has a low, suicidal mood with

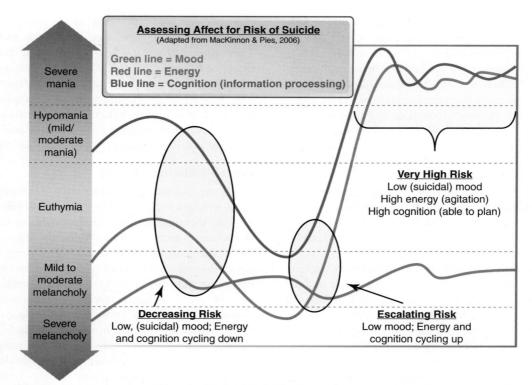

FIGURE 29-3 Assessing Affect for Risk of Suicide. Green line = mood; red line = energy; blue line = cognition. (Adapted from MacKinnon DF, Pies R: Affective instability as rapid cycling: theoretical and clinical implications for borderline personality and bipolar spectrum disorders, *Bipolar Disord* 8:1-14, 2006.)

sufficient energy and cognitive ability to plan and execute a suicidal act or other acts of violence. This person is unlikely to perceive reality accurately, and if mood were elevated here then the individual would be manic and out of control—at risk for dangerous and reckless behaviors such as gambling, violence, and promiscuity. Such individuals are likely to have hallucinations and/or delusions.

Minimum standards of practice by the generalist nurse for managing the potential for suicide and other violence are not well established at this time. In this concept it is recommended that the minimum standard for the generalist nurse in any setting is to assess for violence potential, and when the potential for violence is endorsed the patient should be assessed for acuity.

This is done by asking the patient if he/she has been thinking about suicide or if he/she has any other thoughts of violence. The nurse should remember that talking about frightening thought content is known to provide relief for the patient.[26] It has been consistently demonstrated that talking about suicidal feelings does not increase the likelihood of acting on those feelings at any age. "Nurses talking about suicide directly will not make people more dangerous. In fact, talking about those scary, very threatening thoughts and feelings with someone who is non-judgmental and caring could help keep some patients stay alive" (Becker-Fritz, as cited by Sun and colleagues).[26,p450]

The sudden appearance of unexplained euthymia in a person who has shown persistent affective instability may be an ominous sign of an impending suicidal act. In such cases, the appearance of euthymia results from the relief of making the decision to commit suicide. This decision may be accompanied by gift giving and acts of farewell. Not all suicides are predictable, especially impulsive suicide, but nurses who include assessment strategies discussed in this section will be more effective at recognizing possible mood spectrum disorders, initiating immediate interventions, and referring such patients to collaborative care. Other strategies include noting suicidal situations such as loss.[26] Loss may include the death of a loved one including pets, separation, illness, employment status, and self-esteem. Behavioral signals may warn of suicidal ideation, including writing or creating art about death; giving away prized possessions; and joking about death, dying, suicide, or leaving.[26]

INTERRELATED CONCEPTS

Each of the concepts shown in Figure 29-4 shares functional status impairment as a defining characteristic. That is to say, any individual experiencing affective instability, **Addictions,** or altered **Cognition** (confusion) will also experience functional status impairment. The affective disturbance may assume a variety of presentations such as crying, rage, euphoria, or even flatness during loss of contact with reality, which is typical of confused states whether chronic or acute. Whatever the presentation, the standard of care should be to assess for any deficit in functional status and from that assessment

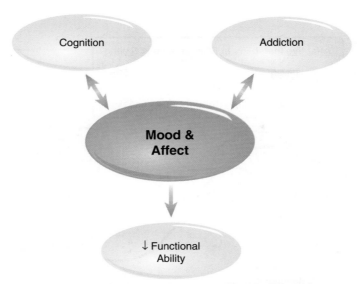

FIGURE 29-4 Interrelated Concepts—Mood and Affect, Addiction, and Cognition.

MODEL CASE

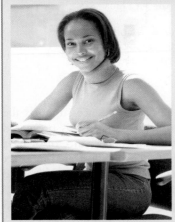

The following case study illustrates how prolonged extreme feelings, functional impairment, and vegetative functioning overlap to form a clinical picture.

Maya Rodgers is a 24-year-old college student whose mood is generally euthymic with stable affect. Her energy level, thinking, and mood fluctuate normally throughout the day. Ms. Rodgers has been struggling academically. She is informed by a course instructor that she must do well on an upcoming major exam or is at risk of failing the course. There is a lot riding on this exam and Ms. Rodgers cannot stop thinking about the exam. Her vegetative functioning is affected, manifesting as insomnia at night and fatigue in the day. On the day of the exam, Ms. Rodgers has a bright affect although her mood is anxious. Her energy and thinking are also elevated, although these fluctuations occur within the euthymic range.

The following day, Ms. Rodgers learns that she has failed the exam and may fail the course (Figure 29-5). Her mood begins to deteriorate through the euthymic range. Eventually, Maya Rodgers feels melancholic and appears affectively unstable. She experiences insomnia because of worried thoughts (elevated cognition) and experiences agitated energy that fluctuates wildly from agitation to lethargy (Figure 29-5).

Case Analysis

This case is an illustration of *exogenous* factors in affective instability. It also illustrates the assessment of the student's mental status. When affective instability is caused by exogenous factors this means there are identifiable causes for the instability, such as failing an exam or having financial or relationship problems. In some therapeutic approaches, the therapist may assist the patient to recognize unidentified exogenous factors. Once they are identified, the patient and therapist can then work to resolve them and hopefully resolve the mood disorder.

Affective instability can also be caused by *endogenous* factors. Endogenous affective instability is very disturbing because mood, energy, and/or cognitive processes fluctuate from neurochemical imbalances. Specifically, the neurotransmitters dopamine, serotonin, and/or norepinephrine become imbalanced for unknown reasons as already discussed. Neurotransmitters may also be affected by hormonal shifts. An individual with endogenous affective instability may, for example, suffer the same or worse agitation as an individual with exogenous instability, but with no externally known cause. This is very frightening and can become extreme, including perceptual disturbances and suicidal ideation.

proceed to establish a nursing diagnosis based on the presence or absence of other defining characteristics. For example, functional status may be impaired by addiction or it can be caused by confusion and it can also be caused by a mood spectrum disorder. Only by a thorough assessment can the nurse differentiate underlying etiologies.

EXEMPLARS

There are a large number of medical/psychiatric conditions with diagnostic criteria (medical defining characteristics) derived using medical reasoning in the *Diagnostic and Statistical Manual of Mental Disorders IV*.[5] These medically defined

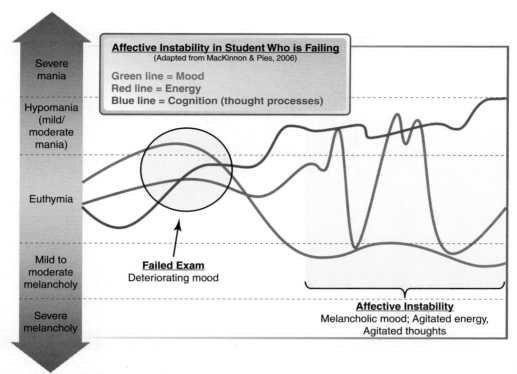

FIGURE 29-5 Affective Instability in a Student Who Is Failing. Green line = mood; red line = energy; blue line = cognition. (Adapted from MacKinnon DF, Pies R: Affective instability as rapid cycling: theoretical and clinical implications for borderline personality and bipolar spectrum disorders, *Bipolar Disord* 8:1-14, 2006.)

conditions provide useful exemplars for the analysis of the mood and affect concept. In medical psychiatry, these conditions are grouped dichotomously as disorders in either the depressive spectrum or the manic spectrum (see Box 29-1).

■■■ **BOX 29-1** **EXEMPLARS OF MOOD AND AFFECT**

Depressive Disorders
- Dysthymic depressive disorder
- Major depressive disorder
- Postpartum depression
- Psychotic depression
- Situational depression
- Suicide

Manic Disorders
- Bipolar I
- Bipolar II
- Cyclothymia
- Suicide

CONCLUSION

The generalist practice nurse who is proficient in the assessment of affective instability plays a key role in detecting mood spectrum disorders and providing patients with opportunities for preventing deterioration in functional status. The most extreme outcome the nurse may prevent is death or

disability by attempted suicide, and evidence supports the idea that when mood spectrum deterioration is prevented in an individual he or she stands a good chance of living a long, happy, and productive life. This is illustrated in an ex post facto review of interviews with individuals prevented from jumping off the Golden Gate Bridge between 1937 and 1978.[27] During that period, 625 people are known to have died of suicide there, and perhaps another 200 possible deaths may have occurred unseen at night or in bad weather. Dr. Seiden carefully followed the 515 "attempters" who were restrained from leaping off the bridge.

Of those who were prevented from suicide by jumping of the Golden Gate Bridge there were higher rates of violent death, but about 90% of those prevented from suicide *did not* die later by violent death. Other data from this study interpreted by Dr. Seiden[27] enabled him to form the following conclusions:

1. The chances are good that a person prevented from suicide will live a long and satisfying life. Ending one's life by suicide overlooks what might have happened—good feelings and good that could have been done.
2. Suicidal people should not be left to handle these emotions on their own. They should receive psychologic help immediately, with at least 6 months of close support.
3. No matter how intense at the moment, the desire to die is temporary in almost all circumstances, negating the notion that "suicide is a choice."
4. Therapy, medication, relatives, friends, and groups all offer hope.

ACCESS EXEMPLAR LINKS ON pageburst

REFERENCES

1. Taber: *Taber's cyclopedic medical dictionary [electronic resource]*, Philadelphia, 2009, FA Davis.
2. Merry SN: Prevention and early intervention for depression in young people: a practical possibility? *Curr Opin Psychiatr* 20(4):325–329, 2007.
3. MacKinnon DF, Pies R: Affective instability as rapid cycling: theoretical and clinical implications for borderline personality and bipolar spectrum disorders, *Bipolar Disord* 8:1–14, 2006.
4. Knight MM: Cognitive ability and functional status, *J Adv Nurs* 31(8):1459–1468, 2000.
5. American Psychiatric Association: *Diagnostic and statistical manual of mental disorders*, ed 4, Washington, DC, 1994, The Association.
6. Cuellar AK, Johnson SL, Winters R: Distinctions between bipolar and unipolar depression, *Clin Psychol Rev* 25(3): 307–339, 2004.
7. Cassano GB, Rucci P, Frank E, et al: The mood spectrum in unipolar and bipolar disorder: arguments for a unitary approach, *Am J Psychiatry* 161:1264–1269, 2004.
8. Angst J, Marneros A: Bipolarity from ancient to modern times: conception, birth and rebirth, *J Affective Disord* 67:3–19, 2001.
9. Harvard School of Medicine: *National comorbidity survey and national comorbidity survey replication*, 2005, Accessed Oct 4, 2010, at www.hcp.med.harvard.edu/ncs/.
10. U.S. Department of Health and Human Services (USDHHS): *Results from the 2007 national survey on drug use and health: national findings*, 2008, Retrieved May 29, 2009, from http://oas.samhsa.gov.
11. Stang P, Frank C, Yood MU, et al: Impact of bipolar disorder: results from a screening study, *Prim Care Companion J Clin Psychiatry* 9(1):42–47, 2007.
12. Shi L, Thiebaudb P, McCombs JS: The impact of unrecognized bipolar disorders for patients treated for depression with antidepressants in the fee-for-services California Medicaid (Medi-Cal) program, *J Affective Disord* 82:373–383, 2004.
13. National Institute of Mental Health: *Symptoms of depression and mania*, 2010. Retrieved Oct 24, 2010, from www.nimh.nih.gov/health/publications/men-and-depression/symptoms-of-depression-and-mania.shtml.
14. Angst J, Cui L, Swendsen J, et al: Major depressive disorder with subthreshold bipolarity in the national comorbidity survey replication, *Am J Psychiatry Advance*, 2010. doi: 10.1176/appi.ajp.2010.09071011.
15. Harkness KL, Monroe SM: Severe melancholic depression is more vulnerable than non-melancholic depression to minor precipitating life events, *J Affective Disord* 9:257–263, 2006.
16. Flaherty JH: Mental status: the 6th vital sign, *Aging Successfully* 17(1):9, 2007.
17. Registered Nurses Association of Ontario (RNAO): *Screening for delirium, dementia and depression in older adults*, Toronto, Ontario, Canada, 2003, Author.
18. United States Preventive Services Task Force (USPSTF): Screening for depression: recommendations and rationale, *Ann Intern Med* 136:760–764, 2002.
19. Sharp LK, Lipsky MS: Screening for depression across the lifespan: a review of measures for use in primary care settings, *Am Fam Physician* 66(6):1001–1008, 2002.
20. National Institute of Mental Health: *Real men, real depression: screening and treatment in primary care settings*, 2010. Retrieved Oct 24, 2010, from www.nimh.nih.gov/health/topics/depression/men-and-depression/healthprovider_may1.pdf.
21. Rollnick S, Miller WR, Butler CC: *Motivational interviewing in health care: helping patients change behavior*, New York, 2008, The Guilford Press.
22. Thase ME: Effectiveness of antidepressants: comparative remission rates, *J Clin Psychiatry* 64(suppl 2):3–7, 2003.
23. National Institute of Mental Health: *Psychotherapies*, 2010, Retrieved Oct 24, 2010, from www.nimh.nih.gov/health/topics/brain-stimulation-therapies/brain-stimulation-therapies.shtml.
24. Taylor DL, Laraia MT: Psychopharmacology. In Stuart GW, editor: *Principles and practice of psychiatric nursing*, ed 9, St Louis, 2009, Mosby/Elsevier.
25. Carey TS, Melvin CL, Ranney LM: Extracting key messages from systematic reviews, *J Psychiatr Pract* 14(suppl 1):28–34, 2008.
26. Sun FK, Long A, Boore J, et al: Suicide: a literature review and its implications for nursing practice in Taiwan, *J Psychiatr Ment Health Nurs* 12(4):447–455, 2005.
27. Seiden R: Where are they now? A follow-up study of suicide attempters from the Golden Gate Bridge, *Suicide Life Threatening Behav* 8(4), 1978.

Anxiety

Jenny Vacek

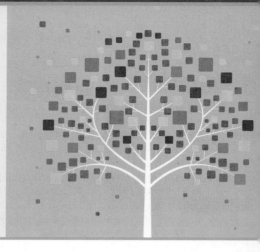

Anxiety is a normal adaptive response to stress that occurs across the lifespan. Anxiety is a subjective experience, with biological and psychodynamic dimensions. At the crux of anxiety is the preservation of biological and/or psychologic integrity—survival of the self. Sullivan[1] asserts that no individual, whether very ill or aged, is ever at a guarantee against any possibility of having anxiety, or fear. Anxiety states can be transient and nonpathologic. However, when anxiety is severe and chronic, and meets other specific criteria, it becomes a diagnosable psychiatric disorder. Any level of anxiety—from mild to severe to panic—warrants medical attention. Nurses who observe objective characteristics of anxiety must confirm these observations with the patient when able, determine the anxiety level, and intervene as necessary.

DEFINITION(S)

Several definitions of anxiety are found within the literature. Peplau describes anxiety as an "unexplained discomfort" such as a frustration, conflict, or need that directs behavior by supplying energy.[2p119] Kneisl and Trigoboff [3] declare that anxiety is a state of wide-ranging degrees of discomfort and uneasiness that is accompanied with fears, doubt, obsessions, and guilt. In addition, when anxiety reaches a point beyond mild, it is described as dread and/or terror. For the purposes of this concept analysis, anxiety is considered as *an alert to the human condition of impending doom, either real or imagined, and is accompanied by autonomic responses that serve as protective.* This classic definition is congruent with current definitions of anxiety.

SCOPE AND CATEGORIES

Scope

Anxiety is a normal response to stress, one that stretches on a continuum ranging from no anxiety to panic. When tolerable, anxiety can be an effective response because it mobilizes biological and psychologic resources.[4] Peplau[2] describes the following four levels of anxiety, and its effects on human action, shown in Figure 30-1.

- *Mild anxiety* is associated with the stress of daily living. During this phase, the individual is alert and the perceptual field, with all its senses, is heightened. Because the body is at work manufacturing energy, this stage is productive in nature, and an effective element of problem solving and growth.
- *Moderate anxiety* is associated with a narrowed perceptual field that permits the individual to concentrate on the imminent problem, so as to "fix" it, and hence mobilize forward.
- *Severe anxiety* can become a clinical problem; it is a very crippling and paralyzing experience. Judgment is extremely impaired; the individual is incapable of processing the problem at hand and synthesizing current feelings with past experiences to cope.
- *Panic,* the last level of anxiety, is clinical in nature and is characterized by striking dread and terror accompanied at times with dissociation, complete loss of control, and associated untoward autonomic physiologic responses; when untreated, panic can be life threatening and cause death.

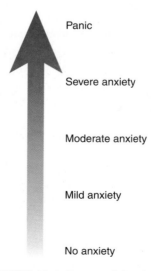

Panic

Severe anxiety

Moderate anxiety

Mild anxiety

No anxiety

FIGURE 30-1 Scope of Anxiety.

Categories

Anxiety translates into clinical pathology when it is out of the realm of what is developmentally appropriate, and/or inconsistent with life situations/circumstances. Classified anxiety disorders, specific substances/withdrawal, certain disease states, and the Cluster C personality disorder comprise this group of mental anxiety related illnesses. Persons with anxiety disorders have impairment in social, occupational, and/or school functioning. Table 30-1 presents the common categories of anxiety.

RISK FACTORS

Anxiety disorders affect all persons across the lifespan; the average age of onset is 11 years.[5] Collectively, anxiety disorders constitute the most prevalent group of mental health illnesses in pediatric, adolescent, and adult populations.[4,6] The 12-month prevalence rate of any anxiety disorder in the United States is 18.1% in adult populations; 28.8% of these cases have lifetime prevalence, 18.1% have 12-month prevalence, and 4.1% have 12-month prevalence classified as severe. The lifetime prevalence rate of any anxiety disorder in the United States for the 13- to 18-year-old age group is 25.1%; the lifetime prevalence rate of severe disorder in this population is 5.9%.[4]

Populations at Risk

Population risk factors include gender, age, and race/ethnicity. In pediatric populations, females have a statistically higher rate of lifetime prevalence of anxiety disorders then males; lifetime prevalence for females is 30.1%, whereas lifetime prevalence for males is 20.3%.[5] In adult populations, females have a 60% higher chance of developing an anxiety disorder than men in a lifetime. The age group with the highest lifetime prevalence of anxiety disorders is between the ages of 30 and 44 years; the age group with the lowest lifetime prevalence is

TABLE 30-1 CATEGORIES OF ANXIETY

CATEGORY	DESCRIPTION
Separation anxiety disorder	Considered a problem when this occurs outside realm of what is developmentally appropriate; it is an extreme response to separation from attachment figures and persistent worry of primary figure being harmed.
Panic and agoraphobia	Panic attack has distinct features; it is a problem that manifests with an abrupt, unexpected period of discomfort whereby cognitive and/or autonomic responses manifest. Agoraphobia occurs when a person feels anxiety about a situation (e.g., the marketplace, bus/trains, crowds) whereby the person perceives escape could cause embarrassment and/or be difficult. These disorders may or may not coexist.
Phobic disorders	This category represents specific and social phobias characterized by a persistent, marked fear of an object or social situation that is unreasonable, excessive, and evokes immediate anxiety. Avoidance is a hallmark characteristic; persons work to keep away from the phobic situation or endure it with extreme distress. Adults have insight into the fear whereas children may not. Children may manifest differently than adults with temper tantrums, crying, shrinking, and/or withdrawal.
Obsessive-compulsive disorder (OCD)	An obsession is a persistent, recurrent thought, impulse, or image that causes distress or anxiety. A compulsion is a repetitive behavior (e.g., hand washing, checking) and/or thought that a person uses to diminish, neutralize, or ward off obsession. Individual usually has insight and works to suppress or ignore the obsession.
Trauma-related anxiety disorder	Individuals suffering from trauma-related anxiety disorders have either witnessed or experienced an event(s) that included real or threatened serious injury or death, and the person felt helpless, intense fear, and/or horror at the time. The emotionally unresolved event triggers distressing biological and psychologic responses such as flashbacks, nightmares, dissociation, and/or psychotic features. Individuals who suffer from this group of disorders avoid trauma-related stimuli.
Generalized anxiety disorder	This group of conditions is characterized by excessive worry and anxiety that occurs more days than not for a minimum of 6 months. Problem is chronic in nature; symptoms may fluctuate, and are exacerbated by stress. Individual struggles to control the worry; fatigue, problems with concentration, irritability, restlessness, sleep disturbances, and/or muscle tension may occur.
Substance-induced anxiety disorder	This category of conditions may manifest with prominent anxiety, generalized anxiety, obsessive-compulsive symptoms, phobic symptoms, and/or panic attacks. This originates during or within 4 weeks of substance intoxication or withdrawal. This problem can occur across the lifespan with usage of certain substances (e.g., drugs, alcohol).
Medical-induced anxiety disorder	This occurs when anxiety is secondary to disease states that are physiologic in nature. Typically, person manifests with prominent anxiety, obsessions or compulsions, and/or panic attacks, and there is evidence from physical examination and/or laboratory findings that the problem is etiologically related to the medical disorder.
Anxiety disorders not otherwise specified	This category is used when anxiety or phobic behaviors manifest that do not meet criteria for other anxiety disorders.
Cluster C personality disorder (PD)	A personality disorder is manifested by a pattern and behavior of subjective experience that deviate from the norm. Cluster C includes three specific PDs that are distinguished by fearful and anxious behaviors.

From American Psychiatric Association: *Diagnostic and statistical manual of mental disorders*, ed 4, Washington, DC, 2000, Author.

60 years and older.[4] Compared to non-Hispanic whites, Hispanics are 30% less likely and non-Hispanic blacks are 20% less likely to suffer from an anxiety disorder in their lifetime.

Individual Risk Factors

Familial and Genetic Risks

Studies of first-degree biological relatives indicate a familial pattern in persons with panic disorders, phobic disorders, and generalized anxiety disorder. Studies with dizygotic and monozygotic twins report a familial pattern in those with obsessive-compulsive disorder (OCD). In addition, the rate of the OCD is higher in the general population in those who have first-degree biological relatives with Tourette's syndrome or OCD.[7]

Current preclinical and clinical investigations in neuroscience have found specific genes that enhance a person's vulnerability to anxiety disorders. Examples of preclinical investigation of genes involved in fear conditioning include *Grp*, γ-aminobutyric acid *(GABA)*, and *GRPR*. The allele of the serotonin transporter is related to elevated reaction of the amygdala to stimuli that evoke fear. Expanded research is needed in precise detection of genotypes related to anxiety disorders.[8]

Environmental Risks

In children, insecure attachment rooted in parental behaviors (deficiency in warmth, overprotected parenting, constant criticism) is likely to contribute to anxiety symptomatology.[6] Exposure to traumatic events can cause trauma-related disorders.[7] A recent study by Macdonald and colleagues reports that multiple exposures to experiencing a potentially traumatic event (e.g., witnessing violence, sexual abuse, physical abuse) were associated with increased chances for developing posttraumatic stress disorder (PTSD).[9]

Medical Conditions

There are a number of medical conditions that may cause anxiety symptomatology. These include various disease processes of the endocrine, cardiovascular, respiratory, metabolic, and neurologic systems[7] (Box 30-1).

BOX 30-1   MEDICAL CONDITIONS ASSOCIATED WITH ANXIETY

- Cancer
- Chronic obstructive pulmonary disease
- Dysrhythmias
- Encephalitis
- Heart failure
- Hyperthyroidism
- Hypoglycemia
- Pheochromocytoma
- Pneumonia
- Vestibular dysfunction
- Vitamin B_{12} deficiency

From American Psychiatric Association: *Diagnostic and statistical manual of mental disorders,* ed 4, Washington, DC, 2000, Author.

PSYCHOLOGIC AND PHYSIOLOGIC PROCESSES AND CONSEQUENCES

Psychologic and Physiologic Processes

Fight or Flight Response

The term fight reflects the aggressive action one would take if confronted with extreme stress; to the contrary, the term flight represents the withdrawal and/or frozen state a person may take. Fight or flight mechanism, first described by Cannon nearly 80 years ago,[10] occurs when one is confronted with very stressful and/or life-threatening situations. Autonomic physiologic responses to stress as seen in anxiety reactions include increased heart rate to facilitate blood to circulate faster, dilation of the airways of the lungs to increase oxygenation of blood, release of glucose from the liver to provide for increased energy, dilation of the pupils to allow more light to enter the eye and increased visual acuity, and inhibition of peristalsis of the gastrointestinal tract to conserve bodily energy.

Selye's Stress Response

Because anxiety is a response to stress, Selye's *General Adaptation Syndrome*[11] is presented. Selye postulates that there is a limited reservoir of energy to cope with stress; and because of this restriction, stress inflicts general wear and tear on the human condition, specifically the body. Both positive and negative stressors are stress experiences. Selye states that how one responds to stressors will either reduce or contribute to bodily responses. Three phases can occur and include alarm (reaction to stress), resistance (organism performs self-repair and stores energy), and exhaustion.

Brain Structure and Neurochemistry

Minimal research has been done in neuroimaging examination of brain structure and function in anxiety disorders. Research studies have shown that several parts of the brain may be involved in the symptomatology of persons with anxiety disorders: the amygdala, hippocampus, bed nucleus of stria terminalis, locus terminalis, and cortical regions.[8] Neuromodulators related to these structures—such as corticotropin-releasing hormone (CRH), cortisol, norepinephrine, and glutamate—can facilitate scientific discovery into effects of fear conditioning and the impact of trauma.

γ-Aminobutyric acid (GABA) is primarily an inhibitory neurotransmitter in the brain. Activation of GABA calms the brain; barbiturates, ethanol, and benzodiazepines bind with GABA. Abnormalities of GABA have been indicated as the probable etiology of anxiety disorders. Changes in the concentrations of the benzodiazepine GABA receptor may be a predisposing factor to anxiety. This hypothesis needs further study and investigation.[12]

Coping Mechanisms

Defense mechanisms are an ego-oriented protective behavior that can fluctuate dependent on the individual's needs. When confronted with anxiety, whether real and/or unknown, threats to the self may trigger untoward coping actions.

Peplau[2] describes obsessions, compulsions, and phobias as defenses against anxiety. A study by Spinhoven and Kooiman compared patients diagnosed with anxiety disorders to those diagnosed with depressive disorders. Compared to the control group, persons with depressive disorder and anxiety disorder scored higher for use of immature (i.e., projection, fantasy, hypochondriasis, passive aggressive) defense styles. Anxiety disorder patients had significantly higher scores for neurotic defense mechanisms compared to patients in the control group and those with depressive disorders. Persons manifesting panic used coping mechanism styles of devaluation, idealization, and somatization. Anxiety was associated predominantly with somatization.[13]

Consequences

Specific consequences of anxiety are largely dependent on the continuum of severity. The consequences of mild to moderate anxiety can have a positive impact because the ability to problem solve and learn is heightened during this stage of anxiety. In many cases severe states of anxiety and panic are, with appropriate nursing intervention, reversible and thus pose no residual threats. However, when intervention does not occur and/or is ineffective, the increased impulsivity, tension, and restlessness and the decreased ability to problem solve place the individual at risk for injury and/or violence to self or others. Fawcett[14] summarizes several studies that correlate high incidence of suicide in persons with severe levels of anxiety and panic attacks. Impulsivity is a risk factor in suicide and severely anxious states can activate impulsiveness. Proactive treatment requires early detection of suicidal risk factors, and intervention in persons with severe anxiety. Anxiety disorders can predict substance use in children and adolescents.[15]

The overall disabling symptomatology of persons who suffer from diagnosable anxiety disorders, when untreated or nonresponsive to treatment, impacts social, occupational, and/or academic function. Persons then may have an impaired ability to complete activities of daily living, sustain relationships, and hold a job, which may result in a life of disability, isolation, and chronic attempts to abate the psychic suffering.

ASSESSMENT

Persons with mild to moderate anxiety may appear asymptomatic to the observer. Assessment of the patient who manifests severe anxiety or panic includes a history, physical examination, and mental status examination. Analysis and interpretation of the assessment data facilitate determination of the etiologic basis for anxiety, whether it is situational or attributable to a psychiatric illness, substance use/abuse, and/or organic illness.

History

The nurse collects data related to past and current medical problems, medication regimen including over-the-counter medications, allergies, appetite and sleep patterns, sexual functioning, toxin exposure, and past or current injuries. Insomnia and problems with sexual functioning may be present. The nurse also elicits a social history that includes assessment of any past or current exposure to stressors and trauma (including interpersonal violence and/or exposure to life-threatening events or death). In addition, appraisal of the patient's coping mechanisms, stressors, and strengths should be addressed. Persons with anxiety may report current stressors and/or past trauma, be socially impaired, and/or demonstrate ineffective coping mechanisms.

Examination

During the process of an assessment, several common clinical manifestations may be observed. Increased or decreased blood pressure, increased perspiration (i.e., diaphoresis), increased respirations, and increased pulse rate may manifest secondary to autonomic responses. Somatic symptoms may occur concomitantly with anxiety (e.g., diarrhea, nausea). Subjective assessment may include asking the patient to rate his or her anxiety level on a scale of 1 to 4, with 1 being the least and 4 being the most severe. Patients who are anxious (when insight is present) often report feelings such as fear, frustration, loss of control, dread, and/or hopelessness. Panic attacks manifest with distinct features that peak at 10 minutes and include palpitations, diaphoresis, shaking/trembling, shortness of breath, feelings of choking, chills/hot flashes, chest pain, nausea, dizziness, derealization or depersonalization, fear of losing control, and/or fear of dying.[7]

A mental status examination (MSE) may reveal several classic findings. These include rapid and/or disorganized speech; trembling or shaking; psychomotor agitation; compulsions; an anxious, fearful, and/or agitated mood/affect; nightmares; hallucinations/illusions (as seen in trauma-related anxiety); obsessions; delusions (as seen in trauma-related anxiety); disorientation or confusion; impaired memory; inability to concentrate and/or problem solve; poor judgment; and/or lack of insight. Because of the high incidence of suicide in persons with anxiety, a suicide screening is an essential component of the MSE.

Diagnostic Tests

Anxiety diagnosis is based on history and physical findings; it is not based on laboratory tests and other diagnostic studies. However, laboratory and other diagnostic tests may be used to determine the underlying pathophysiologic etiology of medical disorders that may manifest with anxiety symptomatology.

CLINICAL MANAGEMENT

Primary Prevention

Well visits across the lifespan are integral to early detection of any disease. Fostering healthy parent-infant/child relationships and providing parental education and guidance regarding facilitating tasks related to specific stages of growth and development are important. Research indicates that evidenced-based programs can significantly decrease early use of alcohol and illicit drugs; these models work by reducing risk factors for substance abuse and addressing protective factors.[16] Crisis intervention may be useful in deterring the impact of trauma-related anxiety disorders. For example, Psychological First Aid (PFA) is a recent preventive approach for persons who survive disasters. Empiric evidence shows that the principles of PFA—calmness, promoting safety, self and community effectualness, social connectedness, and optimism—may alleviate the untoward psychologic distress of anxiety and prevent the development of trauma-related anxiety disorders such as posttraumatic stress disorder.[17]

Secondary Prevention (Screening)

Various screening tools are used to detect anxiety. If substance abuse screening is the suspected cause of anxiety, substance abuse screening is also appropriate. The *Revised Children's Manifest Anxiety Scale* (RCMAS) is a 73-item yes and no answer tool used to evaluate anxiety in children in grades 1 through 12. There are several tools used to screen various types of anxiety in adults. The *Acute Panic Inventory* (API) is primarily a symptom assessment tool to assess a person's characteristics during a panic attack. The *Covi Anxiety Scale* (COVI) is a simple tool to measure the severity of anxiety in three areas: patient's subjective experience, somatic symptoms, and behavior. The *Social Phobia and Anxiety Inventory* (SPAI) assesses the severity of dimensions of somatic symptoms, avoidance, and cognition in persons with agoraphobia and social phobia. The *State-Trait Anxiety Inventory* (STAI) is a self-report tool used to differentiate between acute versus chronic anxiety.[18]

Numerous tools are used for screening PTSD. Examples include the PCL-M (PTSD checklist, military version) screening tool that is used to assess for symptoms related to stressful military experiences and the PCL-C (PTSD checklist, civilian version). The PCL-C is used to assess for symptoms in response to stressful situations; it can be used for any population.[19]

Collaborative Interventions

As noted earlier, there are multiple causes of anxiety; thus the underlying cause (etiology) must be considered in the clinical management plan. Multiple collaborative interventions exist that apply to one or more specific anxiety conditions. These include therapeutic interactions, pharmacologic agents, behavioral therapy and counseling, complementary and alternative medicine, and rehabilitation. Currently access to care and treatment is underutilized in the United States; statistics related to 12-month health care usage in the United States indicate that only 36.9% of those with an anxiety disorder are seeking treatment. Of those receiving treatment, 34.3% are receiving minimally adequate care.[20] Nurses should educate patients and/or families about the importance of seeking care.

Nurse/Patient/Family Interaction

As an energy force, anxiety can be contagious. Peplau[2] stresses the importance that nurses explore their own awareness of feelings about the patient, and observe how the patient reacts to the nurse's behavior, words, or gestures. This can facilitate therapeutic communication and assist the nurse to better help the patient control anxiety. During severe anxiety and panic states, the nurse must remain calm. Vital signs are assessed, and environmental stimuli are kept at a minimum. Communication to the patient should be simple and concrete, and include assuring the patient of security and safety. It is also important for the nurse to assess and/or contain anxiety in family members/visitors because this untoward energy can escalate the patient's anxiety.

Pharmacotherapy

β-Adrenergic receptor antagonists. Administration of medications and assessment of the patient's response to medications is a common treatment for anxiety. Seven major groups of medications are used. This drug classification is prescribed on an as-needed basis for performance anxiety, such as test-taking anxiety, public speaking, and/or stage fright, to facilitate a decrease in tremors and tachycardia. Drugs currently prescribed include propranolol (Inderal) and atenolol (Tenormin). Potential untoward side effects include lightheadedness and fatigue. This medication is contraindicated in persons with heart block, bradycardia, diabetes, and glaucoma.[21]

Benzodiazepines. This classification is prescribed for anxiety disorders on an as-needed basis for performance anxiety. Benzodiazepines can also be prescribed on a regular basis for panic disorder, general anxiety disorder (GAD), and social anxiety disorder. Common benzodiazepines used include alprazolam (Xanax), lorazepam (Ativan), and clonazepam (Klonopin). Potential untoward side effects are dizziness and sedation; alcohol use is contraindicated. Possible areas of concern with these medications include decreased tolerance and abuse.[21]

Selective serotonin reuptake inhibitors (SSRIs). This classification of drugs is prescribed for performance anxiety, OCD, panic attacks, GAD, PTSD, and social anxiety. Examples include sertraline (Zoloft), citalopram (Celexa), paroxetine (Paxil), fluvoxamine (Luvox), and escitalopram (Lexapro). Potential untoward side effects are nausea, diarrhea, lightheadedness, and sexual dysfunction. Medication change should be considered if side effects are intolerable. Efficacy may take at least 8 to 12 weeks. Adjunct therapy, sildenafil (Viagra), can be used to treat sexual dysfunction in males. Evidence shows effectiveness of treatment of SSRIs in children/adolescents with OCD, separation anxiety disorder, and panic disorder.[21]

Serotonin-norepinephrine reuptake inhibitors (SNRIs). Venlafaxine (Effexor) is prescribed for performance anxiety, GAD, and social anxiety disorder. Potential untoward side effects are similar to those of SSRIs, but in some cases patients may experience hypertension. It is imperative that patients taking SNRIs have their blood pressure carefully monitored.[21]

Tricyclic antidepressants (TCAs). This classification of drug is prescribed for panic attacks, panic disorder, and GAD. A common TCA drug prescribed is imipramine (Tofranil). A potential untoward side effect when treatment is first initiated is jitteriness; this eventually resolves itself. Titration of the dose may be necessary to alleviate this symptom.[21]

Monoamine oxidase inhibitors (MAOIs). This classification of drug is effective in treating phobic disorder, GAD, and social anxiety disorder. However, because of the potential side effects of insomnia, hypotension, and weight gain, caution must be used. A challenge for persons taking MAOIs is the need to maintain a diet low in tyramine to reduce the potential risk of hypertensive crisis.[21]

Other anxiolytics. The use of buspirone (BuSpar), a non-benzodiazepine anxiolytic, is limited to treating GAD. Therapeutic efficacy can take several weeks, and sometimes up to several months. Atarax (hydroxyzine) is prescribed for GAD. Gabapentin (Neurontin) is showing promise as a treatment for social anxiety disorder; divalproex (Depakote) may be helpful in treating resistant panic disorders. Other medications effective in the treatment of PTSD are topiramate (Topamax), lamotrigine (Lamictal), and levetiracetam (Keppra).[21]

Behavioral Therapies/Counseling

Family intervention. Family intervention is imperative in terms of psychoeducation, illness management, and overall support. The National Alliance on Mental Illness and Mental Health America are important resources for both patients and families/significant others affected by anxiety disorders. These organizations provide support, public education, advocacy, and research for the mentally ill.[20,22]

Family therapy. This type of therapy assists the family who is living with a person with anxiety disorder; learning coping mechanisms and suggesting ways to improve quality of life are part of this therapy. Family counseling facilitates communication and maintenance of healthy relationships, and provides for psychoeducation regarding the disease process and pharmacologic therapy.

Group therapy. This type of therapy provides a trusting environment whereby patients who have anxiety disorders can express emotions and feelings, receive validation

---

MODEL CASE 1

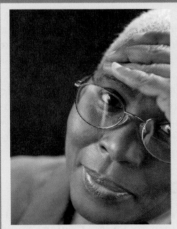

Helen Meyers is a 56-year-old women who came to the emergency department manifesting symptoms of dyspnea, choking sensations, chest pain, and sweating that lasted 30 minutes. A complete medical evaluation was performed including a chest x-ray, electrocardiogram (ECG), and measurement of cardiac enzymes, all of which indicated no signs of pulmonary or cardiovascular problems. Ms. Meyers reported losing her job last week, and she fears that she will not be able to pay her mortgage. She was diagnosed with a panic attack; a referral to a psychiatrist for a follow-up appointment was made. It has been 2 years since the panic attack; no subsequent panic attacks occurred.

Case Analysis

This case exemplifies the concept of anxiety and specifically the exemplar panic disorder. The patient is a female with a recent trigger (loss of job, financial problems) who manifests both cognitive and autonomic responses. The panic attack peaks in 10 minutes, and then subsides.

MODEL CASE 2

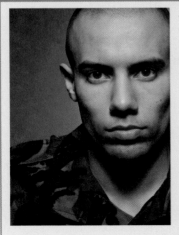

John Williams is a 28-year-old male who returned home from active military combat 8 weeks ago. He awakes in the middle of the night from war-related nightmares and places a gun to his wife's head. The police are called. He is taken to the psychiatric emergency hospital. At the hospital he reports frequent flashbacks about his buddy being blown up in front of him, related nightmares, and recurrent visions of explosives. He reports that he avoids watching the news and communicating with any of his military friends. He has difficulty sleeping and poor concentration and he is hypervigilant. A suicide assessment is completed, and indicates he is at high risk for suicide. John is admitted to the inpatient psychiatric unit, administered Zoloft (an SSRI), and placed on suicide precautions. After a few days the suicidal ideation has subsided. He continues to have flashbacks, nightmares, and intrusive thoughts. Evaluation at discharge indicates John is no longer a danger to himself or others. Discharge includes a prescription for Zoloft, a referral to a psychiatrist, and an appointment for exposure therapy, peer support, and family interventions.

Case Analysis

This case exemplifies the concept of anxiety and specifically the exemplar PTSD. The patient has a history of trauma and symptomatology of flashbacks/nightmares, avoidance, and suicidal ideation. Once treatment is implemented, some symptoms begin to resolve. Follow-up with outpatient treatment is necessary.

and feedback, and obtain reinforcement of coping skills. Examples of types of group therapy include art, exercise, humor, spirituality, psychoeducation, and life skills learning. Play therapy is useful in treating children with anxiety disorders.

Cognitive and behavioral therapy (CBT). This therapy is a tested and effective form of psychotherapy used across the lifespan. Research has shown CBT to successfully treat children/adolescents with separation anxiety disorder, OCD, phobias, and PTSD. In adults it is an effective treatment for panic disorder, agoraphobia, social phobia, OCD, and PTSD.[23]

Prolonged exposure therapy. This specific therapy includes psychoeducation (i.e., common trauma responses, symptomatology), instruction on breathing exercises to decrease anxiety and other techniques to manage short-term distress, and counseling that encourages repeated purging of trauma-related feelings. The expected outcome of exposure therapy is decreased fears related to untoward memories.[24]

Mindfulness. This treatment modality is a way to facilitate persons inflicted with PTSD to think and focus on the present versus past experiences. Mindfulness trains the mind to think in the here and now, and emphasizes attentiveness to all sensations and feelings related to these experiences. Inclusive in this treatment is the need to practice acceptance of one's thoughts without self-judgment.[24]

Eye movement desensitization and reprocessing (EMDR). This treatment is successful in treating PTSD in pediatric and adult populations. This method includes expression of feelings and memories while focusing on other stimuli such as sounds, hand taps, and/or eye movements. It is still unclear how EMDR precisely works; recent studies report it is the cognitive treatment, rather than the accompanied stimuli, that results in positive outcomes.[25]

Peer support. This type of group is led by persons inflicted with mental illness themselves. The intent of peer support is that persons who experience the challenges of mental illness share their own effective wellness tools. Examples of specific peer groups for anxiety disorders include PTSD, agoraphobia, and social phobic support groups.

Complementary and Alternative Medicine

These treatments can prevent and/or alleviate anxiety symptomatology. Examples include meditating, exercising, performing abdominal breathing exercises, listening to music, spending time with a pet, reducing/stopping the intake of caffeine, and/or implementing sleep hygiene measures. The substances kava kava, valerian root, and St. John's wort are natural remedies to reduce anxiety, but must be used cautiously with certain prescriptions. Scientific evidence is still needed to validate the effectiveness of herbal treatments.[21]

Rehabilitation

Psychosocial rehabilitation. This program is designed to maximize patient's strengths, and decrease potential for recidivism. Such programs enable patients to improve communication skills, work on self-care, form and sustain relationships, and use effective coping mechanisms. Patients who receive consistent psychosocial treatment tend to take their medications regularly, have fewer relapses, and show decreased recidivism rates.[4]

Vocational rehabilitation. This program is designed to facilitate job training, resources management, and public resources in mentally ill populations who have difficulty obtaining and sustaining jobs because of cognitive impairment attributable to the disorder.

INTERRELATED CONCEPTS

There are several interrelated concepts that apply to anxiety (Figure 30-2). These include **Stress, Coping, Mood and affect,** and **Interpersonal violence.** Stress refers to the

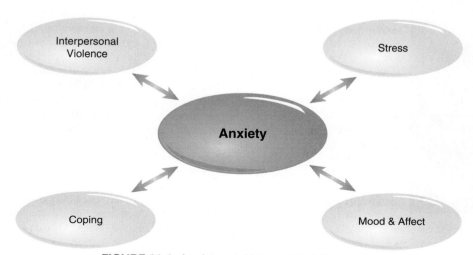

FIGURE 30-2 Anxiety and Interrelated Concepts.

overall wear and tear on the body and can lead to exhaustion/death. Persons with severe anxiety/panic are in stress overload. Increased stress in persons with anxiety can exacerbate or worsen the problem. Coping relates to the use of poor adaptive responses and inability to utilize resources effectively. Mood/affect refers to the patient's emotional state that impacts perceptions and behaviors. Violence refers to behaviors that put the patient and others at risk for emotional or physical harm. Persons who have a fearful/anxious mood, attributable to disorganized thinking and impaired problem-solving abilities, cannot implement previous used coping skills; moreover, the disorganization further impairs coping. Increasing tension, frustration, poor impulse control, and psychotic behaviors (as seen in trauma-related anxiety disorders) place the patient at risk for harming self (i.e., suicidal ideation) and losing control and harming others.

EXEMPLARS

Nine categories of anxiety are used to present anxiety exemplars (Box 30-2). All can occur in pediatric, adult, and geriatric populations. Children may manifest symptoms differently than adults in several of the disorders. Separation anxiety disorder is primarily seen in children. Of high incidence and prevalence is panic disorder (case study 1), which is seen in numerous health care settings such as emergency departments (EDs) and psychiatric units. Posttraumatic stress disorder is currently increasing in prevalence (case study 2). Patients with PTSD may present with symptoms in clinics, EDs, or psychiatric units. Many disorders are successfully treated in outpatient settings and never require hospitalization.

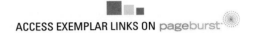

ACCESS EXEMPLAR LINKS ON pageburst

BOX 30-2   EXEMPLARS OF ANXIETY

Separation Anxiety Disorders
- Separation anxiety disorder

Trauma-Related Anxiety Disorders
- Acute stress disorder
- Posttraumatic distress disorder

Panic Disorder and Agoraphobia
- Unexpected panic attack
- Situational panic attack
- Situational predisposed panic attack
- Agoraphobia
- Panic disorder without agoraphobia
- Panic disorder with agoraphobia
- Agoraphobia without a history of panic disorder

Phobic Disorders
- Social phobia (social anxiety disorder)
- Specific phobia (subtypes: animal, natural environment type, blood-injection-injury type, situational type, other type [e.g., space phobia])

Generalized Anxiety Disorders
- Overanxious disorder of childhood
- Generalized anxiety disorder

Obsessive-Compulsive Disorders
- Obsessive-compulsive disorder
- Pediatric autoimmune neuropsychiatric disorder associated with streptococci (PANDAS)

Substance-Induced Anxiety Disorder
- Alcohol
- Amphetamines
- Amphetamine-like substance
- Caffeine
- Cannabis
- Cocaine
- Hallucinogen
- Inhalant
- Phencyclidine
- Phencyclidine-like substance
- Sedative-hypnotic
- Anxiolytic onset during withdrawal

Cluster C Personality Disorders
- Avoidant personality disorder
- Dependent personality disorder
- Obsessive-compulsive personality disorder

Anxiety Disorder Not Otherwise Specified
- Mixed anxiety disorder and depression

REFERENCES

1. Sullivan HS: *The interpersonal theory of psychiatry*, New York, 1953, WW Norton.

2. Peplau H: *Interpersonal relations in nursing*, New York, 1991, Springer, pp 126–128, 146, 159.

3. Kneisl CR, Trigoboff E: Stress, anxiety, and coping. In Kneisl CR, Trigoboff E, editors: *Contemporary psychiatric-mental health nursing*, ed 2, Upper Saddle River, NJ, 2009, Pearson, p 142.

4. National Institute of Mental Health: *Any anxiety disorder among adults*, 2011. Retrieved Feb 2, 2011, from www.nimh.nih.gov/statistics/1ANYANX_ADULT.shtml.

5. National Institute of Mental Health: *Any anxiety disorder among children*, 2011. Retrieved Feb 1, 2011, from www.nimh.nih.gov/statistics/1ANYANX_child.shtml.

6. Charney DS: Anxiety disorders: introduction and overview. In Sadock BS, Sadock V, editors: *Comprehensive textbook of psychiatry*, ed 8, Philadelphia, 2005, Lippincott Williams & Wilkins.

7. American Psychiatric Association: *Diagnostic and statistical manual of mental disorders*, ed 4, Washington, DC, 2000, Author.

8. Charney DS: Anxiety disorders. In Charney DS, Nester EJ, editors: *Neurobiology of mental illness*, New York, 2004, Oxford University Press, p 523.

9. Macdonald A, Danielson CK, Resnick HS, et al: PTSD and comorbid disorders in a representative sample of adolescents: the risk associated with multiple exposures to potentially traumatic events, *Child Abuse Neglect* 34:773–783, 2010.

10. Cannon W: *The wisdom of the body*, New York, 1935, WW Norton.

11. Selye H: *The stress of life*, New York, 1956, McGraw-Hill.

12. Higgins ES, George MS: *The neuroscience of clinical psychiatry. The pathophysiology of mental illness*, Philadelphia, 2007, Wolters Kluwer/Lippincott Williams & Wilkins, p 245.

13. Spinhoven P, Kooiman CG: Defense style in depressed and anxious psychiatric outpatients: an explorative study, *J Nervous Ment Dis* 185(2):87–94, 1997.

14. Fawcett J: Treating impulsivity and anxiety in the suicidal patient. The clinical science of suicide prevention, *Ann N Y Acad Sci* 932:94–105, 2001.

15. Kendall PC, Safford S, Flannery-Schroeder E, et al: Child anxiety treatment: outcomes in adolescence and impact on substance use and depression at 7.4 year follow-up, *J Consult Clin Psychol* 72:276–282, 2004.

16. National Institute of Drug Abuse: *The best strategy*, 2011. Retrieved Jan 11, 2011, from www.nida.nih.gov/science of addiction/strategy.html.

17. Ursano RJ, Goldenberg M, Lei Z, et al: Posttraumatic stress disorder and traumatic stress: from bench to bedside, from war to disaster, *Ann N Y Acad Sci* 1208:72–81, 2010.

18. Sajatovic M, Ramirez LF: *Rating scales in mental health,* ed 2, Hudson, Ohio, 2006, Lexicomp, pp 36, 47, 55, 66.

19. United States Department of Veterans Affairs: *PTSD checklist (PCL)*, 2011. Retrieved Feb 7, 2011, from www.ptsd.va.gov/professional/pages/assessments/ptsd-checklist.asp.

20. National Alliance of the Mentally Ill (NAMI). www.nami.org/.

21. Stein MB: Anxiety disorders: somatic treatment (no pages, electronic). In Sadock BS, Sadock V, editors: *Comprehensive textbook of psychiatry*, ed 8, Philadelphia, 2005, Lippincott Williams & Wilkins.

22. Mental Health America (MHA): *Mission, vision statement of purpose, guiding principles*, 2011. Retrieved Feb 2, 2011, from www.nmha.org.

23. Beck Institute of Cognitive Behavioral Therapy and Research: *What research shows?* 2011. Retrieved Jan 3, 2011, from www.beckinstitute.org/Library/InfoManage/Guide.asp?FolderID=312&Session ID.

24. U.S. Department of Veterans Affairs: *Treatment of PTSD*, 2011. Retrieved Feb 7, 2011, from www.ptsd.va.gov/public /pages/treatment-ptsd.asp.

25. U.S. Department of Veterans Affairs: *PTSD in children and adults*, 2011. Retrieved Feb 7, 2011, from www.ptsd.va.gov/professional/pages/ptsd_in_children_adolescents_overview_for_professionals.

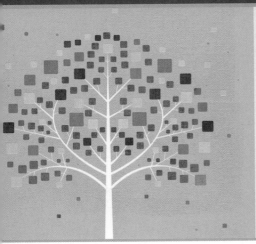

Cognition

Frances D. Monahan

The ability to think has long been considered a defining characteristic of what it means to be human. Attesting to this are the words of the French philosopher Rene Descartes, who said "Cogito, ergo sum," which translates to "I think, therefore I am." Thus the understanding of cognition, a term derived from the Latin verb "to think," is essential to understanding human behavior in health and in disease.

The study of cognition is multidisciplinary in scope with involvement and contributions from psychologists, philosophers, linguists, artificial intelligence scientists, and neuroscientists.[1] Two fields exclusively dedicated to the study of cognition are cognitive psychology and cognitive neuroscience. Cognitive psychology is committed to the study of cognition from an information processing perspective.[1] Cognitive neuroscience is the combined study of the mind and brain.[2]

DEFINITION(S)

Cognition is a comprehensive term used to refer to all the processes involved in human thought.[1] These processes relate to the reception of sensory input, its processing, its storage, its retrieval, and its use.[2] For the purposes of this concept analysis, cognition is defined as *the process of thought that embodies perception, attention, visuospatial cognition, language, learning, memory, and executive function with the higher order thinking skills of comprehension, insight, problem solving, reasoning, decision making, creativity, and metacognition.*[3]

Three related terms—perception, memory, and executive function—are also described here for further clarification. *Perception* is the interpretation of the environment and is dependent on the acuity of sensory input. A related construct is awareness or consciousness, which refers to the ability to perceive or be sensitive to stimuli in the environment and respond to them. Attention is a focus on a particular area of conscious content. It implies selection as well as the ability to direct cognitive effort.[2]

Memory broadly refers to the retention and recall of past experiences and learning. It is not a single, unified mental ability but rather a series of different neural subsystems, each of which has a unique localization in the brain. These different subsystems support different types of memory—namely, declarative episodic memory, declarative semantic memory, immediate memory, working memory, and procedural memory. Declarative memory refers to the ability to consciously learn and recall information. When the information relates to specific events, the terminology used is declarative episodic memory. This is distinct from declarative semantic memory, which refers to memory of knowledge, words, and facts.[4] Declarative memory provides for long-term storage of large amounts of information. Immediate memory or "attention span" allows memory of very small amounts of information, such as a series of six or seven digits, for a very short time.[4] Working memory is analogous to short-term memory. It allows a small amount of information (about four chunks or meaningful units) to be actively maintained and manipulated for a short period of time. Procedural memory refers to the retention and retrieval of motor skills. It requires extensive training and provides for long-term storage of a moderate amount of information. Related to memory is visuospatial cognition, which is the capacity to comprehend, retain, and use visual representations and their spatial relationships.[5]

Executive function refers to the higher thinking processes that allow for flexibility, adaptability, and goal directedness. Executive function determines the contents of consciousness, supervises voluntary activity, and is future oriented.[2]

SCOPE AND CATEGORIES

At the most basic level, cognition may be described as intact or impaired, with intact meaning that an individual exhibits cognitive behaviors that are considered to be within the range of normal for age and culture whereas impaired signifies an observable or measurable disturbance in one or more of the cognitive processes resulting from an abnormality within the brain (Figure 31-1).

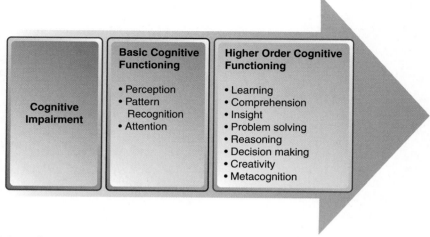

FIGURE 31-1 Scope of Cognition Ranges from Cognitive Impairment to Higher Order Cognitive Functioning.

Within the designation of cognitive impairment, several different cognitive categories exist, and there is little agreement as to which classification system is "correct"; for this reason all three are highlighted and presented in Table 31-1.

One neurologically focused classification of these disorders is into four general categories, which are mental retardation, delirium, dementia, and focal cognitive disorders.[6] A slightly different classification, used in mental health, is that found in the American Psychiatric Association's *Diagnostic and Statistical Manual of Mental Disorders (DSM-IV)*. Categories of cognitive disorders within this classification system include delirium, dementia, amnestic, and cognitive disorders not otherwise specified. With this approach, mental retardation is classified separately as a developmental disorder.[7] A third classification of cognitive disorders combines common elements of both of the aforementioned classifications to include two overarching categories, each with two or more subcategories. These two categories include *global cognitive disorders* (subcategories delirium and dementia) and *focal cognitive disorders* (subcategories include amnesia, aphasic, and cortical vision disorders; hemispatial neglect disorders; and executive function and personal behavior control disorders).

POPULATIONS AT RISK AND RISK FACTORS

Risk recognition for cognitive impairment is essential to preventive intervention aimed at modifiable risk factors. It is also essential for the early identification of cognitive impairment and its subsequent management. Because there are so many different types of cognitive impairment and many causes of each, there is a wide array of risk factors, not all of which apply to every case.

Populations at Risk

Any individual from all population groups is potentially at risk for developing impairment in cognition. Multiple studies have been conducted evaluating characteristics of individuals who developed cognitive impairment compared to the characteristics of individuals who did not. The results of such studies indicate that a primary risk factor for cognitive impairment is advancing age.[8] Thus the primary age group at risk is the elderly population. No differences in impairment have been found across populations based on race, ethnicity, or gender; however, correlated risk factors among women and men differ.[9] Significant risk factors found for women are overall poor health status, dependency, lack of social support, and insomnia whereas significant risk factors specific to men are a history of stroke or diabetes.[9]

TABLE 31-1   CATEGORIES OF COGNITIVE DISORDERS

NEUROLOGICALLY FOCUSED CLASSIFICATION	DSM-IV CLASSIFICATION	COMBINED APPROACH

• Mental retardation
• Delirium
• Dementia
• Focal cognitive disorders
	• Delirium
	• Dementia
	• Amnestic
	• Cognitive disorders not otherwise specified
		• Global cognitive disorders
		  • Delirium
		  • Dementia
		• Focal cognitive disorders
		  • Amnestic
		  • Aphasic
		  • Cortical vision and hemispatial neglect
		  • Executive function and personal behavior control

Risk Factors

There are many individual risk factors associated with impaired cognition. The most common categories of individual risk factors are personal behaviors, environmental exposures, congenital or genetic conditions, and other health-related conditions.

Personal Behaviors

Personal behaviors that predispose to impaired cognition are those related to chemical exposure and risk of traumatic injury to the brain. Specific examples of high-risk behaviors include substance abuse (e.g., alcohol, amphetamines, cannabis, cocaine, hallucinogens, inhalants, opioids, phencyclidine, sedatives, hypnotics, anxiolytics), participation in high-risk activities that could result in traumatic brain injury, or omission of basic safety measures, such as wearing a helmet (e.g., skiing, cycling, motorcycle riding, rock climbing) or wearing a seatbelt (or seat restraint for children) when riding in vehicles. Accidental injuries associated with work, recreation, or violence in the absence of high-risk behaviors can also lead to brain injury and cognitive impairment.

Environmental Exposures

Environmental exposures to toxic substances can negatively impair cognitive function. Despite changes in environmental regulations, lead exposure continues to be a problem because of the presence of lead in the soil and dust as well as old lead-based paint. Lead exposure among young children is particularly concerning because the developing brain is especially vulnerable. Other chemical agents such as pesticides can also negatively impair cognitive function.[10]

Congenital and Genetic Conditions

The term congenital means "present at birth"; genetic conditions differ in that the genetic problem exists at birth, but the condition may or may not be present at birth, manifesting later in life. Many congenital and genetic conditions are associated with impaired cognition. Some are related to maternal conditions (such as fetal alcohol syndrome or cocaine or methamphetamine exposure) and some are caused by birth injuries (such as cerebral palsy). Cognitive impairment also results from many chromosomal abnormalities (such as Down syndrome or fragile X syndrome) or other genetic conditions evident in infancy (such as phenylketonuria, galactosemia)[11] or those that emerge later in life (such as Huntington's disease in which mental deterioration begins typically in the fourth decade of life).

Health-Related Conditions

Many health conditions can lead to temporary or long-term impairments in cognition. Fluid and electrolyte imbalance, systemic or intracranial infection, fever, pain, hypoglycemia, and anoxia can cause delirium that is reversible with treatment of the precipitating cause. Stroke and intracranial tumor can cause irreversible long-term amnestic and other cognitive impairments. Many chronic conditions such as cardiovascular disease, chronic pulmonary disease, and depression have also been found to be significant risk factors for cognitive impairment in both men and women.[12]

Changes in cognition may occur as an adverse effect of medical treatments and medications. This is a particular risk among the elderly population because of decreased physiologic reserve, decline in hepatic and renal function, altered metabolism, presence of chronic disease, and multiple drug regimens. Psychoactive drugs are particularly notorious—these agents can cause delirium or cognitive decline. Examples include sedative-hypnotics (especially the long-acting benzodiazepines flurazepam and diazepam); narcotics (especially meperidine); anticholinergics (such as antihistamines, antispasmodics, heterocyclic antidepressants, neuroleptics, and antiparkinsonians); digitalis glycosides; antidysrhythmics (such as quinine and procainamide); and antihypertensives such as beta-blockers. H_2-antagonists, nonsteroidal antiinflammatory drugs (NSAIDs), corticosteroids, and anticonvulsants as well as over-the-counter sleep aids, cold and sinus medications, and antinausea and acid-reflux preparations can also lead to changes in cognition.[13] Chemotherapy, used to kill cancer cells, has been shown to impair normal brain function—a long-term consequence referred to as chemo-brain.[14]

PHYSIOLOGIC PROCESSES AND CONSEQUENCES

One of the most distinctive features of humans that distinguishes us from all other forms of life on earth is our advanced cognitive abilities. Cognitive development occurs predominantly from infancy through adolescence. Less dramatic development and maintenance of cognition occurs during adulthood. Cognitive impairment or intellectual loss is not a part of normal aging; rather, it is indicative of disease.[13] Older adults have been found to retrieve information from memory more slowly and to learn more slowly but this appears to be an issue of speed not of ability.

Our ability to reason, function intellectually, express personality, and purposefully interact with the external environment is a result of a highly advanced brain. The brain weighs about 3 pounds and has the consistency of thick custard. Optimal brain function depends on the continuous perfusion of oxygenated and nutrient-rich blood. Decreases in oxygen and glucose supply as well as electrolyte and acid-base imbalances significantly impair cognitive function.

The brain is responsible for multiple processes, including those that involve purposeful thought and responses and those that are automated and occur without purposeful thought (such as breathing, heart rate, reflexes, hormonal control, temperature regulation, and sensory regulation). Understanding of cognition and its anatomic and physiologic base is limited although significant insights have occurred in recent years as a result of technologic advancements.[2] The major anatomic areas that have been identified as playing a key role in specific cognitive functions are presented in Table 31-2.[2,15, 16]

Consequences

The consequences of cognitive impairment can be devastating for the affected person and also for family and friends. Delirium is frightening for those close to the patient because of the nature of the symptoms and because of the often life-threatening nature

TABLE 31-2	COGNITIVE FUNCTION AND ASSOCIATED ANATOMIC LOCATION IN THE BRAIN
COGNITIVE FUNCTION	**ANATOMIC LOCATION**
Memory	
• Declarative episodic memory	• Hippocampus
• Declarative semantic memory	• Medial thalamus
• Immediate memory/attention	• Temporoparietal association cortices
• Working memory	• Primary auditory or visual cortex
• Procedural memory	• Lateral frontal cortex
	• Basal ganglia, association neocortices
Language	
• Receptive language function	• Auditory association areas: posterior superior temporoparietal supramarginal gyrus
• Expressive language function	• Lateral inferior posterior frontal lobes
Visuospatial Cognition	• Occipital lobe, inferior temporal and posterior parietal lobes
Executive Function	• Network of brain regions anchored by prefrontal and anterior lobe neocortex

of the precipitating factor. Other types of cognitive impairment impact functional ability and can affect the person's capacity for independent living and normal social interaction. The need for assistive services can range from help with some of the instrumental activities of daily living to constant supervision and complete care. Financial hardship and caregiver role strain can result.

Although understanding of cognitive processes from an anatomic and physiologic perspective is still in beginning stages, observable behaviors associated with altered cognition have been well documented, named, and defined. Common abnormalities of cognition are presented in Table 31-3.[2,5,17,18]

Delirium

Delirium is a disorder of disturbed consciousness and altered cognition. Awareness of the environment is dulled and ability to focus, sustain, and shift attention is reduced. Memory and judgment are impaired and disorientation may occur. Speech is rapid, rambling, and/or incoherent. Sudden, intense emotional swings, hallucinations, vivid dreams, and delusions may occur. Restlessness is common although in some cases activity may be reduced. Onset is rapid, occurring over hours or a few days. Symptoms may worsen in the evening. This phenomenon, known as sundowning syndrome, is most prominent in dementia but also can occur with delirium.

Delirium is the most frequent complication of hospitalization in the elderly population. It may also be the initial sign of life-threatening problems such as pneumonia, urosepsis, or myocardial infarction. Delirium can be reversible with treatment of the precipitating problem and management of related predisposing factors.[13,19,20]

Dementia

Dementia is a disorder in which progressive deterioration of all cognitive functions with little or no disturbance of consciousness or perception occurs over a period of months. Memory, judgment, calculation ability, attention span, and abstract thinking are impaired. Agnosia—a flat affect with slow, incoherent speech—and delusions also occur. Primary dementia is irreversible and not secondary to another disease. Secondary dementia occurs as a result of another disease process.[19]

Focal Cognitive Disorders

Focal cognitive disorders, unlike delirium and dementia, affect a single area of cognitive function. The area involved may be memory, language, visuospatial ability, or executive function.[5] A focal cognitive disorder involving memory is an amnestic disorder in the *DSM-IV*. With an amnestic disorder, a significant decline in the ability to learn and recall new information and to recall previously learned material occurs, resulting in impaired social and occupational function.[20]

ASSESSMENT

Characteristics of normal cognitive status vary with the individual's stage of development. In infants and young children, expected cognitive development is indicated by achievement of developmental milestones and developmental tasks with specialized age-appropriate tests of development used when indicated to determine developmental delays (see Concept 1). During the remaining lifespan, identification of new problems with cognition relies primarily on routine observations of health care providers, self-report, and report of family or others.

History

Assessment of cognitive functioning occurs as part of the health history interview. It begins with assessment of consciousness because unless the patient is fully aware of self and the environment, other cognitive assessments may not be valid. The patient is observed for wakefulness, alertness, and appropriate responses to introductions and to the environment as the health history interview is begun. The patient's speech pattern and content are noted and memory, logic, and judgment are assessed while the interview progresses. Questions related to cognition included in the interview relate to history of intracranial disease or trauma; substance abuse; use of medications that can impair cognition; environmental or occupational exposure to hazards such as lead or insecticides; presence of symptoms such as difficulty in forming words or saying what is meant, headache, behavior changes, or seizures suggestive of a brain disorder; unexplained emotional or behavioral changes; and any noticed change in memory or mental function. If any abnormalities are noted, a more specific cognitive assessment examination is performed.

Examination

Formal assessment of cognition tests attention, memory, judgment, insight, spatial perception, calculation, abstract reasoning, and thought process and content. Adults with normal cognition have an attention span and calculation ability adequate to complete a task such as counting

TABLE 31-3	COMMON COGNITIVE FUNCTIONAL ABNORMALITIES AND DEFINITIONS	
COGNITIVE AREA	**ABNORMALITY**	**DEFINITION**
Memory	Anterograde amnesia	Loss of ability to learn and recall new information in an ongoing basis
	Retrograde amnesia	Impaired ability to retrieve information from the past
Language	Aphasia	Language impairment at the conceptual level; may have difficulty with production or comprehension of language, or both
	Wernicke's aphasia	Impaired comprehension of both written and verbal language even understanding single words. Speech is fluent and person is unaware that words used are incorrect
	Broca's aphasia	Impaired language expression characterized by nonfluent, labored speech. Comprehension of language is intact
	Global aphasia	Both language reception and expression are impaired
	Anomia	Impaired ability to name places or objects. May have difficulty with sentence repetition although comprehension and expression abilities are basically intact
Visuospatial	Alexia	Impaired reading ability
	Agraphia	Inability to write
	Agnosia	Impaired ability to recognize objects or persons through sensory stimuli. May be visual, tactile, auditory, olfactory, or gustatory
	Object agnosia	Impaired ability to recognize visual forms
	Prosopagnosia	Impaired ability to recognize faces
	Simultanagnosia	Impaired ability to integrate complex visual scenes
	Apraxia	Inability to perform purposeful movements or manipulate objects although sensory and motor ability is intact
	Constructional apraxia	Inability to reproduce figures on paper
	Ideomotor apraxia	Inability to translate an idea into action
	Hemispatial (unilateral) neglect	Inability to process and perceive stimuli on one side of the body or the environment despite intact senses; results in a deficit in attention and awareness to the affected side
Calculation	Dyscalculia	Inability to perform calculations correctly
Abstract Reasoning	Conceptual concreteness	Inability to describe in abstractions, generalize, or apply principles
Thought Process and Content	Flight of ideas	Topic of speech changes within a sentence
	Confabulation	Making up answers without regard to facts
	Circumstantiality	Indirect speech characterized by countless details and explanations with resultant prolonged time to reach point
	Echolalia	Involuntary repetition of a word or sentence spoken by someone else
	Clanging	Use of meaningless, rhyming words
	Blocking	Unconscious interruption in the train of thought manifested as a sudden obstruction to the spontaneous flow of speech
	Pressured speech	Frantic, energetic, jumbled speech; speech trying to keep up with thoughts
	Word salad	Meaningless mixture of words or phrases

backwards from 100 by subtracting 7 each time; short-term memory allows functions such as repeating a list of 3 words after 5 minutes of other conversation; and long-term memory allows for correctly responding to questions about events occurring 24 hours or more in the past. Healthy adults can evaluate and respond appropriately in situations requiring judgment; demonstrate a realistic insight into self; state the abstract meaning of a metaphor appropriate to their culture; and exhibit logical, coherent, goal-directed thought processes based on reality. Adults with intact cognitive processes also exhibit spatial perception sufficient to allow copying of a simple shape without difficulty and identify right and left sides of the body. Familiar sounds are able to be identified. Table 31-4 presents the basic techniques used to assess cognitive abilities.

Diagnostic Tests

Diagnosis of cognitive impairment is based primarily on clinical evaluation—that is, on history and physical examination

findings including a Mini-Mental Status Examination. For delirium, a second short screening test called the Confusion Assessment Method (CAM) (CAM-ICU for patients who are unable to speak as a result of intubation) also is used.[13] There are no laboratory tests that diagnose cognitive impairment although laboratory tests are critical in determining the presence of associated disease. Brain imaging techniques such as magnetic resonance imaging (MRI) and positron emission tomography (PET) scans can identify some brain abnormalities such as intracranial tumors, the infarcts associated with vascular dementia, and frontotemporal lobe atrophy. However, their usefulness is limited in the majority of cases of cognitive impairment. Formal neuropsychometric testing by a neuropsychologist is needed for the identification of mild cases of cognitive impairment. Such testing uses more detailed standardized tests of memory and advanced methods of determining visuospatial function and can identify impairments missed on standard clinical evaluation.[5]

TABLE 31-4	BASIC TESTS OF COGNITIVE FUNCTION
COGNITIVE COMPONENT	**METHOD OF ASSESSMENT**
Attention and Immediate Recall	Two numbers are slowly stated and the patient is asked to repeat them as stated and then backwards. The process is repeated with 3 numbers and continues until 5 or 6 numbers are given. If the patient makes an error, a different set of the same number of digits is given. If two errors occur on the same number of digits, the test ends.
Attention and Concentration	The patient is asked to start with 100 and count backwards by subtracting 7 each time. If unable to subtract 7, the patient is asked to subtract 3.
Short-Term Memory	Three items are named and the patient is asked to repeat and remember them. After 5 min of continued conversation the patient is asked to repeat them again. If unable to repeat, a picture of a variety of items including those to be remembered is shown and the patient is asked to pick out the objects in question.
Long-Term Memory	Questions are asked about facts that have been in memory for at least 24 hours such as birth date or spouse's name. The examiner must be sure to have validated the correct answer to the question before asking it.
Judgment	A hypothetical situation, such as "You are driving on the highway when a police car with lights flashing pulls out and follows behind you," is presented and the patient asked what he or she would do. The appropriateness of the answer is evaluated.
Insight	The patient's realistic understanding of self is evaluated by asking a question about general health, life situation, methods of coping.
Spatial Perception	The patient is asked to copy a simple figure such as a circle, triangle, or a diamond. The patient is asked to draw a clock face with the numbers on it. With eyes closed, the patient is asked to identify a familiar sound such as running water or a cough. The patient is asked to identify right and left extremities or other body parts.
Calculation	Starting with 100, the patient is asked to add by 3's to 150.
Abstract Reasoning	The patient is asked to explain the meaning of a proverb or metaphor such as "All that glitters is not gold." The level of concreteness or abstraction of the response is noted.
Thought Process and Content	The patient's thinking as expressed in conversation is evaluated for coherence, relevance, logic, and organization.

CLINICAL MANAGEMENT

Primary Prevention

Promoting a healthy lifestyle—including optimal nutrition, exercise, social activity, regular medical care to prevent and/or manage chronic diseases, and avoidance of substance abuse and other high-risk behaviors—through teaching and community programs is basic to prevention across the spectrum of cognitive impairment. It is essential to healthy pregnancies, growth and development into adulthood, and healthy aging, decreasing vulnerability to delirium and vascular dementia.

Also important to primary prevention of cognitive impairment is genetic counseling related to risk for disorders characterized by impaired cognition. This ranges from pregnancy risks associated with advanced maternal age such as Down syndrome to available genetic testing for inherited disorders such as Huntington's disease, which could affect decisions about having children.

Primary prevention specific to delirium involves educating health care providers about changes in practice that can decrease vulnerability to the disorder. Practices that constitute risk factors for delirium, such as use of sleeping medications, use of urinary bladder catheters, and immobilization, need to be identified along with alternative methods of care.

Secondary Prevention (Screening)

The Mini-Mental State Exam (MMSE) is a standardized cognitive assessment tool commonly used across care settings to screen for dementia and delirium, to detect cognitive impairment occurring during illness, and to monitor response to treatment. The test consists of 11 cognitive tasks that cover the categories of time orientation, place orientation, immediate recall, short-term memory recall, serial 7's, reading, writing, drawing, and verbal/motor comprehension. The test takes 5 to 10 minutes and instructions for administration of the test are simple. The lower the score (out of a total of 30) the more severe the impairment. Individuals who score below 27 should be referred for further evaluation.[13]

Collaborative Interventions

Cognition is a critical consideration in virtually all areas of health care and for all members of the health care team. It is a critical element in communicating with the patient and in the determination of care.[21] It is also critical to discharge planning from acute care facilities and is one determinant of need for home care services or placement in a long term care facility.

Cognitive impairment predisposes to a wide range of adverse health care outcomes. These outcomes include falls, immobilization, dependency, institutionalization, and death. Cognitive impairment also complicates diagnosis and management of disease and requires additional caregivers to ensure safety.[22]

Treatment options are limited for the majority of patients with cognitive impairment. Precipitating trauma or disease is treated when possible but for many types of cognitive impairment, the disease process is not well understood and no treatments or only treatments with limited effectiveness are available. Nonetheless, management of cognitive impairment involves a multidisciplinary effort. Depending on the type and cause of the impairment, one or more of the following services may be required: nursing, medicine, physical therapy, occupational therapy, psychologic intervention, individual and/or family counseling, nutritional consulting, speech and language services, audiology services, home health or homemaker assistance community services such as day care, caregiver support groups, and assistive technologies.

General Management Strategies

Promoting adequate rest, sleep, fluid, nutrition, elimination, pain control, and comfort are essential elements of care for persons with cognitive impairment. Also of great importance is ensuring an appropriate level of environmental stimulation because excessive stimulation can create agitation and confusion whereas a lack of stimulation can result in sensory deprivation effects and withdrawal. If behavior is a problem, attempts should be made to identify and manage environmental triggers and use of physical and pharmacologic restraints should be avoided.[19]

Virtually all patients with cognitive impairment benefit from a predictable routine, consistent caregivers, simple instructions, eye contact, and the presence of familiar people and objects. If needed, sensory aids such as eyeglasses and hearing aids should be used consistently to maximize accurate sensory input. To the extent possible, patients should be involved in self-care and decision making even if the latter is limited to deciding which of two shirts to wear or whether to drink milk or juice. Verbal reorientation to time and place should be provided if needed and a clock and calendar should be within easy vision. For patients with delirium or otherwise agitated, a private room, soft music, relaxation tapes, or massage can be helpful.

Safety is a priority concern for all patients with cognitive impairment. Precise interventions needed vary with the person's age, developmental status, and degree of impairment. Patients should not drive, use machinery, or handle firearms, and the environment should be kept free of potential hazards. Supervision is generally needed with activities such as cooking or taking medications. If the patient wanders, an identification tag or bracelet should be worn or, if appropriate, a wander guard device should be used.

Pharmacologic Agents

In the management of patients with cognitive impairment, pharmacologic agents primarily treat associated diseases and control behavioral alterations such as sleeplessness, anxiety, agitation, and depression.[23] In the management of Alzheimer's disease (AD), however, pharmacologic therapy is aimed at maintaining cognitive function and slowing disease progression by regulating neurotransmitters in the brain. The two classes of drugs used in the treatment of AD are the cholinesterase inhibitors and a glutamate receptor antagonist. The three cholinesterase inhibitors approved by the FDA for the treatment of AD are donepezil (Aricept), rivastigmine

(Exelon), and galantamine (Razadyne). All three of these drugs have been shown to help maintain memory, thinking, and speaking skills for a few months to a few years in *some* patients with mild to moderate AD; donepezil also is used in severe AD. The glutamate receptor antagonist memantine (Namenda) has been shown to delay functional decline in moderate to severe disease.[24]

Caregiver Support

Engaging family members or significant others in goal setting and care planning also is essential. Advanced planning should be encouraged and caregiver needs for education and support should be recognized and addressed. Information should be provided about support groups, respite options, day care, and other community services.

Nursing Interventions

Nursing practice has four major dimensions of concern relative to an individual's cognitive status. The first is recognition of risk for impaired cognition, the second is cognitive assessment, and the third is the planning and delivery of individualized care appropriate to level of cognitive ability. Evaluation of outcomes is the fourth dimension.

The concern of the professional nurse with the patient's cognitive status is underscored by the NANDA-I nursing diagnostic categories related to *Disturbed thought processes, Impaired memory, Acute confusion, Risk for acute confusion,* and *Chronic confusion*[25] as well as the Nursing Outcomes Classification (NOC) outcomes[26] and the Nursing Interventions Classification (NIC) interventions[27] related to each.

INTERRELATED CONCEPTS

The human person is a complex integrated whole that is greater than the sum of its parts. It follows therefore that concepts used to describe aspects of the human person do not represent isolated phenomena but rather phenomena that interrelate with one another. The strength and direction of the impact of one conceptual phenomenon on another varies with the central concept under consideration. Because cognition depends on the interplay of multiple elements within the physical, psychologic, and social dimensions, and because it allows for purposeful interaction with the environment, a multitude of concepts can be identified as influencing and/or being influenced by it. Figure 31-2 depicts the most prominent of these interrelationships. The physiologically focused concepts of **Mobility, Nutrition, Glucose regulation, Gas exchange, Perfusion, Fluid and electrolyte balance,** and **Acid-base balance** have a clearly reciprocal relationship with cognition. These concepts are represented by the ovals surrounding the upper half of the cognition conception and double-headed arrows because of their mutual interaction with it. The concepts of **Functional ability** and **Development** are shown at the very bottom of the figure with arrows pointing from cognition to them because of the primarily unidirectional relationship of these concepts.

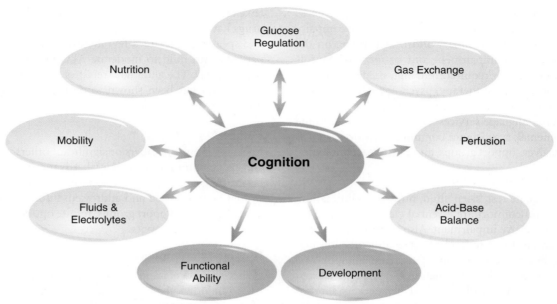

FIGURE 31-2 Cognition and Interrelated Concepts.

MODEL CASE

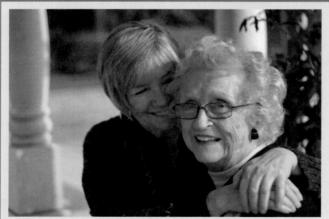

As part of a community health awareness event, a community health nurse has presented a program on problems associated with aging and their management; the nurse is available for meetings with individuals who have questions or concerns. One of the persons requesting a meeting was a middle-age woman named Karen who expressed concern over her mother's condition and asked for guidance. Karen explained that her mother, Ruby Long, is 79 years old and has no known medical conditions. Ruby lives with Karen and has become increasingly difficult to manage over the last 8 to 10 months. Karen states that her mother has become lax in her hygiene, is very forgetful of details of recent events, seems to be only focused on herself and unconcerned with anyone else's needs, is unwilling to try new things or go new places, and has lost interest in activities that she formally enjoyed. Karen also tells the nurse that her mother sometimes makes what appear to be poor decisions, has trouble managing money, and becomes very

upset if any mistakes are mentioned. Upon further questioning, the nurse learns that Ruby Long wears eyeglasses (last eye exam 2 years ago) and has difficulty hearing (but does not use a hearing aid). Ruby has a family physician; her last visit was about 1 year ago. Karen tells the nurse that her grandparents and two aunts on her mother's side had dementia, although she is not exactly sure exactly what caused dementia in her relatives.

The nurse encourages Karen to arrange for Ruby to have a complete physical examination to rule out a physical cause of the behaviors and to determine the presence of any comorbidities, including a hearing and vision examination (to determine if the observed problems are resulting from changes in sensory perception). The nurse stresses the importance of maintaining a safe environment for Ruby. The nurse also discusses with Karen the possibility that she will need to plan for management of life affairs, such as power of attorney and advance directives. Finally, the nurse refers Karen to a local community resource for further education and support for caregivers.

Case Analysis

The behaviors described on the part of the mother are consistent with signs of cognitive impairment. There are two major risk factors present for dementia: advanced age and family history. Current sensory status is uncertain: vision has not been recently checked, hearing has not been tested, and both age and history suggest a possibility of impairment. Sensory input is a determinant of cognition. Physical disease could be responsible for the behaviors; no physical examination has been done in more than 1 year. There is a clear potential for caregiver role strain implicit in the situation and in the daughter's words "increasingly difficult to manage."

EXEMPLARS

Common causes of each of the major cognitive disorders are presented in Box 31-1. It is important to emphasize that there are wide differences in opinion about the best way to categorize impairments in cognition. Box 31-1 includes conditions associated with mental retardation. It is recognized these are commonly considered developmental conditions; however, they are all based on impairments in cognition. Thought disorders are also closely related to the

concept of cognition. Two types of thought disorders are *disorders of form* (which is formal thought disorder) and *disorders of content*, which is delusion. Formal thought disorder is a major symptom of schizophrenia and other psychotic mental illness[28]; these are presented in greater detail in the **Psychosis** and **Mood and affect** concepts within this textbook.

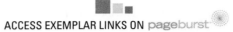

ACCESS EXEMPLAR LINKS ON pageburst

■■■ BOX 31-1   EXEMPLARS OF COGNITION

Delirium
Delirium Attributable to General Medical Conditions
- Dehydration
- Electrolyte or acid-base imbalance
- Brain injury
- Seizure activity
- Infection (systemic or intracranial)
- Hypoglycemia
- Hypotension
- Hypoxia
- Fever
- Pain
- Sleep deprivation

Substance-Induced Delirium
- Alcohol intoxication
- Hallucinogens
- Adverse effect of medications

Dementia
Primary Dementia
- Alzheimer's disease
- Vascular dementia complex
- Pick's disease
- Creutzfeldt-Jakob disease
- Huntington's chorea
- Lewy body
- Dementia attributable to other general medical conditions

Secondary Dementia
- AIDS dementia
- Viral encephalitis
- Pernicious anemia
- Folic acid deficiency
- Korsakoff's syndrome
- Parkinson's disease associated dementia
- Brain injury
- Hypothyroidism

Chemical Exposure–Induced Dementia
- Drug abuse
- Alcohol

- Lead
- Mercury
- Carbon monoxide
- Insecticide

Amnestic Disorders
- Stroke
- Traumatic brain injury
- Brain tumor
- Substance abuse
- Toxins (lead, mercury, pesticides)
- Amnestic disorder not otherwise specified

Aphasic Disorders
- Aphasia
- Broca's aphasia
- Global aphasia
- Anomia
- Ideomotor apraxia

Mental Retardation (Intellectual Disability)
Chromosomal Abnormalities
- Down syndrome
- Fragile X syndrome
- Prader-Willi syndrome

Genetic Conditions
- Galactosemia
- Hunter's syndrome
- Phenylketonuria
- Rett syndrome
- Tay-Sachs disease

Other Conditions
- Encephalitis
- Meningitis
- Congenital rubella
- Congenital toxoplasmosis
- Congenital hypothyroidism
- Fetal alcohol syndrome
- Malnutrition

REFERENCES

1. Wiley J, Jee BD: Cognition: overview and recent trends. In Aukrust VG, editor: *Learning and cognition in education*, New York, 2011, Academic Press/Elsevier, pp 3–8.
2. Baars BJ, Gage NM: *Cognition, brain and consciousness. Introduction to cognitive neuroscience*, ed 2, New York, 2010, Academic Press/Elsevier.
3. Neisser U: *Cognitive psychology*, New York, 1967, Meredith.
4. Magnussen S, Brennan T: Memory. In Baars BJ, Gage NM, editors: *Cognition, brain and consciousness. Introduction to cognitive neuroscience*, ed 2, New York, 2010, Academic Press/Elsevier, pp 85–91.
5. Aminoff MJ: Regional cerebral dysfunction: higher mental functions. In Goldman L, Ausiello D, editors: *Cecil medicine*, ed 23, Philadelphia, 2008, Saunders, pp 2262–2266.
6. Knopman DS: Regional cerebral dysfunction: higher mental functions. In Goldman L, Ausiello D, editors: *Cecil medicine*, ed 23, Philadelphia, 2008, Saunders, pp 2662–2667.
7. American Psychiatric Association: *Diagnostic and statistical manual of mental disorders*, ed 4, Washington, DC, 2000, Author. text revision.
8. Yaffe K: *Arch Neurol* 68:631–636, May 2011. News release, American Medical Association, ©2011 WebMD.
9. Stibich M: *Preventing cognitive impairment: risk factors differ for men and women.* Retrieved from About.com, updated Jan 4, 2010.
10. Brooks M: Long-term pesticide exposure linked to cognitive decline, *Medscape News Today*, Dec 29, 2010. Retrieved from medscape.com>Medscaped Medical News > Neurology.
11. Hockenberry MJ, Wilson DW: *Wong's essentials of pediatric nursing*, ed 8, St Louis, 2009, Mosby/Elsevier.
12. Mild Cognitive Impairment: *Risk factors.* Retrieved from mayoclinic.com/health/mild-cognitive-impairment-1D5005531DSection=risk-factors.
13. Inouye SK: Neuropsychiatric aspects of aging. In Goldman L, Ausiello D, editors: *Cecil medicine*, ed 23, Philadelphia, 2008, Saunders, pp 128–131.
14. *Chemo brain*: Retrieved from mayoclinic.com/health/chemo-brain/DS01109.
15. Goldman L, Ausiello D, editors: *Cecil medicine*, ed 23, Philadelphia, 2008, Saunders.
16. Seidel HM, Ball JW, Dains JE, et al: *Mosby's guide to physical examination*, ed 6, St Louis, 2007, Mosby.
17. Estes MEZ: *Health assessment & physical examination*, ed 4, Florence, Ky, 2010, Delmar CENGAGE Learning.
18. Jarvis C: *Physical examination & health assessment*, ed 5, Philadelphia, 2008, Saunders.
19. Inouye SK: Delirium and other mental status problems in the older patient. In Goldman L, Ausiello D, editors: *Cecil medicine*, ed 23, Philadelphia, 2008, Saunders, pp 131–138.
20. Varcarolis EM, Halter MJ: *Foundations of psychiatric mental health nursing: a clinical approach*, ed 6, Philadelphia, 2010, Saunders/Elsevier.
21. Nursing care for the cognitively impaired—the role of NVC: *J Nurs.* Retrieved Feb 1, 2007 from http://www.asrn.org/journal-nursing/287-nurse-care-for-the-cognitively-impaired-the-role-of-nvc.html.
22. Gottschalk LA: Cognitive impairment associated with acute or chronic disease, *Gen Hosp Psychiatry* 1(4):344–346, 1979.
23. American Association of Geriatric Psychiatry: *Position statement: principles of care for patients with dementia resulting from Alzheimer's disease.* Retrieved from www.aagponline.org/prof/position_caredmnalz.asp.
24. Alzheimer's Disease Education & Referral Center, National Institutes of Health, National Institute on Aging: *Treatment of AD* www.nia.nih.gov/Alzheimers/AlzheimersInformation/Treatment/. Retrieved from updated Dec 8, 2010.
25. NANDA-I: *Nursing diagnoses: definitions and classification, 2009-2010*, Philadelphia, 2009, Author.
26. Moorhead S, Johnson M, Maas M: *Nursing outcomes classification (NOC)*, ed 3, St Louis, 2004, Mosby.
27. McCloskey-Dochterman JC, Bulechek GM: *Nursing interventions classification*, ed 4, St Louis, 2004, Mosby.
28. Barrera A, Berrios GE: Formal thought disorder, *Psychopathology* 42:264–269, 2009.

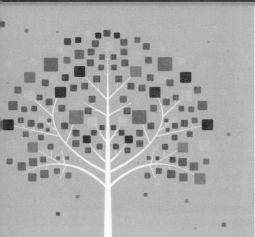

Psychosis

Jenny Vacek

M ental health disorders are among the most common problems in the United States. Psychosis presents in multiple settings and is associated with many mental health problems. Additionally, it can occur secondary to substance use, substance withdrawal, toxin exposure, postpartum states, and medical conditions. For this reason, it is imperative that nurses are aware of conditions placing a person at risk and recognizing when psychosis is developing or has developed so that appropriate interventions are immediately instituted. The purpose of this concept analysis is to present basic elements for application into practice.

DEFINITION(S)

For the purposes of this concept analysis, psychosis is defined as a *change in the brain that disrupts a person's interpretation and/or experience of the world secondary to complex neurobiological changes; hallucinations, delusions, and/or disorganized thinking are hallmark characteristics.*[1,2] A hallucination is a false distortion in perception and can be visual, auditory, gustatory, olfactory, or tactile. A delusion is a false fixed belief. Psychotic episodes can be either acute or chronic dependent on causative factors. Acute psychosis is defined as reversible and may last from weeks to months. To the contrary, chronic psychosis occurs when symptoms are primarily irreversible.

SCOPE AND CATEGORIES

Psychosis is associated with multiple conditions. Five overarching categories are useful to communicate the broad application of this concept. These categories include psychotic disorders, mood disorders, anxiety disorders, substance abuse, and medical disorders and treatments (Figure 32-1). A literature search does not reflect specific incidences of psychosis for each of the categories.

Psychotic Disorders

This is a broad category that includes schizophrenic conditions, psychotic disorders not otherwise specified, and personality disorders.

Schizophrenic Conditions

Schizophrenia is a serious, complex, and chronic neurobiological brain illness. This disorder can affect all persons regardless of ethnic group, race, or gender. Age of onset can occur in childhood and adolescence and varies between men and women. Modal age of onset for men is 18 to 25; modal age of onset for women is 25 to 35.[1] Schizophrenia is defined as having two or more of the following positive or negative features during a 1-month period. Positive symptoms—a distortion or exaggeration of normal behavior—entail

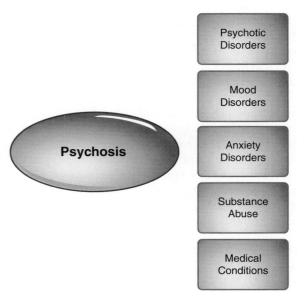

FIGURE 32-1 Categories of Conditions Associated with Psychosis.

hallucinations and delusions. Negative symptoms—a loss or diminution of normal function—consist of disorganized speech, grossly catatonic or disorganized behavior, affective flattening, alogia, avolition, apathy, anhedonia, asociality, and attentional deficit. Five subtypes of schizophrenia are classified according to predominant symptomatology.[1] Several other inorganic-related psychotic disorders with a lower incidence and varying degrees of general psychiatric clinical representation also exist.

Psychotic Disorder Not Otherwise Specified

This type of psychotic symptomatology includes disorders where insufficient or contradictory information does not qualify for a diagnosis that meets the criteria for any other specific psychotic disorder. Psychotic disorders not otherwise specified can occur across the lifespan with the exception of postpartum psychosis, which emerges exclusively during child-bearing years.[1]

Personality Disorder

Personality disorders (PDs) represent "an enduring pattern of inner experience and behavior that deviates markedly from the expectations of the culture of the individual who exhibits it."[1, p685] Schizotypal is a PD that presents with psychosis. General symptomatology comprises eccentric behavior, intense anxiety in interpersonal relationships, lack of close friends, paranormal events, magical thinking, and bizarre fantasies. Hallmark features are perceptual distortions, somatic delusions, bizarre speaking/speech, and paranoid/suspicious ideation.[1]

Mood Disorders

Mood disorders are a group of psychiatric diagnoses in which the underlying disturbance is a persistent emotional state that impacts mood and behavioral and physical responses. Bipolar disorders fluctuate between moods of depression, mania, or mixed depression/mania. Major depressive disorder and bipolar disorder are the primary mood disorders that are at times present with psychosis. Major depressive disorder manifests with symptoms of depressed mood, significant weight loss or weight gain, a decrease in pleasure or interest in most activities, hypersomnia or insomnia, loss of energy or fatigue, psychomotor retardation or agitation, excessive worry, inappropriate guilt, decreased ability to concentrate or think, and/or suicidal behaviors. Bipolar disorder fluctuates between moods of depression, mania, or mixed. Symptoms of mania include affect of extreme elevation, grandiosity, inflated self-esteem, decreased sleep, pressured speech, flight of ideas, excessive participation in pleasurable activities, and/or an increase in goal-directed activity[1] (see Mood and Affect concept for further information).

Anxiety Disorders

Anxiety disorders are characterized by a combination of psychologic, behavioral, physiologic, and cognitive symptoms. Posttraumatic stress disorder (PTSD) is the only one of the anxiety problems that presents with psychotic features.

Posttraumatic stress disorder is the encounter of a significant trauma or stressor that is outside the normal range of experience; it is succeeded by subjective reexperiences of the event. The disorder affects all age groups; however, symptomatology varies in children. Trauma that precedes PTSD involves criminal attacks, interpersonal violence, terrorist attacks, natural catastrophes, and military combat. Symptomatology of PTSD entails flashbacks of intrusive images, perceptions, or thoughts (in children the trauma may be expressed in thematic-related repetitive play); distressing dreams/nightmares of the event (in children the dream may replicate the actual trauma); psychologic affliction when exposed to memories; and/or physiologic hypervigilance when cues trigger a fragment or larger piece of the event. Patients diagnosed with PTSD, if psychotic, may experience hallucinations, illusions (false response and false perception to stimuli), and/or dissociative flashbacks in addition to the aforementioned symptoms.[1]

Substance Abuse
Substance-Induced Psychosis

Psychosis can be associated with substance use (alcohol, illicit drugs, and medications) and exposure to toxins.[1] Diagnosis of this problem occurs with presentation of prominent delusions and/or hallucinations (excluding patient who has insight into the delusion or hallucination) and when a history/physical examination and/or laboratory result validates the symptoms.[1]

Alcohol Withdrawal Syndrome

Alcohol withdrawal occurs among alcoholics who cease drinking and subsequently have a rapid decrease in blood alcohol levels. Mild to moderate symptoms include anxiety, insomnia, coarse hand tremors, and increased heart rate, blood pressure, and body temperature. Approximately 95% of withdrawal is limited to mild to moderate symptoms; however, in 3% to 5% of cases, hallucinations, delusions, and/or convulsions may occur.[3] Hallucinations are transient, and visual, tactile, or auditory in nature. Illusions may also emerge.[1]

Medical Conditions

Multiple medical conditions or treatments can result in psychosis—that is, psychosis can be secondary to disease states that are physiologic in nature or to side effects of medical treatments such as pharmacologic agents. A diagnosis of psychotic disorder attributable to a general medical disorder is made when the presentation of prominent hallucinations and/or delusions and data from the history/physical examination and/or lab findings and/or diagnostic testing confirm that the psychosis is organic in nature. Box 32-1 presents many of the medical conditions and medications with side effects that may manifest with psychosis.

RISK FACTORS

All persons are at risk for psychosis regardless of age, gender, race, and/or ethnicity. Approximately 3% of the population is at risk for any episode of psychosis, acute or chronic.[2] A study

BOX 32-1   MEDICAL CONDITIONS AND MEDICATIONS ASSOCIATED WITH PSYCHOSIS

Medical Conditions

- Brain injury
- Neurologic disease
- Hepatic disease
- Renal disease
- Autoimmune disease
- Fluid/electrolyte imbalances
- Huntington's chorea
- Epilepsy
- Migraines
- Hyperthyroidism
- Hypothyroidism
- Hypoxia
- Hypoglycemia
- Central nervous system infections

Medications

- Analgesics
- Anticholinergics
- Anticonvulsants
- Antihistamines
- Antihypertensives, cardiovascular
- Antimicrobials
- Antiparkinsonians
- Corticosteroids
- Muscle relaxants
- Gastrointestinal medications
- Antidepressants
- Chemotherapeutic agents
- Disulfiram

From American Psychiatric Association: *Diagnostic and statistical manual of mental disorders*, ed 4, Washington, DC, 2000, Author.

by Castagnini and colleagues reported an incidence of acute and transient psychosis to be 9.6% per 100,000.[4] Personal risk factors include impaired physical or mental health, substance and alcohol abuse, stress intolerance, ineffective coping mechanisms, and prodromal states. Psychosis can occur at any age across the lifespan, although the first onset is most likely to occur between 12 and 25 years.[5]

A literature review supports no conclusive predisposing factors for psychosis in general. However, a large body of research regarding predictors of schizophrenia exists. McFarlane[6] identifies genetic predisposition as one risk factor; candidate genes include neuregulin, dystrobrevin binding protein, G72, G30, RGS4, serotonin receptor gene, and dopamine receptor gene. Other biologic and social risk factors have been proposed through research studies: urban residence; trauma exposure; chronic cannabis use; family-rearing problems, such as emotional and communication problems, immigration, and ethnic and racial discrimination; older paternal age (fathers more than 55 years old); maternal issues, such as Rh incompatibility, multiparous births, prenatal maternal infection (rubella, *Toxoplasma*, herpes simplex, influenza, rubella), and birth during the winter.[6]

PHYSIOLOGIC PROCESSES AND CONSEQUENCES

Physiologic Processes

The pathophysiologic process of psychosis is dependent on etiology. Illicit drug use can affect various areas of neurotransmission regulation in regions of the brainstem, limbic system, and cerebral cortex.[7] The precise neurochemical impact is dependent on the substance used. For example, research indicates that psychotic features in cocaine and methamphetamine use are correlated with dysregulation of dopamine; psychotic states in chronic users of cannabinoids are associated with high levels of tetrahydrocannabinol.[7] Psychosis attributable to medical disorders is complicated; etiology is secondary to the disease process itself that results in the interplay of neurobiological, metabolic, immunologic, and/or endocrine changes.

Physiologic processes of schizophrenia are complex and are not well understood. Current biochemical hypotheses suggest involvement of many neurotransmitters as important contributors to the neuropathophysiology of schizophrenia. Dysregulation of each plays a specific role: serotonin, acetylcholine, glutamate, N-methyl-D-aspartate, and γ-aminobutyric acid (GABA). The dopamine theory continues to be one of the most eminent of theories on the cause of schizophrenia; it assumes symptoms of this illness are directly due to the dysfunction of dopamine.[8]

Consequences

Consequences of Acute Psychosis

Specific consequences of acute psychosis are largely dependent on etiologic factors. In many cases acute psychotic episodes are reversible, and pose no residual. However, psychotic states can result in social withdrawal, sleep disturbances, impaired memory, attention deficits, anxiety, decreased motivation, anhedonia, unusual/odd behaviors, difficulty with activities of daily living, diminished sense of smell, decreased tolerance to stress, and increased sensory sensitivity.[2] The risk for violence to self and others is increased in psychotic states. A recent study by Robinson and colleagues reported that persons with first-episode psychosis demonstrate a high risk for suicidal attempts[9]: 21% of participants made a suicide attempt, and of these attempts 19.7% were successful. The risk for violence to others is also increased and may be related to command hallucinations and paranoia. A recent study by Large and Nielssen concluded that a substantial number of patients in first-episode psychosis commit an act of violence—violence, 35%; serious violence, 17%; and severe violence, 6%—before seeking treatment.[10]

Consequences of Chronic Psychosis

Consequences of chronic psychosis are best understood when examining the severe impact of the disease state schizophrenia. Problems occur at the patient, family, and community level. Persons with schizophrenia experience high rates of recidivism, homelessness, incarceration, joblessness, and long-term disability.[11] It is the fifth leading cause of premature mortality and disability.[6] Lifetime expectancy is shortened by 25 years primarily because of cancer, heart disease, and suicide.[6] Injury and risk for violence to self and others is a concern. Ten percent of persons with schizophrenia, specifically young males, have completed suicide.[12] Family members struggle with the burden of caring for these patients. Schizophrenia is costly to society. The lifetime total cost of one case of schizophrenia is estimated at $10,000,000.[6]

ASSESSMENT

Assessment of the patient who manifests symptoms of psychosis includes a comprehensive history and physical examination, mental status examination (MSE), and diagnostic testing depending on the history and clinical manifestations. Analysis and interpretation of data facilitate determination of the etiologic basis for psychosis whether it is due to psychiatric illness, substance use/abuse, alcohol withdrawal, and/or organic illness.

History

The nurse collects data related to past and current medical problems, substance use, medication regimen, allergies, over-the-counter medications, appetite and sleep patterns, sexual functioning, exposure to toxins, and past or current injuries. Depending on the severity of the psychotic state, the patient may be a poor historian; data may need to be collected from other resources. Patients who present in psychotic states may have a history of a psychiatric illness, medical disorder/brain trauma, and/or recent substance abuse/use. A history of general day-to-day functioning may be impaired as evidenced by nutritional deficits, disrupted sleep, and/or deficits in self-care. Patients may report noncompliance with prescribed psychotropic medication because of cognitive impairment and/or untoward side effects. A social history may indicate withdrawal or isolation from family or friends, and/or problems in academic or occupational functioning. Persons with schizophrenia may report profound asociality, avolition (avoidance), and anhedonia (inability to feel pleasure).

Physical Assessment

A physical assessment that incorporates a systems approach is conducted to determine if underlying conditions exist that may explain the psychotic behavior. The systems approach includes neurologic, respiratory, cardiovascular, gastrointestinal, urinary, reproductive, and musculoskeletal systems. Also included is a mental status examination (MSE). The mental status assessment is the cornerstone to assessing psychosis. The MSE is described in detail in this textbook in the Mood and Affect concept.

Psychotic states may be evidenced in patient presentation: disheveled look, unusual attire, inappropriate dress, poor hygiene, poor eye contact, and/or older than stated age. The patient may report his or her mood as being apathetic (as observed in schizophrenia), elated, depressed, angry, anxious, or agitated. Suicidal and/or homicidal ideation may be present. Because of the high incidence of suicide in persons with psychosis, a suicide screening is essential. The nurse

---

BOX 32-2 THOUGHT PROCESS INDICATORS

- **Word salad:** unrelated series of words
- **Thought blocking:** train of thought has a sudden halt during a sentence
- **Perseveration:** excessive involuntary repetition in an activity, idea, or response (e.g., movement, speech)
- **Neologisms:** formation of new words or a mixture of other words
- **Loose associations:** lack of logical relationship between ideas and thoughts, resulting in speech that is unfocused or vague
- **Flight of ideas:** speech is overproductive and manifested by jumping from one topic to another; ideas are fragmented
- **Circumstantial:** speech and thought are related to unwarranted and excessive detail that may or may not be relevant to the question; an answer is eventually provided
- **Tangential:** speech and thought are associated with unnecessary and excessive detail that may or may not be relevant to the question; an answer to the question is not provided

From Stuart GW, Laraia MT, editors: *Principles and practice of psychiatric nursing*, ed 8, p 112, St Louis, 2005, Elsevier/Mosby.

may observe a flat, incongruent, labile, or apathetic affect.[13] A flat affect may be related to the mimic of bradykinesia, an extrapyramidal side effect of psychotropic medication. Psychomotor agitation or retardation, compulsions, hyperactivity, and/or catatonic stupor or catatonic excitability (observed primarily in schizophrenia) may be present. Rate of speech may be slow or rapid, with soft or loud volume. Alogia (observed primarily in schizophrenia), slurring of words, stuttering, or odd accents may be present.[13] Overlapped in Boxes 32-2 and 32-3 are thought content and thought process indicators that reflect variations in delusions and disorganized thought. The patient may report illusions and/or hallucinations. Level of consciousness may be altered; impairment in memory, level of concentration, calculation, judgment, and/or insight may be evident. Attention deficit is also a symptom.[13]

Diagnostic Tests

There are no specific diagnostic tests used to confirm psychosis in the way that other medical conditions can be verified. However, diagnostic tests are useful to detect conditions that contribute to psychosis.

Laboratory Tests

There are many laboratory tests used to identify disorders associated with psychotic features. Infectious disorders can result in psychosis; thus a complete blood count, urinalysis, or a spinal fluid analysis could be used. Blood chemistry tests can uncover an electrolyte imbalance such as hyponatremia that could contribute to acute psychosis. Thyroid, liver, and kidney function studies can confirm multiple conditions associated with organ dysfunction that can lead to psychosis. Immunologic testing and/or serologic screening can identify

BOX 32-3   THOUGHT CONTENT INDICATORS

Delusion

- **Religious:** belief that one is highly favored over others by a higher power, and/or one is sent to do deeds for the higher power
- **Somatic:** belief that parts of or one's entire body is diseased or deranged
- **Grandiose:** unrealistic belief that one holds special powers
- **Paranoid:** unrealistic belief and suspicion that is dominated by mistrust of others; and that others are "out to get them"
- **Thought broadcasting:** belief that others can read one's thoughts
- **Nihilistic ideas:** thoughts of hopelessness and/or feelings of self nonexistence
- **Magical thinking:** belief that one's thoughts make events occur, a distortion in relationship of cause and effect
- **Thought insertion:** belief that others are placing thoughts into one's mind
- **Ideas of reference:** unrealistic misconception that external events have a direct personal reference to oneself
- **Hypochondriasis:** morbid preoccupation with bodily functioning
- **Depersonalization:** the feeling one has of complete loss of self-identity; surroundings are strange, unreal, detached
- **Obsession:** one experiences untoward, unwelcome repetitive thinking of an emotion or impulse
- **Phobia:** intense fear (specific or social) accompanied by anxiety

From Stuart GW, Laraia MT: *Principles and practice of psychiatric nursing*, ed 8, p 112, St Louis, 2005, Elsevier/Mosby.

syphilis and/or human immunodeficiency virus that can cause dementia-related psychosis. Urine and blood drug screening can confirm substance-induced psychosis by identifying the presence of amphetamines, barbiturates, benzodiazepines, cannabinoids, ethanol, cocaine, phencyclidine, and opiates.

Imaging

Neuroimaging techniques used to conform or exclude the presence of organic brain disorder include computed tomography (CT) and magnetic resonance imaging (MRI); both allow for visualization of brain structures. The CT scan and/or MRI can detect cerebral vascular disease, brain tumors and/or trauma, etiology of seizures, intracranial infections, and cerebral changes associated with dementia. Electroencephalography (EEG) studies detect epilepsy and intracranial infections or tumors. Researchers are currently using CT scans, positron emission tomography (PET), and single-photon emission computed tomography (SPECT) to assess neurochemical brain functions in persons with psychotic disorders.[8]

CLINICAL MANAGEMENT

Because psychosis is not a medical condition, in itself, but rather results from multiple conditions the clinical management is directly related to the underlying condition(s). There are, however, general interventions that apply regardless of the underlying condition.

Primary Prevention

Primary prevention involves prevention of disease. For psychosis, primary prevention is aimed at reducing known risk factors for conditions that lead to psychosis. Research indicates that evidence-based programs can significantly decrease early use of alcohol and illicit drugs; these models work by decreasing risk factors for substance abuse and addressing protective factors.[7] In 2007 the Robert Wood Johnson Foundation initiated the national Early Detection and Intervention for the Prevention of Psychosis Program (EDIPPP); this program was designed for screening, consultation, and treatment of children and adolescents showing early symptoms of risk factors.[2]

Prodromal phase of psychotic disorders is a term used restrictively in pediatric and adolescent populations who manifest prodromal symptoms of psychosis that may later evolve into psychotic disorders. Examples of symptoms that occur during the prodromal phase consist of a recent history of social withdrawal, cognitive decline, history of inattentiveness, and psychotic-like symptoms.[14] In general, it can take up to 2 years after the initial signs of the illness to occur before treatment is sought.[15] Early intervention may reduce the sequel of symptoms of psychosis that present, if untreated, after the prodromal phase. Treatment during the prodromal phase includes outreach programs, psychoeducation, screening/referrals, individual/family therapy, school support, employment assistance, and certified peer support.[5] In a recent study, researchers reported that antipsychotics had improved outcomes in youths with a shorter period of untreated psychosis, and were related to fewer patients transitioning from "at risk mental states" into schizophrenia. In addition, the researchers concluded that mood stabilizers, anxiolytics, and antidepressants successfully treat target symptoms in the prodrome.[14]

Secondary Prevention (Screening)

Secondary prevention involves screening for early detection of disease. Screening for substance abuse is essential, and often done among persons who manifest with psychosis. Various screening tools are used in prodromal states. McFarlane[6] cites three specific screening tools for prodromal schizophrenia. Two of these, the Structured Interview for the Prodromal Syndrome and the Comprehensive Assessment for At-Risk Mental States, identify the risk for psychosis in three specific categories: episodes of brief psychosis (1 week to 1 month); attenuated psychotic symptoms; and having a schizotypal PD with recent functional decline and/or a first-degree relative with a psychotic disorder. The Scale for the Assessment of Basic Symptoms is identified as a tool that assesses several elements of a thought disorder (i.e., perseverance, pressure, blockage, interference).[6] The Brief Psychiatric Rating Scale is a reliable and valid tool that assesses a broad range of symptoms seen in psychotic relapse.[16]

Collaborative Interventions

There are several important interventions when caring for patients who are in psychotic states. The nurse should use face-to-face contact, decrease stimuli in the environment, and reorient the patient. It is important not to reinforce hallucinations or delusions; reasonable doubt should be expressed if the patient has hallucinations or delusions. Consistent caregivers are important because of issues of trust. Positive feedback is helpful when the patient's thinking and behavior are appropriate. Self-care neglect is also a problem. The patient's physical needs should be assessed regarding eating, bathing, and dressing. Clear, direct language in a nonhurried fashion is used to facilitate the patient to maintain general health, nutrition, and functional needs. Praise is important, and the nurse should gradually withdraw care as the patient becomes independent. Encouragement of nondestructive means to express feelings and manage tension/anxiety must be done. The patient should be provided opportunities to succeed at tasks, activities, and interactions. The patient should be facilitated to set goals regarding behavior. Positive feedback is important with emphasis on the patient's strengths and abilities.[17] Because of the potential for maladaptive coping, close monitoring is needed is the patient is a danger to self or others. Protocols such as suicide or homicidal precautions need immediate implementation (i.e., one-on-one contact) and seclusion and/or restraints for potentially violent behaviors. Psychotic patients whose agitation is beginning to escalate should be medicated before behavior worsens, as prescribed with as-needed anxiolytics and/or antipsychotics.

Treatment of patients who have chronic psychotic problems such as schizophrenia can be challenging. Schizophrenia has a high recidivism rate. Intervention during the relapse phase is imperative to reduce the severity of psychosis. There are five stages of relapse: stage 1, the overextension phase (patient feels overwhelmed, overloaded, and anxious); stage 2, restricted consciousness (anxiety is accompanied by depression), so withdrawal occurs; stage 3, disinhibition (psychotic features begin to develop); stage 4, psychotic disorganization (psychotic features are clearly noticeable and may intensify); and stage 5, psychotic resolution (psychotic features begin to resolve themselves as a result of prescribed medication).[13]

Pharmacokinetics

Antipsychotic agents are the primary treatment for psychosis when psychiatric illness is the underlying cause. In some cases, antipsychotics are used to treat acute and chronic psychosis secondary to substances or medically related illnesses. Antipsychotics are specifically used to treat positive and negative symptoms. Typical antipsychotics generally improve positive symptoms; atypical antipsychotics improve negative as well as positive symptoms.[13] Antipsychotics are used in pediatric as well as adult and geriatric populations. Extensive patient/significant other psychoeducation is imperative for patients prescribed antipsychotics.

Currently Federal Drug Administration (FDA) approved atypical antipsychotics include aripiprazole (Abilify), clozapine (Clozaril), olanzapine (Zyprexa, Zydis), olanzapine/fluoxetine (Symbyax), risperidone (Risperdal, and the long-acting Consta), ziprasidone (Geodon), and quetiapine (Seroquel). Examples of FDA-approved typical antipsychotics are haloperidol (Haldol), thioridazine hydrochloride (Mellaril), chlorpromazine hydrochloride (Thorazine), trifluoperazine hydrochloride (Stelazine), and fluphenazine (Prolixin).[18]

Side effects of antipsychotics include common side effects and major side effects. Many patients are noncompliant with prescribed treatments because of the nature and complexity of the untoward effects. Common side effects are anticholinergic (constipation, dry mouth, orthostatic hypotension, dizziness, tachycardia, nasal congestion, and urinary retention).[13] Drowsiness, skin rashes, menstrual issues, photosensitivity, weight gain, and metabolic syndrome can occur.[12]

Extrapyramidal side effects (EPS)—parkinsonism, acute dystonia, tardive dyskinesia, and akathisia—are serious and warrant immediate medical attention. Atypical antipsychotics are less likely to cause EPS than typical antipsychotics except when given in high doses.[1] Principle treatment of EPS may include decreasing the dose, adding a drug to treat EPS (e.g., diphenhydramine [Benadryl], benztropine [Cogentin]), using a drug with lower EPS profile, and giving the patient support and education.[13]

Neuroleptic malignant syndrome (NMS) is a potentially life-threatening but rare reaction to antipsychotics and occurs more frequently in high-potency drugs.[13] Onset can occur at any time, but typically occurs during initiation of administration. Symptoms of NMS include elevated temperature, muscle rigidity, diaphoresis, incontinence, changes in level of consciousness, mutism, labile blood pressure, elevated creatine phosphokinase level, and renal failure.[1] Emergent treatment includes immediate discontinuation of the drug and supportive treatment of symptoms (ventilation, hydration, fever reduction, renal dialysis [when indicated]). Bromocriptine or dantrolene is used to treat rigid muscular response. Clozapine can cause agranulocytosis manifested by malaise, fever, sore throat, and leukopenia. Persons taking Clozaril must have weekly complete blood count (CBC) measurements performed. If agranulocytosis occurs, the Clozaril is immediately discontinued; supportive treatment when indicated may include hospitalization with reverse isolation precautions and antibiotic therapy.

Electroconvulsive Therapy (ECT)

Electroconvulsive therapy may be indicated if medication has been ineffective and if psychotic features are present in mood disorders. In persons with schizophrenia, ECT is used in some cases for acute and subacute psychotic events that are refractory to psychotropics.[8]

Behavioral Therapies/Counseling

The following interventions are primarily used for persons with acute or chronic psychosis secondary to substance use and/or psychiatric illness. These interventions are not necessarily used for persons with psychotic disorders attributable to a medical condition, unless a referral is necessary.

Family intervention. Family intervention is imperative in terms of psychoeducation and illness management. Overall support of family members is provided by the National Alliance on Mental Illness (NAMI), which is an important resource for the lives of family members. This organization provides support, public education, advocacy, research, and peer training programs.[19]

Family therapy. This type of therapy assists the entire family to cope and improve quality of life when living with persons with psychotic disorders. Family counseling facilitates empathy, understanding communication, and maintenance of healthy relationships.

Cognitive and behavioral therapy (CBT). This therapy is a tested and effective form of psychotherapy used for the treatment of pre-school and school-age children, adolescents, and adults. CBT is used to treat potentially psychotic-related problems such as geriatric depression, posttraumatic stress disorder, bipolar disorder (combined with medications), substance abuse, personality disorders, and the psychotic disorder schizophrenia (combined with medications).[20]

Group therapy. This type of therapy provides a trusting environment whereby patients who have disorders can express emotions and feelings, receive validation and feedback, and provide reinforcement of coping skills. Examples of types of group therapy include art, exercise, humor, spirituality, psychoeducation, and life skills learning. Depending on the type and length of the therapy session, participation may be contraindicated in persons in severe psychotic states (paranoid, violence to self or others, psychotic agitation).

Tertiary Prevention

Peer support. This type of group is led by persons inflicted with mental illness themselves. The intent of peer support is that persons who experience the challenges of mental illness share their own wellness tools. Examples of such support groups include Schizophrenia Anonymous, Peer Bridger Programs, and the Wellness Recovery Action Plan.

Psychosocial and vocational rehabilitation. This program is designed to maximize patient's strengths and decrease potential for recidivism. Such programs enable patients to improve communication skills, work on self-care, form and sustain relationships, and use effective coping mechanisms. Patients who receive consistent psychosocial treatment tend to take their medications regularly and have fewer relapses and decreased recidivism rates.[12] Vocational rehabilitation facilitates job training, resource management, and public resources in mentally ill populations who have difficulty obtaining and sustaining jobs because of cognitive impairment from the disorder.

INTERRELATED CONCEPTS

There are multiple concepts that are clearly interrelated to the concept of psychosis. Several psychosocial concepts unique to caring for psychotic patients are essential to improving health outcomes. The interrelationships of several professional nursing concepts including many of those featured in this

---

MODEL CASE 1

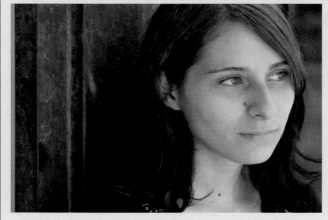

Laura Reyes is a 21-year-old female who is in her junior year of college. She moved away from her family at the age of 19 to attend a university in a nearby state. Recently she has been subjected to increased stressors related to working part time at a retail store while studying for final exams. Laura's housemate found Laura hiding in the closet, crying, screaming, and stating that "if she was to leave her home, the people would capture her, wrap her in Saran wrap, put her in the freezer, and eat her later." When her roommate begins to calm her, Laura becomes agitated and belligerent. Her roommate calls the police. When the police arrive, Laura has scissors in her hand and threatens to stab them. She is handcuffed and taken to the local psychiatric emergency hospital. On arrival, Laura is combative and therefore placed in four-point restraints. An intramuscular injection of Haldol 5 mg/Ativan 2 mg is administered. On this first admission, a MSE is completed and an MRI is ordered; results are normal. Laura is diagnosed with acute psychosis not otherwise specified. She is discharged with a follow-up appointment with psychiatry. One week later she quits taking her medication, in fear of being poisoned. She does not attend her follow-up appointment. Laura continues to hear voices but does not tell anyone. Months later, Laura has auditory command hallucinations that instruct her to kill her mother. She takes a gun from a closet in the home and approaches her mother, telling her she must die. Police are called to the scene, and Laura is rehospitalized in the psychiatric unit. The admission diagnosis now is chronic paranoid schizophrenia.

Case Analysis

This case exemplifies chronic psychosis. The patient has an initial diagnosis of acute psychosis of unknown etiology; it later is confirmed as chronic paranoid schizophrenia. The psychotic agitation, paranoid delusions, and auditory hallucinations in this case are inorganic in nature. The patient is administered antipsychotics; discharge planning includes long-term management of the disorder.

MODEL CASE 2

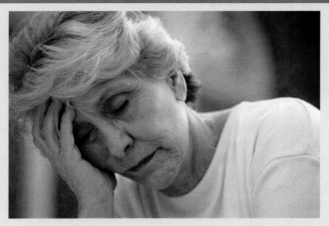

Lucy Barnes is a 58-year-old female who is admitted to the hospital because of stage 2 hepatic encephalopathy secondary to severe alcohol abuse. Vital signs are as follows: B/P 140/90 mm Hg, heart rate regular at 104 beats/min, respirations deep at 12 breaths/min, oral temperature 97° C. Physical assessment is as follows: Mrs. Barnes is agitated secondary to visual hallucinations and disoriented to time and place, speech is slow and slurred, lungs are clear to auscultation, abdomen is distended with abdominal ascites and bilateral 2+ pitting pedal and ankle edema. Laboratory results show: aspartate aminotransferase (AST) and alanine aminotransferase (ALT) levels are normal, decreased total protein level, decreased albumin level, increased serum bilirubin level, increased globulin level, decreased cholesterol level, prolonged prothrombin time, and increased ammonia level. The physician orders lactulose to facilitate elimination of blood ammonia. Twenty-four hours later, Mrs. Barnes is alert and oriented times three; patient reports absence of visual hallucinations.

Case Analysis

This case exemplifies acute psychosis. The patient has a diagnosis of hepatic encephalopathy, with symptomatology of disorientation and visual hallucinations that is organic in nature. Once treated pharmacologically, the symptoms are reversible

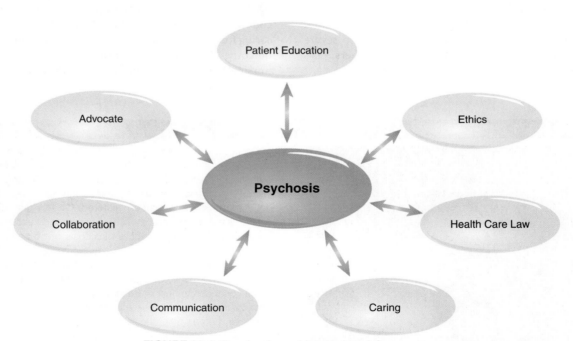

FIGURE 32-2 Psychosis and Interrelated Concepts.

textbook are shown in Figure 32-2. The concepts of **Ethics, Health care law,** and **Advocate** relate to ensuring appropriate use of restrictive treatment interventions (i.e., seclusion, sedation, restraints). In terms of psychiatric commitment, the legal concepts of habeus corpus and justification for involuntary treatment must be respected. Concepts specific to artful therapeutic practice are **Caring** and **Communication.** These concepts are essential to healing the human psyche and for establishing therapeutic relationships. The concept of **Patient education** links to the instruction of treatment protocols, disease processes, and pharmacologic interventions. The concept **Collaboration** is essential for effective treatment and includes a team such as the nurse, psychiatrist, social worker, psychologist, therapist, spiritual counselor, and/or occupational therapist to optimize these specialty-related patient outcomes.

EXEMPLARS

Exemplars of the overarching categories of psychosis are listed in Box 32-4. All exemplars, regardless of etiology, can occur across the lifespan in pediatric, adolescent, adult, and geriatric populations. In addition, psychotic presentation can manifest in any health care setting (e.g., psychiatric, emergency, intensive care, pediatric, obstetric, medical-surgical, oncology, hospice, and community). Because of impairment in emotion, cognition, and behavior, psychotic states impact personal, social, and academic/occupational functioning.

The highest prevalence in the category of inorganic-related psychotic disorders is schizophrenia, with a current 12-month prevalence of 1.1% in the United States.[12] Subtypes are diagnosed depending on clinical picture and most current evaluation.[1] Major depressive disorder and subsets of bipolar disorder are the primary mood states that may present with psychosis. Substance-induced psychosis may resolve quickly[1]; psychotic manifestations vary depending on the type of substance. In some cases substance-induced psychosis may be chronic. Studies indicate methamphetamines, cocaine, and cannabinoid usage can result in a lifelong psychotic presentation that mimics schizophrenia.[21] Psychotic disorder attributable to a medical condition can be reversible or chronic. A case example of acute/reversible psychosis attributable to a medical condition is that of hepatic encephalopathy secondary to elevated blood ammonia levels (see Model Case 2). When blood ammonia levels are treated pharmacologically and reduced to a normal value, psychotic features can resolve within hours to days. A case example of irreversible psychosis attributable to a medical condition is psychotic dementia secondary to Huntington's disease; the psychosis is due to the net effect of cellular loss from caudate atrophy. In this situation, lifetime treatment using antipsychotics may be indicated to alleviate permanent target symptoms of dementia-related psychosis.

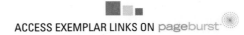

ACCESS EXEMPLAR LINKS ON pageburst

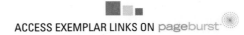

BOX 32-4 EXEMPLARS OF PSYCHOSIS

Psychotic Disorders
Schizophrenia
- Brief psychotic disorder
- Catatonic type
- Delusional disorder
- Disorganized type
- Intensive care psychosis
- Paranoid type
- Persistent auditory hallucinations
- Persistent nonbizarre delusions overlapped with mood episodes
- Residual type

Other Psychotic Disorders
- Schizoaffective disorder
- Schizophreniform disorder
- Schizotypal personality disorder

Not Otherwise Specified
- Shared psychotic feature
- Postpartum psychosis
- Undifferentiated type

Mood-Induced Psychotic Disorders
- Major depressive disorder, single episode with psychotic features
- Major depressive episode recurrent, with psychotic features

- Bipolar I disorder, single manic episode, with psychotic features
- Bipolar I disorder, most recent episode (MRE), manic, with psychotic features
- Bipolar I disorder, MRE depression, with psychotic features
- Bipolar II disorder, MRE, with psychotic features

Anxiety Disorders
- Posttraumatic stress disorder

Substance-Induced Psychotic Disorders
- Alcohol with delusions/hallucinations
- Amphetamine with delusions/hallucinations
- Cannabis with delusions/hallucinations
- Cocaine with delusions/hallucinations
- Hallucinogen with delusions/hallucinations
- Inhalant with delusions/hallucinations
- Opioid with delusions/hallucinations
- Phencyclidine with delusions/hallucinations
- Sedative with delusions/hallucinations
- Anxiolytic with delusions/hallucinations
- Alcohol withdrawal/detoxification

REFERENCES

1. American Psychiatric Association: *Diagnostic and statistical manual of mental disorders*, ed 4, Washington, DC, 2000, Author.
2. Robert Wood Johnson Foundation: *Recognizing and helping young people at risk for psychosis: a professional's guide*, 2009. Retrieved from www.preventmentalillness.org/images/brand/EDIPPP_booklet.pdf.
3. Schuckit MA: Alcohol related disorders. (no pages, electronic). In Sadock BS, Sadock V, editors: *Comprehensive textbook of psychiatry*, Philadelphia, 2005, Lippincott Williams & Wilkins. Retrieved from www.r2libarary.com.libproxy.unm.edu/marc_Frame.aspx?ResourseID=2142005.
4. Castagnini A, Bertelsen A, Berrios GE: Incidence and diagnostic stability of ICD-10 acute and transient psychotic disorders, *Comprehens Psychiatry* 49:255–261, 2008. Retrieved from www.elsevier.com/locate/comppsych.
5. Prevent Mental Illness: *Prevent mental illness with early detection*, 2011. Retrieved from www.preventmentalillness.com/mentalillness.html.
6. McFarlane WR: *Prevention of schizophrenia: a report to the Institute of Medicine*, Portland, Ore, n.d., Author.
7. National Institute of Drug Abuse: *The best strategy*, 2011. Retrieved from www.nida.nih.gov/scienceofaddiction/strategy.html.
8. Hales RE, Yudofsky SC, Gabbard GO, editors: *Essentials of psychiatry*, Arlington, Va, 2011, American Psychiatric Publishing.
9. Robinson J, Harris MG, Harrigan SM, et al: Suicide attempt in first-episode psychosis: a 7.4 year follow-up study, *Schizophrenia Res* 116:1–8, 2010.
10. Large MM, Nielssen O: Violence in first-episode psychosis: a systematic review and meta-analysis, *Schizophrenia Res*, Jan 4, 2011. [Epub ahead of print]. Retrieved from www.ncbi.nlm.nih.gov.libproxy.unm.edu/pubmed/21208783.
11. National Institute of Drug Abuse: *Drugs and the brain*, 2011. Retrieved from www.nida.nih.gov/scienceofaddiction/brain.htm/.
12. National Institute of Mental Health: 2011. Retrieved from www.nimh.nih.gov/statistics/index.shtml.
13. Stuart GW: *Principles and practice of psychiatric nursing*, ed 9, St Louis, 2009, Mosby/Elsevier.
14. White T, Anjum A, Schultz C: The schizophrenia prodrome, *Am J Psychiatry* 163(3):376–380, 2006.
15. Askey R, Gamble C, Gray R: Family work in first-onset psychosis: a literature review, *J Psychiatr Ment Health Nurs* 14:356–365, 2007.
16. Rush JA, First MB, Blacker D, editors: *Handbook of psychiatric measures*, Arlington, Va, 2008, American Psychiatric Publishing, pp 471–493.
17. Schultz JM, Videbeck SL: *Lippincott's manual of psychiatric nursing care plan*, Philadelphia, 2002, Lippincott Williams & Wilkins.
18. Federal Drug Administration: *Atypical antipsychotic drugs information*, 2011. Retrieved from www.fda.gov/Drugs/DrugSafety/PostmarketDrugSafetyInformationforPatientsandProviders/ ucm094303.htm.
19. National Alliance on Mental Health: n.d. Retrieved from www.nami.org/.
20. Beck Institute of Cognitive Behavioral Therapy and Research: *What research shows?* 2011. Retrieved from www.beckinstitute.org/Library/InfoManage/Guide.asp?FolderID=312&;SessionID.
21. National Institute of Mental Health: *Are people with schizophrenia violent?* 2011. Retrieved from www.nimh.nih.gov/health publications/schizophrenia/are-people-with schizophrenia-violent.shtml.

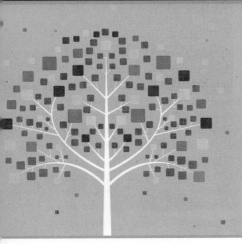

The financial cost of addiction is staggering. It is estimated that addiction costs nearly $1000 a year for every man, woman, and child in the United States,[1] but financial loss does not account for the terrible grief suffered by families as a result of addiction. The purpose of this concept analysis is to develop a generalist nurse conceptual paradigm for the recognition and assessment of addiction on the individual, family, and community levels. A conceptual understanding of addiction will enable nurses to analyze patient data for the planning and implementation of interventions necessary to ensure patient safety during emergency management, and to motivate patients toward successful recovery from addiction during nonemergency management. In addition, it is hoped that this concept analysis will provide nurses with an understanding of their own coping behaviors so they may manage stress in healthy, constructive ways and avoid the unhealthy, destructive ways of addiction.

DEFINITION(S)

Terminology related to the concept of addiction is controversial and subject to debate. For the purpose of this concept analysis, the term addiction is defined as *"a compulsive and maladaptive dependence on a substance (e.g., alcohol, cocaine, opiates, or tobacco) or a behavior (e.g., gambling, Internet, pornography). The dependence typically produces adverse psychologic, physical, economic, social, or legal ramifications."*[2] The American Psychiatric Association (APA) defines a wide selection of mental disorders and their billing codes in the *Diagnostic and Statistical Manual of Mental Disorders (DSM)*, but recent revisions of the *DSM* avoid the term addiction.

Nevertheless, the *DSM* does contain other terminology relevant to nursing practice and establishing addiction as a nursing concept. The terms *abuse* and *dependence* are medical/psychiatric diagnostic terms used in the *DSM-IV*[3] to distinguish two separate but related medical/psychiatric diagnostic models of substance addiction. The application of these models for diagnosis, treatment, and billing uses medical reasoning beyond the scope of generalist nurses; however, because nursing collaborates with medical reasoning practitioners, it is helpful to have some understanding of the medical paradigm and its terminology.

In the medical/psychiatric paradigm defined in the *DSM-IV*, *substance abuse* refers to "a maladaptive pattern of substance use leading to clinically significant impairment or distress"[3,p181] such as legal problems, social problems, or problems at work or school. The *DSM-IV* depicts *substance dependence* as having all the diagnostic characteristics of *abuse* as well as those of *tolerance* and *withdrawal*.

Tolerance is an increasing need for the substance, or a lack of effect by the same dose. *Withdrawal* is a syndrome of symptoms that result from stopping the use of the substance.[3] The terms *tolerance* and *withdrawal* are not medical/psychiatric diagnoses and this concept analysis will use the terms *tolerance* and *withdrawal* as defining characteristics of addiction to facilitate nursing assessment of any possible addiction including behavioral addiction. Impairment or distress will not be used as defining characteristics of addiction in this analysis so that addictive processes may be recognized by nurses before medical/psychiatric diagnostic criteria are met by the presence of impairment.

SCOPE AND CATEGORIES

This analysis will examine the addiction concept within two broad categories of addictions—the substance addictions and the behavioral addictions (Figure 33-1). There is some controversy as to whether behavioral addictions exist, but as new developments take place in understanding brain neurochemistry, it is becoming more evident that substance addictions and behavioral addictions are the result of identical neurochemical processes.[4]

RISK FACTORS

Examples of predisposing risk factors associated with addiction include family history of addiction, burnout, mood disorders, and stress.[5] According to the National Coalition

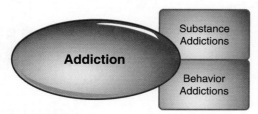

FIGURE 33-1 Categories of Addiction.

for the Homeless,[6] homelessness is also a significant risk factor for addiction. Risk factors identified by the National Institute on Drug Abuse (NIDA) include early aggressive behavior, lack of parental supervision, drug availability, and poverty.[7] Individuals with previous dependence on opiates are at much higher risk for becoming addicted to opioid analgesics.[8] Use of illicit drugs, tobacco, and alcohol is much higher among adults with co-occurring severe psychologic distress,[9] and the unique challenges faced by those with co-occurring disorders will be discussed in the Clinical Management section of this concept analysis.

Prevalence

The National Survey on Drug Use and Health (NSDUH) analyzes data from interviews of more than 67,000 persons; it contains the most recent and extensive information on substance use in the United States.[9] According to the NSDUH the most prevalent abuse of addictive substances used in the United States is alcohol, followed in decreasing order by tobacco products, marijuana, nonmedical use of psychotherapeutics, cocaine, hallucinogens, inhalants, and heroin.[9] Because they are less studied, the prevalence of behavioral addictions is not well established. The more commonly recognized behavioral addictions are gambling, shopping, Internet use, video games, exercise, food addictions, and several subtypes of sex addiction.[4]

More than 50% of all Americans surveyed reported that they drink alcohol, and more than 20% reported binge drinking. Binge drinking is defined by the NSDUH as five or more drinks on one occasion in the 30 days preceding the survey. Heavy drinking is defined as binge drinking on at least 5 days during the 30 days preceding the survey, and 6.9% reported heavy drinking. Among underage persons (defined as ages 12 to 20), 18.6% reported binge drinking and 6% reported heavy drinking. More than 28% of Americans older than age 12 used tobacco within 1 month of the survey, and this included 16.4% of pregnant women.

The NSDUH defines illicit drug use as the unlawful use of a drug within 1 month before the interview, and according to the NSDUH the national rate for illicit drug use in 2007 was 8% of the total population. Almost 10% (9.8%) of individuals between the ages of 11 and 18 used illicit drugs in 2007. Use of illicit drugs among unemployed adults was 18.3%, and 4% of adults interviewed reported driving under the influence of illicit drugs at some time during 2007.

PHYSIOLOGIC PROCESSES AND CONSEQUENCES

Discussions of addiction physiology focus either on the exogenous signs and symptoms of substance abuse or on the endogenous neurochemistry underlying these signs and symptoms (Table 33-1). The neurochemical relationship between addictive behaviors or substances and various neurotransmitters in the brain depends on complex models now being explored on the frontiers of addiction science.[10]

It is believed that neurochemical interactions related to addiction originate in the caudate nucleus, the nucleus accumbens, and the ventral tegmental areas of the brain—otherwise known as the reward centers. The reward centers are affected in different ways depending on which neurotransmitters and other brain areas are involved in various reward pathways. It is evident that the neurotransmitter dopamine plays a key role in many or all addictive processes, whether chemical addictions[10] or behavioral addictions.[4] Dopamine is directly associated with the euphoric reward known as being "high"[10] and other neurotransmitters are associated with dopamine regulation. Examples of other neurotransmitters identified as involved in reward pathways include the endogenous opioids γ-aminobutyric acid (GABA), glutamate, acetylcholine, norepinephrine, and serotonin; there are almost certainly many others that have yet to be identified.

Habituation and Adaptation

Depending on the individual and the particular addiction, the physiologic consequences of addiction are highly variable. However, an understanding of particular neurochemical processes known as *habituation* and *adaptation* forms a conceptual foundation for understanding all addictions. Habituation begins when neurons that receive a repetitive stimulus chemically inhibit their own receptors to restrict the stimulus. Habituation permits the organism to tolerate primal suffering such as hunger pain during a famine, but habituation also facilitates higher order functioning. For example, it allows students to study in the presence of background noise, and as a result of habituation city dwellers are able to sleep in the presence of city sounds such as traffic noise or sirens.

If a repetitive stimulus persists then neurons will *permanently* restrict a sufficient number of their own receptors to permit functioning of the organism in the presence of the stimulus; this is called *adaptation*. In evolutionary terms, adaptation began as a survival mechanism allowing the organism to establish a new equilibrium in the presence of an unceasing, long-term stimulus. *Once adaptation to a repetitive stimulus occurs, the stimulus must be increased to overcome the adaptation for there to be perception of the same stimulus.* A user of cocaine who has adapted to a particular dose, for example, will no longer perceive a high on the same dose; therefore the dose of cocaine must be increased to get high. In turn, the brain neurochemically adapts to the increasing doses of cocaine in an addictive cycle known as *tolerance*. That is to say, habituation and adaptation cause tolerance.

TABLE 33-1 SYMPTOMS AND BEHAVIORS OF ADDICTION

- Fatigue
- Insomnia
- Headaches
- Seizure disorder
- Changes in mood
- Anorexia, weight loss
- Vague physical complaints
- Overabundant use of mouthwash or toiletries
- Appearing older than stated age, unkempt appearance
- Leisure activities that involve alcohol and/or other drugs
- Sexual dysfunction, decreased libido, erectile dysfunction
- Trauma secondary to falls, auto accidents, fights, or burns
- Driving while intoxicated (more than one citation suggests dependence)
- Failure of standard doses of sedatives to have a therapeutic effect
- Financial problems, including those related to spending for substances
- Frequent reference to alcohol or alcohol use indicating preoccupation with and importance of alcohol in the person's life
- Problems in areas of life function (e.g., frequent job changes; marital conflict, separation, and/or divorce; work-related accidents, tardiness, absenteeism; legal problems, including arrest; social isolation, estrangement from friends and/or family)

From O'Brien PG: Addictive behaviors. In Lewis SL, Heitkemper MM, Dirksen SR et al, editors: *Medical-surgical nursing: assessment and management of clinical problems,* ed 7, pp 165–191, St Louis, 2007, Mosby/Elsevier.

Any behavioral reward, such as pleasure, is in fact a neurochemical process mediated by neurotransmitters. Therefore the brain will habituate and adapt neurochemically to repetitive behaviors like gambling in the same way as it will adapt to ingested substances such as cocaine. Gamblers have to gamble more often for higher stakes to overcome the brain's adaptation to the gambling high. All the neurochemical consequences of substance use—whether alcohol, tobacco, cocaine, amphetamines, opiates, or others—apply to nonsubstance addictions such as money, power, relationships, sex, pornography, computer games, television, work, exercise, sports, and even addictive thought patterns like worry or rumination.[4]

The processes of habituation, adaptation, tolerance, and withdrawal are well illustrated by an individual who is too anxious to sleep. The anxiety triggers the release of adrenaline as part of the fight or flight response and insomnia results from the adrenaline. The brain recognizes the importance of sleep and will eventually block the anxiety stimulus so that sleep will occur. Some motor vehicle drivers have experienced this mechanism—the brain chemically overwhelms the alertness necessary to stay awake and accidents occur when drivers fall asleep at the wheel.

Tolerance and withdrawal enter the picture if a sedative is taken to artificially overwhelm the stimulus of anxiety to achieve sleep. In this case, instead of blocking the anxiety stimulus, the brain will block the sedative by signaling the release of more adrenaline. The need for increasing doses of the sedative to overcome the increasing level of adrenaline is tolerance. If the sedative is abruptly discontinued the brain does not immediately stop signaling the release of adrenaline, and therefore the opposite effect of the sedative occurs in the form of restlessness and insomnia even if the original stimulus for anxiety is resolved. This restlessness and insomnia are called the rebound effects of withdrawing the sedative. After one or two nights the neurons will readjust and these rebound effects will cease, but if the sedative is continued to artificially counter the rebound effects, then adaptation will take place and there will be addiction to the sedative.

ASSESSMENT

The first priority of nursing assessment for addictions is aimed at identifying those in need of emergency management so they can be referred immediately to advanced practice care for stabilization. Nonemergency priorities of the assessment are aimed at identifying possible addictions by interview and screening so that treatment options for recovery can be explored. The emergency and nonemergency management of addictions will be discussed in the Clinical Management section of this concept, but the assessment is accomplished during the history and physical examination. The use of screening tools also occurs during the history and physical examination, but will be discussed under Secondary Prevention in the Clinical Management section in this concept.

History and Physical Examination

A routine physical exam may disclose evidence of addiction. Long-term use of toxic substances may harm the liver and result in symptoms of liver failure such as jaundice, fatigue, abdominal discomfort, or ascites. Intravenous drug users may have damaged veins and be at risk for coronary complications that include endocarditis. Opiates and stimulants reduce appetite so users of these substances tend to develop an undernourished, emaciated appearance. Physical signs typical of a withdrawal stress reaction should be noted such as anxiety, palpitations, shakiness, increased heart rate, and diaphoresis. Other physical exam findings are listed in Table 33-1.

Patient history includes exploring the use of prescription and over-the-counter drugs, herbal and homeopathic products, caffeine, tobacco products, alcohol, and recreational drug use. However, the patient may consider the disclosure of addictions to be risky, so it is important to reassure the patient that the information is confidential. Even so, because of the presence of deception in addictive processes, patients are unlikely to accurately disclose addictions.[11] For this reason, it is recommended that the nurse build trust and rapport by using a therapeutic communication technique called motivational interviewing.

The use of motivational interviewing will be discussed further in this concept under Clinical Management because it has been demonstrated to significantly improve recovery.[12]

However, it is also recommended that the nurse use motivational interviewing methods during the assessment to identify the following defining characteristics for addiction: (1) tolerance and withdrawal, (2) deception of the self and others, and (3) relapse processes (loss of willpower). This interview technique allows the nurse to explore the defining characteristics as they arise without loss of rapport. The following discussion of the defining characteristics of addiction is provided to facilitate the assessment.

Tolerance and Withdrawal

Tolerance and withdrawal are the result of the neurochemical processes already discussed: *habituation* and *adaptation*. The nurse can identify tolerance when the patient acknowledges the need for increasingly more of the stimulus to achieve reward. Withdrawal symptoms occur when sufficient quantities are not obtained to achieve reward because of tolerance, or because of reducing consumption. There are two categories of withdrawal symptoms: the stress reaction symptoms and the rebound symptoms. Stress reaction symptoms are mediated by the autonomic nervous system and result from the stress of stopping the addictive behavior. Stress reaction symptoms range from mild uneasiness and irritability to extreme agitation, rapid pulse rate, tremors, and panic.

Rebound symptoms occur when adaptive changes in the brain that counter the effects of the addiction continue despite cessation of the addictive substance or behavior. Therefore the effects of the rebound symptoms are the exact opposite of the effects of the addiction. So, if the addiction is stimulating then rebound symptoms will be sedating and manifest as lethargy. If the addiction is sedating then the rebound symptoms will manifest as agitation. This explains why stimulant addicts experience a "crashing" of mood and energy as a rebound symptom but also have anxiety as a stress reaction symptom. Agitation will be a rebound symptom to stopping the use of substances that are sedating such as alcohol or benzodiazepines, and the agitation may be compounded as a reaction to the stress of stopping the substance.

Deception of the Self and Others (Denial)

Deception of the self and others may be loosely referred to as denial. Sometimes addicts deliberately deceive others to hide their addiction, but they may also deceive themselves. The attention is completely preoccupied by the need to fulfill the addiction and good people will do bad things in pursuit of their addictions. Addicts may commit crimes to pay for the addiction or use the language of love to obtain assistance in maintaining the addiction. Deception underlies much pain and suffering experienced by the families of addicts and explains why addiction is sometimes known as a "family disease."[13]

Relapse (Loss of Willpower)

Relapse processes are invariably linked to addiction, and they are addressed in Clinical Management because they are directly related to recovery.

Diagnostic Tests

Diagnostic tests detect the presence of drug and alcohol metabolites in the blood and urine. Tests may also be ordered to detect addiction-related disorders, such as evidence of hepatitis, liver disease, and smoking-related diseases.

CLINICAL MANAGEMENT

Primary Prevention

To prevent addiction, nurses need to understand the individual and social contexts in which addiction occurs. This section will look at primary prevention from the community perspective and from the individual perspective.

Community Health

Successful models for the prevention of addiction promote healthy families in healthy communities,[14,15] and examples of large-scale community treatment programs shown to be effective in preventing addiction have been implemented in Australia[15] and in Vancouver, British Columbia.[16] In the United States the National Institute on Drug Abuse (NIDA) has established recommendations to support research-based community prevention.[7] The NIDA suggests that a well-constructed community plan first identifies the specific drug problems in the community, and then builds on existing resources to develop short-term goals and projects that include the assessment of outcomes.[7] Numerous examples of educational and community-based programs are offered at HealthyPeople.gov[17] and on the NIDA website.[7]

Individual Positive Coping Strategies

Individual prevention strategies are well illustrated by a general discussion of positive coping strategies aimed at preventing addiction among nurses. The impairment of nurses by substance abuse is documented to have been a problem as long ago as during Florence Nightingale's time in the nineteenth century.[5] The American Nurses Association (ANA) officially addressed the problem of impaired nurses in 1984 and estimates that 6% to 8% of nurses are impaired by substance abuse. The ANA reports that 68% of state board disciplinary actions are related to substance-related impairment, and one descriptive study found that only 3% of nurses in substance abuse recovery had been reported to their respective state nursing boards.[5]

Because stress and burnout have been suggested as risk factors for addiction it may be presumed that effectively managing stress and burnout will reduce the incidence of addiction, but more research is needed to confirm this.[18] Work overload, lack of support, and unreasonable expectations are factors that may lead to burnout, and short-term personal coping strategies that may help mitigate these stressors include participating in simple self-care activities such as exercise, meditation, and journaling; pursuing a personal spiritual orientation; maintaining a sense of humor with positive attitude; and enjoying recreational activities.[18] Long-term personal coping strategies include developing a nursing care philosophy, setting limits at work by saying "no" to unreasonable expectations, debriefing stress through supportive professional relationships, and developing rituals for coping with loss, grief, and death. It is recommended that all nurses reflect upon and further explore ideas for the positive management of stress so that they can experience long and rewarding careers free from addiction.

Secondary Prevention (Screening)

Evidence supports the use of screening to identify adults at risk for addiction; however, there is a distinct lack of research on the role of general practice nurses in screening for addiction.[19] Some evidence endorses the use of the NIAAA Quantity and Frequency Questionnaire and the CAGE questionnaire by generalist nurses.[19] Table 33-2 presents these instruments, and their use to detect possible addictions by nurses is recommended. The CAGE questionnaire in Table 33-2 may also be implemented alone, taking about "one minute."[20,p1530] Initially developed by Ewing in 1984 to screen for alcohol addiction, the reliability and validity of the CAGE questionnaire have been established.[21] It does not distinguish between past and present problems, but it is an expedient and nonthreatening approach to assessing patients for the defining characteristics of any addiction.[19] The CAGE questionnaire is easily adapted for screening of other substances and behaviors by simply referring to them in the CAGE questions.[20]

Collaborative Interventions

The clinical management of addictions and consequences of addictions by the generalist practice nurse consists of emergency management measures to stabilize life-threatening complications and nonemergency measures to facilitate the recovery from substance abuse.

Emergency Management

Generalist practice nurses are likely to encounter many different emergency scenarios related to adverse drug reactions and/or overdose. The primary goal of emergency management is to prevent life-threatening complications that occur as a result of substance consumption or that result as the substance clears the system.[22] Agency-specific protocols should be followed when indicated.

Presenting signs and symptoms depend on the doses of substance or substance combinations that may have been taken, and the nurse should institute basic life support measures as needed until toxicology findings are confirmed and resuscitation efforts are directed by advanced practice personnel. Many agents impact the respiratory system and respiratory management includes monitoring (rate, depth, and oxygen saturation) and support (oxygen administration, ventilation, and medication administration). Cardiovascular support includes monitoring (heart rate, blood pressure, and electrocardiograph) and support (intravenous fluids, medications, and/or resuscitation).

Pharmacologic agents used in emergency management. Opiate overdose risks respiratory arrest, and naloxone is a rapid-acting drug that restores respiratory function by blocking opiate receptors almost immediately. Nurses who administer naloxone should be aware of the potential for violence by the patient attributable to panic and fear as consciousness is restored.

Acute alcohol withdrawal syndrome is a life-threatening condition that may occur unexpectedly whenever long-term, daily alcohol consumption is abruptly discontinued. This may occur in any setting, for example, on admission to the hospital for some other reason. Such patients may deny alcohol use for fear of legal implications or because of shame. Consequently, the nurse may be unprepared for the sudden onset of acute alcohol withdrawal delirium also known as delirium tremens or alcohol withdrawal syndrome.

When it occurs, the onset of alcohol withdrawal syndrome is highly variable, usually beginning within 6 to 9 hours of the last drink.[22] Signs that may lead the nurse to suspect the onset of alcohol withdrawal syndrome are alterations in mental status, tremors, seizures, tachycardia, and hypertension. Late signs such as bradycardia or hypotension are indicative of cardiovascular collapse and the impending need for resuscitation. Other signs of possible alcohol withdrawal syndrome are irritability, depressed mood, impaired concentration, dizziness, hyperreflexia, ataxia, pyrexia, anorexia, and insomnia.[22]

TABLE 33-2	NIAAA QUANTITY AND FREQUENCY QUESTIONS (CONSUMPTION)

1. On average, how many days per week do you drink alcohol?
2. On a typical day when you drink, how many drinks do you have?
3. What is the maximum number of drinks you had on any given occasion during the last month?

CAGE Questionnaire*
In the Last 12 Months:
1. Have you ever felt like you should **C**ut down on your drinking?
2. Have people **A**nnoyed you by criticizing your drinking?
3. Have you ever felt bad or **G**uilty about your drinking?
4. Have you ever had a drink first thing in the morning to "steady your nerves" or get rid of a hangover (**E**ye Opener)?

Screen Positive if:
A positive response on 1 or more questions from CAGE and/or consumption:
- Men >14 drinks/week or >4 drinks/occasion
- Women >7 drinks/week or >3 drinks/occasion
- Over 65 years old >7 drinks/week or >3 drinks/occasion

From National Institute on Alcohol Abuse and Alcoholism: Helping patients who drink too much: a clinician's guide. Washington, DC: Government Printing Office; 2005. Retrieved November 2, 2011 from http://pubs.niaaa.nih.gov/publications/Practitioner/Clinicians Guide2005/guide.pdf.
*The purpose of CAGE is to identify alcohol problems over the lifetime. Two or more positive responses are considered a positive test and indicate further assessment is warranted.

Wernicke's encephalopathy and Korsakoff's syndrome.
Wernicke's encephalopathy and Korsakoff's syndrome are two stages of same emergency problem: heavy alcohol use leads to poor nutritional intake and also inhibits B vitamin absorption (especially vitamin B_1 [thiamine]). This leads to alcohol neuropathy from irreversible brain damage with manifestations of psychosis, ataxia, abnormal eye movements, and death. Therefore, standard treatment for alcohol withdrawal for all patients should also include daily injections of B-complex vitamins.

Substance Abuse Recovery: The Nonemergency Management of Addictions

As stated in the Assessment section, relapse processes are a defining characteristic of addictions managed during the recovery phase. During substance abuse recovery the individual struggles to achieve sufficient willpower to maintain long-term sobriety from addiction. The essence of this struggle is known as the relapse process and an understanding of the relapse process is essential to understanding addiction. For some, addiction recovery may only involve attendance to group support meetings whereas others may have much more complicated rehabilitation needs. Rehabilitation refers generally to a broad spectrum of treatment options that may be inpatient or outpatient, and may include initial detox treatment, group therapy, individual therapy, mental health treatment, psychosocial rehabilitation, and others such as comprehensive community support services.[23]

The term recovery is used to depict an individual who is sober from an addiction and getting the help needed to maintain sobriety.[24] In successful recovery craving is recognized as part of the relapse process and therefore coping strategies are planned in advance to prevent use of the substance or behavior in response to craving. This process is an ongoing struggle as the individual moves through early sobriety from 1 month to 1 year, sustained sobriety from 1 to 5 years, and stable sobriety that begins at about 5 years.[24]

It is a common misunderstanding among many patients and even some clinicians that recovery means simply the absence of addictive behavior, as depicted by line *A* in Figure 33-2. Unfortunately, recovery is complicated by a distinct split between the will for freedom and the will of addiction. Consequently, the recovery from addiction is rarely or never a straight line to freedom, as depicted in line *A* of Figure 33-2.

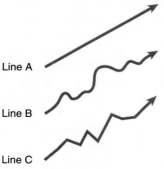

FIGURE 33-2 Recovery and the Relapse Process.

Rather, as soon as anyone suffering from addiction begins to pursue freedom from it, the will of the addiction begins to draw him or her back into it. Therefore recovery is better demonstrated by lines *B* or *C* in Figure 33-2 because lines *B* and *C* depict the two opposing forces of will that pull in one direction down toward addiction and in the other direction up toward freedom. It is important for the person in recovery to understand that this process is normal so that his or her self-esteem can withstand any feelings of failure that may result from the inevitable relapse into craving. The idea of course is that relapse is recognized on the emotional level as craving *before use re-occurs* and therefore use can be prevented by implementing the positive coping strategies as planned. Success in doing this *enhances* self-esteem and strengthens recovery whereas failure to understand this can damage self-esteem and undermine recovery; therefore, it is an important teaching point.

Often it is said that an individual who has been struggling with addiction "has entered rehab." What this means clinically is that to a certain extent the individual has overcome his or her resistance to changing an addictive behavior and is motivated to commit to a treatment program. The overarching goal of any rehabilitation program is to establish and maintain sobriety by helping the patient manage the relapse challenges that will certainly arise. Rehabilitation may also include advanced practice care to manage any mood spectrum problems that emerge as addictive coping subsides. This specialized area of addiction care, which is known as the care for co-occurring disorders or dual diagnosis, will be discussed in more detail later in this section.

Motivational interviewing. It is well-known that in modern health care, individual patient outcomes are greatly influenced by the patient's motivation to change lifestyle behaviors.[12] Yet, it is equally well-known that all too often patients do not change; "patients often resist well-intentioned efforts to persuade them to change."[12,pviii] In fact, there are hundreds of randomized, controlled trials of the motivational interviewing method in health care that endorse this simple truth: *Efforts to persuade patients to change increase their resistance to change.* Clearly, nurses become more effective change agents by "asking patients why they would want to make a change and how they might do it rather than telling them that they should."[12,p9]

Because it has been reliably demonstrated that whatever approach is selected in the treatment of addiction the single most significant factor is the motivation of the patient, motivational interviewing is especially useful in addictions' management.[25] "Virtually every problem drinker we have treated, if allowed to explore it, has felt two ways about drinking...."[12,p8] The underlying "spirit of motivational interviewing"[12,p6] does not involve convincing the patient to do something he or she does not want to do. Rather, it is a collaborative effort that honors the autonomy of the patient to make informed decisions about his or her behavior. In motivational interviewing, the nurse should listen more than talk. The patient will almost certainly have ambivalent feelings about his or her problem behaviors and it is important to understand the ambivalence. In particular, the *benefits* of the addiction should be well understood for any change plan to be effective.

A homeless woman addicted to amphetamines provides a poignant example of the benefits of addiction. In this example, the woman's addiction to amphetamines began when she was sleeping in parks and shelters where her motivation to use the drugs emerged from a need to stay vigilant at night to avoid being raped as she had been once. Besides the benefit of surviving the night, amphetamines were beneficial in providing her with a temporarily enhanced mood in an otherwise bleak and hopeless setting; amphetamines provided her with temporary relief from symptoms of rape trauma syndrome. Once the individual's ambivalent situation is understood in this way, the patient and nurse can then collaborate to resolve the motivations underlying the addiction with a personal plan for recovery that anticipates relapse processes.

To enhance their abilities to do this, nurses are encouraged to participate in motivational interviewing workshops. As a brief overview, when patients are committed to change the nurse should help them to determine the best course of action, but most patients are not initially interested in change or they are ambivalent about changing. When the patient is not interested in changing it is recommended that the nurse remain empathetic, but raise doubt, provide information with permission, and let the patient know that he or she may return if an interest in change develops.[12]

When patients are ambivalent about changing addictive behaviors the nurse should consider ways to tip the balance toward change without arguing because arguing with an ambivalent person will put the person in a defensive position where he or she is resistant to change. One way already discussed to tip the balance toward change is by analyzing the benefits of the addiction so that ideas for meeting the benefits by healthier means can be planned. Another technique is to develop a discrepancy between the patient's present behavior and important goals.

There are compassionate, respectful ways to point out discrepancies, and it is important that the nurse is authentic in his or her style of communication. In the example of the homeless woman who is addicted to amphetamines, lecturing her on the harm of amphetamines is likely only to alienate her and make her defensive. As an alternative, the nurse might ask this patient how she would like her life to be in 2 years. Chances are she would like to have a nice home and a job, providing the nurse with a point of leverage because there is a discrepancy between having a nice home and job while addicted to amphetamines.

The nurse should determine how motivated the woman is to achieve these goals and perhaps chat about how nice it would be to have her own apartment and a job. Patient motivation can be reported on a scale of 1 to 10. This opens the door to establish a discrepancy between amphetamine addiction and having a nice apartment and job. As an example, the nurse might state, "Gosh, it would be really hard to hold down a job and pay rent while supporting an amphetamine addiction, wouldn't it?" Once the discrepancies are established

then resources for relapse prevention and support services can be arranged collaboratively.

Pharmacotherapy in substance abuse recovery. Relapse prevention is improved by reducing craving and withdrawal symptoms; therefore this is the aim of pharmacotherapy in recovery.[23] A complete discussion of the full scope of pharmacotherapy in the routine treatment of addictions is beyond the scope of this concept and there are numerous text sources available for information on this subject.[23]

- *Methadone.* Medications to treat opiate withdrawal either are substitutes for street opiates or are aimed at reducing the symptoms of withdrawal.[23] Methadone is a long-acting opiate that may be prescribed as a replacement; methadone can be gradually tapered once the withdrawal is stabilized.
- *Buprenorphine.* Buprenorphine may be prescribed rather than methadone; buprenorphine is a partial opioid agonist and as such higher doses can be administered with fewer side effects.[23]
- *Suboxone.* Buprenorphine may also be prescribed in a combined preparation with naloxone called Suboxone. Suboxone is taken sublingually, and the addition of the opiate antagonist naloxone in this preparation reduces the potential for abuse of buprenorphine alone by eliminating the opioid euphoria.
- *Clonidine.* The antihypertensive clonidine may also be prescribed for symptomatic relief of opiate withdrawal.
- *Nicotine.* Nicotine gum and nicotine patches may be prescribed to deliver nicotine into the body during withdrawal from tobacco products. These products are intended to alleviate withdrawal symptoms while tapering the dose of nicotine to zero. There are also nasal sprays and inhalers that serve the same purpose but they are less popular.[23]
- *Bupropion.* Bupropion may also be prescribed for nicotine withdrawal; it is a nonnicotine replacement medication that reduces craving.
- *Naltrexone, nalmefene, acamprosate.* Besides the emergency management for acute alcohol withdrawal, there are a number of pharmacologic approaches that may be taken to facilitate the recovery from alcohol addiction. Naltrexone, nalmefene, and acamprosate are all used to reduce cravings for alcohol.
- *Disulfiram.* Disulfiram may be prescribed as *aversion therapy* for alcohol addiction meant to prevent impulsive drinking.[23] The intent of aversion therapy is to extinguish a negative behavior by pairing it with an unpleasant stimulus. Disulfiram works by disrupting the metabolism of alcohol so that toxic blood levels of alcohol metabolites occur in the bloodstream, causing severe headache, nausea, vomiting, palpitations, flushing, tachycardia, chest pain, and dizziness. Severe reactions that include convulsions and death may also occur, but this is rare. Taking disulfiram usually requires written consent to ensure that the patient is fully informed of the risks and aware that he or she must not consume anything containing alcohol. Therefore patient teaching is of critical importance. Such food items as vanilla extract and over-the-counter

preparations of cough medicine and mouthwash often contain alcohol and are likely to induce the side effects of disulfiram and alcohol incompatibility. No form of alcohol should be consumed for at least 2 weeks after discontinuation of disulfiram.[23]

Co-occurring Disorders

Also known as dual diagnosis, co-occurring disorders refer to the unique challenges faced by individuals who are chemically dependent and have serious psychologic distress (SPD). There are two broad etiologies of co-occurring disorders. Persons with mental illness may turn to substance abuse to self-medicate the SPD, or the substance use may cause SPD. In either case, motivational interviewing is recommended as part of a comprehensive treatment approach to unravel the motivations that underlie the problem.[26]

Safe detoxification from the substances of abuse is usually the first step, but motivational interviewing communication skills such as active listening and affirmation will help establish trust so that the etiologies can be understood to avoid years of "revolving door" treatment for these individuals sometimes labeled as "frequent flyers." By doing so, case management can be established to intervene in the underlying causes of the disorder. For example, there are likely to be logical benefits for the use of illicit drugs and alcohol for individuals with SPD.[26] Street drugs may alleviate symptoms of anxiety and psychosis. Intoxication may facilitate social interactions and mask psychosis as substance induced—among the users of street drugs, substance-induced psychosis is socially acceptable whereas psychosis from "being mental" is not. An understanding of all the logical reasons *not to stop* taking street drugs will facilitate the development of treatment plans that are more likely to result in long-term remission by addressing these needs as logical within the patient's social ecology.

There are some contraindications for the use of motivational interviewing in dual diagnosis. The patient might be *too psychotic* to benefit from motivational interviewing.[26] If so, the psychosis will have to be stabilized before motivational interviewing can be of any significant value. These patients may also be *too dangerous* for motivational interviewing.[26] Dangerousness necessitates the removal of freedom and this contradicts the principle of autonomy in motivational interviewing.

For patients who have a degree of orientation to reality despite their confusion or psychosis, the generalist nurse may modify his or her motivational interviewing method by frequently paraphrasing what the patient says to help maintain an organized dialogue. Nurses should try to keep motivational change talk very concrete and target compliance with medications and other treatments. To avoid escalating anxiety, nurses should *avoid exploring despair* and instead explore the patient's motivation for using street drugs. As in the ordinary motivational interviewing method, once the motivation is understood then discrepancy can be established between the drug use and the patient's goals.[26]

INTERRELATED CONCEPTS

Addiction as a concept does not exist in isolation and there are many other interrelated concepts, depending on the specific context of the patient situation. Three common interrelated concepts include **Coping, Family dynamics,** and **Cognition.** When coping, family dynamics, or cognition becomes ineffective the individuals within these systems are at risk for addiction. **Mood and effect** also overlaps with a risk for addiction. Nurses will benefit by mentally applying the defining characteristics of addiction to these interrelated concepts in their own analyses (see Figure 33-3).

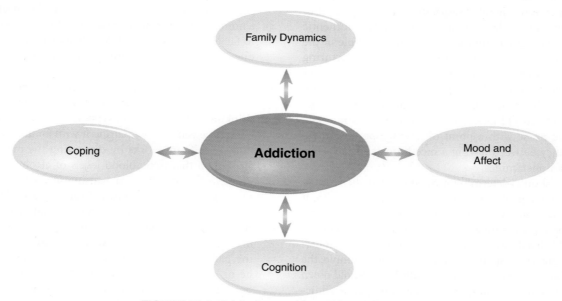

FIGURE 33-3 Addiction and Interrelated Concepts.

MODEL CASE

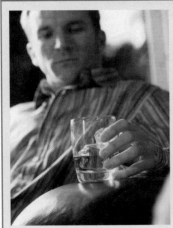

Jim Wright is a 45-year-old White male; he is married to Darla and has two children: 16-year-old Ryan and 9-year-old Jenny. The interview with Jim stemmed from a family therapy meeting to plan Ryan's care in a substance abuse treatment program. Jim is charming, funny, and talkative. His interview began with the CAGE questionnaire and Jim affirmatively acknowledged all four CAGE questions. Jim further acknowledged more than 2 decades of alcoholism and substance abuse. He says he has tried Narcotics Anonymous and Alcoholics Anonymous meetings, "but they didn't help much." He says that after such meetings he and other addicts would go out to drink and use drugs together.

Jim says tearfully that he has tried family therapy as well. "Because of me our whole family is screwed up." Jim has been arrested and incarcerated numerous times for reasons related to drug and alcohol abuse. While in jail, Jim thinks about getting high, he drinks a fermented jailhouse concoction called "pruno" with other inmates, and he plans ways to manipulate his wife Darla back into taking care of him on release. His current plan is to be kind and generous with her at first, and he thinks he "might even have to get a job for a while." In fact, knowing rules of confidentiality Jim admitted that coming in for this interview was part of manipulating Darla.

"Alcoholism runs in the family," Jim says. Like others in his family, Jim has gone through alcohol withdrawal several times. "Withdrawal sucks," he says. "It can last a couple days or more…your skin's all a-crawlin', your heart's a-pounding, and you want that drink so bad…you get all shaky and once in jail I almost died from a seizure. See, you should take some Valium for that but I was in jail and they didn't care. Sometimes you see things…I once saw a six foot rabbit and another time I thought snakes were crawling on me… ."

EXEMPLARS

There are numerous exemplars of addiction, representing both substance addictions and behavioral addictions; some of the most common are presented in Box 33-1. This list is brought to life by the story of a student in an addictions' concept class discussion who mentioned that her boyfriend was addicted to pornography. Inspired to change by the harm his addiction was causing their relationship, he drove to a distant city where he discarded his entire pornography collection in a dumpster. Evidently it became clear to him that he was unable to defeat the will of his addiction without help when he found himself in that same dumpster at 3:00 AM in the morning rummaging for remnants of his precious pornography collection.

Stories like this clearly illustrate tolerance, withdrawal, deception, loss of willpower, and relapse, but interrelated concepts are also clear. The boyfriend's will for freedom was motivated by the harm his addiction had on his family dynamics, mood, and cognition, but his coping abilities were not adequate to withstand the will of addiction. The nurse's role in this story is to recognize how these concepts interrelate so that the boyfriend's motivation to cope can be strengthened with a collaborative plan that will vary, depending on the local resources and the individual's sense of what will work for him.

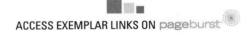

ACCESS EXEMPLAR LINKS ON pageburst

BOX 33-1   EXEMPLARS OF ADDICTION

Substance Addictions
- Alcohol
- Tobacco products
- Marijuana
- Nonmedical use of psychotherapeutics
- Cocaine
- Hallucinogens
- Inhalants
- Heroin
- Opioids

Behavioral Addictions
- Gambling
- Shopping
- Internet
- Video games
- Exercise
- Food
- Subtypes of sex addiction
- Violence
- Relationship addictions
- Sports
- Television

REFERENCES

1. Hopenet™: *Always hope. The elephant in the living room of America.* Retrieved March 22, 2011, from www.hopenetworks. org/addiction/addiction%20facts%20US.htm.
2. *Taber's cyclopedic medical dictionary*, Philadelphia, 2009, FA Davis.
3. American Psychiatric Association: *Diagnostic and statistical manual of mental disorders*, ed 4, Washington, DC, 1994, Author.
4. Holden C: Behavioral addictions: do they exist? *Science* 294:980–982, 2001.
5. West MM: Early risk indicators of substance abuse among nurses, *J Nurs Scholarsh* 34(2):187–193, 2002.
6. National Coalition for the Homeless: *Addiction disorders and homelessness, 2007.* Retrieved April 28, 2011, from www. nationalhomeless.org/publications/facts/addiction.html.
7. National Institute on Drug Abuse: *Preventing drug abuse among children and adolescents, 2010.* Retrieved April 28, 2011, from www.nida.nih.gov/prevention/risk.html.
8. Tedeschi M: Chronic nonmalignant pain: the rational use of opioid medication, *Austr Fam Physician* 35(7):509–512, 2006.
9. U.S. Department of Health and Human Services (USDHHS): *Results from the 2007 National Survey on Drug Use and Health: National Findings, 2008.* Retrieved May 29, 2009, from http:// oas.samhsa.gov.
10. Pettinati HM, O'Brien CP, Rabinowitz AR, et al: The status of naltrexone in the treatment of alcohol dependence specific effects on heavy drinking, *J Clin Psychopharmacol* 26(6), 2006.
11. Stockwell T, Donath S, Cooper-Stanbury M, et al: Underreporting of alcohol consumption in household surveys: a comparison of quantity-frequency, graduated-frequency and recent recall, *Addiction (Abingdon Engl)* 99(8):1024–1033, 2004.
12. Rollnick S, Miller WR, Butler CC: *Motivational interviewing in health care: helping patients change behavior*, New York, 2008, The Guilford Press.
13. Carpenito L: *Nursing diagnosis: application to clinical practice*, ed 13, Philadelphia, 2010, Lippincott.
14. Liddle HA, Rogriguez A, Dakof GA, et al: Multidimensional family therapy: a science-based treatment for adolescent drug abuse. In Lebow JL, editor: *Handbook of clinical family therapy*, Hoboken, NJ, 2005, John Wiley & Sons, pp 128–163.
15. Loxley W, et al: *The prevention of substance use, risk and harm in Australia: a review of the evidence, 2004, Australian Department of Health and Ageing.* Retrieved March 22, 2011, from www.nationaldrugstrategy.gov.au.
16. City of Vancouver: *Preventing harm from psychoactive substance use, 2005.* Retrieved March 22, 2011, from http://vancouver.ca/ ctyclerk/cclerk/20041102/rr1.htm.
17. USDHHS: *Healthy People 2020: educational and community based programs, 2011.* Retrieved April 28, 2011, from http:// healthypeople.gov/2020/topicsobjectives2020/overview.aspx? topicid=11.
18. Maytum J, Heiman M, Garwick A: Compassion fatigue and burnout in nurses who work with children with chronic conditions, *J Pediatr Health Care* 18(4):171–178, 2004.
19. Désy PM, Howard PK, Perhats C, et al: Alcohol screening, brief intervention, and referral to treatment conducted by emergency nurses: an impact evaluation, *J Emerg Nurs* 36(6):538–545, 2010.
20. Mersy DJ: Recognition of alcohol and substance abuse, *Am Fam Physician* 67(7):1529–1532, 2003.
21. Meneses-Gaya C, Zuardi AW, Loureiro SR, et al: Is the full version of the AUDIT really necessary? Study of the validity and internal construct of its abbreviated versions, *Alcoholism Clin Exp Res* 34(8):1417–1424, 2010.
22. Kumar CN, Andrade CA, Murphy PM: A randomized, double-blind comparison of lorazepam and chlordiazepoxide in patients with uncomplicated alcohol withdrawal, *J Stud Alcohol Drugs* 70:467–474, 2009.
23. Taylor DL, Stuart GW: Chemically mediated responses and substance-related disorders. In Stuart GW, editor: *Principles and practice of psychiatric nursing*, ed 9, St Louis, 2009, Mosby/ Elsevier.
24. The Betty Ford Institute Consensus Panel: What is recovery? A working definition from the Betty Ford Institute, *J Substance Abuse Treat* 33:221–228, 2007.
25. Cutler RB, Fishbain DA: Are alcoholism treatments effective? The Project MATCH data, *BMC Public Health* 5(75), 2005. doi:10.1186/1471-2458-5-75.
26. Martino S, Moyers TB: Motivational interviewing with dually diagnosed patients. In Arkowitz H, Westra HA, Miller WR, et al: *Motivational interviewing in the treatment of psychological problems*, New York, 2008, The Guilford Press, pp 277–303.

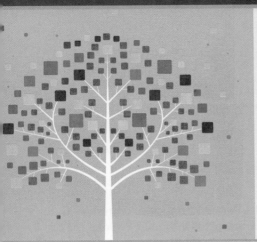

Interpersonal Violence

Pam Schultz

Violence is pervasive and common. It occurs among all people of all ages. There are many facts, relationships, associations, risk factors, and theories about violence. It is a multifaceted problem. Perhaps it is part of the human condition. It is at the very least a destructive behavior. We have legal and moral rules about the use of it. We have cultural traditions, political beliefs, and religious ramifications. It is a quality of humanity. The more we try to understand it the more complicated it becomes. Perhaps we give it more power in the lives of people by compartmentalizing it. However, interpersonal violence is a health concept as well as an elusive human concept. The purpose of this concept analysis is to introduce the concept, including how to recognize it and the role of the nurse as related to interpersonal violence.

DEFINITION(S)

The World Health Organization (WHO) has defined violence as *the intentional use of physical force or power, threatened or actual, against oneself, another person, or against a group or community that either results in or has a high likelihood of resulting in injury, death, psychologic harm, maldevelopment, or deprivation.* Furthermore, they have categorized violence into three subtypes: self-directed violence, collective violence, and interpersonal violence.[1] *Interpersonal violence refers to violence between individuals.* When violence is defined in part as the use of power, then other concepts come into play such as intimidation and bullying. The WHO definition also encompasses the nature of interpersonal violence, for instance, physical, psychologic, sexual, and neglect and/or deprivation. Intimate partner violence (IPV) is recognized as a public health problem but it is also a crime. Assault, battery, homicide, weapon use, kidnapping, and unlawful imprisonment are frequent crimes of domestic violence.[2] This concept will not discuss abuse or violence by strangers, street crime, gang warfare, or military conflict.

SCOPE AND CATEGORIES

Interpersonal violence is a complex concept seen in many forms across the lifespan. In order to fully understand this concept, one must not restrict themselves to the *recipient* of the violence but consider the *perpetrator* as well. They too are part of the public health problem. When considering interpersonal violence one must also consider the *nature* of the violence, the *environment* in which the violence occurs, the *relationship* between the perpetrator and the recipient of the violence, and possibly the *motivation* of the violence (Figure 34-1).

Many categories of interpersonal violence follow the lifespan and include child abuse/neglect, bullying, youth violence, intimate partner violence, and elderly abuse/neglect (Figure 34-2).

Child abuse and neglect encompasses a wide variety of forms of child maltreatment, including physical abuse, sexual abuse, and neglect. The Federal Child Abuse Prevention and Treatment Act (CAPTA), which was amended by the Keeping Children and Families Safe Act of 2003, defined child abuse and neglect as occurring when there is any recent act or failure to act on the part of a parent or caretaker that results in death, serious physical or emotional harm, sexual abuse, or exploitation, or when there is any act or failure to act that presents an imminent risk of serious harm.[3]

Bullying is a form of abuse; it consists of intimidation or domination toward an individual who is perceived as weak. Often the perpetrator does this as a way to establish perceived superiority over another or to get something through coercion or force. Bullying tactics can be physical, verbal, or emotional—often through social and cyber-bullying approaches. Although most prevalent in school-age children and adolescents, adult bullying also exists and is reported in the workplace.

Youth violence refers to harmful behaviors (such as slapping, hitting, or other forms of physical assault with or without weapons) that can start early and continue into young adulthood. The young person can be a victim, an offender,

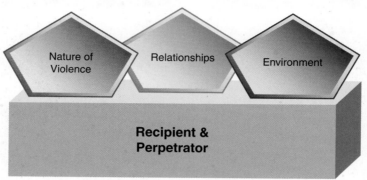

FIGURE 34-1 Scope of Concept.

or a witness to the violence. Patterns of behavior change over developmental stages. During teen and young adult years, violence seems to be most prevalent.

Intimate partner violence (IPV) refers to any behavior within an intimate relationship that results in physical, psychologic, or sexual harm, such as physical aggression, psychologic abuse (which could include intimidation and humiliation), forced sexual coercion, and other behaviors designed to control the recipient of the violence.

Elder abuse refers to abuse to an older person by the older person's family members or caregivers. There is no consensus as to the definition of elder abuse.[4] The age range of the "older person" is not consistent across studies. Abuse can consist of omission or commission and it can be physical, psychologic, sexual, financial, or other forms of maltreatment such as neglect.

Sexual violence is defined by the World Health Organization as any sexual act, attempt to obtain a sexual act, unwanted sexual comments or advances, or acts to traffic (or otherwise direct) a person's sexuality using coercion. It can be committed by any person regardless of his or her relationship to the victim and in any setting, including, but not limited to, home and work. Rape involves any penetration of the vulva or anus with any other body part or object. Rape of a person is considered gang rape if there are two or more perpetrators.[5]

RISK FACTORS

As mentioned previously, interpersonal violence involves all age groups and all races and ethnicities, it is not restricted to any one special interest group or any socioeconomic group, and it can involve all genders. Literally, all individuals have potential risk of experiencing interpersonal violence —either as a recipient or as a perpetrator of violence.

An ecologic model can be used to understand the multifaceted dimension of violence. This model explores the relationships among the individual and contextual factors as well as the multiple layers of risk factors associated with violence. The model distinguishes between individual, relationships, community, and societal levels of factors that contribute to the understanding of violence.[1] Violence has many complex linkages. Some factors are relative to one type of interpersonal violence but in many cases there are commonalities in that violence can share multiple and identical risk factors. For instance, a common factor in most all examples of interpersonal violence involves the use/misuse of alcohol. Alcohol has been reported to be a risk factor in intimate partner violence, child abuse, youth violence, and elder abuse. Interestingly, another commonality is the psychologic consequences of violence, such as depression, anxiety, and posttraumatic stress disorder (PTSD).

Sociocultural Considerations

In North America a sociocultural view of the etiology of intimate partner violence is rooted in the family and society in the form of an historical legacy of oppression and colonization. From the beginning of the colonization of the Americas there has been a stratified caste system based on race, ethnicity, religion, and sexuality.[6] Europeans were privileged over non-Europeans and men over women. Therefore the patriarchy was racialized. At an interpersonal and intrafamilial level, power leads to a culture that breeds violence. Studies have suggested that migration, acculturation, underemployment, undereducation, and economic stress contribute to domestic violence.[6] A high socioeconomic status has generally been considered to be protective against IPV, but not necessarily; generally women living in poverty are disproportionately affected.[7]

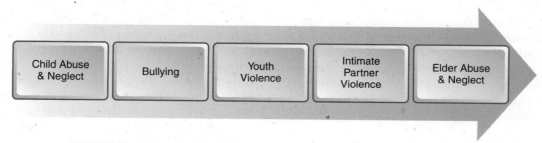

FIGURE 34-2 Categories of Interpersonal Violence Across the Lifespan.

Child Abuse

It is difficult to know exactly the actual figures of child maltreatment. Much of it is unreported. In 2008 the national rate of reports of child maltreatment were 10.3 per 1000 children; Child Protective Services screened 63% of those reported and 772,000 children were confirmed as victims.[8] The U.S. Department of Health and Human Services[9] reported that 71% of these children experienced neglect, 16% were physically abused, 9% were sexually abused, and 12% experienced other forms of abuse. Within the same report it was stated there were more reports of maltreatment for boys versus girls (51% versus 48.3%, respectively) and the ages most affected were from birth to 1 year, with the rate decreasing with increasing age. Most maltreated children were white (45%) and 56% of the perpetrators were women. Another area of potential child abuse involves corporal punishment of children. Its use is widespread and nearly universal, and it has been practiced for generations. In a study done in 1995 in the United States parents were asked how they disciplined their children. An estimated rate of physical abuse of 49 per 1000 children was obtained when the following behaviors were included: hitting the child with an object, hitting the child somewhere other than the buttocks, kicking the child, beating the child, and threatening the child with a weapon.[10]

Bullying

Bullying has become a serious concern and the prevalence is on the rise. Most bullying occurs during childhood and adolescent years, with a peak among middle school children. In most cases, bullying occurs while at school, but this can also occur outside the school grounds, such as on the way to and from school or during extramural youth activities. It is estimated that between 15% and 25% of students are bullied frequently and nearly 20% reported bullying others often. Not surprisingly, there is a direct relationship between being a bully or being bullied and other types of violence (including youth violence).[11]

Youth Violence

Youth violence is a serious worldwide problem and the common quality is that both the perpetrators and the recipients of violence are youths. Worldwide, the highest rates of youth homicide are from Latin America (36.4/100,000 youths) and in the United States this rate is 11/100,000 youths.[12] Multiple studies have shown children exposed to violence are more likely to become violent as adults.[12-17] According to the Centers for Disease Control and Prevention, youth violence is the second leading cause of death among young people between ages 10 and 24 years (see www.cdc.gov/violenceprevention/pdf/YV-FactSheet-a.pdf).

Risk factors for youth violence are varied. Some of the findings reported that pregnancy and delivery complications are associated with future violence; in addition, low heart rates in boys are associated with aggression. Other factors influencing the likelihood of violence are low intelligence, low levels of achievement, poor parental supervision, harsh physical punishment of children, a large number of siblings, low socioeconomic status, income inequality, racism, or the presence of gangs, guns, and drugs in the environment.[12]

Intimate Partner Violence

The overwhelming incidence of IPV is perpetrated by men to women. In the United States approximately one in three homicides of females is committed by an intimate partner, whereas approximately 5% of male homicide victims are killed by intimate partners.[18,19] Factors that have been identified as risk factors for a man abusing his intimate partner include young age, heavy alcohol use, depression, personality disorders, low academic achievement, low income, and witnessing or experiencing violence as a child.[7]

According to 48 population-based studies from several countries, 10% to 69% of women reported being victims of IPV during their lifetime.[19] In the United States the prevalence of IPV in minority women is higher than that in white women, with Hispanic women reporting a greater frequency of rapes and Native American women reporting more violent victimization.[20] It has been reported that IPV exposure causes more severe health consequences than other types of trauma.[21]

Sexual Violence

Sexual violence occurs across the lifespan. The U.S. Department of Health and Human Services[9] reported that 9% of children were sexually abused. In selected population-based surveys between 1993 and 1999, 9% of females reported that their first sexual experience was forced.[5] Older adults also are subjected to sexual abuse within their own homes, nursing homes, or community. Age is not protective; in a study evaluating 284 elders who experienced sexual assault, the mean age was 78.8 years and the age of offenders ranged from 13 to 90 years. The large majority of victims were female. Factors that place elders at risk for sexual abuse include dependence on others (family members, caretakers, agency staff), physical frailty, and cognitive limitations.[22-24] Elder abuse is often associated with physical frailty and/or alterations in mental status.[25] These dependency factors are barriers to detecting elder sexual abuse and can provide for increased risk of abuse with continued low rates of reporting.[26]

Elder Abuse

Like child maltreatment, elder maltreatment can have an element of neglect. Studies from developed countries have reported a 4% to 6% rate of elder abuse with a tendency for there to be a higher incidence in males.[27] There are no national data on the prevalence or incidence of elder abuse. Pillemer and Finklehor reported an overall prevalence rate of 3.2% and a 1 in 14 reporting rate.[28] In a later study by Pillemer[29] it was reported that at least 36% of nursing home personnel witnessed physical abuse within the previous year and 40% admitted to committing an act of psychologic abuse within the preceding year. It is concerning that elder abuse has been largely unrecognized until the 1970s.

Maltreatment by individuals to elders can occur in homes or institutions. Family members who maltreat their elders can continue to maltreat them when they are transferred to an institution. The institution can be abusive and/or neglectful and/or the employees of the institution can be abusive. The elder is restricted in his/her response to abuse by his/her physical and cognitive abilities. Elders can become prisoners to their caregivers and death is often the end result of the abusive cycle. Reduced functional capacity places the elder at risk for maltreatment. Ageism is the stigmatization of older people and is likely an element of the etiology of elder abuse. Negative attitudes towards aging and the glorification of youth may contribute to elder abuse.

Elder abuse situations tend to be more complex than those experienced by intimate partners and children. Elder abuse often concerns multiple forms of abuse, multiple parties, the victim, the perpetrator, neighbors, other family members, and service providers such as nurses, social workers, attorneys, adult protective workers, and physicians.[4] In a study of 730 hospitalized elder patients in Israel, 6% reported that they had experienced elder abuse of varying types. Of those reporting abuse, 25% reported 1 type and the remaining patients reported 2 to 10 types of abuse.[30]

PHYSIOLOGIC PROCESSES AND CONSEQUENCES

In 1995 Johnson[31] proposed a model of intimate partner violence that separated the violence into two types: patriarchal terrorism and situational violence. The first category included cases in which the male partner attempted to dominate and assume control over his partner. The second category occurred when a situation produced an escalation of conflict and the partner initiated physical aggression based in the situational conflict. The first category was considered the most physically violent. Other studies have shown that as physical violence increases, danger of death also increases.[32] When considering the nature of the violence, there can be an overlap among the physical, sexual, and psychologic components, and in children neglect is also often a part of the pattern of violence.

Physical Consequences

Physical consequences of interpersonal violence are completely dependent upon the physical nature of the trauma that results from the violent encounter. There are common patterns that have been identified in the literature,[33-35] primarily headaches, back pain, choking sensations, hyperventilation, gastrointestinal symptoms, chest pain, facial fractures, and other head and neck injuries.[36] It has been reported that 83% of fractures experienced by victims of assault involved the face and 69% of patients with violence-related injuries had involvement of the craniofacial region. Others have reported that the dominant cause of facial fractures in North America is interpersonal violence.[37] Lee[36] reported in his study of more than 2000 patients with craniofacial fractures that those patients whose fractures were caused by IPV were more likely to need surgery. The nature of IPV fractures tends to be different in that the fracture is caused by a punch or kick to the face and prominent points are targeted, such as the cheek, the angle of the jaw, and the nose. Other studies have found an increase in chronic health problems during midlife when previously exposed to IPV.[38]

Sexual violence can occur in the context of child abuse and/or intimate partner violence, or it can occur as an isolated incident. The health consequences depend upon the age of the victim, the relationship between the victim and the perpetrator, the circumstances of the environment, and the severity and/or types of other violence accompanying the incident.

Unintended pregnancy and gynecologic complications—such as bleeding, infection, pain during intercourse, chronic pelvic pain, sexually transmitted diseases, human immunodeficiency virus (HIV) transmission, and urinary tract infections—are associated with sexual violence.[5,39] Violence that occurs during pregnancy can have detrimental effects not only on the mother but also on the fetus. In the United States estimates of abuse during pregnancy range from 3% to 38% and there is increased risk of miscarriage, stillbirth, premature labor and delivery, fetal injury, and low birth weight. There is also an increased risk of maternal mortality.[7]

Mental Health Consequences

Posttraumatic stress disorder (PTSD) is one of the most common mental health consequences of exposure to interpersonal violence, particularly IPV.[20,40-44] The incidence of PTSD among those exposed to IPV varies by study from 33% to 84%. The nature of the violence is predictive of the severity of the symptoms of PTSD. For instance, the use of a weapon and sexual abuse result in more severe symptoms. The characteristic symptoms of PTSD are threefold. *Reexperiencing* includes intrusive and recurrent thoughts, images, and flashbacks of the violence; *avoidance and numbing* include feelings of detachment and persistent avoidance of memories that relate to the violence; and *increased arousal* can include insomnia, difficulty focusing, and hypervigilance.[20] Rape by an intimate partner results in PTSD in many circumstances and is usually associated with greater severity of violence.

Depression is also a common reaction to IPV.[7,38,45] Depression inhibits the ability of abused individuals from formulating a plan to deal with the abuse. This inertia prevents the victim from taking proactive steps to leave the abusive situation. Humphreys and Lee[38] have reported that the presence of social support mitigates the depressive effects of IPV. When an individual experiences depression there is an increased risk of suicide and there are increased suicide attempts in women experiencing IPV.[7]

Studies have shown a link between mental disorders and violence[45] in that there is a high rate of lifetime victimization among psychiatric patients. However, there does appear to be some evidence that suggests that mental illness is exacerbated by exposure to violence and it may also contribute to interpersonal violence. Many of the physical sequelae are associated with mental health disturbances, such as gastrointestinal disorders, headaches, choking sensations, hyperventilation, and other somatic complaints commonly associated with increased physical stress.

Consequences of Child Abuse/Neglect and Youth Violence

As with adults, physical sequelae of childhood abuse are determined by the type of violence done to the child. However, in some cases the social and emotional consequences seem most severe. Windom and Maxfield[46] have reported that a history of childhood maltreatment often results in childhood delinquency and adult criminality; 49% of maltreated children will have been arrested for a nontraffic offense during their adulthood. Children who experience sexual abuse have high rates of PTSD (greater than 34%).[47] Other common consequences of childhood sexual abuse are developmentally inappropriate sexual behavior, such as age-inappropriate knowledge, sexual preoccupation, and excessive masturbation.[47]

The health consequences of childhood abuse have been identified by researchers and seem to be related to specific behavioral risk factors such as smoking, alcohol abuse, poor diet, and lack of exercise. Some of the major adult forms of illnesses include ischemic heart disease, cancer, chronic lung disease, irritable bowel syndrome, and fibromyalgia.[10]

Neglect

Neglect is parental failure to meet a child's basic needs.[48] Erickson and Egeland have described five subtypes of child neglect: physical neglect; psychologic or emotional neglect (these parents typically ignore their child's desire for comfort); medical neglect (not providing medical treatment); mental health neglect; and educational neglect.[49] Studies have shown since the 1970s that neglect has serious consequences for children. Neglected children have learning problems, developmental delays, passivity, low self-esteem, and juvenile delinquency. Aggression has been shown to be associated with neglect before 2 years of age.[49]

Psychologic/Emotional Maltreatment

It is difficult to define psychologic maltreatment and therefore little research has been done to understand the consequences of this form of maltreatment. However, in 1995 the American Professional Society on the Abuse of Children (APSAC) published *Guidelines for Psychosocial Evaluation of Suspected Psychological Maltreatment of Children and Adolescents*[50] and these guidelines defined six subtypes of psychologic maltreatment. These subtypes included spurning, terrorizing, isolating, exploiting/corrupting, denying emotional responsiveness, and mental health, medical, and educational neglect.

Spurning includes verbal and nonverbal acts that reject and degrade a child. Terrorizing is behavior that threatens or is likely to physically hurt, kill, or abandon in dangerous situations. Isolating acts confine the child or place unreasonable limitations on the child's freedom to move or communicate with others. Exploiting/corrupting includes acts that promote inappropriate behaviors from the child, such as criminal, antisocial, or deviant behaviors. Denying emotional responses includes showing no emotion in interactions with the child. Studies have shown multiple emotional problems and social competency problems associated with psychologic maltreatment, for instance, anxiety, depression, low self-esteem, suicidal ideation, impulse control problems, substance abuse, eating disorders, isolating behavior, social phobia, aggression, and violent behavior.[51]

Exposure to Intimate Partner Violence

In homes where IPV occurs, children are exposed to that violence at the very least and often become additional recipients of that violence. IPV usually predates abuse of the child.[52] Studies have shown that younger children seem to have more behavioral problems when exposed to intrafamily violence; for instance, they often have problems with anxiety, depression, and aggression. They often experience many fears and worries that are developmentally inappropriate and PTSD is a concern.[53,54] Associated features of PTSD may be more detrimental than the violence itself. Kletter and colleagues[55] have reported in their study that guilt was highly associated with the severity of PTSD and that resolving the guilt is very difficult because of the child's inability to accept that the violence was beyond his or her control.

Bullying

There is a direct relationship between being a bully or being bullied and other types of violence, including fighting, depression, and suicide.

Youth Violence

Youth violence tends to be regarded mostly as a criminology problem and not a health problem. Most victims of youth violence suffer the physical consequences of the acts but little has been done to study the consequences of that violence in any context other than legally. Consequences of youth violence are usually associated with trauma-related injuries such as cuts, bruises, broken bones, stab wounds, and gunshot wounds. Severe injuries may lead to life-long disability or death.

ASSESSMENT

All health professionals should maintain continuous vigilance for evidence of interpersonal violence with all health care encounters. It is often difficult to differentiate injuries caused by violence from those caused accidentally. Clues are usually present, but only if the astute nurse is keeping an open mind to the presence of signs and symptoms.

History

There are certain elements in the medical history that raise concern for physical abuse. Perpetrators may provide a history of events that are incomplete or inconsistent with injuries seen. Many individuals who experience interpersonal violence are unable or afraid to provide an accurate account of events. Specific examples include a history of trauma that is inconsistent or implausible with the physical examination; a history of no trauma with evidence of injury; a history of self-inflicted trauma that is developmentally unlikely; and serious injuries blamed on siblings or playmates.[56]

One study reported that older adults are exposed to far more abuse than they are willing to admit.[30] Elders were much more likely to report physical and sexual abuse and less likely to report other types of abuse. This creates a serious situation in that direct questioning of elders may not be the best way to determine incidence of abuse. Much more work needs to be done to better understand the pervasiveness of elder abuse and the way it impacts quality of life.

Examination

Examination findings for interpersonal violence range from subtle to obvious. Some may manifest as old or new injuries that may seem mild to more significant (such as cuts, bruises, burns, or fractures) and may not raise concern. For this reason, it is critical to consider the history in relation to injuries seen. The nurse should also maintain a high degree of awareness for injuries that are not typically seen in the context of day-to-day living—such as unusual patterns of bruising or burn marks. In some cases, specific physical injuries are common. Traumatic brain injury usually occurs in infants less than 1 year of age. Shaken baby syndrome is also common in infants and young children. Studies have shown that 15% to 25% of these injuries are fatal and 80% to 90% of the survivors are left with varying degrees of compromise, including learning disabilities, blindness, seizures, and paralysis.[57] Abdominal injuries caused by punching or kicking, which lead to internal bleeding, are the second most common cause of death in child abuse. Burns are a common injury associated with abuse; in fact, it is believed that 10% of all physical abuse cases involve burns, usually with scalding water.[57] Burns with a stocking pattern or circular burn marks always should raise suspicion.

CLINICAL MANAGEMENT

Primary Prevention

The prevention of interpersonal violence is considered a key public health priority. The lead federal organization for violence prevention, established by the Centers for Disease Control and Prevention, is the National Center for Injury Prevention and Control (NCIPC). One of three divisions of the NCIPC is the Division of Violence Prevention (DVP). The strategic directions established by the DVP include reducing rates of various forms of violence (including child maltreatment, intimate partner violence, sexual violence, and youth violence) through individual, community, and societal change. A comprehensive discussion of the national strategic direction for DVP is beyond the scope of this concept analysis, but it is important for nurses to know these directions exist and are readily available on the CDC webpage: www.cdc.gov/Violence Prvention/overview/strategicdirections.html.

Secondary Prevention (Screening)

A large number of screening tools have been developed to screen for various types of interpersonal violence in a number of health care settings. Nurses should be aware of appropriate tools to use in various settings such as emergency departments, school-based clinics, inpatient settings, or community-based clinics, for example. A useful resource for screening tools is the *Intimate Partner Violence and Sexual Violence Victimization Assessment Instruments for Use in Healthcare Settings* published by the Centers for Disease Control and Prevention.[58] This resource presents a variety of screening tools that have been tested and validated for multiple types of interpersonal violence, and among various population groups (age and ethnic/cultural). It is beyond the scope of this concept analysis to describe each screening tool, but nurses are encouraged to become aware of the most appropriate screening tools used in their particular practice settings.

Collaborative Interventions

When interpersonal violence is suspected or identified, the priority intervention is to protect the infant, child, adult, or elder from further abuse. It is the legal and ethical duty of nurses and all health professionals to report suspected abuse. All states have laws for mandatory reporting of child abuse and other forms of violence. When the victim is a child or compromised elderly individual, referrals are made to the state agency child or human welfare departments for a formal investigation; based on these findings the child or elderly person may be left in the home or removed and placed in another setting. Adult victims of intimate partner violence may need a referral to a "safe house" such as a battered women's shelter and/or may need a referral to seek a legal restraining order.

Emotional support and appropriate referrals are also needed for the patient and family. A focus on minimizing the physiologic consequences is needed, particularly helping those who have suffered emotionally to experience and establish positive relationships. Education and counseling are often needed to ensure adequate coping strategies. Nurses can also help patients and families gain access to appropriate community agencies and support groups as available.

Over the last decade much research has been done to draw attention to the problem of IPV. Many studies have shown the serious consequences of IPV. However, there is still an underreporting of IPV; hence there is a lack of formal help-seeking behaviors, which may be a result of sociocultural barriers.[33] Bauer[59] suggested that sociocultural barriers included cultural stigma of abuse, dedication to the family unit, social isolation, and language barriers. When nurses are able to view diversity as an indication of resilience instead of weakness, perhaps help-seeking behaviors will increase.[34] When compared to women with no lifetime exposure to interpersonal violence it was reported that these women were more likely to be unemployed, to have lower incomes, and to be married. It was also found that they had fewer individuals in their support systems.[38]

INTERRELATED CONCEPTS

Many of the sequelae of interpersonal violence result in other health and illness concepts. For instance, interpersonal violence could conceivably involve almost all health and illness concepts depending upon the physical and psychologic effects of the violence. In fact, interpersonal violence sequelae are cumulative and long-lasting beyond the violence events.[21] Figure 34-3 features important interrelationships to consider. Common psychologic consequences of interpersonal violence include **Anxiety, Stress,** and **Mood and affect.** Individuals who experience interpersonal violence rely on **Coping** strategies as part of the response to such events.

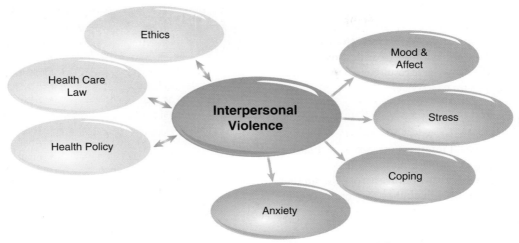

FIGURE 34-3 Interpersonal Violence and Interrelated Concepts.

MODEL CASE

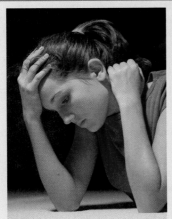

Meredith Long, a 32-year-old female, presents to an outpatient clinic with a chief complaint of headaches and problems sleeping. Yvonne Sanchez, the nurse at the clinic, remembers seeing Meredith in the clinic not long ago. She reviews Meredith's medical record before seeing her and notes that Meredith has been in the clinic four times in the last 5 months, each time with vague symptoms, and each time she is sent home with a nonspecific diagnosis. The nurse reviews Meredith's social history and sees that Meredith is married and has two children, ages 4 and 6; Meredith works as a receptionist. Meredith has no medical conditions and takes no medications other than oral contraceptives.

When Yvonne enters the examination room, she observes Meredith sitting on the examination table with her knees held tightly against her torso and rocking back and forth. Yvonne asks Meredith to describe the symptoms she has been experiencing. Meredith states her headaches have been occurring intermittently for a while, and describes them as "intense" and often keeping her awake at night. As she talks, Yvonne notes a flat affect in Meredith's communication pattern. She also notices bruising to Meredith's neck, just above the clavicle, and on her upper arms. When Yvonne asks Meredith the last time she experienced the headache, Meredith tells Yvonne she cannot remember exactly, but perhaps 1 or 2 weeks ago.

Yvonne suspects Meredith may be experiencing violence. She pulls out the Partner Violence Screening tool, available at her office, and asks Meredith the following three questions:

1. Have you been hit, kicked, punched, or otherwise hurt by someone within the past year? If so, by whom?
2. Do you feel safe in your current relationship?
3. Is there a partner from a previous relationship who is making you feel unsafe now?

Meredith begins to cry and acknowledges she is in trouble. She states her husband has a drinking problem and every couple of weeks he gets drunk and becomes violent. He always feels badly after he becomes sober, but she has become frightened at what he will do to her or the children. She states he has never hurt the children, but they see him regularly hit her. Meredith tells Yvonne she has contemplated leaving, but does not think she can. She explains that her husband controls all of the money, and she has nowhere to go. She is sure she does not earn enough money to support herself and her children, and she is worried that he will track her down anyway. Meredith feels completely trapped and unable to remove herself from the situation.

Case Analysis

This case exemplifies interpersonal violence, or specifically intimate partner violence. Individuals are often reluctant to report this violence; thus the nurse must maintain a keen awareness of the possibility when interacting with every patient. Yvonne first noticed a pattern of frequent clinic visits; she also noted Meredith's flat affect and body posturing as well as the bruises to the neck and arms. Alone, any one of these findings might not seem significant, but together these are indeed concerning. Yvonne used a common screening tool for domestic violence and positively identified this problem.

As a nurse, Yvonne's next steps are to ask Meredith if she would like to speak to a law enforcement officer, to provide Meredith with resources for emotional support, and to direct Meredith to community agencies that can assist Meredith to extricate herself and her children from her abuser. Because of her fear of retaliation it is unlikely that Meredith will want to press charges against her husband.

Interrelationships with several professional nursing concepts also are important to note. Nurses have a *legal* (see **Health care law** concept) and *ethical* (see **Ethics** concept) obligation to report abuses. Because of widespread prevalence, **Health policy** initiatives have resulted in national strategies to address interpersonal violence.

EXEMPLARS

There are many examples of interpersonal violence, many of which have been described throughout this concept analysis. It is important to remember this occurs across the lifespan and it can happen to any individual. Box 34-1 presents common examples of interpersonal violence.

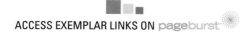

ACCESS EXEMPLAR LINKS ON pageburst

BOX 34-1   EXEMPLARS OF INTERPERSONAL VIOLENCE

- Child maltreatment
  - Physical abuse
  - Sexual abuse
  - Emotional abuse
  - Neglect
- Bullying
- Youth violence
- Intimate partner violence
  - Physical violence
  - Sexual violence
  - Threats
  - Emotional abuse
- Elder maltreatment
  - Physical abuse
  - Sexual abuse
  - Emotional abuse
  - Neglect
  - Abandonment
  - Financial abuse

From Centers from Disease Control and Prevention: *Injury control and violence prevention.* Accessed at www.cdc.gov/violenceprevention/.

REFERENCES

1. Dahlberg L, Krug E: Violence—a global public health problem. In Krug E, Dahlberg L, Mercy J, et al, editors: *World report on violence and health*, Geneva, Switzerland, 2002, World Health Organization.
2. Schaffer B: Male veteran interpersonal partner violence (IPV) and associated problems, *J Aggress Matr Trauma* 19:414, 2010.
3. Giardino A, Lyn M, Giardino E: Introduction: child abuse and neglect. In Giardino A, Lyn M, Giardino E, editors: *A practical guide to the evaluation of child physical abuse and neglect*, New York, 2010, Springer.
4. Anetzberger G: Elder abuse. In Bonder B, Dal Bello-Haas V, Wagner M, editors: *Functional performance in older adults*, Philadelphia, 2009, FA Davis.
5. Jewkes R, Sen P, Garcia-Moreno C: Sexual violence. In Krug E, Dahlberg L, Mercy J, et al, editors: *World report on violence and health*, Geneva, Switzerland, 2002, World Health Organization.
6. Flores-Ortiz Y: Domestic violence in Chicana/o families. In Velasquez R, Arellano L, McNeill B, editors: *The handbook of Chicana/o psychology and mental health*, New York, 2004, Lawrence Erlbaum Associates.
7. Heise L, Garcia-Moreno C: Violence by intimate partners. In Krug E, Dahlberg L, Mercy J, et al, editors: *World report on violence and health*, Geneva, Switzerland, 2002, World Health Organization.
8. DePanfils D: Child protection system. In Myers J, editor: *The APSAC handbook on child maltreatment*, Los Angeles, 2011, SAGE.
9. U.S. Department of Health and Human Services: *Child maltreatment 2007*, Washington, DC, 2007, U.S. Government Printing Office.
10. Runyan D, Wattam C, Ikeda R, et al: Child abuse and neglect by parents and other caregivers. In Krug E, Dahlberg L, Mercy J, et al, editors: *World report on violence and health*, Geneva, Switzerland, 2002, World Health Organization.
11. National Center for Educational Statistics and Bureau of Justice Statistics: *Indicators of school crime and safety*, 2009. Available at http://nces.ed.gov/pubs2010/2010012.pdf.
12. Mercy J, Butchart A, Farrington D, et al, editors: Youth violence. In Krug E, Dahlberg L, Mercy J, et al, editors: *World report on violence and health*, Geneva, Switzerland, 2002, World Health Organization.
13. Slovak K, Carlson K, Helm L: The influence of family violence on youth attitudes,, *Child Adolesc Social Work J* 24:77, 2007.
14. Weaver C, Borkowski J, Whitman T: Violence breeds violence: childhood exposure and adolescent conduct problems, *J Commun Psychol* 36:96, 2008.
15. Xue Y, Zimmerman M, Cunningham R: Relationship between alcohol use and violent behavior among urban African American youths from adolescence to emerging adulthood: a longitudinal study, *Am J Pub Health* 992041, 2009.
16. Legge S: Youth and violence: phenomena and international data, *New Directions Youth Dev* 119:17, 2008.
17. Wilkinson D: Violent youths' responses to high levels of exposure to community violence: what violent events reveal about youth violence, *J Commun Psychol* 36:1026, 2008.
18. Federal Bureau of Investigation: *Crime in the United States:* Washington, DC, 2007, U.S. Department of Justice. Available at www.fbi.gov/ucr/cius2007/offenses/expanded_information/homicide.html.
19. CDC Morbidity and Mortality Weekly Report: *Surveillance for violent deaths—National violent death reporting system, 16 states, 2007,* 59:SS4, 2010.
20. Hien D, Ruglass L: Interpersonal partner violence and women in the United States: an overview of prevalence rates, psychiatric correlates and consequences and barriers to help seeking, *Int J Law Psychiatr* 32:48, 2009.
21. Schumacher A, Jaramillo D, Uribe T, et al: The relationship of two types of trauma exposure to current physical and psychological symptom distress in a community sample of Colombian women: why interpersonal violence deserves more attention,, *Health Care Women Int* 31:946, 2010.
22. Anetzberger G: Elder abuse. In Bonder B, Dal Bello-Haas V, Wagner M, editors: *Functional Performance in Older Adults*, Philadelphia, 2009, FA Davis Company.
23. Marshall CE, Benton D, Brazier JM: Primary care. Elder abuse: using clinical tools to identify clues of mistreatment, *Geriatrics* 55(2):42–44, 47–50, 2000.

24. Wyandt MA: A review of elder abuse literature: an age old problem brought to light. Californian, *J Health Promot* 2(3):40–52, 2004.

25. Swagerty DL, Takahashi PY, Evans JM: Elder mistreatment, *Am Fam Phys*(10)2804–2808, 1999.

26. Nerenberg L: Communities respond to elder abuse, *J Gerontol Soc Work* 46(3-4):5–33, 2006.

27. Wolf R, Daichman L, Bennett G: Abuse of the elderly. In Krug E, Dahlberg L, Mercy J, et al, editors: *World report on violence and health*, Geneva, Switzerland, 2002, World Health Organization.

28. Pillemer K, Finklehor D: The prevalence of elder abuse: a random sample survey, *Gerontologist* 28:51, 1988.

29. Pillemer K, Moore D: Highlights from a study of abuses of patients in nursing homes, *J Elder Abuse Neglect* 2:5, 1990.

30. Cohen M, Levin S, Gagin R, et al: Elder abuse: disparities between older people's disclosure of abuse, evident signs of abuse, and high risk of abuse, *J Am Geriatr Soc* 55:1224, 2007.

31. Johnson M: Patriarchal terrorism and common couple violence: two forms of violence against women, *J Marriage Fam* 57:283, 1995.

32. Gist JH, McFarlane J, Malecha A, et al: Women in danger: intimate partner violence experienced by women who qualify and do not qualify for a protective order, *Behav Sci Law* 19:637, 2001.

33. Amar A, Bess R, Stockbridge J: Lessons from families and communities about interpersonal violence, victimization, and seeking help, *J Forensic Nurs* 6:110, 2010.

34. Alvarez J, Pavao J, Mack K, et al: Lifetime interpersonal violence and self-reported *Chlamydia trachomatis* diagnosis among California women, *J Womens Health* 18:57, 2009.

35. Campbell J: Health consequences of intimate partner violence, *Lancet* 359:1331, 2002.

36. Lee K: Role of interpersonal violence in facial fractures, *J Oral Maxillofac Surg* 67:2009, 1878.

37. Alvi A, Doherty T, Lewen G: Facial fractures and concomitant injuries in trauma patients, *Laryngoscope* 113:102, 2003.

38. Humphreys J, Lee K: Interpersonal violence is associated with depression and chronic physical health problems in midlife women, *Issues Ment Health Nurs* 30:206, 2009.

39. Pallito C, O'Campo P: The relationship between intimate partner violence and unintended pregnancy, *Int Fam Planning Perspect* 30:165, 2004.

40. Astin M, Lawrence K, Foy D: Posttraumatic stress disorder among battered women: risk and resiliency factors, *Violence Victims* 8:17, 1993.

41. Golding J: Intimate partner violence as a risk factor for mental disorders: a meta-analysis, *J Fam Violence* 14:99, 1999.

42. Jones L, Hughes M, Unterstaller U: Post-traumatic stress disorder (PTSD) in victims of domestic violence: a review of the research, *Trauma Violence Abuse* 2:99, 2001.

43. Taft C, Murphy C, King L, et al: Posttraumatic stress disorder symptomatology among partners of men in treatment relationship abuse, *J Abnorm Psychol* 114:259, 2005.

44. Hegadoren K, Lasiuk G, Coupland N: Posttraumatic stress disorder part III: health effects of interpersonal violence among women, *Perspect Psychiatr Care* 42:163, 2006.

45. Meuleners L, Lee A, Hendrie D: Effects of demographic variables on mental illness admission for victims of interpersonal violence, *J Public Health* 31:162, 2008.

46. Windom C, Maxfield M: *An update on the "Cycle of Violence,"* 2001, National Institute of Justice Research Brief, U.S. Department of Justice, Office of Justice Programs. Accessed at www.ncjrs.gov/pdffiles1//nij/184894.pdf.

47. Berliner L: Child sexual abuse: definitions, prevalence, and consequences. In Myers J, editor: *The APSAC handbook on child maltreatment*, Los Angeles, 2011, SAGE.

48. Greenbaum J, Dubowitz H, Lutzker J, et al: *Practice guidelines: challenges in the evaluation of child neglect*, Elmhurst, Ill, 2008, American Professional Society on the Abuse of Children.

49. Erickson M, Egeland B: Child neglect. In Myers J, editor: *The APSAC handbook on child maltreatment*, Los Angeles, 2011, SAGE.

50. American Professional Society on the Abuse of Children (APSAC): *Guidelines for psychosocial evaluation of suspected psychological maltreatment of children and adolescents*, Chicago, 1995, Author.

51. Hart S, Brassard M, Davidson H, et al: Psychological maltreatment. In Myers J, editor: *The APSAC handbook on child maltreatment*, Los Angeles, 2011, SAGE.

52. Stark E, Flitcraft A: *Women at risk: domestic violence and women's health*, Thousand Oaks, Calif, 1996, Sage.

53. Graham-Berman S, Howell K: Child maltreatment in the context of intimate partner violence. In Myers J, editor: *The APSAC handbook on child maltreatment*, Los Angeles, 2011, Sage.

54. Lemmey D, Malecha A, McFarlane J, et al: Severity of violence against women correlates with behavioral problems in their children, *Pediatr Nurs* 27:265, 2001.

55. Kletter H, Weems C, Carrion V: Guilt and posttraumatic stress symptoms in child victims of interpersonal violence, *Clin Child Psychol Psychiatr* 14:71, 2009.

56. Giardet R, Giardino A: Evaluation of physical abuse and neglect. In Giardino A, Lyn M, Giardino E, editors: *A practical guide to the evaluation of child physical abuse and neglect*, New York, 2010, Springer.

57. Reece R: Medical evaluation of physical abuse. In Myers J, editor: *The APSAC handbook on child maltreatment*, Los Angeles, 2011, Sage.

58. Basile KC, Hertz MF, Back SE: *Intimate partner violence and sexual violence victimization assessment instruments for use in healthcare settings: version 1*, Atlanta, Ga, 2007, Centers for Disease Control and Prevention, National Center for Injury Prevention and Control. Accessed at www.cdc.gov/NCIPC/pub-res/images/IPVandSVscreening.pdf.

59. Bauer H, Rodriques M, Quiroga S, et al: Barriers to health care for abused Latina and Asian immigrant women, *J Health Care Poor Underserved* 11:33, 2000.

Professional Nursing and Health Care Concepts

The delivery of safe and effective health care is extremely complex. As the largest group of health care professionals, nurses play an especially important role within health care delivery. Health care delivery represents many critical elements that collectively describe the essence of professional nursing practice. The concepts within Unit 3 relate to these ideas and are closely associated with professional attributes and behaviors desired among all health care providers. As a group, the Professional Nursing and Health Care Concepts represent 19 concepts organized within 4 overarching themes. Unlike the Health and Illness Concepts, these are concepts associated with professional comportment—meaning the identity of nursing as a profession.

The first theme is *Attributes/Roles of a Professional Nurse.* Concepts within this theme represent roles nurses play within health care delivery, and the attributes or characteristics desired of professional nurses; these are the behaviors nurses incorporate into all patient care encounters. Specific concepts represented include *Professionalism, Clinical Judgment, Leadership, Ethics, Patient Education,* and *Health Promotion.*

The second theme is *Care Competencies.* The term competency refers to being competent or well-qualified to complete a skill or task. In the context of nursing and health care, competencies are identified knowledge, skills, and attitudes deemed important for safe and effective care. Specific concepts include *Communication, Collaboration, Safety, Technology and Informatics, Evidence,* and *Health Care Quality.* Although the concepts featured within this theme are not intended to be comprehensive of all competencies, some of the most common to all nurses, regardless of area of practice, are included.

The third theme is *Health Care Delivery.* These concepts represent the context of the application and care delivery situations or models. There are literally thousands of health care delivery models; those included are some of the most important to be aware of and include *Care Coordination, Caregiving,* and *Palliation.*

The final theme is *Health Care Infrastructures.* These concepts are foundational to health care delivery and the practice of nursing. *Health Care Organizations, Health Care Economics, Health Policy,* and *Health Care Law* represent specific concepts within this theme.

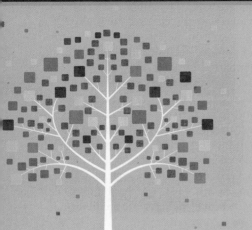

Professionalism

Kathleen DeLeskey

Nurses comprise the largest number of health care professionals in the United States with more than 2.6 million employed in 2008. The number is expected to rise to more than 3.2 million by 2018.[1] Clearly, the work of nurses has an enormous impact on the quality of health care today and will continue to influence the way in which health services are rendered for the foreseeable future.

Through our scope of practice, specialized knowledge, and code of ethics, the discipline of nursing has demonstrated its dedication to improving public health. The integrity and commitment of the profession have not been disregarded by the public. Since 1999, the national Gallup poll has found nursing to be the most trusted of 19 professions, with nurses admired for their honesty and ethical standards. The one exception to this choice was 2001, when firefighters were voted the most trusted profession.

Forming a professional identity and maintaining a professional presence in a highly technological, rapidly changing health care environment can be a challenge. The process demands not only specific knowledge and skills but also the ability to address the challenges and ethical dilemmas that occur on a daily basis. Professional nurses maintain accountability for their work, develop good clinical judgment, strengthen leadership competence, establish high ethical standards, refine therapeutic communication, and educate the public about health issues. Moreover, they constantly aspire to understand and improve their practice.

DEFINITION(S)

Professionalism is a broad concept that applies across disciplines. Professionalism refers to the application of ideal qualities of an individual within a specific professional field. Health care professions share many professional attributes; the unique characteristics for each profession are described through professional identity. Comportment is made up of the knowledge, skills, and attitudes together with values and beliefs of the profession. One might say that professionalism is the comportment that creates professional identity in an individual. Because these attributes are so closely related, they will be discussed together throughout this concept.

Within nursing, professionalism refers to the attributes and behaviors of a nurse as a representative of the profession and as a member of health care professionals. The word *"identity"* is commonly described as a set of definitive characteristics and behaviors that differentiate one individual from another. Personal identity distinguishes the specific uniqueness of each person—it differentiates both how the person perceives and interacts with the surroundings and how the person is perceived by others. Professional identity, on the other hand, is comprised of a compilation of the skills, values, and expertise common to a group of individuals who are part of the same profession. The public recognizes nurses through the fidelity and honesty they exhibit.

Many researchers[2-8] agree that personal and professional identities are closely correlated. Professional identity encompasses personal values, beliefs, and perceptions about the work to be done. The professional identity of a nurse is multilayered and includes knowledge, simple and complex skills, expertise, and curiosity built upon beliefs, assumptions, and values that compose the nurse's identity as a person.[9] It is appropriate then to say that a professional nurse is sensitive to the needs of others but appreciates the significance of understanding personal values, respecting the values of others, and interacting with empathy and discernment in all situations.

The American Nurses Association espouses numerous requirements to assume a professional role, including provision of safe and quality patient care, adherence to the code of nursing ethics, awareness of social policy and standards, competence in the delivery of care, and responsiveness to emerging trends in socioeconomic and political practice arenas. For the purposes of this concept analysis, professionalism is defined as *the assimilation of nursing skills and knowledge integrated with dignity and respect for all human beings, incorporating the assumptions and values of the profession while maintaining accountability and self-awareness.*[4,6-9]

SCOPE AND CATEGORIES

The scope of professional identity in nursing includes *autonomy, knowledge, competence, professionhood, accountability, advocacy, collaborative practice,* and *commitment* (Figure 35-1). These eight elements are described by Baumann and Kolotylo as the sum of professional factors in nursing.[10] Attributes such as education and participation in professional associations are implicit components of the professional elements.

Knowledge and *competence* are the foundation of practice. Knowing and being able to carry out the skills of the profession are the primary components of professional practice. *Collaborative practice* is essential today when patient interaction with the health care system may be extremely time-limited. Nurses practice as members of a health care team in nearly all environments. *Autonomy,* or control over nursing practice, refers to the authority to make decisions related to nursing practice. Determinations are never made without the guidance of ethical and legal regulations; however, a professional nurse is able to make care decisions based on knowledge, experience, and skills. *Commitment* to the profession is demonstrated through continuous learning and professional membership that supports learning. *Accountability* for practice, knowledge, and competence are built into professional practice. *Advocacy* includes endorsement for patients and for the profession and professionals who serve them. Recognizing exceptional activities, supporting colleagues and nursing practice, and seeking to improve care where appropriate all fall within the realm of advocacy. Nurses seeking certification to designate their knowledge, skills, and attitudes in a defined area facilitate in the formation of professional identity. Certification in a practice area is nationally recognized and demonstrates commitment to excellence on the part of the nurse. Seeking and maintaining certification may be illustrated best by the American Nurses Association (ANA) in its mission statement: *Nurses advancing our profession to improve health for all.*[11] The mission implies that a nurse practices at an optimal level using evidence-based practice to improve patient outcomes. The ultimate professional nurse also keeps current on emerging trends in health care, is concerned with world health and political decisions in health care, and upholds the ethical standards of nursing practice.

Nurses view professionalism through the care and advocacy they provide to patients. Even the radical anarchist Emma Goldman found fulfillment in caring for and advocating for the indigent women in New York. She was proud of her nurse training and the relationships she built with her patients. When questioned about her profession, which was to raise public awareness about poverty through radical demonstrations, her pat answer was, "I am a trained nurse." This answer, she recognized, provided her with credibility and respect.[12]

ATTRIBUTES AND CRITERIA

Attributes of nursing professionalism are discussed throughout the literature.[13-18] Professionalism is demonstrated through the accumulation of many attributes. Education, clinical judgment, ethics, comportment, and therapeutic communication are among the most commonly addressed professional attributes. Other important attributes include accountability, leadership, respect, and self-awareness. These are the criteria that guide professional practice and build professional identity. Ethical decision making and respect are paramount in a health care system that has limited resources and differing values. This is emphasized in the 2004 report *Crossing the Quality Chasm: A New Health System for the 21st Century* when the Institute of Medicine mandated that health care workers "respect patients' values and preferences."[19]

Patients view a professional nurse as someone who has good interpersonal skills, good critical thinking, and empathetic, caring practices.[17] Nurses described what they believe to be the best nursing professionals as highly experienced and well-educated with a minimum of a bachelor's degree and certification in their specialty. They also identified the importance of the attributes innovative, active learner, confident, deeply empathetic, and very passionate about nursing.[20]

The picture that begins to develop of a professional nurse is someone who is highly skilled, recognizes patient needs, remains calm and confident, and provides thoughtful, empathetic care to patients. The descriptors comprise behaviors, but professional decorum includes more than behavior. Professional nurses have a unique way of being with others. They adopt a special tone and demeanor in their interactions with others that are observable. Therapeutic interaction validates the "other" and provides an environment that encourages open and genuine communication resulting in a trusting relationship.

The trust and respect toward nurses held by the public validate the strong advocacy role they play. Although nurses are care managers and teachers, they constantly campaign for better patient care. Whether acting in the community, a hospital or nursing home, an academic setting, or a hospice situation,

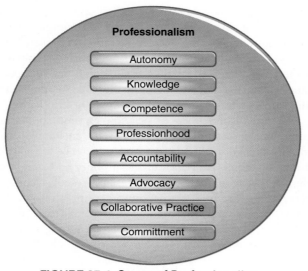

FIGURE 35-1 Scope of Professionalism.

professional nurses continually seek to allay fears, improve treatments, and enhance comfort physically, emotionally, and spiritually while they strive for optimal patient flourishing.

Recent changes in health care have created an environment that demands the use of evidence-based nursing practice. To find and use research evidence to improve practice, nurses have grown more adept at reading, understanding, and conducting research. The role of the professional nurse as "scientist" is growing rapidly as a specialty and providing nursing practice with the evidence that will result in the best patient outcomes.

THEORETICAL LINKS

Social Identity Theory posits that social identity is derived from group membership and that most people work to attain a positive social identity. This, in turn, helps to boost personal self-esteem.[21] A desire to become part of the "group" is apparent even among student nurses as they strive for recognition. New nurses seek acceptance among peers in the work environment. Even seasoned nurses recognize the support that is derived from membership in a professional group.

Social Identity Theory also describes group biases for its members and against non–group members. Even among nurses practicing in the same organization, biases are often seen between accepted social groups. For example, there are differences in identity among nurses who work in a high-acuity specialty care environment (such as the intensive care unit), nurses who work on a general inpatient unit, and nurses who work in outpatient clinics. Each group possesses expertise, yet the tendency is for each group to perceive their work as more important and their own expertise as superior.

As the experience and expertise of a nurse develop, group identity may change. Because there are numerous practice arenas, moving among them is a frequent phenomenon in nursing practice. Professional identity as an operating room nurse may be compelling and therefore further education and exposure to new ideas may lead an experienced operating room nurse to seek skills as a certified registered nurse anesthetist (CRNA), and ultimately a new professional identity with its inherent skills and expertise begins to develop.

Social Identity Theory supports professionalism in nursing. Nurses formulate their own professional identity with and among those with whom they practice. As they form their professional identity, self-esteem is supported and the profession of nursing is underpinned.

CONTEXT TO NURSING AND HEALTH CARE

In order to enter the nursing profession and obtain nursing licensure, an individual must complete a state board–credentialed educational program (thus complete a minimum educational requirement) and successfully pass a common licensure examination. Nurses have argued for decades about the educational level that should be mandated for practitioners. Some believe that all nurses should have a graduate degree to practice, whereas others consider all levels of education as necessary in a diverse profession. There are even arguments over the type of doctorate degree that is acceptable. Regardless, pursuing ongoing education and maintaining clinical competence are expectations of all practicing professional nurses; in many states documentation of continuing education is required for license renewal.

The Institute of Medicine (IOM) in collaboration with the Robert Wood Johnson Foundation has made recommendations in an effort to improve the fractured health care system in the United States. *The Future of Nursing: Leading Change, Advancing Health*[21] recommends that 80% of nurses have a minimum baccalaureate degree by the year 2020.

According to the IOM nurses comprise the largest segment of the health care workforce and provide most of the professional care to patients. Although physicians diagnose and recommend treatments, those treatments are largely provided by nurses. Professional nurses teach, advocate, assess, and nurture patients. As the patient population ages and health care needs among the diverse population become more complex, nurses are collaborating more frequently with other professionals to improve the care and outcomes for patients. Physicians, physical therapists, occupational therapists, social service experts, and home care providers are likely to comprise the health care team that successfully reintegrates patients into the community. Because nurses provide holistic care incorporating physical, social, and spiritual needs of patients, the nurse becomes the team leader who directs the care in a consistent and organized manner as shown in Figure 35-2.

With rapid discharge of patients from the health care system nurses have assumed the role of ensuring that proper follow-up and recovery occur. The IOM rightfully expects nurses not merely to meet those expectations, but also to lead the transformation that will guide America's health care consumers safely through the transition. Nurses must be well educated, highly skilled, and deeply passionate to assume this role.

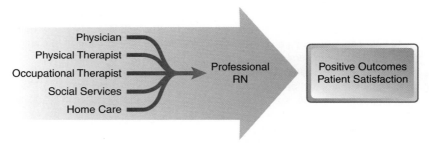

FIGURE 35-2 Team Leader.

INTERRELATED CONCEPTS

The concept of professional identity for nurses is closely related to many other concepts presented in this textbook. Four interrelated concepts that are especially important to emphasize (**Clinical judgment, Leadership, Ethics,** and **Communication**) are described in the following sections and are depicted in Figure 35-3.

Clinical judgment. More than 20 years ago clinical judgment was described by experts[22] as one of the most critical attributes for nurses. It still remains a fundamental skill in the current health care environment of rapidly changing, overwhelming, and complicated nursing assignments. Effective clinical judgment is both demanding and complex. It entails being able to use critical thinking to assess and interpret available data, maintain flexibility, recognize cues from the patient, and respond in a safe and expeditious manner.[23] Part of the knowledge required to make good clinical judgments may be acquired through scientific and theoretical education, but part of it is tacit nursing knowledge gained from experience and familiarity with clinical situations. Studies have shown that as nursing experience increases, the nursing knowledge that is inherent in the role becomes more comprehensive and clinical judgment is enhanced.[24-26]

Leadership. Proficient leadership is a crucial part of maintaining a successful and professional work environment. High-quality leadership can result in retention of nursing staff, better patient outcomes, and fewer costly negative patient events.[27-30] Because nurses possess unique knowledge and maintain relationships with patients, it has become the obligation of the profession to forge stronger advocacy roles on behalf of patients. Passionate and competent leaders are in the best position to influence patient care and policy.

Ethics. The American Nurses Association (ANA) developed the *Code of Ethics for Nurses*. Ethics has become a major challenge in an age of advancement and technology that has enormous momentum. Ethical dilemmas arise that have never before existed. Benner describes that nurses "must maintain ethical comportment, use knowledge and skills appropriately and develop therapeutic relations with patients through communication."[31]

To provide ethical treatment for patients, it is important to recognize personal values. What we value impacts our beliefs, attitudes, and ultimately our behavior and decisions. Patients may have different value systems and nurses must be cognizant of the differences in order to respect patient wishes. Values are not universal. Each individual may have different values as a result of different life experiences, backgrounds, and beliefs.

MODEL CASE

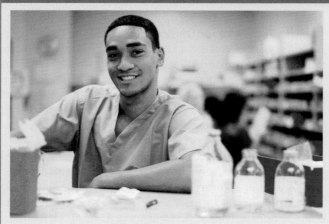

Rob is a 37-year-old former computer programmer. He was previously employed in the technology industry before he was "downsized." Upon his job termination, Rob made the decision to switch to the nursing profession after having observed nursing care when his mother was terminally ill. He initially earned an associate degree in nursing and began working as a medical-surgical nurse. He attended school part-time to earn his bachelor's degree and then his master's degree in nursing.

Rob has been working in the postanesthesia care unit (PACU) in a community hospital for the past 7 years and became manager of the unit 2 years ago. Rob supervises 24 staff nurses and 4 unlicensed assistive personnel (UAP). He communicates clearly with all members of the health care team including the nurses and UAP, anesthesiologists, surgeons, and surgical nurses. He is well respected among all the health care team members for his insight, expertise, and empathetic style of practice. The PACU nurses often seek Rob's guidance with patient care issues because they know he has great clinical expertise and judgment.

Rob belongs to his professional organization and encourages his staff to join. He provides time off for nurses who wish to attend professional educational opportunities. He attends an annual conference in his specialty so he is aware of the professional growth and exposure to new trends and practices. He also reads research and peer-reviewed journals weekly and keeps some on the unit as a source of reference for the staff.

The nursing department in the hospital in which Rob works is governed by several nursing councils. As a manager, Rob is a member of the Nursing Leadership Council and he is also a member of the Nursing Research Council because he is fascinated by nursing research and realizes how important research studies are to creating an environment of evidence-based practice. The PACU nurses are now working to translate an evidence-based guideline for family visitation in the unit into practice under his direction. They are all thrilled to be on the cutting edge of introducing this new guideline into the unit.

Recently, Rob agreed to serve as a mentor for a graduate nursing student. He is grateful for those who supported his education and is honored to be able to meet the needs of another in the profession. He knows as an expert, he has the responsibility to share his skills and knowledge.

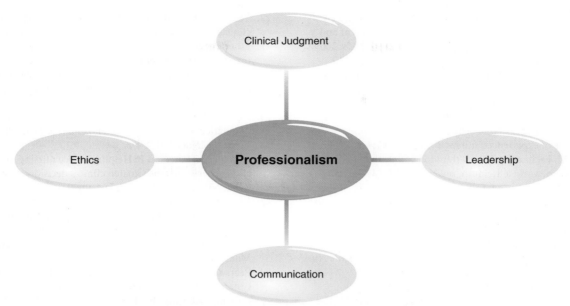

FIGURE 35-3 Professionalism and Interrelated Concepts.

Communication. A strong nurse-patient relationship is the foundation of professional nursing practice. Research shows that novice nurses have difficulty developing trust in the nurse-patient relationship.[32] However, being able to communicate effectively and feel comfortable with a patient helps to strengthen that trust. Strong therapeutic communication skills enhance nursing practice.

Nurses use therapeutic communication to gather and convey information and to promote healing. Therapeutic communication requires attentive listening with requisite positioning and eye contact. It also requires the ability to explore the thoughts and feelings of others. Relationships between nurses and patients are by nature fairly personal. Hospitalized patients may be fearful and dependent. Because nurses spend the most time with patients, it becomes their duty to listen, explore, and reassure while reserving their personal opinions and remaining receptive to patient needs.

EXEMPLARS

There are many examples of professionalism in nursing practice. Box 35-1 presents some of the most common exemplars seen in clinical practice.

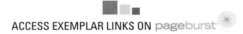

ACCESS EXEMPLAR LINKS ON pageburst

REFERENCES

1. Bureau of Labor Statistics: *U.S. Department of Labor: Occupational outlook handbook.* Accessed Dec 26, 2010, at www.bls.gov/oco/ocos083.htm.
2. Wengstrom Y, Ekedahl M: The art of professional development and caring in cancer nursing, *Nurs Health Sci* 8:20, 2006.
3. Hurley J, Mears A, Ramsay M: Doomed to fail: the persistent search for a modernist mental health nurse identity, *Nurs Philos* 10:53, 2008.
4. Fagerberg I, Kihlgren M: Experiencing a nurse identity: the meaning of identity to Swedish registered nurses two years after graduation, *J Adv Nurs* 34:137, 2001.
5. Randle J: Changes in self esteem during a 3-year preregistration Diploma in Higher Education (nursing) programme, *J Clin Nurs* 12:142, 2003.
6. Callan V, Gallois C, Mayhew M, et al: Restructuring the multi-professional organization: professional identity and adjustment to change in a public hospital, *J HHSA Spring* 449, 2007.
7. Deppoliti D: Exploring how new registered nurses construct professional identity in hospital settings, *J Contin Educ Nurs* 39:255, 2008.
8. Trede F: Professionalism: becoming professional in the 21st century, *J Emerg Prim Health Care* 7:1, 2009.
9. Riddell T: Critical assumptions: thinking critically about critical thinking, *J Nurs Educ* 46:121, 2007.

▪▪▪ BOX 35-1	**EXEMPLARS OF PROFESSIONALISM**

Leadership
- Influential
- Inspired
- Proficient

Clinical Judgment
- Knowledgeable
- Skilled
- Self-confident

Communication
- Therapeutic
- Accurate
- Skilled
- Focused

Ethics
- Morality
- Beneficence
- Respectful
- Truthful
- Honorable

Comportment
- Licensure
- Professional certification
- Lifelong learner
- Self-awareness

10. Baumann A, Kolotylo C: The professional and environmental factors in the workplace questionnaire: development and psychometric evaluation, *J Adv Nurs* 65(10):2216–2228, 2009.

11. Annual Report of the American Nurses Association, 2010.

12. Connolly CA: 'I am a trained nurse': the nursing identity of anarchist and radical Emma Goldman, *Nurs Hist Rev* 18:84–99, 2010.

13. Catlett S, Lovan S: Being a good nurse and doing the right thing: a replication study, *Nurs Ethics* 18:54, 2011.

14. Riley J, Beal J, Lancaster D: Scholarly nursing practice from the perspective of experienced nurses, *J Adv Nurs* 61:425, 2008.

15. Chabeli M: Facilitating critical thinking within the nursing process framework: a literature review, *Health SA Gesondheid* 12:69, 2007.

16. Benner P, Tanner C: Clinical judgment: how expert nurses use intuition, *Am J Nurs* 87:23, 1987.

17. Gallup poll votes nurses most trusted profession, *New Hampshire Nurs News* 34:7, 2010.

18. Wysong P, Driver E: Perceptions of nurses' skill, *Crit Care Nurs* 25:24, 2009.

19. Institute of Medicine: *Crossing the quality chasm: a new health system for the 21st century*, Washington, DC, 2004, The National Academies Press.

20. Brown R: Social identity theory: past achievements, current problems and future challenges, *Eur J Soc Psychol* 30:745, 2000.

21. Committee on the Robert Wood Johnson Foundation Initiative on the Future of Nursing: *Institute of Medicine: The future of nursing: leading change, advancing health, 2010* at www.iom.edu/Reports/2010/A-Summary-of-the-February-2010-Forum-on-the-Future-of-Nursing-Education.aspx. Accessed March 24, 2011.

22. Tanner C: Thinking like a nurse: a research-based model of clinical judgment in nursing, *J Nurs Educ* 45:211, 2006.

23. Etheridge S: Learning to think like a nurse: stories from new nurse graduates, *J Contin Educ Nurs* 38:24, 2007.

24. Harjai P, Tiwari R: Model of critical diagnostic reasoning: achieving expert clinician performance, *Nurs Educ Perspect* 30:305, 2009.

25. Agbedia C, Ofi B, Ibeagha J: Causal model of clinical judgment of practicing nurses in selected hospitals in Delta State, Nigeria, *West Afr J Nurs* 2:11, 2008.

26. Gillespie M, Paterson B: Helping novice nursing make effective clinical decisions: the situated clinical decision-making framework, *Nurs Educ Perspect* 30:164, 2009.

27. Swearingen S: A journey to leadership: designing a nursing leadership development program, *J Contin Educ Nurs* 40:107, 2009.

28. Wong C, Cummings G: The relationship between nursing leadership and patient outcomes: a systematic review, *J Nurs Management* 15:508, 2007.

29. Pearson A, Laschinger H, Porritt K, et al: Comprehensive systematic review of evidence on developing and sustaining nursing leadership that fosters a healthy work environment in healthcare, *Int J Evidence Based Healthcare* 5:208, 2007.

30. Kanste O, Kyngas H, Nikkila J: The relationship between multidimensional leadership and burnout among nursing staff, *J Nurs Management* 15:731, 2007.

31. Benner P, Sutphen M, Leonard V, et al: *Educating nurses: a call for radical transformation*, San Francisco, 2010, Jossey-Bass.

32. Park M: Ethical issues in nursing practice, *J Nurs Law* 13:68, 2009.

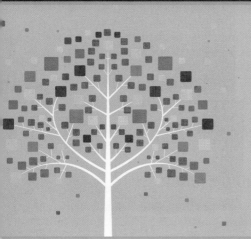

Clinical Judgment

Ann Nielsen and Kathie Lasater

As we entered the twenty-first century, it became clear that the delivery of health care in general and the practice of nursing had become very complex. Larger numbers of patients with complicated medical conditions are cared for in hospital and community-based settings. Health care financing and reimbursement have become major determinants of health care practices; thus patients with interrelated comorbidities are now admitted to acute care settings for shorter periods of time and sicker patients are cared for in community-based settings, such as home health and long-term care.[1] The increased complexity of patients' medical conditions translates to an increased complexity of the nurses' work in all settings. Ebright and colleagues[2] concluded that nurses working in acute care medical-surgical settings must prioritize or "restack" patient care tasks multiple times throughout a shift. This restacking involves a myriad of unexpected events that necessitate reorganizing tasks, such as changes to patient schedules, deteriorating patient conditions, multiple discharges and admissions, and patient care staffing issues. Between the restacked tasks, nurses engage in a thinking process that results in crucial clinical judgments about patient care. The foundation of safe and effective nursing practice is the ability to consistently make good clinical judgments. Clinical judgment as a concept is presented from a theoretical perspective to help the student gain an understanding of the complexities of this process.

DEFINITION(S)

The concept of clinical judgment in general refers to interpretations and inferences that influence actions in clinical practice. Clinical judgment has deep significance to nursing practice. In each clinical encounter inside or outside the hospital, nurses assess patients or populations and their issues that lead to clinical judgments. These judgments impact both safety and quality of care. Definitions, both in generic terms and from the nursing literature, facilitate understanding of this concept.

Two generic definitions of judgment apply most closely to use of the term in health care: one is the *process* of forming an opinion or evaluation by discerning or comparing whereas the second definition denotes *capacity* for judging, discernment, or the exercise of this capacity. A third definition is a proposition stating something believed or asserted, in other words, an *inference, interpretation, and/or decision* about the patient situation. All of these definitions have application to the concept of clinical judgment. The term *clinical,* an adjective, is defined as relating to or conducted in a clinic, involving direct observation of the patient; it may refer to being diagnosable by or based on clinical observation.

Similar to the generic definitions, authors in the nursing literature use the term as an inference or interpretation made in a caregiving setting,[3-7] a process resulting in such an inference or interpretation,[4-7,8-18] or the capacity for making inferences or interpretations about patient care.* The definition we will use for the purpose of this concept analysis is *"an interpretation or conclusion about a patient's needs, concerns, or health problems, and/or the decision to take action (or not), use or modify standard approaches, or improvise new ones as deemed appropriate by the patient's response."*[7,p204]

A related term, *clinical reasoning,* is the thinking process by which a nurse reaches a clinical judgment.[20] It is defined as *"an iterative process of noticing, interpreting, and responding— reasoning in transition with a fine attunement to the patient and how the patient responds to the nurse's actions."*[12,p230] Herein lies the complexity of nursing clinical judgment because it requires that the nurse recognize the unique situation of the patient, including a deep understanding both of the clinical situation and of the nurse's contribution to the patient care situation. Because each patient situation and each nurse are different, so too is the clinical reasoning that leads to clinical judgment.

---

*References 3, 5, 8, 10, 12, 16, 18, 19.

SCOPE AND CATEGORIES

Standards-Based Approach

It is important to recognize that the early research behind clinical judgment focused on trying to understand all the factors involved in clinical judgments about patient care and making them explicit. This resulted in a rules-based or standards-based approach that locates the nurse and the individual needs of the patient outside the caregiving situation, rather than situating the specific patient issue in a context of care. Decision making from this perspective involves selection from options of mutually exclusive possibilities, implying that there is one right decision. This approach often involves use of algorithms, decision trees, and guidelines. These tools provide clear-cut guidance that may standardize approaches to patient care within an institution based on best practices for a given patient population and are important to general patient care quality. Algorithms direct care in emergent situations, such as a cardiopulmonary arrest, that involve numbers of interprofessional personnel. These tools can be very useful, especially for the beginning clinician who lacks knowledge and/or experience. However, their use may or may not result in the best possible care for a particular patient in a given situation. They also may limit options and creative solutions.

A principle that relates decision-making tools to clinical judgment is that if there is a rule that covers the situation, clinical judgment is not required. In fact, more recent research has shown that although standards or guidelines may be useful beginning points, expert nurses rarely use them alone.[7] This is because the expert nurse nuances his or her understanding of the individual patient situation along with knowledge of standards to employ a much more interpretivist approach.

Interpretivist Perspective

Interpretivist approaches originate from the belief that life experiences are culturally bound, that individuals interpret these experiences on the basis of their encounters within a given culture,[21] and that one circumscribed approach is often not appropriate for a large number of patients.[7] The nature of nursing care is not linear, and in fact in numerous situations there are many unknowns; therefore approaches that consider multiple factors in clinical reasoning are often more appropriate.[7] Because there are often no clear-cut answers about nursing care or because of the influence of the individual patient circumstances and context of care, clinical judgments by nurses become very specific to a given patient care situation. Interpretivist approaches situate the nurse squarely in the context of care, and account for what the nurse personally contributes to the caring encounter, including previous experiences, values, and emotions.[12] The creation or construction of understanding the patient and caregiving situation using empirical knowledge, knowledge of the patient, and knowledge of the clinical environment facilitates decisions about care, thereby setting the stage for what the nurse notices and how the nurse interprets and responds.[7,12,15,22]

Reasoning in interpretivist approaches may involve "rule of thumb" methods and be intuitive. It involves understood knowledge,[23] is often inductive in nature, and is referred to by some authors as engaged, practical reasoning.[7,12,16,24] In contrast, rules-based approaches tend to rely heavily on analytic reasoning that requires systematically dividing a situation into parts, examining alternatives, and weighing options.[7] One example of the analytic approach is diagnostic reasoning—considering the evidence that supports each diagnosis.[25]

ATTRIBUTES AND CRITERIA

Using the interpretivist perspective of clinical judgment and clinical reasoning from the nursing literature, clinical judgment has three significant defining attributes that are useful to understand the concept:

1. *Holistic view of the patient situation.* Clinical judgment is inherently complex and influenced by many factors related to the particular patient and caregiving situation, and therefore requires a holistic view.[12,14,16,23] Making excellent clinical judgments requires a willingness to consider all factors involved in patient care, including certain characteristics of the nurse, and is much more than simply a combination of the individual aspects.[7,14]

2. *Process orientation.* Clinical judgment is circular, interactive, and moves fluidly between and among all of the aspects of the process.[6,7,12,15,16] To make clinical judgments, the nurse employs a deep understanding of the individual patient situation and his or her own background, experience, and values. Patients and nurses are unique and bring different backgrounds to the caregiving situation. The nurse notices salient (or relevant) features of a situation based on these factors and intervenes. While the nurse observes the patient response, he or she comes to understand what the next steps are. After the caregiving situation, the nurse connects the patient outcomes in a way that enhances further understanding of future patients' care, utilizing reflection.[7,9,17,22,26] These aspects do not have a linear relationship but rather continuously influence each other in complex ways.

3. *Reasoning and interpretation.* Clinical judgment involves reasoning and interpretation. As described previously, reasoning is the process that leads to clinical judgments. At least three types of reasoning are used: analytic, intuitive, and narrative.[7] The type of reasoning used depends upon the caregiving situation and the nurse's previous experience. When a situation is unfamiliar, the nurse (expert and novice alike) tends to rely on analytic reasoning processes, consider the possibilities, and deduce the solution. At other times the expert nurse may recognize a situation immediately and act intuitively and tacitly. Nurses may also process their reasoning in narrative form, that is, recognizing the significance of the situation at hand to the patient's experience with illness, and engaging in interventions based on this understanding.

THEORETICAL LINKS

The Model of Clinical Judgment[7] is a comprehensive approach to clinical judgment that was developed based on 3 decades of clinical judgment research and through an extensive review of research done primarily with expert nurses in practice. The model (see Figure 36-1) rests on assumptions about complexities in the environment of care and the interplay of multiple factors that affect nurses' clinical thinking. In the Model of Clinical Judgment, four aspects of clinical judgments are described. Influenced by background and contextual factors, the nurse *notices* various things about the caregiving situation—such as clinical assessment findings, lab work, data, patient demeanor, family situation. Through clinical reasoning patterns, collecting additional clinical data as needed, and conferring with colleagues, the nurse develops an understanding of the particular clinical situation, a process called *interpreting*. Based on the interpretation of the situation, the nurse determines appropriate actions, *responding* in the model. The nurse observes the patient's reaction to the nursing action and decides if the action has addressed the primary concerns, if the action needs some refinement to adjust for the particular patient, or if a completely different response is required. This is referred to as *reflection-in-action*. Nursing reflection after the fact, *reflection-on-action,* helps the nurse to connect patient responses with outcomes in a way that contributes to the nurse's further understanding of patient care.[7] Despite the fact that these aspects are described in separate sections, they do not have a linear relationship but rather continuously influence each other in a complex fashion. So the consideration of them as separate aspects may be artificial but is offered here as an in-depth means to better understand the concept.

Noticing

Noticing is most often the impetus for clinical reasoning and is critical to making an effective judgment to address a patient issue. Several important factors impact what the nurse notices. In fact, Tanner[7] asserts that the factors behind the nurse's eyes are as important as what is in front. These include the background of the nurse (including intrapersonal characteristics, ethical grounding for what is right, previous experiences, and theoretical knowledge), the nurse's relationship with the patient, and the context of care (see Box 36-1 for more detail about these precursors to noticing). Influenced by these factors, the nurse develops expectations about potential patient needs that set the stage for *noticing*. Expectations derive from the nurse's experiences with similar patients that allow the nurse to anticipate the patient's appearance and needs, both currently and in the next hours and days. Without these experiences, the nurse uses theoretical, decontextualized knowledge.

The nurse enters the care situation and collects pertinent information and patient data. Broad knowledge based on experience and theoretical understanding as well as understanding a particular context allows nurses to notice what factors are the most salient in terms of caring for a particular patient. Nurses select from a very broad set of data and patient assessment findings, looking for patterns that are consistent with previous experiences and using that information to guide care in the current situation. Less experienced nurses may have difficulty extracting the most important patient data and findings in a particular situation.[12,29]

Knowing the patient (whether it is knowing a given type of patient or knowing a specific patient) in a particular context influences what a nurse notices. For example, a home

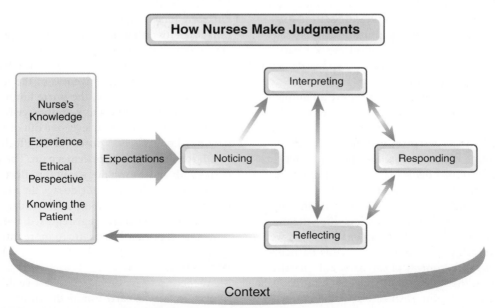

FIGURE 36-1 Tanner's Model of Clinical Judgment. (Adapted from Tanner CA: Thinking like a nurse: a research-based model of clinical judgment, *J Nurs Educ* 45[6]:204–211, 2006.)

BOX 36-1 FACTORS THAT INFLUENCE NOTICING

Intrapersonal Characteristics of the Nurse
- Ethical grounding and personal sense of importance
- Trustworthiness—asking questions/seeking help when unsure
- Developmental maturity in thought and knowing processes; formulates opinions and values relative to the context of learning
- Skill in using various ways of knowing—empirical, experiential, and ethical

Theoretical and Experiential Knowledge of the Nurse
- Novice and less experienced nurses use deductive reasoning, rules, and comparisons of the patient with the textbook in a systematic analysis of the situation
- Expert nurses look at the whole picture and use pattern recognition and intuition derived from their experiences to make judgments

Knowing the Patient
- Knowing the range of patient's pattern of responses
- Knowing the patient as a person, including preferences and desires

Context or Environment of Care
- Setting in which the nurse interacts with the patient
- Unique aspects of nursing practice/patient care needs in a given setting

---

health nurse who has made visits to an older adult patient in his home over several months has a different level of "knowing the patient" than a nurse who sees a patient in an acute care setting. Knowing the older adult allows the home health nurse to know the patient's baseline mental status and to notice subtle changes in cognition or affect. The nurse assuming care for this same patient in an acute care setting might not realize that medication-related confusion demonstrated by the patient postoperatively is not typical for this patient and might make the assumption that the patient has dementia or other cognitive impairment.

Based on what is noticed, the nurse may have an immediate grasp of the situation—recognition of a pattern or cluster of cues that signals one concern. On other occasions, the nurse, despite extensive experience, may have noticed that the situation is not as expected but does not quite have a clear grasp. Depending on this initial understanding, various reasoning patterns may be triggered. Once an issue is noticed, the nurse immediately gathers additional information and draws on his or her background, including theoretical knowledge, past experiences with similar patients as well as his or her relationship and knowledge of this particular patient within the specific context of care, and ethical beliefs about what is right in this situation. Because each individual nurse and patient and the context of care are different, what happens next is also very unique; in many situations, there is no one right way.

Interpreting

Using the particular patient data as well as germane theoretical and experiential knowledge, the nurse begins to assemble all the information to make sense of it. For the expert nurse, certain data carry more weight than others with respect to the patient. For example, in the long term care setting, a patient's age and kidney function may well impact the nurse's clinical judgment about using ibuprofen for pain relief even though the drug may be ordered. The nurse uses reasoning to make that determination.

According to Tanner,[7] expert nurses draw on a variety of reasoning patterns (analytic, intuitive, and narrative) to interpret the meaning of what has been noticed. The types of reasoning used seem to vary with the experience of the nurse.[12] For example, students and novice nurses, or more experienced nurses encountering unfamiliar situations, tend to rely on analytic reasoning based on theoretical knowledge. The nurse makes a hypothesis or best guess about the patient care situation, and then tests the hypothesis. Sometimes this reasoning is not situation specific but based on generalizations. Expert nurses often use intuitive reasoning based on unstated but understood knowledge about the patient, the caregiving context, and their previous experiences.[12,27] A third type of reasoning, narrative reasoning, is a way of making sense of a situation through telling and interpreting stories.[7,28] Narrative reasoning supports deep understanding of caregiving situations.[7,12] Nurses hear patients' stories of their experiences with illness, how they understand their symptoms, what meaning they attribute to their illness, how they cope with it, and what they hope for resolution. This type of reasoning helps nurses understand the patient experience, setting the stage for individualizing care (Christine Tanner, personal communication, July 7, 2011). Nurses may also use narrative reasoning in their own reflections about patient care.

Responding

Once the patient data have been sorted and interpreted, the nurse uses his or her interpretation to respond to the particular patient issue through one or more nursing interventions. Depending on the level of expertise, the nurse may or may not be able to judge the effectiveness of the intervention before initiating it. For example, the nurse knows that the ordered pain medication is likely to help the newly admitted postoperative patient with a pain level of 8 out of 10. What the nurse may not know is what dose will be effective or the level to which it will reduce the patient's pain. The nurse's past experience with and knowledge about the effects of the pain medication will initially direct the dosage the nurse chooses. As the nurse comes to understand the particular patient's response to the medication and dosage required, the reasoning process moves from primarily analytic to more intuitive/narrative.

Reflecting

Many theorists have described reflective thinking and its usefulness. In fact, an early twentieth century educator made the bold statement that "reflective thinking alone is educative."[30,p2] Other theorists consider that reflection and the ability to learn from one's actions are marks of a professional.[31] The clinical judgment model includes two types of reflection: *reflection-in-action* and *reflection-on-action*. Both have significant bearing on clinical judgment.

Reflection-in-Action

Reflection-in-action refers to the nurse's understanding of patient responses to nursing actions while care is occurring.[7] In observations and interactions with the patient, the nurse determines patient status and adjusts care accordingly. It is the thinking that happens in "real time" during patient care. Because of the ambiguous and complex nature of clinical judgments and the particular needs of each patient, reflecting is a critical step in evaluating the patient's reaction to the intervention. To continue the example of the postoperative patient, the nurse chooses a pain medication dose based on many factors; while administering the medication intravenously, the nurse is continually assessing and reflecting on the patient's response to medication. This is an example of *reflecting-in-action*. If the desired response is not achieved, the nurse may need to return to interpreting the data in order to respond with a different intervention.

Reflection-on-Action

Reflection-on-action is consideration of the situation after the patient care occurs. In reflection-on-action, the nurse contemplates a situation and considers what was successful and what was unsuccessful. *Reflection-on-action* is critical for development of knowledge and improvement in reasoning. It is how learning from practice is incorporated into experience. In the previous example, the nurse may take some time at the end of his or her shift to analyze why he or she intervened in a specific way for this particular patient and to consider whether the intervention was successful. *Reflection-on-action* is when significant learning from practice occurs and it is important to the development of increasing skillfulness as a nurse.[28,32] Often, nurses spend more time reflecting on negative results, but it is equally important to consider successful interventions in order to improve nursing practice.

Nurses may use verbal narrative to engage in reflection-on-action, to make sense of their own nursing experiences and to process thinking. Listen to nurses in clinical settings when they talk; they often tell stories about their patients, especially if some aspect of care is perplexing. Telling stories is often a way of problem solving or learning from the experiences of others.

CONTEXT TO NURSING AND HEALTH CARE

All Nurses, All Settings

Clinical judgment is an integral aspect of nursing care of all patients and patient populations. Nurses in all specialty areas and practice settings—whether in public health nursing, community-based nursing, long-term care, or acute care—exercise clinical judgment; thus it is considered an essential skill of the professional nurse.[27] Clinical judgment, however, is not required for every patient care activity or intervention. Some nursing actions are obvious. For example, a postanesthesia recovery nurse knows that it is appropriate to take an immediate postoperative patient's vital signs quite frequently in the first few hours in order to recognize early signs of a problem. This is based on the nurse's knowledge that patients can sometimes have breathing or circulatory difficulties following administration of a general anesthetic and surgical interventions. The nurse also knows that the earlier such a sign or symptom is identified, the better the outcome for the patient.

Environmental Context

As mentioned previously, the context or setting of care influences what a nurse notices. The specific environment of care also has a significant influence on care. Demanding environments of care can add increasing burden to making clinical judgments[2,6,7,22] and can actually interfere with competent clinical judgment.[33] On the other hand, context may also be a boon for easing the burden of clinical judgments. For example, consider the case of a patient experiencing a myocardial infarction in the emergency department, where a wide range of medications, including oxygen, is readily available. Monitoring devices are already on the patient and, in fact, may have signaled an impending life-threatening dysrhythmia. Nurses in this context are trained to respond quickly and confidently; because of the setting, they are anticipating emergent situations. By contrast, consider the nurse who encounters a person experiencing a myocardial infarction in a public setting, such as a park or a church. Very different actions must be employed, including making a decision about what to do first, who should call for help, who should be involved in the resuscitation process, and how long resuscitation should be continued.

Experience, Theoretical Knowledge, and Expertise

Clinical judgment, or thinking like a nurse, requires deep clinical knowledge and several types of thinking. Not surprisingly, deep clinical knowledge provides the nurse with the background needed to recognize patterns and therefore differences when they occur in patients, signaling the need for nursing care. As nurses become more experienced, clinical judgments become more intuitive, with nurses instantly recognizing patterns and grasping the meaning of situations they have previously encountered to immediately know what their response to the situation should be. As such, it may appear that experienced nurses have not engaged in all aspects of clinical judgment, but, in fact, all aspects may occur almost simultaneously and subconsciously.[7] Inexperienced nurses (novices) tend to treat all pieces of information with similar importance. They have difficulty identifying the most important aspects of a given situation. Early in practice, it is more challenging to individualize and contextualize patient care. Expert nurses look at the whole picture and use pattern recognition and intuition derived from their experiences to make judgments whereas those with less experience most often use deductive reasoning, rules, and comparisons of the patient with the textbook in a systematic analysis of the situation.*

---

*References 7, 12, 24, 25, 34, 35.

Consider the experienced nurse in a clinic-based setting, such as an internal medicine clinic. Through honing his or her cardiopulmonary assessment skills over a number of years, the nurse has become familiar with the early signs of impending acute congestive heart failure. A nurse new to that clinic may not as readily recognize the pattern of breathing correlated with patient color, including the nuanced blue tinge of oral mucous membranes, and complaints of increased fatigue with activities of daily living. The outcome of such experience may well be faster initiation of treatment for this patient, thereby preventing a hospitalization.

We have introduced the idea that students and novice nurses rely on theoretical knowledge and analytic reasoning to make clinical judgments. That theoretical grounding is very important to student nurse practice and beyond. Understanding the principles of nursing care, communication, altered states of health, patient teaching, and other aspects of care is fundamental to becoming a nurse. As students and novice nurses acquire more experience, thinking, and clinical judgment, they use previous experiences, along with an understanding of this particular patient, the current context, and the best available, relevant evidence to ground their thinking about patient care. In fact, one study found that preceptors believed that new graduate nurses were ready for independent practice when they were able to integrate multiple sources of knowing and individualize care to the patient.[16] With that in mind, what strategies facilitate clinical judgment development?

Developing Clinical Judgment

Novice nurses and nursing students are often in awe of nurses who possess high-level clinical judgment skills. As mentioned previously, clinical experience is required to develop this expertise. Taking advantage of a wide range of clinical learning opportunities and working closely with experienced nurses foster clinical judgment. Analyzing situations in which appropriate nursing actions are not obvious or clear-cut can enhance development of clinical judgment. Look for factors that impact the judgments that are made—nursing values, theoretical knowledge, previous experiences, knowing the patient, the patient care environment. Consider how these factors influence the situation.

Knowledge or Deep Understanding

Knowing how to respond to a patient issue requires a deep knowledge of the complex interconnected factors that impact the issue.[36] For example, in maternal-newborn nursing, a deep understanding of the birthing process is essential. However, knowledge of interconnected concepts—such as the normal and problematic signs of impending delivery, the physiologic transition of hormonal influences in the immediate postdelivery phase (both physical and psychologic), and also the potential impact of a new member on the family's dynamics—will facilitate the nurse's clinical judgments in that context of care. In this example, the nurse will need specialty-specific knowledge about lab findings, subtle signs of depression, and community resources/supports that are available for new mothers. Deep knowledge provides a basis for focused assessments, including salient factors, and for interpreting findings that lead to appropriate clinical judgments, specific to the patient's needs.

Learning to Recognize Patterns

Pattern recognition of specific conditions is a significant aspect of *noticing and interpreting* patient care needs and leads to a deeper understanding of patient issues. For instance, a patient with septic shock will likely display a pattern of elevated heart rate, poor perfusion, decreased oxygen saturation, low blood pressure, and a left shift on the white blood cell count differential. Knowing this pattern alerts the student or nurse to note what signs or symptoms may be present or absent in order to determine an appropriate response. As students and nurses gain more experience, patterns related to nursing care become more apparent.

Apply Concepts to Nursing Practice

Look for opportunities to learn about patient care concepts; then compare and contrast how the concepts present in various patients in order to see patterns. For example, consider how a particular patient with sepsis matches the pattern of sepsis just described as well as what signs or symptoms are different. Then consider how the context (caregiving situation, your own values, knowing the patient and his or her specific personal qualities and needs, your own past nursing and personal experiences with the concept) impacts the particular caregiving situation. This may help you to recognize how the specific situation influences the nursing response to the individual patient with sepsis.

Another opportunity to do this might occur on a pediatric rotation. In this rotation, you may care for a patient with respiratory problems that require oxygen, perhaps a patient with asthma. Consider why your patient is receiving supplemental oxygen and other factors (physical, developmental, pathophysiologic) that impact oxygenation and oxygen administration to your patient. Then visit another student's patient who is also administered oxygen, perhaps a patient with pneumonia. Consider the same questions for your classmate's patient. Compare and contrast the two patients. What are the similarities? What are the differences? What learning will you apply to future situations?

Reflective Practice

Reflection is a learning activity included in many nursing programs and with good reason. Reflecting helps students to process and consolidate learning about caregiving situations.[28,32] As a student and as a practicing nurse, it is important to reflect on both successful and unsuccessful interventions during a caregiving experience. Nursing students are often acutely aware of their knowledge deficits as well as their shortcomings in performing a particular nursing skill. Although recognizing the need for improvement and analyzing how that will happen are critically important parts of nursing practice, it is important to reinforce in one's mind those things that you did well.

Narrative, Written and Spoken

Telling stories about practice is often a part of clinical postconference and journaling and is integral to reflective learning. By being an active part of this important learning opportunity and considering carefully the patients described by classmates, students multiply their exposure to different patient issues and gain deeper understanding of nursing practice. Questioning each other and expressing different possibilities can help students broaden their thinking about nursing care options.

INTERRELATED CONCEPTS

Several concepts in this textbook are interrelated to the concept of clinical judgment—in fact, all concepts related to patient care activities have this link. Featured in Figure 36-2 are seven concepts that are especially closely related to clinical judgment including **Safety, Health care quality, Leadership, Patient education, Evidence, Professionalism,** and **Care coordination.** These interrelationships are explained further in the following sections.

Safety. Clinical judgment is integral to safe patient care. Consider the situation of an older adult postoperative patient getting up to walk postoperatively for the first time. The nurse may know that particular caution should be exercised because falls are very common in the hospital context, and there may be unit guidelines regarding fall prevention. From theoretical knowledge, the nurse knows that although falling is a danger when ambulating, there are significant dangers associated with immobility and staying in bed. In making the decision to get the patient up, the nurse considers many factors including the patient's level of consciousness, strength, pain control status, and motivation. The environmental context is considered. What physical impediments are in the way (IV poles, rugs, water on the floor, furniture)? The nurse's previous experiences with ambulating older adult patients will significantly inform his or her decisions.

Health Care Quality. The nurse who is committed to high-quality patient care is alert to patterns that may indicate that there are quality concerns in a given hospital unit or agency. Perhaps medications consistently arrive from pharmacy in mid-morning rather than early in the shift. The nurse notices that while other nurses are waiting for medications to arrive, they become involved in other caregiving activities and then forget to administer the medications once they arrive on the unit. Based on theoretical knowledge, the nurse recognizes this as a systems problem. Experiential knowledge of unit culture and organization informs how the nurse takes action to communicate with the unit manager and the pharmacy in order to get medications to the unit on time.

Leadership. Leadership choices are almost always fraught with multiple competing factors. For example, the charge nurse of an adult medical-surgical unit may have to consider the mix of nursing staff needed for a shift, given the patients' acuity. What staffing combination will best serve the needs of the patients on the unit at any given moment? The charge nurse may need to respond by asking for help at a higher level if the staffing mix is inadequate. On the same unit, an individual nurse may delegate certain aspects of more stable patients' care to a certified nursing assistant, allowing greater focus on those more seriously ill. These kinds of leadership choices are dependent on knowing the patient(s) as well as the backgrounds of the nursing staff.

Patient Education. Determining when and how much education a patient and/or family needs frequently requires clinical judgment. A patient newly diagnosed with diabetes needs to know about diet, medication, exercise, and

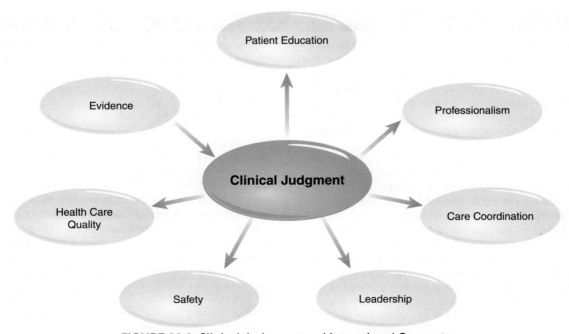

FIGURE 36-2 Clinical Judgment and Interrelated Concepts.

MODEL CASE

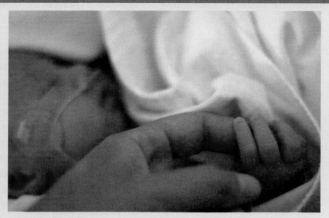

Leon Rowen is a growing premature infant whose 32-year-old mother, Cassandra Rowen, is described by the nurses in the unit as "difficult." The baby is nearing discharge, but Cassandra is reported to be "resistant" to learning about how to feed and care for her infant. She has other children at home, but none of them were premature. A nursing care priority for the day is parental teaching about safe feeding of her premature baby.

Ruth, the nurse assigned to care for Leon, has worked in this unit for 10 years. She observes the entire caregiving situation and sees that Leon's condition is stable. Ruth meets Cassandra and notices she is quiet and sullen. Rather than beginning by explaining how to feed the baby, Ruth asks about Cassandra's other children and shares a little bit about the challenges of parenting her own children who are of similar ages as Cassandra's other children. Cassandra smiles and agrees. As time passes, Cassandra begins to talk about what a frightening experience having a premature baby has been. Ruth acknowledges those feelings. Cassandra smiles and begins to ask questions about how to care for Leon. Ruth answers those questions in a way that is tailored to what the mother has revealed about her family. Cassandra demonstrates feeding Leon in a developmentally appropriate way (side-lying position to prevent aspiration) based on Ruth's teaching. At the end of the shift, Ruth believes Cassandra has made significant progress toward competence in meeting her baby's unique needs. On the drive home, Ruth considers the experience. She realizes that prioritizing getting to know the mother and building a relationship by sharing a bit about herself as a parent helped to create emotional safety and trust so that Cassandra could talk about her apprehension as a first-time mother of a premature baby and then focus on learning infant care.

Case Analysis

In this case study, Ruth's previous encounters with mothers of premature infants and her knowledge of the family experience inform her nursing actions. Experienced nurses incorporate much information simultaneously. Notice that Ruth determines that the baby's physiologic condition is stable while she is beginning to interact with the mother. In this action, she is prioritizing patient safety. While she interacts with the mother, Ruth may interpret Cassandra's behavior as a pattern sometimes displayed by mothers in the NICU. She understands how frightening it is to have a hospitalized newborn and knows from experience that fear can take on many faces. This may be evidence of Ruth's intrapersonal characteristics that value empathy and consider the patient experience. Rather than focusing on Cassandra's negative response to her, Ruth focuses on relationship building before moving on to teaching. This action opens the door to effective teaching. Notice that Ruth takes some time afterward to consider what went well in this challenging situation. This will inform future interactions with mothers of patients.

CONTRARY CASE

Leon Rowen is a growing premature infant whose 32-year-old mother, Cassandra Rowen, is described by the nurses in the unit as "difficult." The baby is nearing discharge, but Cassandra is reported to be "resistant" to learning about how to feed and care for her infant. She has other children at home, but none of them were premature. A nursing care priority for the day is parental teaching about safe feeding of her premature baby.

As is her routine practice, Betsy, the nurse assigned to care for Leon, begins by greeting the mother and assessing the baby. When she is finished assessing the baby and has determined that the baby is stable enough to feed, she hands the baby to Cassandra and provides instructions on how to feed the baby, based on her theoretical knowledge of premature infant development and principles of adult education. Cassandra positions the baby supine for feeding the way she did her full-term children and resists Betsy's attempts to assist her to do otherwise. Leon has an apneic spell during the feeding. The spell resolves in a minute, and Betsy decides to return the baby to his crib and gavage the balance of the feeding. In her documentation, Betsy evaluates her teaching as ineffective and the mother as noncompliant with the feeding plan for the infant. On the drive home, Betsy is exhausted and looks forward to watching a movie that night to relax.

Case Analysis

In contrast to Ruth, Betsy is focused on a single goal, getting the teaching done. Notice that Betsy's care is more stepwise. She assesses the baby first, and then turns her attention to Cassandra. Her personal values of basing care on theoretical knowledge are demonstrated as she uses evidence-based approaches to safe infant feeding. However, she does not consider the context of the situation. She does not notice (or she inaccurately interprets) Cassandra's behavior and does not respond to Cassandra's emotional needs before attempting to teach. Betsy does identify a significant safety concern when Leon aspirates and takes action to complete the feeding in a physiologically safe manner. Betsy draws the conclusion that her nursing care is ineffective, but misses the opportunity to think deeply about the situation after the fact. Thinking about why nursing care was ineffective helps nurses learn from experience and modify approaches in the future.

foot care, for example; in addition, the patient must know how to perform blood glucose monitoring and medication administration. Because it is impossible for a patient to learn everything in one visit, the home health nurse must assess the patient's knowledge and prioritize information. Depending on the patient's ability and ease of learning, the nurse may need to use clinical judgment to refine her teaching to best address the patient's needs. Clinical judgment is exercised throughout the entire learning process—noticing how much the patient remembers from the last visit, how accurately he draws up the insulin for administration, whether he consistently wears adequate shoes inside and outside.

Evidence. In making clinical judgments, nurses consider a variety of evidence. That evidence may come from high-quality research studies, clinical guidelines, and standards of care. The nurse may also use evidence from past experiences with "what works" for patient care within a particular unit culture, as well as practice experiences with a given patient ("knowing the patient") or understanding other contextual factors that impact a caregiving situation. The best available evidence may well impact how the nurse interprets a patient situation and responds to it, but other factors impact nursing actions as well. What happens when a patient has unique needs that depart from the guidelines? Using clinical judgment, values regarding individualizing patient care, and knowledge of the patient, the nurse identifies additional needs and resources, and then advocates for the patient in order to meet the unique needs.

Professionalism. Clinical judgment is applied in situations when the nurse is weighing boundaries in interactions with patients and/or their families. Consider the patient who is newly diagnosed with late-stage lung cancer. The nurse caring for this patient will need to notice the patient's mood and level of interest to determine when the patient needs information about hospice care. The nurse may also have first-hand experience with a family member who had a similar diagnosis. Is there an appropriate opportunity for the nurse to relate to and encourage this patient's family, based on that experience, or is it better with this particular family to focus only on their experience? This situation requires careful noticing and interpretation.

Care Coordination. Determining how best to proceed on behalf of a patient's optimal health care outcomes may require clinical judgment. When planning an older adult patient's discharge after a motor vehicle accident resulting in multiple fractures, the nurse may uncover information that is critical for coordinating the patient's care—information about a patient's home situation that will impact the older adult's recovery (e.g., no help in the home, presence of stairs or other physical barriers, and unavailable home care services). Based on previous experiences with complicated patients, the nurse may request a case conference with the patient's physician, physical therapist, and social worker as well as the patient and family in order to foster the transition for a quality outcome.

EXEMPLARS

Clinical judgment is applied in all areas of nursing practice; thus there are multiple examples. Box 36-2 presents five general areas nurses potentially apply clinical judgment within practice. These include application of clinical skills, recognizing and responding to urgent/emergent situations, communication, medication management, and management of care.

BOX 36-2   EXEMPLARS OF CLINICAL JUDGMENT

Clinical Skills
- Determination regarding size and type of urinary or intravenous catheter
- Decisions about timing and extent of bathing and personal care
- Assessment of a wound
- Selection of an appropriate dressing

Urgent/Emergent Situations
- Detection of subtle signs of sepsis
- Early treatment of patient hemorrhage
- Starting oxygen to respond to decreased saturation levels
- Early recognition of anaphylaxis

Communication
- Content and depth of patient teaching at discharge, pre- and postoperatively
- Advocacy for patient at care coordination conferences
- Communication with distraught or fearful patient or family
- Defusing potentially confrontational interactions

Medication Management
- Selection of dose when a range is ordered
- PRN decisions
- Holding a medication
- Early recognition of adverse reaction or side effect from medication

Management of Care
- Delegation to ancillary nursing personnel
- Prioritization of care among patients
- When to call the physician
- Referral to another health professional (e.g., wound care specialist, dietitian)

ACCESS EXEMPLAR LINKS ON pageburst

REFERENCES

1. Institute of Medicine: *The future of nursing*, Washington, DC, 2010, Author.
2. Ebright PR, Patterson ES, Chalko BA, et al: Understanding the complexity of registered nurse work in acute care settings, *J Nurs Adm* 33(12):630–638, 2003.
3. Lasater K: Clinical judgment development: using simulation to create an assessment Rubric, *J Nurs Educ* 46(11):496–503, 2007.
4. Marshall BL, Jones SH, Snyder G: A program design to promote clinical judgment, *J Nurs Staff Dev* 17(2):78–84, 2001.
5. Rhodes ML, Curran C: Use of the human patient simulator to teach clinical judgment skills in a baccalaureate nursing program, *Comput Inform Nurs* 23(5):256–262, 2005.
6. Samuels JG, Fetzer S: Pain management documentation quality as a reflection of nurses' clinical judgment, *J Nurs Care Qual* 24(3):223–231, 2009.
7. Tanner CA: Thinking like a nurse: a research-based model of clinical judgment in nursing, *J Nurs Educ* 45(6):204–211, 2006.
8. American Association of Critical Care Nurses (AACN): *American Association of Critical Care Nurses (AACN) synergy model*, 2010, . Retrieved from www.aacn.org/wd/certifications/content/synmodel.pcms?pid=1&;&menu=.
9. Becker D, Kaplow R, Muenzen PM, et al: Activities performed by acute and critical care advanced practice nurses: American Association of Critical-Care Nurses study of practice, *Am J Crit Care* 15(2):130–148, 2006.
10. Beecroft PC: Clinical judgment in evidence-based practice, *Clin Nurs Spec* 15(5):191–192, 2001.
11. Benner P, Stannard D, Hooper PL: A "thinking-in-action" approach to teaching clinical judgment: a classroom innovation for acute care advanced practice nurses, *Adv Pract Nurs Q* 1(4):70–77, 1996.
12. Benner P, Tanner C, Chesla C: *Expertise in nursing practice: caring, clinical judgment and ethics*, ed 2, New York, 2009, Springer.
13. del Bueno D: A crisis in critical thinking, *Nurs Educ Perspect* 26(5):278–282, 2005.
14. Di Vito-Thomas P: Nursing student stories on learning how to think like a nurse, *Nurs Educ* 30(3):133–136, 2005.
15. Lin PF, Hsu MY, Tasy SL: Teaching clinical judgment in Taiwan, *J Nurs Res* 11(3):159–166, 2003.
16. McNiesh S: Demonstrating holistic clinical judgment: preceptors perceptions of new graduate nurses, *Holist Nurs Pract* 21(2):72–78, 2007.
17. Pesut DJ: Education: clinical judgment: foreground/background, *J Prof Nurs* 17(5):215, 2001.
18. Roberts K, Lockhart R, Sportsman S: A competency transcript to assess and personalize new graduate competency, *J Nurs Adm* 39(1):19–25, 2009.
19. Bambini D, Washburn J, Perkins R: Outcomes of clinical simulation for novice nursing students: communication, confidence, and clinical judgment, *Nurs Educ Perspect* 30(2):79–82, 2009.
20. Simmons B: Clinical reasoning: concept analysis, *J Adv Nurs* 66(5):1151–1158, 2010.
21. Crotty M: *The foundations of social research: meaning and perspective in the research process*, London, 1998, Sage.
22. Kaplow R, Reed K: The AACN synergy model for patient care: a nursing model as a force of magnetism, *Nurs Econ* 26(1):17–25, 2008.
23. Braude HD: Clinical intuition versus statistics: different modes of tacit knowledge in clinical epidemiology and evidence-based medicine, *Theor Med Bioeth* 30(3):181–198, 2009.
24. Wolf AW: Comment: can clinical judgment hold its own against scientific knowledge? *Psychotherapy* 46(1):11–14, 2009.
25. Croskerry P: A universal model of diagnostic reasoning, *Acad Med* 84(8):1022–1028, 2009.
26. Redding DA: The development of critical thinking among students in baccalaureate nursing education, *Holist Nurs Pract* 15(4):57–64, 2001.
27. Coles C: Developing professional judgment, *J Contin Educ Health Prof* 22:3–10, 2002.
28. Bruner J: *The culture of education*, Cambridge, Mass, 1996, Harvard Press.
29. Benner P: *From novice to expert: excellence and power in clinical nursing practice [commemorative edition]*, Upper Saddle River, NJ, 2001, Prentice Hall.
30. Dewey J: *How we think: a restatement of the relation of reflective thinking to the educative process*, Chicago, 1933, Regnery Publishing.
31. Schön D: *Educating the reflective practitioner: toward a new design for teaching and learning in the professions*, San Francisco, 1987, Jossey-Bass.
32. Schön D: *The reflective practitioner: how professionals think in action*, New York, 1983, Basic Books.
33. Dillard N, Sideras S, Ryan M, et al: A collaborative project to apply and evaluate the clinical judgment model through simulation, *Nurs Educ Perspect* 30(2):99–104, 2009.
34. Burritt J, Steckel C: Supporting the learning curve for contemporary nursing practice, *J Nurs Adm* 39(11):479–484, 2009.
35. Busch F, Schmidt-Hellerau C: How can we know what we need to know? Reflections on clinical judgment formation, *JAPA* 52(3):105–108, 2002.
36. Benner P, Sutphen M, Leonard V, et al: *Educating nurses: a call for radical transformation*, San Francisco, 2010, Jossey-Bass.

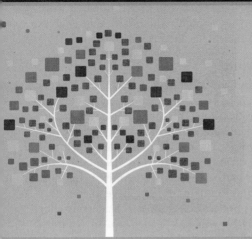

Leadership

Nancy Hoffart

Leadership is an old concept that applies to all aspects of life—from close to home, such as leading a family, to more distant situations, such as leading an international organization. Most people can name leaders in their experiences at school, work, and recreational and volunteer activities. Practical familiarity with the concept of leadership is gained through such experiences.

The focus of this concept analysis is leadership as an essential aspect of the role of the registered nurse (RN). Registered nurses are summoned to be leaders as part of their daily work and most RN competencies delineate leadership as an important capability for professional nurses. Nurses are expected to exhibit leadership when delivering patient care and when working with others to address issues that affect the practice of nursing.[1] Nurses also have been called on to play a leadership role in health policy and in shaping the health care system of the future.[2,3] In this concept you will be introduced to the general principles of leadership and their application in nursing and health care.

DEFINITION(S)

Although there is a vast body of literature on leadership in work settings, a universally accepted definition of the term does not exist. For the purposes of this concept analysis leadership is defined as *"an interactive process that provides needed guidance and direction."*[4,p820] Leadership involves three dynamic elements: a leader, a follower, and a situation. The leader provides guidance to followers, directing them towards a vision or goal, and giving support to enable their success in the particular situation or setting.

TYPES OF LEADERSHIP

Formal and Informal Leadership

A good place to start is with the difference between formal leadership and informal leadership. Individuals who occupy designated administrative or management positions in an organization are considered to hold formal leadership positions. Chief executive officer (CEO), chief nurse executive (CNE), vice president for patient services, and nurse manager are common examples of formal leadership positions in health care. Depending on the location of the institution and type of setting, titles may vary. For example, in some settings titles such as head nurse and nursing supervisor are still used. Another type of formal leadership position is an elected or appointed position in professional nursing associations, such as president or committee chairperson in a specialty nursing association. Informal leadership by individuals who do not occupy a designated administrative or management position also occurs in organizations. Individuals are perceived as informal leaders by their supervisors and peers because of their capabilities and actions. An example would be a senior staff nurse who is recognized as a clinical leader because of her expertise, her willingness to be a spokesperson for other staff, or her involvement in important issues for patient care and nurses. Individuals who are perceived as informal leaders may or may not move into formal leadership positions.

Leadership Styles

Leaders, whether formal or informal, exhibit different styles of leadership. One of the most common leadership typologies describes three styles: autocratic, democratic, and laissez-faire. Another typology for leadership style is transactional versus transformational leadership.[5] Leadership styles from both typologies (shown in Box 37-1) are described, along with a fourth style, shared leadership.

Autocratic Leadership

Autocratic leadership occurs when the leader makes all decisions. Autocratic leaders generally are most concerned with the tasks to be accomplished and maintain distance from their followers. They motivate followers through the threat of punishment and may also offer rewards as incentives. Traditionally autocratic leadership was thought to be effective for leading new employees and large groups and for controlling

BOX 37-1 **LEADERSHIP STYLES**

- Autocratic leader
- Democratic leader
- Laissez-faire leader
- Transactional leader
- Transformational leader
- Shared leaders

work that needs to be coordinated among many departments. It is often used when a decision needs to be made quickly, such as in emergencies.

Democratic Leadership

Democratic leadership occurs when the leader involves followers in the decision-making process. Thus it is also referred to as participatory leadership. Democratic leaders show more concern about followers than do autocratic leaders. Democratic leadership is useful when the followers are experienced workers, and particularly when they have professional education and socialization. It is effective when organizational success requires that followers are committed to the goal. Democratic leadership helps followers develop technical and emotional maturity.

Laissez-Faire Leadership

Laissez-faire leadership occurs when the leader does not interfere with the employees and their work. Laissez-faire leaders stand at a distance, giving followers freedom to make decisions and accomplish their work. They provide minimal information to followers and have little communication with them about their work. Typically laissez-faire leaders wait until a crisis develops to make decisions. This leadership style works best when followers are highly experienced in their work, but often it results in employee apathy, inefficiency, and chaos.

Transactional Leadership

Transactional leaders focus on the daily operations of an organization and develop an exchange relationship with their followers. The transaction entails rewarding followers when they perform, and correcting them when necessary. Transactional leaders focus on getting things done and satisfying their own and their followers' self-interests.

Transformational Leadership

Transformational leadership has been described as a process that changes or transforms individuals. Transformational leaders communicate an organizational vision to their followers, moving them to accomplish more than expected. The focus is long term and involves developing people and organizations.

Shared Leadership

A type of leadership associated with work teams is shared leadership, an approach in which employees are empowered to distribute leadership responsibilities broadly within a group. They lead one another to achieve a goal. Shared leadership

is effective with professionals and with project-focused work groups. Shared leadership is highly interactive and enables employees to develop their skills and professionalism.

Leadership Behaviors

Another common typology categorizes leadership behaviors into two dimensions. The first is socioemotional leadership, also referred to as consideration. This dimension addresses the degree to which a leader shows concern, respect, support, and appreciation for followers. The second dimension is referred to as task leadership, or initiating structure. It addresses the extent to which the leader focuses on work requirements, goal attainment, and accomplishment. Studies have shown that even though followers prefer socioemotional leadership they perform more effectively with task leadership. In contrast, leaders are more satisfied with task leadership but consideration is more strongly related to the leader's job performance.[6]

ATTRIBUTES AND CRITERIA

The concept of leadership has six attributes that must be present for effective leadership to occur. These six attributes are followers, vision, communication, decision making, change, and social power. These attributes are presented in Figure 37-1 and are described in the following sections.

Followers

There are no leaders without followers and no followers without leaders. In fact, most employees spend the greatest part of their work life as followers. Even leaders are followers in some settings, activities, and situations. The effectiveness of leadership and of an organization or department depends on both leaders and followers. Every successful organization must have followers who are enthusiastic, intelligent, and reliable participants in the pursuit of organizational goals. Organizations benefit when followers are confident, honest, credible, committed to the organization, and manage themselves well.[7] Followers can be nurtured by helping them to develop their skills through training, evaluation, and feedback and by recognizing and rewarding their contributions.

Figure 37-1 uses a broken line to show a boundary between leaders and followers. The strength and permeability of the boundary between a leader and followers will depend on the leader's style. Autocratic leaders will maintain more distance from followers, interacting with them less than a leader who employs a democratic style. Transformational leaders also will have high interaction with followers.

Vision

A vision is a leader's ideological statement of a desired, long-term future for an organization. It is the future that a leader wants to create; thus is it something to be worked towards over a period of time. The aim of leadership, as indicated by its definition, is to guide and direct followers towards the organization's vision, or towards goals instrumental for attaining the vision. The importance leaders place on vision will depend on their leadership style. Articulating a clear vision is an essential

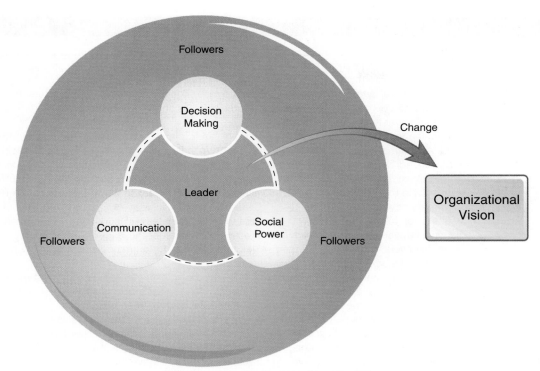

FIGURE 37-1 Attributes of Leadership.

component of transformational leadership, whereas in transactional leadership the leader is focused on performance goals for followers. To move followers towards a vision, a leader will use several processes. Three commonly used processes are communication, decision making, and change.

Communication

Communication is an essential function of effective leadership. In fact, leadership has been referred to as an ongoing conversation between a leader and followers. Leaders communicate with their followers, other leaders, the organization's clients, and people outside the organization to give and receive information. Figure 37-1 depicts communication between the leader and followers as a process that spans the boundary between the two parties. The way in which a leader communicates with followers will depend on the leader's style. Autocratic leaders are more likely to use one-way, top-down communication, but democratic leaders are more likely to use two-way communication, giving and seeking information and feedback from followers. Communication by socioemotional leaders will focus largely on followers' perceptions and feelings. In contrast, task leaders will communicate primarily about the work and means to accomplish it. Laissez-faire leaders will have little communication with their followers.

Decision Making

All leaders make decisions that affect others and organizational success. Good decisions are among the most critical features of good leadership, but good decisions are also among leaders' most invisible actions. Like communication, decision making occurs at the boundary between a leader and followers (Figure 37-1) and varies depending on the leader's

style. Democratic leaders will use a participatory style of decision making. Autocratic leaders are more likely to make decisions without follower input. Laissez-faire leaders generally allow followers to make independent decisions except in a crisis.

Change

Change is the transition process from an old state to a new state. Leaders guide the change process by working with their followers to move the organization or department towards the established vision and goals. A leader's change management skills are vital in the change process. Aspects of leadership that influence change are using effective communication skills, understanding the organizational culture, considering alternate paths to achieve a goal, identifying and dealing with differences among followers, and creating leverage to motivate followers towards the vision.

Social Power

Social power is the potential influence of one individual over another. Leaders derive their social power from a variety of sources, as outlined by French and Raven's Bases of Power model (Table 37-1).[8] A leader's style influences how he/she will use power. For example, formal leaders' power is derived, in part, from the position they hold; autocratic leaders use coercive power and transactional leaders use reward power.

THEORETICAL LINKS

Leadership theory has evolved in waves since the beginning of the twentieth century and new models are still appearing. Each wave includes specific theories founded on common

TABLE 37-1   BASES OF SOCIAL POWER[8]

TYPES OF POWER	DESCRIPTION
Coercive	Uses threat of punishment to get followers to respond. Followers expect to be punished by their leader if they fail to conform to leader's influence. Leader must monitor followers' work in order to allocate punishment. Followers who like their leader are more likely to respond to leader's threats than are followers who do not like their leader. Research also has shown that women are more responsive to coercive power than men.
Legitimate	Recognition that formal leaders have power over their followers because of the position they hold. A legitimate power relationship between two individuals can also be based on reciprocity (i.e., you did "X" for me so I should do "Y" for you), equity (i.e., I have done "X" for you so I have a right to ask you to do "Y" for me), and dependence (i.e., I have an obligation to help others who cannot help themselves). Internalized values dictate the extent to which individuals will respond to legitimate power.
Referent	Results when followers identify with or aspire to be like their leader. It does not require a direct relationship between leader and followers, or action on the part of the leader. Referent power is positive when followers voluntarily mold themselves to the leader. Referent power is negative when followers do not like or want to be like their leader.
Reward	Ability of one person to reward another for compliance with expectations. Leader must monitor the follower in order to give the reward. Like coercive power, reward power is stronger when followers like their leader, and women are more responsive to reward power than men.
Expert	Results when followers respond to their leader's directions because they perceive that the leader knows best. The range of expert power is limited to the leader's area of expertise. For example, one may have expert power as a registered nurse but not as an engineer. Like referent power, there is a negative variation on expert power. In this case followers recognize the expertise of the leader but assume the leader will act in his/her own best interests rather than the followers' interests.
Informational	Based on the leader's ability to influence followers to act by using clear logic, rational argument, and information. Leader may present the information to followers directly or indirectly (e.g., through hints and suggestions). Use of indirect informational power is more effective than direct informational power when followers are trying to influence their leader.

assumptions and incorporates different dimensions. As new waves of theory emerged they have not completely replaced previous waves, but instead added to the understanding about this complex concept. As theory and research have advanced over time the concept of leadership has changed. Leadership is no longer seen as a set of traits; it is now understood as a multifaceted, dynamic process. Today's leaders must know themselves, understand and relate effectively with their followers, and be responsive to varied situational dynamics and needs.

Great Man/Trait Theory

The oldest leadership theories illustrate the "great man" approach and are based on the assumption that leaders are born, not made. These theories hypothesize that when a situation demands leadership, a leader emerges to assume control; prior education or special preparation for leadership does not occur. Another key assumption of these theories is that traits can be used as criteria to select effective leaders. When the great man theory was first proposed leaders were almost exclusively males from aristocratic backgrounds. Research based on the great man approach focuses on identifying traits of great leaders. Historically this included physical characteristics (e.g., height) and demographic traits (e.g., male, aristocratic background). Now this research addresses personality (e.g., self-confidence, decisiveness), intellect (e.g., high IQ, reflection), and social attributes (e.g., friendliness, sense of humor). Gradually the great man approach to

BOX 37-2   AN EXAMPLE OF THE "GREAT MAN" THEORY IN NURSING

Florence Nightingale is internationally recognized as the founder of modern nursing and is well-known for her work in Scutari during the Crimean War, when she led an effort to provide better health care for British soldiers. Like many great man leaders, Miss Nightingale came from an aristocratic background, and although female, she and her only sibling, a sister, were educated and received encouragement from their father to read and study the texts that served as the educational core for men during the Victorian era.[10] Nightingale has been the subject of innumerable biographies, many of which attempt to identify the traits and attributes that made her the leader she became.

leadership came to be termed "trait theory," which is still used to identify characteristics of leaders. Four characteristics commonly identified by respondents around the world who were asked what qualities they look for and admire in leaders are (in rank order) honesty, forward looking, inspiring, and competent.[9] The many biographies of Florence Nightingale illustrate how trait theory has been used to describe her leadership characteristics (see Box 37-2).[10] Recent nursing research shows that trait theory continues to be used to recommend qualities needed by today's nursing leaders.[11,12]

Behavioral Leadership

The second wave of leadership theory concentrates on leader behaviors. The core assumption of this wave is that effective leaders use different behaviors than ineffective leaders. Research using behavioral leadership theories has shown that effective leaders demonstrate high concern for employee needs, feelings, and morale (i.e., consideration) and also address task accomplishment and organizational productivity (i.e., initiating structure). A contemporary behavioral leadership theory popular in nursing is emotional intelligence.[13,14] Emotional intelligence (EI) is comprised of five components: self-awareness, self-regulation, motivation, empathy, and social skill. The theory hypothesizes that to improve their effectiveness, leaders must develop their capabilities in all five components. Emotional intelligence has been used by nurse researchers to study the impact of nursing leadership styles on patient outcomes[15] and nurses' responses to hospital restructuring.[16] EI highlights the importance of knowing one's self, reflection, openness to feedback, and continuous learning in the leadership role.

Situational and Contingency Theory

The third wave of leadership theory, situational and contingency theory, aims to explain why some leadership approaches are effective in one situation and not in another. This wave takes into consideration the subtle and complex ways in which a leader's traits and behaviors, followers' needs and values, and situational parameters interact. It challenges the assumption that there is "one best way" to lead. Education and training to enhance leader effectiveness gained importance during this wave. An application of situational leadership theory in nursing is a leadership development program designed for three levels of nurses—newly appointed unit managers, experienced unit managers, and midlevel managers in the nursing department. The program provided different content and learning activities tailored to the particular knowledge, experience, and job responsibilities at each management level.[17]

Charismatic and Transformational Leadership

The fourth wave of leadership theory is referred to as charismatic and transformational leadership. The underlying assumption is that leaders inspire, intellectually stimulate, and recognize the contributions of their followers. Charismatic leaders influence followers through their personality and charm; they develop an emotional relationship that inspires and motivates followers. Transformational leaders possess similar characteristics and, in addition, convey high expectations to their followers, challenging their assumptions about what can be attained and building their commitment to an organizational vision. Transformational leaders rouse followers to achieve something of significance. They positively affect individual initiative and accomplishment, and encourage trust and performance within work groups.[18] Many have advocated for the use of transformational leadership in nursing[17,19] and studies of charismatic and transformational nursing leadership have shown that they are associated with high nurse satisfaction, low nurse turnover, clarity and empowerment, and high productivity and effectiveness.[20]

Complexity Science and Leadership

A new wave of leadership theory based on complexity science has begun to emerge in nursing. Complexity science is the interdisciplinary study of complex adaptive systems in physical, life, and management sciences. Four main features of complex adaptive systems have implications for leadership in health care. First, complexity science posits that interactions of the parts within a system are more important than the individual parts; thus leaders should look at the system as a whole. Second, complexity science has shown that a few simple rules can stimulate progress towards achieving a difficult goal. Consequently, leaders can initiate problem solving by pointing employees in the right direction, establishing boundaries for the solution, and giving staff the resources and permission to create solutions. Third, complexity science suggests that employees routinely change their behaviors (i.e., self-organize) to cope with changing demands. Thus leaders should search for the factors that attract employees to change, rather than battling their resistance to change. Fourth, leaders can expect variation and uncertainty as features of any complex adaptive system and use these features to their advantage.[21] Nurses are beginning to advocate for the use of complexity science as a way to strengthen nursing leadership and improve patient care and patient outcomes.[22-24]

CONTEXT TO NURSING AND HEALTH CARE

Formal Nursing Leadership

The increasing complexity and rapid change in health care demand effective leadership. The aims of nursing leadership are to ensure quality patient care and to create supportive practice environments for nurses. Nurses who hold executive level leadership positions, such as chief nursing officer or vice president for patient care services, partner with other executives to establish the organizational vision and then align the goals and operations of the nursing department with the organizational vision. Nurses in lower level leadership positions, such as directors and nurse managers, report to the nurse executive. Their focus is to ensure that day-to-day patient care operations meet established standards, to empower staff to participate in improving patient care, and to create work environments that foster professional practice and nurse satisfaction.

The size and complexity of the nursing leadership team depend on the size of the health care agency. For example, a small rural hospital may have only one formal nursing leader—a director who supervises all nursing staff. Home health and public health agencies that have offices in several communities may have designated nurse leaders for each site who report to an executive nurse leader at a central location. Urban quaternary medical centers may have four or five levels of nursing leadership, creating a hierarchy with considerable distance between the nurse executive and nurses who provide direct patient care.

Regardless of the number and levels of formal nursing leaders, all leadership styles and theories discussed earlier can be seen in today's health care agencies. A scan of recently published nursing leadership textbooks and periodic literature, however, reveals that today's nursing leaders are encouraged to use transformational leadership approaches because they have been shown to influence staff satisfaction and patient care in a positive direction (see Association Between Formal Leadership and Outcomes). Leadership practices based on complexity science are also beginning to appear.

Preparation for Formal Leadership

From a review of the literature on nursing leadership and management Jennings and colleagues[25] identified the top categories of competencies recommended for nursing leaders. These are presented in Box 37-3.

Education and training are needed to cultivate these competencies. Academic education is the foundation for nurses who aspire to leadership positions. Current nurse executives identified the educational preparation needed by future nurse leaders. They recommended a graduate degree preferably in nursing administration and/or business (e.g., MSN, MBA, joint MSN/MBA degree) for those preparing for lower level and midlevel leadership roles. Nurses preparing for executive level positions were encouraged to pursue a doctorate degree. They also recommended 2 to 5 years of clinical experience in a specialty field and participation in leadership practicums and internships as part of the academic preparation.[19]

Lifelong learning is required for nurses already functioning as leaders to enable them to stay abreast of continual changes within the health care system and advances in medical therapeutics and leadership theory and to gain understanding of themselves as leaders. Studies have shown that nurses' participation in leadership development programs can result in significant and sustained improvements in leadership skills and competencies.[26]

Many leadership development options are available, including self-study, seminars, workshops, experiential learning, and mentorship from experienced leaders. Programs generally incorporate several components and extend over a period of time. Hospitals, community health agencies, and professional nursing associations often offer leadership

development workshops for new and aspiring leaders. Several well-established national programs sponsored by universities, professional associations, and health foundations enable executive nurses to broaden and deepen their leadership knowledge and competencies.[3] An example of a hospital-based development program is one created by Wolf and colleagues.[17] It was based on transformational leadership theory and designed to prepare nurse leaders to drive change, develop teams, use technology and financial tools for decision making, anticipate medical advances and clinical practice changes, and focus on work redesign and strategic planning. These leader responsibilities are closely tied to the top competencies identified by Jennings and colleagues.[25] The program included a blended, interactive learning environment; didactic sessions; mentoring; and project work. Participants also completed assessments to identify their leadership strengths and personal developmental needs. Evaluation of a 12-month transformational leadership training program for unit level managers in a Belgian hospital showed that the program improved manager communication with staff, which in turn improved job clarify for nurses and increased their sense of empowerment.[27]

Association Between Formal Leadership and Outcomes

There is a small body of research linking formal nursing leadership to outcomes. Investigations have shown that nursing leadership based on consideration and visibility in the clinical setting is positively related to staff nurses' job satisfaction, feelings of empowerment, and autonomy. These studies also showed that visible and considerate leadership is associated with higher work commitment and retention of staff nurses.[20,28] Nursing leadership based on emotional intelligence is positively associated with work environment characteristics that support professional nursing practice, such as more opportunities for staff development, good work relations and teamwork between nurses and physicians, positive work culture, and greater utilization of research in practice.[16,20,29] An investigation of the influence of nursing leadership on patient outcomes showed that hospitals with emotionally intelligent nursing leadership had significantly lower 30-day mortality rates in a population of patients with medical conditions.[15] In an integrated research review positive nurse leadership practices were found to be associated with patient satisfaction, improved patient safety, and reduction of adverse events and patient complications.[30]

Clinical Leadership

A clinical leader is an "expert clinician, involved in providing direct patient care, who influences others to improve the care they provide continuously."[31,p437] Clinical leadership is necessary for the delivery of high-quality nursing care. Historically managers who directly supervised patient care staff were viewed as clinical leaders on the units. Research has identified the behaviors of managers who are viewed by their staff as effective clinical leaders: they are present and available on the patient care unit; support everyday practice by providing

---

BOX 37-3 RECOMMENDED COMPETENCIES FOR NURSING LEADERS[25]

- Personal qualities
- Interpersonal skills
- Thinking skills
- Setting the vision
- Communicating
- Initiating change
- Developing people
- Health care knowledge (clinical, technical, as a business)
- Management skills (e.g., planning, organizing)
- Business skills (e.g., finance, marketing)

information, creating a positive atmosphere, and keeping the unit together; and acknowledge staff through their communications and feedback. They also guard high-quality care and support staff in improving their practice.[32] Nurse managers, however, frequently find it challenging to function as clinical leaders because of the heavy demands of their daily managerial responsibilities (e.g., staffing, budgeting). These responsibilities leave little time for clinical leadership.[11,33,34]

Consequently, clinical leadership is increasingly the purview of staff nurses, clinical educators, and advanced practice nurses. These nurses do not hold formal management positions; instead their colleagues perceive some of them to be clinical leaders because of their specific clinical knowledge. Clinical leaders typically are experienced clinicians involved in direct patient care who serve as visible role models. They are effective communicators and decision makers, motivated, open, and approachable. Regardless of their title, position, or grade, they are passionate about patient care and display their beliefs and values about patient care while fulfilling their responsibilities. They are change agents, guiding other nurses through the change process. They foster teamwork and show respect for others. Clinical leaders use an evidence-based approach to care and are reflective practitioners who learn from their experiences. They stay abreast of advances in clinical care and the standards of practice in their specialty.[2,11,31,33] Consistent with the aforementioned characteristics, their influence in the clinical setting is based on referent, expert, and informational power. A new role, the clinical nurse leader, has been introduced in some health care agencies, but even in those settings staff nurses exercise clinical leadership in their daily work with patients.

Every registered nurse has the potential to be a clinical leader; lifelong learning will enable them to hone the clinical and nonclinical skills needed to fulfill this potential. Clinical leaders in today's practice settings must possess considerable knowledge and skill in their clinical specialty (e.g., adult health, community health) and use expert clinical judgment to apply this knowledge. Their clinical skills also should include use of evidence to guide their practice and quality improvement processes to ensure safe, high-quality care.[31,35]

The nonclinical knowledge and skills that aspiring clinical leaders need to be effective are communication and teaching skills, networking skills, and change management skills.[11,33,35,36] Clinical leaders are encouraged to develop their presentation and professional writing skills, and to learn how to maintain a professional portfolio.[37] They also need knowledge and skills related to teamwork and interprofessional collaboration. George and colleagues[38] grouped these and related skills into five content areas: facilitation, negotiation, accountability, systems thinking, and empowerment.

Learning to be a clinical leader starts in the academic setting through coursework and guided experience.[39] After entering the practice setting, registered nurses can seek clinical leadership development opportunities offered by their employer, continuing education providers, and professional associations. Like development activities for formal leaders, clinical leaders benefit from programs that extend over time and include a variety of learning approaches. Action and experiential learning is particularly important to enable aspiring clinical leaders to link theoretical knowledge with clinical practice. Self-assessment of personal leadership style and behaviors, seeking feedback from supervisors and peers, followed by preparation of personal development goals is encouraged.[27,35,38] Mentorship from experienced clinical leaders, reflection on leadership actions, and feedback on leadership progress are important components of clinical leadership development programs.[31,35,38] Frequent and meaningful contact between leaders and the staff they lead also provides opportunities for aspiring leaders to observe and role model effective leadership behaviors and become more self-aware of their own style.[29,40]

Research on clinical nursing leadership is in its infancy and up to now has focused on understanding the attributes and characteristics of clinical leaders, as reported earlier in this concept analysis. A few studies have been conducted to assess the outcomes of clinical leadership development programs. For example, one comprehensive development program designed to prepare staff nurses for shared clinical leadership showed improvements in self-reported leadership behaviors such as accountability for clinical problem solving, confidence, negotiation skills, and interprofessional team skills. In turn, program participants reported they were better able to meet patient needs and promote their recovery, and thereby positively influence patient satisfaction.[38]

Interprofessional Leadership

Today's health care system requires leadership that goes beyond a specific discipline or health profession. In many health care agencies and health sector businesses nurses have interprofessional leadership responsibilities. For example, countless nurses in executive level leadership positions in hospitals and home health agencies carry titles such as Vice President for Patient Care Services, and in addition to nursing are responsible for other patient care departments such as pharmacy, physical therapy, and chaplaincy. Nurses also move into formal leadership positions in areas such as clinical informatics and quality management. In all of these roles nurses draw on their knowledge and experience as clinicians, their understanding of the health care system, and their leadership training to ensure safe and effective patient care.

Nurse leaders at all levels of the organization, formal and informal, are called on to become full partners in the interprofessional care environment.[3,12,31,41] Interprofessional collaboration reduces the use of redundant services and develops more creative solutions to complex patient care problems. In particular, patients with chronic conditions, patients who are critically ill, and the elderly population benefit from coordinated interprofessional care. Research also has shown that interprofessional collaboration can increase quality, improve patient safety, and decrease the cost of care.[42] Nurses are typically the health care providers who have the most frequent and sustained interaction with patients and their families. Thus it is incumbent on nurse leaders to position the nursing staff to use their close relationships with patients and families

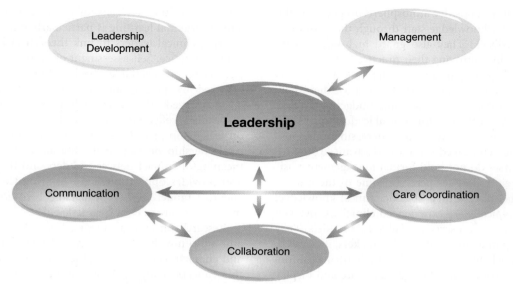

FIGURE 37-2 Interrelated Concepts to Leadership.

as the vantage point for strengthening interprofessional collaboration, and in turn the quality of health care services.

INTERRELATED CONCEPTS

Several concepts within this textbook and two additional concepts are interrelated to the concept of leadership. These are presented in Figure 37-2 and described below.

Leadership development is the "act of expanding the capacities of individuals, groups, and organizations to participate effectively in leadership roles and processes."[4,p841] There is wide agreement that even though some individuals have natural leadership tendencies, the most effective leaders are those who have participated in leadership training. Leadership development is essential for all levels of leadership and for both formal and informal leaders. It is not a single event, but an ongoing and interactive process that enables the leader to learn, apply, and receive feedback that guides further learning.

Management and leadership often are used interchangeably, but they are different. Management is focused on maintaining order in organizations—planning, organizing, staffing, directing, and controlling a work group. Leadership is about change in organizations and is focused on helping followers achieve a vision or goal. Managers always hold formal authority positions in organizations and have operational responsibilities. It is important to note that not all managers and administrators are perceived by others to be leaders. Some, but not all, leaders will hold a formal management or administrative position.

Both management and leadership are needed in organizations and both contribute to organizational success. A study of nursing leadership and management competencies in nursing found that 96% of the competencies identified were common to both leadership and management; only 3% of the competencies identified were unique to leadership. The factor that distinguished leadership from management was

the rank order of the competencies. "Setting the vision" was ranked as the fourth highest competency for leadership, but did not appear in the top 10 competencies for management. Similarly, "developing people" was ranked seventh for leadership, but did not appear in the top 10 for management. For management, "human resource management" and "information management" were ranked eighth and tenth, respectively, but neither of these competencies appeared in the top 10 for leadership.[25]

Because nursing is a practice discipline geared toward the delivery of health care, the coordination of safe and effective patient care falls on the shoulders of leaders. As mentioned previously, there are multiple levels of leadership; thus some leaders are further removed from direct patient care than others. Nonetheless, the efforts of nursing leaders ultimately link to the coordination of patient care. **Care coordination** is one of the distinctive contributions that clinical nursing leaders make in patient care. Care coordination is discussed in more detail elsewhere in the text (Concept 47).

Communication not only is an attribute of effective leaders (described earlier) but also is an interrelated concept found in this textbook. Clear communication is central to effective leadership. Leaders who communicate unambiguous and consistent messages in a timely manner help followers understand the organization's direction, decision-making processes, and changes that may be underway. Listening is an essential aspect of communication. Only by listening to peers, followers, patients, and others will the leader understand all dimensions of a problem or opportunity. Effective leaders additionally provide mechanisms to foster clear communication throughout the organization.

Effective **Collaboration** within and among organizations, and within and across disciplines, is essential to efficient organizations. Skilled nurse leaders encourage and role model this behavior. Effective collaboration enhances communication and delivery of care.

MODEL CASE 1

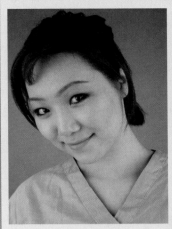

The first case is a model case, told from the perspective of a staff nurse that illustrates clinical leadership by a staff nurse.

We had a very long term patient in our medical/surgical ICU who was with us from early October until January 1 when he died. He had amyotrophic lateral sclerosis and a very aggressive, untreatable cancer, but he and his family were not willing to accept his diagnosis, thus kept him as a Full Code. His mind was intact until the last few days when he developed renal failure.

His wife was very difficult, constantly criticizing our care, constantly "checking him over," looking for a sheet crease or something to pin his deterioration on. She was so difficult, that most nurses gave up trying to even talk to her.

I spoke with my manager, who challenged me to understand her and to have her understand us and his prognosis. I remember telling my manager that I didn't need any more challenges, but I ended up taking it on! I spoke with all his doctors (even those who had "checked off" the case to understand their position[s]), used the Social Services and Case Management teams of nurses/social workers. I finally spoke with him alone to see what his end of life decision[s] were and then I spoke with her alone. He and she both wanted to maintain the Full Code status, so then we discussed his probable course. It took many conferences with her but she came to trust me and eventually called me "his favorite nurse." It taught me that patience is crucial and that was nothing I thought I had in my arsenal!

His room had a small window, but he hadn't been outside in many months other than his transfer from the ambulance from his rehab center to our hospital in October. The respiratory therapist and I decided to take him outside for some sun. We cleared it with the doctors, the charge nurse and finally with the patient. He was terrified and I explained we'd bag him while he was outside and then he could see the life outside. He agreed. It was a major undertaking, but he smiled in the slightly overcast day. We bundled him in warm blankets and he was out there for about 15 minutes, with the wind blowing his hair and he beamed. His wife was thrilled and asked if we could do it again, so we repeated the adventure the following day with her. That day was sunny, so we stayed out longer. We had four to five trips outside over the next two weeks.

His deterioration was substantial after Christmas; his code status was changed to No Code and she asked for a priest to come to give him a final blessing. Eventually, she agreed, on January 1, to take him outside, off the ventilator and allow him to go in peace in the sun where he had enjoyed some last pleasant days. It was a rainy day, but the sun came out for an hour and a half. He breathed for 45 minutes and had his family (real family and hospital family of RNs and 'his' respiratory therapist, who had been with me on our first venture outside) around him when he finally passed away. It was one of the most beautiful experiences of my life and one I've learned a lot from![43,p18] (reprinted with permission)

Case Analysis

This case illustrates clinical leadership. This registered nurse showed her leadership in the following ways: She was a visible role model who demonstrated clinical competence and knowledge. She was an effective communicator, engaging other members of the interprofessional team, the patient, and the patient's family in making decisions about his care. Her care for the patient illustrated her professional values and beliefs, particularly related to patient dignity. Her actions illustrate how she functioned as a care coordinator and empowered, motivated, and opened others to new possibilities in caring for a difficult patient. In writing about this experience she used reflection. This case also illustrates how a nurse manager can empower a staff nurse to become a clinical leader.

MODEL CASE 2

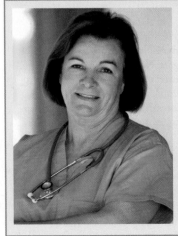

This second case highlights effective leadership by a nurse manager.

The setting for this case is a rehabilitation unit in an 850-bed urban trauma center. The 26-bed unit admits many patients from the neurosurgery ICU, but also from other units and hospitals in the area. The unit employs 14 RNs, 7 LPNs, and 5 nursing assistants. Over the past 2 months a greater than normal number of patients have acquired urinary tract infections (UTIs) during their stay on the unit. This can delay patient recovery and discharge and therefore has serious implications both for the patients and for the unit budget. The nurse manager convenes the unit quality improvement committee and asks them to investigate the problem and devise a plan that will reduce the UTI rate. This empowering approach by the formal leader will enable the unit's clinical staff to use shared leadership to solve the problem of hospital-acquired infections.

CONTRARY CASE

This case study is a contrary case that shows how a nurse manager with a less effective leadership style might handle a similar situation.

The setting for this case is a 12-bed neurosurgery ICU in the same urban trauma center described in Case 2. The unit employs 23 RNs, a nurse manager, and permanent charge nurses on the evening and night shifts. The unit also shares a clinical nurse specialist with the general surgery ICU. Recently the unit experienced an increase in the number of medication errors. The nurse manager meets with the charge nurses and directs them to review the medication error reports. Then she directs the charge nurses to meet with the nurses who have made medication errors to review the medication administration policy and procedure and inform them that if the errors continue notations will be recorded in their personnel files. The autocratic style and use of coercive power by this formal leader is less likely to enable the charge nurses to identify the root cause of the increase in medication errors, making it more difficult in the long term to solve the problem.

EXEMPLARS

There are thousands of clinical exemplars of leadership similar to those presented in the case studies. Box 37-4 presents classic exemplars of leaders. For each type of leader in each setting there are countless examples of situations that are model and contrary to effective leadership.

Leaders are made, not born. Leadership in health care is not an act reserved only for designated administrators and managers. Clinical leaders are needed in every setting to ensure that quality patient care is delivered and that new evidence and research findings are adopted to improve patient care. It is incumbent on nurses who aspire to be leaders, as well as those who are leaders, to embrace opportunities to continue to develop their leadership skills. Although the body of research investigating the outcomes of all types of nursing leadership is small, the findings to date show that leadership development improves leaders' abilities. Research also indicates that people-oriented leadership approaches show promise for improving nurse satisfaction and retention, the nursing work environment, and patient satisfaction with care, and for decreasing patient morbidity and mortality.

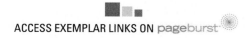

ACCESS EXEMPLAR LINKS ON pageburst

REFERENCES

1. American Association of Colleges of Nursing: *Essentials of baccalaureate education for professional nursing practice, 2008.* At www.aacn.nche.edu/education/bacessn.htm. Accessed June 1, 2011.
2. Holm AL, Severinsson E: The role of the mental health nursing leadership, *J Nurs Manag* 18:463, 2010.
3. Institute of Medicine: Transforming leadership. In *The future of nursing: leading change, advancing health*, Washington, DC, 2011, The National Academies Press. pp 221–254. At www.iom.edu/Reports/2010/The-Future-of-Nursing-Leading-Change-Advancing-Health.aspx. Accessed June 2, 2011.
4. Goethals GR, Sorenson GJ, Burn JM, editors: *Encyclopedia of leadership*, Thousand Oaks, Calif, 2004, Sage.
5. Burns JM: *Leadership*, New York, 1978, Harper & Row.
6. Judge TA, Piccolo RF, Ilies R: The forgotten ones? The validity of consideration and initiating structure in leadership research, *J Appl Psychol* 89:36, 2004.
7. Kelley RE: In praise of followers, *Harvard Business Rev* Nov-Dec 142, 1988.
8. Raven BH: The bases of power: origins and recent developments, *J Social Issues* 49:227, 1993.
9. Kouzes JM, Posner BZ: *The leadership challenge*, ed 4, San Francisco, 2007, John Wiley & Sons.
10. Gill G: *Nightingales: the extraordinary upbringing and curious life of Miss Florence Nightingale*, New York, 2004, Ballantine.
11. Stanley D: In command of care: clinical nursing leadership explored, *J Res Nurs* 11:20, 2006.
12. Upenieks VV: What constitutes effective leadership? Perceptions of magnet and nonmagnet nurse leaders, *J Nurs Adm* 33:456, 2003.
13. Akerjordet K, Severinsson E: The state of the science of emotional intelligence related to nursing leadership: an integrative review, *J Nurs Manag* 18:363, 2010.
14. Goleman D: What makes a leader? *Harvard Business Rev* Nov-Dec 93, 1998.
15. Cummings GG, Midodzi WK, Wong CA, et al: The contribution of hospital nursing leadership styles to 30-day patient mortality, *Nurs Res* 59:331, 2010.

■■■ BOX 37-4   EXEMPLARS OF LEADERSHIP

Clinical Agency—Executive Level
- Chief Nursing Officer
- Vice President for Patient Care Services

Clinical Agency—Operational Level
- Nurse Manager
- Clinical Coordinator
- Director of Nursing Services

Academic Institution
- Dean
- Associate Dean
- Division Director

Governmental Agency or Professional Association
- State Board of Nursing Executive Director
- President
- Chairperson for a Task Force

16. Cummings G, Hayduk L, Estabrooks C: Mitigating the impact of hospital restructuring on nurses: the responsibility of emotionally intelligent leadership, *Nurs Res* 54:2, 2005.

17. Wolf GA, Bradle J, Greenhouse P: Investment in the future: a 3-level approach for developing the healthcare leaders of tomorrow, *J Nurs Adm* 36:331, 2006.

18. Wang X-H, Howell JM: Exploring the dual-level effects of transformational leadership on followers, *J Appl Psychol* 95:1134, 2010.

19. Scoble KB, Russell G: Vision 2020, part I, profile of the future nurse leader, *J Nurs Adm* 33:324, 2003.

20. Cummings GG, MacGregor T, Davey M, et al: Leadership styles and outcome patterns for the nursing workforce and work environment: a systematic review, *Int J Nurs Stud* 47:363, 2010.

21. Plsek PE, Wilson T: Complexity, leadership, and management in healthcare organisations, *Br Med J* 323(7315):746, 2001.

22. Anderson RA, Issel LM, McDaniel RR Jr: Nursing homes as complex adaptive systems: relationship between management practice and resident outcomes, *Nurs Res* 52:12, 2003.

23. Holden LM: Complex adaptive systems: concept analysis, *J Adv Nurs* 52:651, 2005.

24. James KMG: Incorporating complexity science theory into nursing curricula, *Creative Nurs* 16:137, 2010.

25. Jennings BM, Scalzi CC, Rodgers JD III, et al: Differentiating nursing leadership and management competencies, *Nurs Outlook* 55:169, 2007.

26. Cummings G, Lee H, MacGregor T, et al: Factors contributing to nursing leadership: a systematic review, *J Health Serv Res Policy* 13:240, 2008.

27. de Casterlé BD, Willemse A, Verschueren M, et al: Impact of clinical leadership development on the clinical leader, nursing team and care-giving process: a case study, *J Nurs Manag* 16:753, 2008.

28. Germain PB, Cummings GG: The influence of nursing leadership on nurse performance: a systematic literature review, *J Nurs Manag* 18:425, 2010.

29. Cummings GG, Olson K, Hayduk L, et al: The relationship between nursing leadership and nurses' job satisfaction in Canadian oncology work environments, *J Nurs Manag* 16:508, 2008.

30. Wong CA, Cummings GG: The relationship between nursing leadership and patient outcomes: a systematic review, *J Nurs Manag* 15:508, 2007.

31. Cook MJ, Leathard HL: Learning for clinical leadership, *J Nurs Manag* 12:436, 2004.

32. Rosengren K, Athlin E, Segesten K: Presence and availability: staff conceptions of nursing leadership on an intensive care unit, *J Nurs Manag* 15:522, 2007.

33. Christian SL, Norman IJ: Clinical leadership in nursing development units, *J Adv Nurs* 27:108, 1998.

34. Stanley D: Role conflict: leaders and managers, *Nurs Manag* 13(5):31, 2006.

35. Cunningham G, Kitson A: An evaluation of the RCN Clinical Leadership Development Programme: Part 1, *Nurs Stand* 15(12):34, 2000.

36. Cook MJ: The renaissance of clinical leadership, *Int Nurs Rev* 48:38, 2001.

37. Lannon SL: Leadership skills beyond the bedside: professional development classes for the staff nurse, *J Contin Educ Nurs* 38:17, 2007.

38. George V, Burke LJ, Rodgers B, et al: Developing staff nurse shared leadership behavior in professional nursing practice, *Nurs Adm Q* 26(3):44, 2002.

39. Kling VG: Clinical leadership project, *J Nurs Educ* 49:640, 2010.

40. Cunningham G, Kitson A: An evaluation of the RCN clinical leadership development programme: Part 2, *Nurs Stand* 15 (13-15):34, 2000.

41. Sorensen R, Iedema R, Severinsson E: Beyond profession: nursing leadership in contemporary healthcare, *J Nurs Manag* 16:535, 2008.

42. Greiner AC, Knebel E: *Health professions education: a bridge to quality*, Washington, DC, 2003, The National Academies Press. At www.iom.edu/Reports/2003/Health-Professions-Education-A-Bridge-to-Quality.aspx. Accessed June 1, 2011.

43. National Council of State Boards of Nursing: *Report of findings from the post-entry competence study, Research Brief*, vol 38, Chicago, 2009, Author. At www.ncsbn.org/09_PostEntry CompetenceStudy_Vol38.pdf. Accessed June 3, 2011.

38

Ethics

Deb Bennett-Woods

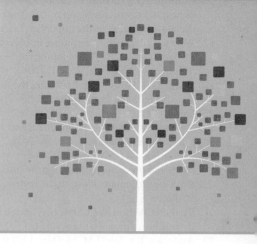

Am I ever justified in withholding the truth from a patient? Should I respect the wishes of the family or the wishes of the patient? Is there a point at which the treatment I am providing causes more harm than good? What do I do when I suspect my best friend is caring for patients while under the influence of alcohol or narcotics? On a shift that is short-staffed, how do I divide my time between too many patients? Is there a limit to how many scarce resources I should provide to any one patient?

These are tough questions and not everyone will agree on the answers. On one level, these are practical problems and decisions that need to be made in order to do a job. However, on a deeper level, they are moral and ethical choices that speak to more than just our formal training and job description. They cannot be answered with simple logic or by referring to a policy or procedure manual. Rather, how you respond to such questions is a reflection of the core values, beliefs, and character that make you the person that you are and, ultimately, the professional that you become. The actions you take in response to ethically challenging situations often require great courage, compassion, or commitment. At the same time, failure to act or respond ethically can lead to serious and even dangerous errors, personal stress, and professional burnout.

Very few of us get out of bed in the morning and wonder "How can I harm someone today?" or "What unethical action should I take to start my day?"[1] In fact, most of us would like to end the day feeling as though we made a positive difference in the world and satisfied that we did our best. We want the respect of our colleagues and patients. Most importantly, we want to feel at home in our own skin. We want a sense of personal and professional integrity—the feeling of wholeness we experience when our actions are consistent with our core beliefs and values. Technical proficiency in nursing is important but not enough, in and of itself, to guarantee this sense of integrity. To achieve the ideal of professional integrity, one also needs the skills and abilities of ethical practice including moral sensitivity, ethical reflection, ethical analysis, and ethical decision making.

DEFINITION(S)

There is no single definition or approach to ethics, although we might all agree that ethical practice is related to how we understand the concepts of right and wrong. Morality is also a broad term without a single commonly recognized definition. Generally, the term *morality* is used to refer to an accepted set of social standards or morals that guide behavior. It should be noted that many authors use the terms ethics and morality, as well as the descriptors ethical and moral, interchangeably. For our purposes, it is helpful to think of the various approaches to ethics as a foundation for morality and moral behavior. Therefore for the purposes of this concept analysis, a simple working definition of *ethics* is *the study or examination of morality through a variety of different approaches.*[2] To understand morality, we must first understand the underlying concepts, assumptions, and methods of the various approaches to ethics.

Ethics is also a process involving critical thought and action. *Ethical sensitivity* helps us recognize when there is an ethical problem or dilemma; *ethical reflection and analysis* enable us to think critically to rank our ethical obligations and priorities; and *ethical decision making* is a method for ensuring that the action we take is well reasoned and can be justified.

Each individual has his or her own moral comfort zone, or sense of personal morality. This comfort zone is influenced by societal concepts of morality but is also unique to the individual and his or her own ethical foundations. It is within this moral comfort zone that ethical reflection and analysis occur. Most of us do not give much thought to our ethical comfort zone. That is, we think of ourselves as being ethical without entirely understanding how we act ethically in practice or why we so often falter ethically when confronted with difficult choices. Knowing and understanding who you are as a moral being, how you think ethically, and why you make certain decisions are critical to ethical practice as a nurse.

The various approaches to ethics begin with *metaethics,* the branch of philosophy that considers fundamental questions about the nature, source, and meaning of concepts such as good and bad or right and wrong. Rather than making judgments about right and wrong, metaethics gives us a foundation for how to think about right and wrong or good and bad. A useful way to describe metaethics is that it provides us with a common language to use when considering the ethical or moral dimensions of a situation.[1]

Normative ethics, on the other hand, deals with very specific judgments about right and wrong in everyday actions. Normative ethics uses the language of ethics, along with factual information, prior experience, commonly held values and beliefs, and acceptable standards of behavior to make practical judgments.[1] Normative ethics is the practical basis for morality.

Finally, when faced with a difficult choice in which there are questions of right and wrong or good and bad, *applied ethics* refers to the process of applying ethical theory and reasoning to daily life. Applied ethics is sometimes also referred to as *practical ethics,*[2] and basically provides the justification for actions taken based upon ethical reflection and reasoning.

SCOPE AND CATEGORIES

The scope of ethics is broad, encompassing many different dimensions of our lives. For example, we all live and work within larger systems, each of which has its own moral dimensions. We are all members of a larger society; we work in organizational settings; and we function within the parameters of a particular profession. To fully understand the scope of ethics, one must consider how each of these dimensions interacts with us, as individuals, in shaping our ethical foundation and behavior (Figure 38-1).

Societal Ethics

If we start at the top, we recognize there are societal ethics that serve the larger community. Issues such as abortion, physician-assisted suicide, embryonic stem cell research, and health care reform are broadly addressed at the societal level in health policy debates and initiatives that are often contentious. However, society provides a strong normative basis for ethical behavior through the legal and regulatory systems. Law is a minimum standard of behavior to which all members of society are held and which, generally, is believed to serve the interests of society as a whole. Laws prohibiting murder, theft, and fraud are all examples of behaviors that society has deemed immoral and unethical. Legal standards such as the clinical standard of care, liability, negligence, and malpractice are examples of legal and ethical obligations owed to patients. Other areas of our professional lives are guided by regulatory parameters such as the practice act that defines educational requirements and your scope of practice as a nurse or the accreditation standards that determine how a health care facility must be organized and managed. Compliance with these minimum standards for practice in health care is expected of nurses, physicians, other health

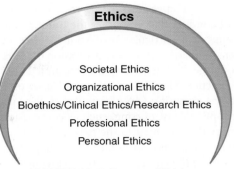

FIGURE 38-1 Scope of Ethics.

care professionals, and the organizations within which they practice.[3] Following the law and other expectations defined by society is the most basic ethical standard required for the privilege of working as a licensed professional in health care. However, even as a minimum standard, law can create moral conflict for nurses, evident in issues such as abortion and physician-assisted suicide where there remains broad disagreement within society.

Organizational Ethics

Organizational ethics involves a set of formal and informal principles and values that guide the behavior, decisions, and actions taken by members of an organization as well as the organizational structures, systems, practices, policies, and procedures developed to ensure ethical operation. The corporate scandals leading to the recent global economic crisis are an example of ethical failures at the level of the organization. Ideally, organizational ethics directs all aspects of an organization from its mission and values, to how it treats both its customers and its employees, to its financial practices, and to how it responds to the needs of the larger community and the environment.[4] A strong ethical climate ideally should support ethical nursing practice; however, nurses may find themselves in conflict with their employer when the ethical practices of the organization are lacking. Even in a strong ethical climate, the nurse may disagree with organizational practices or demands. For example, Catholic hospitals are guided by the *Ethical and Religious Directives for Catholic Health Care Services,* a publication that establishes certain boundaries of practice with which some nurses and other health care professionals may disagree.[5] Examples include directives prohibiting the use of contraception and elective sterilization or restrictions on the management of pregnancy-related conditions in Catholic facilities.

Professional Ethics

Professional ethics refers to the ethical standards and expectations of a particular profession. Because professions have held a privileged role in society, their members are often held to a higher standard in terms of ethics. Therefore ethics becomes a fundamental element of one's professional identity and character as a nurse. As stated by Crigger and Godfrey, "The relationship between the patient and the nurse is, first and foremost, an ethical one."[6,p33] Ethical standards and expectations of practice are often expressed in a code of ethics or code of conduct that embodies the unique demands and philosophies of a particular profession. Unlike the specific minimum standard of the law, professional codes of ethics tend to offer general guidelines that are aimed at the highest ideals of practice. The *Code of Ethics for Nurses* of the American Nurses Association (ANA) establishes clear priorities in the ethical practice of nursing, such as compassion, respect, and primary commitment to the patient as well as advocacy for patient rights.[7] For example, the first principle in the ANA's *Code of Ethics for Nurses* is the following:

> *The nurse, in all professional relationships, practices with compassion and respect for the inherent dignity, worth and uniqueness of every individual, unrestricted by considerations of social or economic status, personal attributes, or the nature of health problems.*

Although this is an admirable ideal, how many of us can say that we live our lives or practice our professions in ways that **always** treat others with perfect compassion and respect, valuing every individual equally, and without any form of bias? Instead, it is the responsibility of the individual nurse to interpret this statement in terms of what it means in each unique situation and how well or poorly it is being demonstrated in his or her professional practice.

Bioethics, Clinical Ethics, and Research Ethics

Bioethics and clinical ethics are separate disciplines in their own right yet closely related to professional ethics. The discipline of *bioethics* deals broadly with ethical questions surrounding the biological sciences and technology, especially as applied in health care, whereas *clinical ethics* is involved primarily with decision making at the bedside and other patient-specific issues. *Research ethics* is a specialized field within bioethics that examines the ethical conduct of research using human subjects and animals.

Personal Ethics

Finally, and perhaps most importantly, personal ethics describes an individual's own ethical foundations and practice. Our personal ethics continuously intersects with these other categories of ethics. Although there is much in common between these various forms of ethics, they do not perfectly overlap so there is also much potential for conflict. Additionally, the sources of our ethics are not static and change over time just as individuals grow and change over time.

SOURCES OF ETHICS

The beliefs, values, and methods that define ethical practice are influenced by a variety of sources. Although not a comprehensive list, the following are common sources of ethical influence within one's own individual ethical comfort zone and are closely aligned with the various categories of ethics described in the previous section. Again, there are natural intersections and places of agreement between the various sources; however, they can also conflict with each other, creating competing beliefs and inconsistency in the way we approach ethical issues (Figure 38-2).

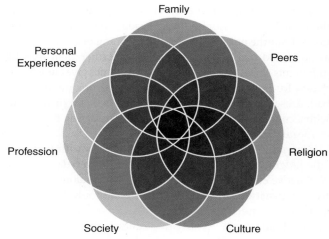

FIGURE 38-2 Sources of Ethics.

Our family is our first and initially most powerful influence on our ethical comfort zone. Many of our earliest memories are of lessons about "right and wrong" as taught by parents and other close relatives. Think about who your moral role models are and you are likely to at least consider a parent, grandparent, or sibling among them. Closely aligned with family is the culture in which we are raised including cultural practices related to our ethnicity, geographic area, and socioeconomic status. These factors shape much of our early identity, so it is not surprising they also influence our experience of ethics and morality. Another strong influence may come from one's faith tradition. Each faith tradition generally teaches basic parameters of morality in the context of religious beliefs and practice. For example, one's views on controversial issues such as abortion or euthanasia may be strongly influenced by the tenets of one's faith tradition or one's culture. Finally, peers become a source of ethical awareness and practice, especially as children move into adolescence, begin to look outside the family for direction, and are exposed to new experiences and decisions in the larger world.

As we mature, other sources begin to contribute to the belief system that shapes our ethical practice. Education, especially college, introduces new ways of thinking about difficult issues. Professional education, such as your nursing program, is charged with both your technical training and your awareness of the ethical practice of the profession. Once in the workplace, your colleagues and the organization where you work may further alter your views and your behaviors. Even the particular focus of nursing practice you select will give you new experience and insights that will further mold your professional identity and ethical priorities.

Each of these sources is filtered through one's own personal worldview and life experience. No two individuals are likely to have exactly the same response to similar life experiences. We are complex creatures and we each assign meaning to our experiences and our lives a little differently. Ultimately, only you can choose how to interpret your experience and translate it into your own ethical practice. If you choose to actively pay attention to all or most of these competing sources, and you make a practice of reflecting on issues and your own response to ethically challenging situations, then you will continue to expand and refine your ethical comfort zone. If you choose not to practice with an awareness of various sources of ethics, or you choose not to take the time to reflect on your own practice, then your ethical comfort zone may not always be prepared to support you when difficult situations arise. For example, you may find yourself in situations in which you are very uncomfortable with certain patient requests or decisions regarding treatment. Addressing your discomfort may require ongoing reflection on these situations to consider how you can balance your own deeply held religious and cultural views with the professional expectation that nurses also respect the religious and cultural views of their patients. Being self-aware and open to reflection in each new situation you confront can help further refine your approach to these difficult conflicts in practice.

THEORETICAL LINKS

The study of ethics can be traced back to philosophers in the ancient world such as Aristotle in the West and Confucius in the East. In medicine, the Hippocratic Oath, although probably not written by Hippocrates himself, is dated to sometime near the fourth century BC.[8] The body of theory in ethics is vast, reflecting the diversity of human thought and action. Nonetheless, there are a few ethical concepts and approaches to ethical theory that tend to describe the essence of our own individual and varied ethical comfort zones. In other words, there are certain elements and assumptions of one or two ethical theories that tend to describe each of us better than others, even though we may not be aware of the theory itself.

Think of each theory or principle as a camera lens. Different lenses have different magnifications and other filters that allow us to look at exactly the same scene but see it from a different angle or in a slightly different light. This body of ethical theory provides the "language of ethics" and allows us to explore situations from many different perspectives and points of view. The perspectives can be quite diverse; therefore most of us are drawn toward one or two theories at most and we may have a very hard time even trying to think in the language of other theories. Ethical conflict occurs between parties when this language fails and each party simply cannot understand the other party's reasoning or point of view.

There are three advantages to being generally familiar with a wide range of ethical theories and principles. First, such familiarity helps you identify your own comfort zone and the areas in which your own analysis is strong. Second, by identifying your strengths in ethical analysis, you are also identifying those areas with which you are not comfortable and may develop an ethical "blind spot" to thinking in those terms. Third, and finally, having an appreciation and understanding of the ethical comfort zones of others can help you mediate ethical conflict. If patients, family members, or colleagues feel as though you truly understand their position, then they will be more willing to consider your position.

Ethical Principles

An ethical principle is a general guide that can be used with judgment to help determine a course of action.[9] A principle might also be described as a basic truth or assumption. Principles have long been used in bioethics and clinical ethics to describe the most common ethical concerns one must consider in most cases. Although all of the principles are important, they can conflict with each other in certain situations. The four principles most often cited are respect for persons, nonmaleficence, beneficence, and justice.[9] Less often considered, but equally important, is the principle of fidelity.

Respect for Persons

Respect for persons simply maintains that human beings have an unconditional moral worth that requires us to treat each individual person with great value, dignity, and respect. In part, the great value of human beings lies in our unique capacity to act as moral agents, which means we are self-aware, capable of moral thought and reasoning, and self-determining.[10] The ethical principle of *autonomy* is an important extension of this principle and suggests that patients must be treated in a way that respects their autonomy and their ability to express their wishes and make informed choices about their treatment.[10] When a nurse advocates for a patient, he or she is often attempting to protect a patient's autonomy when other factors interfere with the patient's ability to act independently. Another ethical principle closely related to autonomy is *veracity* or the principle of truthtelling. A patient is not able to make an informed choice about treatment unless the patient has received the truth about his or her condition and the proposed treatment, with the information presented in a manner that is understandable to the patient.[10]

Nonmaleficence

Nonmaleficence is a complicated term that simply means we should act in ways that avoid harm to others, including even the risk of harm.[10] In health care, the primary focus is on harms such as pain, disability, or death; however, harm is difficult to define and both patients and providers may be concerned about a wide range of perceived harms.[9] Another challenge in health care is that we are often required to inflict some harm and risk in order to benefit the patient and avoid a greater harm. For example, there is always risk associated with surgery or chemotherapy, and both forms of treatment cause patients some level of pain or other discomfort. However, these harms are not avoidable if we are to properly treat the patient. Instead, we are required to carry out such treatments in ways that are unlikely to cause undue risk or needless harm.

Beneficence

Beneficence is an obligation to do good by acting in ways that promote the welfare and best interests of others. Beneficence can be accomplished by promoting good and preventing and removing harm.[9] Patients can reasonably expect that you, as a nurse, will promote their health and well-being. As with nonmaleficence, this principle requires that we weigh the various risks of harm against the benefits of an action. However, much like harm, the concept of good is hard to define.

A patient may define his or her best interests very differently than the nurse or other health care professional.[10]

Justice

The concept of justice is particularly complex and there are no universally accepted definitions of what constitutes justice. However, at minimum, the principle of justice is concerned with treating people equitably, fairly, and appropriately.[9] This means we owe our patients care and treatment that does not arbitrarily discriminate against them as an individual or as a member of a class of individuals. Returning to the ANA's *Code of Ethics for Nurses,* justice is the underlying principle that prohibits a nurse from treating patients differently based on their social or economic status, their personal attributes (such as gender or ethnicity), or the nature of their health problems (such as obesity or self-inflicted harm).[7] Each patient is entitled to the same level of care and consideration without bias. Of particular concern is the concept of distributive justice and the allocation of scarce health care resources. Should all patients receive the health care services they need, or only the services they can afford? Is there a limit to how many resources any one patient should be provided? Do patients who choose unhealthy or high-risk behaviors deserve the same resources as patients who actively attempt to live a healthy lifestyle?

A related concept involves compensation for harm (compensatory justice) such as occurs in a malpractice settlement.[10] Finally, the concept of procedural justice is another aspect of the broad principle of justice. For example, procedural justice dictates the criteria and method by which organs are allocated to people on the waiting list, and patients should be able to trust that they will be treated equitably within the policies and procedures that comprise the organ allocation system.[10]

Fidelity

Fidelity is the principle that requires us to act in ways that are loyal. In the role of a nurse, such action includes keeping your promises, doing what is expected of you, performing your duties, and being trustworthy.[10] Fidelity sounds easy enough but is probably the most frequent source of conflict for health care professionals because they owe loyalty to so many parties. In any particular situation, nurses may find themselves at odds between what they believe is right, what is in their own self-interest, what the patient wants, what other members of the health care team expect, what organizational policy dictates, and/or what the profession or the law requires.

Ethical Theories

As mentioned earlier, there is a vast array of ethical theory. At best, here we can only highlight a few major approaches in very simplified terms. However, you should still be able to recognize your own greater alignment with one or two of these theories than the others. For example, most of us have a preference for either the consistency of rule-based approaches or the flexibility of consequence-based approaches. Likewise, some of us will be more comfortable with the highly contextual and emotionally engaged approach of relational ethics whereas others are more comfortable with a highly rational and detached approach to ethical analysis. In any case, each theoretical approach offers a very different view of the same situation, views that may or may not lead to similar conclusions about an ethical problem or dilemma.

Ethics of Duty

An ethics of duty is based on the ethical approach of deontology. In a deontological theory, moral duties are seen as self-evident, needing no further justification. Moral action is then based on acting according to a specific duty simply because it is the right thing to do.[10] Although the consequences of our actions are important, they are a secondary consideration to duty and our intention to do the right thing. The ethical question one must ask is, "What is my duty?" For example, if a nurse becomes aware that a friend and colleague has been diverting narcotics because she has developed an addiction and the nurse reports her friend to her supervisor because that is what the organizational policy requires, she is complying with her duty to report.

Ethics of Consequences

An ethic of consequences is based on a teleological view that moral actions are defined entirely on the basis of the outcomes or consequences of an action. Deontological theories are often contrasted with teleological theories because, in an ethic of consequences, reaching a particular goal is what defines the ethical justification of an act regardless of your sense of duty or moral intent.[10] It is not enough to just mean well or intend the good. Consequence-based theories often weigh the pros and cons, or the harms and benefits, of different actions in the same situation. Utilitarianism is the most commonly referenced teleological theory. A basic assumption of utilitarianism is that a moral action is one that results in the greatest good for the greatest number. The basic ethical question posed is, "What action will promote the greatest good with the least harm?" For example, if the nurse mentioned previously reports her friend because she is concerned that some patients are being harmed when their pain medications are diverted and all patients are at risk if her friend is practicing under the influence, then her actions are primarily based on a consideration of consequences. Her intention is to protect as many patients as possible, rather than following a particular rule as a matter of duty. In fact, she might choose differently and act outside of the policy if she felt reporting would not result in appropriate action by her supervisor.

Ethics of Character

Theories that emphasize character fall under the general category of virtue ethics. Unlike the ethics of duty or consequences, which use external principles and rules to guide actions, virtue ethics relies on the character of the individual as the primary source of moral action.[10] Character develops over time based on life experiences and our own willingness to reflect on our actions and motives. Virtues are character traits that predispose a person with good intentions to do the right thing. Moral virtues include respect, honesty, sympathy, charity, kindness, loyalty, and fairness, whereas practical virtues include intelligence, patience, prudence, and shrewdness.[11] In general, a moral act must both promote good and intend good based on the moral predispositions of our character. The basic ethical question might be, "What should I intend and what action will serve the good?"

Crigger and Godfrey[6] argue strongly for virtue theory to be the core of nursing ethics, with an emphasis on the virtues of compassion, integrity, humility, and courage. In fact, the concept of virtue has been central to the definitions of professional, professionalism, and professional identity.[6] A common criticism of virtue ethics is that character varies dramatically between individuals, leading to ethical inconsistency. In addition, our choices may change over time on the basis of additional experience and character development. What you might have considered ethical when you were 20 years old may change quite dramatically by the time you are 40. However, a strength of a virtue-based approach to nursing ethics is that it assumes character must be continually developed and refined in practice throughout a nurse's career. Such ongoing development suggests that ethics is a dynamic element of practice that cannot be reduced to simple habits of following rules or weighing outcomes. In the case of our nurse with the impaired colleague, a character-based approach would lead her to act based on a combination of her own good intentions to protect her friend, the patients, and the organization while also seeking the best possible outcome for all. She would be guided primarily by some combination of her own moral and practical virtues, and on the basis of her professional sense of identity, rather than by the externally dictated rules and outcomes.

Ethics of Relationship

Ethical theories that emphasize relationship are focused on the nature and obligations inherent in human relationships and community. With some roots in feminist thought, the ethic of care is generally credited to the work of Carol Gilligan.[12] Gilligan proposed two patterns of reasoning. The first pattern has a focus on justice, rights, and the development of universal rules to ensure fairness, and Gilligan termed this an ethic of justice. The second pattern is focused on emotion and relationships in the context of a particular situation, and Gilligan termed this an ethic of care. In the ethic of care, difficult ethical situations are approached in a context-specific manner that looks for solutions in the particular details of the situation. Universal principles are used only to the extent they can be applied based on the unique circumstances of each situation. Primary attention is paid to preserving relationships, improving communication, enhancing cooperation, and minimizing harm to everyone involved while promoting an ideal of caring.[13] The basic ethical question in the ethic of care might be, "What is the caring response?"

Such an approach is very different from the highly rational, unemotional, and rule-oriented approach of most Western philosophical ethical traditions. On the other hand, it has much in common with virtue ethics, which is also very contextual and rejects the notions of abstract principles and rules. Although duty-based, consequence-based, and, to a lesser extent, character-based approaches have dominated the fields of bioethics, clinical ethics, and medical ethics (physicians), nursing has long embraced an ethic of care as well as feminist theory and other relational approaches. The commitment to a more contextualized approach to ethics is affirmed in the preface to the ANA's *Code of Ethics for Nurses*[7]:

> *There are numerous approaches for addressing ethics; these include adapting to or subscribing to ethical theories, including humanist, feminist and social ethics, adhering to ethical principles and cultivating virtues. The Code of Ethics for Nurses reflects all of these approaches.*

Returning once more to our nurse with the impaired colleague, the ethic of care will direct her first toward gaining a full and empathetic understanding of the context of the situation, including the various relationships that must be protected and preserved if possible. She will seek open communication and a collaborative approach that emphasizes caring and minimizes harm to all parties. For example, she might first approach her friend and offer to accompany her to speak with the appropriate party in the organization to arrange for treatment and address the legal implications of her actions.

Naturally, each of us may use assumptions from any of the four theoretical perspectives in various circumstances, even if we are not consciously aware that this is what we are doing. However, most of us rely more on one or two of these perspectives most of the time. Give some thought to which one or two approaches best reflect your normal response to an ethically challenging situation. Likewise, is there an approach that just does not feel quite as comfortable? Such reflection is a good first step in becoming more familiar with your own ethical comfort zone and how it may influence your nursing practice.

CONTEXT TO NURSING AND HEALTH CARE

Applied ethics addresses the process of ethical analysis and decision making in actual cases or with respect to specific topics. Although the range and complexity of ethical theory can be a little daunting and confusing, applied ethics is fairly straightforward insofar as you have a specific decision that needs to be made and you are free to incorporate any ethical concepts you consider relevant to making that decision. An *ethical problem* is simply a problem with an ethical dimension. Most ethical problems have a reasonably clear solution. If you are busy working on an important project and a patient needs assistance, the proper ethical response will almost always be to offer that assistance either because you have a duty of role fidelity to provide that assistance or because the patient might be harmed if you do not provide assistance. However, if the assistance being requested is to help the patient commit suicide because the patient believes his or her quality of life no longer warrants remaining alive, then you have more than just an ethical problem—you have an ethical dilemma.

An *ethical dilemma* involves a problem for which in order to do something right you have to do something wrong. In other words, it is not possible to meet all of the ethical requirements in the situation. In the case of provider-assisted suicide, you have an ethical obligation to preserve life and to abide by the professional and legal prohibitions that exist, in most states, against directly killing a patient or indirectly assisting in a patient's death. Yet, there are also compelling arguments, supported by an emerging societal consensus, that patients should have the option to choose a compassionate death when faced with a painful and prolonged terminal condition. Similarly, you may personally feel the patient is justified in his request but your religious beliefs prevent you from participating in the action. Finally, you may feel an obligation of fidelity to help the patient in order to prevent the patient from taking action independently that might cause even greater suffering, while also feeling an obligation of fidelity to his family who would not support his decision.

When faced with an ethical problem or dilemma, it is helpful to apply a systematic approach of ethical analysis to the process of making a decision. There are many different methods for ethical analysis.[14] A practical approach is to use some form of decision model, but again, there are a number of different decision models from which you might select.[15] What is important is that the particular method or decision model being used makes sense to you as the decision-maker.

One popular model for clinical decision making is the Four Topics Method of Jonsen, Siegler, and Winslade.[16] The four topics are medical indications, patient preferences, quality of life, and contextual features. Within each topic, questions are posed that clarify factual aspects of the case with an emphasis on the ethical principles of beneficence, nonmaleficence, respect for autonomy, loyalty, and fairness. Answering the various questions provides a framework within which different options for action can be considered.

Any approach to ethical analysis will depend heavily on one's ability to ask good questions. Asking the wrong question or a poorly constructed question will generally get you the wrong answer or a poorly considered answer. An *ethical question* is a question that challenges you to consider a particular ethical concept, principle, or perspective in your analysis. The following are examples of ethical questions:

- Do I have a duty to tell the truth?
- What is the greater harm?
- To whom is my primary loyalty?
- What are the best interests of my patient?

Framing good ethical questions is the key to strong ethical analysis, and the ability to use a variety of concepts and theories naturally expands the range and quality of questions.

Ethical Decision Making in Practice

There will be times when you must assess a situation and make a difficult ethical decision on your own. However, health care decisions are generally not made in a vacuum and the nurse is often participating in ethical decision making as a member of a patient care team or an administrative team. Although there is likely to be some conflict when people with different perspectives are involved, such conflict can be used to enhance the depth and breadth of the analysis by forcing everyone to consider the situation from various viewpoints. Therefore group or team decision making can often result in a more refined solution.

When conflict in the team or between the team and the patient or patient's family cannot be resolved, organizational ethics committees can be consulted to assist with mediating the conflict. Most acute care hospitals and some extended care facilities have an ethics committee onsite or they have access to one. An ethics committee does not make clinical decisions; however, the assigned consult team or the full committee can guide the discussion and act as mediator when there is conflict among the parties.

For organizational issues such as adherence to regulations, safety standards, quality of care, conflict of interest, or billing fraud and abuse, most organizations have a compliance committee or compliance officer, and may even offer a compliance hotline for reporting of suspected violations. When the dilemma involves other professional issues, state and local chapters of professional associations may have similar ethics committees or experts with whom you can consult.

Ethical Issues in Nursing

A study by Fry and Riley (2002) examined (1) the ethical issues encountered by RNs in their practice, (2) the frequency that ethical issues occur in practice, (3) the degree to which RNs are concerned by these issues, (4) the way RNs handle ethical issues, and (5) the types of ethics education topics and resources that RNs perceive helpful to them in practicing ethically.[17] A total of 2408 RNs responded to a mailed survey.

According to study findings, the following are the most frequent ethical issues experienced by RNs:

- Protecting patients' rights and human dignity
- Respecting/not respecting informed consent to treatment
- Providing care with possible risk to the nurse's health
- Using/not using physical or chemical restraints
- Working with staffing patterns that limit patient access to nursing care

Those issues that RNs find most disturbing include the following:

- Coping with staffing patterns that limit patient access to nursing care
- Prolonging the living/dying process with inappropriate measures
- Not considering the quality of a patient's life
- Implementing managed care policies that threaten quality of care, and
- Working with unethical/impaired colleagues.

More than 30% of the respondents reported encountering ethical issues in their practice one to four times per week or daily. In handling their most recently experienced ethical issue, more than 83% reported that they discussed the issue with nursing peers whereas more than 66% discussed the issue with nursing leadership. On the other hand, more than 5% of the nurses reported that they did not deal with the ethical issue at all.[17]

Moral Distress

If ethical practice is the ideal to which all nurses should aspire, what happens when a nurse falls short of that ideal? There has been much research in the field of nursing ethics focused on the concept of moral distress, and there is also growing evidence of moral distress among other health care providers including physicians, respiratory therapists, physical therapists, pharmacists, psychologists, and social workers.[18-24] *Moral distress* occurs when you are unable to act upon what you believe is the morally appropriate action to take or when you otherwise act in a manner contrary to your personal and professional values.[25] In other words, you know what to do but feel like you cannot do it. There can be many barriers to doing what you believe is right. Self-doubt, lack of assertiveness, and the perception of powerlessness are examples of internal barriers that prevent you from taking action when you know you should. In addition, there are also external barriers that can prevent you from doing the right thing, including inadequate staffing, lack of organizational support, poor relationships with colleagues, and policies that conflict with the care needs of patients.[18]

Situations that have been shown to cause moral distress are very similar to the common ethical issues noted earlier. Many of them occur in end-of-life situations and involve what is perceived to be overly aggressive treatment and inappropriate use of resources. Working with other physicians and nurses you consider incompetent is another common situation that has been shown to result in moral distress.[26]

Moral distress is not an experience that simply disappears. The impact of moral distress occurs in two parts.[18] When the situation first occurs, moral distress can result in frustration, anger, guilt, anxiety, withdrawal, self-blame, and other stress-related symptoms. However, the full impact does not stop there. The second part of moral distress is referred to as *reactive distress* or *moral residue,* and is characterized by lingering feelings that can accumulate over time with each subsequent situation in which moral distress is experienced. At least three patterns of response to moral residue have been described. In the first two patterns, health care professionals exhibit one of two almost opposite responses. In the first pattern, a heightened response leads health care professionals to engage in activities of conscientious objection, such as voicing opposition to a plan of care or refusing to follow orders. In the second pattern, they experience a desensitization with a tendency to be passive or to simply withdraw from situations in which they feel ethically challenged. The third pattern is characterized by strong, ongoing physical and psychologic stresses that often lead to burnout and leaving the profession.[18] In all cases, the health care professional's core values, integrity, and professional identity have been undermined.

Because research has continued to demonstrate a strong negative impact of unresolved moral distress on the job satisfaction and retention of nurses and other health care professionals, leaders in health care organizations have become increasingly aware of the need to create an organizational climate in which ethical issues can be openly discussed and resolved.[27] Interventions have included ethics debriefings, more support for ethics committees, and better access to ethics education and other resources.

INTERRELATED CONCEPTS

As evident in Figure 38-3, ethics is closely intertwined with many other concepts related to nursing. **Health care policy, Health care law,** and **Health care economics** can all be the

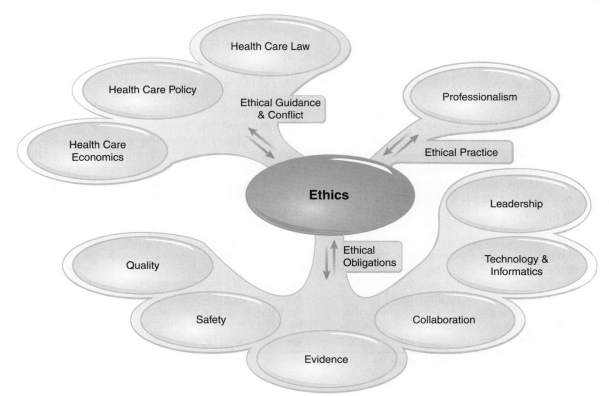

FIGURE 38-3 Ethics and Interrelated Concepts.

MODEL CASE

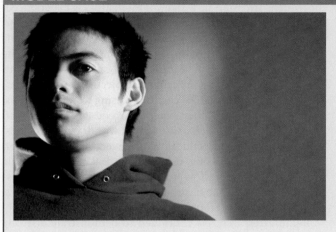

Joshua is a good-natured and intelligent 15-year-old male who was diagnosed with an aggressive bone cancer and underwent a below-the-knee amputation of his left leg. Joshua's cancer metastasized to his chest, skull, and lungs, and he was readmitted a few months later for removal of the remainder of his left leg. Joshua and your son have been friends at school for several years and you had met Joshua many times before his illness. Since then, you have been his nurse on occasion and he has talked to you about his disease. He has told you that talking about it upsets his parents and makes his friends uncomfortable so it is nice to have someone with whom he can be honest. In fact, you have always been impressed with the level of maturity and insight he demonstrates.

Joshua has been readmitted, his prognosis is grim, and he is experiencing a great deal of pain. Although you have not been assigned to care for Joshua during this admission, you are aware that members of the clinical team have been uncomfortable with Joshua's situation throughout his treatment. This is because Joshua's parents have requested that the health care personnel limit the information they share with Joshua. This time, despite the many questions he asks, Joshua has not been told the extent of the metastases or that he will likely die within a few weeks. Members of the care team have frequently omitted information and even lied to Joshua at the insistence of his parents and with the reluctant agreement of his attending physician. Members of the care team have questioned the unit director several times about this policy; however, she continues to instruct them to respect the wishes of the parents to avoid any legal problems. Joshua's parents also insist that he continue to receive every possible intervention and another clinical trial is being considered.

One evening Joshua notices you in the hall and calls you into his room. He confronts you and tells you he knows he is not being told everything. He says he believes he is dying and, although it frightens him, he is ready to die. He has not been able to attend school for several months; his friends no longer come to see him; he knows his younger brother and sister get very little attention because of him; and he is in nearly constant pain. He is tired of pretending to be "strong and brave." He has tried to talk to his parents but they refuse to even listen to him. He says, "I trust you to tell me exactly what's happening and what I need to do to stop treatment, even if it is against my parents' wishes."

Case Analysis

As a nurse who has cared for Joshua in the past and who also knows him personally, you are faced with the practical problem of how to respond to his request to be told the truth of his condition and how to discontinue treatment. The first step in any analysis will be to gather all relevant information so that you are fully informed of the situation and its implications. For example, what are the relevant organizational policies and are there legal requirements that must be considered? Also, you may want to consider your professional code of ethics to clearly identify whether there are particular expectations of you in this situation as a member of the profession.

From this point, how you solve the problem will ultimately depend on the ethical questions you ask and the ethical assumptions you consider. There is no one right solution to the problem. Let us examine some of the ethical questions that could be posed in relation to this case beginning with the ethical principles.

- Should Joshua's autonomy be considered and/or honored with respect to his treatment? (respect for persons)
- Is Joshua being needlessly harmed by withholding information and continuing aggressive treatment? (nonmaleficence)
- Are Joshua's parents and physician acting in his best interests? (beneficence)
- Does Joshua have a moral right to be told the truth of his condition? (veracity)
- To whom do I, as a nurse, owe my loyalty? (fidelity)
- Is Joshua being treated fairly and equitably? (justice)
- Is the health care team caring for Joshua being treated fairly and equitably? (justice)

Similar questions can be posed from each of the theoretical perspectives. An ethic of duty will ask, "What are my duties in this situation and, if in conflict, what duty should take precedence?" An ethic of consequence will ask, "What action(s) will create the greatest benefit and cause the least harm?" An ethic of character will rely heavily on your own moral intuition and ask "What should my intentions be and what actions will serve the good?" Notice that this approach requires you to define "the good" in this particular situation as part of your analysis. Finally, an ethic of relationship will ask, "How can I best advocate for Joshua while considering other important relationships between parents, the physician, and my colleagues?"

Notice that each of the questions posed is highly relevant but quite different in its focus and potential outcome. An ideal solution would address as many of these issues as possible. Unfortunately, Joshua is sitting in front of you expecting an answer now, which is why ongoing practice with ethical reflection and analysis is so important to your practice. You will not always have the luxury of time to explore your options so you need to be able to assess the ethical dimensions of a situation quickly and effectively. How would you respond to Joshua?

source of both ethical guidance and ethical conflict. For example, legal requirements may provide guidance in most situations, yet may create conflict in a specific situation that does not quite fit the context for which the legal requirement was intended. **Professionalism** is contingent upon a conception of ethical practice. The concepts **Health care quality, Safety, Evidence, Collaboration,** and **Technology and informatics** are all grounded in ethical obligations such as preventing needless harm, acting in a patient's best interest, ensuring the best outcomes for the most patients, and serving as a good steward of scarce health care resources. The concept of **Leadership** has additional ethical obligations such as balancing loyalties and the interests of patients, employees, the organization, and the community. Patient care and the process of nursing itself are fraught with ethical problems and dilemmas. Most importantly, the ethical practice of nursing requires that the nurse treat each patient with respect, recognizing and responding to the patient's unique experience of illness and injury.

EXEMPLARS

The scope of ethics in nursing is quite broad as mentioned earlier in the concept. Box 38-1 provides a summary of examples of potential ethical issues faced in nursing practice in three broad categories: clinical ethics and bioethics, organizational ethics, and ethical issues in law and health policy. Although the range is broad, there are a few issues that occur in practice on a fairly regular basis.

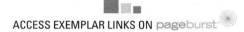

ACCESS EXEMPLAR LINKS ON pageburst

BOX 38-1 EXEMPLARS OF ETHICS

Clinical Ethics and Bioethics

Beginning of Life
- Abortion
- Assisted reproduction
- Child abuse
- Complications of pregnancy
- Emergency contraception
- Genetic enhancement
- Minor consent to treatment
- Prenatal genetic selection
- Prenatal genetic testing
- Severely impaired newborns

Lifespan
- Confidentiality
- Cultural conflicts
- Decisional capacity
- Domestic and elder abuse
- Genetic testing
- Informed consent
- Pain management and addiction
- Patient noncompliance
- Patients as research subjects
- Protecting patient rights

End of Life
- Advance directives
- CPR orders
- Chronically critically ill
- Nonbeneficial treatment

- Organ allocation
- Organ procurement
- Patients without a proxy decision-maker
- Physician-assisted suicide
- Proxy decision making
- Terminal sedation
- Withholding or withdrawal of life support

Organizational Ethics
- Allocation of scarce resources
- Conflict of interest
- Conscience policies
- Disclosure of medical errors
- Fraud and abuse
- Impaired providers
- Inadequate staffing levels
- Patient safety
- Uncompensated care
- Use of restraints

Health Policy
- Abortion
- Allocation of research funding
- Embryonic stem cells
- Health care for the uninsured
- Health care for undocumented immigrants
- Insurance reform
- Privacy of health information
- Rural access to health care
- Tort reform (malpractice)

REFERENCES

1. Bennett-Woods D: *Nanotechnology: ethics and society*, Boca Raton, Fla, 2008, CRC Press.
2. Tubbs JB: *A handbook of bioethics terms*, Washington, DC, 2009, Georgetown University Press.
3. Darr K: *Ethics in health services management*, Baltimore, 2005, Health Professions Press.
4. Boyle PJ, DuBose ER, Ellingson SJ, et al: *Organizational ethics in health care: principles, cases and practical solutions*, San Francisco, 2001, Jossey-Bass.
5. United States Conference of Catholic Bishops: *Ethical and religious directives for Catholic health care services,* ed 5, 2009. Available at http://www.usccb.org/meetings/2009Fall/docs/ERDs_5th_ed_091118_FINAL.pdf.
6. Crigger N, Godfrey N: *The making of nurse professionals: a transformational approach*, Sudbury, Mass, 2011, Jones and Bartlett Learning.
7. American Nurses Association: *Code of ethics for nurses*, 2001. Available at http://nursingworld.org/MainMenuCategories/ThePracticeofProfessionalNursing/EthicsStandards/CodeofEthics.aspx.
8. Devettere R: *Practical decision making in health care ethics*, ed 3, Washington, DC, 2010, Georgetown Press.
9. Beauchamp TL, Childress JF: *Principles of biomedical ethics*, ed 6, New York, 2008, Oxford University Press.
10. Bennett-Woods D: *Ethics at a glance,* Center for Ethics and Leadership in the Health Professions, 2005, Regis University. Available at http://rhchp.regis.edu/HCE/EthicsAtAGlance/index.html2005.
11. Munson R: *Intervention and reflection: basic issues in medical ethics*, ed 9, Belmont, Calif, 2011, Wadsworth.
12. Gilligan C: *In a different voice: psychological theory and women's development*, Cambridge, Mass, 1982, Harvard University Press.
13. Noddings N: *Caring: a feminine approach to ethics and moral education*, Berkley, CA, 1984, University of California Press.
14. Sulmalsy DP, Sugarman J: The many methods of medical ethics (or, thirteen ways of looking at a blackbird). In Sugarman J, Sulmasy DP, editors: *Methods in medical ethics*, ed 2, Washington, DC, 2010, Georgetown University Press.
15. Johnson C: *Meeting the ethical shadows of leadership*, ed 4, Los Angeles, 2011, Sage.
16. Jonsen A, Siegler M, Winslade W: *A practical approach to ethical decisions in clinical medicine*, ed 7, USA, 2010, McGraw-Hill Medical.
17. Fry ST, Riley JM: *Ethical issues in clinical practice: a multi-state study of practicing registered nurses,* Boston: Nursing Ethics Network, 2002. Available at http://jmrileyrn.tripod.com/nen/research.html#anchor195458.
18. Epstein EG, Hamric AB: Moral distress, moral residue and the crescendo effect, *J Clinical Ethics* 20(4):330–342, 2009.
19. Forde R, Aasland OG: Moral distress among Norwegian doctors, *J Med Ethics* 34:521–525, 2008.
20. Hamric AB, Blackhall LJ: Nurse-physician perspectives on the care of dying patients in intensive care units: collaboration, moral distress, and ethical climate, *Crit Care Med* 35(2):422–429, 2007.
21. Schwenzer KJ, Wang L: Assessing moral distress in respiratory care practitioners, *Crit Care Med* 34(12):2967–2973, 2006.
22. Carpenter C: Moral distress in physician therapy practice, *Physiother Theory Pract* 26(2):69–78, 2010.
23. Kalvemark Sporrong S, Hoglund AT, Arnets B: Measuring moral distress in pharmacy and clinical practice, *Nurs Ethics* 13(4), 2006.
24. Austin W, Rankel M, Kagan L, et al: To stay or to go, to speak or to stay silent, to act or not to act: moral distress as experienced by psychologists, *Ethics Behav* 15(3):197–212, 2005.
25. American Association of Critical Care Nurses: *Moral distress [Position Statement]*, 2008. Available at www.aacn.org/WD/Practice/Docs/Moral_Distress.pdf2008.
26. Zuzelo PR: Exploring the moral distress of registered nurses, *Nurs Ethics* 14(3):344–359, 2007.
27. Bell J, Breslin JM: Healthcare provider moral distress as a leadership challenge, *Healthcare Law Ethics Regul* 10(4):94–97, 2008.

Patient Education

Barbara Carranti

Education empowers. Patient education is no exception. Effective patient education allows patients and their families the opportunity to control their own health, reduce risk for illness, improve longevity, and enhance overall wellness. Specifically, the goals of patient education are to learn and adapt by forming connections and associations that will facilitate changes in behavior, resulting in enhanced health and well-being, or improved treatment of illness.[1] Lamiani and Furey point out that the emphasis of patient education frequently focuses on the disease as opposed to the patient, and they stress the importance of incorporating exploration of the patient's illness experience into the educational plan to ensure high-quality care.[2]

The importance of patient education is supported by *Healthy People 2020*. This science-based program, in existence for more than 30 years, has used evidence to establish objectives for the health of the United States. Patient education is key to achievement of the overarching goals of *Healthy People,* specifically increasing the quality and years of healthy life and eliminating health disparities.[3]

DEFINITION(S)

For the purposes of this concept analysis, *patient education* is defined as "*a process of assisting people to learn health related behaviors so that they can incorporate these behaviors into everyday life.*"[4,p11] This is a purposeful process whereby the patient is learning health-related information with the intent of changed behavior. A similar term, *patient teaching,* is used interchangeably. The role of the nurse in patient education is to assist the patient in forming goals; assess patient need, motivation, and ability; plan educational intervention to achieve goals; and evaluate patient outcomes toward goal attainment. In short, nurses empower patients by providing information to enhance wellness and reduce the risk for illness and encourage autonomy by enhancing self-care skills while maintaining a patient-centered approach.

SCOPE AND CATEGORIES

As a concept, patient education represents a wide range of formats and can be described from two perspectives: the delivery approach and educational domains. The process varies depending on multiple variables, including the intended outcome and the characteristics of the learner. For example, is the educational intervention intended to teach the patient a skill or impart knowledge related to a known health problem, increase the probability of successful treatment, prepare for discharge, or to promote a healthy lifestyle and enhance well-being? Thoughtful consideration of intended outcomes will enhance the patient's learning by matching approach to intended goals. The nurse must ask, "What change in the patient is the desired outcome of this activity?" The type of education offered will require that the nurse match the approach, method, and evaluation to this desired outcome.[5]

Educational Approaches

Patient educational approaches can range from formal educational programming such as group lecture settings; to informal, individualized one-on-one teaching; to self-directed learning by the patient that is facilitated by the nurse.[1] Formal patient education courses or classes are useful to address needs common to a group of patients or as individual teaching sessions. Formal courses are often taught using a curriculum/course plan with standardized content. In contrast, informal teaching often occurs in one-on-one sessions with the patient and/or family. It may be planned or spontaneous, but does not follow a specified formalized plan. An informal approach represents a large portion of patient education done by nurses. In fact, the majority of critical education occurs with each patient encounter when medications, diet, or treatment is explained, or simply when answering questions about the patient's issues or concerns. Individual or self-directed education results when a patient or family obtains and/or completes an educational activity independent from the nurse or other health care providers. With the influence of

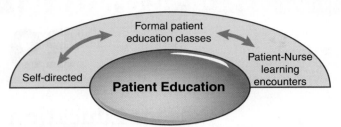

FIGURE 39-1 Scope of Patient Education Concept.

consumerism and the availability of information, a great deal of education can occur through self-directed learning with the use of written material or media (e.g., Internet, video) designed to assist the patient with information about health topics, a particular disease, treatments, or a specific skill[1] (Figure 39-1).

Because of the increasing use of technology in all aspects of life, the use of Internet resources for patient education cannot be ignored. A majority of adults in America use the Internet to find information on many aspects of life, including health, healthy lifestyles, and treatment options.[5] This use of technology expands the role of the nurse in patient education to include teaching on evaluation of Internet sources. Patients should be encouraged to look for information sources that list authors and their credentials and contact information. The source of information should also be listed, and any photographs, charts, graphs, or other graphics should contain helpful understandable information. Any links associated with the site should be functional, active links. It is also important that patients be taught to look for government (.gov), educational (.edu), and nonprofit (.org) sites because they are considered to be the most credible sources of information. Finally, sites chosen for use in gathering information should clearly identify how consumers can contact a site administrator and should be secure sites.[6]

For this discussion of approaches to patient education to be complete, the educated and motivated consumer should be considered. Many patients will be active consumers of health information and use self-directed approaches to education. Patients may present the nurse with articles, computer printouts, and other materials gathered in an attempt to learn about health promotion, symptoms, diagnoses, and treatments. These materials can be incorporated into the nurse's assessment of the patient and the educational plan. The tendency to pursue learning opportunities addresses motivation and presents the nurse with an opportunity to ask the patient to discuss what has been learned. This also gives the nurse the opportunity to teach the patient evaluative skills, looking at sources and content of the material for credibility and reliability.[7]

Learning Domains

Patient education can also be conceptualized from the perspective of learning domains—in other words, in terms of the type of learning a patient will need. The three main domains are cognitive, psychomotor, and affective.[1] Education intended to increase a patient's knowledge of a subject,

for example, is cognitive in nature and using methods such as written material, lecture, and discussion is appropriate. Skill teaching or psychomotor teaching requires that the patient have opportunities to touch and manipulate equipment and practice skills. A patient who must learn to change a dressing over a wound is an example. Education that is intended to change attitudes, such as viewing the lifestyle modifications associated with the treatment of coronary artery disease as a positive change rather than a burden, is known as the affective domain in education.[5]

To illustrate this, consider an example of a patient with a new diagnosis of a degenerative neurologic disorder that will require the patient to self-catheterize. The nurse will need to teach the patient the complex *psychomotor* skill of self-catheterization and the teaching will be successful when the patient is able to competently demonstrate this skill. Part of this teaching will include physiologic information designed to enhance the patient's understanding of the necessity of this procedure (*cognitive* learning) as well as assistance with lifestyle alterations and coping to help the patient to adapt and continue to live fully (*affective* domain).[1]

ATTRIBUTES AND CRITERIA

For patient education to occur there must be an identified need for learning. Although this need may be identified by the nurse, learning will not occur without readiness on the part of the learner. Ultimately, it is patient motivation that determines when, how, and if patient education will occur.[1] In addition to an identified need, the following are other major attributes of patient education:

1. Planning is involved.
2. The outcomes are goal oriented.
3. The patient is motivated to learn.

Like any other teaching-learning process, patient education requires that the teacher (nurse) know the intended audience and plan appropriately. This is a process that must be in place even in the most spontaneous of encounters. There must also be a goal, which is usually a change in behavior or attitude of some sort. The learners (patient and/or significant other) not only should be identified as the target of the teaching plan but also should be motivated by the outcome of the behavioral or attitudinal change. The nurse then develops the plan and evaluation to be consistent with the patient needs.

The nurse must determine the overall appropriateness of patient education. This requires asking, "Is the timing right, are the involved parties ready, and are the goals clear?" Only after these answers are determined can true education of the patient occur.

THEORETICAL LINKS

The goal of all patient education is to produce change. It is helpful to examine theories of behavior and learning in addition to nursing theory to understand patient need and motivation to change.

Theories of Health Behavior

The Health Belief Model was developed by Rosenstock in the mid-twentieth century to help explain individual decisions to use health screening opportunities. It has been adapted many times to explain compliance and behavior as they relate to health.[8] According to the Health Belief Model, individual perceptions of susceptibility to and severity of disease are the primary motivators for making attempts to change health behavior. These motivators are modified by demographic, social, psychologic, and structural variables that may heighten or dampen motivation. The primary motivation of patient perception then allows the patient to be open to cues to act, which of course leads to patient education opportunities.[8]

For example, a patient who is aware that her risk for breast cancer is high because of genetics may be likely to participate in some form of education about risk for the disease. This education can enhance the patient's knowledge level to produce lifestyle changes to reduce this patient's risk.

Simply stated, the Health Belief Model states that for an individual to change behavior related to health and wellness, there first must be a belief that illness can be avoided, and that taking a particular action can reduce risk. Further, the individual must believe that he/she is capable of making the needed change.

Nola Pender's Health Promotion Model (HPM), developed in 1987 and revised in the late 1990s, is "an attempt to depict the multidimensional nature of persons interacting with their interpersonal and physical environment as they pursue health."[9,p88] The HPM is based on the Health Belief Model that was expanded by Pender to include factors that can influence the patient's motivation to change behavior, such as previous experience with behavior changes to address the problem, and the patient's perception of success in these attempts. This model also expands the view of patient motivation by including social supports and competing priorities as factors to consider.

Pender's model is focused on achieving optimum wellness rather than avoiding disease, which Rosenstock's original model stressed as the primary motivator for changing behaviors. Pender points out, for example, that consideration of the patient's prior experience with attempting to change health behaviors is a key factor for the nurse when planning strategy, including educational strategy. An obese patient with comorbidities of coronary artery disease and type 2 diabetes will likely be told to lose weight to avoid serious complications. The Health Promotion Model dictates that part of the nursing assessment would be to ask the patient about prior attempts at weight reduction and perceived success of these efforts. The patient response to these inquiries will assist the nurse in development of educational interventions to address patient need. Pender also emphasizes that how the patient views the benefits and barriers to behavior change as well as the patient's own perception of ability to succeed will impact the nurse's plan for education.[9]

Nursing Theory

In considering nursing theory as it relates to patient education, there are many theories that can be used as a basis for formulation of plans. Dorothea Orem's Self-Care Deficit Theory is based on optimizing the patient's ability to assume responsibility for his/her own care and that motivation is based on the anticipation of resuming this responsibility. Orem defines self-care as a regulatory function that is "a deliberate action to supply or ensure the supply of necessary materials needed for continued life, growth, development and maintenance of human integrity."[10,p134] Orem addresses the role of family and others in the patient's social support system as assuming the responsibility of the patient's care when the patient is unable. Utilization of Orem's theory can assist the nurse to determine if materials are consistent with factors discovered during the assessment process, so that selection can move the patient toward meeting self-care demands.[11]

CONTEXT TO NURSING AND HEALTH CARE

Education of patients is integral to professional nursing practice; this fact is illustrated in multiple documents including the American Nurses Association *Nursing: Scope and Standards of Practice*,[12] each state's Nurse Practice Act, the Institute of Medicine's *Future of Nursing* report,[13] and the *Quality and Safety Education in Nursing* competencies.[14] Nursing practice has been defined as "the protection, promotion, and optimization of health and abilities, prevention of illness and injury, alleviation of suffering through the diagnosis and treatment of human response, and advocacy in the care of patients, families, communities, and populations."[12,p1] These positive patient outcomes are often achieved through education.

Numerous agencies require that patients and families be provided with information required to make decisions about health care and treatment of illness.[15] Modifications in health care in terms of delivery style and financer expectations have also changed the role of the patient in participating in his or her own care. This new level of patient engagement in health care requires that patient education be a priority for the registered nurse in the provision of patient care.[16]

Consumerism has also made more individuals want to take control of their own health and wellness and is promoting more individuals to seek health education opportunities in many venues. Patient education, however, remains the domain of the registered nurse, requiring appropriate assessment, planning, implementation, and evaluation of this often complex process.

The educational process and the nursing process are essentially the same[4] and include learner assessment, planning, implementation, evaluation, and documentation. Each of these steps is discussed in detail.

Learner Assessment

Learner assessment begins with a comprehensive assessment of the patient's learning needs. This may include a formalized written assessment, may be incorporated as part of the health assessment interview, or certainly may be a stated need from the patient. The assessment should include patient resources (education level, literacy level, social support, financial resources), educational resources, and nursing resources. Assessment data should be used to develop a teaching plan that is appropriate for the patient, but also one that will meet the desired goal. To fully individualize the educational plan for a patient, the nurse will consider the age, stage of development, and motivation to change behavior.

Psychosocial Development

Educational interventions must attend to the patient's achievement of developmental tasks. Erikson's Theory of Development is based on an eight-stage process in which each stage requires the achievement of a particular task. Completion of each stage forms the foundation of the next stage.[17] An understanding of Erikson's Theory of Development assists the nurse in patient education by understanding approaches necessary to accomplish the goal. For example, the educational approach taken by the nurse in teaching a patient how to use a metered dose inhaler for delivery of steroids will be different for a school-age child than for a middle-age adult. Using play-type activities to teach the procedure and identifying a celebrity or other role model who may need a similar treatment will appeal to the school-age patient. The middle-age adult is more concerned with fitting this treatment into his or her normal life patterns. Finally, it is critical for the nurse to incorporate the patient's own culture to make the teaching process meaningful.

Pedagogy Versus Androgogy

An appropriate next step to follow when utilizing Erikson's Theory of Development is the differences in learning experienced at different developmental stages. Pedogogy is the methodologies used to assist children to learn, or the strategies of traditional teaching. Androgogy conversely describes adult learning.[5] This implies that the strategies used with great success for teaching children in classrooms may not translate to successful outcomes for the nurse teaching adults. The nurse should attend to the developmental level of the individual and tailor learning activities to account for these differences. In general, learning in the adult is focused at an immediate need to address a personal issue or to solve a problem. The nurse is viewed as one who can facilitate that goal, rather than simply impart knowledge. Any learning should be directed toward what the adult patient needs and all activities should be pertinent to meeting that need. It is also important to note that most adults enter any learning situation with a rich history of experiences that can be, and should be, drawn on by the nurse to enhance present learning.[1] Box 39-1 summarizes adult learning principles.

Hierarchy of Needs

Maslow's Hierarchy of Needs theory is based on a simple premise that for higher level needs to be addressed lower level needs must be met. Maslow, a humanist, concluded that if environmental conditions are appropriate to meet basic needs, then individuals will grow.[18] This is an important

BOX 39-1   ADULT LEARNING PRINCIPLES

Adults learn best when:

Principle 1	Learning is related to an immediate need, problem, or deficit.
Principle 2	Learning is voluntary and self-initiated.
Principle 3	Learning is person-centered and problem-centered.
Principle 4	Learning is self-controlled and self-directed.
Principle 5	The role of the teacher is one of facilitator.
Principle 6	Information and assignments are pertinent.
Principle 7	New material draws on past experiences and is related to something the learner already knows.
Principle 8	The threat to self is reduced to a minimum in the educational situation.
Principle 9	The learner is able to participate actively in the learning process.
Principle 10	The learner is able to learn in a group.
Principle 11	The nature of the learning activity changes frequently.
Principle 12	Learning is reinforced by application and prompt feedback.

From Bastable SB, Gramet P, Jacobs K, et al: *Health professional as educator: principles of teaching and learning,* Figure 5-3, p 174, Boston, 2011, Jones and Bartlett.

concept in all types of teaching and is clear in all levels of education. A school-age child has limited ability to concentrate if the child is hungry. A college student has limited ability to concentrate and learn after an all-night study session. Of course this extends to our patients as well. Inadequate oxygenation, safety deficits, and food, water, and elimination needs, for example, must be addressed before the patient can adequately learn. A patient who needs to learn a complex skill must have the needs of pain management and comfort met before he or she attempts to meet learning needs. The motivation for patient education may also be linked to survival, representing a much more basic level of need. For example, a patient learning to self-administer insulin for the first time may feel a great sense of accomplishment at mastering this complex task, but the ability to self-administer this drug is truly a matter of survival for the diabetic patient.

Generational Differences

Generational differences are also a consideration when approaching patient education. Much has been reported about differences in the learning styles between generations, relating not only to the age of the patient but also to the era in which the individual was raised, as well as the social and political experiences that have been experienced by a group.[19] Educational approaches may need to differ for those born before 1946; members of this age group usually are self-motivated and do not seek feedback for their performance. On the other hand, members of Generation Y are dependent on technology and desire immediate feedback.[20] This factor, perhaps more than any other, will dictate how the nurse approaches patient education.

Literacy Level

The ability to read and understand the written word is, of course, critical if the educational process is to include any written material. Based on the 2003 National Assessment of Adult Literacy 43% of adults in the United States had literacy skills at the basic or below-basic level.[17] It is also important to consider the patient's ability to understand and interpret health-related information and instructions—the individual's level of health literacy.[4] Although assessment of literacy levels can be very difficult in adult patients because of the stigma and shame often associated with limited reading ability, patients may give cues to limited literacy, such as avoiding reading materials provided (the patient may state "I forgot my glasses") or demonstrating repeated inability to follow written instructions. If there is a suspicion that the patient may not be able to read written material or that the information is written at a level that the patient cannot understand, the nurse must use alternate methods of instruction to ensure patient understanding. Although beyond the scope of this text, several methods exist for the nurse to quickly evaluate written material for readability for those with limited reading skills.

Barriers

There are a number of barriers to learning that must be considered as part of learner assessment. The lack of available social support systems, which may impair the patient's motivation to learn or ability to participate in classes or programs, is one common barrier. Lack of support may also limit the patient's ability to practice new skills. Additional patient-related barriers include, cultural differences, lack of financial resources or time, and frequent interruptions. It may be within the patient's or the nurse's ability to control or remove these barriers to enhance patient learning and outcomes.

Barriers on the part of the nurse to participate in patient education include lack of time and multiple competing demands. The role of the professional nurse is often not prioritized because of issues with staffing, payment, and perception of effectiveness of educational efforts. Further, the nurse's professional motivation and confidence in education skills pose a barrier to patient education. Again, assessing the nurse's attitudes can assist in identification of these professional barriers and development of interventions to overcome them.[1]

Planning

Planning is the determination of what methods will be used to meet the educational need. This includes deciding if the outcome is a cognitive (knowledge) change, a psychomotor (performance of a skill) change, or an affective (feeling or attitude) change. This dictates the approach as well as the goal. For example, a patient diagnosed with type 1 diabetes may need to learn about the overall pathophysiology of the disease so that he or she can appreciate the physical and lifestyle impact. However, the patient also needs to develop practical psychomotor skills (e.g., injection, testing) to cope with this disease. The nurse must plan not only to describe what diabetes is but also to demonstrate blood glucose testing and self-injection of insulin, allowing for practice and redemonstration from the patient and perhaps significant others as well. The domain of learning should match the teaching methodology used.

Implementation of Educational Plan

Implementation or carrying out the plan is an area in which flexibility is key. The nurse will need to determine the length of educational sessions, content to be covered, and methodology for teaching. These plans may be influenced by numerous unpredictable factors such as patient condition and competing priorities. The nurse must adjust the teaching session to accommodate the priorities of the patient.

Evaluation

Evaluation of learning outcomes should be consistent with the domain of learning as well. Psychomotor skills, for example, require that the patient be able to *do* something, such as perform a skill. Using a survey or other measurement tool to evaluate a skill will not adequately measure this outcome. Surveys and questionnaires can be used to measure affective behavior change as well as patient satisfaction with the teaching experience. Because the goal of patient education is behavior change, the evaluation of the process may need to be conducted over time and be dependent on multiple sources of data.

Returning to the example of teaching a patient diagnosed with type 1 diabetes, the nurse will likely include cognitive information about disease pathology to appropriately manage the condition. This patient will probably need to master the psychomotor skill of blood glucose monitoring and insulin injection. The nurse will also be concerned with the affective dimension of the diagnosis of chronic disease. Evaluation of all of these dimensions will require that the nurse observe the skills for level of mastery, discuss the "why" of diet and exercise with the patient on multiple occasions, evaluate the impact of the patient's daily decisions on disease management, and use repeated assessment of the patient's acceptance of the condition to fully evaluate behavior change.

No discussion of patient education would be complete without consideration of the issue of noncompliance. An approved nursing diagnosis by the North American Nursing Diagnosis Association International (NANDA-I), noncompliance is defined by Carpenito-Moyet as the "state in which an patient or group desires to comply but factors are present that deter adherence to health-related advice given by health professionals."[21,p429] Carpenito-Moyet stresses that this diagnosis be applied to patients who have the *desire* to comply. This definition is often altered in daily practice to mean that the patient (or family) does not do what they were told. Used properly, this label can communicate to the professional that there are factors that block patient adherence, such as lack of understanding, literacy, financial problems, lack of environmental or interpersonal support, or previous experiences with treatment or self-management failures.[3] These issues should be included in the assessment process and addressed in the educational plan for the patient in an attempt to enhance compliance.

Documentation

To ensure consistency in care, documentation of patient education is included in the patient record. This documentation should be comprehensive and include not only a description of the information that the patient was taught but also an assessment of the patient's motivation, ability to learn (any physical or cognitive issues that may inhibit the process), developmental level, and resources (personal and financial, if appropriate). A detailed plan should be included in the documentation so that other professionals can reinforce the process if education is to be continued across care settings. This should include goals and progress toward them. Finally, the patient response to the educational plan and adjustments to accommodate changes in patient condition or other factors should be included to ensure consistent, successful patient education outcomes.

INTERRELATED CONCEPTS

Patient education as a concept is central to the role of the nurse in the delivery of quality patient care (Figure 39-2). The professional roles and attributes of **Collaboration** and **Communication** are essential in the development, planning, and delivery of patient education, whereas the nurse's role as an educator is central to his or her professional identity (see **Professionalism** concept). The nurse works not only with the patient but also with teams of providers in determining care needs, and quality patient education is one of the results of this skilled collaborative effort. To accomplish this, the nurse's knowledge of **Technology and informatics** along with the ability to teach patients and families the use of health care technology is critical when transitioning care from the acute care facility into the home. The result of current changes in **Health policy** requires the nurse to engage **Leadership** skills not only to assist patients and families but also to prepare the consumer for this evolution of health care.

The role of the nurse in **Health promotion,** an area in which nurses generally take the lead, is also a critical professional dimension that is related to patient education. The nurse's knowledge and skill in recognizing opportunities to improve wellness, health, and function through lifestyle modification is used in all patient encounters and is a critical professional role in the education of patients.

Patient education incorporates the patient's attributes and resources. The nurse approaches each patient encounter as an opportunity to educate. This involves a determination of the patient's developmental level, developmental task accomplishment, functional status, and ability to perform needed skills (**Development** concept) as well as an analysis of the dynamics of relationships (**Family dynamics** concept) to assist in determination of supports and stressors. The patient's desire to learn (**Motivation** concept), cultural background (**Culture** concept), and prior experiences with adherence to prescribed regimens (**Adherence** concept) are also concepts that have a direct relationship to patient education and in fact form the foundation of the assessment and planning process.

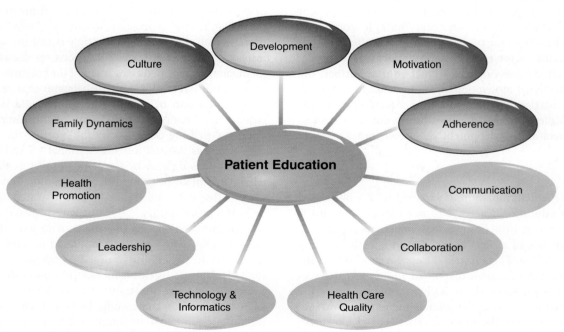

FIGURE 39-2 Patient Education and Interrelated Concepts. Professional nursing concepts are represented in blue; patient attributes and preference concepts are represented in red.

MODEL CASE

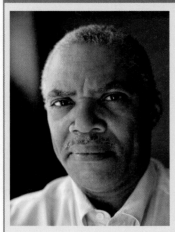

Mr. Jacobs is a 55-year-old college-educated African-American male. Mr. Jacobs was recently diagnosed with colon cancer and opted for surgical intervention with the formation of a colostomy. Before his hospital admission, the nurse is to develop a plan and initiate teaching Mr. Jacobs the self-care required.

During a preoperative visit, the nurse plans to meet with Mr. Jacobs. Before his preoperative visit, the nurse reviews the health record and notes that Mr. Jacobs is well educated and is able to read English. The nurse also learns that Mr. Jacobs is married and has 2 college-age children who are away from home most of the time. Although the patient works in the banking industry he has been unable to work for several months because of his illness but remains insured. Mr. Jacobs' wife works in retail.

During the initial interview, the nurse learns that Mr. Jacobs has been very health conscious his whole life and is somewhat shocked at his current health situation. When asked by the nurse about specific goals for this surgery, Mr. Jacobs responds that he wants to be cured from the cancer and go back to his "normal" life. The nurse asks Mr. Jacobs if he has had any other health challenges before this diagnosis. Mr. Jacobs only mentions a knee injury in college that caused him to stop playing football and give up his athletic scholarship. Mr. Jacobs mentions that he worked full-time during his last 2 years of college to be able to finish his education. The nurse compliments Mr. Jacobs on his perseverance. He notes that he has always been goal oriented and a hard worker, but that he is afraid that this current challenge may be too much for him. The nurse tries to determine Mr. Jacobs' perception of living with a colostomy, noting a comment made by Mr. Jacobs that "it is the one thing I said I would never live with." When questioned about this statement, Mr. Jacobs says that this is an embarrassment and he would like to do everything he can to hide the fact that he has a stoma. He states that he accepts the reality of his situation and is willing to learn to care for it himself. When the nurse asks Mr. Jacobs about involving his family in the teaching, he indicates a preference to master the skills and teach his wife later.

Based on the information gathered the nurse develops a plan to teach Mr. Jacobs one-on-one rather than in a classroom situation. To address the domains of learning, the nurse provides Mr. Jacobs with written materials to address the cognitive information required about colon cancer, anatomy and physiology of the gastrointestinal tract, and alterations presented by having a stoma. The nurse also introduced via written material the options that may be available to Mr. Jacobs to care for the stoma to offer him some control over the care.

To address the psychomotor skills that are required, the nurse planned to meet with Mr. Jacobs to demonstrate how the ostomy appliance is fitted, emptied, and changed. A manikin abdomen with a stoma similar to the proposed placement of Mr. Jacobs' stoma was introduced in the preoperative period to allow Mr. Jacobs to practice with the materials he would be using at discharge. Troubleshooting and "what if" scenarios can be integrated into the teaching after the patient begins to develop mastery of the skill and material handling.

The nurse is concerned about Mr. Jacobs' lack of family involvement in his care and notes his sense of embarrassment. Therefore the nurse begins to address the affective domain by asking Mr. Jacobs to view some videos about individuals who have stomas. In the postoperative period, this can be followed up by a visit from a current stoma patient and support group attendance if Mr. Jacobs is open to those options.

The nurse is careful to attend to Mr. Jacobs' developmental stage of *generativity versus stagnation*[12] when planning for his learning needs as well as principles of adult learning. The nurse also uses multiple sources of information to teach Mr. Jacobs according to his level of education, but also attends to the fact that psychomotor learning is required. By asking about the patient's goals and hesitancy to incorporate family into the teaching process, the nurse attends to the patient's experience of the illness and attempts to fully engage the patient in care.

To evaluate the outcome of the educational intervention conducted, the nurse follows-up with Mr. Jacobs to determine his competency (both actual and perceived) in performing the necessary skills of care and Mr. Jacobs' emotional and attitudinal changes related to the ostomy and his illness. Plans are changed and adjusted according to Mr. Jacobs' progress towards his goals, incorporating family members while Mr. Jacobs becomes ready for this step.

Case Analysis

In this case, the nurse attended carefully to assessment before beginning the educational process. Because the patient was well educated, the nurse could rely on multiple forms of education, including written materials. The nurse did not, however, use print media exclusively. The psychomotor skills would likely not be mastered with written media only.

Although it is ideal to include family members in the educational process, particularly when major changes in routine and lifestyle may affect all members of the household, the nurse honored Mr. Jacobs' request to be allowed to learn the skill on his own before involving his wife and children. This preference may have been culturally related, but is consistent with Mr. Jacobs' traits of perseverance and goal orientation. Including the family members before the patient is ready may hamper education efforts by limiting trust in the nurse-patient relationship.

By asking about goals and listening to Mr. Jacobs' feelings about living with an ostomy before initiating the educational plan, the nurse gathers valuable information about perceptions and attitudes. With this information, the nurse is able to incorporate strategies for addressing the affective domain that will be most effective. The nurse uses video early in the process to "plant the seed" that others live productively with the same condition as Mr. Jacobs, but plans follow-up with actual patients once Mr. Jacobs has had a chance to learn and formulate questions about the impact of the ostomy on his daily routine.

Continued

MODEL CASE—cont'd

The patient's desire to return to his normal life tells the nurse that this patient, in Erickson's stage of *generativity versus stagnation,* wants to resume a productive life as soon as possible, lending to motivation to learn. This could have been further enhanced by incorporating frank discussions about the impact on Mr. Jacobs' sexuality into the teaching plan.

Failing to attend to the patient during assessment would have resulted in failure of the patient's educational experience. For example, if the nurse assumed that the patient would want his wife included from the beginning and arranged the educational sessions with Mrs. Jacobs rather than the patient alone, the nurse would have limited the patient's ability to express his own needs in the educational encounter.

EXEMPLARS

Examples of patient education exist in many formats for a broad range of topics, intended for use in a variety of ways. Box 39-2 represents some common examples. Grouped by the primary focus as well as how the teaching/learning may be accomplished, Box 39-2 highlights the numerous types, venues, and media types that can be considered in patient education.

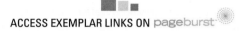

ACCESS EXEMPLAR LINKS ON *pageburst*

BOX 39-2   EXEMPLARS OF PATIENT EDUCATION

Illness Related
Formal Patient Education Programming
- Cancer support groups
- Cardiac education
- Coumadin classes
- Diabetes education
- Disease-specific classes
- Group preoperative teaching
- Ostomy support group

Informal Patient-Nurse Encounters
- Discharge teaching
- Disease-specific diet teaching
- High-tech home care teaching
- Medication teaching
- Symptom control
- Targeted written materials
- Wound care

Self-Directed Patient Education Activities
- Common literature (e.g., magazines, journals, newspapers)
- Instructional videos specific to condition or treatment
- Internet resources (e.g., American Cancer Society, American Heart Association)
- Self-help books (e.g., diet plans, herbal remedies, alternative and complementary treatment, coping with addiction)

Health Promotion
Formal Patient Education Programming
- Childbirth classes
- Drug abuse avoidance
- Elder care classes
- Parenting classes
- Risk reduction activities
- Smoking cessation programs
- Strength/endurance building
- Weight reduction classes
- Wellness education programs

Informal Patient-Nurse Encounters
- Advanced care planning
- Age-specific screening needs
- Breastfeeding
- Counseling
- Genetic screening
- Health counseling
- Immunization teaching
- Preventing sexually transmitted diseases

Self-Directed Patient Education Activities
- Common literature (e.g., magazines, journals, newspapers)
- Exercise videos (e.g., aerobics, yoga, Pilates)
- Instructional videos specific to health-related topic
- Internet resources (e.g., WebMD, Real Age)
- Self-help books (e.g., diet plans, herbal remedies, alternative and complementary treatment, coping with addiction)
- Television (e.g., health-related programming, FIT TV)

REFERENCES

1. Bastable SB, Gramet P, Jacobs K, et al: *Health professional as educator: principles of teaching and learning*, Boston, 2011, Jones and Bartlett.

2. Lamiani G, Furey A: Teaching nurses how to teach: an evaluation of a workshop on patient education, *Patient Educ Couns* 75(2):270–273, 2009.

3. *Healthy People 2020*. Retrieved Oct 30, 2010, from www.healthy people.gov/hp2020/.

4. Bastable SB: *Essentials of patient education*, Boston, 2006, Jones and Bartlett.

5. Clark DR: *Instructional system design concept map*, 2004. Retrieved Nov 14, 2010, from www.nwlink.com/~donclark/ hrd/bloom.html.

6. Anderson AS, Klemm P: The internet: friend or foe when providing patient education? *Clin J Oncol Nurs* 12(1):55–63, 2008.

7. Bradley SM: The internet: can patients link to credible sources? *MEDSURG Nurs* 17(4):229–236, 2008.

8. Richards E, Digger K: In Bastable SB, editor: *The nurse as educator: principles of teaching and learning for nursing practice*, ed 3, Boston, 2008, Jones and Bartlett.

9. Pender NJ, Murdaugh CL, Parsons MA: *Health promotion in nursing practice*, ed 5, Upper Saddle River, NJ, 2006, Pearson Prentice Hall.

10. McEwen M, Wills EM: *Theoretical basis for nursing*, ed 3, Philadelphia, 2011, Lippincott Williams & Wilkins.

11. Wilson FL, Wood DW, Risk J, et al: Evaluation of education materials using Orem's self-care deficit theory, *Nurs Sci Q* 16(1):68–76, 2003.

12. American Nurses Association: *Nursing: scope and standards of practice*, Silver Springs, Md, 2010, Author.

13. Institute of Medicine of The National Academies: *The future of nursing: leading change, advancing health*, Washington, DC, 2010, The National Academies Press. http://books.nap.edu/ openbook.php?record_id=12956&page=232010.

14. *Quality and safety education in nursing*: Retrieved Dec 4, 2010, from www.qsen.org/ksas_prelicensure.php.

15. Nelson JM: In Bastable SB, editor: *Essentials of patient education*, Boston, 2006, Jones and Bartlett.

16. Gruman J, Rovner MH, French ME, et al: From patient education to patient engagement: implications for the field of patient education, *Patient Educ Counsel* 78:350, 2010.

17. Edelman CL, Mandle CL: *Health promotion throughout the lifespan*, ed 6, Philadelphia, 2006, Mosby.

18. Faculty development at The University of Hawaii. Retrieved Nov 14, 2010, from http://honolulu.hawaii.edu/intranet/comm ittees/FacDevCom/guidebk/teachtip/maslow.htm retrieved.

19. Zalenski RJ, Raspa R: Maslow's hierarchy of needs: a framework for achieving human potential in hospice, *J Palliat Med* 9(5):1120–1127, 2006.

20. Moreno-Walton L, Brunett P, Akhtar S, et al: Teaching across the generation gap: consensus from the council of emergency medicine residency directors 2009 academic assembly, *Acad Emerg Med J* 16(12, suppl 2):S19–S24, 2009.

21. Carpenito-Moyet LJ: *Nursing diagnosis: application to clinical practice*, ed 12, Philadelphia, 2008, Lippincott Williams & Wilkins.

40

Health Promotion

Jean Giddens

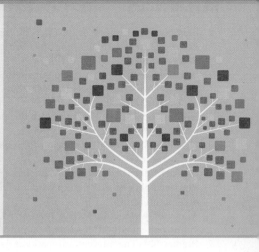

O ver the past century, technological advancements have resulted in dramatic changes in nearly every aspect of our daily lives—particularly in the areas of transportation, communication, food production, and food acquisition. Technological advances have afforded humans with many conveniences incomprehensible 100 years ago. Along with these advances, there have been many consequences. Over time, the lifestyles of people worldwide have changed, resulting in a largely sedentary society with epidemic rates of obesity and many other related chronic diseases. According to the U.S. Department of Health and Human Services (USDHHS), unhealthy lifestyles and unhealthy environments are responsible for a large percentage of morbidity and mortality in the United States.[1]

Early technological advances in medicine fueled an initial interest in developing improved methods for the diagnosis and treatment of disease. As societal changes occurred, it became clear that a focus on health prevention was also necessary. Thus, over the past several decades there has been a significant shift in national attention from the treatment of illness to the promotion of health.

Health promotion has become a national health priority and is foundational to the provision of care for people of all ages; it also influences health policy, economics, and distribution of resources. As the largest group of health care providers, nurses are central to meeting national health promotion goals through interactions with individuals, families, and communities. Not surprisingly, health promotion is a standard of professional nursing practice specifically identified by the American Nurses Association.[2] The purpose of this concept analysis is to introduce health promotion and describe how this concept is applied within nursing practice.

DEFINITION(S)

Initially, the concept of health promotion may seem simple—that is, a focus on improvement of health and prevention of disease. This concept, however, is actually very complex involving multiple dimensions. For the purposes of this concept analysis,

the World Health Organization's definition is proposed: *Health promotion is the process of enabling people to increase control over, and to improve, their health.*[3] Health promotion requires the adoption of healthy living practices and often necessitates a change in behavior. For this reason, long-term success of health promotion efforts is largely dependent on adaptation to change. Disease prevention (also referred to as health protection) is considered a component of health promotion and refers to behaviors motivated by a desire to avoid illness, detect illness early, and manage illnesses when they occur.

To fully understand health promotion, one must have an understanding of various dimensions underlying this concept. Health promotion encompasses health, wellness, disease, and illness. First of all, what is meant by *health*? The World Health Organization defines *health* as "a state of complete physical, mental, and social well-being and not merely the absence of disease and infirmity."[4] Despite the fact that this definition is nearly 60 years old, it remains the most popular definition of health worldwide.[5] A similar term is *wellness,* but unlike health, there is no universally accepted definition. *Wellness* refers to a positive state of health of an individual, family, or community. It is multidimensional, encompassing several dimensions including physical, mental, spiritual, social, occupational, environmental, intellectual, and financial. Wellness is seen as a continually changing state ranging from high-level to low-level wellness. *Disease* is a functional or structural disturbance that results when a person's adaptive mechanisms to counteract stimuli and stresses fail.[6] Although similar to disease, *illness* is seen as the physical manifestations and the subjective experience of the individual. Illness can be present in the absence of disease and it is possible to have no illness when a disease is present. Likewise, many individuals experience wellness in the presence of an illness. As an example, a person who has type 2 diabetes (a chronic illness) can experience high-level wellness. Low-level wellness is seen as an unfavorable state in which illness may result. Over the years, there has been ongoing debate about the relationship between health and illness—as paired entities at opposite ends of a single continuum or as separate entities.[7-9] The complex interrelationship of health, wellness,

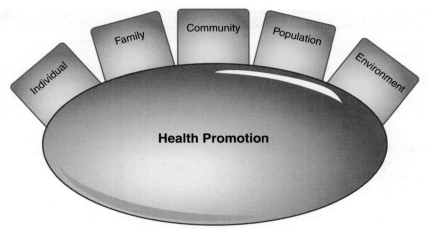

FIGURE 40-1 Scope of Health Promotion.

illness, and disease as components of health promotion would suggest the latter is a more realistic view.

SCOPE AND CATEGORIES

Health promotion is viewed broadly in scope as behaviors that promote optimal health across the lifespan within an individual, family, community, population, and environment (Figure 40-1). Specific recommendations vary according to the unique characteristics of an individual (such as age, gender or race, family history, or medical history), a community, or a population. Health promotion recommendations for population groups often are presented in the context of age groups including infants, toddlers, school-age children, adolescents, adults, and older adults.

Community is a collective group of people identified by geography, common interests, concerns, characteristics, or values.[10] Thus community may be a localized area or may involve groups of people without geographic boundaries. It is also important to recognize the entire world as a global community—meaning that things rarely occur in isolation of one country or region so a very broad perspective of potential impact must be considered.

Three levels of prevention, first defined by Leavell and Clark, serve as a useful framework to describe concept categories and are used throughout this text. The principal categories of health promotion are primary, secondary, and tertiary prevention (Figure 40-2).[6]

Primary Prevention

Primary prevention refers to strategies aimed at optimizing health and disease prevention. The focus is on health education for optimal nutrition, exercise, immunizations, safe living and work environments, hygiene and sanitation, protection from environmental hazards, avoidance of harmful substances (such as allergens, toxins, and carcinogens), protection from accidents, and effective stress management. Specific health promotion strategies are not linked to a single disease entity. As an example, avoiding smoking helps to promote health and reduce the individual's risk for pulmonary,

cardiovascular, and immunologic disease. Also, it is important to understand that a combination of strategies is usually advised for the prevention of specific conditions. As an example, there are many known strategies that prevent or reduce one's risk for developing cardiovascular disease, including implementing a healthy diet, exercising regularly, and avoiding smoking; additional measures may be advised based on other personal risk factors.

Secondary Prevention (Screening)

The goal of secondary prevention is to identify individuals in an early state of a disease process so that prompt treatment can be initiated. Early treatment provides an opportunity to cure, limit disability, or delay consequences of advanced disease. Secondary prevention measures typically involve screening tests. Screenings are typically indicated and recommended if they are safe, cost-effective, and accurate, and if the effort makes a substantial difference in the morbidity and/or mortality of conditions. Screenings are recommended for an individual, family, population, or community based on known risk factors.

To be considered accurate, a screening method must have a high degree of reliability and validity. A screening instrument, test, or method is considered reliable if the approach produces the same results when different individuals (with a similar skill set) perform the test. Validity reflects the ability of the test

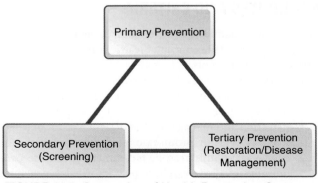

FIGURE 40-2 Categories of Health Promotion Concept.

BOX 40-1   U.S. PREVENTIVE SERVICES TASK FORCE GRADING

Grade A = Strongly Recommends
- There is high certainty that the net benefit is substantial.

Grade B = Recommends
- There is high certainty that the net benefit is moderate or there is moderate certainty that the net benefit is moderate to substantial.

Grade C = No Recommendations for or Against
- There may be considerations that support providing the intervention for an individual patient, but not for the general population. There is at least moderate certainty that the net benefit is small.

Grade D = Recommends Against
- There is moderate or high certainty that the intervention has no net benefit or that the harms outweigh the benefits.

I Statement = Insufficient Evidence to Recommend for or Against
- The current evidence is insufficient to assess the balance of benefits and harms of the service. Evidence is lacking, of poor quality, or conflicting, and the balance of benefits and harms cannot be determined.

From U.S. Preventive Services Task Force: www.uspreventiveservicestaskforce.org/.

---

to accurately detect disease. Ideally, a screening measure will accurately differentiate individuals who have a condition from those who do not have a condition 100% of the time. *Sensitivity* is a measure related to the proportion of those with a condition who are correctly identified. A test with poor sensitivity fails to identify disease in people who actually have a condition—known as a false-negative result. *Specificity* refers to the ability to currently identify those who do not have a condition. If a screening measure has poor specificity, many people who are disease free will have a false-positive test result.

Tertiary Prevention

Tertiary prevention involves minimizing the effects of disease and disability; the focus of tertiary prevention is restorative through collaborative disease management. The aim is to optimize the management of a condition and minimize complications so that the individual can achieve the highest level of health possible. Specific strategies include rehabilitative efforts to increase adherence to medication, nutrition, physical activity, and other disease management strategies. Many strategies used as primary prevention strategies are also used for tertiary prevention. The difference is not the strategy itself, but rather the intent, goal, and context of the strategy. As an example, aerobic exercise is used as a primary prevention strategy to maintain health, but may be a specific weight loss intervention for the obese patient, or be used as a rehabilitation strategy following an acute myocardial infarction.

ATTRIBUTES AND CRITERIA

Attributes are qualities, characteristics, or elements that validate parameters of the concept. Health promotion is characterized by four elements:

1. *Optimization of health.* The focus on optimizing health includes measures to maintain high-level wellness, measures to prevent illness, and strategies for early detection and management of disease when it occurs.
2. *Evidence.* Health promotion guidelines are based on evidence; for this reason, recommendations are periodically updated to reflect new knowledge generated through research efforts. The recommendations are usually disseminated through practice guidelines for health professionals and via consumer-targeted media for the general public. In many cases, recommendations are presented as a matter of priority based on the level of evidence. As an example, the U.S. Preventive Services Task Force (USPSTF) has five levels of evidence; each recommendation statement is accompanied by a recommendation Grade that ranges from A to D or Grade I (Box 40-1). As applied to two examples of cancer screening, USPSTF recommends biennial mammography screening for women ages 50 to 74 (Grade B recommendation)[11] and recommends against routine screening for bladder cancer in adults (Grade D recommendation).[12]
3. *Patient/community centered.* Incorporation of health promotion measures must be valued and desired by the individuals impacted. On an individual level, personal motivation to incorporate the strategies is required. On a community level, leadership from individuals within the community is needed for successful implementation. It is critical that the wishes and desires of the targeted individual(s) are considered and understood. A patient/family/community assessment must be done in order to gain an understanding of the wishes and desires of the individual(s) impacted.[5]
4. *Enculturation.* Designing and implementing health promotion require cultural competence and sensitivity to differences among cultures. Nurses must be willing to listen and learn from patients and communities so that interventions are provided within appropriate languages and within the context of health belief practices.[13] All too often, health care providers make recommendations for actions from their own perspective of what is appropriate and expected behavior—an ethnocentric perspective based on their own set of values and beliefs. Enculturation refers to the full internalization of values of a culture group. To be successful, health promotion plans incorporate the beliefs, attitudes, values, behaviors, and interpersonal dynamics into the planning, implementation, and evaluation of health promotion activities.

TABLE 40-1	MODELS OF HEALTH PROMOTION TARGETING THE INDIVIDUAL
MODEL NAME AND THEORIST	**BRIEF DESCRIPTION**
Health Promotion Model (Pender)	This model shows that healthy behaviors (behavioral outcomes) are influenced by integration of unique characteristics and experiences of an individual (prior behavior and personal factors) and by influences of behavior (perceived benefit and barriers to action, perceived self-efficacy, activity-related affect, and interpersonal and situational influences).
Transtheoretical Model (Prochaska and DiClemente)	This model proposes that health-related behavior progresses through six stages of behavior change on a continuum from motivational readiness to change of a problem behavior. The six stages are precontemplation, contemplation, preparation for action, action, maintenance, and termination. These changes occur regardless of specific behavior change and have been observed both among individuals adopting healthy behaviors and among those stopping an unhealthy behavior (such as smoking).
Theory of Reasoned Action and Planned Behavior (Ajzen and Fishbein)	This theory is built on an understanding of attitudes and subjective norms and the influence these have on changes in behavior. According to the model, the intention to change is driven by the attitude toward the behavior and the subjective norm for the behavior.
Social Cognitive Theory (Bandura)	This is a social cognitive theory used to design individual behavioral change. Self-belief influences behavior; self-beliefs are formed through self-observation and self-reflection. The major concepts within this theory are self-direction, self-regulation, and self-efficacy.
Health Belief Model (Stretcher and Rosenstock)	This model explores behaviors of individuals who take actions to avoid illness and those who fail to take preventive actions and thus has been used to predict which individuals would or would not use preventive measures.

THEORETICAL LINKS

Numerous models and theories of health, health behavior, and health promotion have evolved over the past 30 years as the science and evidence of health promotion have expanded. Two areas of health promotion models include those focusing on the individual as a patient and those focusing on the community.

Individual-Focused Models

Models that focus on the individual typically share common themes including cognition, decision making, motivation, behavior, and environment. Although it is beyond the scope of this concept analysis to detail all the models and theories associated with health promotion, some of the most prominent, contemporary models are presented in Table 40-1.

Community-Focused Models

True community interventions focus on the community as a whole or the majority of the population within a community; this is in contrast to the application of interventions to individuals within a community. Community-focused models share common attributes, including (1) a focus on community values and norms, (2) legitimization of desirable behaviors and environmental changes, (3) participation of community leadership, and (4) a planned change in which community members have control.[14] A number of community-focused models exist for planning and dissemination of health promotion agendas; a few of these are presented in Table 40-2.

CONTEXT TO NURSING AND HEALTH CARE

Nurses have involvement in health promotion on a number of levels including working with an individual or family to enhance health, working with communities and organizations

to enhance health, and participating in the development and implementation of health policy, just to name a few. The most common roles of nurses include the assessment, planning, and implementation of interventions and the evaluation of health promotion strategies for individuals; in fact, nurses have a significant responsibility for enhancing the health of individuals across the lifespan; this occurs in the context of a therapeutic relationship and requires skillful commination by the nurse.

National Health Care Agenda and Health Care Economics

Health promotion is a central focus of health care delivery that has been shown to add quality years of life and to decrease health care costs.[5] National goals and objectives for improving the health of Americans have been outlined in a series of reports beginning in 1979 with the publication of the first of the *Healthy People* series—*Healthy People: The Surgeon General's Report on Health Promotion and Disease Prevention*—and a companion document published in 1980—*Promoting Health/Preventing Disease. Objectives for the Nation.* Since that time the USDHHS has published three additional reports (in 1990, 2000, and 2010) outlining goals and objectives for the upcoming decade. The most current document, *Healthy People 2020*, outlines four national goals for the nation to achieve by the year 2020; these goals are presented in Box 40-2. The 4 goals link to 42 topic areas, each with a set of objectives and target indicators to measure progress.[15]

The support for health promotion and illness prevention services is also demonstrated through the changes in coverage for such interventions by third-party payers. The impact of providing such services is continually evaluated; to maintain support the cost of providing such services (including to those who are uninsured or underinsured) must outweigh

TABLE 40-2 MODELS OF HEALTH PROMOTION TARGETING THE COMMUNITY

MODEL NAME AND THEORIST	BRIEF DESCRIPTION
Social Ecology Models	These are models that emphasize social and cultural contexts of people within an environment—and recognition of multiple variables that influence health behaviors. Consideration for health promotion interventions includes an integration of environmental resources and lifestyles of individuals within that environment.
PRECEDE-PROCEED Model (Green)	This is a nine-stage model designed to guide the planning to health programs by identifying the most appropriate intervention strategies. PRECEDE stands for **p**redisposing, **r**einforcing, **e**nabling **c**onstructs in **e**cosystem, **d**iagnosis, and **e**valuation. PROCEED recognizes forces outside the control of individuals and stands for **p**olicy, **r**egulation, **o**rganizational **c**onstructs in **e**ducation, and **e**nvironmental **d**evelopment.
Diffusion of Innovations Model (Rogers)	This is a model that emphasizes dissemination of health behavior interventions. Rogers' model identifies four steps of diffusion including (1) the innovation, (2) communication channels (spreading the word), (3) time, and (4) social systems. Underlying assumption of adoption is the perceived value placed on the new behavior or innovation.
Social Marketing Models	Social marketing models influence behavior change by influencing adoption of an idea by general public. Foundational to social marketing models are product, price, place, and promotion. When applied to health promotion, the "product" is the desired application; the "price" is the cost (social and economic) to the community as a result of adoption; "place" refers to the location the program(s) is(are) available; and "promotion" refers to strategies used to entice individuals to accept the change through adoption.

BOX 40-2 OVERARCHING GOALS FOR *HEALTHY PEOPLE 2020*

1. Attain high-quality, longer lives free of preventable disease, disability, injury, and premature death.
2. Achieve health equity, eliminate disparities, and improve the health of all groups.
3. Create social and physical environments that promote good health for all.
4. Promote quality of life, healthy development, and healthy behaviors across all life stages.

From U.S. Department of Health and Human Services: *Healthy People 2020*. Accessed at www.healthypeople.gov/2020/about/default.aspx.

the consequences of the absence of such services, particularly in the face of rising health care expenditures. Such issues have been central to health policy debate.

Vulnerable Populations and Health Disparities

Vulnerable populations refer to groups of individuals who are at greatest risk for poor health outcomes. These people are more likely to develop health-related problems and experience significantly worse outcomes when they occur. Vulnerable population groups are often politically marginalized in society; they experience discrimination and intolerance and may not have basic human needs met. Two of the most highly vulnerable populations are persons with low socioeconomic status and persons who are members of ethnic and racial minorities. Health policy to eliminate health disparities aims to increase accessible health services, requiring community involvement. Cultural competence is especially important to the elimination of health disparities because it facilitates integration of culturally appropriate interventions based on the

values and beliefs of the targeted group. Thus, before working with vulnerable populations, nurses must be committed to developing skills in cultural competence.[16]

ASSESSMENT

Health assessment is the foundation for establishing a health promotion plan and the basis for application of health promotion into practice. Assessment can target an individual, family, or community.

Individual Assessment

The primary components of assessment for individuals include a comprehensive assessment of health status, health behaviors, and risk. Advances in genetic research have enhanced the ability to assess risk; thus family history is a critical component of health assessment. Additionally, assessment includes gaining an understanding of personal factors such as health preferences, values, and social relationships. The assessment of health is performed by nurses in nearly all settings and includes conducting a history and physical examination. Effective communication skills are essential to obtain necessary information for a successful health promotion process. The nurse-patient relationship is truly the context of care; the nurse must be sensitive to each person's goals and values.

Family Assessment

A family assessment is necessary to promote health within families. Family assessment includes gaining an understanding of health promotion and disease prevention activities within the family (including risk factors), family strengths, and the relationships among family members—how family members influence behaviors and decision making of others.

A genogram is a useful method to understand family members across multiple generations.[17]

Community Assessment

Community assessment is a necessary component of assessment when developing community-based health promotion strategies—usually in the context of community health nursing and public health nursing. Community assessment is conducted in participation with community representatives and through community data collection strategies including observation, interviews from community residents, and data collection using instruments that quantify data. Additional information about a community typically incorporated into an assessment includes the structure of a community, census, population/demographic statistics, morbidity rates, mortality rates, epidemiologic data, environmental data (such as pollution indices), and community resources such as health care services, government services (fire, police, and other emergency services), schools, and other local government agencies. These data can be collected from a variety of sources including the Internet and city/government offices.

Health Promotion Interventions

Health promotion interventions are planned and initiated on the basis of data gained from assessment. Guidelines for health promotion interventions based on age or other risk factors are readily available for health professionals; nurses should know how to access and interpret the guidelines so these can be incorporated into patient care. The interventions described here are broadly applied to all levels of health promotion (primary, secondary, and tertiary) and can be applied to all targeted groups (individual, family, and community).

Education

Education is a cornerstone for health promotion; this is also one of the most important contributions of nursing. Education intersects with each area of health promotion—as a primary, secondary, and tertiary health promotion strategy. Education is applied to individuals (patient education), families, and communities. Nurses have an opportunity to assist individuals to optimize their health by educating individuals and families about healthy lifestyle choices and encouraging appropriate screening and management of disease when necessary. Teaching involves not only providing information but also helping to align resources and access so health services can be provided. This is especially important among individuals from vulnerable populations.

Immunizations

Edward Jenner is credited with being the father of immunology because he was the first person to successfully develop a vaccination in 1798. Smallpox vaccination was a new and innovative way to prevent disease and provided the foundation for the science of immunology. Since that time, vaccinations have become one of the most effective primary prevention interventions; development and research efforts for new immunizations are ongoing. Nurses are commonly involved in this area of health promotion by providing patient education regarding immunizations, allaying fears of immunizations, identifying those who are in need of immunizations, and administering immunizations. Immunizations are recommended for individuals across the entire lifespan from infancy through geriatric populations. Although it is beyond the scope of this concept analysis to describe all immunizations, nurses should know where to find and interpret current immunization guidelines. The Centers for Disease Control and Prevention, CDC (www.cdc.gov/), is a reliable resource to find current immunization guidelines for all age groups.

Screening

Screening is a secondary prevention strategy; the goal is for disease detection in the early stages of the disease process. Mentioned previously, screening usually involves testing that has high reliability and validity—and screens for important conditions in which early detection is paramount. The benefits must outweigh the consequences and must be feasible from an economic and resource perspective. Specific routine screening guidelines have been developed for individuals across the lifespan. The USPSTF offers reliable screening recommendations as do many other government agencies and organizations such as the CDC, the American Cancer Society, the American Heart Association, and the American Academy of Pediatrics. Screening is also done based on an individual's risk. Genetic screening, as an example, is not routinely performed on all individuals, but is indicated in cases when the history supports the need.

Nutritional Health

It is estimated that more than 60% of all deaths are associated with chronic diseases such as obesity, cardiovascular disease, cancer, and diabetes; a large percentage of these disease are caused or exacerbated by poor or unhealthy nutritional behaviors.[18] According to the National Center for Health Statistics,[19] 18.1% of children between ages 12 and 19 and 19.6% of children between ages 6 and 11 are overweight. Children who are overweight or obese are at significant risk for many health-related problems as adults. For these reasons, one of the most important health promotion interventions is nutrition counseling.

The Dietary Guidelines for Americans, published by the U.S. Department of Agriculture and USDHHS, provides the basis for dietary recommendations and guides state and federal policies related to nutrition.[20] These guidelines are updated every 5 years; the last update was 2010. A consumer-friendly translation of the *Dietary Guidelines,* known as *MyPlate,* serves as a useful tool for dietary teaching and planning and can be found at the following website: www.choosemyplate.gov/.

The promotion of an adequate diet is included in nearly all health promotion plans—either as a primary or as a tertiary prevention focus. For example, a healthy individual whose weight is within normal range may set a goal to increase the servings of fruits and vegetables consumed each day to meet the dietary recommendations found in *MyPlate*. Another individual who is obese and has cardiovascular disease may reduce saturated fats and calorie consumption as a treatment measure with a goal to reduce weight and decrease levels of serum lipids. In addition to improving dietary intake, other topics related to nutrition include dietary supplements, food safety, and nutritional screening.[6]

Physical Activity

The human body was designed to move; therefore it should be no surprise that regular physical activity is an essential component of maintaining optimal physical and psychologic health. Physical activity encompasses any bodily movement involving skeletal muscles and energy expenditure. Physical activity occurs as part of routine daily activities, occupational activities, and recreational activities. Exercise training (purposeful bodily movement with the intention to improve physical fitness) is recommended for individuals across the lifespan and also is an important component to maintaining a healthy weight.

The benefits of physical activity are well documented for individuals across the lifespan. According to the USD-HHS, there is strong evidence that regular physical activity among children and adolescents resulted in improved bone health, improved cardiorespiratory and muscular fitness, improved cardiovascular and metabolic health biomarkers, and increased favorable body composition.[21] For adults and older adults, there is strong evidence that regular physical activity lowers the risk for multiple conditions including coronary heart disease, stroke, hypertension, elevated lipids, type 2 diabetes, metabolic syndrome, breast and colon cancers, weight gain, and depression.[21] There is also a reduced risk for falls and improved cognitive function. In addition to being a primary prevention strategy, physical activity and exercise are also common tertiary health promotion interventions. Examples include physical activity as part of cardiac rehabilitation or following a stroke, and physical therapy following joint replacement surgery.

Specific recommendations and details related to physical activity for each age group are beyond the scope of this concept analysis; however, these are readily available in health promotion textbooks and guidelines such as the USPSTF, the CDC, the National Institutes of Health, and the American Heart Association, to name a few.

Pharmacologic Agents

In addition to immunizations, many pharmacologic agents are useful for health promotion efforts. Details of drugs are primarily discussed in specific concept chapters, but two common examples are provided here.

Drugs used for smoking cessation. Several Food and Drug Administration (FDA)-approved medications are available to assist smoking cessation. Most of these drugs are nicotine replacement therapy for short-term use to reduce nicotine craving and provide relief of symptoms from nicotine withdrawal. These are available in the form of patches, gums, or lozenges.[22]

Drugs used for weight loss. There are four FDA-approved medications for weight loss; three of these (phentermine, diethylpropion, and phendimetrazine) are for short-term use (up to 3 months) in adults as appetite suppressors; the other (orlistat) is a lipase inhibitor that blocks the ability of the body to absorb fat. This is recommended for long-term use (up to 1 year) for adults and children more than 12 years old.[23]

INTERRELATED CONCEPTS

Several important concepts interrelated to health promotion are presented in Figure 40-3. Health promotion actually is linked to every health and illness concept within this book as a matter of prevention, screening, or tertiary care. Interrelationships with the health and illness concepts **Nutrition** and **Mobility** are especially important based on the health promotion interventions discussed in the previous section. Patient attribute concepts **Development, Culture, Motivation,** and **Adherence** are interrelated and form a concept cluster; these impact the type of health promotion interventions and approaches offered, as well as factors that influence the success of behavior change.

Patient education, a professional nursing concept, is based on patient attributes and significantly influences the success of health promotion interventions. Recommended health promotion guidelines are based on **Evidence,** and the effectiveness of health promotion recommendations is evaluated. Because of evidence, health promotion guidelines are implemented through **Health policy,** thus forming a concept cluster (Figure 40-3). An excellent example of health policy as it relates to health promotion and described previously in this concept analysis is *Healthy People 2020.* Health promotion is also interrelated to **Health care economics.** The delivery of health promotion interventions must be financed and these interventions should be cost-effective. Policy influences the payment mechanism for such services.

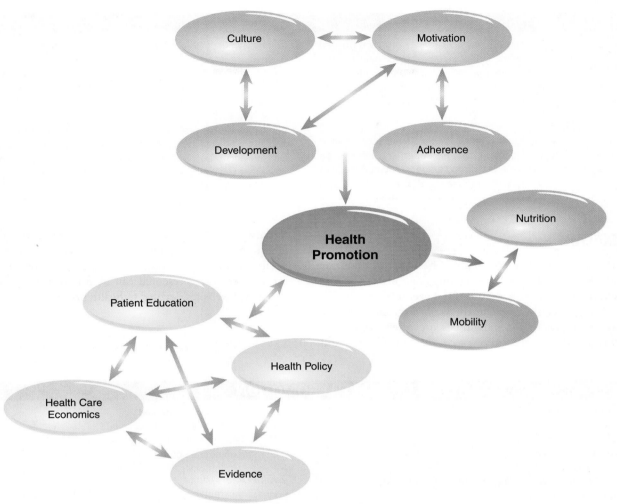

FIGURE 40-3 Health Promotion and Interrelated Concepts. Interrelationships between patient attribute concepts (in blue), health and illness concepts (in purple), and professional nursing concepts (in yellow).

MODEL CASE

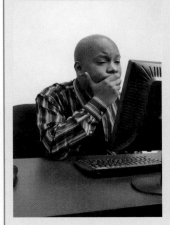

Raymond Brown is a divorced 40-year-old African-American male, and father to three children. He works in the technology industry for a large manufacturing company. Despite the fact that he is a smoker and overweight, Raymond always considered himself to be healthy until the sudden death of his 63-year-old father from a myocardial infarction. Realizing he could have a similar fate, Raymond becomes motivated to improve his health. One of his employee benefits is access to a full-time nurse practitioner who offers occupational health services, including comprehensive health promotion services.

Raymond makes an appointment with the nurse practitioner and shares his concerns. He verbalizes a wish to improve his health by losing some weight and quitting smoking. Based on his history, the nurse learns that Raymond has no known health conditions. He has tried to quit smoking on his own three or four times in the past, but was never successful beyond a few weeks. The nurse also learns Raymond rarely exercises and rarely eats fruits and vegetables. His physical exam findings include normal vital signs, and a body mass index of 28 (overweight). He has slightly elevated lipid levels and his blood glucose screening is within normal limits.

Based on these findings, the nurse evaluates the health promotion practice guidelines and discusses short- and long-term goals with Raymond. Knowing that changing multiple behaviors at the same time can be a challenge, the nurse helps Raymond formulate a plan based on goals most important to him. Because quitting smoking is what is most important to Raymond, he signs up for a smoking cessation class. He also decides that three times a week he will forgo going out to lunch

Continued

MODEL CASE—cont'd

and instead plans to attend a physical activity program offered over the lunch hour at work. On those days he will pack a lunch that will include at least one fruit and vegetable. The nurse suggests that Raymond stop in twice a month for ongoing coaching and tracking progress towards identified goals.

Case Analysis
Raymond has several risk factors for cardiovascular disease including a history of smoking and a sedentary lifestyle as well as being an overweight, middle-age, African-American male with a family history of cardiovascular disease. Important

factors in successful health promotion activities include self-motivation, access, support, and establishment of realistic goals. Raymond demonstrates motivation by initiating the health promoting behaviors. The fact that his employer offers health promotion as part of employee benefits makes accessing services easy—and it demonstrates the importance of such behaviors by his employer. The fact that Raymond has input into his plan and that he plans to attend smoking cessation classes and meet with the nurse practitioner twice a month represent realistic goals and the support needed for long-term behavior changes.

EXEMPLARS

Box 40-3 presents a few exemplars of health promotion for individuals. Considering the recommendations across the lifespan, there are literally thousands of exemplars for health promotion that could be included. Major exemplars for the promotion of health for individuals are often considered in terms of primary prevention, secondary prevention, and

tertiary prevention. It is important to remember that this box is not comprehensive and does not include community or environmental health promotion strategies. Specific details for all exemplars presented can be found in multiple textbooks and websites devoted to health promotion.

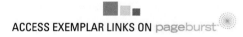

ACCESS EXEMPLAR LINKS ON pageburst

BOX 40-3   EXEMPLARS OF HEALTH PROMOTION

Primary Prevention
Prenatal
- General prenatal care
- Folic acid supplementation
- Vaccinations (e.g., rubella, hepatitis B)
- Abstinence from smoking, alcohol, and other drugs
- Nutrition counseling
- Genetic counseling

Infants/Children/Adolescents
- Injury prevention (e.g., car seats, seat belts, helmets, life jackets)
- Environmental exposures (toxins/poisoning)
- Vaccinations (health protection)
- Physical activity
- Nutrition counseling
- Avoidance of smoking and other substance use
- Oral care

Adults and Older Adults
- Injury prevention (e.g., safety belts, fall prevention measures)
- Physical activity
- Nutrition counseling
- Vaccinations

Secondary Prevention (Screening)
Prenatal
- Ultrasound screening
- Rh factor and antibody screening
- Sexually transmitted infection screening

Infants/Children/Adolescents
- Developmental screening
- Hearing screening
- Vision screening

- Body mass index screening
- Blood pressure screening
- Depression screening
- Substance abuse screening

Adults/Older Adults
- Hearing screening
- Vision screening
- Body mass index screening
- Blood pressure screening
- Depression screening
- Substance abuse screening
- Blood lipid screening
- Cognitive function screening
- Functional assessment screening
- Cancer screenings (e.g., breast, colon, prostate, skin, oral)

Tertiary Prevention
Prenatal
- Diabetes management
- Hypertension management
- Substance use/abuse management

Infants/Children/Adolescents
- Chronic disease management
- Obesity management
- Nutrition counseling
- Physical activity

Adults/Older Adults
- Chronic disease management
- Obesity management
- Nutrition counseling
- Physical activity

REFERENCES

1. U.S. Department of Health and Human Services: *Healthy People 2010*, Washington, DC, 2000, U.S. Government Printing Office.
2. American Nurses Association: *Nursing: scope and standards of practice*, Silver Spring, Md, 2010, Author.
3. World Health Organization: *Ottawa charter for health promotion*, Geneva, 1986, Author.
4. World Health Organization. Accessed at https://apps.who.int/aboutwho/en/definition.html.
5. Pender NJ, Murdoaugh CL, Parsons MA: *Health promotion in nursing practice*, ed 6, Upper Saddle River, NJ, 2010, Pearson.
6. Edelman CL, Mandle CL: *Health promotion throughout the life span*, ed 7, St Louis, 2010, Elsevier.
7. Oelbaum CH: Hallmarks of adult wellness, *Am J Nurs* 74:1623, 1974.
8. Sullivan M: The new subjective medicine: taking the patient's point of view on health care and health, *Social Sci Med* 56:1595–1604, 2003.
9. Dunn HL: *High level wellness*, Thorofare, NJ, 1980, Charles B. Slack.
10. World Health Organization: *Definition of community*. Available at http://www.who.int/hpr/NPH/docs/hp_glossary_en.pdf.
11. U.S. Preventive Services Task Force: *Screening for breast cancer*, 2009. Available at www.uspreventiveservicestaskforce.org/uspstf/uspsbrca.htm.
12. U.S. Preventive Services Task Force: *Screening for bladder cancer in adults*, 2004. Accessed at www.uspreventiveservicestaskforce.org/uspstf/uspsblad.htm.
13. Chinn JL: Culturally competent care, *Pub Health Rep* 115:25–33, 2000.
14. Minkler M, Wallerstein N, Wilson S: Improving health through community organization and community building. In Glanz K, Rimer BK, Lewis FM, editors: *Health behavior and health education theory, research, and practice*, ed 4, San Francisco, 2008, Jossey-Bass, pp 287–312.
15. U.S. Department of Health and Human Services: *Healthy People 2020. Improving the health of Americans*, Washington, DC, 2010, Author. Accessed at www.healthypeople.gov/2020.
16. Giger J, Davidhizar RE, Poole VL: Health promotion among ethnic minorities: the importance of cultural phenomena, *Rehabil Nurs* 22(6):303–307, 1997.
17. Wilson S, Giddens J: *Health assessment for nursing practice*, ed 4, St Louis, 2009, Elsevier.
18. World Health Organization: *The world health report 2002. Reducing risks, promising healthy life*, Geneva, 2002, Author.
19. Ogden C, Carroll M: *National Center for Health Statistics Health E-Stat. Prevalence of obesity among children and adolescents: United States, trends 1963-1965 through 2007-2008*, 2010. Accessed at www.cdc.gov/nchs/data/hestat/obesity_child_07_08/obesity_child_07_08.pdf.
20. U.S. Department of Agriculture and U.S. Department of Health and Human Services: *Dietary guidelines for Americans*, ed 7, Washington, DC, Dec 2010, U.S. Government Printing Office.
21. U.S. Department of Health and Human Services: *Physical activity guidelines for Americans*, 2008. Accessed at www.health.gov/paguidelines.
22. U.S. Department of Health and Human Services: *FDA 101: Smoking cessation products*. Available at www.fda.gov/forconsumers/consumerupdates/ucm198176.htm.
23. National Institutes of Health: *Weight control information network. Prescription medications for the treatment of obesity*. Available at http://win.niddk.nih.gov/Publications/prescription.htm.

CONCEPT

41

Communication

Teresa Keller

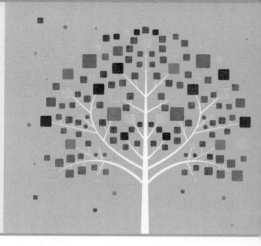

Communication is an essential form of human behavior—so fundamental to human social systems that our world would be barely recognizable without it. As a fundamental behavior, it is so pervasive that the profound impact of communication on our ability to engage with our world cannot be underestimated. Communication is unavoidable within the context of social life.[1] Human social interaction is accomplished through the relationships that develop between people and these relationships are mediated by communication. These relationships vary, from the intimacy of family to the more distant or more formal relationships between members of a community or nation. Yet all of these relationships are dependent upon communication for the creation and coordination of social interaction through the exchange of messages between participants. This exchange of information allows for the creation and coordination of social action, the integration of disparate individuals into social groups, and the subsequent formation of social relationships. Communication is therefore the essential process that ties people together, whether the ties create a family, an organization, a culture, or a nation.

DEFINITION(S)

There are many definitions of communication, and these vary only slightly. Wood defines communication as a distinct interpersonal interaction that is a process for the creation of shared meaning.[1] Samovar and colleagues[2] describe it as a dynamic process whereby participants share their internal states through symbols and symbolic expression. Arnold and Boggs[3] describe communication as a continuous, interactive activity whereas Worley and colleagues[4] describe it as the construction of meaning through symbols.

A synthesized definition would need to include the use of symbols to convey meaning through an interactive process. There is no way to directly communicate, mind-to-mind, with others. For this reason, people must communicate through the use of symbols.[2] Symbols are used to create a message that is transmitted to others, usually through spoken or written language but also through gestures, facial expressions, or body movements.[3] This symbolic interaction between people becomes an expression of mind states and a means to transmit ideas. A simple definition of communication would be that it is *a process of interaction between people where symbols are used to create, exchange, and interpret messages about ideas, emotions, and mind states.*

SCOPE AND CATEGORIES

Communication encompasses all means by which people exchange messages with each other. The scope of the communication concept ranges from effective communication to no communication; ineffective communication lies within this communication. Three primary categories of communication include *linguistic, paralinguistic,* and *metacommunication* (Figure 41-1).

The most obvious form of communication is *linguistic*—the verbal exchange of messages through spoken words and written symbols. Conversing face-to-face, reading newspapers and books, and even cell phone texting are all common forms of linguistic communication. In addition to overt verbal messages, more subtle forms of communication are included in this category. Silence can be a form of communication in the sense that some messages may be eloquently expressed when one or more persons in the communication exchange choose either to withhold messages or to avoid the interaction. Omission and/or avoidance in communication relays a message also, depending on the circumstances of the exchange.

Communication also includes the nonverbal exchange of symbols—*paralinguistics.* Paralinguistics include less recognizable but important means of transmitting messages such as the use of gestures, eye contact, and facial expressions. Paralinguistics are necessary for a complete understanding of the message sent because nonverbal gestures and facial expressions provide important cues about emotions, moods, and/or psychologic states. Nonverbal messages are also conveyed through the use of color, artwork and graphic design,

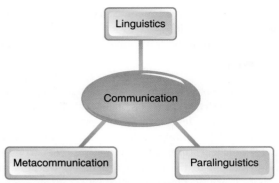

FIGURE 41-1 Categories of Communication.

and dress. Uniforms, for example, provide information about the wearer's social role in a given context.

Metacommunication consists of the factors that compose the context of the message. Because the ultimate goal of communication is to create meaning, the particular context or situation in which the communication act is occurring will have an effect on the meaning derived from the message.[2] Metacommunication factors that affect how messages are received and interpreted would include internal personal states (such as disturbances in mood), environmental stimuli related to the setting of the communication, and contextual variables (such as the relationship between the people in the communication episode).

ATTRIBUTES AND CRITERIA

As defined, communication masquerades as a simple concept that describes the transmission of ideas between people. The concept of communication becomes very complex when studied in depth and is therefore a major field of study for academics and professionals in specialized fields such as speech therapy or linguistics. However, there are some attributes of communication by which it can be distinguished and that form the basis of study in the nursing sciences. The major attributes of communication are that it is a *process* of *complementary exchange* between people and that it occurs in a *context*.[5] Another attribute of communication is that it is a learned skill and, therefore, people are able to achieve not only competence but also sophistication and expertise in communication. This is true whether the communicator is an infant just learning to speak or a nursing student learning the language of professional communication in practice.

Process

Communication occurs through a sequence or series of transmissions between sender and receiver. The sender originates the message and transmits it to another through symbols. The receiver interprets the message and returns another symbolic message. This process could be brief, such as a simple acknowledgment of the other person by saying "Hello," or it can be more complex, such as the back and forth interaction between a nurse and a patient during nursing assessment. The symbols used can vary widely over the range of verbal and nonverbal acts while a message is communicated and then interpreted among the participants in the exchange. During this process, a potential exists for distortion of the message at any point in the series of transmissions.

Complementary Exchange

In the exchange, each participant is, in turn, either a sender or a receiver. In the act of communication, the reception and transmission of messages between participants is iterative, where sustained dialogue serves to support the creation of shared meaning. The sender encodes a message using symbols (both verbal and nonverbal) and transmits the created message to the receiver. As each transmission is completed, the receiver perceives the message, interprets the symbols, and then responds with another act of encoding and transmission of a response to the sender. The implication is that the meaning created for participants during the communication act is negotiated during the exchange while messages are perceived, decoded, and interpreted.[4] Because meaning results from negotiation, effective communication depends on mutual engagement and on the authenticity of each participant's contributions during an exchange. This is why communication by nurses to patients is subject to distortion or misinterpretation when the patient is ill, anxious, or distracted by pain. Communication messages and responses between nurse managers and staff nurses can be misread or negatively perceived if the nurses distrust the manager's intentions or the manager lacks credibility.

Context

The context of communication is relevant because communication cannot occur in a vacuum.[4] The metacommunication aspect, or context of communication, is important to the quality of meaning derived by participants during the process of complementary exchange. Contextual factors are those characteristics of the environment in which the communication occurs that affect perception and subsequent interpretation of messages by participants. Context can include factors such as the relationship between participants, internal mood states, mental and physical condition, experience and education, and external noise emanating from the environment.

Communication between people is both subject to and a reflection of relationships.[5] The relationship could be relatively distant, such as between shopkeepers and customers, or more intimate, as are the relationships between family members. Relationships always affect the communication process.[4] Hierarchical relationships, such as between parents and children or between managers and workers, involve power and status and thus affect the communication between these different types of participants. Children might fear upsetting their parents with some kinds of information because of the consequences of parental reactions. The same holds true with management/staff communication in the workplace. The effect of power and status on communications can be significant, especially if the result is a distortion of meaning that leads to a misunderstanding or a failure to fully appreciate the message being sent.

Other aspects of context that affect communication are both internal and external. Internal factors include personal attributes of the participants, such as culture, experience, education, or physical state. Obviously, people who do not speak the same language will have some difficulty communicating effectively. Related to language are cultural factors that may affect interpretation of messages.[2] Nonverbal gestures acceptable to one culture may be offensive to people from different cultures. Education levels will have an effect on a person's ability to read written communications and to correctly understand the vocabulary used in spoken communications. The specialized languages used among professionals may not be familiar to patients, leading to the potential for misinterpretation of messages sent during communication exchanges. The participant's prior communications' experience will have an impact on his or her perception and interpretation of the symbols used to create a message.

The physical states of participants are also an important factor that affects communication, especially the receiver's perception and interpretation of the message. Illness and anxiety have already been mentioned as important considerations during the exchange of messages in a communication episode. Physical conditions such as diminished eyesight or hearing will have a profound effect on communication, limiting a participant's ability to perceive and interpret messages. Mental health conditions, such as schizophrenia, can also hinder the accurate perception of messages and the ability to distinguish between real versus imagined communications from others.

Physical and mental states could be considered a kind of "noise" that leads to distorted communications. This noise can be both external and internal. External noise is obvious, such as radio transmissions, the sounds of traffic, and the conversations of others. Internal noise is generated within the person, usually distractions caused by worries, emotions, stress, or personal concerns that can affect attention to and interpretation of messages.[4] Whether internal or external, noise inhibits the ability to accurately receive and interpret messages. This leads to message distortion and, ultimately, misinterpretation or misunderstanding within the communication exchange.

Communication as a Learned Skill

Communication is a learned skill that develops over time and through interactions with others. Further, these interactions constitute a complex learning experience that includes the need to understand the meaning of a diverse array of linguistic and paralinguistic symbols. Studies of language acquisition among infants and toddlers indicate that infants receive cues about meaning from the facial expressions of their caregivers during verbal interactions.[6] These verbal and nonverbal cues to children while they learn to communicate are an essential part of growth and development, especially for children with developmental disabilities.[1,7,8]

People continuously learn new ways to communicate throughout their lifetime. For some this might mean the acquisition of a new language, either a spoken language or perhaps a specialized language, such as sign language or the vocabulary specific to a profession. Health care workers use a specific language developed for the purpose of communicating information among members of the group. This specialized language features words and terms that carry specific meanings related to the work for members working in the profession. Learning professional languages integrates people into the specialized social network of health care and helps to create group cohesion while facilitating the coordination of care. Professional nursing has a language developed over time to express and transmit the concepts and ideas relevant to the profession. An example of a term with particular relevance to nursing is *caring*. For nurses, this term is loaded with an array of meanings, some of which are specific to particular patient situations or conditions. Other examples of professional nursing language are the use of a nomenclature for body systems, medications and treatments, and terms that describe patient care practices. Learning this nomenclature is a necessary part of the education of nursing students just as is learning how to communicate in therapeutic relationships. The term *therapeutic communication* probably has little meaning to a layperson, but it is so fundamental to effective function in the nursing role that it is major component of nursing education.

THEORETICAL LINKS

The most basic theory of communication is a linear process model that describes a *sender* transmitting a *message* to a *receiver* (Figure 41-2).[1] The process starts with a sender encoding a message, either verbally or nonverbally, and sending it to the receiver through some medium, such as voice or print. Upon perceiving the message, the receiver decodes and interprets the message, creating meaning from the symbols.

This simplistic representation fails to convey the true richness of the communication exchange as a means to create shared meaning among participants. As noted earlier, there are a great many factors that affect the perception and interpretation of messages. Additionally, this simple model does not reflect the iterative complexity of communication acts where messages are passing back and forth between participants in the exchange.[9] Actual communication episodes involve multiple acts of perception and interpretation as well as the creation of a mutually negotiated meaning. A more accurate representation captures this interactive process and depicts the influence of multiple factors on the meaning created during the interaction between participants.

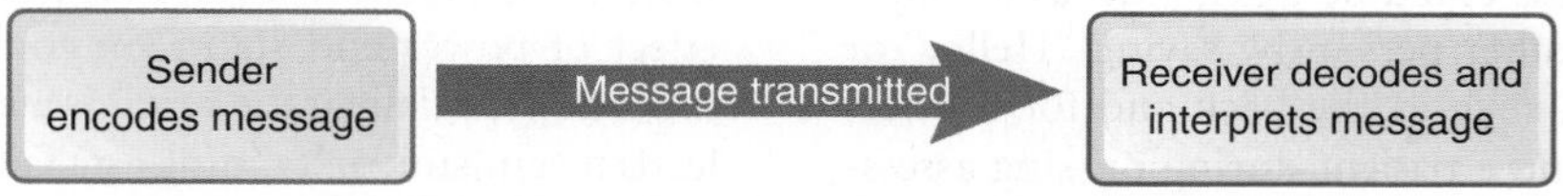

FIGURE 41-2 Basic Communication Theory.

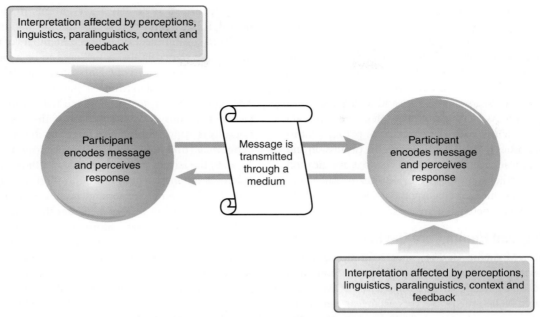

FIGURE 41-3 A Complex Model of Communication.

To be effective, communication needs to have clarity, be goal directed, and possess vigor. In other words, effective communication is vivid and memorable.[10] The negotiation of shared meaning in the communication act is impaired if the purpose of the communication is unclear or the symbols used for expression of ideas are inappropriate. A poorly worded memo can create much confusion or consternation among members of a workgroup because the true meaning of the message is questionable. Course syllabi that fail to provide clear direction because of incomplete information or errors will result in uncertainty for students. For nonnative speakers, the colloquialisms common to any foreign language can be inexplicable and the source of error and embarrassment. In all of these cases, the clarity and goals of the message transmitted are lost and the ultimate meaning of the message is distorted.

Vigor in communication relates directly to clarity and goal.[10] The symbols and medium used to convey a message greatly affect the vigor of the message. Examples are communications meant to be shared among members of a professional group. Communications prepared for members of the health care professions are notable for precision in the use of terminology, an emphasis on appropriate grammar and spelling, and the need for accurate and thorough description. Communication techniques for preparing professional communications are taught to all students of the health professions, including student nurses.

Vigor in communication is also evident in other types of communication. The most common example of memorable and vivid communications is seen in the promotion of consumer products. Advertising campaigns for products such as soaps and foods are colorful, humorous, and often quite memorable. The strategies and techniques utilized by advertisers to create vivid communications about their products can be used to increase the vigor in messages for other purposes. Teaching materials used by nurses are more effective if they feature the judicious use of color and formatting to emphasize important points and if they are age-appropriate as well as culturally sensitive.

CONTEXT TO NURSING AND HEALTH CARE

Health care is a major social activity established for the purpose of helping people with their health concerns. It encompasses a variety of social structures that reflect the myriad of specialized relationships necessary for supporting the delivery of health care services. Nurses can expect to engage in multiple acts of communication daily in their work environments, perhaps even more so than in their personal lives. For nurses, effective communication is critically important. The professional role requires that nurses develop and practice a variety of communication skills that will ensure successful role function as well as the delivery of quality patient care. Because health care is relationship-based, communication competence is highly valued for nurses, whether that communication is with patients or with other members of the health care services environment.

Communication Competence

Communication competence in nursing means that communication is both *effective* and *appropriate*. Effectiveness is achieved when the goals of the communication are met. Appropriate means the communication has been adapted to the people and situation involved in the act of communication.[1] Because communication is a learned skill, instruction begins early in nursing education related to a variety of behaviors and attitudes that produce the framework for communication competence in the nurse. Communication competence among nurses continues to evolve with experience and professional development throughout a nursing career. Professional nurses can expect to be tasked with the need to communicate as a caregiver and as a member of a health care profession, both of which require skill in interpersonal communication. As a caregiver, nurses are expected to effectively and appropriately communicate with patients and families and with members of the health care team. As members of the profession, nurses are expected to competently voice the concerns of patients, families, and communities to others both within the profession and in the larger health services' sector. Achieving communication competence in nursing is important for optimizing safety and quality in health care and for creating the voice and authority needed to advocate for better systems and safer workplaces.

Patient Safety and Health Care Quality

The Institute of Medicine (IOM) captured national attention in 2001 with the report, *To Err is Human: Building a Safer Health Care System.*[11] In this report, the IOM noted that an estimated 98,000 medical errors each year were leading to unnecessary injury and even death for patients in the U.S. health care system. IOM reports since then have critically evaluated the safety and quality problems inherent to our health care systems, especially how these problems are related to the actions of health care professionals, including nurses.[12,13] Communication is a frequently cited cause of errors in the delivery of health care,[14] including being the leading cause of *sentinel events,* defined as unusually serious, unexpected events that occur during episodes of care. Sentinel events—such as wrong-site surgery, adverse drug events, or patient falls—not only result in harm to the patient but also lead to increased health care costs. Consequently, communication competence has become a critical skill that promotes quality of care and patient safety.

One recommendation by the IOM is to educate health professionals to use practices and tools that support effective communication. One tool that supports consistent and accurate communication between professionals is the **SBAR** communication technique. SBAR stands for *Situation, Background, Assessment,* and *Recommendation.* This tool is a structured routine for passing information between team members, most notably between nurses and other health care providers such as physicians and nurse practitioners. When using this tool, the nurse will describe the patient *Situation,* explain the *Background information relevant to the situation,* provide an *Assessment,* and also provide a *Recommendation* for action. This structured approach to communicating patient care information provides the health care provider with the information necessary to make decisions about proposed interventions while also respecting the nurse's status as a member of the care team.[15]

Electronic Health Record

Another fundamental communication skill for nurses is accurate and timely documentation in the patient record. The patient's health care record is a communication tool for documenting progress, treatments, interventions, and patient responses to care. Because many members of the health care team document their care interventions in the health care record, it is an important source of information and a major means of communication between members of the team. The health care record is also considered to be a legal document that records the actions of health care providers and is subject to legal review to determine if standards of care were met. Therefore, clear and accurate documentation of health care provider actions and observation of the patient's response not only is important but also might be the best available evidence that a provider's actions were appropriate and effective.

With the advent of the electronic health record (EHR), the potential for improving communication among health care providers in a variety of settings is enhanced. A digital record of a person's health history facilitates the timely transmission of complete and accurate information between providers. For example, the EHR provides the means by which emergency personnel can access prior history and medical condition for patients who are too ill or too injured to provide a complete medical history. However, the speed of digital transmission and the potential for widespread dissemination of electronic records also create increased concerns related to accuracy and confidentiality. Documentation errors or omissions in the EHR can jeopardize patient safety and the quality of care provided because multiple providers access these records and then make health care decisions based on inaccurate or faulty information. The potential also exists that personal health care information can be accessed by others who do not have a right to access or a need to know this information. Nurses working with an EHR need to be cognizant of these potential threats to the quality of care and patient safety. Access to an EHR has the potential to greatly enhance the delivery of efficient, timely, and patient-centered care but it also increases the requisite for diligence in documentation of that care as well as the need to strictly maintain the confidentiality of the patient's health record.

Advocacy

Communication competence is a necessary component for effective function in the role of advocate. Advocacy is the act of speaking for others to assist them to meet needs and it is an expectation for all who assume the role of professional nurse. The advocacy might be in the form of interceding with members of the health care team on behalf of patients or families, or it could be advocacy on behalf of these same members of the health care team, or it might even be advocacy on behalf of the profession. The ability to speak out assertively, credibly, and authoritatively is a highly valued communication skill that is critical to effective advocacy. Principles of assertive communication are routinely taught in basic nursing education courses with continued refinement of the skill through professional development and graduate education.

INTERRELATED CONCEPTS

Communication is the exchange of information between participants that leads to a negotiated, mutual understanding of a situation or phenomenon. As such, there are related concepts that are closely associated with communication (Figure 41-4).

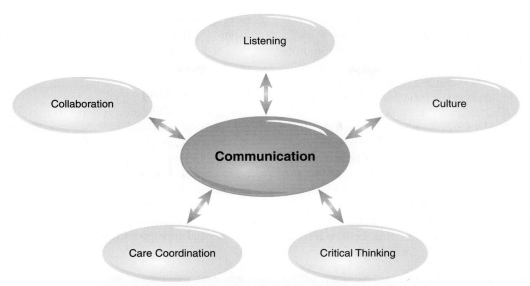

FIGURE 41-4 Communication and Interrelated Concepts.

These interrelated concepts are **Listening, Collaboration, Care coordination, Culture,** and **Critical thinking.**

Listening

An important, but sometimes overlooked, concept related to communication is *listening*. Effective listening is essential to effective communication.[10] Perception of the message is greatly affected by the ability to listen closely and attend to the messages being transmitted by others. All too often people listen with an expectation of the message, anticipating the message to be received and formulating a response. This is a barrier to effective communication because expectations and anticipation can distort the interpretation of the symbols being transmitted in the communication between sender and receiver. The result is an incomplete or inaccurate understanding of the sender's message. Listening for the complete message before responding is a skill that needs to be developed in order to avoid potential distortion. To promote effective communication, nurses should listen carefully for the purpose of the communication, look for themes that emerge from the message, and pay close attention to the paralinguistic and metacommunication factors that might affect the message. *Rhetorical sensitivity* in listening involves understanding the attitudes that people have related to communication and how these attitudes affect the messages exchanged. Rhetorical sensitivity employed during the act of listening is more likely to result in meeting the needs of all parties in the exchange because attitudes are a part the communication context.[4] For example, adolescents may be uncomfortable discussing their health care problems with their parents present. Nurses need to observe the patient and listen for cues that might indicate discomfort because the adolescent is likely to avoid full disclosure of information in this kind of situation.

Collaboration and Care Coordination

Communication is the structure that supports social interaction and social interaction is the primary means for the delivery of health care services. Nurses collaborate with patients and families in the development of a plan of care. Nurses also collaborate with members of the health care team, often functioning as the link between the patient and the rest of the team. As the link, nurses routinely coordinate care to ensure that the care is appropriately and safely delivered and that it is beneficial to patients. The importance of effective collaboration and coordination to quality care and patient safety cannot be overemphasized. It is crucial that communication between the patient and the health care team as well as communication between the members of the health care team be clear, accurate, and timely. Errors, omissions, and gaps in communication can lead to dangerous and costly errors in care.

Culture

Culture and communication exist in a symbiotic relationship. Cultures develop on the basis of an infrastructure of communications. Communications, especially the symbols used in language, dress, and patterns of behavior, are expressions of culture. Behavioral expectations and norms, values and traditions, the way relationships are built and maintained, the definition of personal space as dictated by cultural norms, and even the significance of words and gestures are possible because people are able to transmit ideas, values, emotions, and needs through communication acts.

The relationship between culture and communication has important implications for nurses. As a profession that interacts with people from all cultures, nurses will frequently encounter different, culturally-based communication practices. Nurses need a fundamental appreciation of cultural differences and the potential effect of these differences on care. By recognizing these differences, nurses are able to proactively address potential misperceptions and misunderstandings that might arise during the implementation and evaluation of care.

The appreciation of cultural differences extends beyond the need to think about the language and culture of patients and their families. *Organizational cultures* have a strong impact on nursing practice because most nurses work in some kind of organization, whether a hospital, community health agency, school, hospice, or some other kind of health care unit. Organizational cultures also have norms and values, expectations for appropriate behavior and language, and rituals, symbols, and artifacts. Communications in organizations are both affected by the prevailing culture and also serve to help mold the organizational culture. This is particularly important in health care because of the link between organizational culture and patient safety. Communications and systems for communications must allow for clear, timely, and accurate communications between professionals working together to deliver quality patient care, unimpeded by contextual factors such as power and status. Lessons learned from aviation safety programs indicate that effective communication is fundamental to safe systems, leading to the adoption of improved communication strategies by health care organizations to ensure quality care.[16,17]

Critical Thinking

Effective communication is dependent on the critical thinking skills of participants.[18] Senders and receivers in the exchange must be able to interpret and analyze symbolic messages accurately; otherwise, the meaning of messages can be missed or misinterpreted. Thinking skills related to distinguishing important data and organizing, analyzing, and evaluating information are important components to interpretation and understanding of messages. These skills are also needed to support the development of an appropriate

MODEL CASE

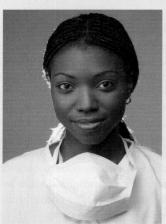

Jenna Wright is a new nurse eagerly anticipating her first day of work. She has obtained a position in the surgical intensive care unit (ICU) of a large hospital in the city near her home. Jenna is very excited to be finished with school and to have her nursing license and a new apartment in the city. She is also pleased that she was chosen to take part in a 6-month residency program for new nurses offered by the hospital.

Jenna reports to her new nursing unit early on her first day. She is dressed in her new scrub suit with a name badge proclaiming her RN status. She appears well groomed, with her hair off her face, her nail polish removed, and her pen and stethoscope at hand. She waits in the nurses' station for her assigned preceptor—a more experienced RN who will help Jenna begin her career as a nurse. Jenna's preceptor, Betty Jones, has 20 years of nursing practice experience and was chosen by the unit manager to be Jenna's preceptor because of her communication skills. Betty is familiar with the "first-day jitters" common with new nurses, so she also arrives a little early and meets Jenna at the nurses' station.

Betty walks directly to Jenna, smiles, and greets her: "Hi, you must be Jenna. I'm Betty and I will be your preceptor during your residency. I have worked on this unit for the last five years and find I really enjoy the challenge of the surgical ICU."

Jenna smiles shyly and nods her head: "I am so excited to be here…it's great to finally be starting out, no longer a student…."

Betty laughs and nods her head: "Oh yeah, I know. Students are fun to have on the unit but I also know there are limits on what they can do. Getting to spread your wings and learn this new role can be very exciting and we want you to be excited. We want you here and we are going to work really hard to get you oriented to the unit and help you get your 'feet on the ground'. We have a great team of nurses on this unit and we expect a lot of each other. We want you to be a part of that team and to learn and grow in the position. After all, that helps all of us, right? So let's find a place for your things and then we will go to report. You know, I think there is another new nurse working in the medical intensive care unit. Let's see if we can arrange to have lunch with her and her preceptor."

Case Analysis

In this small conversation, Betty demonstrates different attributes of effective communication. From her experience, she knows that new nurses are uncertain about themselves and their place in a new workplace. By approaching Jenna directly, Betty creates the first contact needed to begin the acculturation process for new members to the unit. She indicates acceptance of Jenna's uncertainty and uses inclusive language with Jenna, stating that she and the other nurses on the unit welcome a new member. Betty also acknowledges that Jenna is at a legitimate professional transition point, from student to nurse, and she provides Jenna with some information about unit culture and expectations. To support this transition, Betty further assists this new nurse with basic needs, such as finding a place for personal items, and also directs Jenna to an important communication routine on nursing units, the shift report. Betty is also thinking about Jenna's further needs, such as introductions to other staff members, especially another new nurse who might become a social support for Jenna in the future.

In this exchange, Betty also demonstrates a high level of rhetorical sensitivity. She knows that new employees not only are excited by the new situation but also may be experiencing some uncertainty about their acceptance into a new social group. Betty uses verbal and nonverbal communication strategies (inclusive language, smiling, head-nodding) to indicate to Jenna that she is hearing Jenna's message, accepts her as a new member of the team, and is willing to support Jenna while she learns a new culture and grows into professional practice. In addressing the cultural expectations of teamwork and collaboration, Betty is communicating to Jenna the cultural norms for behavior and attitude that will be the foundation of her successful transition to the surgical ICU.

response in the communication exchange. In an incredibly short expanse of time, critical thinkers in a communication exchange are receiving and evaluating information from words, gestures, and context; organizing it into categories and themes; relating this to prior knowledge and experience; and then formulating a response. Without critical thinking ability, communication breakdowns would be frequent and our ability to relate to each other in a meaningful way would be destroyed.

EXEMPLARS

Communication for nurses encompasses a wide range of practices, most of which support effective interactions with others. These communications can be broadly classified as *intrapersonal* or *interpersonal*. Interpersonal communications encompass the dynamic processes of communication between people.[3] Most interpersonal communications in which nurses engage, outside of personal communications with their own friends and families, are with patients and families or with the other professionals with whom they work. Examples of interpersonal communications for nursing are *therapeutic communication* and *interprofessional communication* (Box 41-1).

Therapeutic communication is a form of interpersonal communications taught to health professionals and is an important communication competency for nurses. These communication techniques and strategies form the foundation of the relationship between patients and their health care providers that is necessary for effective diagnosis and treatment. It is the major method for exchanging information between the nurse and patient and the primary means for promoting patient-centered care. Therapeutic communication is largely situated within the social interactions of health care, is directed to the goals and concerns of health, and is individualized to the participants in the exchange.[19] Student nurses are taught language and behavior that are designed to elicit information from the patient regarding the patient's health concerns and also the patient's capacity for engaging in a mutually negotiated plan to address his or her health needs. The principles of therapeutic communication include strategies and techniques that enhance interviewing skills, encourage engagement, facilitate listening, and promote dialogue among participants.

Interprofessional communication is the process of communication between professionals. Nurses are expected to interact daily with a wide variety of professionals either in teams or as members of the health care organization. Health care services delivery is complex and a variety of different professionals are needed to ensure that patients receive the appropriate care services required in a timely and effective manner. Coordination and collaboration in care has never been more imperative than in today's modern health services sector. Daily communications among health care professionals need to be accurate, timely, and coherent. Incomplete, disruptive, or uncoordinated communications between health care professionals inevitably result in conflict and stress, potentially threatening the quality of care. Issues of power and status in the health care workplace complicate the communication process and can lead to unhealthy workplace environments notable for incivility, fear, and the resultant communication breakdowns. Effective communication is an essential part of ensuring the psychologic safety necessary for supporting productivity in a healthy workplace environment. Strategies that support a healthy workplace environment include using assertive communication techniques, developing conflict resolution skills, and promoting organizational policies that sanction disruptive behavior in the workplace.[20]

Intrapersonal communication is an internal process within the individual where ideas and thoughts are entwined with emotions and values. Intrapersonal communication cannot be overlooked as an important strategy that supports professional development and a strong self-identity. *Self-talk* is a form of intrapersonal communications used to address the cognitive distortions that result when internal emotions affect the interpretation of a message.[9] For example, after failing an important exam, a student might believe that a negative approach by the instructor is the cause of the failure or that the student possesses personal flaws that influenced exam performance. Self-talk is a form of behavior therapy that requires the person to choose his or her frame of thinking about the situation. The internal conversation is then directed toward resetting the thinking process to support positive emotional and cognitive responses.[9]

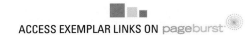

ACCESS EXEMPLAR LINKS ON pageburst

■■■ BOX 41-1 EXEMPLARS OF COMMUNICATION

Interpersonal
Therapeutic Communication
- Interviewing
- Patient/family instructions and teaching
- Conflict management strategies
- Effective listening.

Interprofessional Communication
- SBAR
- Documentation
- Reporting information to other staff during shift report or during patient transfers between units
- Effective listening

Intrapersonal
- Self-talk

REFERENCES

1. Wood J: *Interpersonal communication: everyday encounters*, ed 6, Boston, 2010, Wadsworth.
2. Samovar L, Porter R, McDaniel E: *Communication between cultures*, Boston, 2010, Wadsworth.
3. Arnold E: Theoretical perspectives and contemporary dynamics. In Arnold E, Boggs K, editors: *Interpersonal relationships: professional communication skills for nurses*, St Louis, 2011, Elsevier, pp 1–23.
4. Worley D, Worley D, Soldner L: *Communication counts: getting it right in college and life*, Boston, 2007, Allyn & Bacon.
5. Finkelman A: *Leadership and management in nursing*, Upper Saddle River, NJ, 2006, Prentice-Hall.
6. Green J: Lip movement exaggerations during infant-directed speech, *J Speech Language Hearing Res* 53:1529–1543, 2010.
7. Adamson L, Romski M, Bakeman R, et al: Augmented language intervention and the emergence of symbol-infused joint engagement, *J Speech Language Hearing Res* 53:1769–1774, 2010.
8. McDuffie A, Yoder P: Types of parent verbal responsiveness that predict language in young children with autism spectrum disorder, *J Speech Language Hearing Res* 53:1026–1040, 2010.
9. Arnold E: Self-concept in the nurse-client relationships. In Arnold E, Boggs K, editors: *Interpersonal relationships: professional communication skills for nurses*, St Louis, 2011, Elsevier, pp 62–82.
10. Hattersley M, McJanet L: *Management communications: principles and practice*, ed 3, Boston, 2007, McGraw-Hill/Irwin.
11. Institute of Medicine: *To err is human: building a safer health care system*, Washington, DC, 2000, National Academy Press.
12. Institute of Medicine: *Crossing the quality chasm: a new health care system for the 21st century*, Washington, DC, 2001, National Academy Press.
13. Institute of Medicine: *Keeping patients safe: transforming the work environment of nurses*, Washington, DC, 2004, National Academy Press.
14. Joint Commission Center for Transforming Health Care: *Hand-off communications* n.d. Accessed at www.centerfortransforminghealthcare.org/projects/about_handoff_communication.aspx.
15. Kowalski K: Building teams through communication and partnerships. In Yoder-Wise P, editor: *Leading and managing in nursing*, ed 5, St Louis, 2011, Elsevier, pp 345–371.
16. Weinstock M: Can your nurses stop a surgeon? *Health Hospital Networks*, Sept 2007:39–46, 2007.
17. Pronovost P, Berenholtz S, Goeschel C, et al: Creating high reliability in health care organizations, *Health Services Res* 41(Pt 2):1599–1617, 2006. doi: 10.1111/j.1475-6773.2006.00567.x.
18. Wood J: *Communication in our lives*, ed 6, Boston, 2012, Wadsworth.
19. Arnold E: Developing therapeutic communication skills. In Arnold E, Boggs K, editors: *Interpersonal relationships: professional communication skills for nurses*, St Louis, 2011, Elsevier, pp 175–196.
20. Boggs K: Communicating with other health professionals. In Arnold E, Boggs K, editors: *Interpersonal relationships: professional communication skills for nurses*, St Louis, 2011, Elsevier, pp 452–467.

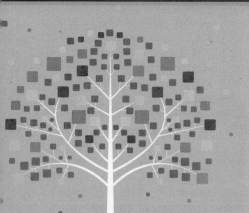

When thinking about the profession and practice of nursing, the words "collaboration" and "nursing" seem inseparable. Nurses work with patients, families, communities, and other professionals in a multitude of settings from state-of-the-art hospitals to remote rural home settings and clinics. Collaboration involves building models of health care using the best ideas of our patients and our partners in the health care setting. Understanding collaboration is perhaps the key component for reducing errors in patient care. Unfortunately, collaboration remains an unclear concept with varying meanings and perspectives among health professionals. Exploration of the concept of collaboration will help to crystallize its meaning and its potential for advancing the nursing profession, and for improving the health outcomes of our patients.

DEFINITION(S)

The word *collaborate* is derived from the Latin word *collaborare,* meaning to labor together. Collaboration usually has the connotation of working with others in an intellectual endeavor. Nurses labor with patients, families, and health care workers such as physicians, pharmacists, social workers, physical therapists, medical assistants, and other lay health workers using knowledge, reasoning, and critical thinking skills to promote or restore health. For the purposes of this concept analysis, collaboration in nursing is the *development of partnerships to achieve best possible outcomes that reflect the particular needs of the patient, family, or community, requiring an understanding of what others have to offer.* Collaboration also involves a joint responsibility for patient outcomes.[1]

SCOPE AND CATEGORIES

Collaboration can be described within four overarching categories—each based on the collaborative with the nurse—including nurse-patient, nurse-nurse, interprofessional, and interorganizational collaboration (Figure 42-1).

Nurse-Patient Collaboration

Nurses are inherent collaborators. The American Nurses Association identifies six standards for nursing practice known as the nursing process: assessment, diagnosis, outcomes identification, planning, implementation, and evaluation.[2] Opportunity for nurse-patient collaboration exists at each level of the process. Nurses particularly collaborate with patients as fully functional members of the health care team in making health care decisions.[3] For example, nurses collaborate with patients regarding health promotion and disease prevention behaviors, treatment strategies and options, lifestyle changes, and end-of-life decision making.

The historical context for nurse-patient collaboration is rich and extensive. Florence Nightingale encouraged collaboration with the patient, assessing what is needed or wanted.[4] In an early use of nurse-patient collaboration, Hildegard Peplau described a component of the working phase of her nursing theory as the patient participating with and being interdependent with the nurse.[5] Also, in her human-to-human relationship model of nursing, Joyce Travelbee defined nursing as an interpersonal process whereby the nurse assists an individual, family, or community to prevent or cope with the experience of illness and suffering and, if needed, to find meaning in these experiences.[6] Through the years many other nurse theorists have examined and defined the nurse-patient relationship with elements of nurse-patient collaboration existing in many of the theories.

Nurse-Nurse Collaboration

Nurse-nurse collaboration, or intraprofessional collaboration, is also important to consider. How do nurses collaborate together? Nurses develop nursing teams on hospital units, in clinics, and in community settings that provide collaboration and support in patient caregiving. Nurses from different fields and with different experiences also collaborate: nurse managers, nurse researchers, nurse educators, advanced practice nurses, as well as novice nurses with expert nurses.[7]

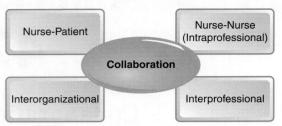

FIGURE 42-1 Categories of Collaboration.

Mentoring

Mentoring is a special type of collaboration, or creative partnership, typically between a novice nurse and an expert nurse, that has been recognized as beneficial to the development of professional nurses.[8] Mentoring is described as purposeful activities that facilitate the career development, personal growth, caring, empowerment, and nurturance that are important to nursing practice and leadership.[9] The purpose of mentoring is to enable a smooth transition from novice nurse to a knowledgeable practitioner who is self-reflective and self-confident, and is able to negotiate both professional and patient relationships.[10] Despite the valuable benefits of mentoring, challenges to successful and constructive mentorships exist. Ketola[11] stated that mentoring needs to go beyond the acquisition of knowledge and skills and include the socialization of a nurse transmitting the values, norms, and accepted modes of behavior for the professional nurse. Jakubik[12] also encouraged mentoring to progress from the traditional approach of fostering support, competency, and job retention to a more modern approach of promoting career development and advancement, similar to mentoring in the business world.

Shared Governance

Shared governance is another type of collaboration found in nursing. Shared governance is a nursing practice model that fosters a decentralized style of management that creates an environment of empowerment.[13] Shared governance is seen as an important component of professional practice and pursuit of Magnet designation from the American Nurses Credentialing Center.[14] The goal of shared governance is to transition from a traditional hierarchical management style to one where nursing staff are more involved in decision-making processes and managers are facilitative rather than controlling.[15] Nurses practicing in a shared governance environment truly labor together and collectively develop collaborative relationships. Collaborating in the shared governance model, nurses can help to improve quality of care and clinical effectiveness, facilitate the development of knowledge and skills, and increase professionalism and accountability.[15] Shared decision making, the cornerstone of shared governance, is an essential element to improve the health care system of the future.[14]

Interprofessional Collaboration

The true essence of collaboration involves working across professional boundaries. With interprofessional collaboration, individual areas of expertise are represented along with diverse perspectives influenced by professional orientation,

experience, age, gender, education, and socioeconomic status.[16] The goal of interprofessional collaboration is the formation of a partnership between a team of health providers and a patient in a participatory, collaborative, and coordinated approach to share in decision making of health and social issues.[17] The scope of interprofessional collaboration is vast and could include professionals from nursing, medicine, pharmacy, occupational therapy, physical therapy, dentistry, social work, education, law, or many others interacting with the patient and family.

Not surprisingly, different professions perceive collaboration in different ways. For example, nurses typically perceive a greater need for collaboration than physicians[18,19]; however, physicians perceive a higher occurrence of collaboration.[20] Makary and colleagues observed that nurses in the operating room setting described collaboration as shared decision making, whereas physicians described it as having their needs anticipated and their directions followed.[21] Interprofessional collaboration involves navigating different professional cultures and specialized languages and understanding different viewpoints and goals, including various measures of success.[16] A growing trend in professional health care curricula is to offer interprofessional courses as a means of facilitating mutual respect, understanding, and commitment to common goals, joint problem solving, mutual give and take, shared accountability, and collegial communication.[17]

How has interprofessional collaboration occurred? Patient rounds are frequently mentioned as a means for collaboration but reviews are mixed if this is an effective strategy for collaboration.[22,23] Team meetings, case conferences, and educational opportunities as well as informal conversations are other ways in which collaboration might occur.

Interorganizational Collaboration

Consideration of interorganizational collaboration is important in today's health care environment. Pooling of resources and information between organizations can benefit patients and communities at regional, national, or international levels. Interorganizational collaboration often takes place in the form of coalitions or consortiums. Nurses have been involved in coalitions addressing health care disparities, diabetes prevention, teen pregnancy, immunization rates, and health care for the homeless, to name a few. Health care consortiums often exist in communities or regions to ensure integrated care delivery, information, and networking among health care deliverers.

ATTRIBUTES AND CRITERIA

The Interprofessional Education Collaborative Expert Panel (a panel representing the nursing, pharmacy, medical, osteopathic, public health, and dental professions) identified four competencies or attributes necessary for effective interprofessional collaboration.[1] These attributes are transferable to intraprofessional collaboration, and represent the ingredients (attributes) needed for successful collaboration. These include (1) values/ethics, (2) roles/responsibilities, (3) communication, and (4) teamwork/team-based practice. These are further described with several specific competencies mentioned for each attribute.

Values/Ethics

Values and ethics, undergirded with mutual respect and trust, are an important component in creating a professional and interprofessional identity. These values and ethics are imbedded in patient-centeredness and strive for safer, more efficient, and more effective systems of care. Demonstration of interprofessional values would be evidenced by professionals working together and applying principles of altruism, excellence, caring, ethics, respect, communication, and accountability to achieve high-level health and wellness in individuals and communities.[1] The ethical principles considering health care as a right and balance in the distribution of resources are also important. Respect for diversity that is found in the individual expertise each profession contributes to care delivery is also considered. Ten competencies were identified for the attribute of values/ethics. The following four are highly pertinent for collaborative practice:

- Embrace the cultural diversity and individual differences that characterize patients, populations, and the health care team.
- Respect the unique cultures, values, roles/responsibilities, and expertise of other health professions.
- Work in cooperation with those who receive care, those who provide care, and others who contribute to or support the delivery of disease prevention and health services.
- Demonstrate high standards of ethical conduct and quality of care in one's contributions to team-based care.

Roles/Responsibilities

Collaboration requires an understanding of how professional roles and responsibilities support patient-centered care. Clearly articulating one's professional role and responsibilities to other professions and conversely understanding other professions' roles is a key element for effective collaboration. Recognizing legal boundaries and limits of professional expertise is also needed. Understanding that roles and responsibilities might change based on a specific care situation is important. The following three competencies are representative of roles and responsibilities in collaboration:

- Engage diverse health care professionals who complement one's own professional expertise, as well as associated resources, to develop strategies to meet specific patient care needs.
- Use the full scope of knowledge, skills, and abilities of available health professionals and health care workers to provide care that is safe, timely, efficient, effective, and equitable.
- Communicate with team members to clarify each member's responsibility in executing components of a treatment plan or public health intervention.

Communication

Communication has been defined as a core aspect of collaborative practice. Health professionals communicate a readiness to collaborate by being available in place and time, as well as being receptive through displaying interest, engaging in active listening, conveying openness, and being willing to discuss.[24] A common language for team communication that avoids professional jargon is considered a key to safe and effective communication. Dismantling professional hierarchies created by demographic and professional differences is also valued in interprofessional communication. All professions and team members are equally empowered to speak up in firm, respectful ways regarding patient care issues. Finally, consideration of health literacy and effective use of communication technologies are viewed as important components of interprofessional communication. The following three competencies are shared as examples of collaborative communication:

- Organize and communicate information with patients, families, and health care team members in a form that is understandable, avoiding discipline-specific terminology when possible.
- Listen actively, and encourage ideas and opinions of other team members.
- Recognize how one's own uniqueness, including experience level, expertise, culture, power, and hierarchy within the health care team, contributes to effective communication, conflict resolution, and positive interprofessional working relationships.

Teams and Teamwork

Learning to be a good team player is an important component of collaboration. Teamwork behaviors involve collaboration in the patient-centered delivery of care, and in coordinating care with other health professionals so that gaps, redundancies, and errors are avoided. Teamwork also involves shared accountability, shared problem solving, and shared decision making. The process of teamwork can occur in microsystems such as hospital units or with increasing complexity between organizations and communities. The following three competencies are representative for collaborative teamwork:

- Describe the process of team development and the roles and practices of effective teams.
- Engage other health professionals—appropriate to the specific care situation—in shared patient-centered problem solving.
- Apply leadership practices that support collaborative practice and team effectiveness.

THEORETICAL LINKS

Kim's theory of *Collaborative Decision-Making in Nursing Practice*[25,26] offers a solid framework for the concept of collaboration. Kim developed her theory in the early 1980s following society's renewed interest in human rights and demand for informed consent. Kim recognized that many different types of nursing care decisions are made for patients that influence their health in various ways and that patients have the resources required to be active participants in making health care decisions affecting the outcomes of nursing care.[25] Collaboration was defined as a process in which two or more individuals work together for the attainment of a goal—a process by which a joint influence on an action is produced. Kim's theoretical framework included the initial context of participant, both the patient and the nurse, and their accompanying role expectations and attitudes, knowledge, personal traits, and definition of the situation. This initial context then influenced the context of the situation, including organizational components of decision making and the nursing care decision type, such as immediate- or long-term effects. Next, the primary outcomes of the decision-making process, the level of collaboration, and the nature of the decision were assessed. Kim stated that collaborative decision making could be assessed on a continuum in which the lowest level of collaboration is expressed as complete domination of decision making by the nurse and the highest level of collaboration is expressed as an equally influencing joint decision making.[25] Finally, the patient outcomes, the result of the primary outcomes, were determined: goal attainment, feelings of autonomy and control, satisfaction, health status, and recovery.

Kim's model specifically addresses collaboration between the patient and nurse but could extend to collaboration with other family members or health professionals at the context of participant level, such as patient, caregiver, and nurse. Kim[25] proposed several research questions to develop a knowledge base for the theory of collaboration in nursing. These questions continue to hold relevancy for collaboration with patients, nurses, and other health professionals. The following is a list of some of these questions:

- Are there opportunities for patients to collaborate in making nursing care decisions?
- Do nurses believe in the value of patients' collaboration in making nursing care decisions?
- What are the relationships between the patients' collaboration in making nursing care decisions and patient outcomes?
- What are the consequences to nurses of patients' collaborations in making nursing care decisions?

The Interprofessional Education Collaborative developed a model that incorporates the four attributes of collaboration as previously described.[1] The model was derived from social theories of learning and complexity theory.[27] These theories recognize the social and experiential nature of interprofessional collaboration and the complex health care environment in which it occurs. The attributes of communication, roles and responsibilities, values/ethics, and teamwork and team-based practice are equally distributed in a fluid circle surrounded by patient- and family-centered care (Figure 42-2). A final outer layer including the importance of community- and population-oriented care is included. A straight arrow representing the learning continuum from prelicensure through practice trajectory is situated at the bottom of the circle.

CONTEXT TO NURSING AND HEALTH CARE

The implications for collaboration and the nursing profession are expansive. The American Nurses Association's *Code of Ethics for Nurses* specifically addresses the importance

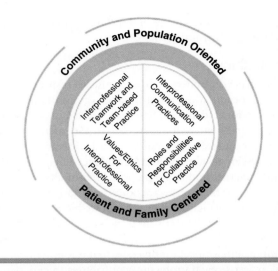

The Learning Continuum pre-licensure through practice trajectory

FIGURE 42-2 Interprofessional Collaborative Practice Domains. (From Interprofessional Education Collaborative Expert Panel: *Core competencies for interprofessional collaborative practice: report of an expert panel,* Washington, DC, 2011, Interprofessional Education Collaborative.)

of collaboration.[28] The code addresses the complexity of health care delivery systems, requiring a multidisciplinary approach with the strong support and active participation of all health professions. The code states that within the context of collaboration, nursing's unique contribution, scope of practice, and relationship with other health professionals needs to be clearly articulated, represented, and preserved. Nurses are encouraged to work together to ensure all relevant parties have a voice in informed decision making and patient care issues. Nurses are also encouraged to promote collaborative planning to ensure the availability and accessibility of quality health services. The code also addresses the importance of intraprofessional collaboration—that is, collaboration of practice nurses with educators, researchers, and administrators—because effective care is accomplished through the interdependence of nurses in differing roles.

The *Quality and Safety Education for Nurses* (QSEN) initiative anticipates that collaboration will have a huge impact on positive patient outcomes and improve quality of care.[29] So far, conclusive results from research have been difficult to determine because of various definitions of collaboration, difficulty in measuring levels of collaboration, and small sample sizes.

There have been hundreds of published narratives and reports involving interprofessional collaboration, but only a few studies evaluated the effects of practice-based interventions occurring as a result of interprofessional collaboration.[30] Daily interprofessional rounds in inpatient medical wards in an acute care hospital had a positive impact on length of stay and total charges but interprofessional rounds had no impact on length of stay in a community hospital telemetry ward.[22,23] In another study, monthly multidisciplinary team meetings improved prescribing of psychotropic drugs for nursing home patients.[31] Videoconferencing, compared to audioconferencing, of multidisciplinary case conferences was found to decrease the number of case conferences per patient and to shorten the length of treatment in another study.[32] Cheater and colleagues[33] reported that multidisciplinary meetings led by an external facilitator, who used strategies to encourage collaborative working practices, had teams using beneficial auditing that improved patient outcomes.

Collaboration also has great potential to benefit nursing and other health professionals. A strong team work culture has been found to promote job retention and to decrease resignation rates.[34] Collaborative practice environments favorable to nursing have shown improved perceptions of registered nurse-physician communication, which was predictive of RN job satisfaction.[35] Other benefits that have been observed include improved communication skills, greater leader satisfaction, improved problem-solving skills,[36] high levels of group cohesion, and increased satisfaction with patient care decisions.[37]

Collaboration has also been shown to benefit health care at the organizational level. A study led by Cowan compared traditional management of general medicine patients with nurse practitioner/hospitalist/multidisciplinary team-based planning. Results showed that length of stay was reduced (5 versus 6 days) and profit to the hospital was higher ($1591 versus $639) in the patients managed with multidisciplinary collaboration.[38]

Lateral Violence in Nursing: What Collaboration Is Not

Lateral violence (LV) is a phenomenon that undermines a healthy collaborative environment. LV is defined as nurse-on-nurse aggression and intergroup conflict.[39] Other terms used for LV include horizontal violence, horizontal hostility, bullying, workplace incivility, and disruptive behavior. The phenomenon of LV seems widespread. Griffin identified the 10 most common forms of LV that nurses use to direct

dissatisfaction toward each another: nonverbal innuendo, verbal affront, undermining activities, withholding information, sabotage, infighting, scapegoating, backstabbing, failure to respect privacy, and broken confidences.[40]

Theories of oppression, powerlessness, and socialization of girls to internalize aggressive feelings have informed the ideas behind LV. Women who internalize anger feel helpless and powerless but those who then externalize anger continue to feel powerless because their anger does effect change.[41] DeMarco and Roberts suggest that powerlessness triggers a cycle of oppressed group behavior among nurses leading to frustration, nonassertive behavior, nonsupport of coworkers, and conflict in the work setting.[42] Nurses socialized in this type of system doubt their ability to depend on others, or to collaborate, to effect change.

Nurses need to be aware of LV as a significant impediment to collaboration. Several interventions have been successful in combatting LV. Griffin[40] successfully used cognitive rehearsal as a strategy with new nursing graduates to shield them from LV. DeMarco and colleagues[43] used group writing as an intervention to decrease negative workplace behaviors. They found that nurses who were provided a venue to discuss and write about important topics developed cohesive and supportive relationships.

INTERRELATED CONCEPTS

Because many closely related concepts exist, collaboration is at times a fluid concept. Figure 42-3 presents these interrelationships. The concepts of **Professionalism, Ethics,** and **Communication** are not only attributes defining the role of nursing but also attributes and antecedents of collaboration. The concept of **Care coordination** and teamwork could be viewed as intertwined/overlapping concepts with collaboration, and the concepts of **Health care quality** and **Safety** could be viewed as outcomes or consequences of collaboration. These concepts are presented in Figure 42-3 and described further.

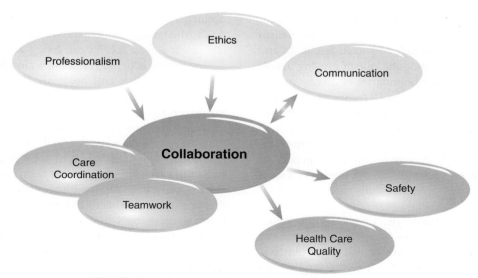

FIGURE 42-3 Collaboration and Interrelated Concepts.

MODEL CASE

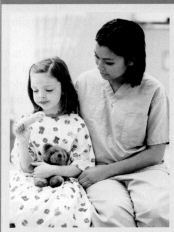

Melanie is a 4-year-old girl with cystic fibrosis and developmental delays. She is from a small rural community. Melanie is presently hospitalized at a large tertiary care center for a "tune-up" consisting of vigorous chest physiotherapy and antibiotics. Kayla is an experienced RN mentoring Janelle, a new graduate nurse who has not worked with patients with cystic fibrosis. Together they are working with Melanie's parents on a nursing plan of care during the hospitalization. The Child Life program has also been included in Melanie's plan of care to assure developmental appropriateness for Melanie's hospital experience.

The pediatric pulmonary team (consisting of the pulmonologist, social worker, nutritionist, nurse practitioner, and nurse educator) meet with Melanie's parents and the pediatric unit nursing staff to discuss the need for a gastrostomy tube because of Melanie's poor weight gain and past aspiration episodes. Via telehealth modalities, Melanie's primary care provider, a pediatric nurse practitioner from Melanie's home town, joins the team conference. Kayla has also linked Melanie's family with a parent advocacy group and has invited a representative to be present at the meeting to ensure understanding of the presented information. Melanie's parents ask many questions regarding the gastrostomy tube placement. The questions are met with open, honest answers using evidence-based information as appropriate. Joint decision making occurs with agreement to have the surgery scheduled. At the end of their shift, Kayla and Janelle hand-off information to the oncoming nurse at Melanie's beside. The parents are present to hear and contribute to the report and plans for Melanie's care. Kayla and Janelle leave work feeling a sense of joy and accomplishment.

Case Analysis

The model case exemplifies many opportunities for collaboration: nurse-patient-family collaboration, intraprofessional collaboration (Kayla mentors Janelle), and also interprofessional collaboration (the interprofessional team meets with Melanie's family). Interorganizational collaboration also occurs when the parent advocacy organization participates with the hospital team and Melanie's family.

The attributes of collaboration are embedded in the case and are the foundation for this hospital unit and for the interprofessional team that meets with Melanie's parents. Values and ethics are displayed in the patient-centered care and in the respect, trust, and accountability that the nurses and team display. The nurses and team appear to truly work in cooperation with one another.

The attribute of roles and responsibilities is particularly exemplified by the nurses when they involve the family and Child Life workers in Melanie's plan of care. The nurses mobilize resources for the family, ensuring that the primary care provider participates in the team meeting as well as the parent advocacy worker. Ensuring that the essential health care professionals were present for the team meeting took time and coordination. This is an important component of collaboration and promotes the most efficient and effective care.

The attribute of communication is apparent in the case. An openness and willingness to discuss and ask questions is evident. Inviting the parent advocate helped to level the field of professional hierarchy and perhaps acted to avoid the use of professional jargon. The use of telehealth was also an effective means to involve and communicate with Melanie's primary care provider. The hand-off of shift information at Melanie's bedside was a safe and effective way to provide information for the oncoming nurse and for Melanie's parents. Teamwork was exemplified as diverse professions, the parent advocate, and Melanie's parents problem solved regarding Melanie's need for a gastrostomy tube.

The attributes/antecedents of collaboration include professionalism, ethics, and communication. **Professionalism** involves use of nursing's full scope of knowledge, skills, and abilities while clearly articulating the role of nursing in collaboration and respecting the boundaries of diverse professions. **Ethics** involves nurses' ethical comportment when working in cooperation with various professions, patients, and families. Altruism, excellence, caring, respect, and accountability are important considerations. **Communication** is also an important ingredient of collaboration because individuals from diverse backgrounds and professions need openness and clear communication skills and strategies for collaboration to occur.

Care coordination is a concept that overlaps collaboration with coordination of care activities occurring simultaneously or in conjunction with collaborative efforts. Care coordination involves ensuring appropriate delivery of services and information as well as coordination of resources to ensure optimal health and care across settings and time. These efforts occur while nurses, patients, and interprofessional teams collaborate to solve a specific caregiving situation.

Teamwork is perhaps the most closely related, overlapping concept with collaboration. Teamwork is a QSEN competency and way to function effectively within nursing and interprofessional teams, fostering open communication, mutual respect, and shared decision making to achieve quality patient care.[29] Teams are actually the individuals who *collaborate* to achieve a common goal.[16] In health care interprofessional teams are defined as individuals from at least two different disciplines who coordinate their expertise to deliver care to patients.[44] These teams are the front-line units that provide the most care to people and are the place where patients and providers of care meet. These small systems, or teams, ultimately determine the overall quality and value of care produced by the larger health care system.[45] The importance of teams for safe and effective health care is paramount. The Joint Commission has cited breakdown in communication among team members as the primary factor in sentinel events.[46] The Institute of Medicine (IOM) also included the ability to work effectively in interprofessional teams as an important professional competency to ensure appropriate exchange of information and coordination of care.[47] Important linkages between interprofessional collaboration, team functioning, and patient safety have been well described.[48] Nurses can develop the capacity to facilitate effective team functioning and to examine strategies that improve systems to support team functioning for quality patient care.[29]

The outcomes/consequences of collaboration include health care quality and safety. **Health care quality** is a desired outcome when collaboration occurs. Serious quality problems continue to plague the health care industry despite highly trained and technically skilled professionals. Error prevention, specifically reducing sentinel events and near-miss events, requires a whole systems' approach that seeks to understand the part and their interactions as well as the broader context in which they are embedded. Questions involving the expectations, assumptions, habits, behaviors, history, and tradition that influenced an adverse situation must be asked. A better understanding of the whole is needed for intelligent leadership and quality results in today's health care organizations. Collaboration with diverse professionals and patient-centeredness can make this happen.

Safety is also a concept that is influenced by collaboration. Multiple threats to patient safety and errors occur at all levels of health care delivery. The IOM, along with the QSEN initiative, has moved from an emphasis on errors to widespread system change to ensure safety. A culture of safety is being promoted. The IOM encourages training programs for effective communication and collaboration including transitions and hand-offs. Collaboration is at the heart of solving safety issues and creating a culture of safety in nursing and health care.

EXEMPLARS

The concept of collaboration with patients, nurses, and other professionals clearly has the potential to improve the safety and quality of health care delivery. Nurses must continue to find ways to clearly articulate the nursing component of health care in collaborative arenas. Involvement of nurses in the development of models of collaboration and development of collaborative interventions is needed. These collaborative strategies will continue to benefit our patients, nursing, other professions, and health care organizations. There are many examples of collaboration within nursing and health care. These are presented as exemplars in Box 42-1 using the concept categories previously discussed.

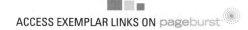

ACCESS EXEMPLAR LINKS ON pageburst

BOX 42-1 EXEMPLARS OF COLLABORATION

Nurse-Patient Collaboration
- Hand-offs (report) at patient's bedside
- Collaboration on plan of care
- Collaboration from time of assessment to discharge plan
- Home care models
- Community partnerships to address identified health and health policy issues
- Community-based participatory research

Nurse-Nurse Collaboration
- Quality improvement project
- Mentoring programs
- Dedicated information exchange: meetings, memos, email
- Shared governance models
- Hand-offs at shift change, with transfer to other units, with transfer to other facilities
- Student nurses: collaboration in group work
- Nurses from various specialties, nurse researchers, nurse educators, nurse managers all collaborating together

Interprofessional Collaboration
- Rapid response teams
- Ethics committees
- Specialty care teams (pediatrics, pulmonology, oncology, palliative care teams)
- Rounding on patients
- Having a structured/dedicated time for information exchange such as team meetings or chart audits
- Quality improvement projects and formats to discuss near-miss or sentinel events
- Use of SBAR (**S**ituation, **B**ackground, **A**ssessment, and **R**ecommendation) to succinctly and safely deliver information about patient care situations

Interorganizational Collaboration
- Regional, national, or international coalitions
- Health care consortiums

REFERENCES

1. Interprofessional Education Collaborative Expert Panel: *Core competencies for interprofessional collaborative practice: report of an expert panel*, Washington, DC, 2011, Interprofessional Education Collaborative.

2. American Nurses Association: *Nursing: scope and standards of practice*, Washington, DC, 2004, Author.

3. The Joint Commission: *The Joint Commission: advancing effective communication, cultural competence, and patient- and family-centered care: a roadmap for hospitals*, Oakbrook Terrace, Ill, 2010, Author.

4. Nightingale FN: *Notes on nursing: what it is and what it is not (Com ed)*, Philadelphia, 1992, Lippincott (original work published in 1859).

5. Peplau HE: *Interpersonal relations in nursing*, New York, 1988, Springer (original work published in 1952, New York, GP Putnam's Sons).

6. Travelbee J: *Interpersonal aspects of nursing*, ed 2, Philadelphia, 1971, FA Davis.

7. Benner P: *From novice to expert: excellence and power in clinical nursing practice*, Menlo Park, Calif, 1984, Addison-Wesley.

8. Metcalfe S: Educational innovation: collaborative mentoring for future nurse leaders, *Creative Nurs* 16(4):167–170, 2010.

9. Wroten S, Waite R: A call to action: mentoring within the nursing profession—a wonderful gift to give and share, *ABNF J*, (20):4:106–108, 2009.

10. Santucci J: Facilitating the transition into nursing practice: concepts and strategies for mentoring new graduates, *J Nurses Staff Dev* 20(6):274–284, 2004.

11. Ketola J: An analysis of a mentoring program for baccalaureate nursing students: does the past still influence the present? *Nurs Forum* 44(4):245–255, 2009.

12. Jakubik L: Mentoring beyond the first year: predictors of mentoring benefits for pediatric staff nurse proteges, *J Pediatr Nurs* 23(4):269–281, 2008.

13. Doherty C, Hope W: Shared governance—nurses making a difference, *J Nurs Manag* 8(2):77–81, 2000.

14. Porter-O'Grady T: Is shared governance still relevant? *J Nurs Adm* 31(10):468–473, 2001.

15. Ballard N: Factors associated with success and breakdown of shared governance, *J Nurs Adm* 40(10):411–416, 2010.

16. Disch J: Teamwork and collaboration competency resource paper, *Quality Safety Educ Nurs*, 2010.

17. Canadian Interprofessional Health Collaborative: *A national interprofessional competency framework*, Vancouver, BC, Canada, 2010, Author.

18. Sterchi L: Perceptions that affect physician-nurse collaboration in the perioperative setting, *AORN J* 86(1):45–57, 2007.

19. Thompson S: Nurse-physician collaboration: a comparison of the attitudes of nurses and physicians in the medical-surgical patient care setting, *MEDSURG Nurs* 16(2):87–104, 2007.

20. Hamric A, Blackhall L: Nurse-physician perspectives on the care of the dying patients in intensive care units: collaboration, moral distress, and ethical climate, *Crit Care Med* 35(2):422–429, 2007.

21. Makary M, Sexton J, Freischlag J, et al: Operating room teamwork among physicians and nurses: teamwork in the eye of the beholder, *J Am Coll Surg* 202(5):746–752, 2006.

22. Curley C, McEachern J, Speroff T: A firm trial of interdisciplinary rounds on the inpatient medical wards, *Med Care* 36(suppl):AS4–AS12, 1998.

23. Wild D, Nawaz H, Chan W, et al: Effects of interdisciplinary rounds on length of stay in a telemetry unit, *J Pub Health Manag Pract* 10(1):63–69, 2004.

24. Baggs J, Schmitt M: Nurses' and resident physicians' perceptions of the process of collaboration in the MICU, *Res Nurs Health* 20:71–80, 1997.

25. Kim H: Collaborative decision-making in nursing practice: a theoretical framework. In Chinn P, editor: *Advances in nursing theory development*, Rockville, Md, 1983, Aspen, pp 271–283.

26. Kim H: Collaborative decision-making with clients. In Hannah KJ, editor: *Clinical judgment and decision-making: the future with nursing diagnosis*, New York, 1987, Wiley, pp 58–62.

27. Sargeant J: Theories to aid understanding and implementation of interprofessional education, *J Contin Educ Health Prof* 29(3):178–184, 2009.

28. American Nurses Association: *Code of ethics with interpretive statements*, Washington, DC, 2001, Author.

29. Cronenwett L, Sherwood G, Barnsteiner J, et al: Quality and safety education for nurses, *Nurs Outlook* 55:122–131, 2007.

30. Zwarenstein MG: Interprofessional collaboration: effects of practice-based interventions on professional practice and healthcare outcomes, *Cochrane Database Syst Rev*, Issue 3: CD000072, 2009. doi:10.1002/14651858.CD000072.pub2.

31. Schmidt I, Claesson C, Westerholm B: The impact of regular multidisciplinary team interventions on psychotropic prescribing in Swedish nursing homes, *J Am Gerontol Soc* 46(1):77–82, 1998.

32. Wilson S, Marks R, Collins N, et al: Benefits of multidisciplinary case conferencing using audiovisual compared with telephone communication: a randomized control trial, *J Telemed Telecare* 10:351–354, 2004.

33. Cheater F, Hearnshaw H, Baker R, et al: Can a faciliated programme promote effective multidisciplinary audit in secondary care teams? An exploratory trial, *Int J Nurs Stud* 42:779–791, 2005.

34. Mohr D, Burgess J, Young G: The influence of teamwork culture on physician and nurse resignation rates in hospitals, *Health Serv Manag Res* 21(1):23–31, 2008.

35. Manojlovich M: Linking the practice environment to nurses' job satisfaction through nurse-physician communication, *J Nurs Schol* 37(4):367–373, 2005.

36. Boyle D, Kochinda C: Enhancing collaborative communication of nurse and physician leadership in two intensive care units, *J Nurs Adm* 34(2):60–70, 2004.

37. Messmer P: Enhancing nurse-physician collaboration using pediatric simulation, *J Contin Educ Nurs* 39(7):319–327, 2008.

38. Cowan M, Shapiro M, Hays R, et al: The effect of multidisciplinary hospitalist physician and advanced practice nurse collaboration on hospital costs, *J Nurs Adm* 36(2):79–85, 2006.

39. Farrell G: Aggression in clinical settings: nurses' views, *J Adv Nurs* 25(3):501–508, 1997.

40. Griffin M: Teaching cognitive rehearsal as a shield for lateral violence: an intervention for newly licensed nurses, *J Contin Educ Nurs* 35(6):1–7, 2004.

41. Thomas S: *Transforming nurses' stress and anger: steps toward healing*, New York, 2004, Springer.

42. DeMarco R, Roberts S: Negative behaviors in nursing: looking in the mirror and beyond, *Am J Nurs* 103(3):113–116, 2003.

43. DeMarco R, Roberts S, Chandler G: The use of a writing group to enhance voice and connection among staff nurses, *J Nurs Staff Dev* 21(3):85–90, 2005.

44. Farrell M, Schmitt M, Heinemann G: Informal roles and the stages of interdisciplinary team development, *J Interprof Care* 15(3):281–293, 2001.

45. Nelson E, Batalden P, Huber T, et al: Microsystems in health care: part 1. Learning from high-performing front-line clinical units, *J Quality Improvement* 28(9):472–497, 2002.

46. The Joint Commission: *Causes of errors and sentinel events*, 2008, Retrieved May 14, 2011, from www.jointcommission.org/SentinelEventsData.

47. Institute of Medicine: *Health professions education: a bridge to quality*, Washington, DC, 2003, National Academies Press.

48. Ingersoll G, Schmitt M: Interdisciplinary collaboration, team functioning and patient safety. In IOM: *Keeping patients safe: transforming the work environment of nurses,* Washington, DC, 2004, National Academies Press, pp 341–383.

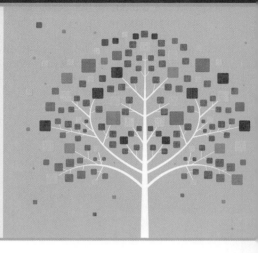

Patient safety has always been fundamental to the delivery of responsible health care but recently new knowledge, skills, and attitudes have redefined how it is understood and operationalized. New theories and frameworks inform current applications of safety science that describe how errors and near misses are recognized and reported, ways to manage the myriad of human factors that impact safe care delivery, and competencies required for health professionals to work in cultures of safety. These undergird an emerging approach to safety first developed in other high-performance industries and now being adapted to health care systems. Important shifts in these advances focus not only on considering personal responsibility and accountability in the delivery of safe care but also on understanding ways to direct efforts to system changes to mitigate the possibility of errors. Nursing has historically focused on maintaining patient safety and integrating new concepts of keeping patients safe; now safety science calls for new knowledge, skills, and attitudes to achieve practice changes identified in national reports from the Institute of Medicine (IOM) (described under Concept Definition). The new focus extends personal responsibility and accountability to incorporate safety from a systems perspective so that analysis of events includes system changes to prevent future occurrences.

DEFINITION(S)

Many of the safety concepts in the health care literature originate from IOM's groundbreaking work in patient safety. Beginning with the publication in 2000 of *To Err Is Human: Building a Safer Health System*, IOM alerted the health care industry and the public to the problem of deaths from preventable errors. In this report, IOM offers a definition of safety as "freedom from accidental injury."[1] An expanded definition of patient safety is offered in this report's appendix: "Freedom from accidental injury; ensuring patient safety involves the establishment of operational systems and processes that minimize the likelihood of errors and maximizes the likelihood of intercepting them when they occur."[1] In *Crossing the Quality Chasm,* IOM defines safe care as "avoiding injuries to patients from the care that is intended to help them."[2] An important emphasis in this IOM report is the expectation of consistent safety in our health care systems: "The healthcare environment should be safe for all patients, in all of its processes, all of the time. This standard of safety implies that organizations should not have different, lower standards of care on nights and weekends or during time of organizational change."[2] In the third report in this series published in 2004, *Keeping Patients Safe: Transforming the Work Environment of Nurses,* safe care is defined as "involve[ing] making evidence-based clinical decisions to maximize the health outcomes of an individual to minimize the potential for harm. Both errors of commission and omission should be avoided."[3]

The National Patient Safety Foundation (NPSF) is an independent, nonprofit organization with a mission to improve the safety of care for all patients. NPSF defines patient safety as the prevention of health care errors, and the elimination or mitigation of patient injury caused by health care errors. To further clarify this definition, NPSF defines health care errors as unintended health care outcomes caused by a defect in the delivery of care to a patient. Health care errors may be errors of commission (doing the wrong thing), omission (not doing the right thing), or execution (doing the right thing incorrectly). Errors may be made by any member of the health care team in any health care setting.[4]

The work of defining safety and safe care by IOM is relevant for all health care professionals, emphasizing safety from the patient's perspective. In nursing, a Robert Wood Johnson Foundation funded national initiative, Quality and Safety for Nurses (QSEN), builds on IOM's work and defines safety: "minimizes risk of harm to patients and providers through both system effectiveness and individual performance."[5] This competency definition is further explicated by the necessary knowledge, skill, and attitude elements to demonstrate safety in one's practice, and can be found at QSEN's website (www.qsen.org).

Levels of errors are important definitions to understand. IOM offers definitions of an adverse event and a near miss,[3] and The Joint Commission offers a definition of a sentinel event:

- *Adverse event:* An event that results in unintended harm to the patient by an act of commission or omission rather than by the underlying disease or condition of the patient.[6,p327]
- *Near miss:* An error or commission or omission that could have harmed the patient, but serious harm did not occur as a result of chance (e.g., the patient received a contraindicated drug but did not experience an adverse drug reaction), prevention (e.g., a potentially lethal overdose was prescribed, but a nurse identified the error before administering the medication), or mitigation (e.g., a lethal dose overdose was administered but discovered early and countered with an antidote).[6]
- *Sentinel event:* A sentinel event is an unexpected occurrence involving death or serious physical or psychologic injury, or the risk thereof. Serious injury specifically includes loss of limb or function. The phrase "or the risk thereof" includes any process variation for which a recurrence would carry a significant chance of a serious adverse outcome. Such events are called "sentinel" because they signal the need for immediate investigation and response.[6]

SCOPE AND CATEGORIES

Types of Errors

In nursing, safety has focused on the safe execution of specific procedures and tasks. However, recent safety work has emphasized the variety of errors that compromise patient safety and the range of variables that impact the occurrence of errors in health care. Understanding types of errors in health care is a vital element in addressing individual practice and improving health care systems. In its early report, IOM cites a pioneer in the field of patient safety, Lucian Leape, who identified the following four types of error[7]: (1) *Diagnostic errors* are the result of a delay in diagnosis, failure to employ indicated tests, use of outmoded tests, or failure to act on results of monitoring or testing. (2) *Treatment errors* occur in the performance of an operation, procedure, or test; in the administration of a treatment; in the dose or method of administering a drug; or in avoidable delay in treatment or in responding to an abnormal test result. (3) *Preventive errors* occur when there are failures to provide any of the following: prophylactic treatment, adequate monitoring, or follow-up treatment. (4) *Communication errors* are another group of errors that occur from failure of communication.[7] In employing a standardized system for classifying different types of errors, best practices can be developed to address safety compromises in health care systems.

Active Versus Latent Errors

Along with types of error, the placement of errors may be described as active or latent. This distinction is important in further understanding the etiology of health care errors, and

appropriate improvements. In health care, active errors are made by those providers (e.g., nurses, physicians, technicians) who are providing patient care, responding to patient needs at the "sharp end" (Figure 43-1).[8,9] Latent conditions are the potential contributing factors that are hidden and lie inactive in the health care delivery system, originating at more remote aspects of the health care system, far removed from the active end.[10] Latent errors—more organizational, contextual, and diffuse in nature, or design-related—are called errors occurring at the "blunt end."[8] A latent failure is a flaw in a system that does not immediately lead to an accident, but establishes a situation in which a triggering event may lead to an error.[11] In distinguishing errors as either active or latent in origin, the part of the system that needs improvement can be more accurately identified. Most bedside nurse clinicians operate at the sharp end of health care, and are involved with active errors, or inherit latent errors that can manifest as active errors. For example, a nurse who administers the incorrect medication because of a failure to check the medication order is involved in an active error. However, a medication error can occur in which a latent error can lead to an active error. For example, a latent error can lead to an active error if a Pyxis (or other medication administration system) is incorrectly stocked with a look-alike, sound-alike medication that a nurse mistakenly administers based on what should have been stocked in a certain Pyxis compartment. As nurses learn about differences between active and latent errors, they can more accurately identify and contribute to processes or systems for improvement.

Culture of Safety

IOM's work in the last decade has facilitated a clearer focus on patient outcomes for health care clinicians and facilities. Historically, a culture of blame has been pervasive in health care. When an error occurred, the focus has often been to identify the clinician at fault and mete out discipline.[12] With greater clarity of focusing on patient outcomes, health care teams now focus on what went wrong rather than just blaming the individual clinician who executed the error. Balancing the historical emphasis on blame within the broader context of a culture of safety is vital to effectively addressing error occurrence. A commonly cited definition of safety

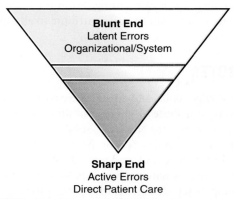

FIGURE 43-1 Scope of Errors: Latent and Active.

culture comes from the Health and Safety Commission of Great Britain, and is utilized by the Agency for Healthcare Research and Quality (AHRQ): "The safety culture of an organization is the product of individual and group values, attitudes, perceptions, competencies and patterns of behavior that determine the commitment to, and the style and proficiency of, an organization's health and safety management."[13] Organizations with a positive safety culture are characterized by communication guided by mutual trust, shared perceptions of the importance of safety, and confidence that error-preventing strategies will work.[14]

From an organizational context, a culture of safety acknowledges the influence of complex systems and human factors that influence safety. In a culture of safety, the focus is on teamwork to accomplish the goal of safe, high-quality care. When errors or near misses occur, the focus is on what went wrong rather than on who committed the error. This shifts the focus from blame to establish fault in order to determine discipline, to a culture in which acknowledging and reporting errors and near misses are used to improve the system. Accountability is a critical aspect of a culture of safety; recognizing and acknowledging one's actions is a trademark of professional behavior.

A 2003 study revealed significant variability in how hospitals address errors with patients.[15] Although the hospitals showed an increase in their reporting of serious patient injuries, the hospitals in the survey that were concerned about malpractice implications or disclosure were less likely to disclose incidents of preventable harm to patients.[15]

A recent review of literature identifies seven aspects of safety culture that contribute to a culture of safety in a health care organization: leadership, teamwork, an evidence base, communication, learning, a just culture, and patient-centered care.[16] This extensive literature search concluded that safety culture is a complex phenomenon that requires support from all of the following: the leadership level, the policy level, and the bedside clinician level.[16] Empowering staff to participate in an error reporting system without fear of punitive action is an important aspect of creating a culture of safety. In surveying nurses and physicians, a barrier to reporting medication errors and near-miss events is the fear of professional or personal punishment.[17-19] Because nurses comprise the largest segment of the health care workforce, they are central to creating and maintaining a culture of safety in any health care setting. From the bedside to the administrative suite, nurses can contribute to all aspects of a culture of safety.

ATTRIBUTES

What knowledge, skills, and attitudes are required for nurses to effectively contribute to safety in health care? The Quality and Safety Education for Nurses (QSEN) project has been the national leader in defining the competency for safety by specifying the knowledge, skill, and attitude objectives for prelicensure students.[5] A national expert panel of thought leaders in each competency used an iterative process to reach consensus on the essential knowledge, skill, and attitude objectives

that all nurses need to contribute to emerging systems of safety in health care.

Knowledge

Historically, the emphasis in nursing has been on the safe execution of discrete skills; however, contemporary nurses need to be knowledgeable in examining human factors and other basic safety design principles as well as making the distinction with commonly used unsafe practices (e.g., work-arounds and dangerous abbreviations). Nurses need to be able to describe the benefits and limitations of selected safety-enhancing technologies (e.g., bar codes, computer provider order entry, medication pumps, and automatic alerts/alarms). Educating nurses in effective strategies to reduce reliance on memory (e.g., checklists) encourages nurses to understand safety as an individual as well as a systems phenomenon. As nurses become more knowledgeable about safety at the systems level, they can delineate general categories of errors and hazards in care (e.g., active versus latent; diagnostic, treatment, and preventive errors). Nurses need to be able to describe factors that create a culture of safety (such as open communication strategies and organizational error reporting systems). Nurses must understand the processes used in understanding the cause of error and allocation of responsibility and accountability through such processes as root cause analysis (RCA) and failure mode effects analysis (FMEA). Nurses participate in national patient safety initiatives; an important facet of nurses' knowledge is their appreciation of the potential and actual impact of national patient safety resources, initiatives, and regulations to effectively use and contribute to these important facets of standardized safe practices.

Skills

Nurses need skills to utilize tools that contribute to safer systems. For example, nurses must develop skills in the effective use of technology and standardized practices that support safety and quality, as well effectively use strategies to reduce risk of harm to self or others. Communication failures are the leading cause of inadvertent patient harm;[20] therefore a vital skill set for nurses is to communicate observations or concerns related to hazards and errors to patients, families, and the health care team. Nurses have the responsibility to use organizational error reporting systems for near-miss and error reporting and to participate in analyzing errors and designing system improvements (e.g., root cause analyses). Nurses are responsible for their own individual practice while also contributing to the development of safer systems. Applying the national patient safety resources for his/her own professional development will also bring the capacity to focus attention on safety in care settings.

Attitudes

Nurses' personal and professional attitudes are instrumental in shaping their nursing practice and recognizing the cognitive and physical limits of human performance. Safety systems utilize principles of standardization and reliability as part of error prevention strategies. Professionals value their own role in preventing errors and realize the difference that one person can make in prevention, even for one patient and family. Developing an attitude of collaboration to work across the health care team to assure safe coordination of care contributes to safe care. It is the collective and shared environmental scanning and vigilance by all team members (e.g., patients, families, and all disciplines and staff) that prevents errors. Because nurse clinicians perceive their own local practice as components of the broader national safety initiatives, patient outcomes can be incrementally improved at the local and national levels.

THEORETICAL LINKS

Theoretical links that further explicate safety include human factors, crew resource management, and high-reliability organizations.

Human Factors

Human factors are adapted from engineering and expanded to address processes in health care by studying the interrelationships between people, technology, and the environment in which they work. Human factors consider the ability or inability to perform exacting tasks while attending to multiple things at once. "Human factors research applies knowledge about human strengths and limitations to the design of interactive systems of people, equipment, and their environment to ensure their effectiveness, safety, and ease of use."[10] Human factors offer a systematic approach to studying process and outcome effectiveness for greater error prevention and greater efficiency. Within human factors' health care research, attention is paid to all levels of care provision: external environment, management, physical environment, human-system interfaces, organizational/social environments, the nature of the work being done, individual characteristics, and aspects of performance.[10]

In applying a human factors' framework to health care, the emphasis is on both supporting health care professionals' performance and also eliminating hazards. Supporting health care professionals' performance in systems design includes physical performance, cognitive performance, and social/behavioral performance.[21] Simultaneously, consideration should be given to designing systems that avoid hazards. A hazard is anything that increases the probability of errors or patient/employee injury.[21] The dual consideration of supporting health care professionals and eliminating hazards is a qualitative shift to the proactive development of systems that do not reactively respond to the occurrence of an error, but work to avoid errors in an anticipatory way through the purposeful design of safer systems, a significant advancement in health care. Reason's Swiss Cheese Model of Accident Causation (Figure 43-2) illustrates how errors occur in spite of a highly skilled health care workforce. The work nurses do is complex with inherent risk in nearly every point in the process. The Swiss Cheese Model shows how errors occur when situational factors align, despite multiple layers of safeguards for prevention.

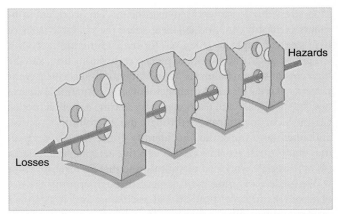

FIGURE 43-2 Reason's Swiss Cheese Model of Accident Causation. (From Reason J: Human error: models and management, *Br Med J* 320[7237]:768–770, 2000.)

A safety culture requires organizational leadership that gives attention to human factors such as managing workload fluctuations, seeking strategies to minimize interruptions in work, and attending to communication and coordination across disciplines, including power gradients and excessive professional courtesy. Effective care coordination uses checklists and other strategies to ensure safe hand-offs between providers or settings.

We need to increase our understanding of the complexity of nurses' work in the acute care environment by applying a human factors' framework to guide research in appreciating and quantifying processes that lead to error. Ebright and colleagues[11] identify eight patterns that relate to complexity of nursing work in the acute care environment, including disjointed supply sources, missing or nonfunctioning supplies and equipment, repetitive travel interruptions, waiting for systems/processes, difficulty in accessing resources to continue care, and breakdown in communication and communication mediums. Using a human factors' paradigm to guide research highlights how work complexity can threaten patient care continuity and contribute to medical error.[11] Nurses are challenged by numerous human factors that impact safety such as multitasking, distractions, complacent attitudes, fatigue, task fixation that limits environmental scanning, and failure to follow-up or follow protocol. Helping nurses understand human factors can inform their understanding of safety and further facilitate nursing's contributions towards the development of safer health care delivery systems.

Crew Resource Management

Crew resource management training was developed in the aviation industry to standardize procedures, standardize communication, decrease errors, and increase efficiency. Within aviation, crew resource management has been defined as a set of instructional strategies designed to improve teamwork by applying well-tested training tools (e.g., performance measures, exercises, feedback mechanisms) and appropriate training methods (e.g., simulators, lectures, videos) targeted at specific content (i.e., teamwork knowledge, skills, and attitudes).[22] Crew resource management emphasizes the role of human factors in high-stress, high-risk work environments. The work environments of health care and aviation share the characteristics of high stress, complexity, the need for highly functioning teams, the importance of accurate and precise communication, and the high cost of system failures.[23] Oriol[24] identifies six critical components of crew resource management as (1) situational awareness by the health care team members sharing a mental model; (2) problem identification through use of voluntary, active, and open communication to identify concerns; (3) decision making through generation of alternative acceptable solutions; (4) appropriate workload distribution so that no team member is overloaded; (5) time management through appropriate use of resources to solve time-critical problems; and (6) conflict resolution by gaining consensus through active listening, focus on issues, and mutual respect. Although crew resource management has been used in improving team functioning in operating rooms, emergency departments, labor and delivery teams, and perioperative teams, there is no standard crew resource management curriculum for health care. Programs are tailored to an individual organization to consider specific human factors that contribute to errors and near misses in that particular environment.[24] Critical reviews of crew resource management training programs in health care indicate the need for further study to validate effectiveness to determine the transfer of the learned behavior to provision of care.[25]

High-Reliability Organizations

High-reliability organizations (HROs) manage work that involves hazardous environments (e.g., nuclear power plants, air traffic control agencies) where the consequences of errors are high, but the occurrence of error is low.[26] AHRQ offers resources for hospitals to adapt and apply the principles and characteristics of HROs.[27] The following five characteristics describe the mindset of HROs:

1. HROs exhibit sensitivity to operations. Beyond policies and manuals, there is a "situational awareness" among HROs in which process anomalies and outliers are quickly identified. Sensitivity to operations both reduces the number of errors and facilitates prompt recognition to avoid larger consequences from errors.
2. HROs are preoccupied with failure and focused on predicting and eliminating errors instead of being in the position of reacting to errors. Near misses are viewed as opportunities to improve current systems by examining strengths and weaknesses and addressing gaps.
3. HROs have a reluctance to simplify. These high-functioning organizations acknowledge the complexity inherent to their work and do not accept simplistic solutions for challenges intrinsic to complex systems. In complex work environments, different team members may have information at different times.
4. Effective HROs exhibit deference to expertise and cultivate a culture in which team members and organizational leaders defer to the person with the most knowledge of the current issue or concern. The team member with the most information may not be the individual with the highest rank, deemphasizing hierarchy.

5. HROs exhibit a commitment to reliance. HROs pay close attention to their ability to quickly contain errors, and return to functioning despite setback.[27]

HROs share power and standardized communication. Especially in the acute care setting, nurses are often the most informed bedside clinician to an emerging error and have an obligation to share critical information. HROs have an explicit value of safety at the organizational level. Organizational leadership helps align safety goals with mission and vision statements so that safety is valued throughout all areas and levels of the system. A hospital is a system, a set of interdependent components that interact to achieve a common goal. Hospitals are comprised of interdependent components such as service lines, nursing care units, ancillary care departments, and outpatient care clinics that interact to achieve a common goal of care delivery. The way in which these separate but united system components interact and work together is a significant factor in delivering high-quality, safe care and the more that clinicians understand the interrelationships the more effectively they can coordinate care. HROs have a multilevel focus on safety; it is pervasive in the culture and all employees must have a mindfulness to observe where the next error may occur and implement prevention strategies.

CONTEXT TO NURSING AND HEALTH CARE
Just Culture

Data about errors have not always been accessible to health care professionals or to health care consumers. To create a culture of safety, adverse events must be reported so they can be analyzed for lessons learned and so that new procedures can be drafted to improve the system. "Just culture" refers to a system's explicit value of reporting errors without punishment. A just culture is one where people can report mistakes or errors without reprisal or personal risk.[27] A just culture does not mean individuals are not accountable for their actions or practice, but it does mean that people are not punished for flawed systems. A just culture promotes sharing and disclosure among stakeholders.[27]

A just culture seeks to balance the need to learn from mistakes and the need to implement disciplinary action.[3] IOM recommends that in most cases front-line workers should be protected from disciplinary action when they report injuries, errors, and near misses, even if they were personally involved, to encourage transparency in the system. These recommendations are based on literature review of other high-risk industries such as aviation safety, nuclear power, and high-reliability military operations. Without such protections, injury reporting rates may drop and thus impede the ability to prevent future injuries. "Such protections reflect an acknowledgement that errors are never intentional, nor are they caused by simple human failures alone."[3] IOM provides exceptions to such protection, however, if an error involves criminal behavior or active malfeasance or in cases in which an injury is not reported in a timely manner.

Transparency in Health Care

IOM recommends new rules to redesign and improve care by increasing transparency in health care.[2] The health care system should make information available to patients and families that allow them to make informed decisions about where and from whom to receive their care. This information should include systems performance on safety, evidence-based practice, and patient satisfaction. The Hospital Compare website, operated as part of the U.S. Department of Health and Human Services (www.hospitalcompare.hhs.gov), is an example that makes Hospital Care Quality Information from the Consumer Perspective (HCAHPS) available to consumers.

More than just making quality information available to consumers, transparency is also defined as open communication and information to patients and their families about their care, including adverse and sentinel events. The value of transparency in communicating errors to patients and families is confirmed by patient satisfaction in knowing the truth of what happened and that steps are taken to avoid future occurrences. A 2006 consensus statement of the Harvard Hospitals Collaborative provides helpful, specific guidance for health care professionals to learn what is meant by transparency in health care, and why transparency is advantageous to patients, families, and the health care team.[28] Timely, open, honest communication with patients and families about adverse events helps restore trust. Professionals trained in the principles and practice of transparency, usually risk management staff, communicate with the patient and family as soon as an adverse event is recognized and the patient is ready physically and psychologically to receive this information, usually within 24 hours. There are specific recommendations to help health care professionals understand how transparency can be operationalized in a health care system and fit within the framework of a just culture. Patients should be told what happened and those involved should take responsibility, apologize, and explain how the organization will respond and what will be done to prevent future events.[28]

INTERRELATED CONCEPTS

Safety is a multidimensional term as applied to health care with several interrelated concepts (Figure 43-3). Interrelated concepts with safety include **Quality,** a just culture, and a culture of safety, human factors, **Vigilance,** teamwork and collaboration, high-reliability organizations, and regulatory mandates. The connections between safety and a just culture, a culture of safety, human factors, and high-reliability organizations have already been discussed.

Safety and Quality

Safety and quality are interrelated concepts that overlap; it is difficult to achieve outcomes in one without working on the other. Quality is basically defined as identifying the gap that occurs between ideal care and actual care delivered. Quality improvement is an approach to practice that measures the variance in ideal and actual care and implements strategies to close the gap. Quality measures include benchmarks from other areas of the same institution or from peer institutions across the health care industry, such as comparisons of the National Database of Nursing Quality Indicators (NDNQI), led by the American Nurses Association.[29]

Safety may be considered a part of creating a quality culture by focusing on how to eliminate discrepancies in care that are the result of provider actions in delivering care. In 2001 IOM[2] described the characteristics of quality care with the acronym STEEP: quality care is **s**afe, **t**imely, **e**ffective and **e**fficient, **e**quitable, and **p**atient centered. Safety interfaces quality in such areas as error prevention. Applying principles and strategies from quality improvement, one can measure the rate of medication errors occurring in a given setting. The data may be compared with data from a peer unit or industry

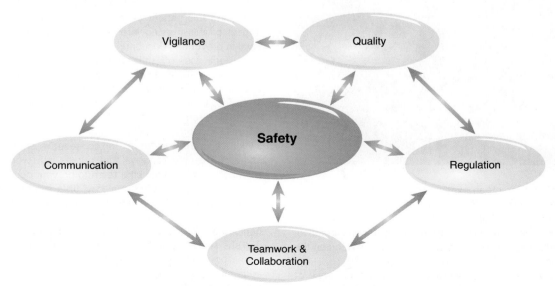

FIGURE 43-3 Safety and Interrelated Concepts.

benchmark. Through root cause analysis or another strategy, the reasons for errors in medication administration can be mapped to ascertain points in the system in which changes could be implemented to prevent or lessen the possibility of the occurrence of errors.

Vigilance

Vigilance is another concept related to safety. Nurses have responsibility for constant surveillance of patients in acute care as well as in outpatient settings. Yet, individual vigilance is not sufficient to maintain a culture of safety that expands to include the system perspective. Professional nursing has historically recognized the role of the nurse in observing, reporting, and responding to patients' responses to their health state; safety includes the examination of actions from a system perspective to minimize the possibility of the occurrence of mistakes. Nurses are the professional most often at the point of care and have responsibility for constant surveillance of patients in inpatient settings. The proximity to patients provides nurses with the opportunity to collect critical data for use across the health care team and is vital for safe care delivery.

Teamwork, Collaboration, and Communication

How well health care professionals work together accounts for as much as 70% of health care errors.[1] Ineffective communication, hierarchy, and disruptive behavior are challenges to patient safety. Coordinating complex care requires cross-disciplinary communication, knowing scope of responsibility, and organizational support for communicating when safety is compromised. Teamwork begins with self-development based on emotional intelligence to monitor appropriate reactions and responses to team members. Nurses need skills in problem solving, conflict resolution, and negotiation to be able to coordinate safe care across interprofessional teams. Team STEPPS (team strategies and tools to enhance performance and patient safety) is a multimedia training program for health professionals from a safety perspective. The curriculum includes knowledge, skills, and attitudes that can be used for all disciplines so there is a common language and shared mental model for safe care. Standardized communication can ensure safe hand-offs between providers or between settings, provide clear direction in seeking and sharing information between providers, and instill collaborative behaviors for communicating to prevent the occurrence of errors. Shared leadership based on the provider most expert in the situation is consistent with HROs.

Regulatory Mandates

Many of the improvements in our health care systems are the result of regulatory mandates from groups such as The Joint Commission, which grants institutional accreditation. The Joint Commission updates annual National Patient Safety Goals to provide guidance for highly vulnerable problem areas when evidence-based solutions become available. Based on data from IOM reports, The Joint Commission has helped to foster safety solutions through continued regulatory mandates to help lead organizational change. Most recently The Joint Commission issued regulations requiring organizations to establish policy regarding disruptive behavior among health care professionals. Organizations are required to develop a code of conduct to define acceptable and inappropriate behavior and identify a process for managing such behaviors.

MODEL CASE

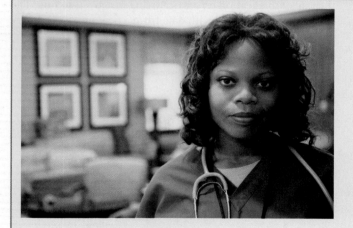

Gloria considers herself an expert nurse on her medical/surgical unit. She has been an RN on this unit for 12 years, and has seen some important changes in how care is provided. Keeping up with these changes is an important part of Gloria's practice, and many RNs look to Gloria for guidance in understanding the latest evidence.

Lately, Gloria has been concerned about the occurrence of decubitus ulcers on her unit. She knows that there are several strategies that must be employed to effectively address this deleterious patient outcome.[31] When caring for JB, a postoperative spinal stenosis patient, Gloria knows that at the individual practice level it is important that she establish a schedule of turning this patient every 2 hours. Evidence supports the impact of this nursing intervention at the individual clinician level in preventing decubitus ulcers.[32]

As Gloria goes off shift after caring for JB, she thinks about the importance of clear communication with the rest of the health care team about decubitus ulcer prevention for JB. Therefore to address safety at the health care team level, Gloria posts a reminder above JB's bed for all health care team members to turn JB every 2 hours.

While Gloria cares for JB for consecutive shifts, she thinks about the variety of ways that nurses can work with other members of the health care team to prevent decubitus ulcers. On JB's second postoperative day, JB's surgeon mentions to Gloria that because JB has been prescribed steroids, she is at especially high risk for developing decubitus ulcers. Gloria decides to address this safety concern for JB at the unit level, and she seeks input on JB's care from the physical therapist to learn about skin protection products and from the dietitian to address nutritional strategies to help prevent decubitus ulcer prevention in JB.

MODEL CASE—cont'd

When speaking with the physical therapist and dietitian about decubitus ulcer prevention for JB, both colleagues mention the increase in occurrence of decubitus ulcers on this medical/surgical unit. Gloria decides to work with her manager and the quality improvement department to track the decubitus ulcer rate on her medical/surgical unit for the previous 6 months. Once Gloria has gathered these data, she plans on comparing this rate with state and national quality benchmarks for decubitus ulcer prevention. She is also aware that there are many studies published by the Institute for Healthcare Improvement (www.ihi.org) on best practices for decubitus ulcer prevention. Once Gloria has retrieved the data from her own unit to compare to other benchmarks, she will collaborate with her manager and RN colleague to identify some systematic strategies that can be adopted on her unit. Gloria understands that safety needs to be addressed at the individual clinician level as well as at the systems level.

Case Analysis

Any source of potential injury to patients can be examined on a continuum from an individual practice perspective to a safe systems perspective. Therefore nurses need to understand all levels of evidence-based, effective interventions to keep their patients safe. Teaching nurses what they can do in their individual practice is an important component in improving patient safety outcomes. Similarly, teaching nurses about evidence-based system approaches to safety will also improve patient safety outcomes. The previous case provides several levels of instruction to improve patient safety outcomes.

Safety is a multilevel phenomenon. However, in nursing, safety has been traditionally understood as primarily the responsibility of the individual nurse clinician. Until recently, safety was considered only the individual nurse's responsibility to prevent medication errors, to prevent a patient from falling, or to prevent decubitus ulcers. Applying principles from safety science to health care systems offers a broader understanding of safety with several levels of implementation. Gloria's decisions in her own nursing practice to prevent the development of a decubitus ulcer for JB exemplify individual clinician strategies that are important and effective. Additionally, Gloria's work in collaborating with other members of the health care team and comparing unit level data to system, state, and national data are valuable strategies in addressing patient safety from a larger perspective. To improve patient safety outcomes, compromises to safety need to be addressed on many levels simultaneously.

EXEMPLARS

Because multiple exemplars exist for safety and injury prevention within health care, it is impossible to list them all. Box 43-1 presents the most common safety issues at the "sharp end" (i.e., the point of care delivery) and the "blunt end" (i.e., the systems level). Because safety issues are multifactorial, specific exemplars fit in both categories and within those categories multiple variables exist so that these are, in fact, more of a continuum of events than a list. Thus it is important to emphasize that the exemplar box is an oversimplification of exemplars for this concept.

Medication errors are a widely studied adverse event. Although review of the seven rights of medication administration (right patient, right medication, right route, right time, right dose, right education, and right documentation) is paramount, there are more contemporary approaches to medication administration from a systems level. For example, the Institute for Safe Medication Practices (ISMP) endorses the adoption of Tallman lettering by the pharmaceutical industry. Tallman lettering is a term coined by ISMP and describes the practice of using unique letter characteristics of similar drug names known to have been confused with one another. Tallman lettering is used to differentiate products with look-alike names such as predniSONE and prednisoLONE. Highlighting a portion of the drug name with different size lettering can help to draw attention to the dissimilarities between look-alike drug names as a prevention strategy.[33]

ISMP also offers recommendations for clinicians in evidence-based, effective approaches to standardizing medication order sets. The standard order set should include the following:

- Drug name (generic name followed by brand name when appropriate)
- Metric dose/strength
- Frequency and duration (if appropriate)
- Route of administration
- Indication
- Frequency and details regarding necessary patient assessments
- Drug administration precautions
- Specific drugs to discontinue during therapy
- Instructions to address known potential emergencies

ISMP recommends that the following elements be excluded from standardized medication orders:

- Drugs prescribed only by volume
- Number of tablets
- Number of vials, ampules, etc.
- Range orders without objective measures to determine correct dose

---

BOX 43-1 EXEMPLARS OF SAFETY

Point of Care
- Prevention of decubitus ulcers
- Medication administration
- Fall prevention
- Invasive procedures
- Diagnostic workup
- Recognition of/action on adverse events
- Communication
  - With patients/families
  - With other health care providers

Systems Level
- Care coordination
- Documentation/electronic records
- Team systems
- Work processes
- Communication process
- Environmental systems
- Error reporting/analysis systems
- Regulatory systems
- National quality benchmarks

- Nonformulary medications or drugs withdrawn from the market
- "If…then" orders
- Overlapping parameters
- Contraindicated or dangerous combinations of drugs
Standard order sets reduce variation and oversight through standard formatting and clear presentation of the orders, and decrease the potential for medication errors by incorporating safety alerts and reminders.[34]

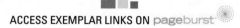

ACCESS EXEMPLAR LINKS ON pageburst

REFERENCES

1. Kohn L, Corigan J, Donaldson M, editors: *To err is human: building a safer health system,* Committee on Quality of Health Care in America, Institute of Medicine, Washington, DC, 2000, National Academies Press.
2. Institute of Medicine: *Crossing the quality chasm,* Washington, DC, 2001, National Academies Press.
3. Institute of Medicine: *Keeping patients safe: transforming the work environment of nurses,* Washington, DC, 2004, National Academies Press.
4. National Patient Safety Foundation: *Our definitions.* Retrieved on July 3, 2011, at www.npsf.org/au/mission_definitions.php.
5. Cronenwett L, Sherwood G, Barnsteiner J, et al: Quality and safety education for nurses, *Nurs Outlook* 55(3):122–131, 2007.
6. The Joint Commission: *Sentinel events,* n.d. Retrieved July 4, 2011, from www.jointcommission.org/assets/1/6/2011_CAMBHC_SE.pdf.
7. Leape L, Lawther AG, Brennan TA, et al: Preventing medical injury, *Quality Rev Bull* 19(5):144–149, 1993.
8. Cook R, Woods D: Operating at the sharp end: the complexity of human error. In Bogner M, editor: *Human error in medicine,* Hillsdale, NJ, 1994, Lawrence Erlbaum Associates.
9. Reason J: *Managing the risks of organizational accidents,* Burlington, Vt, 1997, Ashgate.
10. Henrickson K, Dayton E, Keyes MA, et al: Understanding adverse events: a human factors framework. In Hughes RG, editor: *Patient safety and quality: an evidence-based handbook for nurses,* Rockville, Md, 2008, Agency for Healthcare Research and Quality (AHRQ), Pub No. 08-0043.
11. Ebright PR, Patterson ES, Chalko BA, et al: Understanding the complexity of registered nurse work in acute care settings, *J Nurs Adm* 33(12):630–638, 2003.
12. Barnsteiner JH: *Safety competency resource paper,* Washington, DC, 2010, American Association of Colleges of Nursing QSEN Education Center.
13. Health and Safety Commission Advisory Committee on the Safety of Nuclear Installations: *Organizing for safety: third report of the ACSNI study group on human factors,* Sudbury, UK, 1993, HSE Books.
14. Gadd S, Collin AM: *Safety culture: a review of the literature, definition of 'safety culture' as suggested by ACSNO, HSE, 2002.* Retrieved July 4, 2011, at www.hse.gov.uk/research/hsl_pdf/2002/hsl02-25.pdf.
15. Lamb RM, Studder DM, Bohmer RM, et al: Hospital disclosure practices: results of a national survey, *Health Affairs* 2:73–83, 2003.
16. Sammer C, Lynken K, Singh K, et al: What is patient safety culture? A review of the literature, *J Nurs Schol* 42:156–165, 2010.
17. Cohoon BD: Learning from near misses through reflection: a new risk management strategy, *J Healthcare Risk Manag* 23(2):19–25, 2003.
18. Schmidt CE, Bottoni T: Improving medication safety and patient care in the emergency department, *J Emerg Nurs* 29(1):12–16, 2003.
19. Bullock LM: Transform into a culture of safety, *Risk Manag* 42(7):14–15, 2011.
20. Leonard M, Graham S, Bonacum D: The human factor: the critical importance of effective teamwork and communication in providing safe care, *Quality Safety Healthcare* 13: I85-I90, 2003.
21. Karsh BT, Holden RJ, Alper SJ, et al: A human factors engineering paradigm for patient safety: designing to support the performance of the healthcare professional, *Quality Safety Healthcare* 15(Supp 1):I59–I65, 2006.
22. Salas E, Prince C, Bowers C, et al: A methodology for enhancing crew resource management training, *Hum Factors* 41:161–172, 1999.
23. Rivers RM, Swain D, Nixon WR: Using aviation safety measures to enhance patient outcomes, *J AORN* 77(1):158–162, 2003.
24. Oriol MD: Crew resource management, *J Nurs Adm* 36(9): 402–406, 2006.
25. Salas E, Wilson KA, Burke CS, et al: Does crew resource management training work? An update, an extension and some critical needs, *Hum Factors* 48(2):392–412, 2006.
26. Baker DP, Day R, Salas E: Teamwork as an essential component of high-reliability organizations, *Health Serv Res* 41(4):1576–1598, 2006.
27. Agency for Healthcare Research and Quality: *Becoming a high reliability organization: operational advice for hospital leaders* Rockville, Md, 2008, U.S. Department of Health and Human Services. Last retrieved July 4, 2011, at www.ahrq.gov/qual/hroadvice/hroadvice.pdf2008.
28. Harvard Hospitals: *When things go wrong: responding to adverse events,* Burlington, Mass, 2006, Massachusetts Coalition for the Prevention of Medical Errors.
29. American Nurses Association: *The national center for nursing quality indicators.* Retrieved July 10, 2011, at www.nursingquality.org/.
30. Dolansky M: Teaching and measuring systems thinking in a quality and safety curriculum, *Proceedings of the 2011 QSEN national forum,* in Milwaukee, Wisc. 2011.
31. Soban LM, Hempel S, Munjas BA, et al: Preventing pressure ulcers in hospitals: a systematic review of nurse-focused quality improvement interventions, *Jt Comm J Quality Patient Safety* 37(6):245–252, 2011.
32. Lyder CH, Ayello EA: Pressure ulcers: a patient safety issue. In Hughes RG, editor: *Patient safety and quality: an evidence-based handbook for nurses,* Rockville, Md, 2008, Agency for Healthcare Research and Quality (AHRQ), Pub No. 08–0043.
33. Institute for Safe Medication Practices: *Look-alike drug names with recommended tallman letters,* n.d. Retrieved July 4, 2011, from www.ismp.org/Tools/tallmanletters.pdf.
34. Institute for Safe Medication Practices: *ISMP's guidelines for standard order sets,* n.d. Retrieved July 4, 2011, from www.ismp.org/Tools/guidelines/StandardOrderSets.asp.

Technology and Informatics

Helen Connors, Judith Warren, and Sue Popkess-Vawter

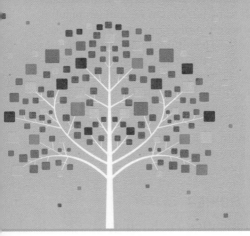

From the beginning of patient care, those providers responsible for health care delivery have gathered information to provide the best care possible. Over time, new devices and technology have provided more accurate and timely information about patients. For several decades, computer technology has evolved to the point of playing a significant role in managing health information. With the emergence of this new technology, a new discipline referred to as informatics was born. Health providers with expertise in specialty areas or practice, along with a background in computer and information science, became focused on furthering and broadening their specialty area of practice with informatics. This new focus created a wide range of informatics specialty areas frequently referred to as domains of informatics. Nursing informatics is one of those domains (Figure 44-1).

Throughout the world, health care has been transformed significantly through the widespread use of information and communication technologies. In April 2004 President George W. Bush issued the Executive Order *Incentives for*

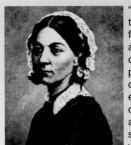

"In attempting to arrive at the truth, I have applied everywhere for information, but in scarcely an instance have I been able to obtain hospital records fit for any purposes of comparison. If they could be obtained they would enable us to decide many other questions besides the ones alluded to. They would show the subscribers how their money was being spent, what amount of good was really being done with it, or whether the money was not doing mischief rather than good."
Florence Nightingale (1863).

Longman, Green, Longman, Roberts and Green: Notes on Hospitals, 1863, London, p. 176

FIGURE 44-1 The First Nurse Informatician.

the Use of Health Information Technology and Establishing the Position of the National Health Information Technology Coordinator.[1] The goal of this order was to provide leadership for the development and nationwide implementation of an interoperable health information technology (health IT) infrastructure. The promise of this national health IT infrastructure is to improve the quality, safety, and efficiency of health care as well as to ensure that the health records of a *majority* of Americans are available in electronic format by 2014. Shortly after this order was executed by President Bush, the Secretary of Health and Human Services, Tommy Thompson, appointed Dr. David Brailer to the role of National Coordinator of Health Information Technology. Dr. Brailer was charged with implementing the strategic plan outlined in Secretary Thompson's report titled *The Decade of Health Information Technology.*[2] This strategic plan was updated in 2008 and continues to be advanced through the Office of the National Coordinator (ONC). In 2009 President Barack Obama escalated the health IT effort by calling for electronic health records (EHRs) for *all* Americans within the next 5 years.[3] Congress passed the Health Information Technology for Economic and Clinical Health (HITECH) Act[4] as part of the American Recovery and Reinvestment Act (ARRA) in 2009 and appropriated $20 billion for health IT projects. The HITECH Act and its funding positioned informatics and the use of health information technologies front and center in all health care arenas, including academia. The field of health IT and informatics is rapidly advancing and must include a workforce prepared to meaningfully use these evolving technologies. There is a growing requirement for practicing nurses, nurse educators, nurse researchers, and nurse administrators to ensure that expected competencies in informatics are met. Despite widespread use of the term informatics, few seem to understand exactly what it means. The purpose of this concept analysis is to define and analyze health information technology (health IT) and health informatics as it relates to the profession of nursing.

DEFINITION(S)

Technology is a broad concept that describes the knowledge and use of tools, machines, materials, and processes to help solve human problems. It can be applied to a specific discipline such as education technologies, medical technologies, or health technologies. Technology is the product of creative human action and it is sustained by human action.[5] For the purpose of this concept analysis, the focus is on *health information technology (health IT)* as the essential antecedents for health informatics. In today's world, you cannot have health informatics without health IT.

Health IT provides the umbrella framework to describe the comprehensive management of health information and its secure exchange between consumers, providers, government and quality entities, and insurers. Health IT is generally viewed as the most promising tool for improving the overall quality, safety, and efficiency of the health delivery system.[6]

Informatics, like technology, also is a broad concept and is derived from the French word *informatique*—it is the science that encompasses information science and computer science to study the process, management, and retrieval of information.[7] In this concept, the focus is on *health informatics*.

Health informatics is a discipline in which health data are stored, analyzed, and disseminated through the application of information and communication *technology* (Box 44-1). It involves the use of technology and information systems to support the health care industry. Today, the term informatics as it relates to health care is ubiquitous and ambiguous because of the many health professions and related disciplines that use health data. Health informatics encompasses the interprofessional study of the design, development, adoption, and application of IT-based innovations in health care services delivery, management, and planning.[8] Health informatics is a rapidly growing field in health care and can be divided into discipline-specific categories, according to the various branches of health and health care practices. Common categories are discussed later in the concept and presented in the exemplar box.

TYPES AND CATEGORIES

Types of Health Information Technology

The electronic health record (EHR) is the central component of the health IT infrastructure. An EHR is an individual's official, digital health record and is shared among multiple facilities and agencies. The other essential elements of the health IT infrastructure are the electronic medical record (EMR), which is an individual's health record within a health care provider's facility; the personal health record (PHR), which is an individual's self-maintained health record; and a Regional Health Information Organization (RHIO), which oversees communication and exchange of information among providers and across geographic areas.

The concepts of health information technology and health informatics intersect with the science of health to provide powerful tools and processes for advancing health practices. Health IT is a precursor or antecedent to health informatics; therefore the concept analysis of health IT is summarized in the Table 44-1. The defining characteristics and consequences of health IT also are reflected in the analysis of health informatics.

Categories of Health Informatics

Health informatics refers to the way in which health data are captured, organized, stored, retrieved, and shared for the purpose of health care. Health informatics facilitates optimal use of health data for problem solving and decision making and is closely tied to information and communication technologies. A summary of discipline-specific categories of health informatics is presented in the following sections. All categories integrate computer science and information science to manage and communicate data, information, and knowledge; however, they differ in the integration of the discipline-specific science and discipline-specific practice. The field of informatics has recently grown to reflect the substantive contribution of the various health disciplines to the generation and usage of health care data and related information, which has helped to differentiate the often confusing terminology.

Health informatics is new enough that in some disciplines, their definition and standards are a work in progress. Although there is no universally accepted taxonomy for the major domains of informatics today, for the purposes of this concept analysis, the American Medical Informatics

TABLE 44-1	HEALTH INFORMATION TECHNOLOGY SUMMARY	
ANTECEDENTS	**DEFINING CHARACTERISTICS**	**CONSEQUENCES**
• Need for a tool, machine, materials, and/or processes to improve health care • Information science • Computer science • Health discipline science (e.g., nursing, medicine) • Information technology specialist	• Technology (hardware and software) that supports discipline of health informatics (e.g., EHR) • Clinical point of care tools • Interoperable • Evolutionary and updated to provide new functionality	• Improves health provider's workflow • Improves health care quality • Prevents medical errors • Reduces health care costs • Increases administrative efficiencies • Decreases paperwork • Improves disease tracking • Creates cultural, social, organizational, and intellectual change • May be used in unintended ways

Association's (AMIA) domains of informatics will be used. These domains include the following:

1. Clinical informatics (including health care, research, and personal health management)
2. Public health/population informatics
3. Translational bioinformatics

The domains overlap in various ways and are not exclusive to one another.[9] In the discussion that follows, each domain is defined and the major subtypes, if applicable, are described.

Clinical Informatics

Clinical informatics is the application of information and communication technologies to the delivery of health care services. Despite some variations, informatics, when used in health care delivery, is essentially the same regardless of the health professional group involved whether they are dentists, pharmacists, physicians, nurses, or other health professionals. According to AMIA, clinical informatics has two subdomains: clinical health care informatics and clinical research informatics.

Clinical health care informatics. Clinical health care informatics seeks to transform health care and enhance human health through a creative and innovative use of informatics. This transformation will be accomplished through a well-educated and properly trained informatics workforce, an enhanced performance of health care processes and systems, appropriate public policy, and a relevant research agenda. Clinical health care informatics includes the development of direct approaches to patients and their families and even to individuals who are not yet patients (consumers) who desire to seek the use of information and communications technology support to preserve and/or improve their health status.

A subset of clinical health care informatics is *nursing informatics (NI)*. As defined by the American Nursing Association, nursing informatics "is a specialty that integrates nursing science, computer science, and information science to manage and communicate data, information, knowledge, and wisdom in nursing practice. NI supports consumers, patients, nurses, and other providers in their decision-making in all roles and settings. The support is accomplished through the use of information structures, in formation processes, and information technology."[10,p1]

Another subset of clinical health care informatics is **consumer health informatics (CHI)**. Consumer health informatics is defined by the American Medical Informatics Association as a form of health information technology geared towards delivering better health care decision making based upon the consumer's perspective.[9] It is well recognized that consumer informatics stands at the crossroads of other disciplines, such as nursing informatics, public health, health promotion, health education, library science, and communication science, and is perhaps the most challenging and rapidly expanding field in health informatics. CHI is paving the way for health care in the information age and advancing the medical home concept and the use of personal health records. CHI includes technologies focused on patients as the primary users of health information.[11]

Clinical research informatics. Clinical research informatics relates to informatics whose objective is to advance the biomedical/health sciences through the humane and ethical use of informatics. Included are issues relating to the use of information and knowledge as well as the sound and socially appropriate collection and maintenance of person-specific and/or de-identified patient data. Electronic health records will enhance the availability of clinical data for research and quality improvement initiatives.

Public Health Informatics

Public health informatics (PHI) and its corollary population informatics are the application of information, computer science, and technology to public health science to improve the health of populations. Application of the principles and practices of public health informatics leads to the development of new tools and methodologies that enable the development and use of interoperable information systems for public health functions such as biosurveillance, outbreak response, and electronic laboratory reporting.

Translational Bioinformatics

AMIA refers to translational bioinformatics as the development of storage, analytic, and interpretive methods to optimize the transformation of increasingly voluminous biomedical and genomic data into proactive, predictive, preventive, and participatory health. Translational bioinformatics is the intersection where bioinformatics meets clinical medicine. Translational bioinformatics is a relatively new term that supports the National Institutes of Health (NIH) roadmap for medical research. The end product of translational bioinformatics is newly found knowledge from integrative efforts that can be disseminated to a variety of stakeholders, including biomedical scientists, clinicians, and patients.

ATTRIBUTES AND CRITERIA

The results of the health IT and informatics concept analysis suggest several attributes related to these two concepts. These attributes are hardware and software, data standards and terminology, policies and procedures, privacy and security, informatics workforce, and organizational skills.

Hardware and Software

Health IT is the application of information processing involving computer hardware, computer software, communications, and networking technologies that enables the storage, retrieval, sharing, and use of health care data, information, knowledge, and wisdom for communication and decision making.[2] Certified *clinical information systems (CIS)* offer the best set of tools for achieving quality outcomes and are at the heart of health care information technology and informatics. CIS consist of information technology that is applied at the point of clinical care. They include electronic health records, clinical data repositories, decision support programs, handheld devices for collecting data and viewing reference material, imaging modalities, and communication tools such as electronic messaging systems. Increasingly, care is provided in multiple settings, thus creating a need for clinicians to share data with providers at other locations. Advances in computer networking and broadband and wireless communication technologies have now made it possible for clinicians to access these data from any location—whether it is in the office, the hospital, at home, or even when traveling out of town.

Standardized Information Systems and Terminology

The proliferation of clinical information systems has created a pressing need for standardization of patient information systems and terminology. Standardized terminology within the electronic health record is critical for communicating care to the interprofessional team and exchanging health information. The universal requirement for quality patient care, efficiency, and cost containment makes it imperative to express data, information, and knowledge in a meaningful way that can be shared across disciplines and care settings.[12] EHRs must use consistent, codified terminology to eliminate ambiguity and confusion, and ensure interoperability. The many different ways of organizing data, information, and knowledge are built on taxonomies and nomenclature developed over decades using a clear coding scheme. The terminologies recognized by the American Nurses Association are listed in Table 44-2.

Policies

Responsibility for developing an overall policy infrastructure that supports health IT and health information exchanges (HIE) primarily lies with the Office of the National Coordinator for Health IT (ONC). ONC has worked closely with the Centers for Medicare & Medicaid Services (CMS) to assist in establishing policies related to Medicare and Medicaid payment for "meaningful use" of EHRs. ONC rules specify the standards, implementation specifications, and other criteria for EHR systems and technologies to be certified whereas CMS rules specify how hospitals, physicians, and other eligible professionals must demonstrate their meaningful use of these technologies in order to receive Medicare and Medicaid payment incentives.[13] In addition to meaningful use criteria and certification standards, the ONC health IT policy committee has issued recommendations regarding health information extension centers, workforce training, and privacy and security. Once the policies are established at the federal level, states, professional organizations, and institutions adopt and adapt these fundamental practices at the local level to reduce barriers to health information exchange.

Privacy and Security

A major concern with health care information, as with other highly sensitive personal data, involves privacy and security. The privacy and security rules issued under the Health Insurance Portability and Accountability Act (HIPAA) of 1996, along with multiple state laws, create a complex network of laws and regulations that address patient privacy and consent for the use of identifiable personal health information. Recent reports have indicated that these laws need to be changed to reflect new technologies and to enhance personalization and the quality of health care.[14,15] Building and maintaining the public's trust in health IT requires comprehensive privacy and security protections that establish clear rules on how patient data can be accessed, used, and disclosed. The public cares very deeply about the privacy of health information, and failure to protect privacy will impair adoption of health IT systems and data exchanges.

Informatics Workforce

An informatics workforce with the right skill set is critical to the advancement of health IT and informatics. Over the past decade, a great deal of work has been done in nursing and other disciplines to define informatics competencies; however, currently there is no single consolidated list of competencies. Several professional organizations are working toward identifying nursing informatics competencies, such as the American Medical Informatics Association (AMIA), the Health Information Management Systems Society (HIMSS), the National League for Nursing Task Group on Informatics Competencies, and the Technology and Informatics Guiding Education Reform (TIGER) initiative.[10,14] Through the work of these groups, it is becoming evident that with the rapid technological changes and proliferation of information and knowledge, informatics competencies will be evolutionary and essential for all nurses to some degree. These informatics

TABLE 44-2 ANA-RECOGNIZED TERMINOLOGIES

ANA-RECOGNIZED TERMINOLOGIES	TERMINOLOGY URL	NURSING PROCESS WITHIN TERMINOLOGY	DATE RECOGNIZED BY ANA	INTEGRATED WITHIN OTHER TERMINOLOGIES
CCC Clinical Care Classification	www.sabacare.com/	Diagnoses, interventions, and outcomes	1992	NLN-UMLS SNOMED CT
ICNP International Classification of Nursing Practice	www.icn.ch/icnp.htm	Diagnoses, interventions, and outcomes	2004	NLN-UMLS SNOMED CT
NANDA NANDA International	www.nanda.org	Nursing diagnoses	1992	NLM-UMLS SNOMED CT PNDS HL7
NIC Nursing Interventions Classification	www.nursing.uiowa.edu/cnc	Interventions	1992	NLN-UMLS SNOMED CT HL7
NOC Nursing Outcomes Classification	www.nursing.uiowa.edu/cnc	Outcome indicators	1998	NLM-UMLS SNOMED CT HL7
Omaha System	www.omahasystem.org	Problem classification scheme Intervention scheme Problem rating scale for outcomes	1992	NLM-UMLS SNOMED CT HL7 LOINC
PNDS Perioperative Nursing Data Set	www.aorn.org/PracticeResources/PNDSAndStandardizedPerioperativeRecord/PNDSResources/	Diagnoses, interventions, and outcomes	1999	NLM-UMLS SNOMED CT HL7
SNOMED CT Systematic Nomenclature of Medicine Clinical Terms	www.cap.org/apps/cap.portal?_nfpb=true&_pageLabel=snomed_page	Assessment concepts, diagnoses, interventions, and outcomes	2002	NLM-UMLS

competencies are along a continuum from basic informatics knowledge and skills that all nurses should possess to advanced competencies for informatics nurse specialist or nurse informatician. Certification as an informatics nurse is available through the American Nurses Credentialing Center (ANCC).[10]

Informaticians are informatics specialists with advanced education and training who collaborate with other health care professionals and information technology specialists to enhance and support patient-centered quality health care.[10] Informaticians use their knowledge of patient care (e.g., nursing, medicine) combined with their understanding of informatics concepts, methods, and tools to analyze, design, implement, and evaluate information and communication systems that enhance individual and population health as well as provide efficient administrative services.[16] The hallmark of nursing informatics practice is its cross-disciplinary nature, with nurse informaticians often leading the team to create practical informatics solutions for use by many disciplines.[10]

Peopleware and Organizational Skills

Informatics is not limited to the hardware and software; it includes people and organizational skills. When talking about widespread use of health IT and informatics, technical skills alone are not sufficient for implementation success.

Peopleware, a key component of successful implementation, is a term used to refer to anything that has to do with the role of people in the development and use of computer hardware and software systems. Peopleware involves the sociologic side of informatics implementations and includes issues such as productivity, teamwork, group dynamics, project management, organizational factors, human interface design, and human-machine interaction. When introducing new technologies into an organization, the peopleware issues become as important and at times more important than the technological issues. Learning to manage people is crucial to managing technological change.[17] Table 44-3 summarizes the concept analysis of health informatics and its impact on nursing practice and consumer/patient health.

THEORETICAL LINKS

Classic theories that underpin the concept of informatics are from information science and computer science. Other sciences that play a role in the implementation of informatics are cognitive science and organizational science. Discipline-specific science, such as nursing science or medical science, is what differentiates informatics in the specialty areas of practice or domains of informatics and provides the fundamental building blocks for knowledge and wisdom.[10,18]

Information Science

Information science is a branch of applied mathematics and electrical engineering that involves the quantification of information. It is a collection of mathematical theories, based on statistics, concerned with methods of coding, transmitting, storing, retrieving, and decoding information. Its application includes the design of systems, such as clinical information systems, that are involved with with data transmission, encryption, compression, and other information processing techniques. Recent advances in health information technology and health information exchange have resulted in an enormous increase in health care data requiring large storage capacities, powerful computing resources, and accurate data analysis algorithms. Every clinical decision is based on this availability of the information that is transmitted. If the exchange of information works well, clinical care is solidly based upon best evidence, whereas poor transmission of clinical data can lead to poorly informed decisions.[18]

Computer Science

Computer science is the study of the theoretical foundations of information and computation as these techniques relate to implementation and application of computer systems. It is frequently described as the systematic study of algorithmic processes that create, describe, and transform information. Computer science is a broad field of study that focuses on computation, algorithms and data structures, programming methodology and languages, and computer elements (hardware, software, networks) and architecture. It also includes fields such as software engineering, artificial intelligence, computer networking and communications, database systems, and human-computer interaction.[19]

TABLE 44-3   HEALTH INFORMATICS CONCEPT SUMMARY*

ANTECEDENTS	DEFINING CHARACTERISTICS	CONSEQUENCES FOR STAFF NURSE	CONSEQUENCES FOR PATIENT
Certified health IT hardware and software (CIS and computer applications)	Interoperable EHR and tools that allow for formal representation of data/information/knowledge	Clinical decision support tools at point of care Reduces duplication of services Evidence-based practice Opportunity for shared learning environment	Consumers adopt personal health record Decreased cost of health care Patient-centered, personalized health care and user-generated data
Standard terminology for data collection and electronic exchange of health information	Data structure that allows for uniform input and retrieval of health data Algorithms that support evidence-based clinical decision making and provide safety checks	Mechanism to determine costs of nursing and other health care services Accurate, timely, and up-to-date information at point of care	Better understanding of health care benefits and services Improved quality of health care and reduce medial errors
Policies for data transmission and use	Policy framework for development and adoption of health IT infrastructure and information exchange	Ensures security and privacy of health information and exchange	Confidentiality of health data
Broadband capacity for widespread electronic data transmission and download	Sufficient bandwidth requirement to achieve full functionality of health IT applications	Ability to transfer health data among providers and across health care systems	Health data available at point of care
Persons with specialized education in informatics	Informatics specialist as team member	Maximize use of clinical information system	
Persons with technical knowledge and skill	Health information management and health IT professionals as team members		
End users with basic informatics competencies and discipline-specific knowledge and wisdom	Clinicians (nurses) with knowledge of phenomena of nursing in their area of practice as a team member	Broad-based team approach to patient care to support clinical judgment and meaningful use	
Organizational culture that supports a learning health care system	Dynamic interprofessional team oriented digital culture focused on peopleware and organizational skills	Use of data to inform clinical care and support research and knowledge development	Improved patient education, self-management, and health literacy

*Working definition: Health informatics is a discipline that sorts, enhances, processes, operates on, organizes, makes usable, and retrieves information related to human health and illness through the application of technology for the purpose of sharing information, knowledge, and wisdom among health providers, among consumers, and across organizations.

Cognitive Science

Cognitive science is the interprofessional study of mind, intelligence, and behavior from an information processing perspective. It encompasses how people think, understand, remember, synthesize, access, and respond to stored information and knowledge. Cognitive science provides the scaffolding for the analysis and modeling of complex human performance in technology-mediated settings. Theories from cognitive science inform and shape design, development, implementation, and assessment of health information systems. The mind is frequently compared to a computer and experts in cognitive science try to model human thinking using the artificial networks of the computer.[18]

Organizational Science

Organizational science is an emerging field that focuses on behavior of organizations and includes a wide variety of topics such as individual, group, and organizational decision making; the management of human resources; and the design of organizations and interorganizational networks. Understanding an organization and particularly understanding how culture, behavior, and social change impact an organization are essential requirements for successful implementation of health IT and health information exchange within and among organizations.[17] Health care has been determined to be a complex adaptive system and as such involves patients, providers, and policymakers alike to ensure that every health care decision is guided by timely, accurate, and comprehensive health information to guarantee patient-centered care in a timely, efficient, and equitable manner. Informatics specialists with knowledge and skills in analyzing organizational culture, planning change within the organization, building and working in interprofessional teams, and leading information system development and implementation are key resources for the organization. In order for health care professionals and health care systems to embrace and meaningfully use informatics and other emerging technologies, a change in culture is critical.[20]

MODEL CASE

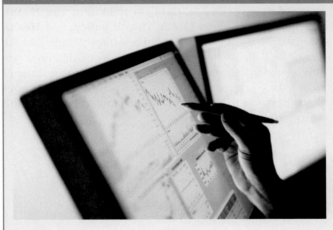

The Jayhawk Medical Center uses an electronic health record certified by the Office of the National Coordinator of Health Information Technology. To demonstrate nursing's contribution to patient care, the chief nursing officer supports the Council for Nursing Informatics and provides trained informatics nurses to help the Council achieve the goals of safe patient care and quality nursing data. Jayhawk Medical Center is a Magnet hospital and is actively engaged in a patient safety program, including National Database for Nursing Quality Indicators (NDNQI) quality metrics. Ellipse Wrigglesworth, MSN, RN, is one of the informatics nurse specialists. Her current informatics project is to design and implement a falls risk management protocol in the electronic health record that also collects data to submit to NDNQI. She first meets with the nursing staff to determine the evidence supporting falls risk management. Based on this evidence they select a falls risk assessment tool and other data that need to be collected to document and manage the falls risk. They determined the levels of risk are none, moderate, and high risk and defined order sets for each risk level. Next, Ellipse interviews and observes the staff to determine the workflow surrounding the assessment, documentation, and management of a falls risk. With this information, she begins to design the screens for the assessment and order sets to facilitate accurate data entry and present the information in a way that all clinicians can understand and make accurate clinical judgments about the care of the patient at the point of care. As she evaluates the evidence, she determines the data elements and their values (assessment questions and possible patient observation) and the appropriate data types (e.g., numeric, free text, coded response list). This is the first step in representing the data for both data input and data retrieval. For each question and coded response list, she matches each concept to a standardized language. She selects the appropriate standardized language from a list that has been approved as HIPAA code sets and in the "meaningful use" criteria. Next she ensures that the design reveals the nursing process and maps each component to the Reference Information Model of Health Level Seven, an electronic message standard required for health information exchange as specified in the HITECH Act of 2009. She adds a decision support rule that states: "When the falls risk assessment score indicates a risk, Falls Risk is added to the patient problem list and an order set for the indicated risk level is presented to the nurse for approval." Finally, she determines the staff members who may view and interact with the protocol to ensure confidentiality. After Ellipse completes the implementation of the protocol, she meets with the nursing staff again to evaluate whether the protocol meets their needs and represents the evidence for falls risk management. After the final approvals for the protocol, she builds the screens in the electronic health record and implements a training program for the staff. Three months after implementation, Ellipse evaluates the protocol and its use by the staff. The number of falls has been reduced by 15%, all of the NDNQI falls metrics were collected electronically (saving money on data collection from charts), nurses loved the decision support that saved them time by automatically adding the risk to the problem list and entering orders, and patient satisfaction increased by 10% with free text comments about the staff's thoughtfulness in keeping them safe.

Nursing Science

Nursing is one example of a discipline-specific science within the broad category of clinical informatics. McGonigle and Mastrian[18] defined nursing science as the "ethical application of knowledge acquired through education, research and practice to provide services and interventions to patients in order to maintain, enhance, or restore their health, and to acquire, process, generate and disseminate nursing knowledge to advance the nursing profession."[18,p6]

CONTEXT TO NURSING AND HEALTH CARE

The future is bright for health information technology and informatics. Great strides over the past decade have been taken to move health records into the twenty-first century. Widespread and meaningful use of fully functional electronic health record systems combined with a robust infrastructure for broad-based health information exchange has the potential to improve the quality, safety, and efficiency of health care for all Americans. As more organizations adopt electronic health records, health professionals will have greater access to patient information, allowing faster and more accurate diagnoses and treatment. Patients too will have access to their own information and will have the choice to share it with family members securely, over the Internet. This will allow better coordination of care for themselves and their loved ones. Electronic health records are becoming increasingly widespread across the health care system because of their efficiency in disseminating knowledge and promoting safe

patient care. The future looks bright, but the vision cannot become a reality without first laying the infrastructure. The Health Information Technology for Economic and Clinical Health (HITECH) Act set aside close to $20 billion to develop that infrastructure. As the incentive programs from this Act are distributed over the next few years, we will see a rapid increase in the adoption and implementation of health IT across all health settings including consumer health, population health, and health workforce education and training programs.

INTERRELATED CONCEPTS

There are many interrelated concepts that bear some relationship to health information technology and health informatics but do not necessarily share the same set of attributes. Related concepts identified here included data, information, knowledge, wisdom, trust, health, health care, meaningful use, bandwidth, and interoperability.

Interrelated concepts that are found in this book include **Clinical judgment, Leadership, Communication, Collaboration, Safety, Evidence, Care coordination,** and **Health care quality** as well as **Ethics, Health policy,** and **Health care law** (Figure 44-2). It also is important to note that the *Health and Illness* concepts in Unit Two of this book are interrelated concepts in that they provide the substance for the data, information, knowledge, and wisdom components that form the framework for meaningful use of health informatics.

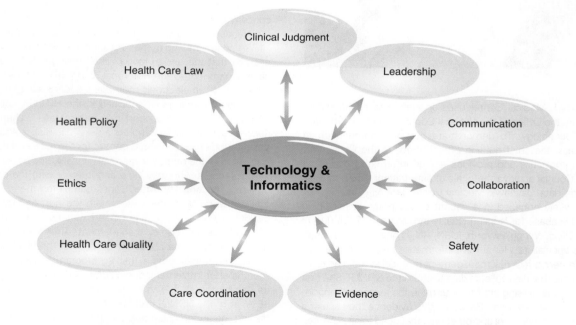

FIGURE 44-2 Technology and Informatics and Interrelated Concepts.

■■ BOX 44-2   EXEMPLARS OF TECHNOLOGY AND INFORMATICS

Clinical Informatics
Clinical Health Care Informatics
- Consumer informatics
- Dental informatics
- Medical informatics
- Nursing informatics
- Pharmacy informatics
- Physical therapy informatics

Clinical Research Informatics
- Biostatistics
- Clinical investigation
- Data management

Public/Population Health Informatics
- Community health informatics
- Global health informatics
- Population health informatics
- Public health informatics

Translational Bioinformatics
- Biomedical informatics
- Biomolecular computational informatics
- Genetic informatics
- Imaging informatics
- Proteomics informatic

EXEMPLARS

Box 44-2 displays common exemplars within the domains of informatics as previously described in the section Types and Categories of Health Informatics.

SUMMARY

Figure 44-3 displays a summary concept model of health informatics that incorporates the overlapping components of health IT and demonstrates the outcomes on nursing practice and patient care.

■■ ACCESS EXEMPLAR LINKS ON pageburst

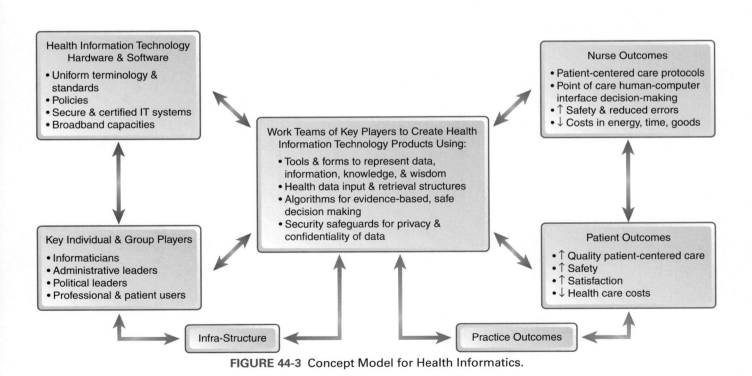

FIGURE 44-3 Concept Model for Health Informatics.

REFERENCES

1. Executive Order No. 13335: *Incentives for the use of health information technology and establishing the position of the national health information technology coordinator,* Federal Registry 24059, 2004.
2. Thompson TG, Brailer DJ: *The decade of health information technology: delivering consumer-centric and information-rich health care. Framework for strategic action*, Washington, DC, 2004, U.S. Department of Health and Human Services.
3. American Recovery and Reinvestment Act. Accessed March 4, 2011, at http://frwebgate.access.gpo.gov/cgi-bin/getdoc.cgi?dbname=111_cong_bills&docid=f:h1enr.pdf.
4. Health Information Technology for Economic and Clinical Health Act. at www.hipaasurvivalguide.com/hitech-act-text.php. Accessed March 4, 2011.
5. Definition of technology: *Merriam-Webster* at http://mw1.merriam-webster.com/dictionary/technology. Accessed Feb 14, 2011.
6. Chaudhry B, Wang J, Wu S, et al: Systematic review: impact of health information technology on quality, efficiency, and costs of medical care, *Ann Intern Med* 144:744, 2006.
7. Saba VK: Nursing informatics: yesterday, today, and tomorrow, *Int Nurs Rev* 48:177, 2001.
8. *eHow.* at www.ehow.com/facts_5672206_definition-health-informatics.html. Accessed Feb 2, 2011.
9. American Medical Informatics Association (AMIA): *Domains of informatics*. Retrieved from www.amia.org/inside/initiatives. Accessed Jan 12, 2010.
10. American Nurses Association: *Scope and standards of nursing informatics practice*, Washington, DC, 2008, American Nurses Publishing.
11. Brennan PF, Greenes RA: Consumer health informatics. In Shortliffe EH, Cimino JJ, editors: *Biomedical informatics: computer applications in health care and biomedicine*, New York, 2006, Springer.
12. Lundberg CB, Warren JJ, Brokel J, et al: Selecting a standardized terminology for the electronic health record that reveals the impact of nursing practice on patient care, 2008. *Online J Nurs Informatics*. Accessed Jan 2, 2011, at http://ojin.org.
13. President's Council of Advisors on Science and Technology (PCAST): *Report to the President and Congress designing a digital future*. Available at www.whitehouse.gov/sites/default/files/microsites/ostp/pcast-nitrd-report-2010.pdf. Accessed Dec 21, 2010.
14. *Technology and Informatics Guiding Education Reform (TIGER)*. Available at www.tigersummit.com. Accessed Dec 21, 2010.
15. Institute of Medicine (IOM): *Digital infrastructure for the learning health system*. Available at www.iom.edu/Reports/2010/Digital-Infrastructure-for-a-Learning-Health-System.aspx. Accessed Dec 20, 2010.
16. Gardner RM, Overhage M, Steen LB, et al: Core content for subspecialty of clinical informatics, *J Am Informatics Assoc (JAMIA)* 16:153, 2009.
17. Lorenzi NM, Riley RT: *Organizational aspects of health informatics: managing technological change*, New York, 1995, Springer.
18. McGonigle D, Mastrian K: *Nursing informatics and the foundation of knowledge*, Boston, 2009, Jones and Bartlett.
19. Shortliffe EH, Blois MS: The computer meets medicine and biology emergence as a discipline. In Shortliffe EH, Cimino JJ, editors: *Biomedical informatics: computer applications in health care and biomedicine*, New York, 2006, Springer.
20. Walker PH: Strategies for culture change. In Ball M, Douglas JV, Walker PH, editors: *Nursing informatics: where caring and technology meet*, ed 4, New York, 2011, Springer.

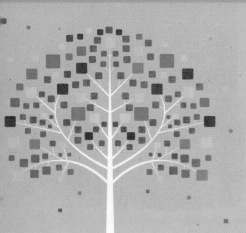

Evidence

Ingrid Hendrix

Evidence has become a ubiquitous term in health care and society as a whole. Public fascination with forensics and police and legal proceedings has proliferated in the media. Evidence uncovered at crime scenes or in autopsy rooms is vital to solving cases. Evidence can describe the course of events leading to a crime or a death and can solve the riddle of who committed the crime. An emphasis on evidence also permeates every aspect of health care. Evidence serves a similar function in health care as it does in the legal system. It provides proof of the usefulness of an intervention, the projected course of a disease, or the link between environmental insults and illness.

The phrase 'evidence-based' is applied to every health discipline: evidence-based practice, evidence-based health care, evidence-based medicine, and evidence-based nursing. But what is evidence? This concept analysis examines evidence broadly and includes how the term is defined, describing the various forms of evidence, and the way it is used in health care. Understanding approaches to recognize and codify evidence in clinical or educational situations aids in incorporating evidence in useful and meaningful ways.

DEFINITION(S)

General Definitions of Evidence

The concept of evidence is probably most closely associated with law and the sciences. In the legal system, evidence is used to establish guilt or innocence. In the sciences, evidence establishes benefit or harm. Evidence is defined as a testimony of facts tending to prove or disprove any conclusion or something that furnishes proof. When used as a verb, evidence means to attest or prove. These definitions describe most aptly why evidence-based practice (EBP) is so fundamental to health care. Evidence supports or disputes the efficacy of a treatment, the use of a diagnostic tool, the transmission of a disease, or any number of scenarios relevant to health care. Similarly in the legal arena, evidence is a highly regarded and essential element in judging a situation. Evidence is "Information, whether in the form of personal testimony, the language of documents, or the production of material objects, that is given in a legal investigation, to establish the fact or point in question."[1] Distilling this definition into its key elements, evidence is information given to establish fact. Synonyms for evidence further clarify this definition and include affirmation, attestation, confirmation, corroboration, data, documentation, information, substantiation, and testimony. However, evidence is more than just data or documents. Aikenhead[2] states that evidence, as opposed to data, is scrutinized by comparing it with other information and thus is more credible than raw data. Examples of this definition of evidence in forensic and legal arenas can be witness testimony, phone records, toxicology reports, or DNA samples. In clinical practice and health research, it is usually exemplified by research studies. Clinical experience and expert opinion can be considered as evidence, but these forms of evidence are usually given less value because of their subjective nature.

Origins of Evidence in Health Care

Examining the origins and definitions of the phrase 'evidence-based' is useful in determining the meaning of evidence within the context of health care. Although there has been a recent emphasis placed on the use of evidence in clinical practice, this is not a new phenomenon. Examples of evidence-based medicine and evidence-based nursing can be found throughout history. One example is the link between an absence of hand washing and the transmission of infection. In the 1800s, Ignaz Semmelweis, a physician, was alarmed by the high rate of childbed (i.e., puerperal) fever in women delivered by physicians as compared to those attended by midwives.[3] Semmelweis questioned the cause of this disparity, an essential element in uncovering the evidence to prove or disprove his theory. He observed that the women dying of this fever were being attended by physicians and students who had just finished working in the dissection lab. These physicians and medical students did not wash their hands after working on cadavers and so were spreading infections from the cadavers to the laboring women. The women who had a lower rate of puerperal fever were not attended by these physicians. Semmelweis did not purposely randomize the women, but rather discovered the difference between the two groups through observation. Unfortunately, his discovery was not met with immediate acceptance; in fact, his colleagues were hostile and insulted by the suggestion that they were at fault. Semmelweis was forced to move to another city, where he implemented hand washing techniques and reduced the prevalence of puerperal fever significantly.[4] He questioned existing and entrenched practices, examined the variables involved, discovered the difference in hand washing, and then changed his practice based on the evidence he uncovered.

Florence Nightingale is well-known for her work in establishing the nursing profession and being instrumental in hospital reform. Her work and writings provide a classic example of the practice of evidence-based nursing. She used observations and statistics as evidence to support her demand for improved hospital conditions to reduce infections and mortality.[5] Nightingale began evidence-based reporting during her work in the Crimean war, but continued throughout her career to incorporate evidence in her lobbying for hospital design reform, patient record systems, nursing care, and patient outcomes.[6]

The more recent emphasis on using evidence to guide practice came from Dr. Archie Cochrane, a British epidemiologist, who called on the medical profession to incorporate more evidence, in the form of randomized controlled trials, into the care of patients. He was disturbed that many health care professionals were not implementing information that could improve patient care and instead turned to colleagues for information or relied upon historical methods of treatment. He also advocated for a regularly updated database of randomized controlled trials, which later developed into the *Cochrane Database of Systematic Reviews*.[7]

Defining Evidence in Nursing

Although medicine has been one of the early adopters of evidence-based practice, nursing has joined the movement within the last 18 years.[8] Nursing defines evidence in a slightly different way. Evidence-based nursing has been defined by Sigma Theta Tau International as *"an integration of the best evidence available, nursing expertise, and the values and preferences of the individuals, families and communities who are served."*[9] Scott defines evidence-based nursing as "an ongoing process by which evidence, nursing theory and the practitioners' clinical expertise are critically evaluated and considered, in conjunction with patient involvement, to provide delivery of optimum nursing care for the individual."[8] A commonality among all of these definitions is the use of evidence to guide practice while incorporating key elements of patient involvement and the expertise of nurses.

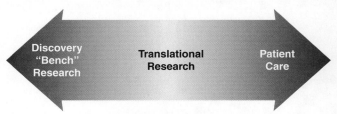

FIGURE 45-1 Scope of Evidence. Scope extends from the discovery of evidence to the application of evidence into patient care through patient care standards.

SCOPE AND TYPES

Scope

From a very broad perspective, the scope of evidence can be thought of as a range from the discovery and generation of evidence on one end of the spectrum to the delivery of care at the bedside on the other end (Figure 45-1). Discovery of evidence is often referred to as "bench" research when discovery is on a molecular or cellular level. Moving bench evidence to studying the application in clinical practice is known as translational research. This is a bidirectional process because the focus of bench research is based on clinical problems observed, and advances in clinical practice are dependent upon bench research. In health care, research can be done by an individual, but more recently a greater emphasis and value is placed on collaborative and interprofessional research, particularly with translational research efforts.

Types

An expectation of the professional nurse is the incorporation of evidence into his or her practice. Evidence can present in many ways; thus it is important to recognize and understand the various types when encountered. Essentially, there are two ways evidence appears: as primary literature and as secondary literature.

Primary Literature

Primary literature constitutes original research studies upon which the secondary literature is based. Two broad types of primary literature represent research studies that are the building blocks of evidence: quantitative research and qualitative research.

Quantitative research. Quantitative research has been defined as being "focused on the testing of a hypothesis through objective observation and validation."[10] The types of studies that make up this category include randomized controlled studies, cohort studies, longitudinal studies, case-controlled studies, and case reports (Figure 45-2).

Randomized controlled double blind studies are considered the 'gold standard' for quantitative research. The reason is that the methods used to conduct these types of studies introduce the least amount of bias. Patients are randomly assigned to the experimental or control group and both researchers and subjects are 'blind' to the intervention. Minimal bias in research studies allows the user of this information to have more confidence in the evidence created by that research. As

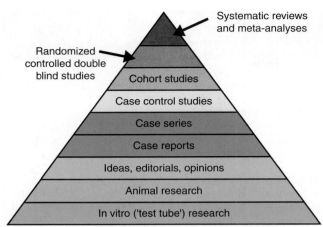

FIGURE 45-2 Types of Quantitative Studies. (From Image Source: SUNY Downstate Medical Centre: *Guide to research methods.* Accessed at http://library.downstate.edu/EBM2/2100.htm.)

Gugiu explains, "by 'credible evidence' we mean results for which the study design, conduct, and analysis has minimized or avoided biases that would otherwise raise doubt in their veracity beyond a reasonable doubt."[11] Other study designs further down the pyramid introduce more variables and thus the potential for more bias. For example, case reports look at only one subject, making it difficult to draw meaningful conclusions to other patients based on the findings.

Qualitative research. Qualitative research answers questions that cannot be answered using a quantitative study design. Qualitative research focuses on a person's experience and uses analysis of textual, or nonnumeric, data, such as interviews, surveys or questionnaires. Morse[12] argues that more attention and funding needs to be paid to qualitative research because these types of research studies answer questions essential to health care, and are of particular interest to nurses. Examples of qualitative studies are ethnography, phenomenology, grounded theory, and case reports.

Mixed design research. Increasingly, mixed design studies are being conducted that feature both quantitative and qualitative approaches. Gilgun[13] suggests that the melding of the two methodologies of qualitative and quantitative research complement each other and provide a holistic approach to the research question. As Gilgun points out, the quantitative study may prove the efficacy of a drug, but not address patient compliance if the patient considers the side effects of the drug too harsh. The compliance issue can be addressed by examining the patient's response to treatment and barriers to compliance and therefore increase the usefulness of the treatment.[13]

Secondary Literature

Busy professionals tasked with providing evidence-based care are faced with an enormous body of literature to guide their practice. This information explosion in the health sciences has led to the development of several types of secondary literature. Three categories of secondary literature include evidence summaries, systematic reviews and meta-analysis, and practice guidelines.

Evidence summaries. Evidence summaries are considered secondary literature because they summarize original research studies. Summary publications have emerged in recent years to address the problem of busy clinicians trying to deal with the explosion of information. Publications such as *Evidence-Based Nursing, WORLDviews on Evidence-Based Nursing,* and *ACP Journal Club* review individual studies and summarize the results for their readers.

Systematic reviews/meta-analyses. Systematic reviews and meta-analyses have been referred to as synthesis of the evidence.[14] Systematic reviews collect the available evidence on a topic in the form of randomized controlled trials that are summarized using a systematic methodology. Rather than conducting one very large study, the results of many studies can be evaluated and a conclusion can be drawn about the effectiveness of a particular treatment. Because creation of a systematic review is very labor-intensive—exhaustive searches of the literature and the complex methodology used to evaluate each study included in the review—there are only a few of these types of publications available. Their number is expanding with initiatives such as the Cochrane Collaboration, the Campbell Collaboration, and the Joanna Briggs Institute. As a result, the topics found in a systematic review tend to focus on areas of research that would be of the most interest to the greatest number of practitioners. Meta-analyses, similar to systematic reviews, summarize evidence from multiple studies. What differentiates a meta-analysis from a systematic review is that it combines the statistical results of numerous randomized controlled trials and analyzes that evidence.

Practice guidelines. Practice guidelines are another type of summary publication. They are designed to summarize findings of the research and advise practitioners in their care of patients. Ideally, guidelines result in a faster integration of new evidence into practice and address issues of cost and variation in practice. Guidelines are often developed by government agencies or societies, such as the U.S. Preventive Services Task Force, the American College of Obstetricians and Gynecologists, or the National Association of Pediatric Nurse Practitioners. They create guidelines by using evidence from the literature, research studies on the topic of the guideline, and expert opinion to craft the publications. These publications are then referred to as the standard of practice for a particular treatment. Unlike systematic reviews or meta-analyses, practice guidelines are less structured in their design. One source for guidelines is National Guideline Clearinghouse (www.guideline.gov/), a searchable database of available guidelines provided by the Agency for Healthcare Research and Quality (AHRQ).

ATTRIBUTES

An attribute is a quality or characteristic that is associated with the concept that helps to clarify or confirm the concept. Several attributes of evidence exist. Major attributes of evidence include replicability, reliability, and validity. Evidence is built on research findings and findings can only be verified if they can be repeated. Evidence must also be consistently and accurately measured.[2] Even clinical experience, as a form of evidence, demonstrates the same treatment applied to similar patients over time leads to similar outcomes. Minor attributes of evidence include that it is publicly available, understandable, and usable. Furthermore, there should be no doubt about its veracity.[15]

Levels of Evidence

Unfortunately, not all evidence produced is equal. Conclusions drawn from research are not necessarily valid just because they originate from a study. For this reason, levels of evidence have been created to help the busy practitioner determine the quality of a study. These are tables that arrange study types in a hierarchy based on how much trust can be placed in the results of a study design. Unfortunately, although these levels were originally designed to help clinicians evaluate evidence, there has been no standardization and therefore different organizations have created their own versions. Initiatives such as GRADE (Grading of Recommendations Assessment, Development, and Evaluation) are attempting to consistently measure the quality of research studies.[16] Basically, this system classifies studies as strong or weak based on the methodology of the study—such as sample size and blinding of the researchers and/or study subjects. For quantitative studies, there are numerous websites showing detailed tables of what has become known as levels of evidence.[17,18] Attempts have been made to create levels of evidence for qualitative studies, but these efforts have been less successful.[19] The nature of qualitative studies makes them less well suited for such categorization.

Another level of evidence is applied to secondary literature, particularly practice guidelines. In this context, a grade or level is assigned to a recommendation to help a health care professional understand how well the recommendation is supported by the collective research. As an example, the U.S. Preventive Services Task force has a grading of evidence A, B, C, D, and I (Box 45-1).

Evidence on the Internet

Levels of evidence are designed to be applied to original research studies—the primary literature. How is information on the Internet evaluated? Because of the accessibility of information on the Internet, many health care professionals look to search engines such as Google to find the information that they need. This can be a risky practice. Anyone can post information on the Internet and create very authoritative appearing websites, even if the information provided is false or misleading. As with levels of evidence, criteria have been developed to use with information found online, especially health information. Organizations have created checklists of criteria to use when surfing the Web.[20] First, determine the author and sponsor of the information. This is not always easy to discern. Looking at the *About Us* or *Contact Us* page of a website can provide clues. But as with research studies,

---

BOX 45-1 U.S. PREVENTIVE SERVICES TASK FORCE GRADING OF EVIDENCE

Grade A = Strongly Recommends
- There is high certainty that the net benefit is substantial.

Grade B = Recommends
- There is high certainty that the net benefit is moderate or there is moderate certainty that the net benefit is moderate to substantial.

Grade C = No Recommendations for or Against
- There may be considerations that support providing the intervention in an individual patient, but not for the general population. There is at least moderate certainty that the net benefit is small.

Grade D = Recommends Against
- There is moderate or high certainty that the intervention has no net benefit or that the harms outweigh the benefits.

IStatement = Insufficient Evidence to Recommend for or Against
- The current evidence is insufficient to assess the balance of benefits and harms of the service. Evidence is lacking, of poor quality, or conflicting, and the balance of benefits and harms cannot be determined.

From U.S. Preventive Services Task Force: www.uspreventive servicestaskforce.org/.

---

information found online should limit bias as much as possible. For example, if the information about a particular drug is provided by the pharmaceutical company selling that product, it would be prudent to evaluate that information with such a bias in mind. Looking at a website's domain can help determine the source of the information, for example, **.edu** for educational institutions or **.gov** for a government website. In addition, determine who is providing the content of the website. Is it a health care professional, a concerned individual, or a government agency? Content on a website should be validated with evidence, such as references to research studies. Otherwise, the information should be considered opinion. Currency is another important element of information found on the Web, especially in regards to health information. Organizations, such as the Health on the Net Foundation (www.hon.ch/), provide a seal of approval to websites adhering to their standards of quality. This seal provides a quick visual that the information on the site has met certain criteria.

THEORETICAL LINKS

Various models of evidence-based nursing (EBN) have been developed to help nurses understand how to incorporate evidence into practice on a routine basis. Some models address evidence-based nursing from the standpoint of an individual, others from an organizational point of view. Two such models that facilitate the use of evidence into practice are the Johns Hopkins Nursing EBP Model and Guidelines and the Iowa Model of Evidence-Based Practice. The Johns Hopkins

Nursing EBP Model and Guidelines provides a systematic method for applying evidence in the clinical, research, and educational settings.[21] This model, developed in collaboration with clinical and academic nurses, uses a mentored, stepwise approach to evidence-based nursing. It addresses the three common barriers to implementing EBN—lack of knowledge, overwhelming amounts of information, and time constraints. Staff nurses are provided with educational opportunities and tools to facilitate gathering and evaluating evidence. The key to this model is the individual mentoring and support from nursing leadership.

The Iowa Model of Evidence-Based Practice[22] takes a broader and more institutional approach to implementing evidence-based practice. The flowchart of the model begins with either of two types of triggers—problem focused or knowledge focused. These triggers are initiated by events such as clinical problems, risk management or quality improvement data, organizational guidelines, or new evidence from the literature. What is unique about the Iowa Model is that it identified triggers beyond just a clinical question that arises from practice. Nurses can easily follow the steps of the flowchart to identify if there is a sufficient evidence base to guide a change in practice, to determine steps to take if there is insufficient evidence, and to establish outcomes to monitor after initiating a change. Another unique element of this model is that it examines the relevance of the question to the organization, which in turn guides the level of support that can be expected when piloting, adopting, and instituting the projected change and evaluating outcome data. The 2001 revision of the model provides even more feedback loops and gives very detailed instructions for incorporating evidence-based practice.

CONTEXT TO NURSING AND HEALTH CARE

To provide safe, quality care, nurses must base their practice decisions on evidence. The context of evidence in nursing is through conducting research and by using the available evidence.

Nurses as Researchers: Evidence Discovery

Many nurses are involved in research. Involvement may include leading a research study as a principal investigator, being a collaborating investigator on a study, or contributing to a study through data collection. Leading research studies requires a specific skill set that is acquired by completing graduate education at the doctoral level and by following research protocols outlined by an institutional oversight committee, such as an institutional review board. Most researchers are affiliated with an academic health sciences center, private organizations and foundations with dedicated research departments, or government agencies dedicated to research.

Nurses as Consumers of Evidence

All nurses must be skilled as consumers of the evidence. Understanding research designs and learning to incorporate high-quality evidence into practice can make creating nursing research a less daunting endeavor. For nurses, being a consumer of the evidence generally assumes two forms: practice policies and procedures, and findings solutions to practice problems.

Policies and Procedures

All health care agencies have policy and procedure manuals that outline the practice standard for various care activities; nurses are expected to follow policies and procedures for the agency in which they practice. Policies and procedures should be regularly updated to reflect the current evidence and standards of practice and are approved by a committee charged with this oversight. Nurses have a role in developing and maintaining policy and procedure guidelines by serving on such committees or volunteering to participate in updates. In this context, nurses must be skilled research consumers in order to make accurate and efficient recommendations for policy updates.

Finding Solutions to Practice Questions or Problems

There are many occasions when practicing nurses identify practice-related problems that require solutions. As consumers of evidence, nurses should use available evidence to find solutions or answers to clinical questions. To facilitate the use of evidence, steps have been developed to systematically approach a question of patient care. The steps are outlined as follows:

1. Develop an answerable question.
2. Search the literature to uncover evidence to answer the question.
3. Evaluate the evidence found.
4. Apply the evidence to the practice situation.
5. Evaluate the outcome.

Develop an answerable question. The first step in finding evidence is determining a question to ask. This may seem straightforward and obvious, but this step is often a stumbling block for many people. The reason is that most people start looking for information, or evidence, with only a vague idea of what they are seeking. It would be similar to looking for someone's house and only knowing they are in the southeast part of town. One could spend hours or even days trying to find the exact location with such vague directions—and the person would probably quit the search without success. To find the most direct route, one must start with a good map. And a good map begins with the question, "Where do you want to go?" The best way to find evidence is to be clear about what information is needed. The question needs to be specific or answerable, without being too vague or so specific that the probability of finding information about the topic would be unlikely. Entering a search query such as 'breast cancer' or 'diabetes' would lead to an overwhelming abundance of information. What particular aspect of breast cancer or diabetes is of interest: treatment; supportive services; prevention strategies? Before searching for the evidence, define the question to be answered and map a strategy to get there.

One formula that can be helpful in designing an answerable question is the PICO formula. The acronym stands for

Population, Intervention, Comparison, and Outcome. Using these elements clarifies the formulation of a question. An example of a PICO question would be, "For inpatients (P), is turning every 2 hours (I) more effective than air mattresses (C) for preventing pressure ulcers (O)?"

There are two types of questions to consider: background and foreground questions. Background questions are those that provide foundational knowledge. An example of a background question would be "What is scleroderma?" These types of questions can most easily be answered by a textbook, review article, or a reputable website. Foreground questions address issues of a more specific nature, such as "Is drug x more effective that drug y in treating scleroderma?" These questions are best answered by searching the primary literature, which is found in databases indexing research studies.

Search the literature. Once a question is developed, the next step is searching the literature. With a question mapped out, it is easier to determine which keywords will be used in the search. Most databases accept quotes to search for phrases, such as 'kangaroo care'. Without quotes around the phrase, the search engine will look for the words 'kangaroo' and 'care' but not necessarily next to one another. This may lead to retrieval of studies unrelated to this particular type of care of newborns. Additionally, it is a good strategy to think of synonyms for any keywords used. This saves time and frustration. For example, a search on the topic 'AIDS' will result in articles discussing hearing aids or walking aids, for example, in addition to articles on the disease itself. Searching the phrase 'acquired immunodeficiency syndrome' will retrieve only articles focused on the disease. If retrieval is too limited, remove a keyword of less importance to the question. A large retrieval can benefit from limits such as language, age groups, or dates of publication.

It is virtually impossible to keep current with new findings and different approaches to patient care. On the topic of evidence-based nursing alone, in the PubMed database the number of articles has expanded from 1 in 1996 to 2220 in 2011. Bibliographic databases have been designed to help access and catalog the rapidly expanding body of literature. However, it is an imperfect system. There are many databases that cover different topic areas and each has a different search engine, or interface, to learn. As a result, many clinicians resort to Google or Wikipedia because of its fast, user-friendly interface. But there are drawbacks to using search engines such as Google. The amount of information retrieved is usually quite large. Shultz found that PubMed was much more precise than Google Scholar, commenting that "...efficient retrieval of the best available scientific evidence can inform...protocols, recommendations for clinical decisions in individual patients, and education which minimizes information overload."[23] Both Shultz[23] and Anders[24] noted in their comparison of searches in PubMed and Google Scholar that Google Scholar returned more articles that were not relevant to the search. More importantly, the quality of that information can be questionable. Using databases specifically focused on health care research is much more efficient, but requires some training. Most searchers use only keywords, but using the subject heading search feature of a database can significantly narrow

a search and yield far more precise results. Consulting with a medical librarian or using tutorials provided by the database producer saves valuable time in locating evidence to guide practice. Searching the literature is more an art than a science and requires creativity and perseverance. As with any skill, practice will increase satisfaction with the outcome.

Evaluate the evidence found. Once information has been located to provide the evidence for a change in practice, that information should be evaluated for its quality and applicability to a particular patient situation. The following questions are most commonly used to evaluate studies: Are the results of the study or systematic review valid? What are the results, and are they meaningful and reliable? Are the results clinically relevant to my patients? Many articles have been published in the nursing literature to help nurses assess the quality of the information found in research studies.[25-31] The American Medical Association has also published the book *Users' Guides to the Medical Literature,* which is a compilation of articles from *JAMA* covering topics on how to read and understand the information found in published studies. As stated previously, not all evidence is created equal and nurses need to be critical consumers of the information they uncover. By reading the articles just referenced,[25-31] nurses can improve their skills in critically evaluating the literature.

Apply the evidence found. If sufficient evidence is found to guide a change in practice, the next step of evidence-based practice is to apply that evidence to a particular patient situation. Although evidence provides proof of the validity of a course of action, it is not the sole arbitrator of treatment decisions. A key element in any practice situation is the incorporation of patients' preferences for their health outcome: "The active involvement of patients, integrated with the clinical expertise of practitioners, is considered fundamental to the whole enterprise of nursing."[15] A patient should be provided with the evidence and advice of a well-informed health care professional to support his or her decision to move forward with the care he or she desires. It is the responsibility of the health care professional to use the most appropriate and current evidence to guide his or her practice and optimize the care of his or her patients.

Evaluate the evidence. To complete the process, the nurse evaluates the outcome. Evaluation includes appraisal of the degree of success of the intervention and the patient's satisfaction with the outcome in addition to assessment by the nurse of the efficacy of the evidence. Repeatedly following the steps of evidence-based nursing will facilitate its use.

INTERRELATED CONCEPTS

There are many concepts that relate to and work in synergy with evidence; in fact, nearly everything in health care is impacted by evidence. In addition to guiding individual practice, evidence also impacts health care on a more global scale. Four concepts featured in this textbook have an especially important interrelationships: **Safety, Health policy, Technology and informatics,** and **Health care economics.** Figure 45-3 illustrates the multidirectionality of evidence. The arrow pointing out illustrates how evidence provides the foundation and evolution for these concepts. The arrow pointing back towards evidence indicates that these concepts provide evidence to their efficacy; thus their connection to the evidence is not static. Outcomes inform future research to update previous evidence and thus a constant flow of evidence is maintained.

Safety

In 2003 the Institute of Medicine released its report *Keeping Patients Safe: Transforming the Work Environment of Nurses.*[32] As stated in their activity description, the Institute of Medicine used evidence from a variety of industries, other IOM reports, and expert testimony to create the report. In the report the IOM makes policy recommendations related to nurse/patient ratios, work hours, and overtime, all factors that influence the delivery of safe patient care. As the report notes, because nurses spend the most amount of time with patients, they are the ones who can have the most impact on patient safety. Patient safety initiatives and the pursuit of quality health care are all built upon the foundation of evidence. If accidental falls are an issue on a unit in the hospital, a nurse practicing evidence-based care would develop a question such as, "Do nursing rounds every 2 hours prevent accidental falls in an inpatient setting?" Prepared with the question, the nurse would then search the literature, assess the evidence, and institute a change in practice. Such a practice based on evidence would increase the quality of care provided because it had a proven, validated approach to care.

Health Policy

Another factor influencing the integration of evidence into policy is the high cost of health care. The benefits of new treatments and diagnostic tests need to be evaluated by examining the evidence proving their efficacy for policymakers to approve their use. Policies developed to guide practice are based on evidence found in the literature. Other factors

affect guideline development, what Oxman[33] describes as 'local evidence'. "This includes evidence of the presence of modifying factors in specific settings, the degree of need (e.g., the prevalence of disease or risk facts or problems with delivery, financial or governance arrangements), values, costs and the availability of resources."[33] Federal agencies and other health care agencies not only use evidence to create policy decisions but also promote the use of evidence to improve patient outcomes and education of health care professionals.[33]

Technology and Informatics

Technology and informatics is another concept related to evidence. Technology has revolutionized health care; imaging, monitoring, drug delivery, and the electronic medical record are just a few areas that have changed dramatically because of advances in technology. Technology in the context of evidence has also changed the way health care is delivered. It allows for increased access to the literature through online databases, Web content, electronic books, and online journal articles. Sophisticated search engines provide end users with increasingly intuitive interfaces that are faster and more powerful than computers of previous generations. PDAs and smartphones allow information to be distributed from anywhere the user is located—whether at the patient's bedside or in an airport waiting area. Evidence also influences technology in that new technology is not incorporated into practice until it has been tested for its validity and utility, such as positron emission tomography (PET) scans or new indwelling catheter devices.

Informatics allows researchers to manipulate large data sets to discern trends in health care and link clinical data systems and evidence. As with evidence-based practice, every discipline has its own definition of informatics. The American Nurses Association defines nursing informatics as "the specialty that integrates nursing science, computer science and information science to manage and communicate data, information and knowledge in nursing practice."[35]

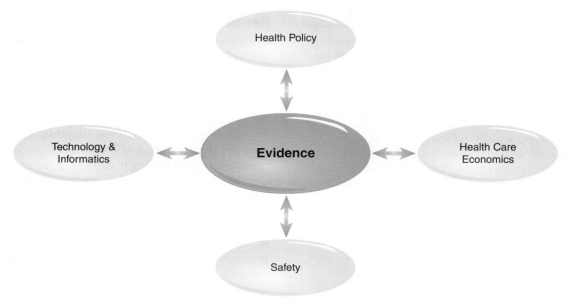

FIGURE 45-3 Evidence and Interrelated Concepts.

Informatics has been the driving force behind such innovations as the development of the electronic medical record (EMR). Increasingly, the EMR is becoming more sophisticated and is projected to provide portable personal health data to allow patients to carry their information with them to any health care facility. The integration of the electronic medical record with clinical decision support tools is a perfect example of the evolution of technology and informatics and evidence. In such a model, a summary of the clinical evidence relevant to a patient's problem would be part of the information within the patient's record.[14] Further, it would be continually updated with the best current evidence.

MODEL CASE

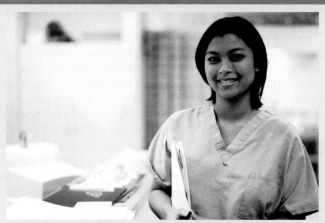

Susan Ryan, a registered nurse working in the neurosurgical intensive care unit (NSICU), observes that many of the patients under her care need to be transferred from their beds to wheelchairs. However, most of these patients have very little motor control and are unable to assist the nurses with transfers. As a result, she observes more absences among her coworkers attributable to back injuries. Susan realizes there is a need for change and is curious about how other similar units address this issue. She asks her coworkers who have worked in other units if they have seen a solution to this problem. No one reports a satisfactory solution.

Susan turns to the evidence from the published literature to see if anyone has conducted a study to address this problem. The question she develops is, "In intensive care units, specifically neurosurgical ICUs, is there a method of transferring patients that doesn't cause injury to the nurse?" She starts her search in the PubMed database and types in the keywords 'neurosurgical icu' and 'patient transfers' and 'nurses'. This yields a few hits, but nothing very useful. So she decides to broaden her search to include any ICU and this time spells out 'intensive care unit' and tries the keyword of 'lift*'. By using an asterisk, Susan retrieves articles that use the word *lift* or *lifts* or *lifting* or *lifted*. She omits the word 'nurse' because she decides if the article refers to other health care employees she can still use that information. She finds a few articles that she wants to examine in more depth, so she links to the full text of the articles and prints them. Later that evening, when it is quieter on the floor, she reads the articles. Susan learns that many hospitals have developed 'no lift' policies and have also purchased a moveable lift that can be used throughout the unit. One article discusses the cost-effectiveness of using the lift versus dealing with staff absences attributable to back injuries and workers' compensation claims. Susan then looks at how many employees in her unit in the past year have missed work because of injuries caused by transfers. Armed with this information, she approaches the unit manager to request that the hospital purchase a lift that can be rolled from room to room. Based on the evidence that she provided to prove her point—both from the literature and from hospital injury reports—Susan's request is approved and a lift is purchased. Not only has she won the thanks of her coworkers, but also she has saved the hospital substantial money in lost time from occupational injuries.

CONTRARY CASE

In an outpatient pediatric clinic, the nurse sees an infant for a 2-month well-baby checkup. The child has not received current immunizations. The mother says she is afraid her child will get autism from the shots. The physician counsels the mother to have the immunizations to prevent any life-threatening illnesses. After seeing the physician, the mother pulls the nurse aside, saying she is still afraid her child will get autism and asks the nurse to tell her what she would recommend. The nurse asks the mother to wait a moment while she looks up the information. The nurse accesses the Internet and types the keywords 'autism' and 'immunizations'. She finds a site that confirms that immunizations cause autism so she prints the page and gives it to the mother, confirming the mother's fears. What the nurse did not realize was that the website she used had a **.com** address and was published by an individual who was using the website to further his own agenda linking autism and immunizations. A similar search in PubMed would have led to numerous studies that were not able to prove a link between autism and immunizations.

Health Care Economics

Evidence plays a vital role in cost containment in health care. With allocation of resources driving health care decisions, policymakers, governments, institutions, and the public are all demanding evidence to support decisions. One example of evidence resulting in cost savings is the recommendation by the American Diabetes Association of using hemoglobin A_{1c} measurements for diabetes diagnosis. Because this test does not require fasting, it is conceivable more people will take the test, thus leading to earlier diagnosis. Early diagnosis could in turn reduce health care costs if people adopt lifestyle changes to avoid serious complications.[36-37] Another example of the relationship between economics and evidence is that care provided by nurse practitioners has been shown to be more cost-effective in certain situations than that of physicians, a significant issue in an era of health care reform.[38]

EXEMPLARS

An exemplar is a specific example of a concept and there are literally thousands of evidence exemplars. Although research studies, practice guidelines, and expert opinions are general categories of evidence exemplars, the studies or practice guidelines themselves are the exemplars. As an example, in the category of practice guidelines alone, there are more than 7000 practice guidelines listed in the National Guidelines Clearinghouse. Box 45-2 presents common exemplars linked to this concept.

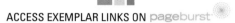

ACCESS EXEMPLAR LINKS ON pageburst

BOX 45-2 EXEMPLARS OF EVIDENCE

Quantitative Research Studies
- Randomized controlled trial
- Cohort study
- Case-controlled study
- Case study
- Longitudinal study

Qualitative Research Studies
- Ethnography
- Phenomenology
- Grounded theory
- Case study

Practice Guidelines
- Standards of medical care in diabetes (American Diabetic Association)
- Lipid screening and cardiovascular health in childhood (American Academy of Pediatrics)
- Guideline for human papillomavirus (HPV) vaccine use to prevent cervical cancer (American Cancer Association)

Expert Opinion/Commentaries
Health Care Policies
- Healthy People 2020

REFERENCES

1. Evidence: In *Oxford English dictionary*, 2010. Available at www.oed.com/search?searchType=dictionary&;q=evidence&_searchBtn=Search.
2. Aikenhead GS: Science-based occupations and the science curriculum: concepts of evidence, *Sci Educ* 89:242, 2005.
3. Lane HJ, Blum N, Fee E: Oliver Wendell Holmes (1809-1894) and Ignaz Philipp Semmelweis (1818-1865): preventing the transmission of puerperal fever, *Am J Public Health* 100:1008, 2010.
4. Best M, Neuhauser D: Ignaz Semmelweis and the birth of infection control, *Qual Safety Health Care* 13:233, 2004.
5. Aravind M, Chung KC: Evidence-based medicine and hospital reform: tracing origins back to Florence Nightingale, *Plast Reconstr Surg* 125:403, 2010.
6. McDonald L: Florence Nightingale and the early origins of evidence-based nursing, *Evid Based Nurs* 4:68, 2001.
7. Shah HM, Chung KC: Archie Cochrane and his vision for evidence-based medicine, *Plast Reconstr Surg* 124:982, 2009.
8. Scott K, McSherry R: Evidence-based nursing: clarifying the concepts for nurses in practice, *J Clin Nurs* 18:1085, 2009.
9. Sigma Theta Tau International: *Evidence-based nursing position statement.* Accessed Nov 11, 2010, at www.nursingsociety.org/aboutus/PositionPapers/Pages/EBN_positionpaper.aspx.
10. Hamer S, Collinson G: *Achieving evidence-based practice: a handbook for practitioners*, ed 2, Edinburgh, 2005, Baillìere Tindall Elsevier.
11. Gugiu PC, Gugiu MR: A critical appraisal of standard guidelines for grading levels of evidence, *Eval Health Prof* 33:233, 2010.
12. Morse JM: Reconceptualizing qualitative evidence, *Qual Health Res* 16:415, 2006.
13. Gilgun JF: The four cornerstones of qualitative research, *Qual Health Res* 16:436, 2006.
14. Haynes RB: Of studies, summaries, synopses, and systems: the "4S" evolution of services for finding current best evidence, *Evid Based Nurs* 8:4, 2005.
15. Closs SJ, Cheater FM: Evidence for nursing practice: a clarification of the issues, *J Adv Nurs* 30:10, 1999.
16. Guyatt G, Oxman AD, Akl EA, et al: GRADE guidelines: 1. Introduction-GRADE evidence profiles and summary of findings tables, *J Clin Epidemiol* 64:383, 2011.
17. American Academy of Family Physicians: *Levels of evidence in AFP.* Accessed Dec 15, 2010, at www.aafp.org/online/en/home/publications/journals/afp/afplevels.html.
18. Phillips B, Ball C, Sackett D, et al: *Levels of evidence.* Accessed Dec 5, 2010, at www.cebm.net.
19. Cesario S, Morin K, Santa-Donato A: Evaluating the level of evidence of qualitative research, *JOGNN* 31:708, 2002.
20. Medical Library Association: *A user's guide to finding and evaluating health information on the web.* Accessed Nov 18, 2010, at www.mlanet.org/resources/userguide.html.
21. Newhouse R, Dearholt S, Poe S, et al: Evidence-based practice: a practical approach to implementation, *J Nurs Adm* 35:35, 2005.
22. Titler MG, Kleiber C, Steelman VJ, et al: The Iowa model of evidence-based practice to promote quality care, *Crit Care Nurs Clin North Am* 13:497, 2001.
23. Shultz M: Comparing test searches in PubMed and Google Scholar, *J Med Libr Assoc* 95:442, 2007.
24. Anders ME, Evans DP: Comparison of PubMed and Google Scholar literature searches, *Respir Care* 55:578, 2010.
25. Stillwell SB, Fineout-Overholt E, Melnyk BM, et al: Asking the clinical question: a key step in evidence-based practice, *Am J Nurs* 110:58, 2010.
26. Fineout-Overholt E, Melnyk BM, Stillwell SB, et al: Critical appraisal of the evidence: part III: the process of synthesis: seeing similarities and differences across the body of evidence, seventh article in a series, *Am J Nurs* 110:43, 2010.
27. Fineout-Overholt E, Melnyk BM, Stillwell SB, et al: Evidence-based practice step by step. Critical appraisal of the evidence: part I: an introduction to gathering, evaluating, and recording the evidence, fifth in a series, *Am J Nurs* 110:47, 2010.
28. Fineout-Overholt E, Melnyk BM, Stillwell SB, et al: Evidence-based practice, step by step. Critical appraisal of the evidence: part II: digging deeper—examining the "keeper" studies, sixth article in a series [corrected] [published erratum appears in *Am J Nurs* 110(11):12, 2010], *Am J Nurs* 110:41, 2010.

29. Stillwell SB, Fineout-Overholt E, Melnyk BM, et al: Evidence-based practice, step by step: searching for the evidence, *Am J Nurs* 110:41, 2010.

30. Melnyk BM, Fineout-Overholt E, Stillwell SB, et al: Evidence-based practice: step by step. The seven steps of evidence-based practice: following this progressive, sequential approach will lead to improved health care and patient outcomes, *Am J Nurs* 110:51, 2010.

31. Melnyk BM, Fineout-Overholt E, Stillwell SB, et al: Evidence-based practice: step by step. Igniting a spirit of inquiry: an essential foundation for evidence-based practice: how nurses can build the knowledge and skills they need to implement ERP, *Am J Nurs* 109:49, 2009.

32. Page A, editor: *Committee on the work environment for nurses and patient safety. Transforming the work environment of nurses,* 2004. Accessed Jan 10, 2010, at www.nap.edu/openbook/php? isbn=030909-679.

33. Oxman AD, Lavis JN, Lewin S, et al: SUPPORT tools for evidence-informed health policymaking (STP) 1: What is evidence-informed policymaking? *Health Res Policy Syst* 7(suppl 1):S1, 2009.

34. Committee on Quality of Health Care in America: Institute of Medicine: *Crossing the quality chasm: a new health system for the 21st century*, Washington, DC, 2001, National Academy Press.

35. American Nurses Association: *Scope and standards of nursing informatics practice*, Washington, DC, 2001, American Nurses Publishing.

36. Barclay L: New guidelines issued on optimal hemoglobin A1C targets for type 2 diabetes, *Medscape Medical News,* Dec 20, 2009. Retrieved from, www.medscape.org/viewarticle/562889.

37. American Diabetes Association: Standards of medical care in diabetes—2011, *Diabet Care* 34(suppl 1):S11, 2011.

38. Bauer JC: Nurse practitioners as an underutilized resource for health reform: evidence-based demonstrations of cost-effectiveness, *J Am Acad Nurse Pract* 22:228, 2010.

Health Care Quality

P.J. Woods

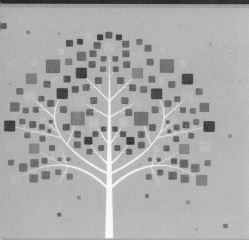

Health care organizations have a duty to the communities they serve for maintaining the quality and safety of care. Health care quality applies within the realm of healthcare delivery in any public or private setting. Whatever structures, systems, and processes an organization establishes, it must be able to show evidence that standards are upheld. Nurses are a crucial link in meeting the needs of patients and ensuring patient safety, medication safety, and communication as part of the health care team. The concept of health care quality is presented here, including concept definitions, concept attributes, error prevention and management, the role of oversight and regulatory bodies, quality plans and philosophies, and the use of health information technology to enhance patient safety.

DEFINITION(S)

The term *quality* in health care has 19 definitions on a single quality dictionary website (http://dictionary.reference.com/browse/quality). This includes definitions from the general meaning that it is merely an attribute of something (like soft or hard), to more specific meanings associated with the degree of excellence or superiority (which, for the purpose of this concept analysis, applies more to how the term is used in health care evaluations).

The importance of quality dates back to Florence Nightingale when she assessed for quality by measuring patient outcomes.[1] Defining quality is difficult because the meaning of "quality" can vary based on context, expectations, and requirements. The expectations of patients, providers, and managers may be different. For example, according to Meade[2] quality care to the patient is determined by the patient's perception of whether he or she received extraordinary service. This is the "wow" factor that makes the organization and the care, according to patients' perspectives, unique and unparalleled among competing facilities. An additional benefit to having superb overall quality according to patients' perspectives is that it leads to improved clinical outcomes.[3]

The provider might consider quality as the effects of medical interventions and scientific knowledge resulting in successful and cost-effective recovery without complications. The nurse at the bedside might view quality as the delivery of safe, caring, and competent care, whereas the nurse manager might see quality as a ratio of volume of care in relation to the available resources, or the score on a patient satisfaction survey. Regardless, the focus should be on providing patients excellent services via competent health care, comprehensive communication, interprofessional teamwork, and cultural sensitivity.[4]

Quality is also both tangible and intangible. The care delivered can be technically perfect, but if the patient does not improve, according to realistic expectations, or is very dissatisfied with the care, it is useless. Although quality can be a perception, a feeling, or an impression, it can also be something measured. Quality health care is competent and cost-effective. It meets the needs of the patient and utilizes the hospital's resources in a cost-effective way. It meets and/or exceeds an established standard. At times, it seems an impossible goal, but one for which we continually strive. For the purposes of this concept analysis, the Institute of Medicine (IOM)[5] definition of quality will be used. The IOM defines quality of care as *the degree to which health services for individuals and populations increase the likelihood of desired health outcomes and are consistent with current professional knowledge.*

SCOPE AND CATEGORIES

Clearly articulating the scope of quality is challenging because of the abstract nature of this concept. However, as a starting point, it might be helpful to think about the scope of quality on a continuum ranging from consistently poor quality and poor outcomes, to perfection—that is, always delivering error-free, high-quality care, resulting in optimal outcomes for every patient (Figure 46-1).

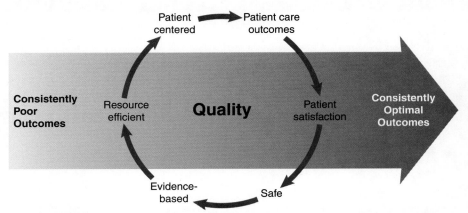

FIGURE 46-1 Scope of Quality: A Continuum of Quality Consistency.

Embedded within this continuum are multiple variables that collectively impact the overall quality including:

- Patient care outcomes
- Patient satisfaction
- Delivery of care based on latest evidence
- Delivery of care that is safe
- Delivery of care that is patient centered
- Effective resource utilization

These variables are highly interrelated, adding to the complexity of this concept. Achievement of expected or benchmarked quality measures is a high-stakes priority for health care recipients and everyone who works in the health care industry.

Quality is a culture that has to begin with leadership and the mission and vision of the organization. The organization's mission and vision should clearly reflect responsibility and accountability for delivering high standards and quality of care and be transparent to the public.[6] Transparency should be viewed as a means to an end. The "end" is a culture of safety in a learning organization that heeds lessons from preventable deaths, adverse harmful events, and performance not consistent with evidence-based standards of care.[7] Transparency is a powerful catalyst for change and serves as a continual feedback loop for improving outcomes in patient care.

Complex, high-reliability organizations (HROs) refer to organizations or systems that operate in hazardous conditions but have fewer than their fair share of adverse events. Examples of these include aviation, air traffic control, nuclear power plants, petrochemical processing, and naval aircraft carriers.[8] These HROs have successfully developed reporting and fixing systems that lead to serious accidents and important near misses. Although none of these industries offers a perfect template for the health care industry, the health care industry must pursue a carefully studied paradigm that eliminates serious injuries.[9] As noted in the 2001 IOM publication *Crossing the Quality Chasm: A New Health System for the 21st Century,*[5] accountability to the public is a quality goal needed to build trust through disclosure. The IOM notes that being transparent is not in conflict with confidentiality nor does it involve open disclosure of errors, but fear of discipline and malpractice suits can impede this goal. The goal of transparency is to have information flow freely for the purpose of mitigating potential errors and allowing patients to make decisions based on all the available information.

ATTRIBUTES

A fundamental attribute inherent in the concept of health care quality is that you cannot improve what you cannot or do not measure. In the same way that nursing students track their grade point averages to determine how well they are doing in school, the health care system uses measures to gauge progress and improve results. Measurement identifies gaps in performance and allows us to gauge the quality of care we deliver. Publicly reporting the results of measurement provides valuable information for patients choosing high-quality providers, purchasers and insurers shaping payment policies based on rewarding quality and efficiency, physicians making referral decisions, and patients recommending a specific health care system to their friends and family.[10]

It is difficult, if not almost impossible, to list or rank all of the many attributes that can identify health care quality or to integrate them to identify a single measure that identifies quality. However, ways to define, categorize, and measure quality have become increasingly important concerns in the era of managed care and cost containment. Most attempts at developing quality indicators have been based on the development of outcome measures.[11] The U.S. Department of Health and Human Services *National Healthcare Quality Report* published in 2009[12] identifies quality health care as a delivery of services that diagnose, treat, and result in improvement of physical and mental well-being of patients of all ages in a way that is safe, timely, patient-centered, efficient, and equitable. The IOM's report *Crossing the Quality Chasm*[5] defines the attributes for quality health care as safe, effective, timely, patient-centered, efficient, and equitable. In *Crossing the Quality Chasm* the IOM states, "The health care environment should be safe for all patients, in all of its processes, all the time."[5,p45] The major criteria associated with these attributes are safe, effective, and efficient care. These major attributes are shown in Table 46-1.

TABLE 46-1   MAJOR ATTRIBUTES OF HEALTH CARE QUALITY

SAFE	EFFECTIVE	EFFICIENT
• Demonstrates knowledge base on health/illness status of individual/groups • Provides sound decision making in care of individuals/groups • Avoids injuries from care that is intended to help your patient • Acts within scope of practice of license or certification • Conforms to standards of practice for both self and patients	• Offers services that address most important • Addresses health problems of most vulnerable groups • Integrates curative and preventive services • Attains high population coverage	• Ensures that transitions between providers, departments, and health care settings are respectful, coordinated, and efficient • Routinely uses information for decision making • Same work is performed with fewer resources • Reduces length of hospital stays (result of increased safety and better scheduling and coordination) • Monitors costs and delivers most effective, cost-effective interventions

In addition, health care quality has minor attributes that include being timely, patient centered, and equitable. When health care is delivered in a timely manner, wait times and harmful delays for both the patient and the provider of care are reduced and care is offered before unnecessary complications occur. Patient-centered care is care that is respectful of and responsive to individual patient preferences, needs, and values and ensures that patient values guide all clinical decisions. It also means treating patients with respect and dignity, focusing first on the patient, caring about the patient, and treating the patient the way you would like to be treated. Equitable care is providing care that does not vary in quality because of gender, ethnicity, geographic location, and socioeconomic status; it strives to serve the underserved and is delivered in a system that allows for exemptions.[5]

THEORETICAL LINKS

Avedis Donabedian[13] defined quality as values and goals present in the medical system and defined outcomes as a validator of the quality and effectiveness of medical care. He stated that examining care processes instead of focusing on outcomes provided a more reliable indicator of the quality of medical care. Donabedian believed there was a framework that included all the various definitions and specifications, including how variations in care occur, or relate to one another, and the consequences they have on measuring, monitoring, and developing quality measurements in health care. This model is depicted in Figure 46-2.

The model identifies ways to define, categorize, and measure quality. This has become increasingly important in the era of managed care and cost containment. Most attempts at developing quality indicators have been based on the development of outcome measures. The framework in the Donabedian model is founded on quality using a three-part procedure: *structure, process,* and *outcomes. Structure* is defined as the attributes of settings where care is delivered. These include the adequacy of facilities, equipment, supplies, staff training, provider knowledge and attitudes, and supervision. The context (structure) in which care is delivered affects processes and outcomes. For example, if the facility is lacking in amenities, wait times are too long, or the providers

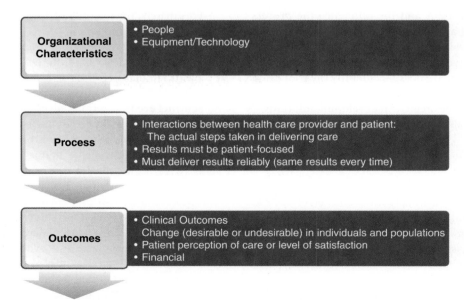

FIGURE 46-2 Donabedian Model of Structure-Process-Outcomes.

and staff are not adequately prepared, people will prefer to avoid the facility. Service *process* dimensions include the services offered, the technical quality of the services (i.e., the staff and providers perform the technical aspects of the task or job), the quality of interpersonal relations, and the adequacy of patient education, access, safety, and promotion of continuity of care (i.e., appropriate referral, follow-up). *Outcomes* are the impact of structure and process on the patient's satisfaction; perceptions of quality, knowledge, attitudes, and behavior; and health outcomes. For example, if a provider or facility is unavailable or if patients do not have accessibility, then the outcome will be a direct result of inadequate access.[13]

The Donabedian model is the most common quality-of-care framework employed and it has been universally accepted and used as the basis for much of the work addressing quality and outcome.[14,15] In the Centers for Medicare & Medicaid Services *Premier Hospital Quality Incentive Demonstration Project*, there are multiple examples that document the positive outcomes that result from implementing certain process-oriented outcome measures.[16]

CONTEXT TO NURSING AND HEALTH CARE

Delivering quality health care and monitoring its outcomes are inherent in all nursing practice environments, and all nurses are responsible for delivering safe, effective, and efficient care. Nurses are the front-line defense against actual and potential risks to patients; this requires an understanding of, and willingness to participate in, measures that promote and ensure the health and safety of patients. This includes being able to identify unsafe practices and respond appropriately to ensure a safe outcome for patients, clients, oneself, and others.

Quality is evaluated on the basis of process and outcomes. Process components include how health care is provided and how the system works. Outcome components include health status and the difference the process made. The following are some of nurses' key objectives in providing quality health care: remember that improving health care quality is your responsibility and that measurement and improvement are possible; identify the root cause before making changes; be proactive and prevent errors before they occur; and be creative in developing solutions.[17] Several aspects of quality, as they apply to nursing practice, are discussed next.

Error Reduction

In health care the stakes are extremely high, more so than any other profession. A seemingly innocuous error such as forgetting to wash your hands or leaving a unit drug cabinet unlocked can have dire, even life-threatening consequences. Obviously, it is not possible to eliminate all errors, but quality efforts are geared to minimize errors. Nurses are central to quality efforts.

According to the IOM,[18] tens, if not hundreds of thousands, of errors occur every day in the U.S. health care system.

BOX 46-1   CLASSIFICATIONS OF SAFETY EVENTS

Never-Miss Event
- Mild variation in standard of care
- Caused by human or system error
- Does not reach the patient
- Does not cause harm
- Use FMEA to analyze causes

Adverse Event
- Moderate variation in standard of care
- Caused by human or system error
- Reaches the patient
- Minimal or no harm
- Use FEMA to analyze causes

Sentinel Event
- Severe variation in standard of care
- Caused by human or system error
- Reaches the patient
- Death or major harm
- Use RCA to analyze causes

A medical error or adverse event is defined as the failure of a planned intervention or action to be completed as intended and includes a variation from the standard of care. This is referred to as an error of execution. These adverse events are caused by someone on the health care team or by a system failure, rather than by the underlying disease or condition of the patient. Another type of error is using the wrong plan to achieve an outcome, which is an error in diagnosis, planning, or delivery of care. As shown in Box 46-1, errors are classified in the following ways:

- **Near miss:** A near miss is an error that could have caused harm to a patient, but did not, as a result of chance, prevention, or some intervention that mitigated the impact. Fortunately, the majority of adverse events that occur are considered near misses.
- **Adverse event:** Some errors result in moderate to severe harm to a patient. One of the most common adverse events familiar to nurses involves medication administration and these are called adverse drug events (ADEs).
- **Sentinel event:** A serious adverse event is called a sentinel event when a patient dies or has a serious, undesirable, and largely avoidable outcome as a result of the error.[19]

Plsek and Greenhalgh[20] define complex adaptive systems (CAS) as a collection of individuals who have freedom to act in ways that are not always predictable and who are interconnected so that small changes can affect other individuals in the CAS. Our current health care system is a perfect example of a CAS. There are multiple relationships that are organized and evolving together to meet patient needs. These relationships are often nonlinear and dependent on individual behavior. Because our health care system is a CAS, medical errors occur as a result of human fallibility compounded by poor system designs that allow for error. It is important to emphasize that medical errors are rarely the result of personal negligence or criminal activity. Whatever the cause, medical errors can have devastating emotional and physical consequences for the patient, the nurse, the health care provider, and the agency or system as a whole.

Quality measures are used to gauge how well a health care entity provides care to its patients. Measures are based on scientific evidence and can reflect guidelines, standards of care, or practice parameters. A quality measure converts medical information from patient records into a rate or percentage that allows facilities to assess their performance (CMS hospital quality indicators, 2007).[21] Error prevention and management quality analysis tools are used to analyze and report quality measures and these include analyzing errors and near misses as well as preventing adverse events in the first place.

Root Cause Analysis

Traditionally, adverse event reporting systems have focused on past events, logging serious events and facilitating root cause analysis (RCA) and the formulation of system improvements. By using RCA, the team can help define the problem, identify risks and protective factors, develop and test prevention strategies, and ensure widespread adoption of system improvements. An RCA is used when a patient has been seriously harmed or has died as a result of a medical error. The importance of RCA is for the team to thoroughly investigate each level of the adverse event in order to identify problems that affect the entire system. Dlugacz and colleagues[6] identified a series of specific questions that dissect the causes of an event to uncover the fundamental flaws in the process, which is important in determining risk points. The RCA is a critical tool to identify the systems that failed during the course of a given patient's care.

Failure Mode Effective Analysis

Failure mode effective analysis (FMEA) is designed to prevent the occurrence of errors or system failures. For example, an FMEA strategy can assist in producing positive results when the goal is decreasing the number of catheter-related bloodstream infections, which is one of the patient safety goals of The Joint Commission (TJC), the American Nurses Association (ANA), and the National Database of Nursing Quality Indicators (NDNQI).[1] The first step is to define the critical problem: maintaining sterile technique with both central line insertion and line maintenance.

- **Potential failure modes** include inappropriate skin preparation, compromised equipment, and outdated procedures and nursing protocols.
- **Analyze causes** of the system failure, such as a break in sterile technique, inadequate size of the sterile field, or lack of standardized catheter insertion kits and/or equipment.
- **Solutions to the problem** can include designing custom catheter insertion kits, providing catheter insertion carts, developing central line insertion checklists,

informing nurses to stop the insertion procedure when there is a break in sterile technique, avoiding the femoral site, standardizing maintenance supplies, requiring daily documentation of need for central line, implementing a central line team, and providing extensive education.[22]
- **Evaluate the results.** Examples include utilizing a central line team review procedure for catheter insertion and maintenance documentation and communicating results of central line infections per 1000 central line days.

Regulatory Agencies

Health care quality has multiple oversight bodies and regulatory agencies that exist to ensure the safety of the public. These regulatory agencies are legitimized through their power to withhold reimbursement such as Medicare or Medicaid if the delivery of patient care does not meet national quality standards. They also license facilities for operation (e.g., specific state licensing regulations) and can fine organizations or restrict services and suspend operations. The agencies you will encounter most often are the Centers for Medicare & Medicaid Services (CMS), The Joint Commission (TJC), and the Occupational Safety and Health Administration (OSHA). In addition to these, examples of other important regulatory agencies that ensure health care quality are the Department of Health and Safety of the U.S. Food and Drug Administration (FDA), the Department of Justice (DOJ), the Office of the Inspector General (OIG), and the Drug Enforcement Administration (DEA), which is part of the DOJ.

Centers for Medicare & Medicaid Services (CMS)

CMS regulates organizations, not nurses specifically. CMS has quality oversight for Medicare and Medicaid reimbursements. The Centers for Medicare & Medicaid Services (CMS) program for Reporting Hospital Quality Data for Annual Payment Update (RHQDAPU) now includes a focus on measuring nursing quality. Beginning October 1, 2010, the CMS requirement includes hospital reporting on whether or not your health care entity participates in a systematic clinical database registry for nursing-sensitive care and will eliminate additional Medicare payments for eight preventable hospital-acquired conditions.[23]

The Joint Commission

Since its founding in 1951, The Joint Commission (TJC)[24] has been acknowledged as the leader in developing the highest standards for quality and safety in the delivery of health care, and evaluating organization performance based on these standards. TJC is also the only accrediting organization with the capability and experience to evaluate health care organizations across the continuum of care. TJC accreditation and certification is recognized nationwide as a symbol of quality that reflects an organization's commitment to meeting certain performance standards.[24] In order for a health care organization to participate in and receive payment from the Medicare and Medicaid programs, it must be certified as complying with the conditions of participation (CoP), or standards, set forth in the CMS regulations. TJC has aligned their scoring practices with these regulations. If an organization does not meet a condition of participation (e.g., restraint and seclusion), they will receive a condition-level deficiency and TJC will conduct a follow-up TJC survey (unannounced). Failure to clear a condition-level deficiency after the second survey results in notification of CMS, and affects the accreditation decision and funding from Medicaid and Medicare if the deficiency is not resolved.[25]

In 2002 The Joint Commission (TJC) established its National Patient Safety Goals (NPSGs) program and the first set of NPSGs was effective January 1, 2003. The NPSGs were established to help accredited organizations address specific areas of concern in regards to patient safety. Development and annual updating of the NPSGs are overseen by an expert panel comprised of patient safety experts, as well as nurses, physicians, pharmacists, and risk managers, for example. The panel of experts works with TJC staff to undertake a systematic review of the literature and available databases to identify potential new NPSGs. The 2011 NPSGs cover nine health care delivery systems and each of these main systems has specific patient safety goals. Examples in ambulatory health care include (a) identify the patient correctly, (b) use medicine safely, (c) prevent infection, and (d) check patient medicines. In each of these goals there are specific measures that the organization must attain. The goals for hospitals are the same as those for ambulatory health care facilities, but also include improve staff communication and identify patient safety risks.[26]

In addition to TJC, students should be aware there are many agencies that provide regulatory oversight such as those identified here. Many facilities have elected to use an alternative agency for accreditation. The following organizations survey and accredit hospitals and health care organizations in the United States. A number of these also have the power to implement Medicare and Medicaid reimbursement.

- Healthcare Facilities Accreditation Program (HFAP)
- The Joint Commission (TJC)
- National Committee for Quality Assurance (NCQA)
- Community Health Accreditation Program (CHAP)
- Accreditation Commission for Health Care (ACHC)
- The Compliance Team, "Exemplary Provider Programs"
- Healthcare Quality Association on Accreditation (HQAA)
- Accreditation Association for Ambulatory Health Care (AAAHC)

Advisory Bodies
The Institute of Medicine

The Institute of Medicine (IOM) is an independent, nonprofit organization that conducts studies and provides unbiased and authoritative advice to improve the nation's health.[18] Many of the studies that the IOM undertakes begin as specific mandates from Congress whereas others are requested by federal agencies and independent organizations. The IOM is best known by nurses for its landmark study *To Err Is Human: Building a Safer Health System,*[27] which may have resulted in increased awareness of U.S. medical errors. The report was followed in 2001 by another widely cited report, *Crossing the Quality Chasm: A New Health System for the 21st Century.*[5] This report urgently mandated change to the health care system processes to improve the level of quality. It analyzed this dilemma, and explored potential ways in which change could be implemented in the health care system to improve outcomes.

The National Quality Forum (NQF)

The NQF is a unique, multistakeholder organization that has been instrumental in advancing efforts to improve quality through performance measurement and public reporting. NQF is a private, nonprofit membership organization with more than 375 members representing virtually every sector of the health care system. NQF has become the "gold standard" for health care performance measures. Major health care purchasers, including CMS, and the ANA rely on NQF-endorsed measures to ensure that the measures are scientifically sound and meaningful and to help standardize performance measures used across the industry. To date, NQF has endorsed more than 500 measures including many of the NDNQI measures.[28]

Nursing-Specific Advisory Bodies

Licensed registered nurses (RNs) are critical participants in our national effort to protect patients from health care errors because the nature of the activities nurses typically perform provides an indispensable resource in detecting and remedying error-producing processes in our health care system. Regulatory agencies recognize the critical nature of the nurse's role in health care quality and there are now oversight and regulatory agencies that specifically track nursing quality performance and outcomes.[29]

The National Database for Nursing Quality Indicators (NDNQI)

The mission of the NDNQI is to aid the registered nurse in patient safety and quality improvement efforts by providing research-based national comparative data on nursing care and its relationship to patient outcomes. NDNQI Indicators® (NDNQI®) is a proprietary database of the American Nurses Association. NDNQI is the only national nursing database that collects and evaluates unit-specific nurse-sensitive indicators and provides quarterly and annual reporting of structure, process, and outcome indicators to evaluate nursing care at the unit level.[30] Table 46-2 shows these specific indicators.

Participating facilities receive unit-level comparative data reports to use for quality improvement purposes. Linkages between nurse staffing levels and patient outcomes have already been demonstrated through the use of this database. Currently more than 1100 facilities in the United States contribute to this growing database, which can now be used to

TABLE 46-2	**NDNQI QUALITY INDICATORS**
Patient Falls (NQF)	RN Education and Certification
Patient Falls with Injury (NQF)	Pediatric Pain Assessment, Intervention, Reassessment (AIR) Cycle
Pressure Ulcers	Health Care–Associated Infections
• Community Acquired (NQF)	• Ventilator-Associated Pneumonia (VAP) (NQF)
• Hospital Acquired (NQF)	• Central Line–Associated Bloodstream Infection (CLABSI) (NQF)
• Unit Acquired	• Catheter-Associated Urinary Infection (NQF)
Skill Mix (NQF)	Pediatric IV Infiltration Rate
Nursing Hours per Patient Day (NQF)	Psychiatric Patient Assault Rate
RN Surveys: Job Satisfaction	Restraint Prevalence (NQF)
Practice Environment Scale (NQF)	Nurse Turnover (NQF)

Data from ANA: *The national database of nursing quality indicators,* 2011.

show the economic implications of various levels of nurse staffing.[1]

The National Center for Nursing Quality (NCNQ)

Created by the American Nurses Association, the NCNQ addresses patient safety and quality in nursing care and nurses' work lives. The center advocates for nursing quality through quality measurement, novel research, and collaborative learning. Issues such as the nursing workforce shortages and impact on patient outcomes are tackled through innovative initiatives, which include the National Database for Nursing Quality Indicators (NDNQI) and Safe Staffing Saves Lives, among others.[29,30,31]

Quality Plans and Philosophies

Health care agencies deliver health care within the context of a quality plan or philosophy designed to reduce the chance of causing harm to a patient. An integral part of these quality systems are error prevention and management strategies. Health care organizations strive for an error-free environment. To develop and maintain the goal of zero errors, many organizations are adopting a culture of safety to ingrain this as their fundamental philosophy of care. The Centers for Disease Control and Prevention (CDC) has defined a culture of safety as the shared commitment of management and employees to ensure the safety of the work environment. The safety of patients and employees is paramount. In a comprehensive literature review, seven subcultures of patient safety culture were identified. They were (a) leadership, (b) teamwork, (c) evidence-based, (d) communication, (e) learning, (f) just, and (g) patient-centered.[32] A culture of safety acknowledges the inevitability of error, and proactively seeks to identify latent threats.[33] The following are characteristics of such a culture:

- Acknowledgment of the high-risk, error-prone nature of an organization's activities
- A blame-free environment where individuals are able to report errors or close calls without fear of reprimand or punishment
- An expectation of collaboration across ranks to seek solutions to vulnerabilities
- A willingness on the part of the organization to direct resources for addressing safety concerns

Plan-Do-Study-Act

All health care entities will have a quality plan or model that they follow. A common model students may see is the plan-do-study-act (PDSA). The original model was developed by Deming and helps a health care team determine if changes they are making will lead to quality improvement. The PDSA cycle includes developing a plan to test the change (plan), trying out the change (do), analyzing what happened from the change (study), and determining what was learned (act). The team then refines the change based on what was learned and then this cycle is repeated. The PDSA cycle is usually done on a small scale so the health care team can quickly find what will provide the best results before they implement a change on a large scale.[34]

Leapfrog Group

The goal of the Leapfrog Group is to make health care safer. It is composed of more than 150 public and private organizations that provide health care. The Leapfrog Group works with medical experts throughout the United States to identify and propose solutions designed to reduce medical errors. It has proposed specific best practices that health care systems can adopt to reduce errors. These include computer physician order entry (CPOE), evidence-based hospital referral, and ICU physician staffing standards.[35] Leapfrog Group has adopted a "never events" policy. Never events are categorized as events that should never occur in the delivery of health care.[35] Leapfrog Group's never events policy requires hospitals to do the following:

- Apologize to the patient and/or family affected by the event.
- Report the event to at least one of the following agencies: The Joint Commission; state reporting program for medical errors; or a patient safety organization.
- Agree to perform a root cause analysis, consistent with instructions from the chosen reporting agency.
- Waive all costs directly related to a serious reportable adverse event.
- Make a copy of the organization's policy available to patients and payers upon request.

Health Information Technology (HIT)

HIT enables organizations to mine the data collected in the delivery of patient care and track performance against established benchmarks more quickly and economically than with manual systems. This speeds adjustments to improve outcomes, regardless of whether they are clinical nursing outcomes, workforce outcomes, patient and consumer outcomes, or organizational outcomes. The RAND Foundation estimates that widespread adoption of various Health Information Technologies could save up to $77 billion annually.[36] HIT structural measures are intended to help providers assess the efficiency and standardization of current HIT systems and identify areas where additional HIT tools can be used.[5] Examples of HIT include the electronic health record (EHR), computerized physician order entry, and medication administration systems.

In *Crossing the Quality Chasm,* the Institute of Medicine[5] emphasized the importance of using HIT to accomplish the following:
- Design care processes based on best practices.
- Translate new clinical knowledge and skills into practice.
- Support the work of multidisciplinary teams.
- Enable the coordination of care across patient conditions, services, and settings.
- Measure and improve performance.

According to the Leapfrog Group in the IOM report *Preventing Medication Errors* one of the survey's main questions concerns whether a hospital utilizes "computer physician order entry." CPOE[35] is an electronic prescribing system that intercepts errors when medications are ordered—before they reach the patient. With CPOE, rates of serious errors can be reduced by nearly 90%[5] because this type of system provides immediate information to physicians (for example, warning them about a potential adverse reaction with the patient's other drugs) (RAND). CPOE is described in *Crossing the*

Quality Chasm as the use of technology to support health care in order to ensure safe and effective care, and the potential for improvement is very significant because "there is growing evidence that automated order entry systems can reduce errors in drug prescribing and dosing."[5] Although CPOE is focused on the physician, the role of the nurse is critical in avoiding errors, especially early in the system's implementation. Berger and Kichack[37] describe an increased number of potential life-threatening errors that were "intercepted" by nurses just before administration that were attributed to "bugs" in the CPOE system's mechanism for ordering potassium infusions (the problem was eliminated after the system was repaired). Examples like this one emphasize the importance of the nurse's adherence to the five rights of medication administration.

INTERRELATED CONCEPTS

This concept represents areas that relate to health care quality. Several concepts featured in this textbook have a relationship with this concept. Health care policy (see **Health policy** concept) is used to provide overarching goals and set priorities for the allocation of valuable health resources. **Health care economics** is concerned with issues related to the scarcity of resources in the allocation of health and health care. **Health care organization** and delivery systems provide the framework for the delivery of health care. The concept **Safety** examines how we prevent accidental injury or harm to patients, and **Technology and informatics** provides tools to help deliver quality health care. These interrelationships are depicted in Figure 46-3.

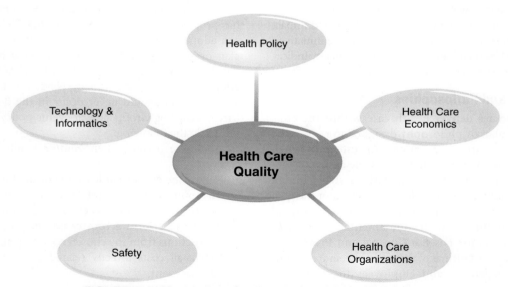

FIGURE 46-3 Health Care Quality and Interrelated Concepts.

MODEL CASE

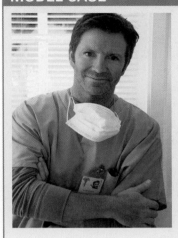

Matt had been assigned the task of creating a program to take the primary responsibility for cardiac monitoring away from the nursing units by creating a centralized monitoring station. This decision was made following a root cause analysis conducted for a death on one of the subintensive nursing units attributable to a missed lethal cardiac rhythm. This miss resulted not only in the loss of the patient but also in the near mental breakdown of the secretary and RN involved. As if these outcomes were not bad enough, the hospital was striving for a culture of safety and believed in transparency; therefore the policy was to inform the patient or family when a mistake had occurred. This rightfully resulted in a lawsuit that was quickly settled for the maximum allowable limits per state law.

Because of the severity of the outcome as well as the cost to the organization, a root cause analysis (RCA) was done. The root cause analysis determined the central monitor screens for the cardiac units were at the nurses' stations, giving them primary responsibility for oversight. However, the RNs were so busy that the unit secretaries were eventually trained to watch the monitors because they sat at the desk where the monitors were located.

The unit secretaries were also very busy taking orders, answering phones, accessing lab results, and performing the other duties of their jobs. This made having a constant eye on the cardiac monitors impossible, resulting in inconsistent monitoring, reporting, and follow-up related to monitor alarms. During the root cause analysis it was determined that the nurses did not intend the secretaries to be the only pair of eyes on the monitors and had every intention of being closely involved. To that end, the secretaries were instructed to notify the RN of any monitor alarm and it was the nurse's responsibility to respond.

When the nurses assigned the responsibility to the secretaries, they became complacent of their primary responsibility to ensure someone observed, reported, and responded to any alarm. In the case of the death, the secretary had learned to silence the monitors once she had alerted the nurse because the noise was overwhelming at the already noisy nursing station. During the root cause analysis, the secretary reported, "I had seen the nurses do it all the time because they often complained that patients turning over could cause the alarms to go off." This statement was corroborated by the nursing staff and they admitted they often instructed the secretaries to, "Shut it off," based on their having just been in the patient's room several times for monitor alarms and the patient was fine.

On this particular day, the monitor was alarming and the secretary told the nurse as usual, but on her way to the patient's room, the nurse was called to an emergency at the other end of the hall. This prevented her from checking the patient immediately. The alarm had continued to alert, but the secretary silenced the alarm on two subsequent times once she had notified the nurse, thinking it had been addressed. The patient had been in ventricular fibrillation and died before the nurse returned to the room. A root cause analysis also looks at problems from a system-wide perspective, and reviews all incident reports for any related cases. During the investigation, it was discovered there had been an additional five other incident reports filed for similar problems over the past 2 years, including two near-death cases.

In a review of these incident reports, it was documented that the solution to the early problems had been to train the secretaries as a backup because the nurses and patient care technicians (PCTs) were often in the hallways or in patients' rooms. Therefore, they saw or heard the majority of alarms first hand. It was believed that having someone who was always near the monitors and who could watch them and report alarms to the nurses would solve the problem. It became clear, based on the recent death, that a more drastic solution was needed. The committee analyzed several proposed solutions, and decided that having a centralized monitor room separate from the nursing station monitors was the best solution. It would be staffed with monitor techs 24 hours a day, 7 days a week; these techs would serve as first eyes, leaving the unit secretary and RNs as backup second eyes. In addition to the centralized monitor room, the ability to silence a monitor was removed from the central unit at the nurses' station, so the alarm could only be silenced by an RN at the patient's bedside to ensure someone had seen the patient before silencing the alarm. Finally, in the event of a lethal alarm, the monitor room techs would call a code blue before phoning the nursing unit.

Case Analysis

This model case illustrated a system failure that did not meet the major attributes of health care quality of being safe, effective, and efficient. In addition, according to Figure 46-2 this error would be classified as a sentinel event because there was a severe variation in the standard of care caused by both human error and system error. This error reached the patient and resulted in death. Finally, an RCA was done to analyze the causes and corrections were made to ensure this could not happen again.

◼◼◼ BOX 46-2   EXEMPLARS OF QUALITY

Regulatory Agencies
- Centers for Medicare & Medicaid Services (CMS)
- The Joint Commission (TJC)

Advisory Bodies
- Association for Healthcare Research and Quality (AHRQ)
- Institute of Medicine (IOM)
- National Center for Nursing Quality (NCNQ)
- National Quality Forum (NQF)

Quality Plans and Philosophies
- Baldrige
- Culture of safety

- Magnet designation
- Plan-do-study-act (PDSA)
- Six sigma
- Total quality improvement

Error Prevention Management
- Failure mode effective analysis (FMEA)
- Root cause analysis (RCA)

Health Information Technology
- Computerized physician order entry (CPOE)
- Electronic health records (EHRs)
- Medication administration systems

EXEMPLARS

In the United States, nurses can expect to encounter health care quality in any setting and whenever they interact with a patient. Nurses will encounter regulations and standards that their health care entity must meet along with nurse-sensitive indicators for which they are personally responsible. All health care entities will have an error prevention strategy and tool to classify and manage errors, will be based on quality plans and philosophies, and will be involved in the use of health information technology to enhance patient safety. A sample of some of the more visible and relevant examples of these categories that direct and influence care delivery by nurses is listed in Box 46-2.

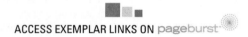

ACCESS EXEMPLAR LINKS ON pageburst

REFERENCES

1. Montalvo I: The National Database of Nursing Quality Indicators (NDNQI), *OJIN: Online J Issues Nurs* 12(3), 2007, manuscript 2, Sept 30.
2. Meade C: *Alliance for health care research organizational change processes in high performing organizations: in-depth case studies with health care facilities, 2003.* Retrieved Feb 20, 2011, from www.studergroup.com/content/ahc_research/associated_files/ahcr_study_final.pdf.
3. Chilgren A: Managers and the new definition of quality, *J Healthcare Manag* 53(4):221–229, 2008.
4. Wharam JF, Sulmasy D: Improving the Quality of Health Care, *JAMA* 310(2):215–217, 2009. doi: 10.1001/jama.2008.964.
5. Institute of Medicine: *Crossing the quality chasm: a new health system for the 21st century, Committee on Quality of Health Care in America,* Washington, DC, 2001, National Academies Press.
6. Dlugacz YD, Restifo A, Greenwood A: *The quality handbook for health care organizations,* San Francisco, Calif, 2004, Jossey-Bass.
7. Swensen SJ, Cortese DA: Transparency and the "End Result Idea," *Chest* 133(1):233–235, 2008.
8. Reason J: Human error: models and management, *BMJ* 320(7237):768–770, 2000.

9. Paterick ZR, Paterick BB, Waterhouse BE, et al: The challenges to transparency in reporting medical errors, *J Pt Safety* 5(4):205–209, 2009.
10. National Quality Forum: *Measuring performance, n.d.* Retrieved Jan 7, 2011, from www.qualityforum.org/.
11. McCabe S: Academy for Health Services Research and Health Policy. Meeting, *Abstr Acad Health Serv Res Health Policy Meet.* 2000; 17: UNKNOWN.
12. U.S. Department of Health and Human Services: Agency for Healthcare Research and Quality, *National Healthcare Quality Report,* 2009. AHRQ Pub No. 10–0003. Retrieved from www.ahrq.gov/qual/nhqr09/nhqr09.pdf.
13. Donabedian A: Quality assessment and monitoring: retrospect and prospect, *Eval Health Prof* 6(3):63–75, 1983.
14. Donabedian A: *The methods and findings of quality assessment and monitoring: an illustrated analysis,* Ann Arbor, Mich, 1985, Health Administration Press.
15 Donabedian A: The quality of care: how can it be assessed? *JAMA* 260(12):1743–1748, 1988.
16. Centers for Medicare & Medicaid Services: *Hospital quality initiatives,* 2007. Retrieved Jan 7, 2010, from www.cms.gov/hospitalqualityinits/01_overview.asp20.
17. Duke University Medical Center: *Patient safety-quality improvement. What is quality improvement?* 2005. Retrieved Jan 17, 2011, from http://patientsafetyed.duhs.duke.edu/module_a/module_summary.html.
18. Institute of Medicine: *About the IOM,* 2010. Retrieved Jan 15, 2011, from http://iom.edu/.
19. Aspden P, Corrigan JM, editors: *Patient safety: achieving a new standard for care,* Washington, DC, 2003, IOM, National Academies Press.
20. Plsek P, Greenhalgh T: The challenge of complexity in health care, *Br Med J* 323(7313):625–628, 2001.
21. U.S. Department of Health and Human Services, Centers for Medicare and Medicaid Services: *Hospital Quality Initiatives, Quality Measures.* Retrieved Oct 30, from https://www.cms.gov/HospitalQualityInits/20_OutcomeMeasures.asp.
22. Bereholtz SM, Pronovost PJ, Lipsett PA, et al: Eliminating catheter-related bloodstream infections in the intensive care unit, *Crit Care Med* 32(10):2014–2020, 2004.
23. Kurtzman E, Buerhaus P: New Medicare payment rules: danger or opportunity for nursing? *Am J Nurs* 108(6):30–35, 2008. Retrieved Feb 13, 2011, from www.nursingcenter.com/library/JournalArticle.asp?Article_ID=798117.

24. The Joint Commission: *About The Joint Commission.* Retrieved Jan 4, 2011, from www.jointcommission.org/about_us/about_the_joint_commission_main.aspx.

25. Brown A: Deciphering TJC condition-level findings, *Hosp Accred Compl J,* May 19, 2011. Retrieved from www.compass-clinical.com/hospital-accreditation/2011/05/deciphering-tjc-condition-level-findings/.

26. The Joint Commission: *National patient safety goals,* 2011. Retrieved Jan 2, 2011, from www.jointcommission.org/standards_information/npsgs.aspx.

27. Institute of Medicine: *To err is human: building a safer health system, Committee on Quality of Health Care in America,* Washington, DC, 2001, National Academies Press.

28. National Institute of Standards and Technology: *Health care criteria for performance excellence.* Retrieved Feb 14, 2009, from http://www.baldrige.nist.gov/PDF_files/2009_2010_HealthCare_Criteria.pdf.

29. Centers for Medicare & Medicaid Services, Office of the Actuary, National Health Statistics Group: *Historical data from CY 1960–2008; projected data from NHE projections 2009–2018.* Available at www.cms.hhs.gov/NationalHealthExpendData/.

30. ANA: *The national database of nursing quality indicators,* 2011. Retrieved Jan 8, 2011, from www.nursingworld.org/MainMenu Categories/ANAMarketplace/ANAPeriodicals/OJIN/TableofContents/Volume122007/No3Sept07/NursingQualityIndicators.aspx.

31. ANA: *Safe staffing saves lives—ANA's national campaign to solve the nurse staffing crisis,* 2011. Retrieved Jan 8, 2011, from www.safestaffingsaveslives.org/.

32. Sammer K, Lykens K, Singh K, Maines D, Nuha L: What is a patient culture? A review of the literature, *J Nurs Scholarsh* 42(2):156–155, 2010.

33. Pizzi L, Goldfarb D, Nash D: *Making health care safer: a critical analysis of patient safety practices. Committee on Quality of Health Care in America,* Washington, DC, 2001, IOM National Academies Press.

34. Institute for Healthcare Improvement: *Plan-do-study-act (PDSA) Woorksheet.* Retrieved June 2, 2011, from www.ihi.org/IHI/Topics/Improvement/ImprovementMethods/Tools/Plan-Do-Study-Act%20%28PDSA%29%20Worksheet.

35. The Leapfrog Group: *Time to recommit to preventing "never events,"* 2010. Retrieved Jan 8, 2011, from www.leapfroggroup.org/news/leapfrog_news/4783929?o4750968=.

36. RAND Foundation: *Health information technology: can HIT lower costs and improve quality?* 2005. Retrieved Jan 6, 2011, from www.rand.org/pubs/research_briefs/2005/RAND_RB9136.pdf.

37. Berger RG, Kichack BA: Computerized physician order entry: helpful or harmful? *Am Med Informatics Assoc* 11(2):100–103, 2004.

47

Care Coordination

Janet Prvu Bettger

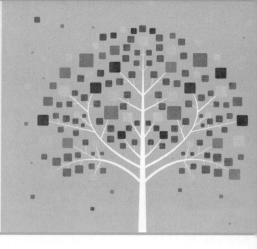

Care coordination is a central component of service delivery because of its role in attaining optimal patient outcomes and health care quality. It is recognized as essential for organizing care and information around patients' needs and preferences.[1,2] Although it is now a focal point of health care policy and research, care coordination was not as prominent before the turn of the century. Implementation of the advances in technology and renewed commitment to patient-centered and family-focused care have increased the visibility of this concept. Care coordination is now a top priority for health system redesign.[3] However, the concept in practice is still evolving and, in some settings, still emerging. Without the adoption of care coordination models, fragmented service delivery, cost inefficiencies, and poor health outcomes will continue. This concept analysis explores the defining characteristics, attributes, and theory supporting care coordination, highlighting clinical exemplars and other related concepts.

DEFINITION(S)

A 2007 systematic review of care coordination published by the Agency for Healthcare Research and Quality identified more than 40 definitions of care coordination and related terminology.[4] A universally accepted definition of care coordination does not yet exist. However, several professional organizations and consensus bodies have endorsed definitions to guide practice and measurement. As a professional organization, the American Academy of Pediatrics made one of the earliest efforts to define this concept.[5] With a focus on children with special health care needs, care coordination was presented as a process connecting both services and resources and involving patients, providers, and families, with the goals of both optimal health care and optimal patient outcomes. These core themes provided an important foundation for definitions developed in the years to follow.

Definitions of care coordination in the peer-reviewed and gray literature vary by the population and care environments

of focus. Several are provided here as examples. The National Coalition on Care Coordination was formed in 2008 to promote better coordinated health and social services for older adults with multiple chronic conditions; the emphasis of their definition is on a "client-centered and assessment-based interdisciplinary approach" across settings and providers to coordinate medical and supportive services over time.[6] Discussions of care coordination for persons with mental illness suggest services also be coordinated across people and sites, functions, and activities.[7] From the perspective of the Veterans Health Administration, care coordination is meant to match every veteran's disease-specific needs with the resources available.[8] For the purposes of directing measurement, the National Quality Forum endorsed a definition focused on patient's needs and preferences for health services over time but also explicitly acknowledged the role of information sharing across people, functions, and sites of care.[9]

Review of the definitions of care coordination developed thus far reveals several core components. The identification of these is important to be able to consider the types and attributes of care coordination and the theory that supports this concept in practice. Guided by the 2007 systematic review and the evolution of the concept to date, care coordination can be defined as *a set of activities purposefully organized by a team of personnel that includes the patient, to facilitate the appropriate delivery of the necessary services and information to support optimal health and care across settings and over time.*

SCOPE AND CATEGORIES

Several variations of care coordination models have emerged to improve care, promote health and independence, and reduce unnecessary service utilization. To understand and evaluate the different types, it is important to recognize that people—our patients and consumers—live and have needs beyond the health care system. Health care services are just one component in our society of services supporting health. Care coordination for some people may also require the knowledge and organization of social services such as those in sectors of education, employment, and the community from housing to utilities, transportation, or insurance of all types. When considering a person's needs that may fall in these different arenas, the different care coordination models include social models, medically oriented models, and integrated models of both social and medical services (Figure 47-1). Each model type is described next, and although social and medically oriented models are distinctly separate from one another, integrated models incorporate aspects of both models and can be differentiated by the level of influence of each model.

Social Models

Care coordination models first emerged to manage home and community-based services and usually did not address medical care. For children and teens the model would include school-based services. Adults also occasionally require these or other traditional vocational programs when returning to work. Elderly individuals or financially disadvantaged families may require utilities assistance programs or have other housing needs that range from finding a home to making the home arrangement safe and accessible. Food and meal services are organized at the community level from shelters, to drop-in programs, to home delivery, or can be facilitated at the state level with vouchers and food stamps. State programs also support local organization and facilitation of transportation, insurance, and disability-related services. Health care needs are sometimes also addressed by a variety of community programs, particularly for people who have become disconnected from a regular source of care. However, the care provided in social models is usually to support activities of daily living rather than skilled care. Although services in a social model vary based on need, the models are organized to offer information, referral, screening and assessment, planning, authorization, and monitoring.[10]

Leadership and organizing responsibility for social models of care coordination can be at the local or state level. For example, Area Agencies on Aging are often designated as coordinators and administrators of care coordination programs that can then be standardized at some level across a state. County social service agencies also assume care coordination responsibilities and are often able to serve as a single entity for multiple funding sources such as waiver services, block grants, state-funded services, and Medicaid. Having a single entity coordinate all relevant social services can reduce the likelihood of redundancy and duplication of efforts. Advances in technology and electronic social networking interfaces will continue to facilitate opportunities for partnership and referral to social services. Social models of care coordination are an important part of promoting health and independence in the community.

Medically Oriented Models

Medical models coordinate medical services and were traditionally designed to be diagnosis specific. As health systems have evolved, so have medical models of care coordination. New models have emerged as payers and providers of health services are needed by individuals for coordination of multiple treatments and visits for multiple conditions. The infrastructure and attributes vary more because of funding and financing than because of locale and geography, as seen with community and social programs. Financing medical models further challenges the ability to coordinate care across settings (e.g., hospital to skilled nursing facility to assisted living) as well as over time. Managed care has been the most stable vehicle to support coordination across settings and payers, particularly for individuals with complex conditions that increase the risk of hospitalization and adverse outcomes.

Provider initiatives for Medicare beneficiaries are most common in the literature on medical models of care coordination.

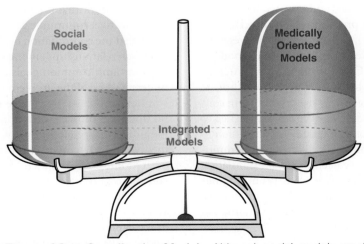

FIGURE 47-1 Types of Care Coordination Models. Although social models are distinctly different from medically oriented care coordination models, integrated models address both the social and the medical or health needs of individuals. Some integrated models support a greater focus on health needs and others are more socially focused, tipping the scale of service coordination to one side or another. This balance may be driven by person and family need, by resource availability, or by the structure and organization of the care coordination model.

There are several types and most are limited models targeting either a specific disease or patient population, a specific setting of care, or a prespecified amount of time. Examples of these include pharmacist-supported models focused on medication management,[11-14] and self-management programs designed to empower patients to actively manage their own health needs.[15] Models more common in practice and with a stronger evidence base include disease management programs that supplement primary care for ambulatory-based conditions such as heart failure or diabetes,[16] and case management models that collaborate with primary care to support patients in navigating available services.[17] Although each of these provider-driven medical models is supported with randomized controlled trials yielding positive patient and health service outcomes, providers and patients have come to realize the limitations of addressing only the medical needs of patients and their families.

Integrated Models

Models committed to the integration of health care, social support, and community clinical and nonclinical services are still evolving. They offer significant promise for supporting holistic, patient-centered, family-focused care, but building bridges between services and settings is fraught with barriers. In the United States, most challenges stem from having the different service types financed from different sources. Coordination is only further complicated by the scope of authority for managing the different services and the level of involvement of each agency or organization. An example might be the need to coordinate services across community programs supported philanthropically, social services supported with government financing, and medical services supported by a health system. It can also be difficult to determine the setting in which the coordination should reside and ultimately the relationship or nature of the partnership that should exist between agencies and service organizations. Fully integrated models need to be able to coordinate a full range of services across settings and over time; they should also be funded and financed by different entities and inclusive of service providers (both clinicians and nonclinical community leaders), patients, and their caregivers.

A well-documented example of a fully integrated model is the Program for All Inclusive Care for the Elderly (PACE).[18] The PACE program is provider based and integrates both acute and long-term health care and social services. Working in contract with Medicare and Medicaid, the program is designed to support people age 55 and older who qualify for admission to a nursing home but prefer to continue residing in the community. Other integrated models have been tested but translation to practice will take time because evidence is promising but limited. These include interprofessional primary care models, outpatient comprehensive geriatric assessment programs, and geriatric evaluation and management programs.[19]

ATTRIBUTES AND CRITERIA

Analysis of this concept yielded a definition of care coordination that states a set of activities be purposefully organized by a team of personnel that includes the patient, to facilitate the appropriate delivery of the necessary services and information to support optimal health and care across settings and over time. This definition facilitates the discussion of attributes into specific components as outlined in Table 47-1.[4-7,10,20-23] Although evidence is mounting in favor of care coordination programs benefiting patients, the 2007 technical review for the Agency for Healthcare Research and Quality found evidence about key intervention components to still be lacking.[4] Intervention descriptions from randomized controlled trials and consensus recommendations in the gray literature converge on five key attributes of care coordination:

- An interprofessional team of personnel that includes the patient
- A proactive plan of care
- A targeted set of purposeful activities
- Proactive follow-up
- Communication

THEORETICAL LINKS

The literature on organizational theory provides useful insights for addressing the interactions and relationships among organizations that are required for effective delivery of care coordination in complex situations. An exhaustive review of relevant theories is less important than understanding the applicability of organizational theory in supporting the concept of care coordination. Perhaps most useful is review of a theory that captures the primary attributes for the concept and describes how these attributes relate to one another.

Relational Coordination Theory is a relatively new theory that originated from studies of aviation. Independent of an industry, the theory guides understanding of the "relational dynamics of coordinating work" reliant on task integration.[24] It stresses the importance of the interaction of two distinct aspects of work that are very relevant for care coordination to be effective: communication and relationships. The theory states that the coordination of work is most effectively carried out when relationships among participants are respectful, oriented around common goals, and function with a common understanding of the problem and knowledge of the goals. In addition, processes to achieve these goals are most successful when communication among and between participants in the process is frequent, timely, and accurate.[25,26] In Gittell's theory, it is hypothesized that the *relational* dimensions (shared knowledge, shared treatment goals, mutual respect, and shared problem solving) are influenced and reinforced by *communication* dimensions (frequency, timeliness, and accuracy of communication between and among participants in the care delivery process). Although several health service studies have explored the relational aspects of coordination, these have focused on specific populations or providers.[27-29] The theory is, however, emerging as an important foundation for supporting the translation of care coordination trials to practice. Empirical studies of care coordination interventions are often not funded to undergo extensive evaluation

TABLE 47-1   ATTRIBUTES OF INTEGRATED CARE COORDINATION MODELS AND A BRIEF DESCRIPTION

ATTRIBUTE	DESCRIPTION
Interprofessional team of personnel that includes patient	• Team based and interprofessional • Inclusive of patient and ideally patient's designated supports • Trusting interaction among "team" members • Shared and appreciated understanding of roles • Clinical integration and interdependence • Central point of contact (a person, partnership of providers, agency or organization) responsible for continuity of care and management of all other attributes • Primary or designated "coordinator" either as centralized contact or as point of access: randomized controlled trials have identified nursing as most common clinical discipline in this role, followed by social workers and pharmacists
Proactive plan of care	• Created, documented, executed, and updated with every patient • Comprehensive: includes community and nonclinical services as well as health care services that respond to patient's needs and preferences and contribute to achieving patient's goals. • Developed and shared across providers and patient's network of support • Revise as needed
Targeted activities	• Identify patients most likely to benefit* • Patient-centered and family-focused • Individual's needs, preferences, and risks assessed • In-person and telephone contact • Following evidence-based standards of care including evidence-based referrals • Shared decision making • Clear goals and shared goal setting • Teach and coach patient to promote self-care skills and independence • Link service systems with patient and caregivers • Avoid duplication and unnecessary cost • Health care includes health promotion, acute and chronic conditions
Proactive follow-up	• Systematic process of surveillance, evaluation, and monitoring of both patient and process, including follow-up assessments, tests, treatments, or services and informed by plan of care
Communication	• Information exchanged across services and members of team before and after each interaction • Standardized communication template of a minimal set of core data elements accessible to patient, caregivers, and all providers during transitions of care • Electronic record system to allow timely access to plan of care and data for all involved and at all points in time with efficient and effective integration of patient information, laboratory data, imaging results, referrals, medications, social and community services, and self-management support; support for quality improvement and safety; evidence-based decision support tools; provider alerts; and patient reminders
Coordination across settings, hand-offs	• Comprehensive in-hospital planning, home-based visits, and telephone follow-up to ensure continuity over transitions in care

*Explained more fully under Context to Nursing and Health Care.

and documentation of the interactions, communication, and relationships. Thus, planning translation and investigating implementation using relational coordination theory as the foundation will help identify the specific processes that facilitate positive outcomes.

CONTEXT TO NURSING AND HEALTH CARE

Care coordination is important for everyone. Over the life course, everyone will have at least a temporary need for improved coordination and communication between providers, settings, or periods of time during an illness. Thus, everyone is at risk for, at a minimum, an episodic illness with at least temporary needs for care coordination. However, the structure of health care in the United States today and the workforce supporting it does not allow for everyone to be supported by a fully integrated care coordination program or model of service delivery.

The general population needs to be stratified based on risk and need (Figure 47-2). To best support those in greatest need, care coordination may need to be reserved for those individuals particularly vulnerable to fragmented, uncoordinated care on a chronic basis and at highest risk of negative health outcomes. At this time, as evidence amounts and the translation, adoption, adaptation, and implementation of care coordination models is accepted across the country, the priority population will need to be those most vulnerable and frail. This may include a targeted

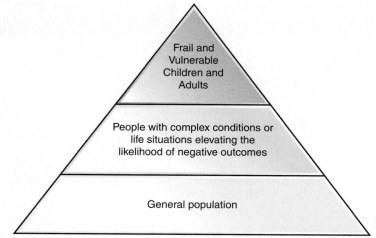

FIGURE 47-2 Stratification of the Population by Need and Likelihood of Positive Outcomes.

focus on serving children with special health care needs, the frail elderly population, and people at the end of life before other high-risk populations. People in the second tier of risk and need for care coordination are those individuals with complex conditions or life situations elevating the likelihood of negative outcomes, including people with cognitive impairments, complex medical or mental health conditions, disabilities, low incomes, or unstable health insurance coverage. Unfortunately, it is only a matter of time before the latter high-risk group will also become vulnerable and in greater need and the risk increases for people in the general population.

The paradigm shift in health care financing and delivery of holistic patient-centered, family-focused care is facing resistance, and as a result people in need are not benefiting from a structured model of care known to produce positive outcomes. It will take time and continued research to fully implement care coordination for everyone, at all levels of need and in all communities. Until then, care coordination is best reserved for those most likely to benefit: vulnerable and frail children and adults.

INTERRELATED CONCEPTS

Care coordination is a generic term that is sometimes used interchangeably both with specific types, such as case or disease management, and with related concepts that share a subset of defining attributes. The most closely related concepts and the ways they distinctly differ from care coordination are discussed next and illustrated in Figure 47-3.

Collaboration is an important interrelated concept of care coordination but the precise overlap is unclear. Defined as trusting interaction among providers, and in some cases extended to include patients and families, collaboration can only be fully realized when these interactions include a shared understanding of goals and roles, supported with effective communication that stimulates shared decision making.[7] Each of these elements is important for care coordination but other attributes are also

necessary. Collaboration is a concept presented in greater detail in this textbook.

Interprofessional. Another important attribute of care coordination is for the care to be team based and interprofessional. Use of the term "interprofessional" does not specify the composition of the team or that the team be formal, informal, or virtual. It instead implies an underlying process that people representing two or more disciplines communicate frequently with each other in an effort to provide comprehensive care.[19] These elements are especially important to the care coordination concept because they direct attention to both the likely need of several disciplines and also the interdependence among disciplines. Although also related to collaboration, interprofessional alone is not enough to support care coordination.

Transitional Care. The defining characteristics of transitional care interventions are all recognized as specific attributes of care coordination. The major factor distinguishing the two concepts is time. Transitional care, defined as "a set of actions designed to ensure the coordination and continuity of health care as patients transfer between different locations or different levels of care within the same location," is a time-limited intervention that does not include extensive follow-up.[30] This particular type of care supporting transitions and hand-offs is a component or subpart of care coordination.[31]

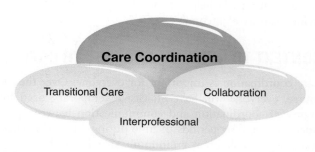

FIGURE 47-3 Care Coordination and Interrelated Concepts.

MODEL CASE

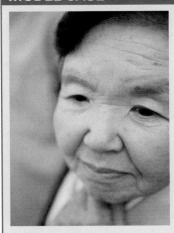

Mrs. Haung is an 83-year-old-widow who lives alone in a rurally located one-level home. Her daughter, a single mother of three, lives nearby and visits weekly. It is mid-winter and Mrs. Haung has been indoors more than usual because of cold weather. She has been experiencing more generalized arthritis pain, which has changed her functional level and usual daily activities. The increased pain in her hands gives her trouble opening cans and bottles and holding a fork. Mrs. Haung no longer cooks, and when she makes her own meals she generally eats soup, toast, and fruit. Her daughter usually delivers hot meals but the seasonal road conditions have interfered. Mrs. Haung also has increased pain in her hips, knees, and back, resulting in changes in her mobility. Somebody at her church suggested using a cane. She tried her husband's old cane with some success but he was a taller person than Mrs. Haung. She recently ran out of her prescription for Lasix. She called to get it refilled but has not been able to get to the store to pick it up and does not want to bother anyone else. No delivery service available.

A neighbor noticed the newspaper still on the driveway one morning, and after no response at the front door, he used the hidden key to go inside to check on Mrs. Haung. She was found on the floor, just outside of the bathroom, lying in a pool of urine. Mrs. Haung was awake, but frightened, embarrassed, and annoyed. She clearly communicated that she had tripped and fell on the way to the bathroom during the night and could not get up. She decided to sleep on the floor because she "hurt all over" and had trouble with her right leg when she tried to move. The neighbor called the daughter and then emergency medical services for transport to the local community hospital.

An advanced practice nurse (APN) with training in geriatric syndromes visited Mrs. Haung in the emergency department while she was waiting for x-rays. The APN teamed with a social worker to fully assess the acute and chronic situation and develop a plan of care. A hospital admission was averted with a visit by physical therapy to assess for assistive mobility devices and with a referral for a home safety evaluation in the next 24 hours by occupational therapy to determine Mrs. Haung's level of functioning in the home and her need for durable medical equipment. The social worker organized home-based services including companion care, meal service, and transportation to the area's senior center and church. Medications were ordered by the APN in bulk to be sent by mail and a home visit by a primary care provider from the local clinic was to take place within the week. Mrs. Haung's daughter drove her home and the social worker called later that evening to follow-up. Contact between the social worker and APN with Mrs. Haung continued daily for the first week until all new services and arrangements were in place. A lifeline system was installed in Mrs. Haung's home should she fall again and need to contact someone more easily, now from the wristband she wore. Contact tapered to monthly until the APN noticed in the electronic health record that Mrs. Haung had not renewed her prescription and cancelled transportation to church the previous Sunday. A quick call revealed that Mrs. Haung had indeed forgotten to renew the prescription and did not attend church because she was out of town.

Case Analysis

This model case illustrates how Mrs. Haung's preferences and needs are recognized in a plan of care and met by a team of providers and services spanning health care and community-based programs supported by ongoing communication and follow-up. The case highlights the involvement of Mrs. Haung's family and social network even before the hospitalization—for example, the daughter providing hot meals when possible, the neighbor knowing where a key was hidden to gain access and fortunately find Mrs. Haung, and Mrs. Haung expressing some affiliation with a place of worship. Although her age, social isolation, pain, and functional decline had not previously alerted health care providers of the need for coordinated care, the emergency department visit provided access to an existing model of care delivery organized by the community hospital and led by an APN with training in geriatric syndromes who worked in conjunction with a social worker.

This case presents an integrated care coordination model that spans across settings, from the emergency department and into the community. Although this appears to be an APN/social worker team model that addressed both social and medical needs, other clinical specialists were accessible and involved in this case to prevent a hospital admission and support the transition back home. Community services were newly engaged to facilitate improved social and spiritual connectedness, adequate nutrition, and medication compliance. Each service filled a preexisting need but had not been referred or provided under the traditional model of primary care available and accessed by Mrs. Haung.

Communication was a key component of this case and needs to be in care coordination models. Not only were the APN and social worker in contact with one another and routinely in contact with Mrs. Haung but also an electronic health record was actively monitored for deviations from her plan of care and a device was added to the home to increase accessibility to emergency responders. Although not all attributes are fully presented in Mrs. Haung's case (Table 47-1), it is clear that this model of care delivery better suits her needs, particularly while she is at high risk for negative health outcomes.

> ### ■■■ BOX 47-1   EXEMPLARS OF CARE COORDINATION*
>
> **Social Models**
> - Adult vocational programs
> - Area Agencies on Aging
> - Disability-related services
> - School-based services
>
> **Medically Oriented Models**
> - Pharmacist-supported models[11-14]
> - Self-management programs[15]
> - *Disease management[16,32]
> - Patient navigation services[17]
>
> **Integrated Models**
> - Program for All Inclusive Care for the Elderly (PACE)[18]
> - *Guided care[33]
> - *Geriatric Resources for Assessment Care of Elders (GRACE)[34,35]
> - *Nurse case management[36,37]
> - *Senior life management[38]
> - Patient-centered medical home[39]

*Any of these models may employ a nurse as the designated "coordinator." The models indicated with an asterisk, however, are evidence-based nurse-led models tested in randomized controlled trials.

EXEMPLARS

Effective models of care coordination continue to emerge but the translation into practice has been slow. Few models developed in practice have rigorously evaluated the impact of care coordination on outcomes. Informal caregiving is one particular example of care coordination that may function as any one of the three types described in this concept but has little empirical research to confirm the presence of specific attributes of care coordination models. For this reason it is not explicitly listed in the exemplars of Box 47-1. The exemplars in Box 47-1 are organized to provide examples of each model type: social, medically oriented, and integrated. Randomized controlled trials with positive outcomes resulting from care coordination models led by nurses are also specifically noted.[32-38]

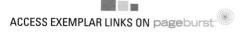

ACCESS EXEMPLAR LINKS ON pageburst

REFERENCES

1. Davis K: *Transformation change: a ten point strategy to achieve better health care for all*, New York, 2004, The Commonwealth Fund.
2. Institute of Medicine: *Crossing the quality chasm: a new health system for the 21st century*, Washington, DC, 2001, National Academies Press.
3. Adams K, Greiner AC, Corrigan JM: *The first annual crossing the quality chasm summit: a focus on communities*, Washington, DC, 2004, National Academies Press.
4. McDonald KM, Sundaram V, Bravata DM, et al: Care coordination, Vol 7. In Shojania KG, McDonald KM, Wachter RM, et al, editor: *Closing the quality gap: a critical analysis of quality improvement strategies, Technical Review 9*, Rockville, Md, 2007, Agency for Healthcare Research and Quality.
5. American Academy of Pediatrics Committee on Children with Disabilities: Care coordination: integrating health and related systems of care for children with special health care needs, *Pediatrics* 104:978, 1999.
6. Brown R: *The promise of care coordination: models that decrease hospitalizations and improve outcomes for Medicare beneficiaries with chronic illnesses*, New York, 2009, National Coalition on Care Coordination.
7. Horvitz-Lennon M, Kilbourne AM, Pincus HA: From silos to bridges: meeting the general health care needs of adults with severe mental illnesses, *Health Affairs* 25:659, 2006.
8. Perlin JB, Kolodner R, Roswell RH: The Veterans Health Administration: quality, value, accountability, and information as transforming strategies for patient centered care, *Am J Manag Care* 10:828, 2004.
9. National Quality Forum (NQF): *NQF-endorsed definition and framework for measuring care coordination*, Washington, DC, 2006, Author.
10. Mollica RL, Gillespie J: *Care coordination for people with chronic conditions*, Baltimore, 2003, Partnership for Solutions Johns Hopkins University.
11. Lee JK, Grace KA, Taylor AJ: Effect of a pharmacy care program on medication adherence and persistence, blood pressure, and low-density lipoprotein cholesterol: a randomized controlled trial, *JAMA* 296:2563, 2006.
12. Lopez C, Falces S, Cubi Q, et al: Randomized clinical trial of a postdischarge pharmaceutical care program vs regular follow-up in patients with heart failure, *Farm Hosp* 30:328, 2006.
13. Wu JY, Leung WY, Chang S, et al: Effectiveness of telephone counselling by a pharmacist in reducing mortality in patients receiving polypharmacy: randomised controlled trial, *BMJ* 333:522, 2006.
14. Spinewine A, Swine C, Dhillon S, et al: Effect of a collaborative approach on the quality of prescribing for geriatric inpatients: a randomized, controlled trial, *J Am Geriatr Soc* 55:658, 2007.
15. Clark NM, Janz NK, Becker MH, et al: Impact of self-management education on the functional health status of older adults with heart disease, *Gerontologist* 32:438, 1992.
16. Holtz-Eakin D: *An analysis of the literature on disease management programs*, Washington, DC, 2004, Congressional Budget Office.
17. Chen A, Brown R, Archibald N, et al: *Best practices in coordinated care*, Princeton, NJ, 2000, Mathematica Policy Research.
18. Boult C, Wieland GD: Comprehensive primary care for older patients with multiple chronic conditions: "nobody rushes you through, " *JAMA* 304:1936, 2010.
19. Boult C, Green AF, Boult LB, et al: Successful models of comprehensive care for older adults with chronic conditions: evidence for the Institute of Medicine's "Retooling for an Aging America" report, *J Am Geriatr Soc* 57:2328, 2009.
20. National Quality Forum: *Preferred practices and performance measures for measuring and reporting care coordination: a consensus report*, Washington, DC, 2010, Author.
21. Bodenheimer T, Berry-Millett R: *Care management of patients with complex health care needs, Research Synthesis Report No. 19*, Princeton, NJ, 2009, Robert Wood Johnson Foundation.

22. Peikes D, Chen A, Schore J, et al: Effects of care coordination on hospitalization, quality of care, and health care expenditures among Medicare beneficiaries: 15 randomized trials, *JAMA* 301:603, 2009.

23. Antonelli RC, McAllister JW, Popp J: *Making care coordination a critical component of the pediatric health system: a multidisciplinary frame work*, publication no. 1277, New York, 2009, The Commonwealth Fund.

24. Gittell JH: *Relational coordination: guidelines for theory, measurement and analysis*, 2011 at www.jodyhoffergittell.info/content/rc.html. Accessed Jan 10, 2011.

25. Gittell JH: Relationships between service providers and their impact on customers, *J Serv Res* 4:301, 2002.

26. Gittell JH, Seidner R, Wimbush J: A relational model of how high-performance work systems work, *Organiz Sci* 21:490, 2010.

27. Weinberg DB, Lusenhop W, Gittell JH, et al: Coordination between formal providers and informal caregivers, *Health Care Manag Rev* 32:140, 2007.

28. Pfefferle S, Gittell JH, Hodgkin D, et al: Pediatric coordination of care for children with mental illness, *Med Care* 44:1085, 2006.

29. Weinberg DB, Gittell JH, Lusenhop W, et al: Beyond our walls: impact of patient and provider coordination across the continuum on outcomes for surgical patients, *Health Serv Res* 42:7, 2006.

30. Coleman EA, Boult C: Improving the quality of transitional care for persons with complex care needs, *J Am Geriatr Soc* 51:556, 2003.

31. National Transitions of Care Coalition Measures Working Group: *Transitions of care measures*, Little Rock, Ark, 2008, Author.

32. Kasper EK, Gerstenblith G, Hefter G, et al: A randomized trial of the efficacy of multidisciplinary care in heart failure outpatients at high risk of hospital readmission, *J Am Coll Cardiol* 39:471, 2002.

33. Boult C, Reider L, Frey K, et al: Early effects of guided care on the quality of health care for multimorbid older persons: a cluster-randomized controlled trial, *J Gerontol A Biol Sci Med Sci* 63A:321, 2008.

34. Counsell SR, Callahan CM, Clark DO, et al: Geriatric care management for low-income seniors: a randomized controlled trial, *JAMA* 298:2623, 2007.

35. Counsell SR, Callahan CM, Tu W, et al: Cost analysis of the geriatric resources for assessment and care of elders care management intervention, *J Am Geriatr Soc* 57:1420, 2009.

36. Gary TL, Batts-Turner M, Yeh H, et al: The effects of a nurse case manager and a community health worker team on diabetic control, emergency department visits, and hospitalizations among urban African Americans with type 2 diabetes mellitus: a randomized controlled trial, *Arch Intern Med* 169:1788, 2009.

37. Hiss RG, Armbruster BA, Gillard ML, et al: Nurse care manager collaboration with community-based physicians providing diabetes care: a randomized controlled trial, *Diabetes Educ* 33:493, 2007.

38. Martin DC, Berger ML, Anstatt DT, et al: A randomized controlled open trial of population-based disease and case management in a Medicare Plus Choice health maintenance organization, *Prev Chronic Dis* 1:A05, 2004.

39. McAllister JW, Presler E, Cooley WC: *Medical home practice-based care coordination: a workbook*, Greenfield, NF, 2007, Center for Medical Home Improvement, Crotched Mountain Foundation and Rehabilitation Center.

Caregiving

Sharon L. Lewis, Lyda C. Arévalo-Flechas,
and Denise Miner-Williams

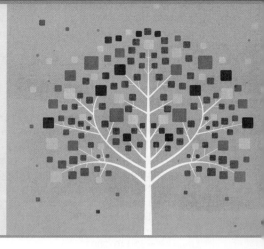

There are only four kinds of people in the world—those who have been caregivers, those who are currently caregivers, those who will be caregivers, and those who will need caregivers.

Rosalyn Carter

An estimated 65.7 million Americans provide unpaid care for an adult or child with functional and/or cognitive limitations. These dedicated caregivers provide between 80% and 90% of the long-term care provided at home. About 66% of caregivers are women and 34% are men.[1] Many caregivers of older people are also older adults. Of those caring for someone older than age 65, the average age of the caregiver is 63 years; one third of those receiving care are in fair to poor health. One third of caregivers provide care for two or more people.[1,2]

The need for family caregivers will escalate dramatically in the coming years because of our aging population, increased longevity, and an overwhelmed formal health care system. People with chronic, debilitating diseases are being treated more effectively and they are living with rather than dying from these diseases. It is important for nurses to be aware of the role that caregivers have in health care delivery, the impact of this role on the lives of caregivers, and supportive interventions that can be provided to caregivers.

DEFINITION(S)

Caregivers are people who care for others who cannot care for themselves. A person becomes a caregiver when he or she provides direct care for children, older adults, or people who have acute or chronic illnesses or disabilities. Nurses and other health care professionals are *paid caregivers* who assist in the management of a person's illness or disability. However, the responsibility of day-to-day caregiving falls on the family. Family caregivers are sometimes called *informal caregivers* or *unpaid caregivers* because they provide care without pay, usually in a home or community setting. The

focus of this concept analysis is on the family caregiver. For the purpose of this concept analysis, the definition of a caregiver is *a lay individual (e.g., family member or significant other) who provides direct care to another individual with a health-related condition (e.g., elderly person or one who has a chronic illness)*.

Alzheimer's disease is the most common reason that someone becomes a family caregiver. The incidence of Alzheimer's disease is increasing steadily. There are now more than 5.4 million people in the United States with the disease. It is estimated that someone in America develops Alzheimer's disease every 69 seconds.[3] In addition to the increasing number of people with Alzheimer's disease, care is required for people with this disease for an extended period of time. The range of time from diagnosis until death is often from 8 to 20 years, which is why Alzheimer's disease is often called the long, lingering death. The demands of caregiving over that long period of time can cause an incredible amount of stress for the caregiver.

SCOPE AND CATEGORIES

The scope of the caregiving concept ranges on a continuum from a temporary/limited caregiving role for an individual with an acute illness or condition to a long-term or permanent caregiving role (Figure 48-1). Caregiving roles may be shared among family members so that the caregiving role may also be episodic.

Caregivers are often categorized by their relationship to the person receiving care (care recipient). Although some caregivers may not have a familial relationship, the most common types of caregivers are spousal caregivers, adult children caregivers, grandparent caregivers, and parent caregivers.

Spousal Caregivers

In the United States spousal caregivers are the most common family caregivers. Many of these caregivers are older themselves, and now find themselves in the role of caring for

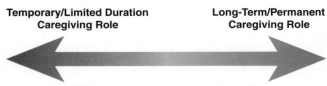

FIGURE 48-1 Scope of Caregiving Role.

someone with physical and/or cognitive disorders. Most commonly, family caregivers are older women who have their own chronic health problems and/or disabilities and are poor.[4]

With the increase in military war casualties, there is a new population of very seriously wounded service members who require extensive care and rehabilitation. Young spouses are now becoming caregivers for their husbands or wives with multiple physical injuries, including traumatic brain injuries. In addition to the physical injuries, the emotional "wounds" related to war, combat stress, and the effects of the injuries are challenging these young families.

Spousal caregivers have to face the reality that they have lost the husband or wife that they once knew. They have "lost" their partner because of physical, mental/emotional, or cognitive disabilities, and sometimes all of these reasons.

Adult Children Caregivers

Adult children are often caregivers for their elderly parents. With people living longer, adult children are more frequently assuming the role of primary caregiver for their aging parents who have multiple chronic illnesses.

The impact of the caregiving role can be overwhelming for adult children caregivers who have to assume multiple roles and responsibilities while juggling employment and family responsibilities. They have to change their lives to meet the needs of their parent(s). Most adult children caregivers are in the "sandwich generation"— they are parents to their children as well as "parents" to their own parents. Commuting between their own homes and the homes of their parents can be very difficult. Often they ultimately end up moving their parents into their home or move themselves near or into their parents' home to take care of them. The move may involve geographic relocation from one area of the country to another. Financial strain and consequences often accompany their caregiving role. Adult children caregivers also experience many forms of loss, including:

- Loss of their parent(s) as they knew them before the illness
- Loss of their jobs (or needing to cope with job changes)
- Change in their social networks

It is also very stressful to realize the "loss" of their own lives. A term that can be used to characterize the adult children caregiver is *role captivity*—a feeling that one has unwittingly become captive of an unwanted role.

Grandparent Caregivers

Today, many grandparents are raising their grandchildren and providing care in a variety of ways. Approximately 5.8 million grandparents live with a grandchild. More than 6.5 million children across the country live in households maintained by grandparents or other relatives. In about one third of these homes no parents are present.[5] Most grandparents had not planned on this role because they have already raised their own children. The most common reasons that grandparents become the primary caregivers are that their own children (1) have died, (2) have abandoned the grandchildren, (3) are mentally ill or substance abusers, or (4) are in prison. Grandparents are often overwhelmed in the role of caring for their grandchildren. This feeling of being overwhelmed may occur because they are:

- Raising their grandchildren on a fixed income and facing financial hardships
- Experiencing the effects associated with normal aging and/or the health problems that make caring for their grandchildren difficult
- Worrying about who will be the caregivers when they die or are physically unable to provide the care
- Raising children who may have mental, behavioral/emotional, or physical problems

In addition, a more subtle stressor occurs when grandparents become primary caregivers of children. When the parenting role is assumed, they lose the special relationship and unique role of a grandparent. However, these grandparents gladly accept the challenges, often at great personal sacrifices to their own physical, emotional, and financial well-being. They may neglect their own health issues because the grandchildren become their priority. Grandparents may also be challenged with needing legal assistance and guardianship rights for their grandchildren in order to register them in school, apply for affordable housing, qualify for special community resources, and obtain medical care.

Parental Caregivers

A primary role of parents is the provision of care for their children. However, parents become "caregivers" for their children when the children are at an age when they would normally be expected to care for themselves. This can be due to a disability such as severe physical limitations or mental retardation. It can also happen later in life from an accident (such as a spinal cord injury), a debilitating illness, or severe trauma experienced in military combat (physical and/or emotional).

Stressors of parent caregivers of children will be unique to their situations. For parent caregivers of children with lifelong disabilities, stressors may include the fear of what will happen to their children when they outlive their parents. Parents of adult children who have experienced severe trauma or illness may suddenly be thrust into the parenting role again. Then these parents must decide how and when to relaunch their children into independence under a new context.

ATTRIBUTES

Concept attributes are identified characteristics that enhance a shared understanding and meaning to those discussing, observing, or experiencing the concept. Stated another way, attributes are the structural elements of a concept that are consistently described or observable. Attributes of caregiving include an unpaid family member (e.g., spouses, children, grandchildren, other relatives) or friend who provides the following type of care:

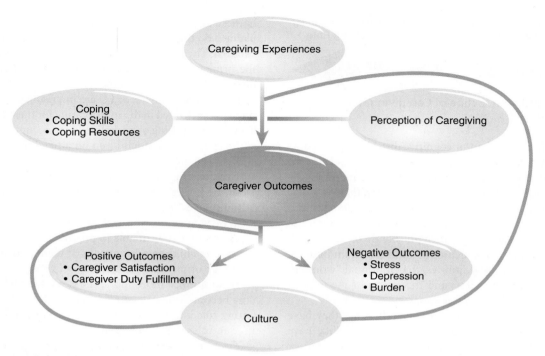

FIGURE 48-2 Concept of Caregiving. (Adapted from Arévalo-Flechas LC: Factors influencing Latino/Hispanic caregivers' perception of the experience of caring for a relative with Alzheimer's disease, *Dissert Abstr Int,* DAI-B 69/06 [UMI 3311328], 2008.)

- Give and/or assist with activities of daily living.
- Provide emotional and social support.
- Manage and coordinate health care services.

THEORETICAL LINKS

Lazarus and Folkman proposed a theoretical model highlighting the concepts of stress, appraisal, and coping. Stress is defined as a stimulus that can serve as a positive drive or a negative event. Stressors can be acute (sudden onset or time-limited) or chronic. Prolonged caregiving is a chronic stressor. Psychologic stress is a particular relationship between the person and the environment that is appraised by the person as taxing or exceeding his or her resources and endangering his or her well-being.[6,7]

Judging a situation as stressful relies on the cognitive ability of appraisal. Appraisal is the process of categorizing or evaluating a situation with respect to its significance for well-being. *Primary appraisal* is done by a person when some of these questions are asked: Am I in trouble? Is this a good or a bad thing? Does this make me happy? Is this a challenge? Can this have positive or negative consequences? *Secondary appraisal* is taking place when the person asks the question: What, if anything, might and can be done? Secondary appraisal takes into account the possible coping strategies that can be used to manage a situation.

CONTEXT TO NURSING AND HEALTH CARE

Caregiving, the act of assuming responsibility for another person, involves daily demands that become the caregiver experiences for the caregiver.[8] It is essential that nurses understand the caregiving experience from the perspective of caregivers in order to provide appropriate interventions.

Caregiver Experiences and Perspectives

How the caregiver deals with the experiences (stressors) associated with caregiving determines the caregiver's response and the outcomes to the caregiving experience. Important factors influence how caregivers react and respond to the challenges of caregiving. One factor that influences their response is their perception of the experience. Another important factor affecting their response to caregiving is their ability to cope and the coping resources that they have available. Culture also affects how a caregiver will cope and perceive the caregiving experience. Caregiver outcomes can range from experiencing satisfaction and a sense of duty fulfillment to becoming stressed or depressed and feeling burdened (Figure 48-2).

Caregiver Experiences

As caregivers assume responsibilities for another person, they experience a tremendous amount of change in their lives. Caregiving involves unique experiences that may not be what most people expected during their lifetime. The realities of caregiving can produce a negative effect on the caregiver's physical and emotional health. On the other hand, it may be an opportunity for positive changes and rewards.

Difficult journey. Caregiving is challenging, and can often be viewed as a difficult journey, one for which most people are not prepared. In the beginning a daughter may say she will take care of mom for a few weeks, not realizing that those few weeks will extend into years. Eventually the emotional and physical tasks of caregiving can become overwhelming.

BOX 48-1   CAREGIVER STRESSORS

- Change in roles and relationships within family
- Lack of respite or relief from caregiving responsibilities
- Juggling day-to-day activities, decisions, and caregiving
- Change in living conditions to accommodate family member
- Conflict in the family related to decisions about caregiving
- Lack of understanding of the time and energy needed for caregiving
- Inability to meet personal self-care needs, such as socialization, sleep, eating, exercise, and rest
- Financial depletion of resources as a result of a caregiver's inability to work and the increased cost of health care
- Inadequate information and/or skills related to specific caregiving tasks, such as bathing, drug administration, and wound care

Adapted from Lewis SL, Dirksen SR, Heitkemper MM, et al: *Medical-surgical nursing: assessment and management of clinical problems*, ed 8, St Louis, 2011, Mosby/Elsevier.

Some common caregiver stressors are listed in Box 48-1. Family caregivers perform an incredibly valuable service for their family member. However, they do so at a considerable cost to themselves emotionally, socially, financially, and/or physically.

Uncertainties about present and future. Caregivers face uncertainties about the present and future. Caregivers simply do not know what is going to happen. For example, dementia is a roller coaster disease, with the patient's behaviors often changing daily. There can be many fluctuations in the disease, especially early in its course. Sometimes the person can seem quite cognitively intact with no noticeable indication that anything is wrong. Then there may be other days when the person is combative and barely able to function. Many caregivers will say that they never feel prepared to deal with the challenges of caregiving.

Inadequate understanding of the disease. Frequently caregivers have an inadequate understanding of the disease. In Alzheimer's disease memory loss is the most widely known symptom. However, as the disease progresses there are often many changes in the person's personality and behavior. These behavior changes are very challenging to address. The caregiver may become confused and hurt by the strange and/or difficult behaviors. Caregivers who do not understand the disease or manifestations of the disease may feel that there is something wrong with them (e.g., person with dementia verbally lashing out). This can result in caregivers feeling guilty. They may express feelings such as, "If I love her more, if I could be more patient, she would not be so combative." However, that is not the situation. Caregivers need to understand that it is the disease that is causing their loved one to act in a certain way, and the caregiver usually has no or little control over it.

Financial consequences. Caregivers often experience negative financial consequences. The majority of family caregivers work full-time or part-time. Nearly 60% of those caring for an adult over the age of 50 are working, with the majority working full-time.[9] Many of these caregivers have to make adjustments in their work life to accommodate their caregiving responsibilities. They report late for work or leave early, need to take time off because of their caregiving responsibilities (e.g., to take their loved one to physician's appointments), reduce their hours or take a less demanding job, decline a promotion, alter work-related travel, quit their job entirely, or take an early retirement. Grandparents find their retirement funds dwindle rapidly to cover the unexpected costs of raising their children's children.

Many older adults do not have long-term-care insurance so the financial responsibilities of their care need to be paid for by the family. The caregiver may need to sell the family home to pay for health care or long-term care for the person with the disease. Many caregivers see their life savings quickly depleted.

Social isolation. When caregiving responsibilities for those with progressive illness increase and demand an increased amount of time, caregivers may become isolated and removed from family and friends. The caregiver's world revolves around the person with the disease, and the caregiver cannot be away from the individual with the disease. For example, it may be difficult to transport the patient with a stroke or Parkinson's disease. Just transferring the person from the wheelchair in and out of a car is a limiting factor in how often the caregiver takes that person out of the house.

Time commitments, fatigue, and, at times, socially inappropriate behaviors of the patient contribute to social isolation. For patients with dementia the caregiver may be embarrassed to take them out in public because of the behaviors they might exhibit. They may say or do inappropriate things such as touching children. The end result is that caregivers have limited leisure activities and their social network changes. Caregivers sacrifice time with family and friends, and they give up their vacations, hobbies, social life, and sense of self as their caregiving responsibilities become more intensive.

Family relationships. An illness experienced by one family member will affect the entire family and alter family interactions. Family relationships change when a chronic disease, especially a debilitating one, enters into the family picture. An important issue among adult children is who will care for mom or dad. Even with the best of intentions, families can struggle. Preexisting patterns in the family, such as a history of disagreements or unresolved issues, influence how a family responds after a person is diagnosed with a disease and requires caregiving. If problems such as poor or bad relationships existed before the disease, they are probably going to worsen after the diagnosis of the disease.

Many different situations exist with regard to how care is provided within a family. Some families share the responsibilities. Most often, primary care will fall to (or be designated to) one person with or without helpful (or often unhelpful) input from other family members. These other family members may not be willing to be involved in the care, but their comments can be very stressful to the person who has become the primary caregiver. A common situation with spousal caregivers is that they find that their children do not help with the caregiving of their father or mother. Children may distance themselves because they cannot emotionally handle seeing their parent in a "sick" role. Parents may feel that their children are very busy with their own lives (career and children) and they cannot expect them to do anything. Spousal caregivers may feel it is their responsibility and they do not want to seem overbearing or demanding of their children.

Families frequently do not communicate with each other about the needs of the patient or other important issues such as the delegation of responsibilities. Also, families frequently communicate very little about the emotions related to the issues. This results in tension, which results in stress for the caregiver.

Changing roles and relationships. The original roles of the patient can no longer be managed after the person has been diagnosed with diseases such as a severe stroke, Parkinson's disease, or Alzheimer's disease. Roles and relationships need to be restructured. A woman who has never managed finances may now need to balance the checkbook. She may also need to learn to do home and car repairs. Men who have never used a kitchen may now need to learn to cook and clean. The family patriarch may no longer be able to fulfill that role and the family struggles to find a new leader. Grandparents may be unfamiliar with the different roles of children being raised in today's world, which may be quite different than their past child-rearing experiences. In addition, they may experience difficulty resolving legal issues and obtaining medical care for their grandchildren.

Perception and Coping

How caregivers deal with the experiences and realities of caregiving depends on their perception of the experience and their coping abilities. *Perception* is the mental process of viewing and interpreting a person's environment. The caregiver experiences (potential stressors) are not stressful unless the individual *perceives* them as stressful. Events or circumstances themselves are not stressful. They only become stressful when the person *perceives* them as stressful. That is why what is stressful for one person may not be stressful for another.

Coping is a person's efforts to manage stressors. Coping can be either positive or negative. Positive coping includes activities such as exercising and spending time with friends and family. Negative coping may include substance abuse and denial. Ultimately, whether coping is positive or negative depends on how well it addresses the problem. For instance, it may be good for the caregiver to have some free time and go shopping, but if this involves spending excessive money then this would become a negative coping mechanism.

Influence of Culture on the Caregiving Experience

Culture is the conglomerate of morals, values, beliefs, norms, customs, and meanings that a group of people share and communicate from one generation to the next. Culture profoundly influences how a caregiver perceives and copes with this role. Culture permeates every aspect of the caregiving experience, from the initial demands placed on the caregiver to the final perception of the overall experience and the outcomes for the caregiver.[10]

The culture in which the caregiver was socialized as a young person determines how caregiving duties are assumed, managed, and perceived. People from a culture that values individualism, competition, and independence may see the role of being a caregiver differently from people who come from collectivistic cultures in which interdependence and family take precedence over individual achievement. Although becoming a caregiver is an expectation in some cultures, caregivers in other cultures may feel captive in their role and perceive only the negative aspects of caregiving.

A value shared in some cultures (e.g., Hispanic/Latino culture) is *familism*. This value refers to the central role of family in an individual's life, and the individual's reliance on family as a priority. Some cultures value familism whereas others place greater value on the individual's independence and success.[10] The sense of duty and responsibility towards family members, especially parents, may determine whether a caregiver feels caregiving is an honor, a duty, an obligation, or a burden. The meaning attached to the caregiving experience is greatly influenced by cultural values.[8]

Similarly, the support and resources that caregivers seek are largely determined by cultural values. The stressors in the caregiving experience are common to the vast majority of caregivers regardless of racial or ethnic background. However, how the caregiver perceives the situation and whether and when resources are mobilized to cope with the demands of caregiving are influenced by the cultural meaning given to the situation. Support of caregivers needs to be tailored to the cultural meaning that the caregiver is giving the experience. The nurse needs to be first aware of the caregiver's view of family, health, caregiver role, and traditions. Take into consideration the influence of culture in the caregiving experience if you want to incorporate the caregiver as a full partner of the health care team.

Caregiver Outcomes

Caregiving can have both positive and negative outcomes. One half of caregivers of individuals living with Alzheimer's disease or dementia surveyed found an equal balance of positive and negative experiences in their caregiving. One third indicated that their caregiving experience is more positive than negative.[11]

Positive caregiver outcomes. How caregivers perceive their caregiving experience may influence their ability to focus on the positive aspects of caregiving. Focusing on the positive aspects can create meaning for caregivers and even improve the relationships between caregivers and the person for whom they are providing care. Caregivers need to be assured that they are taking good care of the person that they love and keeping that person happy, comfortable, and safe. Feelings of accomplishment result when caregivers realize that they are able to assume another person's role. For women this may mean managing the finances and the house and car repairs. For men this may involve cooking and cleaning. For adult children caregivers they may have a feeling of satisfaction in helping their parents who provided and sacrificed for them.

Another positive aspect of caregiving is the intimacy of the caregiving relationship that helps a person gain insight into another person and strengthens the bonds of that relationship. Caregivers can live with a sense of peace that they cared for the person that they loved.

For some caregivers just thinking about the positive aspects can "reframe" their role and help it seem more manageable. Caregiving may be difficult for those people who were emotionally, physically, or sexually abused by the person for whom they are now caring. Through reframing and/or forgiveness, these caregivers may be able to come to terms with the situation and find positive aspects in their role of caregiver.

Negative caregiver outcomes. It is common for caregivers to become physically, emotionally, and financially overwhelmed with the responsibilities and demands of caring for a family member. Caregivers often sacrifice their own health to care for a loved one dealing with a debilitating disease. Caregiving stress has many causes, particularly the need to provide constant supervision and handling communication and behavior problems. The stress of caregiving can increase because of a perceived lack of support from family and friends and criticism from other family members. The stress of caregiving may result in emotional problems such as depression, anger, and resentment. Caregivers may reach the point in which the daily demands exceed their ability to mobilize resources and cope. Signs of caregiver stress include irritability, inability to concentrate, fatigue, and sleeplessness. Stress can progress to burnout and result in negligence and abuse of the family member by the caregiver.

Nursing and Caregiver Support

Caregiver Assessment

How does a nurse know when caregivers need help? The Alzheimer's Association has developed 10 signs of caregiver stress (Table 48-1). These are indicators that if the caregiver is not helped, the person can develop more serious health problems. Caregivers are frequently unaware that they have

reached a breaking point. The first step in helping family caregivers is to identify persons as caregivers—either by health care professionals or by the caregiver him/herself. Initially, caregivers may not identify with the term "caregiver." They may only see themselves as carrying out family responsibilities. Helping them to understand and respect the important role that they have undertaken is a critical first step to allow caregivers to accept help.

They must first be identified either by health care professionals or self-identified. Caregivers have been referred to as "hidden patients" because a common characteristic of caregivers is primarily having concern for their loved one and personally ignoring their own needs or being ignored by health care professionals.[12,13]

When you assess a patient, include an assessment of the caregiver. As a nurse, you are a key person in this process. Areas that should be assessed are presented in Box 48-2. Listen attentively to the caregivers' stories. They provide clues as to what their lives are like, and these clues should be explored.

Identifying and Accessing Resources

Caregivers who provide intense care often need outside assistance and have difficulty asking for help because they do not want to be a burden on others; are afraid of being rejected if they ask for help; may be embarrassed or feel guilty for having a sick person in the family, especially when the disease has cognitive, memory, or behavior components; or believe it is their duty to be the single provider of care.

Many caregivers suffer in silence because they may not know *how* to ask for help or *where* to look for help, or they do not know that help is available for them. Nurses should encourage caregivers to seek and accept the support of family, friends, and community resources when needed. It is important for

TABLE 48-1 SIGNS OF CAREGIVER STRESS

SIGNS	DESCRIPTION	WHAT THE CAREGIVER MAY SAY
1. **Denial**	About the disease and its effect	I know that Mom is going to get better.
2. **Anger**	At the person with the disease or others	If he asks me that question one more time, I will scream.
3. **Social withdrawal**	From friends and family that once brought pleasure	I don't care about getting together with the neighbors anymore.
4. **Anxiety**	About facing another day and what the future holds	What happens when he needs more care than I can provide? What happens if I'm not here to provide his care?
5. **Depression**	Begins to break the spirit and affects the ability to cope	I don't care anymore.
6. **Exhaustion**	Makes it nearly impossible to complete necessary daily tasks	I'm too tired to do anything.
7. **Irritability**	Leads to moodiness and triggers negative responses and reactions	Leave me alone!!
8. **Sleeplessness**	Caused by a never-ending list of concerns	What if she wanders out of the house, falls, and hurts herself?
9. **Lack of concentration**	Makes it difficult to perform familiar tasks	I was so busy, I forgot we had an appointment.
10. **Health problems**	Begin to take their toll both mentally and physically	I can't remember the last time that I felt good.

Adapted from the Alzheimer's Association. Available at www.alz.org/national/documents/brochure_caregiverstress.pdf.

BOX 48-2   ASSESSMENT OF FAMILY CAREGIVERS

Assess family caregivers using the following questions:

1. What is your level of stress?
2. What are you doing to cope and how well are you coping?
3. How well do you maintain your own nutrition, rest, and exercise?
4. What is your level of social interaction vs. social isolation?
5. How much support do you get from outside sources (e.g., other family members, friends, church members)?
6. How well are you taking care of your own health care needs (especially those with chronic illnesses of their own)?
7. Are you aware and do you use community and Internet resources (e.g., community resources, such as disease-specific professional organizations [e.g., Alzheimer's Association, American Heart Association], local adult day care centers, and Internet sites such as www.caregiver.org)?
8. Do you know about resources available for respite (someone caring for your loved one while you have time to yourself)?
9. What kind of help or services do you think you need now and in the near future?

Adapted from Lewis SL, Dirksen SR, Heitkemper MM et al: *Medical-surgical nursing: assessment and management of clinical problems*, ed 8, St Louis, 2011, Mosby/Elsevier.

caregivers to understand that exhaustion and burnout are common consequences if they attempt to do everything for themselves. Nurses can help caregivers by finding out what specific types of help they need and helping them access appropriate resources.

Caring for the Caregiver

Another way nurses can assist caregivers is to help them to understand and cope with the stressors of caregiving. You can communicate a sense of empathy to the caregiver by allowing discussion about the burdens and rewards of caregiving.

Monitor the caregiver for indications of declining health and emotional distress. A strategy to reduce stress is to help caregivers acknowledge feelings of stress and plan self-care activities. Caregiver support can be accomplished in a number of ways. Discuss with the caregiver the potential that support groups, networks of family and friends, and community resources have for reducing stress.[14] Support groups provide self-help by sharing experiences and information, offering understanding and acceptance, and suggesting solutions to common problems and concerns. Encourage the caregiver to seek help from the formal social support system regarding matters such as respite care, housing, health care coverage, and finances. Respite care, which is planned temporary care for the patient, can allow the caregiver to regain a sense of equilibrium. Respite care includes adult day care, in-home care, and assisted living services. Additionally, caregivers need to be encouraged to take care of themselves in all aspects of life, as stated next.

Physically. Eating a healthy diet at regular times, exercising to help relieve stress, and obtaining adequate sleep are essential.

Emotionally. Keeping a journal can help the caregiver express feelings that may be difficult to express verbally. Humor is important, and its use from time to time in some situations can provide distraction and relieve stress-filled situations. Maintenance of regular activities, interests, and hobbies is also important to help the caregiver.

Socially. Physical contact with others provides emotional support and acknowledgment of the caregiver's own need for comfort and assurance.

Cognitively. Encourage the caregiver to appraise his or her perception of situations and try to maintain a positive perspective.

Spiritually. Maintain a sense of awe in life. Connect with the transcendent. Encourage religious involvement if that is important to the caregiver.

INTERRELATED CONCEPTS

Multiple concepts presented within this textbook are interrelated to the caregiving concept. Four concepts with particularly important interrelationships include **Stress, Coping, Family dynamics,** and **Culture.** These interrelationships are presented in Figure 48-3.

Stress

Stress is the inability to cope with a perceived (real or imagined) threat to one's mental, emotional, and spiritual well-being. This results in a series of physiologic responses and adaptations.[15] The emotional and physical strain is caused by a person's response to pressure (stressors) in the environment. It leads to rapid changes throughout the body affecting almost every system.

Coping

Coping is the process through which a person manages the demands placed on the person-environment relationship and the emotions generated by a given situation. Lazarus and Folkman view coping as a dynamic process specific to the presenting situation and to the stage of the encounter. Coping is not merely a response to stress or tension. Coping is influenced by a person's cognitive appraisal of an event and one's cognitive appraisal subsequently influences emotional arousal.[6,7]

Family Dynamics

Caregiving can trigger many changes in family structure and family roles. Family members relate to each other in a variety of ways. Family members take part in different experiences that can affect the family as a whole. Culture influences a person's definition of family and the relationships among family members.

Culture

Culture is a set of behaviors, attitudes, and policies that come together in a system to enable effective work in cross-cultural. Health care services that are respectful of and responsive to the health beliefs, practices, and cultural and linguistic needs of diverse people can help affect positive health outcomes.

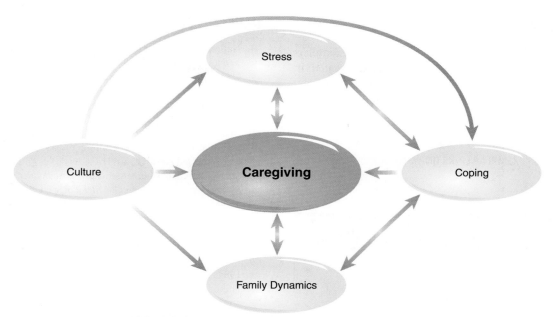

FIGURE 48-3 Caregiving and Interrelated Concepts.

MODEL CASE

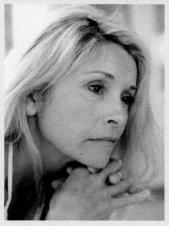

Barbara, age 45, recently moved from Kentucky to San Antonio to take care of Melinda, her 3-year-old granddaughter. Laura, age 19, who is Barbara's daughter and Melinda's mother, was recently sent to prison for selling drugs. Barbara, her husband Jeff, and their 17-year-old son Ben moved into a doublewide mobile home. After their move it took Jeff about 4 weeks to find a job delivering supplies for a tool supply company. Ben, who protested the move, just started his senior year in high school.

About 1 month after their move, Barbara's parents, who live near Dallas, called Barbara to tell her that their house had sold and they wanted to move in with Barbara. Barbara's father Steve is 85 years old and was diagnosed about 3 years ago with Alzheimer's disease. Steve is very irritable and controlling. Barbara has spent much of her life resenting the control that her father has over the entire family. Barbara's mother Shirley is very passive and spends much of her time reading to avoid dealing with Steve.

Living with Steve and Shirley is their youngest daughter Nancy, age 41, who had a liver transplant 3 years ago. After the liver transplant, her husband filed for divorce and moved to Oklahoma with their children. Shortly after the divorce, Nancy had a mental breakdown from which she never recovered.

Barbara's father with dementia, her passive mother, and her sister with both medical and emotional problems moved into Barbara's 3-bedroom doublewide mobile home 3 months ago.

At first the merged family of 7 managed to cooperate and be civil. Then Barbara found out that her father Steve had lost all of his finances through a scam. That left the family of 7 living on Jeff's meager salary and Nancy's disability checks.

Barbara spends as much time as possible in her bedroom with the door closed watching TV. She has gained about 10 pounds from eating junk food while she watches TV. Her granddaughter is allowed to roam the house as she desires. Barbara is worrying that Ben may be involved in drugs because of his change in attitude and appearance. Barbara is afraid to discuss any concerns with her husband Jeff because all of the stress is being "caused" by her family. Meals are spent in silence since everyone is afraid to make Steve angry if they say the wrong thing.

Case Analysis

Barbara is in an incredibly stressful situation. She appears to avoid dealing with the issues by watching TV or maintaining silence. In her current situation, Barbara has limited coping resources. She needs to find support outside of her home environment. A first step for Barbara to take would be to contact the Alzheimer's Association so she can access local resources that may be helpful. A family meeting with an outside person as leader/mediator may help the family initiate problem-solving strategies. Finding a senior day care center for her parents would be beneficial for both Barbara and her parents. Barbara and her husband need some respite care for the rest of the family so they can get away and renew their marriage. Melinda would benefit from a preschool or nursery where she can interact with children her own age. Barbara should try to get involved with a caregiver support group.

EXEMPLARS

Although it is impossible to list all possible exemplars of caregiving, some common examples are presented in Box 48-3. Many exemplars represent situations requiring temporary caregiving and others represent long-term caregiving responsibilities.

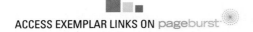

ACCESS EXEMPLAR LINKS ON pageburst

BOX 48-3   EXEMPLARS OF CAREGIVING

Temporary/Limited Duration Caregiving
Acute Illness or Condition
- Acute myocardial infarction
- Burns
- Influenza
- Pneumonia
- Surgery
- Traumatic injury

Long-Term/Permanent Caregiving
Chronic Illness or Condition
- Alzheimer's disease
- Cancer
- Chronic kidney disease
- Chronic obstructive pulmonary disease
- Diabetes mellitus
- Handicapped /disability
- Heart failure
- HIV/AIDS
- Mental illness
- Multiple sclerosis
- Parkinson's disease
- Stroke

Social Situations
- Grandparenting

REFERENCES

1. National Alliance for Caregiving: *Executive summary: caregiving in the U.S. 2009.* Available at www.caregiving.org/data/Caregiving USAllAgesExecSum.pdf. Accessed April 18, 2011.
2. National Family Caregiving Alliance: *Fact sheet.* Available at www.caregiver.org/caregiver/jsp/content_node.jsp?node id=2313. Accessed April 18, 2011.
3. Alzheimer's Association: *2011 Alzheimer's disease facts and figures* at www.alz.org/alzheimers_disease_facts_and_figures. asp. Accessed April 18, 2011.
4. Shriver M: Alzheimer's Association: *Alzheimer's in America: the Shriver report on women and Alzheimer's*, Chicago, 2011, Simon and Shuster.
5. Generations United: Grandfacts: *data, interpretation, and implications for caregivers*, Washington, DC. at www2.gu.org/ OURWORK/Grandfamilies.aspx. Accessed April 18, 2011.
6. Lazarus RS, Folkman S: *Stress, appraisal, and coping*, New York, 1984, Springer.
7. Folkman S, Lazarus R: The relationship between coping and emotion: implications for theory and research, *Soc Sci Med* 26(3):309, 1988.
8. Arévalo-Flechas LC: Factors influencing Latino/Hispanic caregivers' perception of the experience of caring for a relative with Alzheimer's disease, *Dissert Abstr Int*, 2008. DAI-B 69/06 (UMI 3311328).
9. MetLife Mature Market Institute & National Alliance for Caregiving: *The MetLife caregiving cost study: productivity losses to U.S. business, 2006.* Available at www.caregiving.org/data/Care giver%20Cost%20Study.pdf. Accessed April 18, 2011.
10. U.S. Department of Health and Human Services: Office of Minority Health: *What is cultural competency?* at http://min orityhealth.hhs.gov/templates/browse.aspx?lvl=2&lvlID=11 Accessed April 18, 2011.
11. National Alliance for Caregiving: *What made you think Mom had Alzheimer's?* at www.caregiving.org/data/NAC%20 Alzheimers0411.pdf. Accessed April 18, 2011.
12. Saban KL, Sherwood PR, DeVon HA, et al: Measures of psychological stress and physical health in family caregivers of stroke survivors: a literature review, *J Neurosci Nurs* 42(3):128, 2010.
13. Van Vliet D, De Vugt ME, Verhey FR, et al: Impact of early onset dementia on caregivers: a review, *Int J Geriatr Psychiatry* 25(11):1091, 2010.
14. Lewis SL, Miner-Williams D, Novian A, et al: A stress-busting program for family caregivers, *Rehabil Nurs* 34(4):151, 2009.
15. Seaward BL: *Managing stress: principles and strategies for health and well-being*, ed 7, Boston, 2011, Jones and Bartlett.

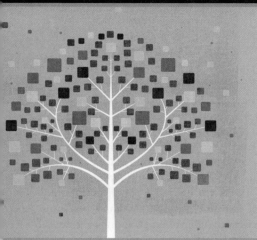

Palliation

Kim K. Kuebler and Michelle A. Cole

The issues affecting the care of patients with chronic disease are expected to intensify over the next several decades. It is predicted that by the year 2030, for the first time in history, the old will out-number the young.[1] In 2010 the oldest of the baby boomers reached 65 years of age. Not only will there be older Americans, but it is predicted that they will live with debilitating diseases much longer.[2] A century ago, most people died of infections, accidents, and other rapidly lethal disease states. Now the leading causes of death in the United States include cardiovascular disease, cancer, stroke, chronic obstructive lung disease (COPD), and dementia.[3]

DEFINITION(S)

Palliation is the relief or management of symptoms without providing a cure. To *palliate* is to reduce the severity of an actual or potential life-threatening condition or a chronic debilitating illness. Palliation is not equivalent to cure but is the reduction of undesirable effects resulting from the incurable disease or condition.

In 2002 the World Health Organization (WHO) expanded and broadened the definition of palliative care outside of the disease of cancer and suggested its use and integration into the symptomatic management of chronic diseases (e.g., congestive heart failure [CHF], chronic obstructive pulmonary disease [COPD]). This newer definition promotes the earlier integration and use of palliative interventions into the clinical management of chronic disease. As disease progresses and further treatment is no longer effective, appropriate, or desired, palliative care increases in intensity and is used during the end of life. The definition of palliative care by the WHO recognizes that:

Palliative care is the active total care of patients whose disease is not responsive to curative treatment. Control of pain, of other symptoms, and of psychological, social and spiritual problems is paramount. The goal of palliative care is achievement of the best quality of life for patients and their families. Many aspects of palliative care are also applicable earlier in the course of illness in conjunction with therapies such as anticancer treatment.[4]

Palliative care can further be defined as specialized care that is used to reduce the severity of a disease or slow its progression rather than providing a cure for the disease.[5] Palliative care is appropriate for those patients who are living with symptomatic incurable diseases such as severe chronic renal failure, COPD, or CHF and for those patients for whom there is no cure or reversibility to their underlying disease pathophysiology. Palliative care can be used to improve symptoms and promote patient quality of life. The following are some goals of palliative care:

- Prevent or treat as early as possible the symptoms of a disease or the associated side effects caused by treatment of the disease.
- Prevent or treat the psychologic, social, and spiritual problems related to the disease or its treatment.
- Help patients with chronic or life-threatening disease to live more comfortably.[4]

If optimally delivered, palliative care can provide patients with aggressive symptom management while helping to restore and promote function and engage patients and families with earlier and supportive discussions about advance care planning.[6] Palliative care requires a marked shift in the goals of care when symptom management is exchanged for curative care.

SCOPE AND CATEGORIES

Palliative care, symptom management, supportive care, comfort care, end-of-life care, and hospice care are terms that are frequently used interchangeably. However, hospice and end-of-life care are distinctly different from the others. Hospice and end-of-life care are parts of palliative care and/or supportive and comfort care; the reverse is not true.[6] However, because palliative care is more than end-of-life care or hospice care, where does it begin and end in the care of the patient living with symptomatic disease? In recent years, the trend has been to initiate palliative care practices and principles earlier into the management of advanced disease.[6] The WHO definition of palliative care supports this trend—and the idea of providing palliative care for all patients with advanced disease regardless of their underlying diagnosis has increased in awareness.[4,6]

Symptom Management

Effective symptom management requires the use of the best possible evidence to support the specific pharmacologic interventions to manage the multiple symptoms that frequently accompany chronic disease and the dying process. Symptom management is considered a multidimensional approach of care—meaning that many health care professionals (e.g., physicians, nurses, social workers, spiritual advisors, nutritionists) become involved in the holistic approach of the patient. Symptom management differs from supportive care and comfort care in that it is all-encompassing and not specific or limited in use to the end of life or to the oncology patient population.

Supportive Care

Supportive care is the least well-defined area of care that is used in the management of symptoms and palliation.[6] Supportive care employs the use of medical interventions to prevent, control, and/or relieve the complications of disease and the associated side effects of specific therapies.[6,7] Supportive care is similar to comfort care and palliative care because it is used to improve the patient's quality of life. Supportive care is frequently used in the oncology setting and is primarily based upon the medical interventions used to support the cancer patient, such as providing blood transfusions, managing fluid replacement therapy, or administering bone marrow stimulating agents. Supportive care includes specific interventions and is not viewed as a holistic approach to the patient because the focus is predominantly medical and interventions are used to return the patient to a stable hemodynamic state.

Supportive care in the oncology setting refers to those aspects of medical care focused on the physical issues that accompany cancer. Supportive care may consider the psychologic and spiritual needs of the patient and his or her family in the broader sense of cancer management. Therefore supportive care for the oncology patient is used to manage the adverse effects caused by antineoplastic therapies through the utilization of what is considered the broad rubric of palliative interventions.[8]

Comfort Care

Comfort care is an approach to the care of the dying that emphasizes the relief of discomfort rather than the cure of illness or prolongation of life. Physical, social, and emotional needs are the first priority, even when treatment such as high-dose pain medication may have the effect of hastening death.[9] Comfort care is a term that is often used by physicians and nurses in the context of the dying, terminally ill, or seriously ill and dying patient. Yet, comfort care is predominantly used by nurses who attend to the dying patient and family by providing physical comfort measures such as repositioning and oral and skin care, while valuing the ongoing medical management of the patient's symptoms. Comfort care can be multidimensional, such as providing attention to the patient's emotional and spiritual dimensions along with their physical care needs.[9,10] Comfort measures are predominantly carried out in the actively dying phase of life. Comfort care is not symptom management, but describes the nursing interventions used to promote comfort—comfort care provides important interventions to support the patient and family at the end of life. Hospice nurses utilize comfort care and symptom management during the terminal stages of disease—this is often viewed as palliative care.

End-of-Life Care

End-of-life care is more often than not used synonymously with hospice care and identifies a time-defined aspect of care.[6] End-of-life care is somewhat evident in its use and terminology in that it is the care the patient and family receive in the actively dying, terminally ill, or near-death phase of life (Table 49-1).[11] The Medicare hospice benefit is available to patients when they receive a prognosis for survival of 6 months or less—patients who receive this type of care are expected to die. Death is considered the final outcome in hospice care and the services provided for the patient and family at the end of life include comfort and palliative care (symptom management).

Concept Discussion

Palliative experts believe that palliative care should not be used synonymously or confused with the term end-of-life care.[5] Proclaiming that palliative care is caregiving for the dying person reinforces that primary care providers consider

TABLE 49-1   SCOPE OF PALLIATION

EXEMPLAR FOCUS	COMFORT CARE	SUPPORTIVE CARE	END-OF-LIFE CARE	HOSPICE CARE
Focus of care	Terminal illness	Cancer	Terminal illness	Terminal illness
	Dying	Malignancy	Dying	Dying
Provider of care	Nursing	Medical	Health team	Health team
Intervention focus	Comfort measures	Hemostasis	Comfort care	Comfort care
	Palliation	Symptom management	Symptom management	Symptom management
		Palliation	Palliation	Palliation
Timeframe	Weeks to days of life	Acute management	Weeks to days of life	Prognosis of 6 months or less

palliative care only for the actively dying patient.[12] Reserving the use of palliative care interventions for symptomatic patients at the end of their life prevents the use of effective symptom management in the care of patients living with chronic disease states.

End-of-life care is a quantitative term, and limits the opportunity to expand the use of palliative care into the management of chronic disease.[5] Using the term end-of-life care to describe palliative care does not adequately describe the complex problems and high case mix of patients who require the skills of effective palliation (e.g., chemotherapy, radiation therapy, or blood transfusions). End-of-life care in the form of hospice care utilizes palliative care for the imminently dying by introducing a team of health care professionals at the end of the patient's life. This type of care delivery often promotes a discontinuous model of care rather than a coordinated continuous delivery of patient care.[5,13]

The premise of palliative care is to promote the optimal management of symptoms that are common to chronic disease states in a coordinated manner.[6,13] Optimal symptom management promotes improved physical functioning and patient-perceived quality of life.[14,15] Despite the symptom burden associated with the most common chronic diseases, patients with nonmalignant diseases are often underrepresented in palliative care populations.[14,16]

As mentioned previously, because most clinicians perceive palliative care to be terminal or end-of-life care only, there is often a withdrawal of active treatment as compared with the active management of the disease process. Because of this, the management of distressing symptoms and the provision of psychosocial and spiritual support that accompany comprehensive palliative care are often reserved for the last weeks and days of life.[17,18]

ATTRIBUTES

Palliation is the reduction of symptoms without elimination of the cause. Palliative care refers to the provision of care for patients who are diagnosed with a disease or condition without a cure. This approach encompasses:
- A focus on the care of the patient, not on the cure of the disease or illness
- A supportive role, including symptom management
- An interprofessional approach to the delivery of care
- Individualized holistic care that addresses the unique needs of the patient and family
- Collaborative communication among patients, providers, and families to determine realistic goals
- A focus on the quality of life versus the length of life
- Care provided early in the course of disease that extends into the end of life

THEORETICAL LINKS

The Macmillan nurse model, familiar in the United Kingdom (U.K.), is used as the conceptual framework for this concept. Since 1975, Macmillan nurses have been instrumental in the development of specialist palliative care services across therapeutic settings throughout the U.K.[19] The Macmillan nurse's advanced practice and specialty training promote an in-depth knowledge of advanced disease pathophysiology as well as the psychologic, social, and spiritual needs of the patient living with advanced disease.[20-23] Components defined and developed by the Macmillan nurse are expert practitioner, consultant, educator, researcher, and leader.[20,24] The Macmillan nurse, as a member of the palliative care team, integrates seamless palliative interventions early into the course of a patient's disease and follows the patient and his/her family several years before death. Macmillan nurses recognize that palliative care is applicable and relevant when disease is no longer curable or when attempting to treat a chronic disease that may involve years of disability before death.

Macmillan nurses are not reserved for time-limited interventions, such as those familiar to end-of-life care of hospice services, but rather integrate palliative care throughout the clinical course of the disease from diagnosis until death.[24] Community-based Macmillan nurses work in collaboration with a general practitioner (GP) in providing expert pain and symptom management for patients with advanced diseases for several years before death. Macmillan nurses recognize when to make specific referrals to support the needs of the patient and family. Most specifically, they know when it is appropriate to refer patients into hospice care, which in the U.K. is an inpatient setting for patients to spend their last days of life.[21] Macmillan nurses demonstrate how effective palliative care is integrated into the care and management of patients living and dying from advanced chronic diseases in which symptoms intensify as the disease progresses.

CONTEXT TO NURSING AND HEALTH CARE

Millions of Americans are living with 1 or more chronic debilitating diseases, and 7 out of 10 Americans can expect to live with their diseases several years before dying.[25,26] When coupled with the advancing age of the 8 million baby boomers who now qualify for Medicare, this will soon create a huge demand on health care resources and community-based services. These demands will force changes in patterns of care for those patients living for several years before dying from chronic disease and its associated complications. The current health care system spends the majority of U.S. dollars during the last 6 months of life, when patient care is often fragmented between multiple providers and care settings.[25] The Institute of Medicine (IOM) identified U.S. health care as costly and disenfranchised and made recommendations for a coordinated and continuous care delivery model.[27] Changes in care models will require attention to the cost-effective management of chronic diseases and their associated symptoms.[2]

Nurses spend more time with patients during the advancing stages of their diseases than any other health care discipline.[28] An increasing number of nurses will be required to support the needs of the growing and aging patient population. An aging population can benefit from the integration of skilled palliative care interventions used to support the management of symptomatic chronic disease. Optimal symptom management can enhance quality of life and help to maintain ideal physical functioning.[4,6]

Advances in medical therapies and treatments have created a higher quality of life and lower rates of disability and mortality. In the early 1980s mortality rates for colon cancer began to decline; breast, prostate, and lung cancers soon demonstrated similar patterns in the early 1990s.[22] The most noted improvements in morbidity and survival, however, came from advances in the treatment and prevention of cardiovascular diseases.[29]

The Face of Advanced Disease

Despite the advancements in modern medicine, the rates of chronic diseases are steadily increasing and, if left unchecked, may begin to threaten and negate the gains.[29] The past 2 decades have witnessed a dramatic growth in the percent of the population diagnosed with diabetes and cardiovascular disease, driven in large part by increased rates of obesity.[29] The incidence of stroke, pulmonary disease, and mental disorders, such as depression, is also rising, mostly related to an aging population.[29]

Health Policy

The U.S. Department of Health and Human Services (USDHHS)[2] has recently commissioned a task force to recommend and produce a strategic framework to improve the health status of Americans who are living with concurrent multiple chronic conditions (MCCs). The USDHHS aims to change the culture or produce a paradigm shift and implement new strategies that will provide a foundation to support and maintain optimal health and quality of life for patients with MCCs.[2] To achieve this vision, the following four overarching goals have been identified:

1. Provide better tools and information to health care and social service workers who deliver care to individuals with MCCs.
2. Maximize the use of proven self-care management and other services by individuals with MCCs.
3. Foster health care and public health system changes to improve the health of individuals with MCCs.
4. Facilitate research to fill knowledge gaps about individuals with MCCs.[2]

Because millions of Americans are currently living with unmanaged symptoms such as pain, depression, and dyspnea, this shift of legislation will provide an opportunity to advance the use of palliative care into the management of chronic diseases instead of reserving effective symptom management for those patients in the last days and weeks of life.

Palliative Care Delivery

Palliation is not an isolated concept. To fully appreciate the concept, other principles should be considered as necessary constructs that link to the definition and provide for a richer understanding of palliation as something more than symptom management. Palliative care should be integrated into the management of chronic symptomatic disease that increases in its intensity and use as the patient approaches death. At times there is a fine line between palliation and a curative approach to disease management.

Because Americans are living longer with chronic advanced disease the following discussion can provide some grounding principles that provide a context for palliation that is integrated into the management of chronic disease. The principles of curative care, disease trajectory, and the interprofessional team are presented in the sections that follow.

Curative Care

The biomedical approach to chronic disease management is typically overseen with a curative rather than a palliative focus. Health care providers often approach chronic disease management in an aggressive manner, seeking a cure or a recovery or investigating contributing factors associated with disease and disability. The focus of care in a curative approach remains on the cure and rehabilitation of disease. Care is often planned on the basis of routine protocols and delivered through the traditional medical model. The goal of care is to alter or attempt to eradicate the disease process despite disease futility and symptom burden. Care is largely determined by diagnosis and medical specialty services. Curative care is evidence based and traditionally and historically practiced in routine health care, and provides the familiar and expected approach to disease management.

Disease Trajectory

The trajectory of disease can be viewed from three different perspectives. The patient who is diagnosed with cancer will often have an obvious decline in physical functioning, and there are clear prognostic indicators that can help the health care provider identify when the patient is beginning to decline and approaching the dying phase. This trajectory of disease can be identified as a short period of evident decline.[30] The cancer patient typically maintains function for a substantial period of time; then as the disease becomes overwhelming, the patient's status declines rapidly in the final months and days of life.[30] The hospice care model was initially based upon the cancer disease trajectory—in which there are clear and obvious indications of decline based upon the effects of metastatic disease and its associated therapies (Figure 49-1).

Patients who live and die from chronic disease states, such as congestive heart failure (CHF) and chronic obstructive pulmonary disease (COPD), often experience disease exacerbations that insidiously lead toward a poor prognosis. This trajectory of disease follows a long-term limitation with intermittent exacerbations and sudden dying—typical of organ system failure.[30] Patients who follow this disease trajectory often live for several years with their chronic disease and may have minor functional limitations in activities of daily living. Occasionally, some physiologic stress overwhelms the body's reserves and leads to a worsening of serious symptoms. Patients often survive these episodes of acute exacerbations. Patients who follow this disease trajectory will typically die suddenly from a complication or an acute exacerbation.[30]

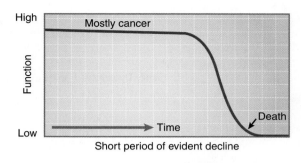

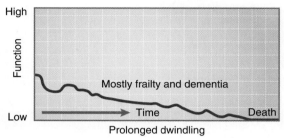

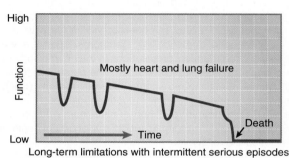

FIGURE 49-1 Disease Trajectories.

Each time these patients encounter an exacerbation of their disease and enter into the acute care setting, their disease is gradually progressing and physiologically unresponsive to curative measures (see Figure 49-1).

The third disease trajectory is what is known as prolonged dwindling—this is seen in patients with dementia or Alzheimer's disease, disabling stroke, and frailty.[30] Patients who follow this disease trajectory do not have cancer or chronic disease states that lead to organ failure—these patients are more likely to die at older ages.[30] Patients who reside in long-term care settings are most likely following this type of disease trajectory where the prolonged insidious decline in function will eventually lead to multiple organ failure and death.

Interprofessional Team

An interprofessional team approach involving health care professionals from different disciplines is central to optimal palliative care practice and quality outcomes. In contrast, a multiprofessional approach is one in which several subspecialists independently make patient care consultations and recommendations to the patient's plan of care. In palliative care, a team addresses the needs of both the patient and the family—biological, psychologic, emotional, social, and spiritual. Interprofessional care is further characterized by a collaborative effort that includes information exchange and coordinated care planning; it places the patient and family at the center of team deliberations and maximizes the unique contributions of each member.[31] The palliative care team is composed of the following disciplines:

- *Nursing*—The nurse caring for the patient and the patient's family recognizes the multidimensional needs and aspects that surround advanced disease and death. The nurse assesses and evaluates the ongoing needs of the patient's physical, emotional, and spiritual well-being as well as advocates and provides referrals to the other disciplines of the team.
- *Social services*—Social workers often bridge the gap between physical and psychologic care for the patient and family, helping to identify areas of need such as communication and isolation issues and assisting in reducing the emergence of crises surrounding unfinished business. Social workers can connect the patient and family to resources, helping them prepare not only for the death event but also for the grief and bereavement process.
- *Physician*—The medical leader directs the medical management of the patient. The physician should provide patient evaluation and assessment of clinical manifestations, diagnostics, and interventions.
- *Spiritual care*—Members of the clergy and other spiritual advisors provide spiritual counseling and support for the patient and his/her family. Spiritual issues often are intertwined with other symptoms and can be masked by both physical and psychoemotional responses. The spiritual advisor's approach should be consistent with the patient's and family's beliefs and desires.
- *Ancillary services*—Based on the goals of care, other members of the team can help support the care of the patient and needs of the family. These roles include volunteers, nursing assistants, physical and occupational therapists, art and music therapists, pharmacists, psychologists, and psychiatrists.

The successful palliative care team collaborates on providing "best practice" to address the multiple needs of the patient and family. This is accomplished through the development and maintenance of an integrated, individualized plan of care. The plan of care is based first on the patient's and family's realistic expectations and goals, and second on the team's assessment, recommendations. and support. The primary medical provider is considered a part of the team and should not be regarded as directing the medical care and management of the patient, but rather participating with the efforts of the team striving to meet the individual needs of the patient and family.[30]

INTERRELATED CONCEPTS

There are several concepts discussed in this book that are interrelated to palliation and include **Evidence, Ethics, Safety, Family dynamics,** and **Culture.** The use of evidence supports high-quality interventions that are used in optimal symptom management. Ethical considerations are used to minimize harm and improve quality of life in fragile and

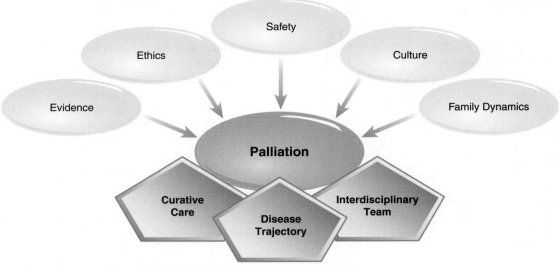

FIGURE 49-2 Palliation and Interrelated Concepts.

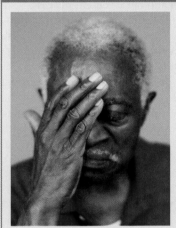

Mr. Carl Stevens is a 76-year-old African-American male and retired accountant who was diagnosed with chronic obstructive pulmonary disease (COPD) by his primary care physician (PCP) 4 years age. He is a 40 pack-year smoker and has continued to smoke half a pack of cigarettes daily despite requests by both his primary care provider and his wife to quit. His recent pulmonary function test suggested that his disease has progressed from mild to moderate staging (FEV_1 <70% predicted). Carl's recent laboratory analysis revealed normal values for his complete blood count and chemistries. He has a significant weight loss of 12 pounds over the past 6 months. Carl complains of severe dyspnea, weakness, insomnia, and depression. He states that his symptoms are all interrelated and he has become homebound and no longer enjoys socializing with his former colleagues and friends. He describes how these symptoms have impacted his physical functioning and that he is no longer able to walk to the end of his driveway to retrieve his mail or early morning newspaper. Because Carl is unable to sleep in his bed, he has been sleeping upright in his armchair throughout the daytime and watching television during normal hours of sleep, which has disrupted his wife's sleep.

Carl states that he has not been using any of his medications according to his physician's directions and was hospitalized last year for an exacerbation that eventually led to pneumonia, requiring extensive intravenous antibiotic and systemic corticosteroid therapy. Carl's PCP has made a recent referral for a skilled nursing home visit to evaluate Carl's needs attributable to his debilitating dyspnea and inability to carry out activities of daily living (ADLs).

Given Carl's concomitant diseases and associated symptoms, his PCP is planning a palliative approach to his disease management. The home care nurse informs the PCP that Mr. Stevens has not been taking his medications because of financial issues and his depressed mood. The nurse further informs Carl's physician that Mr. Stevens has been caring for his wife, who recently developed dementia-like symptoms. His wife was responsible for all the meal preparations in their home and now can no longer use the stove and oven. The nurse facilitates a social worker, dietitian, and spiritual advisor referral for additional assessment and supportive recommendations.

The PCP encouraged the home care nurse to ensure Mr. Stevens follows a pharmaceutical management regimen that included the following:

- Long-acting bronchodilator (maintenance medication) used for COPD and dyspnea
- Short-acting bronchodilator (rescue medication) for immediate dyspnea relief
- Short-term titrated systemic corticosteroid medication to improve breathing, and initially affect his mood and appetite
- An antidepressant to be used at bedtime, which could also improve Carl's insomnia

The nurse recommended a hospital bed until Carl's symptoms improved; this would allow Carl to sleep in a bed and restore normal day-night sleeping patterns.

After 1 month of ongoing home nursing visits, the nurse informed the PCP that Carl had improved from his medical management regimen and no longer complains of dyspnea. Carl has increased his ability to walk to the end of his driveway without being short of breath. He is sleeping throughout the night, has gained 5 pounds, and has been actively involved in working with his social worker to obtain community support for his wife. The multilevel approach to this patient has improved his symptoms, his quality of life, and his ability to gain control and improve his functioning and sense of well-being.

Case Analysis

The model case illustrates the effects that chronic disease has on a person's life. Mr. Stevens' symptoms, including insomnia, dyspnea, depression, and weakness, prevented him from participating in his activities of daily living. Using an interprofessional approach the goal is to reduce the symptoms associated with COPD. Treating his symptoms does not provide a cure for his illness, but does allow for improved quality of life.

CONTRARY CASE

Baby Janella is a 6-month-old former 32-week infant who presents to the emergency department with cough, irritability, and rhinorrhea. Baby Janella's symptoms started 2 days ago and the patient's mother stated "I see the baby's ribs every time she breathes." The patient's mother also reports the baby has not been feeding well and "has not wet her diaper since last night." The patient's mother states, "She finally started growing and now she is sick. Will she be ok?" Baby Janella has been thriving since her discharge from the neonatal intensive care unit. The patient's mother is very concerned about her daughter's disinterest in feeding, possible weight loss, and new onset of illness.

The infant was admitted to the inpatient unit for monitoring and with a diagnosis of bronchiolitis. Baby Janella's physical assessment findings include fever, tachycardia, tachypnea, intercostal retractions, and mild hypoxemia. Cool mist oxygen is administered to maintain adequate oxygenation. Chest physiotherapy is used every 4 hours to assist with secretion mobilization. Acetaminophen has been administered as needed as an antipyretic. Baby Janella continues to be irritable and is refusing oral intake. IV fluids are ordered. A topical anesthetic is first applied to Baby Janella's skin before IV insertion and then hydration is initiated. The parents are aware of the current treatment plan and despite their exhaustion they plan to actively participate and collaborate with the health care team to provide curative care for Baby Janella.

After 3 days of receiving supportive and symptomatic care for the treatment of bronchiolitis, Baby Janella is ready for discharge. The baby is tolerating oral feeds, although requiring smaller, more frequent feedings. Her weight remains stable without further weight loss. The parents, despite being well-informed throughout the admission, are anxious to care for the baby at home. They voice concern and worry that she may relapse and are apprehensive about Baby Janella's inability to tolerate her previous feeding schedule. The nurse reviews the disease trajectory and informs the parents that most infants with bronchiolitis fully recover within 1 to 2 weeks. The parents are educated on bulb syringe suctioning and feeding techniques to reduce the baby's fatigue. A follow-up appointment with their pediatrician is scheduled in 2 days to evaluate Baby Janella's condition and the effectiveness of treatment.

Case Analysis

This case does not represent palliation because Baby Janella, was diagnosed with bronchiolitis, a condition that affords a cure. A variety of symptomatic approaches were utilized in the treatment of Baby Janella. The duration of illness is short-term and it is expected that the baby will return to her previous state of wellness. Despite having symptomatic treatment, the goal of treatment for Baby Janella is curative. The type of illness and associated goals determine the approach to patient care— whether it is palliative or curative in nature.

---

dependent patients—the use and utilization of ethics can also be applied to patient safety. Maintaining optimal symptom control and comfort promotes patient safety and satisfaction. The patient and family are at the core of palliation; the care is individualized based upon disease and disability. The family serves as a member of the interprofessional care and often takes an active role as caregiver. Culture cannot be isolated from the individualized care that is considered for each patient in the palliative setting. Beliefs, values, and practices are integrated and considered in the care of the patient, especially as death approaches and rituals are used in the final days of life. It is the nurse who is able to integrate all of these concepts into the care and management of the patient who is living with and dying from chronic symptomatic disease.

EXEMPLARS

There are multiple clinical examples of palliation that are seen in diverse clinical settings. Box 49-1 identifies exemplars of the terms described in this concept analysis and helps to differentiate the manner in which they are used based upon where the patient falls along the path of his or her disease trajectory. It is beyond the scope of this concept analysis to describe each exemplar in detail—but it is important that nurses recognize the concept of palliation with each exemplar. There are multiple nursing textbooks and other resources that provide details of the exemplars presented in Box 49-1.

◼◼ BOX 49-1 EXEMPLARS OF PALLIATIVE CARE

Palliative Care (Not Actively Dying)
- Aggressive symptom management such as dyspnea, fatigue, anxiety, depression
- Prevention of disease exacerbations
- Promote activity, increasing physical functioning
- Rehabilitation

Comfort Care (Actively Dying)
- Interventions for symptom management
- Provide patient and family reassurance
- Reduction in physical functioning

Supportive Care
- Aggressive use of laboratory analysis
- Blood transfusions
- Bone marrow stimulating factors
- Referral to specialty physicians to manage pulmonary disease and symptoms
- Used in lung cancer patients undergoing oncology care

End-of-Life Care
- Admission into hospice care
- Do not resuscitate order
- Expectation that death will occur within 6 months of admission into hospice care
- Patient no longer seeks aggressive disease management
- Symptom management

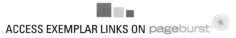

ACCESS EXEMPLAR LINKS ON pageburst

REFERENCES

1. U.S. Department of Health and Human Services: *Healthy People 2020*, 2010, at www.healthypeople.gov. Accessed Jan 11, 2011.
2. U.S. Department of Health and Human Services: *Multiple chronic conditions—a strategic framework: optimum health and quality of life for individuals with multiple chronic conditions*, Washington, DC, Dec 2010, Author.
3. Centers for Disease Control and Prevention: *Healthy aging improving and extending quality of life among older Americans. Chronic disease prevention and health promotion*, 2009, at www.cdc.gov/NCCdphp/publications/aag/aging.htm. Accessed Jan 2, 2010.
4. World Health Organization: *National cancer control programmes. Policies and managerial guidelines*, ed 2, Geneva, Switzerland, 2002, Author.
5. Davis M, Walsh D, LeGrand S: End-of-life care: the death of palliative care, *J Palliative Med* 5:813, 2005.
6. Kuebler K, Lynn J, Von Rohen J: Perspectives in palliative care, *Semin Oncol Nurs* 21:2, 2005.
7. Berger A, Shuster J, Von Rohen J: Foreword. In Berger A, Shuster J, Von Roenn J, editors: *Principles and practice of palliative care and supportive oncology*, ed 3, Philadelphia, Pa, 2007, Lippincott Williams & Wilkins.
8. Berger A, Portenoy R, Weissman D: Preface. In Berger A, Portenoy R, Weissman D, editors: *Principles and practice of palliative care and supportive oncology*, ed 2, Philadelphia, 2002, Lippincott Williams & Wilkins.
9. Wenger N: Response to the UCLA medical center ethics committee, *HEC Forum* 6:315, 1994.
10. Kolcaba KY: The art of comfort care, *J Nurs Schol* 27:287, 1995.
11. Krinzbrunner B: Palliative care perspectives. In Kuebler K, Davis M, Moore C, editors: *Palliative care perspectives: an interdisciplinary approach*, Philadelphia, 2005, Elsevier.
12. Woodruff R: The problem of definitions, *Prog Palliative Care* 10:17, 2002.
13. Davis M, Kuebler K: Palliative and end-of-life care perspectives. In Kuebler K, Heidrich D, Esper P, editors: *Palliative and end-of-life care clinical practice guidelines*, ed 2, St Louis, 2007, Saunders/Elsevier.
14. Brooksbank M: Palliative care: where have we come from and where are we going? *Pain* 144:233, 2009.
15. Webber J: A model response, *Nurs Times* 90:66, 1994.
16. Barnes S, Gott M, Payne S, et al: Prevalence of symptoms in a community-based sample of heart failure patients, *J Pain Symp Manag* 32:208, 2006.
17. Corcoran A, Casarett D: Improving communication and rethinking hospice care, *Chest* 137:1262, 2010.
18. Gwyther L, Bremmem F, Obs D, et al: Advancing palliative care as a human right, *J Pain Symp Manag* 62:1, 2009.
19. Seymour J, Clark D, Hughes P, et al: Clinical nurse specialists in palliative care. Part 3. Issues for the Macmillan nurse role, *Palliative Med* 16:386, 2002.
20. Bullen M: Macmillan nurses: fighting cancer with more than medicine, *RCN Nurs Update* 6:3, 1994.
21. Kuebler K, Moore C: The Michigan advanced practice nursing palliative care project, *J Palliative Med* 5:752, 2002.
22. Scott G: Challenging conventional roles in palliative care, *Nurs Times* 91:38, 1995.
23. Webber J: A model response, *Nurs Times* 90:66, 1994.
24. Astin F, Closs S, Hughes N: Macmillan nurses' education and development needs: a documentary analysis, *J Clin Nurs* 10:2008, 1949.
25. Wennberg J, Fisher E, Goodman D, et al: Tracking the care of patients with severe chronic illness, *Executive summary: the Dartmouth atlas of health care*, 2008.
26. Grant M, Elk R, Ferrell B, et al: Current status of palliative care clinical implementation, education, and research, *CA Can J Clin* 59:327, 2009.
27. Institute of Medicine: *The 1st annual crossing the quality chasm summit: a focus on community*, Washington, DC, 2003, National Academies Press.
28. Foley K, Gelband H: *Improving palliative care for cancer*, Washington, DC, 2001, National Academies Press.
29. DeVol R, Bedroussian A: *2007; An unhealthy America: the economic burden of chronic disease charting a new course to save lives and increase productivity and economic growth*, Milken Institute at www.milkeninstitute.org. Accessed Jan 8, 2011.
30. Lynn J, Adamson D: *Living well at the end of life: adapting healthcare to serious chronic illness in old age, White Paper*, RAND Health, 2003.
31. Kuebler K, Froelich S: Palliative care perspectives. In Kuebler K, editor: *Palliative nurses continuing education modules*, 2010. Retrieved Feb 25, 2011, from wwwgeorgianurses.org.

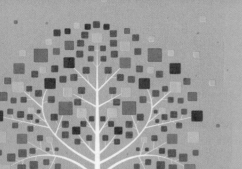

Health Care Organizations

Teresa Keller

To describe health care organizations as complex is to understate their fluid and dynamic nature. The delivery of health care services in the United States is driven by the need to provide a broad spectrum of care in a variety of settings to diverse consumers. The delivery of these services requires a highly specialized, professional workforce, financed by a mix of private and public funding, and subject to oversight and regulation by many different public and private authorities. Whether they are rural clinics catering to migrant laborers, large teaching hospitals in urban environments, or integrated health systems providing a spectrum of services across the nation, health care organizations (HCOs) face challenges that require them to adapt and innovate or face extinction. The result is new service delivery arrangements, new kinds of health care workplaces, new types of service providers, and new treatments and services hardly imagined in prior times.

The variety of organizational forms and the services that evolve are ultimately only a reflection of the dynamic nature of the human social interaction and collaboration required to meet the health care needs of a society. HCOs are social systems created by people and managed by people; therefore the HCO is a socially created entity with no meaning outside of the collective actions and aspirations of the people involved. The significance of this perspective of the organization is that all people involved with an HCO have the capacity to create, innovate, and make meaningful contributions toward producing the dynamic, living social system recognized as an HCO.

DEFINITION(S)

Organizations can be defined as a group of people who come together for a purpose[1] or as a collection of people brought together for a predetermined purpose in a defined environment.[2] Common to both of these definitions is that organizations are composed of people and have a purpose. Organizations could be further defined as having a socially determined structure provided by formal properties such as rules, policies, and procedures, and by informal properties such

as customs, norms, and values.[1] A more robust definition for organizations is that they are structured social arrangements that use systematic strategies to combine and coordinate a mix of resources (people and capital) to provide specific products or services. For the purposes of this concept analysis, the definition of HCO is *a purposefully designed, structured social system developed for the delivery of health care services by specialized workforces to defined communities, populations, or markets.*

SCOPE AND CATEGORIES

The scope of the HCO concept is broad and complex with numerous variables to consider when examining different types and categories of HCOs. There are so many different ways to organize an HCO that the result is a large variety of distinctive organizations in the U.S. health care sector—an estimated 535,000 HCOs![3] Because they are purposely designed to meet the need for health care services in a community or population or market, HCOs vary widely in their form and function. There are HCOs specifically designed to deliver health care services, such as hospitals and clinics, and those that are designed for a health-related purpose but not to deliver services, such as pharmaceutical companies or manufacturers of medical equipment.

Obviously, a discussion of the concept of the HCO can be quickly complicated by all the different possible purposes and forms of organization. The variety of distinctive organizations with specific purposes meant to meet the needs of a particular community or population defies simple classification. For the purpose of establishing an initial understanding of this complex concept, the scope of the HCO will be limited to those organizations that provide a range of health care services for health promotion, illness, and wellness care. This would include a variety of organizations including (but not limited to) hospitals, ambulatory care centers, home health agencies, clinics, nursing homes, provider offices and organizations, and long term care facilities of all types. To further limit complexity for this discussion, HCOs can be broadly classified by their *mission, financial classification,* and *ownership.*

Focus of Mission

HCOs have an organizational mission in the health services sector. These missions may be specific or general but each mission is always related to the delivery focus. For example, research and teaching hospitals are large HCOs usually associated with academic health centers whose mission includes the education of health professionals as well as the delivery of health care services. Community hospitals, on the other hand, offer general medical and surgical services to a surrounding community but most will not have a research or teaching mission.[3] Hospice is a type of HCO with a specific mission—to provide end-of-life services to patients and their families. Other HCOs with highly specialized purposes include U.S. Department of Defense HCOs that provide health care services to military members and their families or Indian Health Services HCOs that provide health care services for Native American populations.

Financial Classification

Another way to classify HCOs is by their financial purpose as either for-profit or not-for-profit entities. The difference between the not-for-profit versus the for-profit HCO is not the profits generated but how the profits are distributed. For-profit HCOs are designed to generate profits for shareholders while also providing health care services. Not-for-profit HCOs also generate profits but these are used for organizational purposes, such as building additional facilities, providing improved services, or acquiring new equipment.

In reality, this distinction between for-profit and not-for-profit HCOs is less clear because any HCO must pay attention to financial viability. The need to generate revenues to meet expenses is important to all organizations, whether for-profit or not-for-profit, because the failure to cover expenses creates risks to the HCO's continued existence. Unprofitable HCOs that collect less revenue than what is required to meet expenses—even if they are publicly supported—will eventually have to close or be reorganized.

Ownership

Health care organizations, in addition to their mission and financing, can also be classified as publicly or privately owned.[2,3] Publicly owned HCOs are commonly seen as community organizations that are supported by government funding. The typical example of this type of ownership is the tax-supported county or state hospital that provides generalized health care services or specific health services such as behavioral and mental health. State and local public health departments could also be considered a publicly owned HCO. Investor-owned corporations would be considered privately owned, but private ownership could also include HCOs owned by religious or social organizations. Privately owned HCOs are not generally supported by public funding.

The major classifications of mission, finance, and ownership noted earlier can be combined to create a myriad of HCOs designed to meet the challenges of the health care environment. The variety seen in HCOs can be illustrated using hospice as an example. Hospice services provide specialty care to a specific population—the terminally ill and their families. As an HCO, (1) the hospice might be a for-profit institution, privately owned (by investors) HCO, where any profits generated by services are returned to the investors in the form of dividends; or (2) the hospice might be nonprofit and privately owned by a religious organization and any profits realized are returned to the HCO to improve the quality of services and infrastructure or to sustain other services offered by the organization. Both of these types of hospice provide the same unique service and play a distinct role in the health care community, although they vary by ownership and by profit status. Further, a hospice could also be a part of an integrated, national network of HCOs delivering a full spectrum of coordinated health care services. Regardless of the structure and institutional arrangement, as an HCO the hospice must be ready to manage costs and maintain services while evolving as the health services environment changes. Table 50-1 provides an illustration of mission, financing and ownership for selected types of organizations.

ATTRIBUTES

All organizations have defining attributes. Each has a purpose, a structure, and members who do the work of the organization. HCOs are no different from other kinds of organizations in this regard. As social systems, HCOs are situated within an environment from which resources are obtained and from which challenges are presented that require an organizational

TABLE 50-1	SELECTED CATEGORIES OF HEALTH CARE ORGANIZATIONS		
EXAMPLES	**MISSION**	**FINANCIAL PURPOSE**	**OWNERSHIP**
State/county hospitals	Provide services for geographic area or specialized population but especially for poor or underserved residents	Nonprofit/tax supported	State/local governments
Shriners hospitals	Provide services for no to minimal cost to burn patients and children with orthopedic needs	Nonprofit	Shriners International, private philanthropic organization
Hospital Corporation of America® (HCA)	Network of HCOs that provide range of medical and surgical services nationally	For-profit	Investor-owned corporation
Good samaritan	Network of HCOs that provides range of health care services for elderly nationally	Nonprofit	Good Samaritan Society,® religious philanthropic organization

response. In daily operations, HCOs must be able to acquire resources, produce services, and change as necessary to sustain their existence within the challenging U.S. health care services sector.

Major Attributes

HCOs are distinguished from other types of organizations by their unique *purpose,* by their *specialized workforce,* and by a level of *public trust* that these institutions are primarily designed to help others achieve and maintain optimal health and/or well-being.

Purpose

The purpose of HCOs is to help others by providing health care services. This distinguishes an HCO as a service-oriented organization distinct from other organizations with health-related purposes. The primary purpose of companies that sell health insurance is to sell an insurance product. Schools for health professions have a primary educational purpose. The purpose of accreditation and public regulatory agencies is to support the work of the HCO, but these organizations do not directly deliver health care services. An HCO provides health care services to manage illness or promote health, whether that service is childhood immunizations, surgical interventions, diabetes education, family planning advice, or any of a wide variety of other health care services offered to individuals, families, and communities. This purpose remains the same—to provide health care services—regardless of profit status or ownership arrangements.

The purpose of an HCO can be determined by the organization's mission, vision, and values.[2] Mission statements issued by HCOs describe the organization's purpose based on a vision of what the HCO hopes to achieve. Mission statements also describe the values that drive the work of the organization, such as quality and excellence. Even if the HCO is a for-profit, privately owned corporation that pays dividends to shareholders, the mission statement will reflect values commonly associated with helping others, such as service and professionalism. Because mission statements reflect strategic vision, they focus and drive the work of the HCO toward organizational goals. Mission statements that reflect values that primarily benefit shareholders, such as seeking higher profits, would drive the work of the HCO in a direction that is inconsistent with the goal of helping others with their health care needs. Mission statements that prominently feature service ideals and values and that promote assistance and support to others serve to sustain the primary purpose of the HCO.

Specialized Health Care Workforce

HCOs are notable for the highly specialized workforce needed to deliver health care services. The work produced in an HCO is complex, variable, and at times urgent in nature. The margin for error is narrow with little tolerance for mistakes that can lead to life-threatening and costly consequences.[1] Health professionals who work in HCOs undergo extensive education and experiential learning. The knowledge and skills that these specialized workers bring to the HCO are necessary for the effective delivery of services in an ambiguous, challenging work environment. The compelling need for this specialized workforce increases the costs for HCOs but it also benefits the organization in terms of maintaining standards and ensuring quality service outcomes. An additional benefit is that the strong professional ideals of these workers promote and strengthen the service values that support the purpose of the HCO.

Further, the work of managing the health of humans is not easily divided because people present with health problems that affect the whole person, their families, and perhaps the entire community. The need to treat a person, rather than a disease or problem, centers the work of health care professionals and creates an interdependence among these workers that is another notable characteristic of HCOs.[1] Although labor might be divided among numerous specialized personnel, the need to address the person or patient as a whole means each of these professionals is dependent upon the knowledge and skills of others. An interprofessional approach to the treatment of human health problems not only is a distinguishing feature of the HCO but also serves to increase the complexity of the organization.

Although the HCO is uniquely defined by its specialized workforce of health care professionals, a discussion of the health care workforce is not complete without reference to the numerous other personnel essential to the effective function of the HCO. For example, the human resource department of any large HCO provides critical services necessary for the daily operations of the HCO since most health care professionals expect to receive a salary and benefits. Dietary and housekeeping personnel provide important services within the HCO that support the work of health care professionals, as do the administrators responsible for ensuring adequate supplies and other resources. Because the HCO is a specialized organization with unique functions, all of these workers could be considered a part of the specialized health care workforce.

Public Trust

The historical development of HCOs demonstrates a long record of service to others. Early organizations were created by religious orders or by social service groups to provide services to a society's most vulnerable members—the ill and infirm. The work of these early organizations gained the confidence of the public that their altruistic purpose was to serve others by providing care and comfort, regardless of personal circumstances. These laudable efforts helped to establish a social contract between the public and the HCO, one from which HCOs have benefited in both financial terms and public regard.

Currently, the level of public trust in HCOs has eroded with the growth of managed care, national corporate chains of for-profit HCOs, and allegations of fraud and abuse by health care providersa.[4] Yet people still turn to their physicians and nurses for help and advice and they still seek the services offered by HCOs when they need help with health issues. This indicates that the social contract is still intact, if a little worn. As such, HCOs are still distinguished by their relatively positive image of institutions designed to provide valuable and needed services to others. As mentioned earlier, all organizations must generate income to remain viable so the for-profit/not-for-profit status of the HCO is less important than managing the tensions created by financial issues versus the need to preserve altruistic values. HCOs that provide quality health care services and are good corporate citizens will be able to maintain their positive image and their part of the social contract, regardless of their profit status.

Minor Attributes

The minor attributes of HCOs differ from major attributes in terms of the HCO's relationship to other kinds of organizations. The major attributes of HCOs discussed in the preceding section are identified with health care and the health care services sector. The minor attributes of an HCO are attributes that define them as forms of purposeful organizations and are features they share in common with other types of organizations.

Structure

Structure is the collective of formal rules and policies that govern organizational practices and that promote the effective management of materials and resources. Structure also creates the various roles and associated responsibilities that are required for organizational function. Different organizational roles carry varying levels of authority for decision making relative to the assigned responsibilities of those roles. Organizational rules, policies, and authority are necessary for the integration of diverse functions and activities across the organization into a coordinated system capable of supporting the purpose of the organization. However, too much structure can be stifling, causing the HCO to be so encumbered by rules and regulations that meaningful action is hampered. An organization needs sufficient structure to support important processes and operations; otherwise, it will disintegrate into anarchy. A balance needs to be maintained that provides the structure necessary for sustaining the HCO while not producing unnecessary constraints.[5]

The requirement for supportive structures that minimize constraints is especially important for HCOs because of the type of personnel seen in these organizations. As noted earlier, the workforce of HCOs is comprised of a large number of health care professionals. These professionals possess valuable knowledge and skills that are critical to the delivery of health care services. These professionals also have a strong allegiance to a set of professional values. Most health care professionals possess a state-licensed authority to manage their own practice and are responsible for the outcomes of their work.

For an HCO, this means management authority and control is relatively weak in relationship to professional authority[1] because decision making related to practice is not subject to control by those outside the profession. This requires additional lines of authority to be established within the HCO,

for example, nurses are accountable to nursing officers and physicians are accountable to medical executives. This is true for most of the institutional arrangements that create authority within an HCO. Professional control of licensed practice is the basis for the interdependency between health professionals in the HCO but it can also fuel the typical conflicts and "turf wars" seen in an HCO.

The result of these divided lines of authority is that management control by those outside of the profession is limited to those work activities that lie outside the professional's scope of practice. For example, nurses can expect that their professional practice will be directed and evaluated by other nurses and that they will be accountable for maintaining the standards of the profession, However, they can also expect that they will need to meet the requirements established by nonnursing administrators for other expected work behaviors such as reporting to work on time.

Organizational Environments

Organizations possess both an internal environment as well as an external environment with which they interact. The internal environment of the HCO consists of an integrated web of factors such as organizational culture (where culture is defined as a set of values, beliefs, and practices), systems such as information systems or the human resources management system, and structural elements such as role responsibilities, rules, and practices. All of these factors affect the decisions and responses of the HCO to demands and challenges encountered during daily operations.[6]

The external organizational environment consists of those external forces, conditions, or events that affect the organization, such as economic trends or new laws and government regulation.[3] An example of external environmental forces would be a widespread economic recession or government funding changes that affect HCOs. These kinds of forces in the external environment provide resources and/or feedback as inputs to the organization and are major factors that drive organizational change.

There is an interplay between the internal and external environments of the HCO, where organizational decisions and operations are affected by perceived forces from the external environment. Organizations integrated into their environments will also change those environments in some ways, adding to the complexity of the relationship. For example, a national economic recession can prompt workers to expand their work hours, either by increasing the hours they work or by seeking additional employment. This holds true for nurses. If experienced professional nurses are working more hours or seeking additional employment, the effect on the HCO could be human resources changes that mean fewer new and inexperienced nurses are hired. The drop in demand for new nurses has the potential to affect the admission decisions of nursing schools or the funding decisions made by government organizations that support nursing education. As these resources are curtailed, there are fewer new nurses prepared and, subsequently, fewer new nurses for the HCO to hire to replace nurses who leave or retire.

Before the twentieth century and the rise of organized health care delivery, the health care industry was unregulated, health care workers were less knowledgeable, and health care markets were small and relatively simple.[7] Currently, multiple interacting forces in the health care environment have profound effects on HCOs, especially as they increase uncertainty and create instability. While HCOs evolve to meet the challenges presented by their environments, they are still expected to maintain the service orientation that is fundamental to their purpose. An example of the internal pressures created by external environmental demands is tying government reimbursements to HCOs to meeting selected standards for care and for ensuring optimal patient safety. Meeting quality and safety standards is highly desirable yet it is also costly in terms of training personnel, providing additional staffing and building work processes that support quality care and patient safety. This creates tensions within the HCO while workers seek to meet expectations for safe and effective care with limited additional resources.

HCO policies created to meet environmental challenges might conflict with professional values or with legal guidelines, requiring actions to negotiate and resolve the conflict. New technologies might need to be adopted that require a shift of resources from one part of the organization to another. The need to change (rapidly in some cases) in response to environmental effects means that HCOs are complex and their work environments are notably ambiguous.

THEORETICAL LINKS

Organizational theories have developed over about the last 100 years, fueled by the growth of manufacturing during the Industrial Revolution. As organizations have grown they have also become the vehicle through which many different kinds of human activity are organized and coordinated. This prompted social scientists to study the phenomenon of purposive, organized systems and to create theories to explain these systems. A complete description of the organizational theories of the last 100 years is beyond the scope of this concept presentation. Instead, an overview of the major directions in theory development related to organizations is useful to understanding the HCO concept.

Bureaucracy

Early conceptualizations of the organization were that they were closed systems and were a rational, machine-like collection of components to be coordinated and controlled through effective management. Max Weber, German sociologist and economist, developed the first theoretical model of bureaucracy in the early twentieth century. Weber described the principles of organization that created efficiency in work design and were thought to be the most effective way to organize work. He also described the distribution of authority in bureaucracies, noting that authority grounded in position and divided into hierarchies was preferable to authority derived from personal characteristics. Weber viewed the bureaucracy

of the organizational design as the one most likely to create the stability needed to sustain an organization.[8]

Bureaucratic design was common to the large organizations that developed during the Industrial Revolution because the manufacturing and distribution of goods required a rational system of centralized control to effectively acquire resources and efficiently convert them to a finished product.[9] Bureaucratic organizations were made of functional parts, or divisions, all welded together through management control made possible by hierarchical authority. These organizations were believed capable of achieving a high degree of coordinated precision in production, leading to the common metaphor of a well-oiled machine."

The drawback to this model of rational efficiency is that it takes little account of the organization as a social system within an environment. Bureaucratic theory mainly focuses on authority and control to achieve efficient production within a closed system. The human dimension of the organization is not well-defined outside of the role of management. Other organizational theorists of that time attempted to describe and explain the social dynamics of organizations, but the main theoretical approach taken was mechanical and emphasized the role of management in attaining maximal productivity from workers through planning and control.[8] The effects of environmental factors on the production and efficiency of an organization were also not considered by these early theorists. The bureaucratic organization was a self-contained, closed system.

Systems Theory

The view of organizations as social systems had an early beginning with the human relations school of organizational theorists. This group focused their study on the needs and desires of people who work in the organization. From this field of study grew an understanding that the organization has social components that interact and that these components are affected by factors from the outside environment.[9] These social components (people, relationships, roles) interact with environment, technology, and organizational structure in an integrated fashion to create a unified, dynamic system.[2,10] This open systems perspective paved the way for interesting new theories that not only intrigue organizational theorists but also provide for new ways to organize and new ways to empower the people who work in these systems (see Figure 50-1).

Complex Adaptive Systems

Current organizational theory describes the organization as having biological characteristics that allow the organization to react and change when stimulated. This understanding of the organization defines a new way of viewing organizations as organic and lifelike entities that are open to the environment and capable of transforming themselves in light of perceived opportunities and threats. The organizations can "read" and interpret the environment[5] and they can adjust and adapt through the coordinated action of their interdependent parts. The changes that occur within an organization

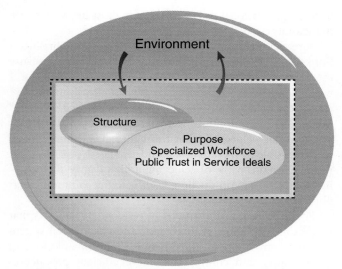

FIGURE 50-1 Health Care Organizations: Open Systems Model.

in response to environmental stimuli are necessary for sustaining the organization, just as metabolic processes within the human body change to allow the body to adapt to environmental challenges. In the case of the HCO, the need for change and adaptation requires that all organizational members be engaged and motivated to meet the organization's goals. Viewing the organization as a living social system recognizes the creative energy of the people who innovate to produce desirable products and services in uncertain, changing environments. Understanding the HCO as a complex, adaptive system is probably the most realistic of the organizational theories developed so far because it is able to account for the complexity created by interrelated and interdependent social systems responding to environmental stimuli.

CONTEXT TO NURSING AND HEALTH CARE

The nursing profession in the United States is the largest health professional group. Nurses are working throughout the health services sector and in all HCOs because their knowledge and skill is integral to the delivery of health care services.[11] Nurses are a major workforce within HCOs, especially those HCOs that directly deliver health care services. However, nursing contributions to successful HCOs go beyond providing bedside patient-focused care to include roles in management and administration as well as collaboration with their professional colleagues in other departments or network entities for the purpose of improving care or conducting research. Nurses work as case managers, infection control specialists, managers of information technology, human resources specialists, and quality/risk managers. Further, professional nursing affects the environments of HCOs by creating partnerships with other institutions, educating future nurses in universities and community colleges, and working with public policy decision makers to create policies that enhance health services environments. It is likely that professional nurses will be associated in some way with HCOs for most, if not all, of their professional nursing careers.

INTERRELATED CONCEPTS

Other organizational concepts are important to understanding the HCO as a dynamic and social system. These concepts are **Leadership, Power,** and **Learning organizations** (Figure 50-2).

Leadership

Bureaucratic structures require authoritative leadership capable of controlling all aspects of the organization. The concept of leadership, however, has changed with this new era

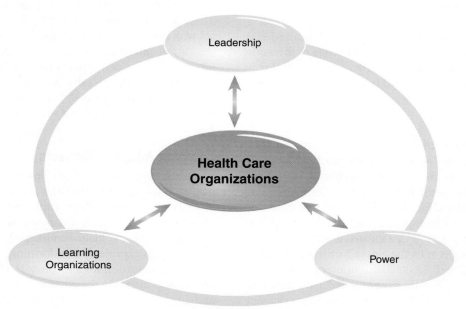

FIGURE 50-2 Health Care Organizations and Interrelated Concepts.

of organizational thinking where organizations are viewed as fluid, adaptive, and dependent on an engaged and activated workforce.[5] A new kind of leadership is required for these organizations, including the HCO, a leadership that creates inspiration, is able to sustain motivation to achieve results, and that values the contributions of all members. These leaders have to be able to "read" the environment and interpret the trends or changes for others. They must be able to lead others through turbulent and uncertain environments and must be able to adapt to change as readily as their followers.[5] Therefore, leadership styles developed to work in older, more static organizations will be less effective in the complex HCOs seen today.

Power

The concept of power in the organization has also evolved as the understanding of how organizations operate has changed. Power is commonly defined as the ability to influence others or to control events or circumstances. Much of this power was in the form of the decision making that supported control of organizational operations. In older hierarchical organizational models, power is seen as a part of structure and assigned to particular roles.

Power is now seen as a more diffuse, even infinite, phenomenon in that much power resides in the individual or within teams in the complex adaptive system.[5] It is no longer an exclusive tool of management because much decision

MODEL CASE

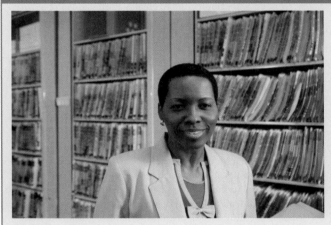

The model case of an HCO with integrated, interactive components and one that is open and receptive to environmental signals is the Magnet© organization. Magnet organizations are those HCOs, primarily hospitals, who have adopted organizational practices that promote excellence in nursing practice. The HCO that adopts Magnet principles is committing to an organizational design and structure that empowers nursing staff to achieve higher levels of performance through engagement and participation. The Magnet designation is only obtained after a process of learning and self-evaluation followed by changes to the organization's structure.[12] These design changes provide a decentralized authority structure created to support participative management and professional autonomy for nurses.[13,14] Nurses working in Magnet facilities are expected to be active participants in organizational processes, to govern themselves, to collaborate with other professional colleagues, and to be both responsible and accountable for the outcomes of nursing care.

Magnet designation is an empowerment model that captures the main features of the complex adaptive system. Adopting Magnet principles meant to attract and retain excellent nurses is, fundamentally, recognition that professional nursing is a valuable and scarce resource essential to the effective function of the HCO. Nurses are not simply workers in the system but are instead a critical component of the organization that makes substantial contributions to the success of the HCO. To achieve this recognition an HCO must be able to demonstrate the full integration of professional nursing into its operations through authority structures that move decision making, power, and control of practice to nurses throughout the organization. This is usually accomplished through the creation of governance councils in which all nursing staff are able to voice their concerns with care issues and then make decisions that will affect how care is delivered in that facility. Professional decision making is no longer the exclusive domain of the nursing executive and directors. Instead, there is a flattening of hierarchical relationships related to authority and control over practice with more of the responsibilities for care outcomes being assumed by nursing staff.

The HCO must also demonstrate that appropriate processes are in place that allow for the development of innovative care strategies and that nurses can implement and review the results of their innovation efforts. Quality management in Magnet organizations is robust and nurses are fully involved in creative activities that encourage continuous quality improvement and the achievement of excellence in nursing care. These facilities promote the continuing professional development of their nurses by supporting education and career-ladder programs.[14]

Although Magnet designation is specific to nursing, the adoption of a Magnet design by an HCO has the potential for and is intended to have spillover benefits for the entire organization. Because the HCO is an integrated system and professional nursing is the largest workforce in most of these organizations, there is a great potential to positively influence other members and other components of the HCO. Engaged and empowered nurses can act as transformative agents in the Magnet structure, leading efforts to improve the quality of care and inspiring others in the organization to join in the effort to create better systems and improved HCO outcomes. In the end, the HCO with Magnet designation benefits from increased collaboration, self-determination, and participation by nurses because this increases the capacity of the organization to adapt to uncertainty and change.

making and action is the responsibility of those who function outside of the management structure. Individuals and teams, empowered to make decisions and work collaboratively, are able to create and innovate in ways that would not have been possible in older command and control organizational structures.

Learning Organizations

Intelligent, living systems perceive, respond, and adapt. In an organization, changing and adapting are the result of learning—perceiving stimuli, organizing a change response, and then reviewing the results of the change to determine if a satisfactory outcome was obtained. The lessons learned from reviewing feedback are then used as the basis for adjustments to the adaptive response and for consideration in future actions. Learning organizations are those that are receptive to their environments, are open to change, and have adopted processes that allow their personnel to experiment, make changes, risk mistakes, and take responsibility for their decisions.[5] A culture of learning is important for HCOs because professional judgment and decision making are central to the delivery of health care services in destabilized, uncertain environments. The capacity to learn from mistakes and to use this learning to improve performance is the basis of the recommendation by the Institute of Medicine (IOM) that all HCOs adopt the principles of the learning organization to improve patient safety and health care outcomes in the United States.[15]

EXEMPLARS

Examples of HCOs are numerous. As defined earlier, an HCO can be any type of organization developed for a purpose, employing health professionals and directed by a mission to deliver health care services. These would include hospitals, ambulatory care centers, provider offices, nursing homes, community health agencies, and hospice facilities (Box 50-1). These are the more familiar types of HCOs where nurses are likely to be employed. These facilities can be classified by ownership, financial purpose, and services delivered, but, when combined with their organizational mission and purpose, the potential for an unknown variety of HCOs is endless. The importance of the basic concept, however, cannot be discounted because HCOs are the major work arenas for the nursing profession.

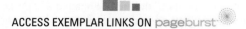
ACCESS EXEMPLAR LINKS ON pageburst

BOX 50-1   EXEMPLARS OF HEALTH CARE ORGANIZATIONS

- Ambulatory care facilities
- Community hospitals
- Federally qualified health centers
- Nurse-managed centers
- University-based teaching hospitals

REFERENCES

1. Shortell S, Kaluzny A: Organization theory and health services management. In Shortell S, Kaluzny A, editors: *Health care management: organization design and behavior*, ed 5, Clifton Park, NY, 2006, Delmar, pp 5–41.
2. Mancini M: Healthcare organizations. In Yoder-Wise P, editor: *Leading and managing in nursing*, ed 5, St Louis, 2010, Elsevier, pp 116–136.
3. Longest B, Darr K: *Managing health services organizations and systems*, ed 5, Baltimore, 2008, Health Professions Press.
4. Zazzali J: Trust: An implicit force in health care organization theory. In Mick S, Wyttenbach M, editors: *Advances in health care organization theory*, San Francisco, 2003, Jossey-Bass.
5. Porter-O'Grady T, Malloch K: *Quantum leadership: advancing innovation, transforming health care*, ed 3, Sudbury, Mass, 2011, Jones and Bartlett.
6. Ledlow G, Coppola N: *Leadership for health professionals: theory, skills, and applications*, Sudbury, Mass, 2010, Jones and Bartlett.
7. Scott K, Mesnick J: Creating the conditions for breakthrough clinical performance, *Nurse Leader* 8(4):48–52, 2010.
8. Olden P, Diana M: Classical theories of organization. In Johnson J, editor: *Health organizations: theory, behavior and development*, Sudbury, Mass, 2009, Jones and Bartlett, pp 29–46.
9. Diana M, Olden P: Modern theories of organization. In Johnson J, editor: *Health organizations: theory, behavior and development*, Sudbury, Mass, 2009, Jones and Bartlett, pp 47–62.
10. Cummings T, Worley C: *Organization development & change*, Mason, Ohio, 2009, South-Western Cengage Learning.
11. Buerhaus P, Staiger D, Auerbach D: *The future of the nursing workforce in the United States: data, trends and implications*, Sudbury, Mass, 2009, Jones and Bartlett.
12. Sportsman: Care delivery strategies. In Yoder-Wise P, editor: *Leading and managing in nursing*, ed 5, St Louis, 2011, Elsevier, pp 249–271.
13. Folse V: Managing quality and risk. In Yoder-Wise P, editor: *Leading and managing in nursing*, ed 5, St Louis, 2011, Elsevier, pp 389–409.
14. Gormley D: Collective action. In Yoder-Wise P, editor: *Leading and managing in nursing*, ed 5, St Louis, 2011, Elsevier, pp 372–388.
15. Institute of Medicine: *Keeping patients safe: transforming the work environment of nurses*, Washington, DC, 2004, The National Academies Press.

Health Care Economics

P.J. Woods

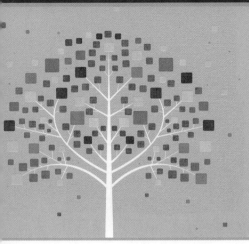

Health care touches all of our lives. Everyone visits a physician, nurse practitioner, or dentist and many of us have needed emergency or hospital services. The future of our health care system consistently surfaces as one of the most important issues facing the United States. There is great passion when we discuss health care. Determination of those who qualify for health care and the amount they should receive is both a moral and a practical challenge to our society and of personal interest to us all. We do not want to become ill, but we want to receive quality care if we do. However, there is a shortage of facilities, equipment, providers, nurses, and health care workers in general to provide quality health care, leading to resource challenges.

A foundational element in this discussion is the concept of health care economics. Economics as a discipline can provide insight into the issues of the distribution of health care because the fundamental problem of scarcity requires making choices. Even if our preference is to spend more on health care, there are clearly limits regarding how much individuals, employers, and the government can spend on its provision. Health care economics is concerned with both efficiency (getting the most out of a fixed amount of resources) and distribution (determining who receives resources and who will be denied). Moreover, sellers of medical goods and services are motivated by economic interests as well as patient needs.[1]

DEFINITION(S)

All definitions of health care economics in one way or another are focused on how people deal with a finite resource and scarcity. Consequently, people are constantly juggling how to get the most out of life and health by choosing how they use resources available to them. These resources include the time and talent people have available; the land, buildings, equipment, and other tools on hand; and the knowledge of how to combine these resources to deliver high-quality health care services.[2]

For the purpose of this concept analysis, health care economics is defined as a behavioral science that begins with two propositions about human behavior. First, human behavior is purposeful or goal directed, implying that persons act to promote their own interests. Second, human desires and demands are unlimited, especially for something like health care; however, resources are limited and cannot meet unlimited demands. Thus, the basic problem addressed by health care economics is how to allocate limited resources among unlimited demands and how to pay for these resources.[3]

SCOPE AND CATEGORIES

Health care economics represents the availability (or scarcity) of health care resources and financing, or payment mechanisms, to pay for these resources. Whether or not there is payment influences utilization of resources, regardless of the availability and distribution of health care. These categories and their interrelationships are shown in Figure 51-1.

In addition to these relationships, health care economics is highly influenced by government, public, and private agencies as they define and control payment for health care services. This is the foundation of health care economics.

Availability of Resources

According to Leavitt and colleagues, "an effective political strategy must take into account the resources that will be needed to move an issue successfully. Resources include money, time, and intangible resources. [Additional resources include] sharing available resources, such as space, people, and expertise."[4] Individuals of lower socioeconomic status are more likely to report unfulfilled health care needs. Cultural and linguistic factors often contribute to the aforementioned issues of unmet health care needs stemming from decreased access.[5]

The most tangible and notable outcome of a lack of available resources is seen in health disparities. Health care disparities exist in the United States. The Agency for Healthcare Research and Quality's (AHRQ) *National Healthcare Disparities Report*[6] defines health care disparities as "the differences

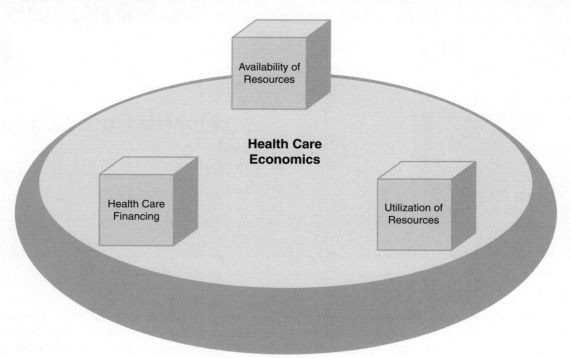

FIGURE 51-1 Categories of Health Care Economics.

or gaps in care experienced by one population compared with another population"[6] and reports differences related to access, use, and patient experience of care by racial, ethnic, socioeconomic, and geographic comparison. The disparities within different groups in the United States are a result of access to care, provider biases, poor communication of important health information to patients by providers, poor health literacy, and numerous other factors.[7] Many population groups in our country experience health disparities, including racial and ethnic minorities, residents of rural areas, women, children, the elderly population, and persons with disabilities.[8]

According to the Kaiser Commission on Medicaid and the Uninsured,[9] individuals without health insurance are more likely to postpone medical care, to deny themselves needed medical care, and to forego prescription medicines. Compared to whites, minority groups in the United States lack insurance coverage at higher rates. In addition, without access to a regular source of care, patients have fewer physician visits and greater difficulty obtaining care and prescription medications. Compared to whites, minority groups in the United States are less likely to have a physician they see on a regular basis and are more likely to use emergency departments and clinics as their regular source of care.[10]

One of the greatest health care challenges is reducing disparities. Within the United States, minority populations exhibit a higher incidence of chronic diseases, diminished health outcomes, and increased risk for mortality. In this effort, the National Center on Minority Health and Health Disparities (NCMHHD) strives to lead, coordinate, support, and assess the effort of the National Institutes of Health (NIH) to reduce and ultimately eliminate health disparities.

Research is currently being conducted and policy changes are being implemented with the intention of eliminating these problems.[11]

Health Care Financing

The U.S. health care system is funded by a patchwork of health insurance programs. In contrast to most other nations where the government finances health care for the majority of its residents, private, employer-sponsored insurance is the primary source of insurance in the United States. This system is expensive and complex, resulting in a complicated array of participants, including insurance companies, employers, and regulators. Insurance coverage also affects patients' interactions with the health care delivery system, particularly in terms of the type of care and the providers they can see along with the out-of-pocket costs they may spend.

The United States spends more money on health care than any other nation; in fact, by 2017 it is estimated that $13,000 per person will be spent on health care, according to the annual projection by the Centers for Medicare & Medicaid Services (CMS). Annual health care spending in the United States is estimated to surpass $4.2 trillion in 2018, representing 19% of the gross domestic product by 2018.[12]

Payment mechanisms are needed to cover these costs. Approximately 60% of Americans have employer-provided health care insurance (including military health care) and 9% self-pay for their health insurance. For many employees, the growth in health care premiums is displacing wage increases. For other employees, high health care costs mean their employers cannot offer coverage at all. Among businesses with less than 10 employees, only 46% offer health care coverage to their workers.[13]

It is estimated that 17% of Americans have no health care insurance and this number has been growing steadily over the past decade.[14,15] Although many of the uninsured are covered by government programs (such as Medicare or Medicaid), 56% of the uninsured are ineligible for public programs and cannot afford coverage, whereas another 25% are eligible for public programs but not enrolled. Several health care payment mechanisms help Americans cover health care costs, including Medicaid, Medicare, U.S. Department of Veterans Affairs insurance programs, military programs, and State Children's Health Insurance Programs (SCHIP).[16]

The rising health care costs, coupled with a growing number of uninsured Americans, has caused increasing concern among the general public. This underscores the importance health care financing plays in health care economics.

ATTRIBUTES AND CRITERIA

There are three main attributes associated with health care economics. These are cost-effectiveness, efficiency, and value. A discussion of the economic laws of supply and demand is necessary as a framework in understanding the main attributes associated with health care economics.

The relation between supply and demand is an economic model of how prices are determined in a market. In a competitive market like the United States, the unit price for a particular good will vary until it settles at a point where the current price will equal the quantity supplied by producers. This results in an economic equilibrium of price and quantity. The two important concepts to understand are the laws of supply and demand. For supply, this means that when the selling price of an item rises, more people will produce the item because they can make a profit. The law of demand states that when the price of an item is reduced, the demand for it increases. This means there is a balance that as a price increases demand decreases, and vice versa. Generally, supply reflects demand as individuals would not continue to develop a product or supply a service for which demand has dropped, nor would they buy something when the price is too high.[17] Regardless of where the market is in terms of supply and demand, long-term sustainability of health care entities hinges on delivering care that is cost-effective, is efficient, and has value.

Cost-Effectiveness

Health economics aims to find the best way to satisfy the increasing demand for health care given the limited resources. The resources used to provide care services are scarce, and decisions about the services that will be provided and who will be eligible to receive these services usually have resource and cost implications. The overall aim of economic evaluation is to aid decision makers to make efficient and equitable decisions about the allocation of resources by comparing the cost-effectiveness and benefits of health care interventions.[18] Cost-effectiveness analyses of health care interventions have become one of the focal points in the decision-making process in health care. The introduction of any health technology, whether it is a new drug or a new medical device, is often associated with an increase in health care costs and can limit the funding available for other interventions. Using health economics and measuring the cost-effectiveness helps policymakers, health care providers, and insurance companies determine whether the new intervention is cost-effective in comparison to other options.[19]

Efficiency

We typically think of efficiency in the delivery of health care as avoiding waste (including waste of equipment, supplies, and people) or as using health care resources to get the best value for the money. The definition of efficiency used by economists was formulated after the Italian economist Vilfredo Pareto. He said that an allocation of resources is efficient when no one can be made better off without making someone else worse off.[7]

Today, health care system financial resources in the United States are less frequently controlled by physicians and nurses and more often by administrators, financial managers, third-party payers, and politicians. These people view reduced illness and death as a reasonable goal, but also seek objective evidence that this goal is achieved with fiscal efficiency (i.e., by the least expenditure of increasingly scarce financial resources).[20] Economic analysis is based on the fundamental notion of efficient use of available resources. Two basic points are that economics is about resource allocation and efficiency in resource use (getting the most from available resources).[3]

Value

Cost-effective and efficient delivery of health care is needed to achieve value, and thus is a critical attribute of economics in health care. The best way to drive system progress is rigorous, disciplined measurement and improvement of value. Yet, value in health care remains largely unmeasured and misunderstood.[21] Achieving high value for patients must become the overarching goal of health care delivery, with value defined as the health outcomes achieved per dollar spent. This goal is important for patients and unites the interests of all who interface with the system. If value improves, patients, payers, providers, and suppliers all benefit and the economic sustainability of the health care system increases. Because value depends on results, not inputs, value in health care is measured by the outcomes achieved, not the volume of services delivered, and shifting focus from volume to value is a central challenge. Nor is value measured by the process of care used; process measurement and improvement are important tactics, but in economics they are not substitutes for measuring outcomes and costs.[22] The interrelationship between these attributes is shown in Figure 51-2.

Attribute Relationships

The interrelationship of how these attributes build on one another is represented as a bull's-eye because the "target" for the concept of health care economics is to have cost-effective care; thus it is in the center of the bull's-eye. Close to the center of the bull's-eye is efficiency in delivery of care; even if the care is cost-effective, if you are inefficient you waste resources and the system becomes unsustainable. At the outer rim of the

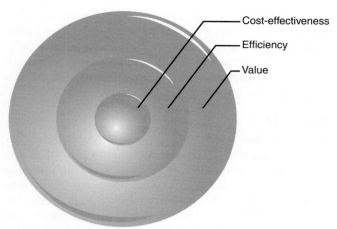

Cost-effectiveness

Efficiency

Value

FIGURE 51-2 Relationship Between Attributes of Health Care Economics.

bull's-eye is value. If you fire at the target and hit value, you will still be contributing economic benefits to the health care delivery system, but without the others, value alone cannot sustain the system. As an example, if a patient were to spend a full hour with a primary care provider during a routine visit that normally would be a 20-minute visit, the patient would likely perceive value. However, the time involved is not efficient, cost-effective, or sustainable. Alternatively, if no value is perceived by the patient, the system is still not sustainable; thus these attributes are interrelated.

THEORETICAL LINKS

The Transaction Cost Theory (TCT), developed by Williamson,[23,24] was an attempt to use economic principles to define a framework for health care that is comprised of the multiple complex sequences of transactions among patients, providers, and other stakeholders. The framework identified that health care transactions serve one of two functions: (1) the production or delivery of care (e.g., treating or laying on of hands to a patient) or (2) the coordination of that care (e.g., scheduling, logistics). It is critical that coordination of all the transactions that occur before, during, and after a patient interfaces with the health care system is executed seamlessly and efficiently.[25]

This theory sheds light on firm boundaries and the conditions under which it is better to arrange activities within a hierarchy rather than interacting in a market with suppliers or other contractors. Governance arrangements are evaluated by comparing the patterns of costs generated for planning, adapting, and monitoring production and exchange.[26] Vertical integration (i.e., unified ownership) permits details of future relations between suppliers (including employees), producers, and distributors to remain unspecified; differences can be changed as events unfold. This pools the risks and rewards of various activities undertaken by the organization, and can facilitate the sharing of information, the pursuit of innovation, and the attainment of a culture of cooperation. An example of the application of this theory can be seen in the new vertically integrated accountable care organizations.

These organizations are specifically organized to deal with increasing health care costs resulting from patient and staff frustration with the rising cost of care and lack of continuity in a complicated health care system coupled with employer reluctance to provide traditional managed care offerings. This has led to a larger proportion of patients and staff with complex health problems electing to remain (unmanaged) in costly indemnity products.[25]

The advantage of applying the TCT to the health care market is based on the fact that health care is delivered via complex sequences of transactions among patients, providers, and other stakeholders. Sometimes these transactions are concrete and easily identified. For example, a surgery is performed or a medication is administered. However, most of the time the transactions are intangible and abstract, such as providing patient teaching, offering care or comfort, and giving advice. Using this theory from the economic viewpoint, the potential exists for additional transaction costs at every juncture where information flows, at every hand-off in the process of care, and in all aspects of organizing and delivering care, including who is providing the care, where it is provided, and how it is reimbursed. Without purposeful integration and management of all transactions these costs remain unchecked, and care is fragmented rather than producing lower expenditures, better health outcomes, higher satisfaction levels, and improved quality of life for patients, providers, employers, and staff alike.[25] The model is shown in Figure 51-3.

As seen in Figure 51-3 situation **A,** the health care entities are integrated within a single firm and are linked by scope and geographic area. In situation **B,** the health care entities are independent firms that have a similar scope and are in the same geographic area. It is apparent that the transaction costs associated with the delivery of health care are going to be less in the integrated system than in the independent system, thus reducing the overall economic impact because the costs of care are less in situation **A.**

CONTEXT TO NURSING AND HEALTH CARE

Patient Protection and Affordable Care Act (Public Law 11-148)

Health care economics affects all professional nursing practice environments as well as the individual nurse and his or her family. One of the biggest impacts overall is the Patient Protection and Affordable Care Act (PPACA).[27] This legislation has elicited much debate among policy experts and the public alike. No one knows exactly how this new complex law will evolve, and objective evaluation of its effects is important.[27]

The American College of Physicians hopes that the legislation will advance key priorities on coverage, workforce, and payment and delivery system reform. The goal of the PPACA is to help provide affordable health insurance coverage to most Americans and to improve access to primary care. What remains to be seen is to what extent the PPACA will ensure affordable coverage or sufficient numbers of primary care physicians.[28]

The current PPACA is expected to cover an estimated 32 million uninsured Americans.[29] Without the PPACA, the

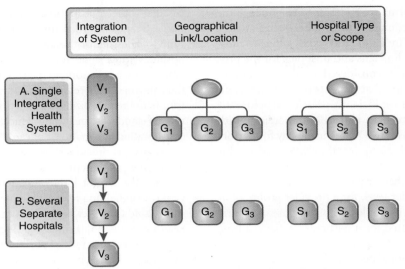

FIGURE 51-3 Transactional Cost Theory Model.

Census Bureau projects that the number of uninsured persons will increase to more than 60 million, or one out of five U.S. residents.[30] The Congressional Budget Office (CBO) estimates that 95% of legal U.S. residents, as compared with 83% currently, will be covered under the legislation, including the aforementioned 32 million who otherwise would have been uninsured.[31] According to the Kaiser Foundation,[32] the following are some of the law's major provisions:

- The requirement that most U.S. citizens and legal residents have health insurance by 2014
- The creation of state-based exchanges through which individuals can purchase coverage, with subsidies available to lower-income individuals
- A major expansion of the Medicaid program for the nation's poorest individuals
- The requirement for employers to cover their employees or pay penalties, with exceptions for small employers
- New regulations on health plans in the private market requiring them to cover all individuals, regardless of health status
- Establishment of a national, voluntary insurance program for purchasing community living assistance services
- Increases in payments for primary care services
- Greater support for prevention, wellness, and public health activities

Accountable Care Organizations

The 2010 Patient Protection and Affordable Care Act (PPACA) has provided a mechanism, an Accountable Care Organization (ACO), which has sown the seeds for a major reorganization of the U.S. health care delivery system. As defined by the PPACA, an ACO is an organization of health care providers that agrees to be accountable for the quality, cost, and overall care of Medicare patients, for whom they provide the bulk of primary care services.[33] ACOs must have defined processes for promoting evidence-based medicine, reporting data with which to evaluate the quality and cost of care and coordinating

care. ACOs that meet specified quality standards will receive a share of the savings if Medicare's cost for the care of their assigned patients is below a certain benchmark.[34] ACOs, along with bundled payments and other payment innovations, are intended to transform the health care delivery system both by replacing fee-for-service payments, which tend to increase utilization, and by boosting collaboration among providers so as to reduce costs and improve quality.[35]

In almost every region of the country, hospitals and physicians are in the process of forming accountable care organizations (ACOs) and entering into other arrangements designed to integrate care, manage chronic conditions, and enhance the use of evidence-based practices.[33] Critical to the achievement of these ACOs are the regulations and guidance soon to be issued by the Centers for Medicare & Medicaid Services (CMS) and the Federal Trade Commission (FTC). One of the most important judgments these agencies will be asked to make entails determining how best to ensure that ACOs foster, not hinder, competition in health care markets.[36]

ACOs offer a much-needed vehicle for integrating health care delivery and reducing the well-documented shortcomings of the system that are attributable to payment and organizational features that reward high volume rather than low cost or high quality. However, studies have shown that development of ACOs could foster more disparities because dominant hospitals and specialty physician practices can reorganize into ACOs more easily than sparsely populated areas, resulting in the attainment of high levels of reimbursement that are not attributable to differences in quality, case mix, or demographic factors.[37] Nurses will be impacted by ACOs because many health care organizations where professional nurses are employed will be transitioning to these integrated delivery care systems in the future.

Pay for Performance

Current health policy initiatives to reduce market distortions are directed at both the supply and the demand side of the market. Pay for performance is designed to enhance the communication and coordination of care between patients, providers, and clinicians (including nurses) by offering additional reimbursement to clinicians and hospitals for the provision of health care services considered appropriate and of high quality. This will ensure that patients receive important care that may not have been sufficiently prioritized before the program's existence. More than half of commercial health maintenance organizations (HMOs) are using pay for performance, and recent legislation requires the CMS to adopt this approach for Medicare.[38]

There is much debate whether pay for performance should be at the individual provider level, for a provider group, or at an organizational level. An example of this is the use of generic drugs. Unless contraindicated for a particular patient, a provider who prescribes a generic drug is saving the health care system money; thus they should be rewarded. One of the struggles with pay for performance is how to develop performance reporting on both cost and quality measures, and then to use the same performance data to calculate financial rewards. Many current pay for performance programs offer rewards for high relative performance (being among the top 10% of physicians) rather than absolute performance. Rewarding only the top providers creates competition and can stretch a small bonus pool. On the other hand, competition may limit collaboration and sharing of best practices and may create or sustain quality gaps between high- and low-performing providers.[39]

Nurses are indirectly part of pay for performance with new Medicare reimbursement guidelines. Starting in 2009, Medicare will not cover the cost of preventable hospital-acquired conditions, mistakes, and infections that can occur during a patient's hospitalization. For example, if a patient admitted to a hospital develops a pressure ulcer during his or her hospital stay, Medicare will not pay for the extended admission related to acquiring the pressure ulcer. Other nurse-sensitive indicators included in Medicare's new ruling are falls from bed, catheter-associated urinary tract infections, blood incompatibility mistakes, and

vascular catheter–associated infections. This is placing an additional financial burden on hospitals because nurses need the time to assess all of these indicators on an ongoing basis and hospitals must code for infections and other conditions as "present on admission" so they are not liable for a reduction in their payment. Therefore, staff nurses have the ability to contribute to the organization's efforts in achieving pay for performance standards, including education, documentation, team collaboration, and patterns of care.[40]

Nursing is the largest segment of the nation's health care workforce. With more than 3 million members who often provide the largest bulk of patient care, nurses can play a vital role in helping realize the objectives set forth in the 2010 Affordable Care Act, legislation that represents the broadest health care overhaul since the 1965 creation of the Medicare and Medicaid programs. Working together with government, businesses, health care organizations, professional associations, and the insurance industry, nurses can play a vital role in assuring that health care is equitable and accessible to all and leads to improved health outcomes.

INTERRELATED CONCEPTS

This concept represents areas that relate to health care economics. Several concepts featured in this textbook have a relationship with this concept. **Health policy** is used to provide overarching goals and to set priorities and values for the allocation of health resources. **Health care quality** is concerned with issues related to ensuring standards of care and outcomes are achieved in the delivery of health care. **Health care organizations** provide the framework for the delivery of health care. **Health care coordination** involves the marshalling of personnel and other resources needed to carry out all required patient care activities. **Health care law** affects health care economics because it governs the insurance industry and is illustrated in the application of health care funding and reform. These interrelationships are depicted in Figure 51-4.

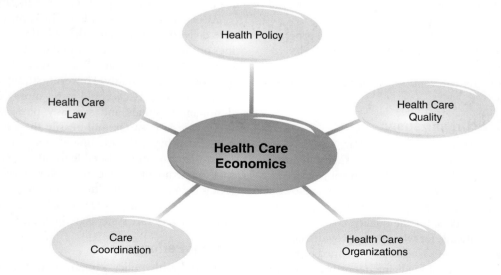

FIGURE 51-4 Health Care Economics and Interrelated Concepts.

MODEL CASE

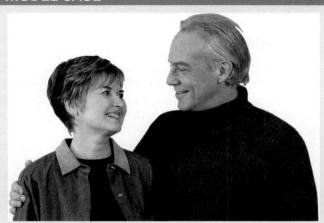

Raymond Wiley operates a small business in a small town in a rural area of the United States. There is a 10-bed hospital in his community that has a 2-bed intensive care unit (ICU). Most individuals with serious health conditions are transferred to a large hospital in a city located approximately 100 miles away.

Mr. Wiley became ill with a fever and cough. Because his regular physician was out of town, he went to the emergency department at the local hospital, where he was diagnosed with pneumonia and admitted. Mr. Wiley received supportive care, but after 3 full days with no apparent improvement, the admitting physician decided to transfer him to the city hospital for a referral with a pulmonologist.

The Wiley's wanted to drive to the city hospital in their private vehicle, as opposed to having Mr. Wiley transported by ambulance. Their rationale was based on the fact that Mrs. Wiley could drive, Mr. Wiley was stable, and their insurance did not cover ambulance transport unless it was a medical emergency. Up to this point, Raymond had only received supportive care; his IV had been capped and he was taking oral antibiotics. Their request to drive him was refused and he was transported by ambulance; they were charged $1300 for the transport. They were quite upset because it was unclear if this decision was based on a necessity or whether it represented inefficiency or resulted from legal issues.

Once Raymond arrived at the city hospital, it took 2 days for the pulmonologist and thoracic surgeon to see him because the admitting unit "got his name mixed up with another patient." The Wiley's were told the hospital had faced budget cuts and the nurse to patient ratio was cited at 9 or 10 patients per nurse, and mistakes happen. A CT scan was completed, which revealed he had a large mass and pleural effusion. Mr. Wiley

was then seen by a thoracic surgeon, who scheduled him for a thoracotomy the next day—a Sunday. This required assembling an on-call surgical team at the higher weekend rate.

Following surgery, Raymond was in the intensive care unit. He experienced several postoperative complications, many of which were precipitated by the initial delay in correct diagnosis and treatment. On postop day 11, an order was written to transfer Mr. Wiley out of ICU to the medical unit, but because of a shortage of nursing staff on the medical unit, he remained in the ICU for 2 additional days. Raymond was transferred to a floor bed on day 13 and discharged home later that day. The Wiley's were shocked to find out that the ICU charged $2800 per day, and were particularly upset because the last 2 days Raymond spent in the ICU were because the hospital was short staffed and could not transfer him to the medical unit.

Mrs. Wiley spent 10 months of her time (along with hours of hospital and insurance company time) fighting many of the charges because her husband's care had been delayed by the medical team, causing his complications and extensive hospitalization. In addition, the Wiley's felt they should not be charged and held responsible for the 3 days in the rural hospital, the 2 days in the city hospital before Mr. Wiley was seen by the specialist, and the 2 days spent in the ICU because the hospital was short staffed. The insurance company and hospital finally agreed upon how much the insurance company would pay for the $136,000 worth of services billed. This was somewhat less than $60,000, leaving the hospital to write-off the remainder of the bill. However, Raymond had paid nearly $5000 in co-payments during the course of his illness.

Case Analysis

This model case illustrates the three attributes of health care economics: cost-effectiveness, efficiency, and value. Mr. Wiley's care was not cost-effective because there were many delays that were costly both from a systems viewpoint and from the exacerbations to the seriousness of his illness. The hospital eventually was forced to write-off nearly half of the billed charges, which will eventually result in higher charges across the system to compensate for these and other losses. Mr. Wiley's story highlights how a lack of communication and resulting lack of effectiveness in timely treatment continue to haunt health care, affecting the quality of patient care and outcomes as well as patient costs. Finally, the third attribute—value—was not attained because Mr. Wiley's care was delayed in both the rural and the tertiary care hospitals and the Wiley's did not receive value for their health care dollars.

EXEMPLARS

Nurses work lives and ability to deliver patient care will be affected by a wide variety of categories involved in health care economics. This includes the factors that constitute our health care markets, including the distribution of health care that results in health disparities and the principles of free market and supply and demand, and the influence these have

on creating health care that is efficient, is cost-effective, and has value. In addition, health care financing, which includes government-sponsored care, managed care, and private insurance, is the driving force behind health care economics. Payment mechanisms dictate the use of care and this influences the availability and scarcity of resources. These exemplars are shown in detail in Box 51-1.

■■■ BOX 51-1 **EXEMPLARS OF HEALTH CARE ECONOMICS**

Health Disparities
- Distribution of health care
- Free market approach
- Supply and demand

Health Care Payment Mechanisms
- Insurance
- Managed care organizations
- Medicaid
- Medicare

Medicaid and SCHIP

Medicaid is the nation's major public health insurance program for low-income Americans, financing health and long-term care services for more than 52 million people, including children and many of the sickest and poorest in our nation. Since its enactment in 1965, Medicaid has improved access to health care for low-income individuals, financed innovations in health care delivery, and functioned as the nation's primary source of long term care financing. Medicaid is now one of the centerpieces of expanding coverage in the national health reform bill.[41] By 2019 the program is expected to cover nearly one in five Americans. The State Children's Health Insurance Program (SCHIP) was enacted in 1997 to provide coverage to uninsured low-income children who did not qualify for Medicaid.[16] Medicaid and SCHIP are jointly funded by state and federal governments and Medicaid and SCHIP eligibility is determined by income and need. State sources of Medicaid funding include legislative appropriations, intergovernmental transfers, certified public expenditures and permissible taxes, and provider donations. Medicaid payments are only paid to qualified hospitals, nursing facilities, and home health agencies and cannot exceed a reasonable estimate of the amount Medicare would pay for the same services.[42]

Medicare

Medicare provides health care coverage for all people ages 65 and older, people who are permanently disabled, and individuals 65 and older with end-stage renal disease. It is a federal health insurance program that individuals or their spouses paid into through employment or self-employment taxes.[43] Medicare includes hospital insurance (Part A), supplemental medical insurance (Part B), Medicare Advantage plans (Part C), or outpatient prescription drug coverage (Part D). Part A includes hospital coverage and Part B includes outpatient coverage and is optional; the recipient must contribute a premium each month to preserve coverage. Patients with Part A may opt to add Part B, which covers 80% of the fees for outpatient services.[44]

Managed Care Organizations

In managed care, health care providers and insurance companies assume a part of the financial responsibility for health care. Patients pay a monthly premium for health care insurance. Medicaid and Medicare have incorporated managed care into their health plans. Patients can choose from several different plans under the managed care system, including preferred provider organizations (PPOs) and health care maintenance organizations (HMOs), and patients may receive health care from a list of providers who participate in the PPO or HMO.[45] Current trends show more insurance companies have multiple health care plans that they manage for different employers. The health care services that these plans cover are determined by the employer and not the insurance company. Insurance payment varies according to geographic region and depends greatly on the type and plan of coverage. This may often leave the patient with unpaid medical expenses or the need to obtain prior authorization before seeking treatment or medication.[45]

Private or Indemnity Health Insurance

Private health insurance may be purchased on a group basis (e.g., by a firm to cover its employees) or purchased by individual consumers. Most Americans with private health insurance receive it through an employer-sponsored program. According to the U.S. Census Bureau[15] nearly 60% of Americans are covered through an employer, whereas about 9% purchase health insurance directly. An example of private indemnity health insurance that can be purchased either by an employer for its employees or by an individual themselves is the Blue Cross Blue Shield Association (BCBSA). The BCBSA consists of 39 separate health insurance organizations and companies in the United States. Combined, they directly or indirectly provide health insurance to more than 98 million, or 1 in 3, Americans.[46]

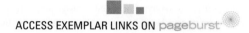

ACCESS EXEMPLAR LINKS ON pageburst

REFERENCES

1. Wells DA, Ross JS, Detsky AS: What is different about the market for health care? *JAMA* 298(23):2785–2787, 2007.
2. American Economic Association: *What is economics?* 2008. Retrieved Jan 26, 2011, from www.aeaweb.org/students/WhatIs Economics.php.
3. Solomon S, McGowan J Jr: Applying economic principles to health care, *Emerg Infect Dis* 7(2):282–295, 2001.
4. Leavitt JK, Cohen SS, Mason DJ: Political analysis and strategies. In Mason DJ, Leavitt JL, Chaffee MW, editors: *Policy and politics in nursing and health care*, St Louis, 2007, Saunders/Elsevier, pp 94–109.
5. Betancourt JR, Green AR, Carrillo JE, et al: Cultural competence and health care disparities: key perspectives and trends, *Health Affairs* 24(2):499–505, 2005. Retrieved Jan 27, 2011, from http://web.ebscohost.com.libproxy.u nm.edu/ehost/pdfviewer/pdfviewer?hid=119&sid=7cd6 8bf6-9ca7-45ae-909a-e6606be70312%40sessionmgr114& vid=3.
6. Agency for Healthcare Research and Quality: *National healthcare disparities report*, 2003. Retrieved from www.ahrq.gov/qual/nhdr03/nhdrsum03.htm.

7. Agency for Healthcare Research and Quality: *Addressing racial and ethnic disparities in health care—fact sheet*, 2008. Retrieved from www.ahrq.gov/research/disparit.htm.

8. MedlinePlus: *Health disparities*, 2011. Retrieved from www.nlm.nih.gov/medlineplus/healthdisparities.html.

9. Kaiser Commission on Medicaid and the Uninsured: *The uninsured and their access to health care*, 2003. Retrieved June 8, 2011, from http://www.kff.org/uninsured/upload/The-Uninsured-and-Their-Access-to-Health-Care-Fact-Sheet-6.pdf.

10. Fryer GE, Dovey SM, Green LA: The importance of having a usual source of health care, *Am Fam Physician* 62:477, 2000.

11. National Center on Minority Health and Health Disparities (NCMHHD). Retrieved from www.nimhd.nih.gov/.

12. Centers for Medicare & Medicaid Services, Office of the Actuary, National Health Statistics Group: *Projected data from NHE projections, 2009-2018*. Retrieved from www.cms.hhs.gov/NationalHealthExpendData/.

13. U.S. Census Bureau: *Income, poverty, and health insurance coverage in the United States*, 2008. Retrieved March 10, 2011, from www.census.gov/prod/2008pubs/p60-235.pdf.

14. Agency for Healthcare Research and Quality: *Health care efficiency measures*, 2008. Retrieved Jan 27, 2011, from www.ahrq.gov/qual/efficiency/hcemch1.htm.

15. U.S. Census Bureau: *Health insurance coverage: 2007*, 2007. Retrieved Jan 26, 2011, from www.census.gov/hhes/www/hlthins/hlthin07/hlth07asc.html.

16. Pulcini J, Neary S, et al: Health care financing. In Mason DJ, Leavitt JK, Chaffee MW, editors: *Policy and politics in nursing and health care*, St Louis, 2002, Saunders/Elsevier.

17. Besanko D, Braeutigan DS: *Microeconomics*, ed 2, Hoboken, NJ, 2005, Wiley and Sons.

18. Ratcliffe J, Laver K, Couzner L, et al: *Age Ageing* 39:426–429, 2010. Retrieved Jan 26, 2011, from http://ageing.oxfordjournals.org.libproxy.unm.edu/content/39/4/426.full.pdf+html.

19. Giang N: *The role of health economics*, 2009. Retrieved Jan 26, 2011, from www.brighthub.com/health/technology/articles/6763.aspx.

20. McGowan J Jr: Cost and benefit in perioperative antimicrobial prophylaxis—methods for economic analysis, *Rev Infect Dis* 13, 1991.

21. Porter M: What is value in health care? *N Engl J Med* 363:2477–2481, 2010. Retrieved Jan 17, 2011, from www.nejm.org.libproxy.unm.edu/doi/full/10.1056/NEJMp1011024.

22. Porter M, Teisberg E: *Finding health care: creating value-based competition on results*, Boston, 2006, Harvard Business School Press. Retrieved from http://px7gv7gt2n.search.serialssolutions.com.libproxy.unm.edu/?V=1.0&pmid=21239947.

23. Williamson O: Transaction-cost economics: the governance of contractual relations, *J Law Econ* 22(I233):261, 1979. Retrieved Jan 26, 2011, from www.nek.lu.se/NEKAHA/hemsida/Williamson.pdf.

24. Williamson O: *The economic institutions of capitalism: firms, markets and relational contracting*, New York, 1985, Free Press.

25. Stiles R, Mick S, Wise C: The logic of transaction cost economics in health care organization theory, *Health Care Manag Rev* 26(2):85–92, Spring 2001. Retrieved Jan 26, 2011, from http://px7gv7gt2n.search.serialssolutions.com.libproxy.unm.edu/?V=1.0&pmid=11293015.

26. Williamson OE: The economics of organization: the transaction cost approach, *Am J Soc* 87(3):548–577, 1981.

27. Affordable Care Act: HR 3590(2010). Retrieved Jan 26, 2011, from www.ncsl.org/documents/health/HlthWrkfrceProvHR3590.pdf.

28. Doherty RB: The certitudes and uncertainties of health care reform, *Ann Intern Med* 152(10):679–682, 2010. Retrieved Jan 26, 2011, from www.ncbi.nlm.nih.gov.libproxy.unm.edu/pubmed/20378676.

29. Dubay L, Holahan J, Cook A: The uninsured and the affordability of health insurance coverage, *Health Affairs* 26(1):22–30, 2007. (published online). Retrieved Jan 29, 2011, from http://content.healthaffairs.org/content/26/1/w22.abstract.

30. U.S. Census Bureau: *Health insurance: current population survey, annual social and economic supplement*, 2009. Retrieved Jan 19, 2011, from www.census.gov/hhes/www/hlthins/hlthins.html.

31. Congressional Budget Office: *Preliminary estimate of the direct spending and revenue effects of an amendment in the nature of a substitute to H.R. 4872, the Reconciliation Act of 2010*, 2010. Retrieved Jan 26, 2011, from www.cbo.gov/ftpdocs/113xx/doc11355/hr4872.pdf.

32. Kaiser Foundation: *Health policy education: health reform*, 2010. Retrieved Jan 26, 2011, from www.kaiseredu.org/Topics/Health-and-Government.aspx.

33. McClellan M, McKethan A, Lewis J, et al: A national strategy to put accountable care into practice, *Health Affairs* 29:982–990, 2010. Retrieved from www.ncbi.nlm.nih.gov.libproxy.unm.edu/pubmed?term=a%20naional%20strategy%20to%20put%20accountable%20care%20into%20practice.

34. Thomas L, Greaney JD: Accountable care organizations—the fork in the road, *N Engl J Med* 364:e1, 2011. Retrieved Jan 6, 2011, from www.nejm.org.libproxy.unm.edu/doi/full/10.1056/NEJMp1013404.

35. Robert F, Leibenluft R: ACOs and the enforcement of fraud, abuse, and antitrust laws, *N Engl J Med* 364:99–101, 2011. Retrieved from www.nejm.org.libproxy.unm.edu/doi/full/10.1056/NEJMp1011464.

36. Sinaiko A, Rosenthal M: Patients' role in accountable care organizations, *N Engl J Med* 363:2583–2585, 2010. Retrieved from www.nejm.org.libproxy.unm.edu/doi/full/10.1056/NEJMp1011927.

37. Williams C, Vogt W, Town R: *How has hospital consolidation affected the price and quality of hospital care?* Princeton, NJ, 2006, Robert Wood Johnson Foundation. Retrieved from www.rwjf.org/files/research/no9policybrief.pdf.

38. Rosenthal M, Dudley R: Pay-for-performance: will the latest payment trend improve care? *JAMA* 297(7):740–744, 2007.

39. Belshe K: But pay for performance is unlikely to be a panacea. California's role in ensuring that the potential of health reform becomes reality, *JAMA* 298(23):2785–2787, 2007.

40. Bedrock J, Mion L: Pay for performance in hospitals: implications for nurses and nursing, *Care Qual Manag Health Care* 17(2):102–111, 2008.

41. Centers for Medicare & Medicaid Services (CMS): *Community services and long term supports*, 2010. Retrieved from www.cms.gov/CommunityServices/15_Balancing.asp#TopOfPage.

42. U.S. Department of Health and Human Services: *Overview state plan Medicaid service reimbursement*, 2011. Retrieved Jan 19, 2011, from www.cms.gov/MedicaidRF/.

43. U.S. Department of Health and Human Services: *Centers for Medicare & Medicaid Services*, 2009. Retrieved Jan 4, 2011, from www.cms.gov/HospitalAcqCond/downloads/HACFactsh eet.pdf.

44. Pulcini JA, Hart MA: Financing health care in the United States. In Mason D, Leavitt J, Chaffee M, editors: *Policy and politics in nursing and health care*, St Louis, 2007, Saunders/ Elsevier.

45. Kreitzer MJ: Successes and struggles in complementary health care. In Mason DJ, Leavitt JK, Chaffee MW, editors: *Policy and politics in nursing and health care*, ed 5, St Louis, 2007, Saunders/Elsevier, pp 336–344.

46. Blue Cross and Blue Shield: *About the Blue Cross Blue Shield Corporation*, 2011. Retrieved March 3, 2011, from www.bcbs. com/about/.

Health Policy

Teresa Keller and Nancy Ridenour

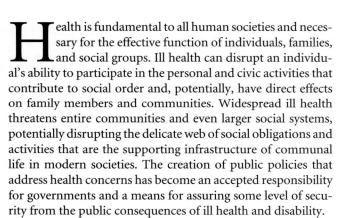

Health is fundamental to all human societies and necessary for the effective function of individuals, families, and social groups. Ill health can disrupt an individual's ability to participate in the personal and civic activities that contribute to social order and, potentially, have direct effects on family members and communities. Widespread ill health threatens entire communities and even larger social systems, potentially disrupting the delicate web of social obligations and activities that are the supporting infrastructure of communal life in modern societies. The creation of public policies that address health concerns has become an accepted responsibility for governments and a means for assuring some level of security from the public consequences of ill health and disability.

In the United States, decisions about health policy are dispersed among many levels of government and among political institutions.[1,2] Health policy is determined through laws, regulatory actions, judicial decisions, and the administrative actions of government agencies.[3] Health policy decision making in the United States is also affected by the numerous cultural and social trends that arise from technological change, shifting demographics, economic pressures, and consumer demands.[4] The results are health policies that support a decentralized health services sector where there is no single source of decision-making power. Instead, health policies are formulated at the federal, state, and local levels of government and are subject to the pressures of organized interest groups and business as well as concerned individuals and advocacy groups. The health care policies created within this dynamic environment are meant to address policy goals distilled through a political process of negotiation and compromise, subjected to public review and comment, and, ultimately, acceptable to the widest possible majority of interested parties. However, the outcome of widespread, decentralized health policy decision making can also be that the policies are fragmented, complex, contradictory, and even unconstitutional.

This slow and sometimes cumbersome process reflects the realities of the health care environment in the United States.

A mix of private and public systems, the health care environment is constantly changing and constantly creating new opportunities for innovations that are both a part of and in response to the political and cultural values of Americans. It is also this type of health policy environment that provides opportunities for nurses to intervene in the interests of their patients, families, and vulnerable populations as well as for the interests of the nursing profession. To effectively participate and advocate in the health policy decision-making process, nurses should have a clear understanding of the concept of health policy, including its definition, major characteristics, and ways it is differentiated from related concepts.

DEFINITION(S)

A clear definition of health policy needs to account for the variety of ways that health policy is determined and controlled in the public sector. Initially, health policy can be defined as a form of public policy, differentiating it from other kinds of decision making. A classic and basic definition of public policy is what governments decide to do or not to do.[5] Public policy can also be defined as the choices made by a society or social entities that relate to public goals and priorities as well as the choices made for allocating resources to those goals and priorities.[6] Health policy would therefore be the result of choices and resource allocations made to support health-related goals and priorities. Public policy is further defined as "authoritative guidelines that direct human behavior toward specific goals,"[7] so health policy is also authorized and directed toward health goals. Longest and Darr[3] define health policy as public policies pertaining to health that are the result of an authoritative, public decision-making process. A realistic definition of the concept health policy is *goal-directed decision making about health that is the result of an authorized, public decision-making process*. Health policy is further defined as *those actions, non-actions, directions, and/or guidance related to health that are decided by governments or other authorized entities.*

Examples of this definition of health policy include decisions related to federal subsidies for the education of health professionals, state regulations that cover insurance benefits, and court decisions that overturn these same state regulations based on constitutional arguments. This definition would also include a variety of other health policies related to Medicare reimbursements to nurse practitioners, state-mandated immunizations for school children, and the decisions of a state or federal court that establish the rights of families to make health care decisions for their children or for elderly parents. This definition also provides for government *inaction,* as is the case when a legislative committee defers a decision on a health-related matter or when a proposed health program is not adopted by a government agency because of resource restraints. All of these examples demonstrate the public, goal-oriented, and authoritative nature of health policy decision making. They are also examples of the divided nature of health policy decision making in the United States.

SCOPE AND CATEGORIES

Health policy as a concept can first be differentiated by locating it within the realm of public decision making by political authority including executive order, legislation, judicial process, or regulatory rule-making agencies. Health policy determined through a presidential executive order or by legislation is easily recognizable as the legitimate responsibility of elected leadership. Health policy that is the result of regulatory actions or results from the administrative decisions of government agencies is not as easily identified. Yet, the decisions made in these other policy arenas may have significant impact on the distribution and quality of health care services.

Scope

The scope of health policy is wide and as varied as the numerous entities responsible for decisions, funding, enactment, and oversight as well as the many populations and individuals who are affected by these decisions. Health policy decisions can have both macro-level (Medicare program funding) and micro-level effects (co-payments for episodes of care) and can be made on the basis of economics, social justice, political trends, and/or changing social values. Health policy can also be the source of much political conflict because it has the potential to affect a large number of people, depending on the health policy goal.

Categories

Because health policy, as defined earlier, is the result of authoritative, public decision making, then a simple way to categorize it is to use the major types of political institutions established in the United States for politically determined decisions. These major government institutions decide, implement, and regulate policies, including health policy, and are legally authorized to do so by constitutional arrangements. Each of these authorities uses a public process for decision making. The major public authorities operating at the federal, state, and local levels are (1) state and national

legislatures, (2) state and national as well as local courts and judiciary, (3) the executive branches of federal and state governments, and (4) regulatory agencies.[3,7]

Legislatures

The United States Congress and state legislatures are deliberative bodies that establish laws to serve some policy goal. Along with the authority to create laws, legislatures are also tasked with determining the appropriate funding for a legislative act and for providing oversight for policies that are administered by government agencies. Health policy that results from law is legally binding as long as it is consistent with the authorizing constitutional framework.[3] The multiple perspectives embodied by the independently elected representatives to legislatures ensure the consideration of a diversity of different values in the political process.[2]

Courts and Judiciary

Health policy is the result of the political integration of values and interests. The enactment of new health laws can result in the establishment of new rights related to health programs or benefits. At the same time, it might be necessary to ensure preservation of previously established rights. Court systems play an important role in the development of health policy because the federal and state courts are often the staging ground for determining rights in health policy disputes through judicial review. Judiciary review can be addressed to widely varying concerns, including challenging unreasonable government action, supporting the establishment of newly created rights through legislation, and ensuring protections provided by health care law.[8]

Executive Branch

The executive branch of federal and state governments is responsible for the execution of laws passed by legislatures. Government executives, such as state governors and the U.S. President, oversee a vast apparatus of agencies and personnel tasked with the implementation of laws. The chief executive plays a large leadership role in health policy because of the legitimate powers of the office. Chief executives develop and implement institutional budgets, control the vast resources of the executive branch, and are usually able to use veto authority to influence policy changes. The office is also a clearly identified leadership position that provides the chief executive with a stage from which to influence the direction of health policy goals and decision making.

Regulatory Agencies

Regulatory agencies either can be a part of the executive branch or may be independent or semi-independent organizations. These agencies are established by legislatures to implement and enforce laws through a rule-making process.[3] The rules developed by these agencies are made through public administrative processes and have the force of law. Health care is a highly regulated industry so many health policies are established through administrative rule making by regulatory agencies. Decisions related to nursing licensure by state boards of nursing are an example of administrative rule making.

ATTRIBUTES AND CRITERIA

Health policies relate to a health concern or issue and are meant to address a public policy goal. Health policies result from a public decision-making process that directs the action or inaction of governments. The following are the major attributes of health policy:

1. Decisions are made by authorized government institutions such as legislatures or courts or by government-authorized entities.
2. The decision-making process is subject to public review and public input.
3. Health policies address a public policy goal.

Minor attributes of health policy include the following:

1. Health policies are subject to ongoing review by governing institutions and by the public.
2. Health policy goals change according to changes in political and social values, trends, and attitudes.

THEORETICAL LINKS

The attributes described above provide one means for understanding the concept of health policy. The concept can be further understood by developing an understanding of the process by which health policy is made. Anderson[9] provides a simple framework for understanding how health policy is created through sequential stages of activities. In the first step or stage, *agenda setting,* a health-related issue is identified, usually as a problem. Nurses can be especially effective in this stage by helping to frame the issue. Framing the issue means creating a particular perspective for the issue, for example, that assisted suicide is ethically justified because patients have a right to make their own health care decisions.

Once defined and framed, an issue is refined through a political process that involves negotiation and debate as well as the mobilization of support from interested politicians and interest groups. The next stage is *policy formulation,* in which different policy interventions are proposed and considered. *Policy adoption* is the next stage; during this stage a proposed intervention is selected. Selection is followed by *policy implementation* (carrying out the proposed intervention) and the process ends with *policy evaluation* or determining if the policy achieved the desired policy goals (see Figure 52-1).

This simple process model does not fully describe the complexities of health policy but it does provide a structure to begin to build a conceptual understanding. As defined earlier, health policies result from political processes. A basic understanding of health policy is impossible without consideration of key political concepts that affect policy development and implementation in the United States. These concepts are basic to the operations of constitutionally-grounded governments in the United States and are necessary for assuring health policies that account for the myriad of perspectives present in a multicultural, democratic society. These include the dynamics of intergovernmental relationships, the social expectations created by a system of participative governance, and the effect of dominant cultural values on political processes.

Intergovernmental Relationships

The United States consists of 50 sovereign states and a federal government, united by a mutually agreed upon constitution. The U.S. Constitution provides for a division of power between the federal government and the states that seeks to balance one against the other. The result is divided and limited government powers that create the need for political collaboration through systems of intergovernmental relations. The concept of *federalism* explains the dynamics of these intergovernmental relationships. Since 1965, federal funding for health policy initiatives has increased significantly. Policy initiatives requiring collaborative federal-state relations may result in state governments ceding some of their decision-making authority in return for federal funding. The reverse can also be true; the federal government may devolve more decision-making responsibility for health policy to state governments. This results in a complex mix of collaborative strategies supported by a web of shared responsibilities between state and federal governments.[10] The effect on health policy can be profound, leading to ongoing policy changes as authority and discretionary power shift.

Participative Governance

State and federal constitutions also provide for governments to operate through *consent of the governed.* Government power, especially in the United States, is limited to that allowed by the governed, U.S. citizens. Representatives of the governed are elected through a public voting process to conduct the business of government and to be accountable to voters for their decisions. Citizens are also expected to attend to the actions of government and participate in the political process. Paying attention and participating includes a range of activities, from the simple act of voting in elections to more active political participation such as lobbying or running for office. Participative governance is fundamental to American democratic

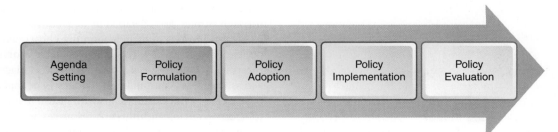

FIGURE 52-1 The Policy Process.

institutions because government powers are limited and subject to the will of the governed. It is a necessary check on government power that promotes the interests and values of the citizenry rather than a few elected officials. Health policies created by governments but that do not engender support from the governed do not enjoy much prolonged success.

Values

The dynamic relationship between the levels of government and sustained participative governance provide for the negotiation of diverse values through the political process. All health policy in the United States should be viewed as a product of negotiated values. Fairness and efficiency are the two competing values that are at the heart of most public policy decisions.[11] These values are decision drivers and the source of much health policy conflict because decision makers must be accountable for prudent use of public funding while also considering the needs of different constituencies. The values of fairness and efficiency are subject to interpretation and highly influenced by time, social trends, cultural expectations, economic priorities, and political situations. To ensure fairness in health policy might mean that legal rights are preserved, whether that is an individual right or communal rights established by law. Fairness might be interpreted as equitable distribution of health resources or as improved access to those resources. Establishing a fair policy might mean a trade-off with efficiency. Less efficient health policies may be more impartial but they are also more costly. The additional costs must be balanced against the benefits to be derived from the policy. American democratic institutions are uniquely crafted to provide the mechanisms for negotiating values through open, clearly identified political processes.

Dynamic Tension

Federalism, participative governance, and the need to negotiate values produce a dynamic tension between competing health policy interests at the intersection of access, cost, and quality (Figure 52-2). Providing access to care for uninsured Americans, for example, will require increased government expenditures and increases the need for tax revenue. Depending on state and national policy goals, increasing access to health care for the uninsured would bring into play the forces of federalism, politics, and negotiation. Current national concerns with the quality of health care are another major

focus of U.S. health policy since the publication of two Institute of Medicine (IOM) reports that emphasized the morbidity and mortality caused by medical errors.[12,13] In an effort to address the issue of quality care while also managing costs, the federal government has issued new Medicare and Medicaid guidelines that provide incentives for quality outcomes while reducing reimbursements to providers for poor quality outcomes. Improving access to quality care while decreasing overall costs again involves the forces of federalism, negotiation, and the politics of a variety of interested parties including state and federal government agencies, legislatures, professional provider organizations, and advocacy groups.

CONTEXT TO NURSING AND HEALTH CARE

Health policy and its effects are evident in all professional nursing practice environments. The most obvious are health policies that affect the scope and standards of professional nursing practice. The licensing and regulation of health professionals, including nurses, are the responsibility of state governments. States create laws that establish professional practice acts meant to regulate health professionals. A state regulatory agency and a politically-appointed board of nursing are tasked with the implementation and administration of nurse practice acts, including issuing licenses to individuals to legally practice nursing. Some state regulatory boards are specifically created for nursing and some boards are tasked with regulation of several health care professions, but all of these regulatory boards establish the scope of legally licensed practice and minimum standards for professional performance under that license. Regulatory boards have authority delegated by the state legislature to make rules and these rules have the force of law. Professional practice errors that violate the provisions of the practice act are subject to disciplinary action by boards and are adjudicated by the regulatory agency through established disciplinary procedures. Boards have the authority to revoke licenses for unsafe practice as defined by the practice act, including actions or behavior by the nurse that lies outside of the scope and standards of practice established by the license.

Related to professional licensing are health policies that govern professional negligence, or malpractice. Professional negligence occurs when the actions of the nurse are judged as substandard to what is expected in "reasonable and prudent" standard of practice and that result in harm to others. Whether a nurse is in violation of these standards is dependent on the minimum standards for practice set by the relevant state board of nursing, by practice standards published by professional societies, and by standards established through similar cases decided in state courts.

Health policies and the economic consequences of these policies are everyday realities for most working nurses, regardless of their specialties or their workplace. As noted, access to care is a national health policy issue that is driven, in part, by economics. Americans with health insurance are able to access available health care resources with relative ease. Uninsured Americans either do not seek care or they obtain care through federal- and state-sponsored clinical facilities or

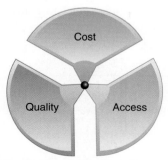

FIGURE 52-2 The Dynamic Tension Between Cost, Quality, and Access.

in the nation's emergency departments. The lack of secured access to primary care or to needed tertiary care results in a chaotic and costly health care system where financial incentives drive health behavior and health outcomes. Nurses encounter a variety of patient care dilemmas caused by economic factors in daily practice. These situations can be the source of frustration and moral distress for many professional nurses although they can also be the motivation for nurses to engage in the political processes that produce health policies.

In addition to engaging in the political process, nurses have a profound influence on health policy through their actions in everyday practice. Lipsky[14] introduced the concept of "street-level bureaucracy" to define the impact of frontline workers on public policy. He demonstrated that these frontline workers, such as police officers and social workers, have great influence in implementing policy at the "street-level," or where the policy meets its intended beneficiaries. Street-level decision making works to ensure that *policy intent* becomes the *policy as experienced*. Nurses work very closely with the patients and families that are the intended recipients and beneficiaries of health policies; therefore nurses are "street-level" workers who have the potential to greatly impact the implementation of policy at the bedside as well as in the community. Nurses deal with policy issues daily while assuring the confidentiality of patient information, allocating health care resources through staffing assignments, or teaching patients about their health care rights—these actions all have a health policy impact for patients and their families that can be traced back to an authorized decision-making process. In addition, the clinical expertise of nurses can be used to influence policy at local, state, national, and international levels. Nurses are always engaged in health policy at many different levels, whether as a frontline worker or as a policy advocate in the regulatory, legislative, judicial, and executive arenas.

INTERRELATED CONCEPTS

Health policy is not an autonomous concept. To fully appreciate the concept, other related concepts should be considered as necessary constructs that link to the definition and provide for a richer understanding of health policy as something more than government decisions. Health policies are negotiated through a political process. The potential is always present that some interests will be disadvantaged compared to the interests of others as a result of the competition of ideas and values that is the American political process. Because health policies, especially at the national level, have the potential to affect large portions of the public, there must be some grounding principles that provide a context for policy development and that help to integrate the interests of many into policy goals and directions. These principles could be explained through the interrelated concepts of social policy, institutional policy, markets, and advocacy.

Social Policy

Social policy, in its broadest sense, relates to decisions that promote the welfare of the public.[6] Social policy can be directed at a wide variety of social concerns and issues where the primary policy goal is not necessarily health but it still has an impact on health. For example, government policies related to a social policy goal that addresses obesity may result in legislation or regulation that governs the sale of high-fat/high-sugar content foods available in public schools. A state or federal law might govern WIC (Women Infants and Children) payments for healthy foods at farmers' markets. A linked health policy goal would be directed at assuring Medicare/Medicaid payments for exercise and weight loss programs.

Institutional Policy

Social policies are also not always public policies that result from political decision making. Institutional policies govern the workplace.[6] Nurses are often familiar with the policy and procedure manual of their unit or clinic or home health agency. An organization might have specific institutional policies developed for their workforce that relate to the prevention of obesity, such as providing exercise facilities onsite. Nurses also work with institutional policies that govern nursing practice, such as professional job descriptions. Social policies also take the form of organizational position statements established by professional organizations and advocacy groups. The student nurses association (SNA), for example, might adopt a resolution supporting exercise classes for nurses.

Markets

The U.S. health care system is situated within an economic system that emphasizes capitalism and markets. In capitalism, markets function to assure efficient distribution of resources to those goods and services that are the most desirable among many options. A major assumption of market systems is that the exchange of goods and services takes place among knowledgeable participants in a transparent and equitable process. This ideal is not always present in the sophisticated and expensive U.S. health care markets. Most Americans are dependent on the expertise of health care professionals to help them manage serious health problems. If they also lack adequate health insurance, they might have limited access to necessary health services if they cannot afford to pay for their care out of their own pockets.

Market ideals under these circumstances break down as the pursuit of efficient resource allocation results in resources being directed away from important social needs. An example is over-allocation of health care resources to relatively lucrative health markets such as cardiovascular care in the hospital but limiting resources for childhood immunizations. This creates a need for government interventions to direct resources to goods and services that serve some public interest, provide for equity in market transactions, or subsidize care for vulnerable or neglected populations. In the complex U.S. health care system, the marriage of governments and markets is inevitable as policy goals shift between the twin values of efficiency and equity.[15]

Advocacy

Advocacy is another related concept. Nurses support and advocate for their patients and for the profession. Advocacy is integrating the support provided to others on an individual basis and rallying that support to a cause. Nursing interest groups might unite for the purpose of advancing national health policy reform that assures greater access to health care for all Americans. In another example, nurses can advocate for nurse-managed centers to be eligible for Federally Qualified Health Clinic (FQHC) status. Nurse practitioners working in an FQHC are eligible to receive a higher rate of reimbursement. Nurse-managed centers have a long history of providing primary health care to underserved patients. By advocating for FQHC status, nurses can support increased access to quality care at an affordable cost.

Nurses are in a unique and pivotal position to impact the cost/quality/access equation through advocacy. A recent IOM[16] report developed in collaboration with the Robert Wood Johnson Foundation provides a roadmap for nurses to become active in health policy at the local, state, and national levels. This report calls on all health professionals, regulatory bodies, and policymakers to improve health care by removing scope of practice barriers and increasing education, leadership, and standardized workforce data collection and analysis (Box 52-1).

Other Interrelated Concepts

Several additional concepts discussed in this book are also interrelated: **Evidence, Ethics, Safety, Health care quality, Health care economics,** and **Health care law** (Figure 52-3). Data and research are used to generate support and interest for a specific health policy agenda. This use of evidence supports advocacy. Distribution of scarce resources and policy development to enhance the greater good while minimizing harm require use of ethical decision making. Negotiation of diverse values in the context of balancing the competing values of fairness (ethics) and efficiency (economics) epitomizes

| BOX 52-1 | **EIGHT RECOMMENDATIONS FROM *THE FUTURE OF NURSING* REPORT[17]** |

1. Remove scope-of-practice barriers.
2. Expand opportunities for nurses to lead and diffuse collaborative improvement efforts.
3. Implement nurse residency programs.
4. Increase proportion of nurses with BSN degree to 80% by 2020.
5. Double the number of nurses with a doctorate by 2020.
6. Ensure that nurses engage in lifelong learning.
7. Prepare and enable nurses to lead change to advance health.
8. Build an infrastructure to collect and analyze health care workforce data.

the challenge of designing and implementing successful health policy. The tension described earlier between cost, quality, and access highlights these competing values. Nurses are in a unique position to combine their advocacy role of ensuring patient safety and quality with the ethics and health economics values of fairness and cost efficiency. In some contexts it may be difficult to distinguish health policy from health law. Health professionals often respond to the laws and regulations that have been promulgated as a result of health policies. For example, the Health Information Portability and Accountability Act of 1996 (P.L.104-191 HIPAA) was developed with the policy intent to limit the ability of employers to deny health insurance coverage to their employees based on preexisting medical conditions. Another policy intent was to preserve the privacy of patients by limiting access to health care records.

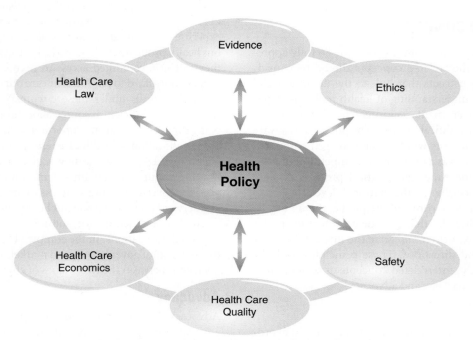

FIGURE 52-3 Health Policy and Interrelated Concepts.

MODEL CASE

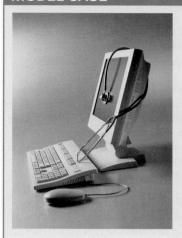

As described, any given health policy is the result of political and social interactions that result in health policies that integrate many interests while addressing some policy goal. One example of this is the protection of confidential health care records afforded by the provisions of HIPAA. The confidentiality of medical information became an *agenda* item for Congress when electronic data systems became widely adopted throughout the United States. The increased use of computers in health care had created the capacity for critical health care information to be efficiently shared among health care providers and among insurance companies. Advocates for patient confidentiality and information privacy argued that the ease of information sharing through electronic transmission of records would result in personal health information becoming available to a wide variety of interested parties. Access to this information could result in a variety of actions, including denial of coverage through employer-sponsored plans to individuals or family members with chronic or debilitating conditions. Other unfavorable outcomes from the unrestricted sharing of private health information could also result, such as the sale of mailing lists of individuals with particular medical conditions to companies with a commercial interest in obtaining those lists.

The policy intent of this federal statute was to limit the ability of employers to deny health insurance coverage to their employees based on preexisting medical conditions. In the *formulation* of a policy response, the intervention chosen by Congress was to limit access to health care information to only those parties with a legitimate role in the financing and delivery of services, specifically health care providers, insurance companies, and third-party contractors.[17] Through HIPAA, Congress directed the United States Department of Health and Human Services (USDHHS) to *implement* the policy by developing privacy rules that protect electronically transmitted health information. These rules cover any entity that must have access to this information for legitimate purposes and provide guidelines for determining access to and disclosure of protected health information. Criminal and financial penalties are provided for proven HIPAA violations, including federal prison sentences for perpetrators and fines of up to $250,000. Investigations and prosecutions of HIPAA violations are the responsibility of the United States Department of Justice.[18]

One of the federal agencies tasked with public review and reporting for federal policies is the United States Government Accounting Office (GAO). The GAO has published different reviews of HIPAA at the request of government officials over the years since passage of the statute and these reports are publically available on the GAO website. A recent review[19] documents the ongoing issues of implementation of this widespread policy that governs the electronic transmission of health care information. HIPAA provides broad guidelines for the protection of patient information that must be interpreted for implementation. Covered entities targeted by the statute are expected to develop HIPAA-compliant policies that govern the treatment of protected health information in their organizations and during transactions with contracted third parties. The GAO report notes there is still much guidance to be issued by USDHHS to assist these entities in complying with HIPAA guidelines. This guidance will be created through USDHHS rule-making authority and will be publicly available for comment and feedback by affected organizations and the general public during the rule-making process.

CONTRARY CASE

Not all policies in health care settings are health policies. Health care organizations formulate their own policies to support processes, resource management, and production functions. For example, a clinic, hospital, or clinical unit may decide to institute a policy related to types of scrubs or uniforms for employees. This is an institutional policy, but not a health policy. Other institutional policies that are similar to health policy are policies that govern workplace behavior, scheduling and staffing, infection control measures, performance evaluation, and professional development. These are all policies and are subject to changes in the organization, but they are not created by government authorities, subjected to ongoing public review, or created through a political negotiation process.

EXEMPLARS

In the United States, nurses can expect to encounter a wide variety of health policies that have a direct impact on their work. These policies are determined through laws, regulatory actions, judicial decisions, and the administrative actions of all levels of government. A sample of some of the more visible and relevant health policies that shape the environment of nursing is listed in Box 52-2.

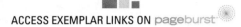

ACCESS EXEMPLAR LINKS ON pageburst

BOX 52-2 EXEMPLARS OF HEALTH CARE POLICY

Federal
- Access to Emergency Medical Services Act of 2009
- Americans with Disabilities Act of 1990
- Emergency Medical Treatment and Labor Act (EMTLA) of 1986
- Health Information Technology for Economic and Clinical Health Act of 2009 (electronic health records)
- Health Insurance Portability and Accountability Act of 1996
- Patient Protection and Affordable Care Act of 2010
- Patient Safety and Quality Improvement Act of 2005
- Patient Self-Determination Act of 1998
- Promoting Health/Preventing Disease: Objectives for the Nation, *Healthy People 1990, 2000, 2010, 2020*
- Social Security Act of 1965 (Medicare and Medicaid)
- The Mental Health Parity and Addiction Equity Act of 2008
- U.S. Preventive Services Task Force (USPSTF)

State
- Scope of practice and licensing for nurses as defined by state professional practice acts
- State public health programs and policies related to infectious diseases
- State public health regulations that govern health care facilities
- State statutes and case law related to professional negligence and malpractice

Local
- City and county fire codes that govern safe occupancy limits in health care facilities
- City and county ordinances that govern facility maintenance, signs, utilities, parking, and/or traffic around hospitals and other health facilities
- City and county tax districts for publicly supported facilities

REFERENCES

1. Cummings T, Worley C: *Organization development & change*, Mason, Ohio, 2009, South-Western Cengage Learning.
2. Peterson M: Congress. In Morone J, Litman T, Robins L, editors: *Health politics and policy*, ed 4, Clifton Park, NY, 2008, Delmar, pp 72–94.
3. Longest B, Darr K: *Managing health services organizations and systems*, ed 5, Baltimore, 2010, Health Professions Press.
4. Shortell S, Kaluzny A: Organization theory and health services management. In Shortell S, Kaluzny A, editors: *Health care management: organization design and behavior*, ed 5, Clifton Park, NY, 2006, Delmar, pp 5–41.
5. Dye T: *Understanding public policy*, ed 7, Englewood Cliffs, NJ, 1992, Prentice Hall.
6. Mason D, Leavitt J, Chaffee M: Policy and politics: a framework for action. In Mason D, Leavitt J, Chaffee M, editors: *Policy and politics in nursing and health care*, St Louis, 2007, Saunders/Elsevier, pp 1–16.
7. Hanley B, Falk N: Policy development and analysis: understanding the process. In Mason D, Leavitt J, Chaffee M, editors: *Policy and politics in nursing and health care*, St Louis, 2007, Saunders/Elsevier, pp 75–93.
8. Betts V, Keepnews D, Gentry J: Nursing and the courts. In Mason D, Leavitt J, Chaffee M, editors: *Policy and politics in nursing and health care*, St Louis, 2007, Saunders/Elsevier, pp 825–834.
9. Anderson JE: *Public policymaking: an introduction*, ed 7, Australia, 2010, Wadsworth Cengage Publishing.
10. Thompson F, Fossett J: Federalism. In Morone J, Litman T, Robins L, editors: *Health politics and policy*, ed 4, Clifton Park, NY, 2008, Delmar, pp 153–172.
11. Stone D: Values in health policy: understanding fairness and efficiency. In Morone J, Litman T, Robins L, editors: *Health politics and policy*, ed 4, Clifton Park, NY, 2008, Delmar, pp 24–36.
12. Institute of Medicine: *To err is human: building a safer health system*, Washington, DC, 2000, The National Academies Press.
13. Institute of Medicine: *Crossing the quality chasm: a new health system for the 21st century*, Washington, DC, 2001, The National Academies Press.
14. Institute of Medicine: *The Future of Nursing: Leading Change, Advancing Health*, Washington, DC, 2010, The National Academies Press.
15. Lipsky M: *Street level bureaucracy. Dilemmas of the individual in public services*, New York, 1980, Russell Sage Foundation.
16. Rice T: Markets and politics. In Morone J, Litman T, Robins L, editors: *Health politics and policy*, ed 4, Clifton Park, NY, 2008, Delmar, pp 37–48.
17. Institute of Medicine: *The future of nursing: leading change, advancing health*, Washington, DC, 2011, The National Academies Press.
18. Flores J, Dodier A: HIPAA: past, present and future implications for nurses, *Online J Issues Nurs*, 2005. doi: 10.3912/OJIN.Vol10No02Man04.
19. Harman L: HIPAA: a few years later, *Online J Issues Nurs*, 2005. doi:10.3912/OJIN.Vol10No02Man02.

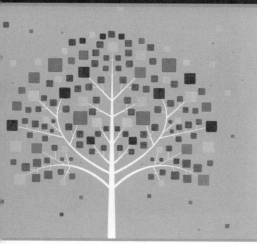

Health Care Law

Yvonne Masters

Health care is becoming exponentially more complex every day. As a society, our response to this complexity has been to legislate, regulate, and litigate. The societal rules that result from these activities tell us who we can or must treat, how we must treat them, and how much we can charge or who will pay. Health care law is a fundamental concept for all health care professionals. Nurses must be aware of health care law as it applies to health care, in general, and the specific impact on professional nursing practice.

DEFINITION(S)

A law is a rule enacted by a government or government agency that details how an individual or group must behave in a given circumstance. A law may be *prescriptive*—it defines something that must be done—or *proscriptive*—it defines something that must not be done. Laws also may describe the rules of dealing with certain conflicts, such as laws that prioritize surrogate decision makers if the patient has not assigned a health care surrogate. Some laws have a financial incentive attached to them to encourage compliance. This incentive may be in terms of a fine that is paid if something is done that the law has proscribed, such as the fines that are attached to breaches of the Health Insurance Portability and Accountability Act of 1996 (HIPAA). Some laws may describe how certain monies will be spent as long as specific criteria are met; an example of this would be Medicare legislation, which determined that when an individual reaches the age of 65 or becomes disabled the government will provide health insurance that pays for health care and hospitalization. Some laws, in particular criminal laws, may impose a harsher incentive, such as incarceration or death, to encourage compliance. For the purposes of this concept analysis, *health care law* is defined as *the collection of laws that have a direct impact on the delivery of health care or on the relationships among those in the business of health care or between the providers and recipients of health care.*

SCOPE AND CATEGORIES

As a concept, health care law is very complex and represents a wide spectrum in both creation and application. To gain a better understanding of the scope of health care law, it is important to have an understanding of the source of many of these laws.

Many different government bodies and agencies can create laws that affect the delivery of health care in the United States. These entities exist at both the federal and the state levels of government. The primary source of power for these government entities is the U.S. Constitution. Power may also be derived from state constitutions, from the executive or judiciary branches of federal and state governments, and from the laws themselves. Laws can be created through legislation, through regulatory activities by government agencies, and through the process of litigation.

These law-making activities foster a continuing evolution in health care law. There is no true linear process by which these activities function. Laws may evolve by a legislature identifying an issue and drafting a law that addresses that issue. Within that legislation authority may be given to an existing federal agency to draft rules that support compliance with the policy goals of the initial law. A situation may arise that does not completely fit within the law as drafted by the legislature or an individual affected by the law may believe that the law is unconstitutional or in conflict with other laws; this can lead to a legal challenge in court. Sometimes the judicial ruling will stand alone as a law and sometimes the legislature will revise a law to be consistent with the court's ruling. Sometimes, a legal challenge will precede the legislation and the legislature may or may not decide to make a formal declaration of law. These processes are interwoven or braided together to continually revise and refine the law (Figure 53-1).

Legislation

The powers of the federal government are specifically defined in Article I Section 8 of the U.S. Constitution. These powers include such things as the power to coin money, the power

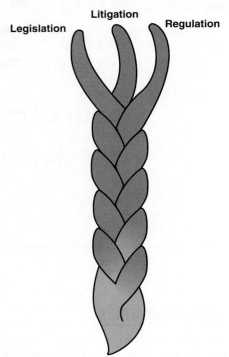

Legislation   Litigation   Regulation

FIGURE 53-1 Scope of Health Care Law.

to establish a uniform rule of naturalization, the power to declare war, the power to tax and spend, and the power to regulate interstate commerce. None of the powers specifically given to the federal government has a direct relationship to health care, so the federal government must find a link or relationship to the Constitutional powers when drafting health care laws. Federal laws are considered the highest source of law and trump all state or local laws.

The Tenth Amendment to the Constitution states, "The powers not delegated to the United States by the Constitution, nor prohibited by it to the States, are reserved to the States respectively, or to the people." This means the powers of the state government include anything and everything that is not specifically described as being a power of the United States. This includes the power to license professionals, provide and regulate public education, and provide for public health and safety.

Although the state powers do have a more direct relationship to health care than the federal powers, the federal government often usurps the state power through its power to tax and spend and its power to regulate interstate commerce. Medicare and Medicaid were enacted through the spending powers as the federal government collects the taxes and then spends them as distributions to the states to subsidize their Medicaid programs or directly to hospitals and providers as Medicare payments. The Health Insurance Portability and Accountability Act of 1996 (HIPAA) was enacted through the federal government's power to regulate interstate commerce. Congress found, "provisions in group health plans and health insurance coverage that impose certain pre-existing conditions impact the ability of employees to seek

employment in interstate commerce, thereby impeding such commerce."[1]

Regulation

There are some government agencies that also have the power to make laws in the form of regulations. Sometimes when Congress passes a law, the law contains only a broad framework for an overall policy goal. Congress will then delegate power to a specific federal agency that is tasked with creating the specific rules for promoting and enforcing the legislative policy. These agencies are often under the control of the executive branch; they act as an agent for the President to protect the public interest. The rules that have the effect of law are compiled in a set of documents known as the *Code of Federal Regulations*.

An example of a regulatory agency that has an effect on health care law is the U.S. Department of Health and Human Services (USDHHS). "The Department of Health and Human Services (HHS) is the United States government's principal agency for protecting the health of all Americans and providing essential human services, especially for those who are least able to help themselves."[2] The Secretary of USDHHS is a member of the President's Cabinet. There are 11 divisions within USDHHS; these include the Centers for Disease Control and Prevention (CDC), Food and Drug Administration (FDA), National Institutes of Health (NIH), Agency for Healthcare Research and Quality (AHRQ), and Centers for Medicare & Medicaid Services (CMS). CMS has been given broad authority to draft the *Medicaid and Medicare Conditions of Participation for Hospitals*. When CMS became concerned regarding the death of patients while in restraints or seclusion, they enacted a regulation that delineates specific rules regarding the use of restraints and seclusion for hospitals that participate in Medicaid and Medicare. This regulation also requires hospitals to report any deaths that occur during or are reasonably assumed to have resulted from restraint or seclusion.[3] These regulations are now a part of the restraint policy for any hospital that participates in Medicare and Medicaid funding.

Litigation

Litigation is the process of filing a lawsuit and seeking the help of the courts to redress a perceived wrong. Individuals or groups may seek redress for harm caused by the negligence of another or for breach of contract; they may also seek to challenge or resolve a situation to which the laws do not apply or to address a situation in which they think the applicable law is wrong. These cases may be decided by a jury, especially when deciding whether someone committed a crime or whether someone behaved negligently and caused harm to another person. Some cases may be decided by judges (known collectively as the judiciary); these are usually cases in which the challenge brought by the parties involves the validity or application of the law in question.

The role of the judge or the judicial branch of government is to interpret the law, but often their interpretation leads to law itself. This type of law is referred to as case law or common law. The job of the judiciary is to look at all the statutory laws (laws that have been enacted by a legislative body), applicable regulations, and all the precedents (what have courts decided to do in similar situations in the past); they apply these to the situation as it exists now, and make a decision or establish a rule. Sometimes that rule is limited to the exact facts of the case, sometimes the rule is limited to a specific state or area of the country, and sometimes the rule impacts the country as a whole. Sometimes one area of the country may not have addressed a question that another area of the country has already answered in the courts and may adopt the ruling of another area without going through the process of litigating the question in the courts.

In the case of *In re Quinlan*[4] the court ruled that if the attending physician and the hospital "Ethics Committee" agreed that there was no reasonable possibility of Karen Ann Quinlan returning to a cognitive, sapient state then her present life support system could be withdrawn without risk of civil or criminal penalty. Although this was a decision of the New Jersey Supreme Court, the decision prompted hospitals in states all over the country to establish hospital ethics committees to help them address the question of removing life support.

ATTRIBUTES

To be considered a health care law, the law or rule must have been created by a government agency with appropriate authority. There are some health care rules that may define expected behavior, but if these rules were not created by a government entity with legal authority then they are not health care laws.

Major Attributes

A rule established by a government body such as a legislature, agency, or judiciary is one type of major attribute. Another example would be a law or rule that defines the expected behavior of persons in the business of health care or in health care relationships.

Minor Attributes

In a minor attribute, the law or rule may have a financial or other incentive attached to encourage compliance.

THEORETICAL LINKS

Unlike other areas of the law that have historical roots that date back to medieval England, classical Rome, and ancient Persia, the field of health care law is a relatively new invention of the latter half of the twentieth century. It is a rapidly evolving discipline. Furrow has identified five major concerns that form the basis for health care law and provide a foundation for theoretical understanding: "oversight of the quality of health care, control of the cost of health care, assurance of equitable access to health care...protection of the person of the patient...[and]the structuring of business relationships among the institutions and professionals that provide health care."[5]

To address these concerns health law relies on many of the traditional legal disciplines (Figure 53-2). Constitutional law and tort law are the two legal disciplines from which most health care laws are derived. Clauses within the Constitution are the vehicles with which our society has been able to ensure access to health care for our poor and elderly. The due process clause of the Fourteenth Amendment was the legal principle under which the Supreme Court decided the landmark case

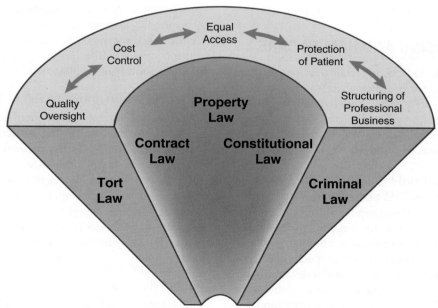

FIGURE 53-2 Theory of Health Care Law.

of *Roe v. Wade,*[6] which legalized first-trimester abortions, and the case of *Cruzan v. Missouri,*[7] which clarified the law of living wills. The Tenth Amendment to the Constitution is the legal principle under which those who challenge the mandate to buy insurance under the newly enacted Patient Protection and Affordable Care Act of 2010 are arguing that the federal government has overstepped its bounds.[8]

Tort law has been responsible for shaping and defining many of our patient care quality parameters. Tort is the area of law under which cases of negligence, including malpractice cases, are argued. When malpractice cases are argued, the standard against which negligence is measured is set by the profession (see Malpractice). Sometimes the response to a trend in malpractice cases is to reevaluate and refine the standard. Often these new standards come in the form of new regulations (e.g., *CMS Standard: Seclusion or Restraint*). Other rules, such as The Joint Commission's *National Patient Safety Goals,* also promote the health care industry's continued focus on improving patient safety and decreasing the risk for harm. Tort cases can also help to refine our understanding of health care law as it applies to different health care situations (see the Model Case discussion of EMTALA).

Other areas of the law such as contract, property, and even criminal law have also addressed the concerns of and helped to shape health care law. To some degree routine conditions of admission and consent forms represent a contract between the patient and the health care facility or the physician. Principles of contract are also used to define the work agreements of those who provide the services of health care. Property claims have been asserted in some unique cases such as *Moore v. UCLA*[9] in which a patient asserted he had a property interest in a cell line that was derived from cells taken from his body. Criminal penalties are now emerging as enforcement tools for some health care laws. Under HIPAA, purposeful breaches of protected health information can cause an individual to be subject to fines as well as jail time.[10]

CONTEXT TO NURSING AND HEALTH CARE

Many laws at both the federal and state level have been enacted with the intent to directly impact the business or relationships of health care. Some laws have evolved with time. Other laws may not have been enacted with the intent to directly affect health care, but they may have an effect on the business of health care, nonetheless.

Federal Laws that Directly Impact Health Care
Social Security Act of 1965 (Medicaid and Medicare)
The Social Security Act of 1965 amended the existing Social Security law and created two major health care programs: Medicaid and Medicare. Because most health insurance was and still is attached to employment, Congress sought to create a form of health insurance for those who by definition did not have jobs to provide their insurance—retired individuals and the unemployed. The 1965 Act created a trust fund for Medicare and grants to the states for the support of Medicaid programs.[11]

Reimbursement under the Medicare program has seen many changes since it was initially enacted in 1965, and health care organizations have worked hard to meet the requirements of all these changes. One of the most significant changes was the adoption of the diagnostic related group (DRG) in 1983, which abolished the traditional fee-for-service payment and instead provided prospective payment based upon a patient's diagnosis.[12] Because Medicare reimbursement has set the standard for all public and private reimbursement, the implementation of DRGs not only affected Medicare patients but also was quickly adopted by insurance companies as a means to compensate health care organizations for the care of those patients.

The creation of the Medicare program has given the federal government increased influence in the realm of health care law; many federal laws that have been enacted since 1965 find their legitimacy as added requirements for health care organizations that participate in Medicare reimbursement. In other words, because the federal government is spending money on the Medicare program they can decide what rules the health care organizations must follow if they wish to participate. These rules apply to the treatment of all patients by the health care organization, not just Medicare patients.

Consolidated Omnibus Budget Reconciliation Act and Emergency Medical Treatment and Active Labor Act of 1986

The Emergency Medical Treatment and Active Labor Act (EMTALA) was a provision of the Consolidated Omnibus Budget Reconciliation Act (COBRA) of 1986.[13] COBRA was an enormous piece of legislation that addressed, among other things, deficit reduction and social security trust funds and modified the student loan program. EMTALA required that any hospital that operated an emergency department and received Medicare funds provide an appropriate screening exam to anyone who presented and stabilize any emergency medical condition before transfer to another facility.[14] COBRA also contained a provision that allowed individuals to continue group medical insurance provided by an employer after termination of employment.[15]

Patient Self-Determination Act of 1991

Under the provisions of the Patient Self-Determination Act, health care organizations that participate in Medicare programs are required to (1) give patients information regarding advance directives (medical power of attorney and living will) and advise patients of their right to participate in their medical decisions and (2) document in the medical record whether or not a patient has completed an advance directive.[16] Because this information must be shared upon admission to the hospital, it is usually provided by the admitting personnel.

Health Insurance Portability and Accountability Act of 1996

The Health Insurance Portability and Accountability Act (HIPAA) was an uncelebrated milestone in health insurance reform. It was intended to provide individuals with preexisting medical conditions, who might otherwise be denied health care coverage outright, affordable access to health insurance. The law gives tax incentives to states and companies that create high-risk pools to provide coverage for these individuals with preexisting medical conditions.[17] The problem has been that the cost of insurance through a high-risk pool remains high and out of reach of most who need it.

The provision of HIPAA that has garnered much more attention is *Title II—Preventing Health Care Fraud and Abuse; Administrative Simplification; Medical Liability Reform.* This portion of the law did provide some basic medical liability reform in terms of creating a standard statute of limitations and limiting damage awards. This is also the provision responsible for creating the broad health information privacy requirements with which all in the business of health care must contend. These privacy provisions were included in the bill because of the concern that improper sharing of health information could reveal the existence of health conditions that could result in the denial of individual or employer-sponsored health coverage.

Patient Protection and Affordable Care Act of 2010

The Patient Protection and Affordable Care Act was the primary health care agenda item of the Obama presidential campaign. Provisions within the law include subsidies for high-risk pools to enable Americans with preexisting conditions to more easily afford insurance, the creation of health insurance exchanges that will make insurance coverage more accessible and affordable for individuals and small businesses, and the elimination of insurance co-pays for preventive care. The law also requires that every American have minimum essential health insurance beginning in 2013.[18] This is the most controversial provision of the law and it has already been litigated in some jurisdictions; those jurisdictions are not in agreement regarding whether or not it is constitutional for the government to compel individuals to purchase insurance.

Other Federal Laws

There are a myriad of other laws whose primary intent may not have been to directly affect the business or relationships of health care but continue to have some impact on health care. These include federal drug laws (prescribing and dispensing of narcotics), federal anti-kickback laws (prohibiting gifts or compensation for promoting the services of another to a government payer such as Medicare), the Americans with Disabilities Act, the Common Rule for Protection of Human Research Subjects, and even federal employment laws.

State Laws that Directly Impact Health Care

Because each of the 50 states has independent legislative bodies, the laws that are enacted by the states may vary in title, but the underlying concept of the law is the same. Because the U.S. Constitution did not specifically reserve for the federal government the power to legislate for the general health and welfare of the people, states have broad authority to legislate on health care matters.

Licensing of Professionals—Scope of Practice

The area of health care law that has the most direct impact on health care providers is state licensing laws. These laws, referred to as practice acts, establish the requirements necessary to obtain a license and the scope of practice for those with that license. For nursing this means that the state legislature sets minimum education standards for applying for a nursing license, examination and endorsement guidelines, and criminal background check guidelines, as well as establishes the legal authority for nursing practice. Under these practice acts states also create regulatory bodies, such as a state board of nursing, which are responsible for creating and enforcing rules that are consistent with the state practice act.

The scope of practice for professional nursing is the range of permissible activity as defined by the law; in essence it defines what nurses can and, sometimes more importantly, what nurses cannot do. Historically, medicine was the first profession to have a legally defined scope of practice. Generally, the scope of practice for medicine is broadly defined to include diagnosis and treatment, offers of advice, prescription or administration of drugs, and penetration of human tissues. Under these definitions are provisions that also make it illegal for anyone who is not licensed to practice medicine to undertake any of the described activities. Traditionally, this general definition gave medicine exclusive legal authority to treat all possible human conditions and has allowed the physicians the continued authority to supervise and control the activities of other medical professionals. Every other health care practice has defined their scope of practice by "carving out" exceptions from this all-inclusive definition of medical practice.[19]

Because the scope of nursing practice is defined by state legislation, there is great variation from state to state both in specificity and in the range of activities that are legally authorized. Many state legislatures have enacted very specific scope of practice statements whereas others have drafted very vague and broad scope of practice statements and have left the job of describing the specific activities to the state board of nursing. Some state scope of practice statements are very restrictive, whereas others allow a much broader range of activities. Although there is general consistency for the scope of practice for the professional registered nurse (RN), there is significant variability for the scope of practice of licensed practical or vocational nurses (LPN/LVN) and even more variability for the scope of practice for advanced practice nurses (nurse practitioners, midwives, anesthetists, collectively called APRN).[20] Thus it is very important that a nurse become very familiar with the practice act and the scope of practice as defined by the legislature or the state board of nursing of the state in which he or she is practicing.

In *The Report on the Future of Nursing: Leading Change, Advancing Health,* the Institute of Medicine[20] has identified the variability of scope of practice for advanced practice nurses as one of the barriers to transforming practice and meeting the health care needs of the twenty-first century. Because of the restrictive nature of the scope of practice statements of many states, all APRNs are not able to practice to the full extent of their education and training. There is, however, evidence to suggest that when nurses play an integral role in the delivery of primary care there are improvements in quality, access to care, patient satisfaction, and value. Allowing nurses to practice to the full extent of their education and training would likely benefit patients and the health care system as a whole.

Licensing of Health Care Institutions

In addition to licensing individual practice, states also have the authority to license and regulate health care institutions, again determining necessary requirements in terms of building size, structure, safety requirements, staffing requirements, duties of the administrators, and types of services that can be offered. These requirements can become entangled with municipal (city) building and fire codes as well as federal laws such as CMS regulations that outline requirements hospitals must meet in order to participate in Medicare and Medicaid services.

Laws Relating to Public Health and Disease Prevention/Control

Promoting the public's health is a prime responsibility of the states. This includes determining appropriate immunizations required to enter school, providing surveillance and treatment for certain infectious diseases, ensuring that institutions preparing food for public consumption are clean and sanitary, and providing the infrastructure that supports the sanitary utility services we enjoy.

Consent

Consent laws have been largely shaped by the common law, but many states now have statutory laws that designate who can consent or make decisions for a patient if the patient has not already designated someone. The concept of consent arises from the ethical principle of autonomy and the policy that patients have a right to be involved in decisions about their health care. It is also a protective response to the tort of battery, which is the purposeful, unwelcome, harmful touching of another. Performing a procedure without patient consent could constitute battery even if the procedure was done competently and the outcome was good.

To be valid, information for consent must be given by the provider who will be performing the procedure and the information given must include a description of the procedure, an explanation of the risks and benefits of the procedure, and a discussion of any alternatives to the proposed procedure. Consent by the patient must be voluntarily given and the person who consents must have the capacity to consent. Capacity can be determined by the health care provider and may be affected by drugs or the current/underlying medical condition. In short, the provider must be sure the patient understands the information provided and the consent is voluntarily given. If the patient is unable to give consent directly, he or she may designate a person who can give consent on his or her behalf. If such a person is not designated by the patient, most states provide a statutory solution, a law that lists "statutory surrogates," individuals who based on their relationship to the patient would be given priority to consent on the patient's behalf.

Advance Directives

All states have laws that provide guidelines for the execution and enforcement of health care directives. These directives include living wills, medical power of attorney for health care decisions, and prehospital do not resuscitate orders. These directives identify how a patient wishes to be treated in the event of certain medical conditions and also identify who the patient wants to make decisions on his or her behalf in the event that the patient was unable do so. These laws encourage compliance with the patient's directive by giving health care providers who act in reliance on these documents immunity from civil or criminal liability, and some states impose criminal liability if a patient's advance directives are not followed.

Physician-Assisted Suicide

In the late 1990s in the midst of the "right to die" movement, Oregon enacted physician-assisted suicide legislation.[21] Washington passed a similar initiative in 2008.[22] Known as the Death with Dignity Acts, these laws allow physicians to write a prescription for a lethal dose of medication that the patient can use to end his or her life if the patient is expected to have less than 6 months to live. Safeguards within the law require a waiting period between the initial request for medication and the receipt of the prescription, referral to counseling if the patient seems depressed, and referral to a second physician who concurs with the terminal nature of the patient's condition. In 2009 the Montana Supreme Court ruled that it was not against public policy for a physician to aid in dying by prescribing a lethal dose of medication.[23] With this decision, Montana became the third state to allow physician-assisted suicide.

Negligence
Malpractice

Malpractice or the law of medical liability is actually a special section of the area of law known as tort law. Most of the rules of tort law are found in the common law, meaning the law has developed through centuries of court decisions and is not codified in statutes. For tort liability to attach, four elements must be satisfied: duty, breach, causation, and harm. Duty arises from a special relationship; most notably, in relation to health care law, the physician-patient relationship is traditionally seen as a special relationship that gives rise to a duty. Health care providers breach that duty when they fail to follow the standard of care that a similarly situated provider would follow when caring for a similar patient. That breach of care must be the direct or proximate cause of the harm that the patient experienced; in other words, if the breach had not occurred there would not be any harm. The resultant harm must be real, physical, measurable harm. In other words, a patient cannot recover from emotional harm alone without an accompanying physical disability.

The term *standard of care* is widely used in hospitals to mean the standard way of doing business, but it is really a legal term that defines the liability standard as established by the profession. When a patient presents with a certain condition, the standard of care defines all the treatment and care that a provider with similar education and training would provide in a similar setting. From a legal standpoint, the nurse in a rural setting would be held accountable to a different standard of care than the nurse in an urban, tertiary care setting. Likewise, a nurse is held accountable to a different standard of care than other health professionals (such as a physician), and nurses with different areas of expertise or specialty practice are held accountable to different standards of care as well. The standard for liability is defined from within the profession and the specialty; this is one of the very unique characteristics of medical malpractice. Although these standards used to be based on the prevailing practice ("the way we do things"), more are now evidence based for best outcomes.

Employer/Employee Liability

Professional liability can also attach to an employer for the acts of its employee. This is known as vicarious liability and it arises from the common law doctrine of *respondeat superior,* a Latin term that means "let the master answer." Under vicarious liability, an employer can be liable for the acts of its employee if the employee was acting as the agent of the employer and the actions that resulted in injury occurred within the scope of employment. Thus, an employer would not be liable for injury that happened while the employee was not at work or injury that resulted from activities that were outside of the employee's scope of practice. This is one reason why hospitals are so concerned about validating that their staff have been properly trained in the scope of their duties. Hospitals require annual training in many areas such as clinical competencies and HIPAA not only to meet federal requirements but also to demonstrate that employees have the appropriate skills training, and can thus be held accountable. Similarly, policies and procedures are developed and updated by employers as a mechanism to document standard of care expected by an employee.

Criminal Liability

There are specific situations in which the act of negligence was so egregious or done with such disregard that the act may be considered criminal. As described previously, professional liability can occur when there is a breach in the duty one owes to a client and that breach causes harm. In contrast to professional liability, criminal liability looks at the act and not necessarily the resultant harm; criminal liability can attach even when there is no resulting harm. Criminal liability can result when that breach is not the result of negligence, but instead the result of reckless behavior or even worse—purposeful behavior. An example of reckless behavior would be showing up for work under the influence of alcohol and inadvertently giving a medication that led to injury. There was not a purposeful intent to give the wrong medicine or harm the patient,

but a reasonable person would expect that if a provider came to work under the influence of alcohol there would be a much greater chance for a mistake to occur. (Remember, too, that just the act of driving to work under the influence is a crime even if no one is injured.) Health care workers have also been found guilty of criminal neglect or abuse when they have shown extreme indifference to the needs of their patients, such as restraining patients and then ignoring their cries for help or needs for repositioning, toileting, or other care. In Arizona, a physician was found guilty of manslaughter for refusing to return to attend to a patient after she developed complications from an elective procedure.[24]

Seeking a Change in the Law—Political Advocacy

Sometimes in their day-to-day business nurses may encounter a situation in which they feel a law is needed to protect their profession or their patients. These things may range from mandating nurse to patient staffing ratios, to funding full coverage for prenatal care, to imposing harsher penalties for workplace violence against health providers. The first step, before addressing the issue with a legislator, is to research the current state of the law and determine if a law already exists at the state or federal level. If a law exists, determine what changes would make the law more favorable. If a law does not exist, determine which legislator at which level of government (state or federal) would be best able to address the issue. Federal legislation packs a sweeping punch, but the powers of the federal government to legislate in the area of health care are limited to the powers given in the Constitution. When writing to a legislator be specific about the issue, cite any relevant evidence that supports the issue, and state specifically what should be done about the issue. If a bill of interest has been introduced in the state or federal legislature, take the time to show support through letter writing or in-person testimony. As skilled patient advocates nurses are well qualified to advocate or lobby for health care legislation.

Initiatives and Propositions

Although the traditional political process has been to lobby a legislator to support a cause and draft a bill that is then voted on by the legislature as a whole, many laws are enacted through the initiative process. Through this process an interested party creates a proposition and then collects signatures to have the proposition appear on a ballot; the population as a whole, not just elected representatives, then have the opportunity to vote on the proposition and decide if they want to enact the proposed law. This is the means by which the Oregon and Washington Death with Dignity Acts were adopted as well as state Medical Marijuana Laws.

INTERRELATED CONCEPTS

Health care law, Health policy, and **Ethics** are all interrelated and sometimes indistinguishable concepts. At its most basic level, a law is a set of rules that is designed to help meet a specific policy or goal. Analogizing to the nursing process, health care policy is the goal or expected outcome and health care laws are the interventions that are intended to effect the expected outcome. Health care ethics are the framework or boundaries in which many of those policies and laws are made. To look at this another way, adherence to an ethical principle may drive a desire to adopt a policy and create laws that promote the policy.

Another concept that is closely interrelated is **Health care economics.** As previously described many laws have a financial incentive to compel compliance with the law. There are organizations and departments within health care organizations whose job it is to ensure compliance with many health care laws and regulations. Within a health care organization or hospital this job may be the responsibility of the compliance officer or compliance department. The job of the compliance officer is to monitor the organization's activities so

that the organization can continue to receive payments from the government and is not subject to any fines.

The Joint Commission (TJC) is an independent organization that accredits health care organizations (hospitals) so that they can maintain their ability to bill Medicare for their services. Accreditation through TJC is not the only means of maintaining the ability to bill Medicare, but it is a common means used by many organizations. The requirements of TJC are not laws; however, because a large majority of hospitalized patients are older than age 65 and because 97% of those older than age 65 receive health benefits through Medicare, hospitals are very dependent upon their ability to continue to receive Medicare payments for patient services.[25] Thus, within the health care organization TJC rules can seem to have the effect of law. Many activities associated with quality management and quality improvement are organized around

MODEL CASE

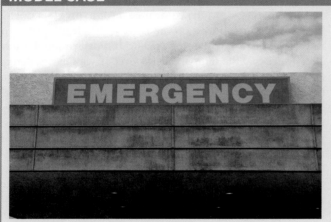

In 1996 Congress passed the Emergency Medical Treatment and Active Labor Act (EMTALA) requiring all hospitals that operate emergency departments and participate in Medicare payment systems to (1) provide basic screening exams to all patients who presented for emergency treatment and/or active labor needs and (2) render all medical care necessary to stabilize the patient prior to transfer to a lower level of care. This law was enacted in a response to the public perception that individuals were being turned away from hospital emergency departments or were being transferred to public hospitals in unstable condition if they could not pay for services up front. The underlying policy is that hospitals that have emergency departments hold themselves out as providing these services to all members of the public and owe the public a duty to render such care to those in need. Hospitals can be fined by the government for EMTALA violations.

EMTALA has also had the effect of providing patients with another avenue for malpractice claims, especially when state laws might place caps on the maximum damage award. Take for example the case of *Power v. Arlington Hospital Association*.[26]

In this case a young woman presented to a hospital emergency department with complaints of hip, back, and leg pain accompanied by rigors and chills. She was seen by a physician, given a prescription for pain medication, and sent home. She returned the following day in apparent septic shock and was admitted to the ICU. She remained in the hospital for more than 4 months, during which time she had both legs amputated and lost the sight in one eye. In this case Power contended that the hospital failed to give her an adequate screening exam when she first presented to the hospital. Medical experts testified that she did not receive a blood test that was necessary for adequate screening of a patient who presented with her symptoms and that such a test would have most likely revealed an infection that could have been properly treated before becoming so widespread. The court agreed with Power, stating that because she had been treated differently than other patients who would have presented with the same symptoms, she had not received an adequate medical screening and she could pursue recovery under the EMTALA statutes.

Contrast this case with the case of *Cleland v. Bronson Methodist Hospital*.[27] In Cleland, a 15-year-old boy was brought to the hospital with complaints of abdominal pain and vomiting. He was observed for 4 hours in the emergency department; diagnosed with gastroenteritis, dehydration, and hypoglycemia; and sent home. Cleland died within 24 hours of discharge; autopsy showed he suffered an intussusception. His parents brought an action under EMTALA stating that the emergency department physicians failed to provide an appropriate screening exam that would have adequately diagnosed Cleland's condition and failed to stabilize him prior to him home. In this case the court did not sustain the EMTALA claim, noting instead that the screening exam provided to Cleland was no different than would have been offered to any other patient who presented with the same symptoms. The court found what the Power court later stated—there is no requirement of EMTALA that a screening exam result in a correct diagnosis.

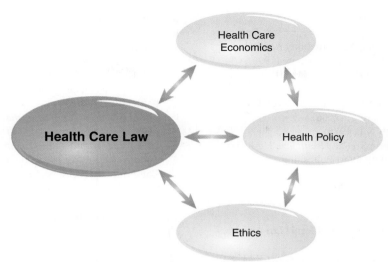

FIGURE 53-3 Health Care Law and Interrelated Concepts.

meeting the requirements of TJC. TJC rules (especially those associated with patient safety) can also have the effect of becoming standards under which malpractice cases can be argued. Figure 53-3 presents these concepts.

EXEMPLARS

There are a multitude of exemplars of health care law—so many, in fact, that it would be impossible to list them all. However, the most common and important exemplars of health care law are presented in Box 53-1. Some exemplars are listed in more than one category; this illustrates the intertwined nature of the source of laws.

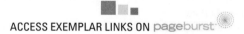

ACCESS EXEMPLAR LINKS ON pageburst

BOX 53-1 EXEMPLARS OF HEALTH CARE LAW

Federal Statutes
- Social Security Act of 1965
- Social Security Amendment of 1983
- Emergency Medical Treatment and Active Labor Act of 1986
- Patient Self-Determination Act of 1991
- Health Insurance Portability and Accountability Act of 1996
- Patient Protection and Affordable Care Act of 2010
- Americans with Disabilities Act of 1990

State Statutes
- Licensing of professionals (state board of nursing)
- Scope of practice/education requirements (state board of nursing)
- Licensing of health care institutions
- Immunization
- Public health and safety—disease surveillance, sanitation
- Consent/statutory surrogates

- Advance directives
- Physician-assisted suicide

Administrative Regulations
- *Conditions of Participation for Hospitals* (CMS)
- *The Common Rule for the Protection of Human Research Subjects*
- State board of nursing (scope of practice/education requirements)

Common Law/Case Law
- Right to die (Quinlan)
- Abortion rights (Roe)
- Advance directives (Cruzan); later codified in all states
- Elements of a malpractice case
- Elements of consent
- Physician-assisted suicide (Baxter)

REFERENCES

1. Health Insurance Portability and Accountability Act. Pub. L. No. 104–191 § 195(a)(1), 42 U.S.C. § 300gg note (1996).
2. U.S. Department of Health and Human Services. Retrieved from www.hhs.gov/about/.
3. Conditions of Participation for Hospitals, Standard: Restraint or Seclusion, 42 CFR § 482.13 (e-g) (2006).
4. In re Quinlan, 355 A.2d 647 (N.J., 1976).
5. Furrow B, Greaney T, Johnson S, et al: *Health law: Hornbook series*, ed 2, St Paul, Minn, 1995, West Publishing.
6. Roe v. Wade, 410 US 113 (1973).
7. Cruzan v. Missouri, 497 US 261 (1990).
8. Florida v. U.S. Dept. Health and Human Services, No. 3:10-cv-91-RV/EMT (2011).
9. Moore v. Regents of the University of California Los Angeles, 739 P.2d. 479 (Cal., 1990).
10. Health Insurance Portability and Accountability Act, 42 U.S.C. § 1320(d)(6) (1996).
11. Social Security Act of 1965, Pub. L. No. 89-97, 79 Stat 285 (1965).
12. Social Security Amendments of 1983, Pub. L. No. 98-21, 97 Stat. 65 (1983).
13. Consolidated Omnibus Budget Reconciliation Act of 1986, Pub. L No. 99-272,100 Stat 82 (1986).
14. Emergency Medical Treatment and Active Labor Act, 42 U.S.C. § 1395dd (1986).
15. Consolidated Omnibus Budget Reconciliation Act, 29 U.S.C. § 1161–1168 (1986).
16. Patient Self-Determination Act (42 U.S.C. § 1395cc(f) (1991).
17. Health Insurance Portability and Accountability Act, Pub. L. No. 104-191, 110 Stat. 1936 (1996).
18. Patient Protection and Affordable Care Act. Pub. L. No. 111-148, 124 Stat.119 (2010), as amended by the Health Care and Education Reconciliation Act of 2010, Pub. L. No. 111-152, 124 Stat. 1029(2010).
19. Safriet BJ: *Federal options for maximizing the value of advanced practice nurses in providing quality, cost-effective health care*, 2010. Paper commissioned by the Committee on the RWJF Initiative on the Future of Nursing, at the IOM (Appendix H).
20. Committee on the Robert Wood Johnson Foundation Initiative on the Future of Nursing: *Institute of Medicine: The future of nursing: leading change, advancing health*, Washington, DC, 2011, The National Academies Press.
21. Oregon Death with Dignity Act: *Ore Rev Stat* 127:800-995, 1994.
22. Washington Death with Dignity Act: *Rev C Wash* 70:245, 2008.
23. *Baxter v. Montana, 2009 MT 449 (2009)*.
24. Sowers C: *Doctor guilty in abortion death: jurors convict Biskind, assistant*, Feb 21, 2001. The Arizona Republic, pp A1, A4.
25. Moon M: What Medicare has meant to older Americans, *Health Care Finance Rev* 18(2):49–59, 1998. (winter).
26. Power v. Arlington Hospital Association, 42 F.3d 851 (4th Cir., 1994).
27. Cleland v. Bronson Methodist Hospital, 917 F.2d 266 (6th Cir., 1990).

Page numbers followed by *f* indicate figures, *t*, tables, *b*, boxes.